AF515720

# SKIN

## Clinical Dermatology

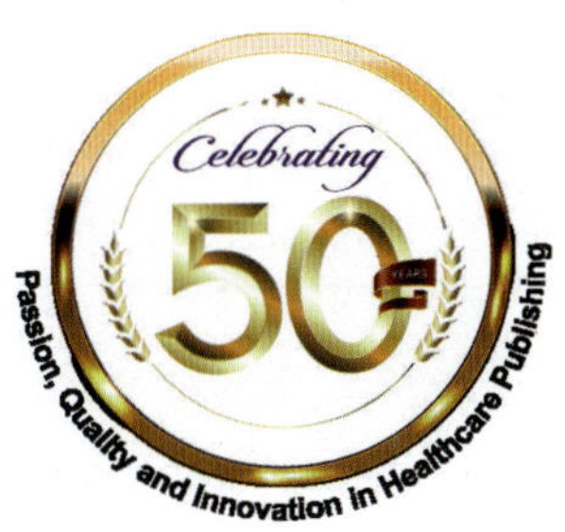

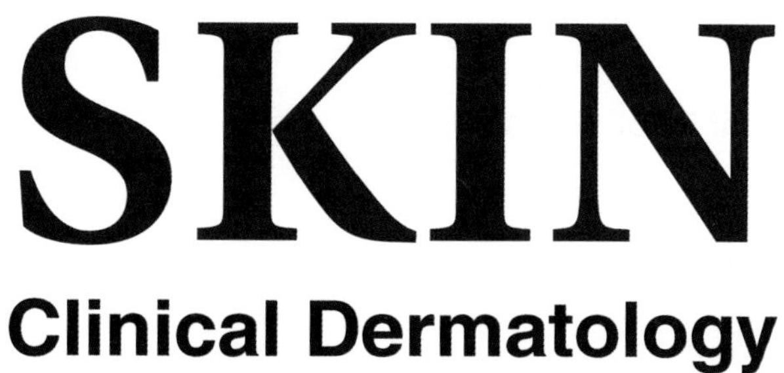

# SKIN

## Clinical Dermatology

*Editor-in-Chief*

**Nilendu Sarma** MD FAAD
Associate Professor and Head
Department of Dermatology
Dr BC Roy Post Graduate Institute of Pediatric Sciences
Kolkata, West Bengal, India

*Assistant Editors*

**Sayantani Chakraborty** MD
Assistant Professor
Department of Dermatology
RG Kar Medical College
Kolkata, West Bengal, India

**Joyeeta Chowdhury** MD
Assistant Professor
Department of Dermatology
Nil Ratan Sircar Medical College
Kolkata, West Bengal, India

*Foreword*

**Howard I Maibach**

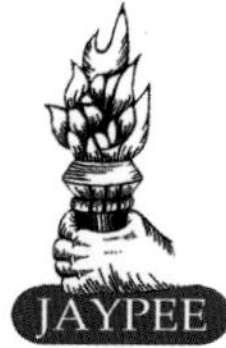


JAYPEE BROTHERS MEDICAL PUBLISHERS
*The Health Sciences Publisher*
New Delhi | London | Panama

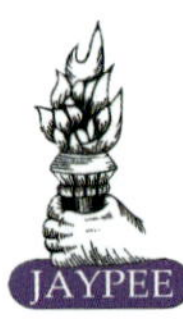

**Jaypee Brothers Medical Publishers (P) Ltd**

### Headquarters

Jaypee Brothers Medical Publishers (P) Ltd
4838/24, Ansari Road, Daryaganj
New Delhi 110 002, India
Phone: +91-11-43574357
Fax: +91-11-43574314
Email: jaypee@jaypeebrothers.com

### Overseas Offices

J.P. Medical Ltd
83 Victoria Street, London
SW1H 0HW (UK)
Phone: +44 20 3170 8910
Fax: +44 (0)20 3008 6180
Email: info@jpmedpub.com

Jaypee-Highlights Medical Publishers Inc
City of Knowledge, Bld. 235, 2nd Floor, Clayton
Panama City, Panama
Phone: +1 507-301-0496
Fax: +1 507-301-0499
Email: cservice@jphmedical.com

Jaypee Brothers Medical Publishers (P) Ltd
Bhotahity, Kathmandu, Nepal
Phone: +977-9741283608
Email: kathmandu@jaypeebrothers.com

Website: www.jaypeebrothers.com
Website: www.jaypeedigital.com



**Inquiries for bulk sales may be solicited at:** jaypee@jaypeebrothers.com

***Skin: Clinical Dermatology*** / Nilendu Sarma, Sayantani Chakraborty, Joyeeta Chowdhury

*Cover Design*: Dr Nilendu Sarma

*First Edition*: **2019**

ISBN: 978-93-86322-27-2

*Printed at: Samrat Offset Pvt. Ltd.*

**Dedicated to**

*My parents and mama*
*Dr AK Singh, who taught me dermatology, personality, and humanity and Dr Subrata Malakar, who inspired me to dream*
*Rakhi, Sonai, Rivu, and my sisters*
*The readers, my friends, colleagues, and my patients*

# AUTHOR COUNTRIES

Germany

India

Italy

Mexico

Singapore

Thailand

The Netherlands

United Kingdom

United States of America

# CONTRIBUTORS

## EDITOR-IN-CHIEF


**Nilendu Sarma** MD FAAD
Associate Professor and Head
Department of Dermatology
Dr BC Roy Post Graduate Institute of Pediatric Sciences
Kolkata, West Bengal, India


## ASSISTANT EDITORS


**Sayantani Chakraborty** MD
Assistant Professor
Department of Dermatology
RG Kar Medical College
Kolkata, West Bengal, India

**Joyeeta Chowdhury** MD
Assistant Professor
Department of Dermatology
Nil Ratan Sircar Medical College
Kolkata, West Bengal, India


## CONTRIBUTING AUTHORS


**Ishad Agarwal** MD
Consultant Dermatologist
Kolkata, West Bengal, India

**Uma S Agarwal** MD
Senior Professor
Department of Dermatology
SMS Medical College and Hospital
Jaipur, Rajasthan, India

**Puneet Agarwal** MD
Assistant Professor
Department of Dermatology
SMS Medical College and Hospital
Jaipur, Rajasthan, India

**Sarah A Ahmed** PhD
Senior Researcher
Department of Medical Mycology
Westerdijk Fungal Biodiversity Institute
Utrecht, The Netherlands

**Aurora Alessandrini** MD
Dermatologist, Fellow Researcher
Department of Specialized, Experimental and Diagnostic Medicine
University of Bologna
Bologna, Italy

**Attila S Antal** MD
Department of Dermatology and Allergy
Ludwig Maximilian University of Munich
Munich, Germany

**Amanjot Kaur Arora** MD DNB MNAMS
Senior Resident
Department of Dermatology
Postgraduate Institute of Medical Education and Research
Chandigarh, India

**Nirmal B** MD FRGUHS
Department of Dermatology
Christian Medical College
Vellore, Tamil Nadu, India

**Pradeep Balasubramanian** MD
Assistant Professor
Department of Dermatology
Andaman and Nicobar Islands Institute of Medical Sciences, Port Blair, Andaman and Nicobar Islands, India

**Priya Bishnoi** MD
Clinical Associate
KK Women's and Children's Hospital
Singapore

**Riti Bhatia** MD
Assistant Professor
Dermatology and Venereology
All India Institute of Medical Sciences
Rishikesh, Uttarakhand, India

**Alexandro Bonifaz** MD PhD
Professor and Senior Researcher
Department of Dermatology and Mycology Services
Hospital General de México "Dr Eduardo Liceaga"
Mexico City, Mexico

**Sayantani Chakraborty** MD
Assistant Professor
Department of Dermatology
RG Kar Medical College
Kolkata, West Bengal, India

**Monica Chahar** MD
Consultant Dermatologist and Hair Transplant Surgeon
AK Clinics
New Delhi, India

**Somodyuti Chandra** MD
Consultant Dermatologist
Kolkata, West Bengal, India

**Joyeeta Chowdhury** MD
Assistant Professor
Department of Dermatology
Nil Ratan Sircar Medical College
Kolkata, West Bengal, India

**Anupam Das** MD
Assistant Professor
Department of Dermatology
KPC Medical College
Kolkata, West Bengal, India

**Nilay Kanti Das** MD
Professor
Department of Dermatology
Bankura Sammilani Medical College
Bankura, West Bengal, India

**Dipti Das** MD DNB
Consultant Dermatologist and Cosmetologist, Dr Marwah's Skin Clinic
Mumbai, Maharashtra, India

**Dipankar De** MD
Associate Professor
Department of Dermatology
Postgraduate Institute of Medical Education and Research
Chandigarh, India

**Sandipan Dhar** MD DNB FRCP
Professor and Head
Department of Pediatric Dermatology
Institute of Child Health
Kolkata, West Bengal, India

**Deepashree Daulatabad** MD DNB
Senior Resident
Department of Dermatology and STD
University College of Medical Sciences and GTB Hospital
New Delhi, India

**Samujjala Deb** MD
Post-doctoral Fellow
Department of Dermatology
St. John's Medical College Hospital
Bengaluru, Karnataka, India

**Atul Dongre** MD
Associate Professor
Department of Dermatology
Seth GS Medical College and KEM Hospital
Mumbai, Maharashtra, India

**Nagaraju Donthula** MD DVL
Consultant Dermatologist
Shweta Dental, Skin and Hair Clinic
Hyderabad, Telangana, India

**Paschal V D'Souza** MD
Director Professor and Head
Department of Dermatology, Venereology and Leprology
Employees State Insurance Post Graduate Institute of Medical Science and Research
New Delhi, India

**Gan Yiping Emily** MRCP MMed
Consultant Dermatologist and Pediatric Dermatologist, Dermatology Service
KK Women's and Children's Hospital
Singapore

**Shilpa Garg** DNB
Assistant Professor
Department of Dermatology
Army College of Medical Sciences
Base Hospital
Delhi, India

**Vinita Garg** MD
DM Resident Doctor
Department of Nephrology
SMS Medical College and Hospital
Jaipur, Rajasthan, India

**Aparajita Ghosh** MD
Associate Professor
Department of Dermatology
KPC Medical College and Hospital
Kolkata, West Bengal, India

**Parasar Ghosh** MD DM
Professor
Department of Rheumatology
Institute of Post Graduate Medical Education and Research and SSKM Hospital
Kolkata, West Bengal, India

**Sanjay Ghosh** MD
Professor and Head
Department of Dermatology
MGM Medical College and LSK Hospital
Kolkata, West Bengal, India

**Boon Kee Goh** BSc MBChB MRCP FRCP FAMS
Director and Consultant
Skin Physicians
Mount Elizabeth Medical Centre
Singapore

**Tarang Goyal** MD
Professor and Head
Department of Dermatology, Venereology and Leprosy
Muzaffarnagar Medical College
Muzaffarnagar, Uttar Pradesh, India

**Lalit K Gupta** MD
Senior Professor
Department of Dermatology
RNT Medical College
Udaipur, Rajasthan, India

**Somesh Gupta** MD DNB
Professor
Department of Dermatology and Venereology
All India Institute of Medical Sciences
New Delhi, India

**Vishal Gupta** MD
Senior Research Associate
Department of Dermatology and Venereology
All India Institute of Medical Sciences
New Delhi, India

**Sushila Hansda** MD
Senior Resident
Skin and Venereal Disease
Indira Gandhi Institute of Medical Sciences
Patna, Bihar, India

**Ravi Hiremagalore** MD
Consultant
Department of Pediatrics and Dermatology
Manipal Hospitals and Centre for Human Genetics
Bengaluru, Karnataka, India

**Sybren de Hoog** PhD
Professor
Department of Medical Mycology
Westerdijk Fungal Biodiversity Institute
Utrecht, The Netherlands
Senior Scientist
Department of Medical Microbiology
Center of Expertise in Mycology of RadboudUMC/CWZ
Nijmegen, The Netherlands

**Arun C Inamadar** MD DVD FRCP
Professor and Head
Department of Dermatology, Venereology and Leprosy
Shri BM Patil Medical College, Hospital and Research Center
Vijayapura, Karnataka, India

**Anuradha Jindal** MD
Senior Resident
Department of Dermatology
Kasturba Medical College, Manipal Academy of Higher Education
Manipal, Karnataka, India

**Rajiv S Joshi** MD DVD DNB
Consultant
Department of Dermatology
PD Hinduja Hospital and Medical Research Centre
Mumbai, Maharashtra, India.

**Ann M John** MD
Resident Physician, PGY-3
Department of Dermatology
Rutgers Robert Wood Johnson Medical School
Newark, New Jersey, USA

**Sujay Khandpur** MD DNB MNAMS
Professor
Department of Dermatology
All India Institute of Medical Sciences
New Delhi, India

**Uday Khopkar** MD
Professor and Head
Department of Dermatology
KEM Hospital and Seth GS Medical College
Mumbai, Maharashtra, India

**Vinay Kulkarni** MD DNB FAMS AAHIVS
Head, Department of Dermatology
Deenanath Mangeshkar Hospital
Pune, Maharashtra, India

**Piyush Kumar** MD
Associate Professor
Department of Dermatology
Katihar Medical College and Hospital
Katihar, Bihar, India

**Rajesh Kumar** MD
Associate Professor
Department of Dermatology
Grant Medical College
Mumbai, Maharashtra, India

**Shashi Kumar BM** MD DVL FRGUHS
Associate Professor
Department of Dermatology
Mandya Institute of Medical Sciences
Mandya, Karnataka, India

**Saurav Kundu** MD FAAD
Associate Professor
Department of Dermatology
MGM Medical College and LSK Hospital
Kishanganj, Bihar, India

**Eswari Loganathan** MD DVL FRGUHS
Assistant Professor
Department of Dermatology
Bangalore Medical College and Research Institute
Bengaluru, Karnataka, India

**W Clark Lambert** MD PhD FAAD
Professor and Associate Head
Dermatology
Professor of Pathology
Chief, Dermatopathology
Rutgers New Jersey Medical School
Newark, New Jersey, USA

**Ramesh Bhat M** MD DVD DNB
President IADVL (National)-2018
Professor
Father Muller Medical College
Mangaluru, Karnataka, India

**Sendhil Kumaran M** MD DNB MNAMS
Additional Professor
Department of Dermatology
Postgraduate Institute of Medical Education and Research
Chandigarh, India

**Imran Majid** MD FRCP
Consultant Dermatologist
Cutis Institute of Dermatology
Srinagar, Jammu and Kashmir, India

**Abhay Mani Martin** DVD MD DNB FIMSA
Senior Consultant and Head
Department of Dermatology
Baby Memorial Hospital
Kozhikode, Kerala, India

**Yogesh S Marfatia** MD
Professor and Head
Department of Skin-VD
Baroda Medical College
Vadodara, Gujarat, India

**Tess McPherson** MA MBBS MD FRCP
Consultant Pediatric Dermatologist
Oxford University Hospitals
London, United Kingdom

**Debdeep Mitra** MD
Assistant Professor
Department of Dermatology
Base Hospital
Delhi, India

**Nadia Zakir Mian** MD
Senior Registrar
St. Stephens Hospital
New Delhi, India

**Amiya K Mukhopadhyay** MD PhD DNB (Derma) DNB (Derma and Vener) MNAMS
Consultant Dermatologist
PRANAB
Asansol, West Bengal, India

**Rochelle C Monteiro** MD
Assistant Professor
Father Muller Medical College
Mangaluru, Karnataka, India

**Brijesh Nair** MD
Consultant Dermatologist
Military Hospital
Jaipur Cantonment
Jaipur, Rajasthan, India

**Smita Nagpal** MD
Consultant Dermatologist
Anya Skin Clinic
Ahmedabad, Gujarat, India

**Shekhar Neema** MD
Assistant Professor
Department of Dermatology
Command Hospital
Kolkata, West Bengal, India

**Vivek V Pai** MBBS DVD FCGP FAMSc
Director
Department of Leprosy and Dermatology
Bombay Leprosy Project
Mumbai, Maharashtra, India

**Aparna Palit** MD
Professor
Department of Dermatology, Venereology and Leprosy
Shri BM Patil Medical College, Hospital and Research Center
Vijayapura, Karnataka, India

**Tanmay Padhi** MD
Associate Professor
Department of Dermatology
VSS Institute of Medical Sciences and Research
Sambalpur, Odisha, India

**Saumya Panda** MD
Professor and Head
Department of Dermatology
KPC Medical College and Hospital
Kolkata, West Bengal, India

**Bianca M Piraccini** MD PhD
Associate Professor and Head
Department of Specialized Experimental and Diagnostic Medicine
University of Bologna
Bologna, Italy

**Swetalina Pradhan** MD
Senior Resident
Department of Dermatology
All India Institute of Medical Sciences
Bhubaneswar, Odisha, India

**Kumar Satya Prakash** MD
Associate Professor
MGM Medical College and LSK Hospital
Kishanganj, Bihar, India

**Indrashis Podder** MD DNB
Senior Resident
Department of Dermatology
College of Medicine and Sagore Dutta Hospital
Kolkata, West Bengal, India

**Poonam Pund** MD DNB
Consultant Dermatologist
Pratibimb Skin and Hair Clinic
Ahmednagar, Maharashtra, India

**Reena Rai** MD
Professor
Department of Dermatology
PSG Institute of Medical Sciences and Research
Coimbatore, Tamil Nadu, India

**Raghavendra Rao** MD DNB
Additional Professor
Department of Dermatology
Kasturba Medical College
Manipal Academy of Higher Education
Manipal, Karnataka, India

**Raghunatha Reddy R** MD DVL FRGUHS
Consultant Dermatologist
Dr Raghu's Mathapitha Skin Clinic
Bengaluru, Karnataka, India

**Siba P Raychaudhuri** MD FAAD FACP FACR
Professor, Department of Dermatology
Rheumatology and Clinical Immunology
School of Medicine
University of California Davis
Davis, California, USA

**Smriti K Raychaudhuri**
Sacramento VA Medical Center
Department of Veterans Affairs
Northern California Health Care System
Mather, California, USA

**Suravi Raychaudhuri**
School of Medicine
University of California
San Francisco, California, USA

**Sanjay K Rathi** MD
Consultant Dermatologist
Dr Rathi Skin Clinic
Siliguri, West Bengal, India

**Tanumay Roychowdhury** MD
Consultant
Tata Medical Center
Kolkata, West Bengal, India

**Thomas Ruzicka** MD PhD
Chairman
Department of Dermatology and Allergy
Ludwig Maximilian University of Munich
Munich, Germany

**Savitha AS** MD DNB FRGUHS
Assistant Professor
Department of Dermatology
Sapthagiri Institute of Medical Sciences and Research Centre
Bengaluru, Karnataka, India

**Abhijit Saha** MD
Consultant
Department of Dermatology
Rita Skin Foundation
Kolkata, West Bengal, India

**Wendy WJ van de Sande** PhD
Associate Professor
Department of Medical Microbiology and Infectious Diseases
Erasmus MC
Rotterdam, The Netherlands

**Rashmi Sarkar** MD MNAMS
Professor
Department of Dermatology
Maulana Azad Medical College
New Delhi, India

**Nilendu Sarma** MD FAAD
Associate Professor and Head
Department of Dermatology
Dr BC Roy Post Graduate Institute of Pediatric Sciences
Kolkata, West Bengal, India

**Robert A Schwartz** MD MPH DSc FRCP FAADV
Professor and Head
Department of Dermatology
Professor of Pathology
Rutgers New Jersey Medical School
Newark, New Jersey, USA

**Archana Singal** MD MNAMD
Director Professor
Department of Dermatology and STD
University College of Medical Sciences and GTB Hospital
New Delhi, India

**Rajeev Sharma** MD FAAD
Consultant Dermatologist
Bishen Skin Centre
Aligarh, Uttar Pradesh, India

**Vanaja P Shetty** MSc PhD
Senior Mentor
The Foundation for Medical Research
Mumbai, Maharashtra, India

**Sahana M Srinivas** DNB DVD FRGUHS
Consultant
Department of Pediatric Dermatology
Indira Gandhi Institute of Child Health
Bengaluru, Karnataka, India

**Vijay Vanchinathan** MD FAAD
Assistant Clinical Professor
Department of Dermatology
Medical College of Wisconsin - Central Wisconsin
Wausau, Wisconsin, USA

**Biju Vasudevan** MD
Professor
Department of Dermatology
Base Hospital
Lucknow, Uttar Pradesh, India

**Vishalakshi Viswanath** MD DNB DDV
Professor and Head
Department of Dermatology
Rajiv Gandhi Medical College and Chhatrapati Shivaji Maharaj Hospital
Thane, Maharashtra, India

**Vesarat Wessagowit** MD PhD
Head
Department of Molecular Genetics
Advisor to Director (Academic)
Institute of Dermatology
Bangkok, Thailand

**Vijay Zawar** MD DNB DVD FRCP
Professor
Department of Dermatology
Dr Vasantrao Pawar Medical College
Nashik, Maharashtra, India

# FOREWORD

This textbook will be an important academic and clinical success.

The universe of dermatologic textbooks may be divided into those that are encyclopedic, middle-sized, and the highly concise textbooks—mainly oriented for students. Our group purchases all the encyclopedias and most of the middle-sized books, as well as several of the smaller varieties. The encyclopedias include Rook (United Kingdom), Fitzpatrick (USA), Bolognia (USA), and Bergdorf (Germany). The middle-sized version most widely used is the original Andrews (USA), and many smaller versions exist in many countries.

The power of the Sarma text consists of its balance—it is not the enormous tome of the encyclopedias nor is it the highly concise version for students.

The book is structured in a highly reasoned manner so that the reader can find the question of interest in seconds; what follows is a structured, easy-to-read and comprehend understanding of our current knowledge, all tailored for the clinical domain.

It is not only concise and accurate, but also well illustrated.

This book will help not only the medical student, but also the residents throughout the English-reading world and the experienced dermatologist.

I predict that this edition, and many to come, will be widely used.

**Howard I Maibach** MD
Professor
Department of Dermatology
University of California Medical School
San Francisco, California, USA

# PREFACE

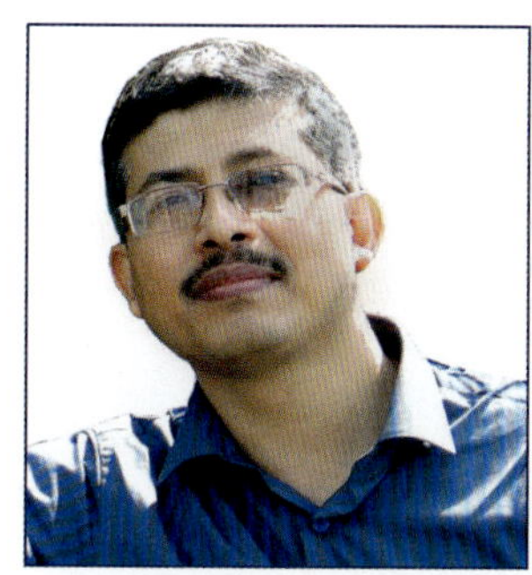

**Nilendu Sarma** MD FAAD
Associate Professor and Head
Department of Dermatology
Dr BC Roy Post Graduate Institute of Pediatric Sciences
Kolkata, West Bengal, India

Skin: Clinical Dermatology is a concise yet comprehensive book of dermatology that has been meticulously prepared with updated and relevant information.

Between the cover, entire dermatology has been covered in 21 sections, 80 chapters. Management section has been extensively covered in three chapters. Two chapters have been dedicated for "emergencies in dermatology," a highly necessary section for these days. "Skin and genetics, environmental and occupational dermatology, dermatology in ages, skin diseases in systemic disorders, and dermatoses with specific histological reaction patterns" are few notable sections in addition to all the other regular sections.

Leading experts in the field from all over the world have penned their extraordinary knowledge in the form of written words. Great care has been taken to provide numerous images that are relevant, informative, and of high quality. Numerous images from different parts of the globe with patients from varied racial and ethnic background will provide unique opportunity to learn the diverse nature of dermatological manifestations.

It took more than 4 years for a successful completion. This was not unusual for the painstaking job required for the first edition of a massive project like this as perfection was the only objective.

Despite all the efforts, I cannot claim that this volume is error-free. I expect comments and valuable suggestions from the reader on how this book can achieve its target of being the preferred book.

# ACKNOWLEDGMENTS

I thank the authors for their outstanding pieces of writing for the book. I must extend my heartfelt thanks to Dr Sayantani Chakraborty and Dr Joyeeta Chowdhury for their commendable job as the assistant editor and unstinted cooperation. My students and my friends have always been the source of continuous stimulation.

The entire team lead by Shri Jitendar P Vij, Group Chairman and Mr Ankit Vij, Managing Director, M/s Jaypee Brothers Medical Publishers (P) Ltd. New Delhi, India, and the perfect leader, Dr Neeraj Choudhary, Senior Acquisition Editor-Corporate along with Ms Neha Bhatia and Mr Sabyasachi Hazra have paved a seamless way for this admirable job being done. Their role has been appreciable.

During these long 4 years, my family silently accepted my absence from so many vital moments of their life. I sincerely acknowledge their role in making of this book.

# CONTENTS

## Section 6: Urticaria, Mastocytosis and Flushing Disorders



## Section 7: Acne, Rosacea and Related Disorders



## Section 8: Blistering Disorders of Skin



## Section 9: Pigmentation Disorders



## Section 10: Papulosquamous Disorders and Arthritis

# 1 SECTION Approach to Diagnosis

# 1 CHAPTER Principles of Clinical and Laboratory Diagnosis in Dermatology

*Nilendu Sarma*

## INTRODUCTION

Dermatological diagnosis is primarily dependent of clinical assessment of the eruption, commonly referred to as "lesion". Such lesions are described with specialized terms. Knowledge of such terms is necessary for understanding the descriptions.

Changes in the skin are often subtle. Meticulous examination under sufficient illumination is of paramount importance. Diffuse day light is the best light source. Examination of large body surface is required in many occasions. A trained attendant of same sex, as that of the patient is important to gain confidence of the patient and also necessary to avoid legal consequences.

Examination of a skin lesion is done to elicit changes in the following parameters:

- *Elevation/thickness:* Skin lesions can be elevated or palpable or flat or nonpalpable
- *Color change:* Erythema, hypo- and hyperpigmentation with variable shades
- *Margin:* Well defined, ill defined
- *Shape and pattern:* Annular (round), (Fig. 1) circinate (shape that originates after multiple circles are merged), irregular, linear, serpiginous, and segmental
- *Surface:* Smooth, shiny, rough, scaly, oozing, lichenification, etc.
- *Contour:* Convex, concave, some areas like central part depressed and margin elevated (like saucer)

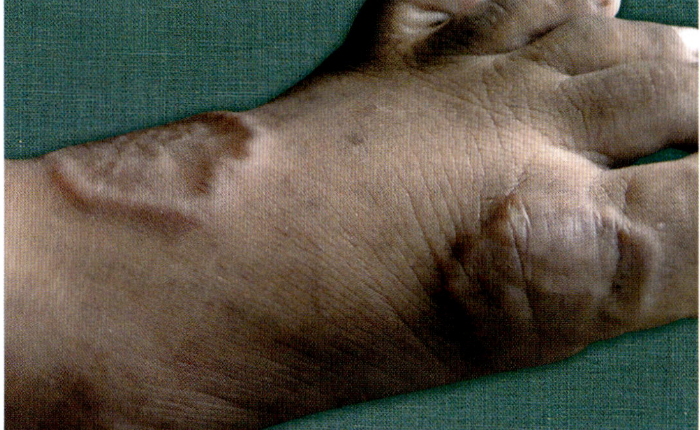

**FIG. 1:** Annular lesion with beaded margin in granuloma annulare.

- *Consistency:* Soft, firm, hard, cystic, and fluid-filled (assess type of fluid)
- *Infiltration:* Thickening/sclerosis and atrophy
- Additional features on surface like presence of ulcer, discharge, and scar.

## TERMINOLOGIES IN DERMATOLOGY

It is important to know the different standard terminologies used to describe a skin lesion.

Based on the above mentioned parameters, each individual lesion can be classified into following type of lesion. The terms used in description of dermatological lesions dermatology are unique. Readers must be well versed with the different dermatological terminologies and their definitions (Box 1).

## CLINICAL AND ADVANCED DIAGNOSTIC TOOLS AND METHODS

Dermatology is one subject in medical science that is well-known for tremendous dependence on clinical accuracy for diagnosis. Tools are less often used as a necessary diagnostic aid. Diagnosis is often made during the first inspection in most of the cases. It is often said, in a lighter vein that "dermatological diagnosis, not made during inspection, is difficult to arrive ". This may be an oversimplified comment, but not absolutely wrong as well. This indicates the prime role of clinical diagnosis in dermatology.

Despite the high dependence on clinical acumen, diagnosis in dermatology has been significantly enriched with remarkable progress in the technology especially in the field of molecular and genetic diagnosis. However, these are still beyond the reach of most of the dermatologists. Description of these advanced diagnostic methodologies is also beyond the scope of this book. Simple tools like a torch, glass slide, pin, nylon monofilament, cotton and spirit, and a quality hand lens are basic necessary instruments. Some traditional diagnostic techniques like biopsy, slit skin smear, and Tzank smear are still considered highly important procedures for diagnosis in day to day practice. Since last few years, dermatoscope has also become a very common and useful instrument in everyday practice. Some of these instruments and techniques are overviewed here.

**BOX 1 Basic dermatological morphology**

- Macule: Flat lesion upto 1 cm
- Patch: Flat lesions more than 1 cm
- Papules: Elevated lesions upto 1 cm (Fig. 2)
- Plaque: Elevated lesions more than 1 cm
- Nodule: This is an elevated/ raised lesions more than 1 cm. They may also be situated within the skin. Thus palpation is required to identify them (Fig. 3)
- Vesicle: Fluid filled lesion less than 1 cm (Fig. 4)
- Bulla: Fluid filled lesion more than 1 cm
- Pustule: Pus filled lesion
- Cyst: Encapsulated lesion filled with semisolid or soft material
- Erythema: Reddish color
- Hypopigmentation: Less pigmentation than that of surrounding skin
- Hyperpigmentation: More pigmentation than that of surrounding skin
- Depigmentation: Complete absence of pigmentation. This appears white
- Dyschromia: Presence of both hypo- and hyperpigmentation
- Poikiloderma: Presence of hypo- and hyperpigmentation, telangiectasia and atrophy.
- Petechiae: Hemorrhagic lesion, size upto 4 mm
- Purpura: Hemorrhagic lesion, size 5–9 mm
- Ecchymosis: Hemorrhagic lesion, size ≥1 cm
- Circinate shape: Shape that develops from merging multiple circles
- Crust: Crust is the dried-up exudates (Fig. 5)
- Lichenification: Thickened skin surface with exacerbated skin markings (Fig. 6)
- Telangiectasia: Presence of dilated capillary
- Verrucous: Rough surface like wart
- Atrophy: Decrease in the skin thickness. This may involve epidermis, dermis and subcutaneous tissue and clinically appear as thin, wrinkled and transparent skin

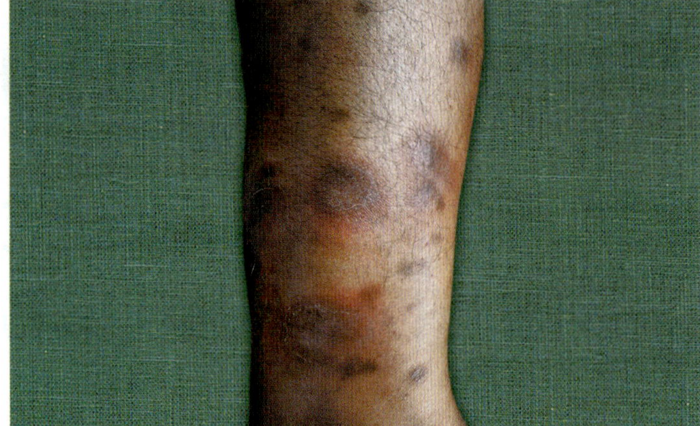

**FIG. 3:** Deeper nodules in erythema nodosum.

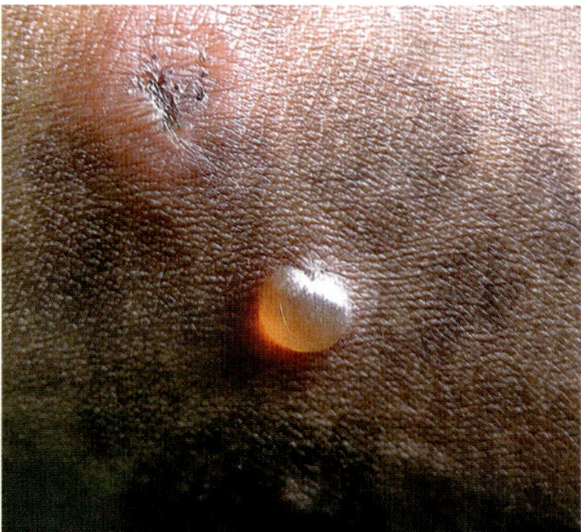

**FIG. 4:** Vesicular eruption along with erythematous plaque in bullous pemphigoid.

**FIG. 2:** Widespread tiny papular eruptions in keratosis pilaris.

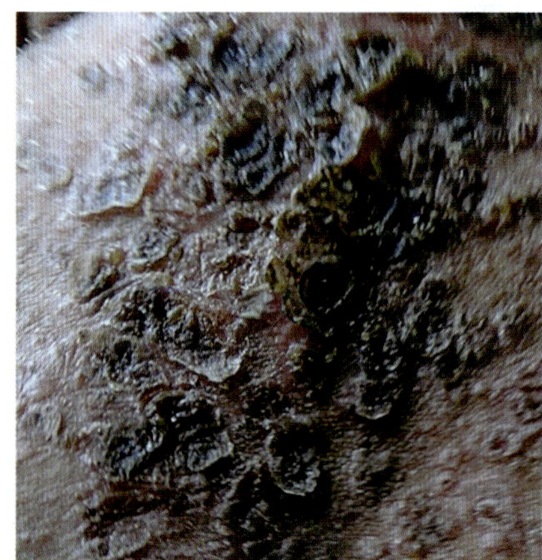

**FIG. 5:** Crust in impetigo contagiosa.

## Dermoscopy

Dermoscopy, also known as epiluminescence microscopy is one relatively new tool being increasingly used in clinical practice. Dermatoscope or dermoscope is a handheld instrument with inbuilt light source is a useful instrument in clinical practice.

Light falls on the skin at an angle of 20° and penetrates inside the skin and is reflected back to eye. To prevent scattering, polarized lights are used that has helped to achieve a better clarity. Interface liquid are used to further reduce the scattering. Water, alcohol-gel, glycerin, ultrasonography gels, and liquid paraffin can be used for this purpose.

Standard handheld dermoscope supports a magnification of 10-20x. Digital (video) dematoscopes are attached with computer can offer much higher magnification but resolution is lower.

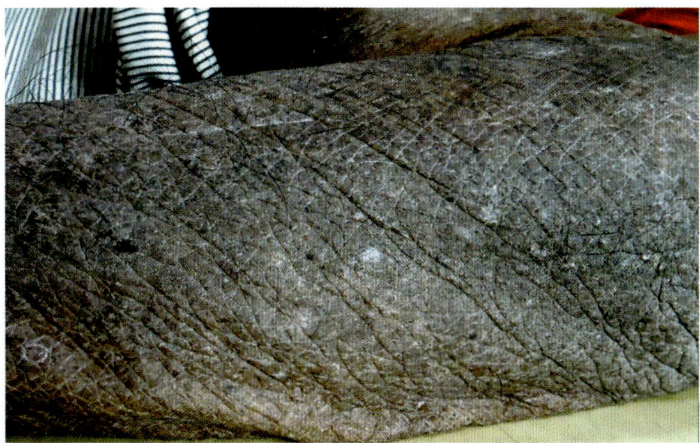

**FIG. 6:** Thickened skin with prominent skin markings (lichenification).

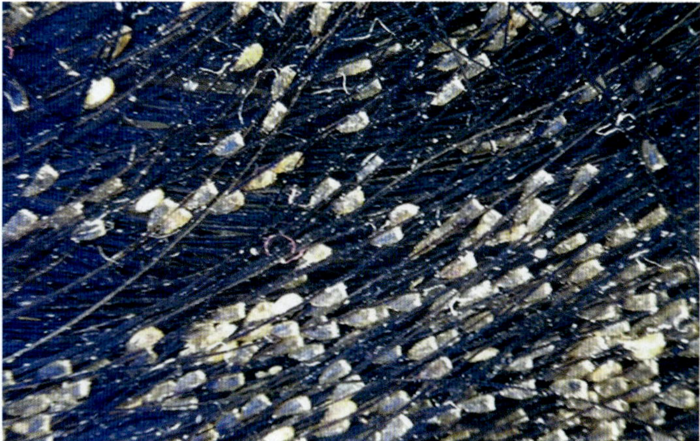

**FIG. 7:** Pediculosis capitis (nits) seen under dermoscope (10x).
*Courtesy*: Dr Sayantani Chakraborty, Assistant Professor, Department of Dermatology, RG Kar Medical College, West Bengal.

Images can be taken with normal hand held digital camera and saved for future use and comparison.

Appearance of normal skin depends on the surface textures, rete patterns, dermal tissues, and vasculature. Diagnosis of skin conditions with dermoscopy requires knowledge of the specific appearance of the condition under dermoscope.

The most wide-spread use of dermoscopy is in fact for the evaluation of suspected moles and differentiation from malignant melanoma. However its use has expanded to incorporate large number of other neoplastic conditions and inflammatory skin conditions (Box 2).

Knowledge of the normal pigmentary network that varies depending on the area of the body is important. Melanin in the epidermal keratinocytes in association with variable thickness of the skin and presence of rete leads to formation of pigmented network like appearance of the skin. Many diseased conditions, particularly pigmented diseases feature alteration of the pigmented network.

Color of pigmentation formed by melanin is dependent on its depth. When melanin is present in superficial epidermis, it appears black, when in dermoepidermal junction, it appears as light to dark brown, melanin in papillary dermis appears a gray, and when in reticular dermis, it appears as bluish. Hemoglobin in blood appears as red and fibrosis appears as white color.

There are many proposed methods and algorithms to identify a malignant melanoma and differentiating it from benign moles like "seven-point checklist", "Menzies scoring method", "three-point checklist", "ABCD algorithm", "The CASH algorithm", and "chaos and clues". The basic principles followed in most of these are identifying gross abnormality in pattern (chaos) and finding the abnormality in detailed examinations (clues). Asymmetry, loss of normal pigmented network, blue-white lesions, structureless areas, and margins are important parameters to differentiate melanoma from benign lesions.

**BOX 2 Uses of dermoscopy in dermatological conditions**

- Pigmentary disorders and melanoma
- Alopecia and other hair disorders
- Tumors
- Inflammatory disorders
- Infection and infestations (Fig. 7)
- Nail and nail fold capillary alterations (Fig. 8)
- Granulomatous disorders
- Vascular lesions

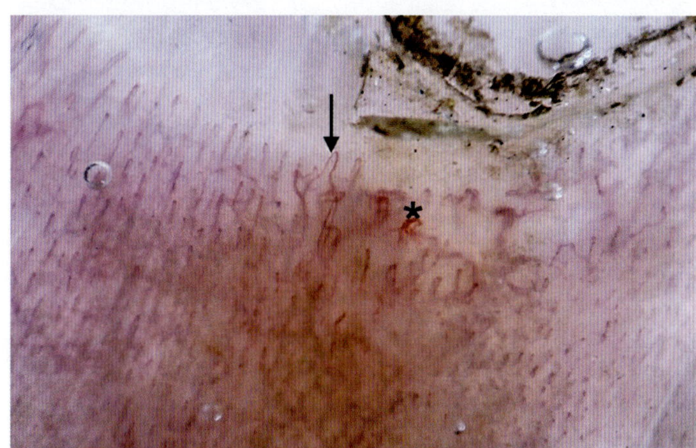

**FIG. 8:** Nailfold capillary under polarized light dermoscopy (Dermlite 4, 10x,) in systemic sclerosis showing normal hairpin loops in the left side, irregular and widened loops (arrow), larger efferent loops and areas of absent capillary (capillary loss) (star) in the right side.

Blood vessels are tiny structure that requires higher magnification than the standard magnification available with most dermoscope, i.e., 10x. Thus visualization of prominent vessel may indicate abnormality. Layout of the vessel like vertical versus horizontal, tortuosity, thickness, depth, and regularity are important while evaluating the disease. Nail fold capillary examination is one of the most important uses of dermoscopy.

Dermoscopy reduces the necessity of skin biopsy for evaluation of scarring and nonscarring alopecia. Alopecia areata and trichotillomania share many identical features. Chronic telogen effluvium and androgenic alopecia also share some common features. But dermoscopy can be of great help in differentiation of these conditions.

Table 1 shows some of the important and known dermatoscopic changes in some diseases. However, it has to be remembered that dermatoscopic diagnosis is not based on finding a "diagnostic" finding. Features known to be characteristic of a disease may be absent in particular cases or are also present in some other conditions. Thus, presence of constellation of features and differentiating of other closely similar conditions makes the diagnosis.

**TABLE 1: Important dermatoscopic signs**

| Dermatoscopic findings | Suggested diagnosis |
|---|---|
| Reticulated pigmentation | Normal skin |
| Cerebriform pigmentation | Seborrheic keratosis |
| Moth-eaten border, fingerprint pigmentation | Seborrheic keratosis, solar lentigo |
| Vessels in 'string of pearls' pattern | Clear cell acanthoma |
| Solitary or multiple flesh colored facial papules | Sebaceous hyperplasia |
| Crown vessels | Sebaceous herplasia, basal cell carcinoma |
| Pustules, absence of follicular units, tufted folliculitis, neovascularization (Fig. 9) | Folliculitis decalvans |
| Peripheral pseudonetwork and prominent central scar-like area | Dermatofibroma |
| Spoke-wheel pigmentation | Basal cell carcinoma |
| Leaf-like areas | Basal cell carcinoma |
| Superficial arborizing vessels (Fig. 10) | Basal cell carcinoma |

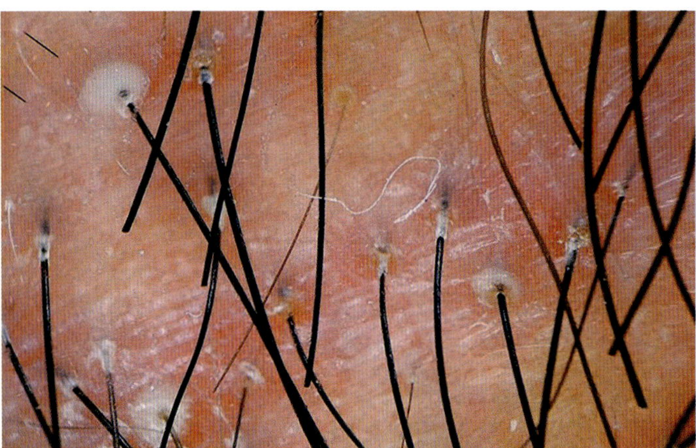

**FIG. 9:** Pustules, loss of follicular units in folliculitis decalvans.

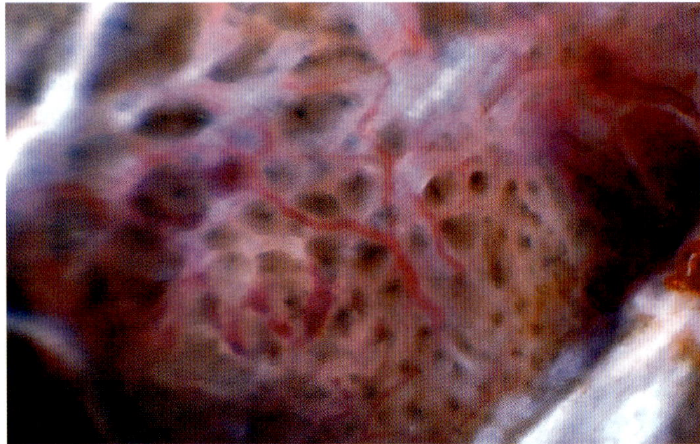

**FIG. 10:** Arborizing vessels in basal cell carcinoma (dermoscopic view).

## Tzank Smear

### Principle and Uses

This is a method of cytology. This has its known importance in dermatology. The most common use of Tzank smear is in the diagnosis of pemphigus and herpes virus infection. However, it has been used in many other conditions (Table 2). However, many of the findings mentioned below may not be present in all cases (low sensitivity).

### Method

When an intact bulla is present, it should be precisely cut at one side and the blister roof folded over the other part exposing the base of the bulla. The base is then scraped gently with a scalpel blade and the material is placed on glass slide, spread and air dried.

Erosive lesions, ruptured bulla can be directly scraped. Crust can be removed to scrape the surface of a lesion.

**TABLE 2: Important findings in Tzank smear**

| | |
|---|---|
| Pemphigus vulgaris | • Acantholytic cells (most common)<br>• Streptocytes: Chains of white blood cells<br>• Sertoli rosette cells: Groups of cells with epithelial cell at the center surrounded by a ring of leukocytes |
| Bullous pemphigoid | Eosinophils |
| Herpes infection | Acantholytic and multinucleated giant cells (Fig. 11) |
| Herpes zoster | Intranuclear inclusions (Cowdry A body) |
| Candidiasis | Pseudohyphae |
| Bullous impetigo | Dyskeratotic acantholytic cells, neutrophils, and cocci |
| Staphylococcal scalded skin syndrome (SSSS) | Dyskeratotic acantholytic cells (Fig. 12) |
| Spongiotic dermatitis, contact dermatitis | Tadpole cells |
| Darier's disease | Corps ronds and grains |
| Hailey-Hailey disease | Acantholytic cells |

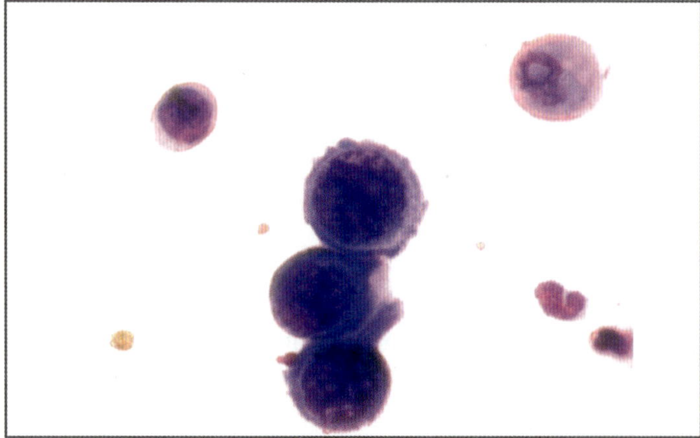

**FIG. 11:** Multinucleated giant cells, round cells with smooth surface in herpes simplex infection.

*Courtesy*: Dr Abhay Mani Martin, Senior Consultant and Head, Department of Dermatology, Baby Memorial Hospital, Kozhikode, Kerala.

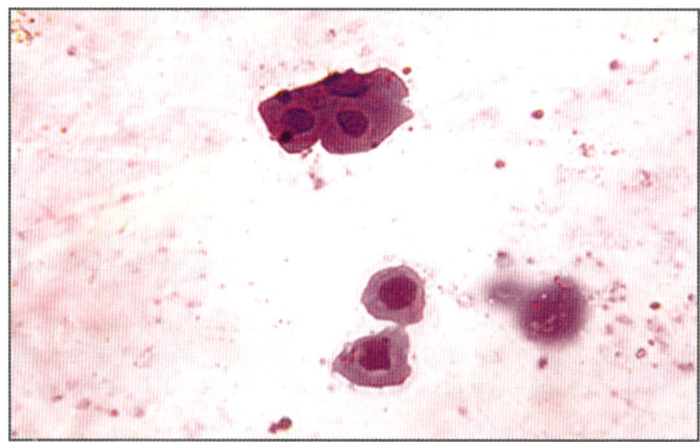

**FIG. 12:** Acantholytic cells in staphylococcal scalded-skin syndrome (SSSS).

*Courtesy*: Dr Abhay Mani Martin, Senior Consultant and Head, Department of Dermatology, Baby Memorial Hospital, Kozhikode, Kerala.

Usefulness of Tzank smear can be increased by proper staining. Following stains can be helpful for diagnosis:

- May-Grünwald-Giemsa stain is commonly employed
- Methylene blue for suspected candidiasis
- Gramm's stain for infective bacilli and cocci
- Direct immunofluorescence (DIF) can be done for autoimmune bullous disease.

The slide is then examined under microscope with higher magnification.

## Skin Biopsy and Tissue Processing

Histopathological examination (HPE) of the tissue has been the gold standard and most sought after investigation in dermatology. Dermatopathology on the other hand is one of the toughest subjects. Nondescript nature of the histopathological findings in many occasions invariably requires more intimate interaction between a pathologist and dermatologist for proper evaluation of the sections. Except for some conditions that have specific and characteristic histopathological findings, a large number of conditions share similar histopathological alterations. Thus, it is always a good practice for the dermatologists to get trained in dermatopathology.

Dermatopathology is beyond the scope of this book. Some important technical points on skin biopsy will be discussed here.

### Timing of Biopsy

Timing of biopsy is important. Bullous disease may develop keratinocyte necrosis when older making differentiation from toxic epidermal necrolysis (TEN) difficult (Table 3).

**TABLE 3: Timing of biopsy**

| Condition | Preferred timing of biopsy |
|---|---|
| Autoimmune bullous disease | Fresh lesion |
| Epidermolysis bullosa (Mechanobullous disease) | New lesion less than 12 hour old |
| Vasculitis | • Well-developed lesion (>3 days) for routine HPE.<br>• Fresh lesion for DIF studies |
| Discoid lupus | Well-developed, persistent but active lesion (few months old) |

HPE, histopathological examination; DIF, direct immunofluorescence.

### Thickness and Depth of Biopsy

Biopsy should generally include deeper tissue like subcutaneous fats except when typical changes are expected in the upper part of skin. Biopsy in panniculitis, morphea requires deeper biopsy so that subcutaneous fats are included. TEN has features of satellite necrosis of epidermal keratinocytes. Bowen's diseases have diagnostic features in epidermis. However, it has to be remembered that even in conditions where superficial skin can be diagnostic, differentiation from some other conditions may need a deeper biopsy especially when clinical diagnosis suggests these differential diagnoses to be ruled out. Differentiation of extensive bullous fixed drug reaction from TEN necessitates a deeper biopsy to show the alterations in infiltrations around deeper vessels.

### Punch or Incision

Biopsy is most commonly done with a disposable punch. However, when the pathology is in subcutaneous fat as in panniculitis, when excision of the base appears difficult, when there is chance of missing the affected deeper tissue, or when the tissue is friable, excision biopsy is preferred over punch technique.

### Size of Punch

Ideally punch should be 4 mm or above for highest yield. Biopsy on the face may be done with 3 mm punch to avoid visible scar. When evaluating hair or follicular plugging, size at least 4 mm is considered necessary.

### Site of Biopsy for Direct Immunofluorescence

Biopsy of skin lesions for DIF has to be selected according to the disease. In case of suspected autoimmune bullous disease, normal appearing nonbullous skin is chosen. Study has shown that the site yields highest positivity if it is within 1 cm skin of a bulla. Trunk is also shown to be better than limbs. This is in contrast to discoid lupus where lesional skin (not the perilesional skin) is to be taken from an established lesion (>6 months old).

### Difficulty in Performing Biopsy in Bullous Disease

Getting the intact bulla in case of bullous disease with the punch is difficult. Roof of the bulla is frequently lost during processing. Selection of a small vesicle is ideal. Punch or saucerized shave biopsy are often required and considered best.

In case of epidermolysis bullosa (EB), in absence of bulla, normal appearing area can be rubbed with cotton swab, pencil eraser, or even a gloved-finger before taking the biopsy. A firm downward pressure followed by a twisting movement at 180° is exerted. This is continued until erythema is developed (usually 1 minute). Biopsy should be done after some time so that fluid can accumulate. Best site for biopsy in such cases is junction between erythematous and normal skin.

### Transport Medium

Initially, Michelle's medium was considered mandatory for DIF study in autoimmune bullous disease. Now it has been shown that sample can be transported in normal saline for DIF. It has also been reported that normal saline may result in better immunofluorescence.

### Biopsy for Hair Disease

Punch direction should be oblique along the hair to avoid sectioning of the hair and to get highest number of full length hair per punch biopsy. As discussed, punch should be at least 4 mm in size. However, more important is tissue sectioning with microtome and making the slide. Androgenetic alopecia and telogen effluvium is best diagnosed with horizontal sections that show proportion of anagen, catagen, and telogen follicles as well as relative proportion of terminal and vellus hairs. Most other diseases are best diagnosed with longitudinal sections where full-length hair is seen. There are two known techniques for sectioning of the hair called HoVert technique and Tyler technique. It is better to take two biopsies. One is sectioned horizontally and serial longitudinal sections are done. Another tissue is bisected horizontally at the level of 1 mm above dermal-subcutaneous junction. The freshly cut side of the both the tissues are placed facing downward and then serial horizontal sections are made.

## Staining of Tissues

Staining of the histology section is important as it can effectively differentiate different component of the tissues in the section. It is the primary job of the dermatologist to suspect some disease and ask for specific tissue stain so as to diagnose or rule out that disease. Some commonly used stains and the tissues that are stained by them are mentioned in table 4.

**TABLE 4: Commonly used stains in histopathology**

| | |
|---|---|
| Melanin | Silver nitrate, Fontana masson, DOPA |
| Iron (hemosiderin) | Perl's Prussian Blue |
| Calcium | Von Kossa, Alizarin red |
| Fibrin | Martius Scarlet blue (MSB) |
| Collagen | Masson trichrome |
| Elastic fibers | Verhoeff-Van Geisen for reticular dermis, Pinkus orcein for papillary dermis |
| Reticulin fiber | Silver nitrate |
| Mucin (mucopolysaccharides) | Mucicarmine, periodic acid Schiff (PAS) for neutral mucin, Giemsa, colloidal iron, and alcian blue for acid mucin |
| Fat | Scarlet red, Oil red O |
| Amyloid | Congo red |
| Mast cells | Giemsa, toluidine blue |
| *M. leprae* | Wade Fite |
| Spirochetes | Warthin-Starry stain |
| Fungi | PAS, Grocott/Gomori methenamine silver (GMS) |

DOPA, dihydroxyphenylalaline.

## Ultrasonography

Ultrasonography is a relatively new tool in dermatology. This works on a principle of sound waves reflected from tissues is converted into images. B-mode scanning is the preferred method in dermatology, analyze "brightness" values on a gray scale.

Ultrasonography uses low and high frequency waves. Increasing the frequency increases the resolution but decreases the depth of penetration. Thus high frequency is used for superficial like epidermal tissue.

Most high resolution images of epidermis and dermis are obtained with 20–25 MHz. For subcutaneous tissues, 5–12 MHz is used. For clearer images of epidermis, 50–100 MHz can also be used.

Epidermis and dermis appears hyperechoic and subcutaneous tissue appears hypoechoic. Tumors appear hyperechoic.

Ultrasonography is being used increasing in dermatology for a large number of conditions. Skin thickness assessment has been one of the earliest and useful indications. It has been used to assess steroid induced skin atrophy, and psoriasis plaque thickness.

Many other newer and experimental indications have been explored.

It is useful in assessment of cyst, benign, and skin malignancy and many other conditions. It has been shown to be of use in depth of penetration as well as marginal extension in tumors. Thus, it helps in differentiation of malignant tumors from benign one. It can also help in differentiating seborrheic keratoses, and benign nevi from melanoma.

Doppler ultrasonography is being used extensively in dermatology. It can assess vascularity in verruca and this can be correlated with depth of penetration and thus resistance to standard treatment. Similar principal has been utilized in malignancy and lymph nodes. Reactive and metastatic lymph nodes have been differentiated with vascularity pattern.

It can discriminate between lichen sclerosis et atrophicus from morphea and evaluation of severity and aggressiveness of systemic sclerosis.

## Immunohistochemistry

Immunohistochemistry (IHC) is a technique through which presence of antigen in tissues is identified with specific antibody. Antigens are components of cells or other body tissue and may range from benign to malignant or infiltrating inflammatory cells. Thus a wide array of disease can be diagnosed with IHC and the number of conditions is expanding fast.

Two methods are employed—immunofluorescence and immunoenzyme method. The latter is advantageous on certain grounds; it allows the tissue to preserve longer for examination and electron microscopy can be done simultaneously.

Initially, the test was done of fresh, frozen tissue. Now, formalin fixed paraffin-embedded tissue block are used for most of the markers.

Immunohistochemistry follows a principle of indirect staining where antibodies against specific antigens are used. Then another antibody labeled with an enzyme (peroxidase or alkaline phosphatase) along with a chromagen is added (Box 3). This makes the reaction visible.

**BOX 3 Chromagen**

- Diaminobenzidine (DAB): Brown color
- Fast red and aminoethyl carbazole (AEC): Red color

## Polymerase Chain Reaction

Polymerase chain reaction (PCR) is a method of amplification of target DNA sequence (generally less than 10 kb). Essentially unlimited number of copies of that DNA can be made. Kary Mullis received part of the Nobel Prize in Chemistry in 1993 for his invention of the PCR.

### Method

The process starts with a template that can be small or very large. Two different primers called reverse and forward are designed that can bind to the complementary regions of the target DNA. The primers are short DNA fragments that have a sequence that is complementary to the two ends of the target DNA. The process of binding of the primers with the target DNA sequence is called hybridization or annealing.

Primers are added to the template along with deoxynucleoside triphosphate (dNTP) precursors (dATP, dCTP, dGTP, dTTP) and one buffer. This is then heated at 95°C. Double-stranded DNA of the organism is denatured to single strand. When cooled to 55–65°C, primers bind to the template.

DNA polymerases are added to synthesis of complementary DNA from the primers from both the target DNA strands.

The same process can be repeated multiple times for increasing the number of amplicons.

Detection of the amplicon requires staining that can be done through staining of the amplicon after the PCR process or staining of the nucleotide or the primer before the process. Ethidium bromide is commonly used for staining of amplicon and fluorescent dyes (fluorophores) are used to label the nucleotide.

Detection is done most commonly through agarose gel electrophoresis. DNA products are characterized on the basis of size and charge and compared with standardized set of DNA products with known sizes.

The standard method of PCR is called specific PCR. Simultaneous detection of multiple organisms in a single sample is called multiple PCR.

### Use

Most important indication is diagnosis of infectious disease. There exist other methods for this nucleic acid target amplification like ligase chain reaction (LCR), transcription-mediated amplification (TMA), nucleic acid sequence-based amplification (NASBA) but PCR is the most commonly used method.

### Advantage and Disadvantages

In contrast to DNA cloning that also amplifies DNA primers, PCR is more sensitive and much faster.

However, the main disadvantage is the necessity for a primer and information of the sequence of the target DNA. Secondly, PCR can amply a target DNA upto 40 kb. These are major limitations.

## Reverse-transcriptase PCR

In reverse-transcriptase PCR (RT-PCR), the starting point is RNA (or mRNA) instead of DNA. The RNA is first converted to cDNA, which is then amplified.

- This is a three step process, cDNA is synthesized with a primer and an enzyme called reverse transcriptase
- cDNA is then amplified
- PCR products are then analyzed with gel electrophoresis.

## Real-time PCR

This method can even assess the increase in the amount of DNA as it is amplified. Thus it is aptly called real-time PCR. Here also, the starting point is RNA. This is thus a quantitative method.

## Enzyme-linked Immunosorbent Assay

### Principle

Enzyme-linked immunosorbent assay (ELISA) uses the principle of radioimmunoassay. This is a method to detect the antigens in a sample. The basic principle of identifying the antigen is to bind the antigen in liquid form with an antibody which is then bound to a secondary antibody coupled with an enzyme. This enzyme is added with a chromagen for colorimetric analysis of the antigen-antibody complex. Fluorogenic substrates offer higher sensitivity and help in accurately measuring the levels of antigen concentrations in the sample.

### Method

As mentioned, the antigen in this case has to be in liquid state. This is added in the well in which the antigens adhere to the wall of the well. The "capture" antibody immobilizes the specific antigen among the mix of various antigens.

Four different methods are available

1. Indirect ELISA
2. Sandwich ELISA
3. Competitive ELISA
4. Multiple and portable ELISA.

## T-cell Receptor Gene Rearrangement Studies

### Principle

This is a sophisticated method primarily used for diagnosis of cutaneous T-cell lymphoma (CTCL). The principle of the test is dependent upon understanding the T-cell receptor (TCR) and the TCR gene rearrangement.

Each T-cell has one unique antigen receptor on its surface. This acts like a specific marker or fingerprint for that particular T-cell and its clonal progeny. So, if this T-cell becomes neoplastic, this TCR becomes the tumor marker for that cell.

TCRs are protein heterodimers that are composed of either α, β, or γ, δ chains. The first pair is much common than the later. Each chain is composed of four regions called variable (V), joining (J), diversity (D), and constant (C).

These chains and its individual segments are encoded by specific set of genes. Specific combinations of these genes are arranged during development at thymus by a process called somatic recombination. During maturation of T-cell, there is further rearrangement of the gene segments. The final gene arrangement is thus highly exclusive for each TCR.

## Method

T-cell receptor gene rearrangement analysis is done with PCR technique. For various technical reasons, γ chain is analyzed. This is done from the formalin-fixed paraffin-embedded tissue or fresh-frozen samples. The later is preferred and is more sensitive. Genomic DNA is extracted and is amplified through PCR. Gel electrophoresis method is used to separate the PCR products as mentioned earlier.

Source of the tissue can be affected skin, blood (Sezary syndrome) or lymph node.

## SUGGESTED READINGS


1. Argenziano G, Fabbrocini G, Carli P, et al. Comparison of the ABCD rule of dermatoscopy and a new 7-point checklist. Arch Dermatol. 1998;134(12):1563-70.
2. Durdu M, Baba M, Seckin D. The value of Tzanck smear test in diagnosis of erosive, vesicular, bullous, and pustular skin lesions. J Am Acad Dermatol. 2008;59:958-64.
3. Elston D. The "Tyler technique" for alopecia biopsies. J Cutan Pathol. 2012;39:306.
4. Elston DM, Stratman EJ, Miller SJ. Skin biopsy: biopsy issues in specific diseases. J Am Acad Dermatol. 2016;74:1-16.
5. Kleinerman R, Whang TB, Bard RL, et al. Ultrasound in dermatology: principles and applications. J Am Acad Dermatol. 2012;67(3):478-87.
6. Menzies SW, Ingrar C, McCathy WH. A sensitivity and specificity analysis of the surface microscopy features of invasive melanoma. Melanoma Res. 1996;6(1):55-62.
7. Nachbar F, Stolz W, Merkle T, et al. The ABCD rule of dermatoscopy. High prospective value in the diagnosis of doubtful melanocytic skin lesions. J Am Acad Dermatol. 1994;30(4):551-9.
8. Nguyen JV, Hudacek K, Whitten JA, et al. The HoVert technique: a novel method for the sectioning of alopecia biopsies. J Cutan Pathol. 2011;38:401-6.
9. Pariser RJ. Diagnosis of spongiotic vesicular dermatitis by Tzanck smear: the "tadpole cell". J Am Acad Dermatol. 1983;8:519-22.
10. Rallan D, Harland CC. Ultrasound in dermatology–basic principles and applications. Clin Experiment Dermatol. 2003;28:632-8.
11. Vodegel RM, de Jong MC, Meijer HJ, et al. Enhanced diagnostic immunofluorescence using biopsies transported in saline. BMC Dermatol. 2004;4:10.
12. Zalaudek I, Argenziano G, Soyer HP, et al. Three point checklist of dermoscopy: an open internet study. Br J Dermatol. 2006;154(3):431-7.

- *Uniparental disomy:* When a person receives two copies of chromosomes from the same parent, due to any error in meiosis.

## CUTANEOUS MOSAICISM

Mosaicism refers to the presence of two or more genetically different populations of cells originating from one genetically homogeneous zygote.

### How to Recognize Mosaicism of Skin

Mosaicism is usually present in different shapes and patterns. They typically follow lines of Blaschko or may have flag-like patterns with a sharp superior and inferior border and midline separation. Other patterns include checkerboard, phylloid, block type, zosteriform or dermatomal and garment-like. Figs 1 to 4 shows the various patterns of hypopigmented patterns of mosiacism. Figs 5 to 7 shows the hyperpigmented patterns. Archetypal patterns are more likely to have extracutaneous involvement than nonarchetypal patterns. Another example of cutaneous mosaicism is incontinentia pigmenti as shown in Figs 8 to 10.

## GENETIC MECHANISM

Mosaicism can be due to:

- *Genetic*: Mutations occur during embryonic development
- *Epigenetic*: This happens due to modifications in gene expression.

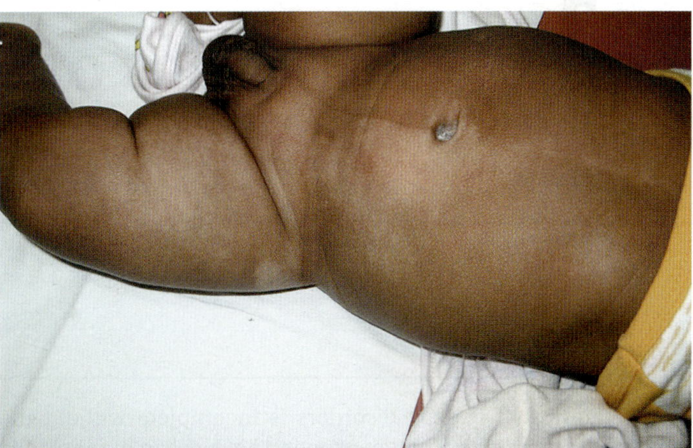

**FIG. 3:** Flaglike pattern with sharp midline cut-off.

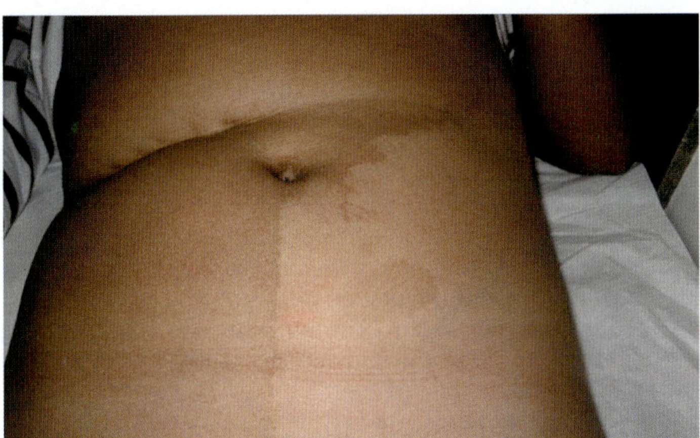

**FIG. 1:** A large nevus depigmentosus.

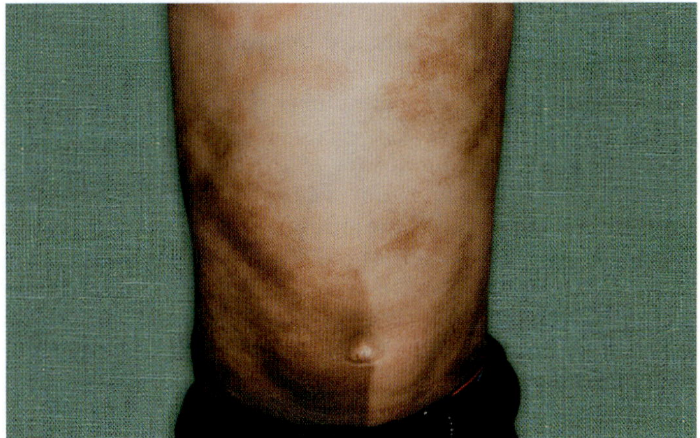

**FIG. 4:** Block like patterns seen on the anterior chest and abdomen.

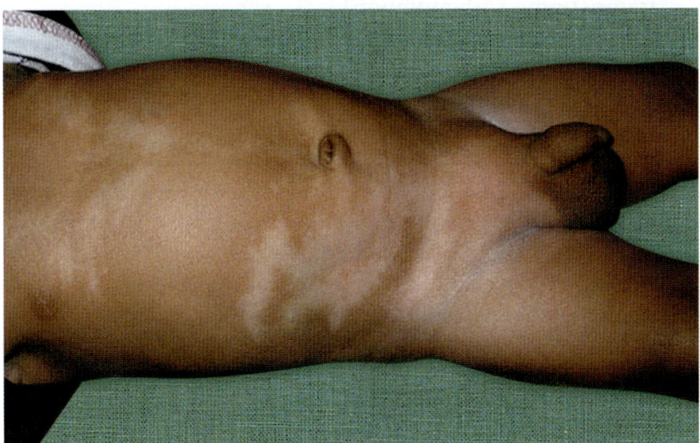

**FIG. 2:** Phylloid pattern of pigment mosaicism.

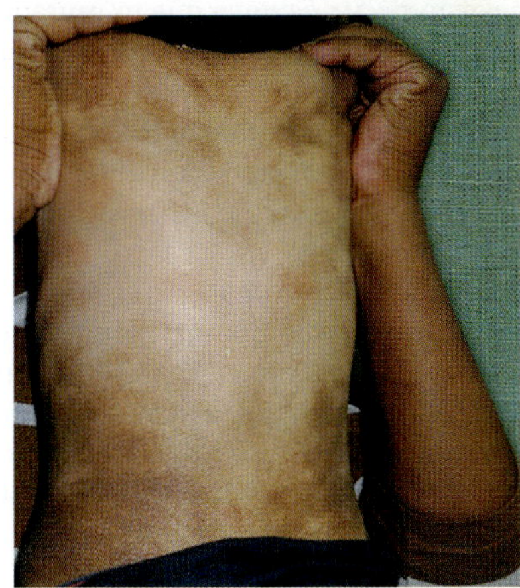

**FIG. 5:** Blaschkoid pattern on the back.

2

SECTION

# Skin and Genetics

2

CHAPTER

# Principles of Genetics

*Priya Bishnoi, Ravi Hiremagalore*

## INTRODUCTION

Understanding of genetic disorders is incomplete without the basic understanding of human genetics. Each cell in human body has a nucleus which contains the essential information in the form of genes, which is required for the normal functioning of cells. Genes are made up of DNA, which are made up of a unique sequence of bases. All the information in DNA is transcribed into mRNA which later gets translated into proteins. Chromosomes are linear structures in the nucleus which are made up of genes. Every cell has diploid number of chromosomes that is two pairs of 23 chromosomes each (44 autosomes and two sex chromosomes). The reproductive cells in an individual undergo cell division (meiosis) and from male and female gametes which fuse together to give rise to the offspring. Every gene exists in two or more forms known as alleles and thus individuals can have the same alleles *(homozygous)* for a particular character or they can have two different alleles *(heterozygous)*. If only a single allele is required for expression of a particular character, then this allele is the dominant allele and if two similar alleles are required, then this allele is the recessive allele for that character.

## GENETIC DISORDERS

Genetic disorders can be either inherited from one generation to the other or they can occur *de novo* due to mutations. Inherited genetic diseases can be due to single gene defects, multiple gene defects, or can even be due to chromosomal anomalies. These disorders can be classified according to the type of inheritance:

- Autosomal dominant—affected individuals are heterozygous for the defective allele and both males and females are affected
- Autosomal recessive—both males and females are affected and affected individuals are homozygous for the defect
- X-linked recessive—defect lies on X chromosome and thus only males are affected and females are always carriers
- X-linked dominant—defective allele is present on X chromosome and this allele is dominant. Both males and females can be affected but in males the mutation is lethal and hence only females are seen with this group of disorders.

Mutation is an irreversible change anywhere along the DNA sequence which causes defective flow of genetic information. If a mutation occurs in the reproductive cells, it is known as *germ line mutation* and can be passed on to the next generation. Germ line mutations again can be heterozygous, homozygous, or even compound heterozygous (both alleles are mutated but with a different mutation in both the paternal and maternal alleles). If the mutation occurs in somatic cells, it is known as somatic mutation and is not passed on further. Mutations can be of many different types:

- Point mutation occurs if a single base in the sequence is replaced by another base. The consequence of a point mutation depends on the type of point mutation and it need not always be disastrous. Types of point mutation are as follows:
    - *Nonsense mutation:* When the mutation results in a codon which does not translate into a functional protein
    - *Missense mutation:* When mutation results in a stop codon and results into truncation of protein
    - *Silent mutation:* Mutation does not lead to any abnormality, either because the mutation is in the noncoding area or the base mutated does not cause any alteration in the amino acid
    - *Neutral mutation:* Due to the mutation the amino acid formed is different but chemically similar to the original amino acid.
- *Insertions*: Insertion of a base would cause either alteration in splicing of mRNA (splice mutation) or shift in the reading frame (frame-shift mutation)
- *Deletions*: It is due to removal of a base from the sequence and thus could lead to a shift in the reading frame.

## FEW TERMINOLOGIES IN GENETICS

- *Genetic heterogeneity:* When diseases with very similar phenotypes are a result of various different alleles, e.g., ichthyosis, epidermolysis bullosa, psoriasis
- *Pleiotropy:* Single defective gene is responsible for multiple phenotypic expressions in a single disease. This could be because the gene could code for a product which is required by various different types of cells for their function, e.g., albinism
- *Genomic imprinting:* This is a very rare phenomenon where inheritance does not follow the Mendelian laws and is rather dependent on the parent of origin. Only one of the genes would be expressed depending on the paternity, e.g., Angelman syndrome, Prader-Willi syndrome

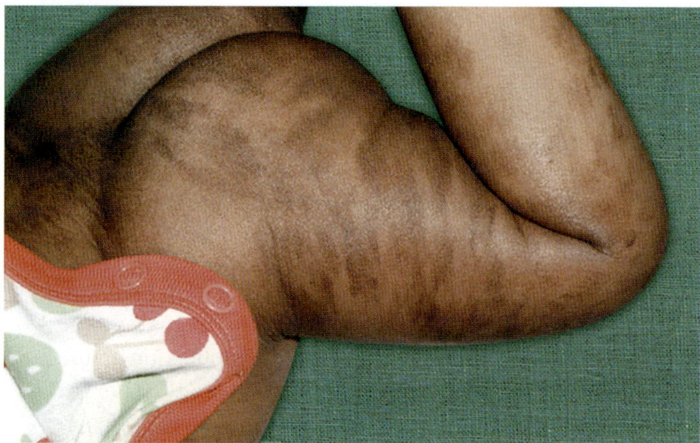

**FIG. 6:** Hyperpigmented variant in a zosteriform distribution.

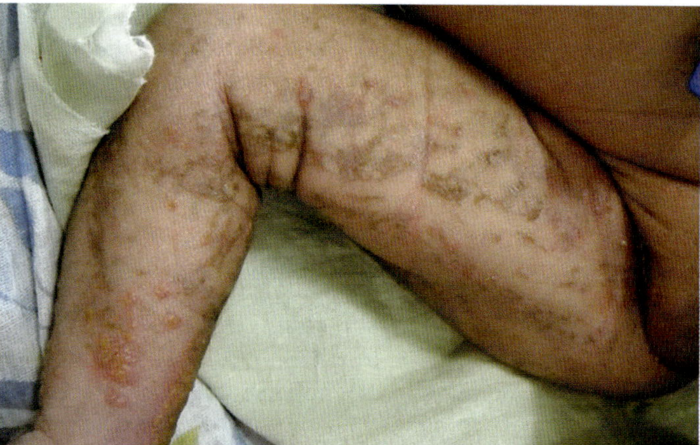

**FIG. 9:** Incontinentia pigmenti in papular stage showing some vesicles and hyperpigmentation.

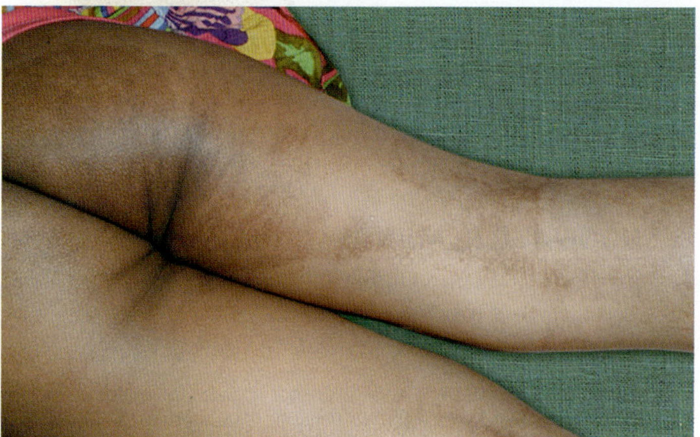

**FIG. 7:** Hyperpigmented variant in blaschkoid distribution.

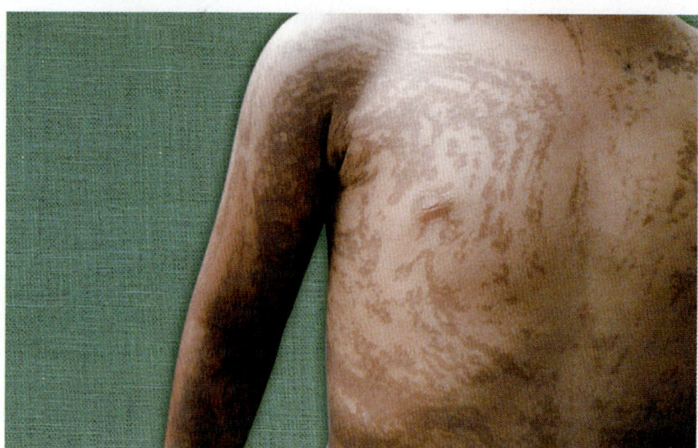

**FIG. 10:** Final stage of incontinentia pigmenti showing whorled pattern of hyperpigmentation.

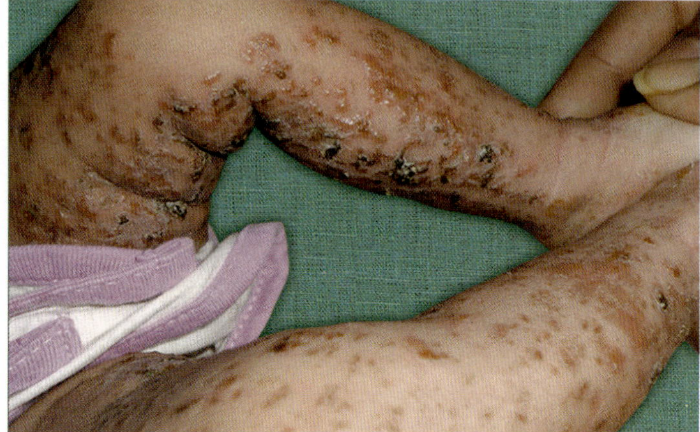

**FIG. 8:** Incontinentia pigmenti in the vesicular stage.

## Genetic (Somatic) Mosaicism

Mutational event occurs in the embryo stage. Lethal autosomal mutations can survive secondary to mosaicism. Keratinocyte epidermal nevus syndrome is an example of this type of mosaicism. Likewise, lethal autosomal recessive mutations appear in a normal carrier heterozygous individual due to mosaicism. This can be secondary to loss of heterozygosity resulting from a second mutation or a loss of normal allele during embryo development.

Nonlethal autosomal dominant mosaicism can be of two types:

1. *Type 1:* This is usually a postzygotic new mutation and can have a generalized counterpart. A parent with a linear epidermal nevus of the epidermolytic hyperkeratosis type, can have a child with bullous ichthyosiform erythroderma due to mosaicism
2. *Type 2:* A heterozygous embryo with a generalized disease can have an areas of skin far more severely affected. This is due to loss of heterozygoisity.

Mosaicism can be seen in polygenic inflammatory disorders secondary to loss of heterozygosity during the development of embryo. The common disorders with this pattern include psoriasis, lichen planus and vitiligo.

## PROGRESS IN MOLECULAR GENETICS

With the techniques of polymerase chain reaction (PCR) and sequencing, it has been possible to identify the genes that are mutated in more than 350 genodermatosis. Developments in molecular analyses have enabled genotype-phenotype correlation. This has helped in understanding the pattern of inheritance. For example, previously it was difficult to determine if a child with moderately severe blistering and scarring, born to unaffected parents was due to sporadic autosomal dominant inheritance or an autosomal recessive trait.

### DNA-based Prenatal Diagnosis

The major immediate benefit of advances in molecular analysis is prenatal diagnosis to couples in whom there is an increased risk of recurrence of a particular genodermatosis. This is accomplished by obtaining fetal DNA from chorionic villus sampling (CVS) between 10 and 12 weeks of gestation. The first step involved in DNA based prenatal diagnosis is to identify the pathogenic mutation in the proband. This is accomplished by direct sequencing the target gene which is a very laborious process. In the case of large genes like collagen VII A 1 (Col 7A1), it is preferable to have an algorithm for testing by screening for the hot spots first and then proceed to whole gene sequencing if no known mutations are identified. This is followed by sequencing the parents DNA for this specific mutation. This strategy establishes the pattern of inheritance which thereby helps in counseling. Finally, the fetal DNA taken from CVS would be tested for the mutation and parents are again counseled regarding the possibilities and thus a rationalized decision can be taken. The most common skin disorder for which a DNA based prenatal testing has been established is Hallopeau-Siemens recessive dystrophic epidermolysis bullosa (EB) and Herlitz junctional EB. In the conditions where there is considerable genetic heterogeneity, like junctional EB and lamellar ichthyosis, it is pertinent that the mutation is accurately identified in the proband. This problem can be approached by recent advances in techniques like Next-gen sequencing and exome sequencing. This involves screening the entire genome or exome which generates enormous data that require training in bioinformatics to interpret accurately.

### Ethical Issues in Prenatal Diagnosis

The development of DNA based prenatal testing has raised several ethical issues. With the advances in molecular genetics, it is not only possible to do DNA-based prenatal testing for severe phenotypes of certain genodermatosis but also in milder forms, which is considered unjustified by some health care personnel. On the contrary, society perceive that every couple at risk have the right to know the options available and hence the right to prenatal diagnosis with termination of an affected pregnancy. Such decisions are often complex and very personal and may vary with the region and religion.

### Gene Therapy

Advances in molecular genetics have been responsible for the initiation of research in gene therapy. Classically, EB has been the most common genodermatoses where gene therapy has been studied. There are two approaches.

1. *Ex vivo:* In this strategy, cells are harvested from the patient and they are propagated in a vector and gene corrected and cells are expanded in a culture and finally transplanted back to the patient. This approach has been tried in junctional EB. The major limitation is carcinogenesis
2. *In vivo*: This approach involves topical application or injection of gene therapy compound into the skin.

## CONCLUSION

Genodermatoses form a major part referral to pediatric dermatology services. Hence understanding of some of the basic terminologies in genetics is imperative. Cutaneous mosaicism is common and awareness amongst dermatologists is necessary for early diagnosis and alleviate patient anxiety and to avoid unnecessary use of topical medications. Advances in molecular genetics have enabled DNA-based prenatal diagnosis and evidence-based genetic counseling.

## SUGGESTED READINGS

1. Engel E. A new genetic concept: the uniparental disomy and its potential effect, the isodisomy. J Genet Hum. 1980;28:11-22.
2. Eyre-Walker A, Keightley PD. The distribution of fitness effects of new mutations. Nat Rev Genet. 2007;8:610-8.
3. Fassihi H, Eady RA, Mellerio JE, et al. Prenatal diagnosis for severe inherited skin disorders: 25 years' experience. Br J Dermatol. 2006;154:106-13.
4. Fraser GR. Genetics and medicine I. Br Med J. 1966;2:345-7.
5. Fraser GR. Genetics and medicine II. Br Med J. 1966;2:397-9.
6. Happle R. Mosaicism in human skin: understanding the patterns and mechanisms. Arch Dermatol. 1993;129(11):1460-70.
7. Leech SN, Moss C. A current and online genodermatosis database. Br J Dermatol. 2007;156:1115-48.
8. Mavillo F, Pelegrini G, Ferrari S, et al. Correction of junctional epidermolysis bullosa by transplantation of genetically modified epidermal stem cells. Nat Med. 2006;12:1397-402.
9. Millington GM. Genomic imprinting and dermatological diseases. Clin Exp Dermatol. 2006;31:685-8.
10. Uitto J, Pulkkinen L. Molecular genetics of heritable blistering disorders. Arch Dermatol. 2001;137:458-61.
11. Wells RS, Kerr CB. Genetic classification of ichthyosis. Arch Dermatol. 1965;92:33-55.
12. Williams JC. Pleiotropy, natural selection and senescence. Evolution. 1957;11: 398-411.

# 3 CHAPTER Genomic Stability Disorders

Nilendu Sarma, Indrashis Podder

## INTRODUCTION

Human DNA is constantly exposed to various noxious environments of exogenous and endogenous origin. Exposure to ultraviolet rays, ionizing radiation (X-rays and gamma rays), heat, plant toxins, mutagenic aromatic chemicals, and viruses are important exogenous substances that can incur damage to the DNA. Endogenous metabolic process can also damage the DNA. Even the routine replication and recombination process during cell division generates many errors. Reactive oxygen species (ROS) are considered one of the prime mechanisms for DNA damage. Endogenous mechanisms for DNA damage are oxidation, alkylation, hydrolysis, bulky adduct formation, mismatch of bases, and monoadduct and diadduct formation. The rate of development of new molecular lesions may be as high as 10,000–1,000,000 per cell per day.

There are many protective mechanisms in our body that constantly protect the DNA and maintain the integrity in it.

The result of insults depends on many factors like cell type, severity and type of damage, and existence and capacity of effective repair mechanisms.

Final outcome of damage in DNA from various kinds of endogenous and exogenous factors are:

- The formation of pyrimidine dimers
- Methylation (of guanine bases)
- Replication errors—mismatch
- Depurination
- Bulky adducts formation
- Cross-link
- Single strand damage
- Double strand breaks: This is highly deleterious and can lead to chromosomal rearrangements.

## MECHANISMS FOR DNA REPAIR

Human body is equipped with complex and effective mechanisms to protect from cancers that may result from abnormal DNA. The defense mechanism induces cell cycle arrest to allow the repair system to get activated. There are various repair mechanisms as discussed later. In case of irreparable damage, the cell undergoes programmed death (apoptosis).

There exist different mechanisms for immediate repair of DNA damages. These are:

- *Direct reversal*: It does not require any template and the defect is correct directly
- *Excision repair*: In case of single strand damage, the normal strand is used as template. There are three mechanisms for excision repair, e.g.:
    - Nucleotide excision repair (NER)
    - Base excision repair (BER)
    - Mismatch repair
- *Double strand break*: There are three mechanisms that repair double strand break, called:
    - Homologous recombination (HR)
    - Nonhomologous end joining (NHEJ)
    - Microhomology-mediated end joining (MMEJ).

### Mismatch Repair

Replication error during normal cell division is a common event. These errors are corrected by proofreading genes. Any replication errors that are missed also by proofreading genes are repaired by a mechanism called "mismatch repair system".

### Nucleotide Excision Repair

Nucleotide excision repair is one of the most effective mechanisms in repair of defective DNA. It removes a wide range of structurally-unrelated defects, including UV photoproducts and single strand damage. The mechanism of damage by UV rays is formation of cyclobutane pyrimidine dimers (CPDs) and 6–4 photoproducts (6–4 PPs). This is repaired by NER. NER has three sub-pathways called global genome repair (GGR/GG-NER), transcription-coupled repair (TCR), and transcription domain-associated repair (DAR).

Global genome-nucleotide excision repair can remove damaged DNA located anywhere throughout the genome and included actively transcribed as well as inactive regions of DNA double helix. TC-NER on the other hand, recognizes actively transcribed genes. Once recognized, the subsequent repair involves common processes like unwinding of the damaged DNA, dual incisions, excision of damaged oligonucleotide, synthesis in the resulting gap, and ligation of the repair patch.

Diseases that result from defect in NER are xeroderma pigmentosum (XP), Cockayne syndrome (CS), trichothiodystrophy (TTD), and UV-sensitive syndrome (UVSS). All of these manifest photosensitivity. Only XP has increased tendency to cancer development.

Both CS and UVSS involve same genes. In both these, there is defect in recovery of RNA synthesis after UV irradiation (RRS) and a defect of TCR of UV damage but have a normally functioning GGR.

## DISEASES RESULTING FROM ABNORMALITIES IN DNA REPAIR

Damage to the DNA can lead to formation of mutation and can induce different diseases. In slowly dividing cells, accumulated abnormal proteins from unrepaired damaged DNA may lead to early senescence and degenerative process. Once mutation sets in, it becomes irreparable and heritable. This is because, mutations are alterations in the base sequence of the DNA and are not identified by the enzymes. Harmful mutation can progress to cancer formation in rapidly dividing cells.

Defective capacity for repair of DNA damage (genomic instability) leads to chromosomal structural alterations or alteration in numbers (aneuploidy). Genome instability typically manifests with premature aging, photosensitivity, neuro-degeneration (e.g., amyotrophic lateral sclerosis), neuromuscular disease (e.g., myotonic dystrophy), cognitive decline, immuno-deficiency, growth retardation, and high prevalence of cancer (Table 1).

### Genomic Instability and Cancer

As discussed, diseases with DNA instability may manifest with increased risk of cancer. Here is a list of cancers and pathway involved:

- Nucleotide excision repair—XP
- Mismatch repair—Muir-Torre syndrome (a subtype of the hereditary nonpolyposis colorectal cancer syndrome)
- Homologous recombination—Bloom syndrome (*BLM*, RecQ helicase-like), and breast cancer (BRCA1, 2)
- Nonhomologous end joining—Werner syndrome, Nijmegen breakage syndrome
- Microhomology-mediated end joining—cancers of the breast, prostate, neuroblastomas, pancreatic, and lung.

**TABLE 1: Diseases with genomic instability**

| Disease | Defective pathways |
|---|---|
| Xeroderma pigmentosum (XPA-G, XPV) | NER |
| Cockayne syndrome (CSA, CSB, XAB2) | NER |
| Trichothiodystrophy (ERCC2, ERCC3, or GTF2H5) | NER |
| Down syndrome | NER |
| Triple-A syndrome | NER |
| Huntington's disease | BER |
| Parkinson's disease | BER |
| Down syndrome | BER |
| Amyotrophic lateral sclerosis | BER |
| Ataxia telangiectasia (ATM) | DSB repair |
| Nijmegen breakage syndrome (NBS1) | NHEJ (DSB repair defect) |
| Werner syndrome (WRN) | NHEJ (DSB repair defect) |
| Fanconi anemia (FANC-A, B, C, D1, D2, E, F, G) | HR, repair of inter-strand crosslink |
| Rothmund-Thomson syndrome (RTS) | – |
| Bloom syndrome (BLM) | Homologous recombination defect |
| Alzheimer's disease | DSB repair |

NER, nucleotide excision repair; BER, base excision repair; DSB, double-strand break; NHEJ, nonhomologous end joining.

### Genomic Instability and Premature Aging Disorders

There are many diseases that manifest with different features aging (Box 1). However, complete phenotype of aging is hardly ever seen. Thus, these are often called segmental progeria.

### Xeroderma Pigmentosum

Xeroderma pigmentosum is a rare, autosomal recessive DNA repair disorder, described in 1874 by Moriz Kaposi, characterized clinically by significant photosensitivity, high prevalence of cancer in the exposed skin, and also the mucous membranes of the eyes and mouth. There is an autosomal dominant type too. It is sometimes (in 25% of cases) associated with progressive neurological degeneration. Incidence ranges from 1 per 100,000 live births in the West to 1 per 40,000 live births in Japan.

#### *Pathogenesis*

UV radiation exposure leads to development of several types of stable dipyrimidine nucleotide photoproducts, cyclobutane pyrimidine dimer being the major one. These photoproducts are premutagenic and are repaired by NER pathway that is defective in XP.

The DNA polymerase may stop replication at this unrepaired photoproduct resulting in cell death or may incorporate a incorrect nucleotide (T instead of C). The resulting C to T mutation, commonly known as "UV signature mutations" is frequently detected in XP.

There are seven complementation groups in XP (XPA to G) and a variant group called XP-V. Genes for XPA to XPG are involved in NER and the gene in XPV (POLH) encodes for DNA polymerase-η that causes replication of UV-damaged DNA. Recently, a new DNA repair factor has been implicated called TFIIH in yeasts and human beings.

#### *Clinical Presentation*

Disease manifests during infancy to early childhood. Photo-sensitivity is variable. Severely affected patients develop acute photosensitivity with redness and blistering on slight exposure. Patients with less severe photosensitivity never burn. Usual manifestation in these patients is freckling on the exposed areas. Freckle that often develops before the age of 2 years is highly characteristic feature of XP.

**BOX 1 Diseases presenting with premature aging due to DNA repair defect**

- Bloom syndrome
- Cockayne syndrome
- Ataxia telangiectasia
- Fanconi's anemia
- Progeria
- Rothmund-Thomson syndrome
- Trichothiodystrophy
- Werner syndrome

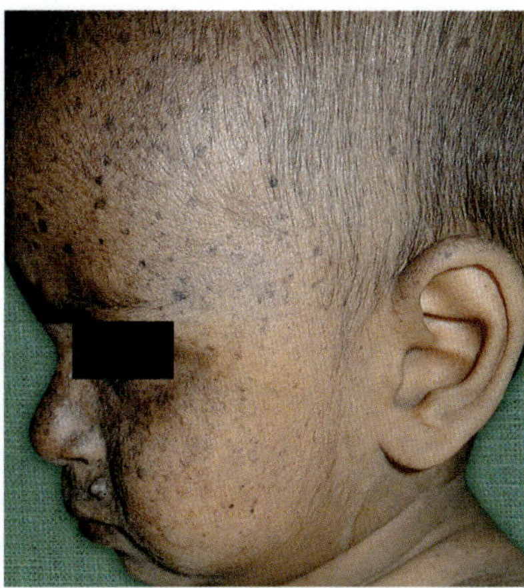

FIG. 1: Extensive freckles and lentigines in a case of xeroderma pigmentosum.

Xeroderma pigmentosum is characterized by epidermal involvement. Thus, it develops different epidermal signs of photo-aging like xerosis, atrophy, tightened skin, telangiectasia, and poikiloderma (hyperpigmentation, hypopigmentation, atrophy, and telangiectasias). It characteristically lacks dermal alterations like skin laxity, wrinkles, sagging and cutis rhomboidalis nuchae is not seen. These are found typically in solar elastosis (Fig. 1).

Persistent photophobia may lead to permanent eye damage in the form of conjunctivitis, keratitis, corneal vascularization, ectropion, entropion corneal opacity, and visual impairment.

Lens protects inner eye from the damaging effects of UV rays. Malignant growths are commonly seen in anterior eyes.

Cancer is highly prevalent on lips, central nervous system, and other internal organs. Benign tumors like angioma and keratoacanthoma are also more common.

Xeroderma pigmentosum increases the risk of cancer to many folds. Cancers develop at very early life. The risk is 10,000-fold higher for nonmelanoma skin cancer (NMSC), 2,000-fold higher for melanomas, 1,000-fold higher for eye (sun-exposed areas), and a 100,000-fold higher for tongue cancers before the age of 20 years. NMSC develops earlier (median age 9 years) than melanoma (median age 22 years). Prevalence of cancer is also high on lips. Melanoma is common on the extremities.

Progressive neurological impairment that starts soon after birth and manifests with delayed developmental milestones is sometimes seen. Dwarfism, microcephaly, spasticity, lack of coordination (ataxia), areflexia, difficulty in swallowing, sensorineural hearing loss, and slurred speech are noted in some cases.

### *Diagnosis*

Xeroderma pigmentosum needs to be differentiated from other diseases with photosensitivity like CS and TTD (brittle hair, short stature, hypogonadism, and ichthyosis) and neonatal lupus. Freckles and lentigines are not present in these.

De Sanctis-Cacchione syndrome has features of XP along with dwarfism, inadequate gonadal function, and neurological abnormalities.

Laboratory diagnosis is done with amniocentesis (prenatal). Genetic analysis to detect the defect can be done. *In vitro* methods to show UV-induced DNA photoproduct and impaired repair of DNA damage in lymphocytes and fibroblasts are done in some referral centers.

### *Management*

Lifelong and strict sun protection is most important. Genetic counseling, early detection, and removal of neoplastic tumors are also very important. Calcium and vitamin D supplementation have to be provided if deemed necessary.

Management of malignant and premalignant conditions (actinic keratosis, squamous cell carcinoma, and basal cell carcinoma) is also important. Topical application of bacterial DNA repair enzyme (T4N5) in liposomal drug delivery system is currently under trial.

## Bloom Syndrome

This is one of the five human disorders due to defects in RecQ family of helicases, the other two important conditions being Werner syndrome caused by mutation in *WRN (also known as RECQL2*) and Rothmund–Thomson syndrome (RTS) (*RECQL4).* All these three diseases have increased cancer risk. Bloom syndrome is transmitted as an autosomal recessive disorder.

### *Pathogenesis*

Bloom syndrome, RecQ helicase-like, occurs due to mutation in *BLM* gene (*RECQL3*) that encodes BLM protein (more than 70 mutations in the *BLM* detected). This lies in chromosome 15 (15q26.1). Genomic instability that results from this abnormality is the key mechanism involved in Bloom syndrome including the increased cancer risk. Thus, cancer in this disorder has a different mechanism than that involved in XP (carcinogenic effect of UV rays) (Box 2).

There may some phenotypic and genotypic link between Bloom syndrome and Fanconi anemia indicating some additional pathomechanisms being involved in Bloom syndrome.

### *Clinical Presentations*

Bloom syndrome is particularly common in Eastern European Ashkenazi Jews. Disease manifests within few months of life with growth retardation that actually starts in the intrauterine period.

Patient develops a typical facies with prominent nose, dolichocephaly (long head), and smaller mandible and maxilla. Longer, disproportionate limbs and hands, feet with quick bird like movement of the limbs are also characteristic.

Skin manifestations take few years to develop. Photosensitivity that may be of variable degree is common and starts in early childhood. Telangiectasia develops early over malar area. This is a very characteristic sign. This can also develop on dorsal aspect of hands and sclera.

Pigmentary alterations (hypo and hyper) that may develop both exposed and covered areas. Café-au-lait spots are also seen.

**BOX 2 Helicase and DNA instability disorders**

During cell division, two chromosomes (sister chromatids) are formed. Some amount of error is natural during this process. These are corrected through DNA exchange between the sister chromatids. This sister chromatid exchange (SCE) is a necessary protective mechanism to assist removal of errors. Helicase (known as "caretakers of the genome") is a protein that unwinds the double helix of DNA and plays an important step in DNA repair. Bloom syndrome has defective RecQ helicase and shows a very high level of SCE (>10 times).

Eyes develop conjunctivitis, bilateral optic nerve hypoplasia, and sectoral iris pigment in additional to sclera telangiectasia.

Other findings are recurrent bacterial infection [otitis media, respiratory, and gastrointestinal (GI)], diabetes, chronic obstructive pulmonary diseases, syndactyly, polydactyly, and sterility.

There is increased risk of malignancy like lymphomas, leukemia, oral, and GI tract cancers.

### Diagnosis

This has to be differentiated from CS and RTS (much early onset of poikiloderma and cataracts).

Genetic analysis and chromosomal ultrastructural analysis under electron microscope aid in the diagnosis. Quadrilateral configuration of chromosomes in lymphocytes and fibroblasts is a diagnostic feature.

### Management

Symptomatic management in the form of strict photoprotection is mandatory. These patients need regular follow-up for early detection of malignancy.

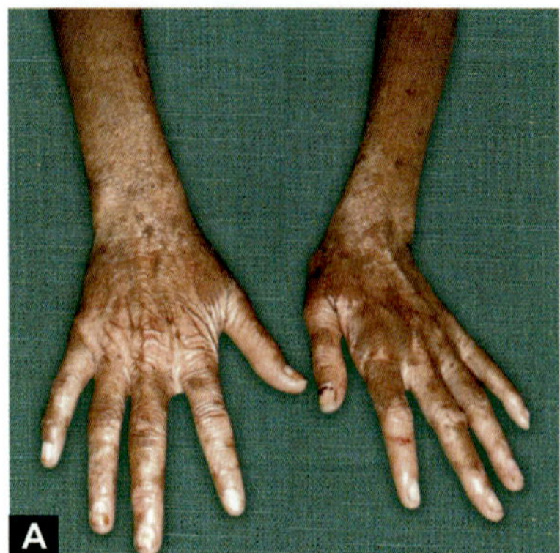


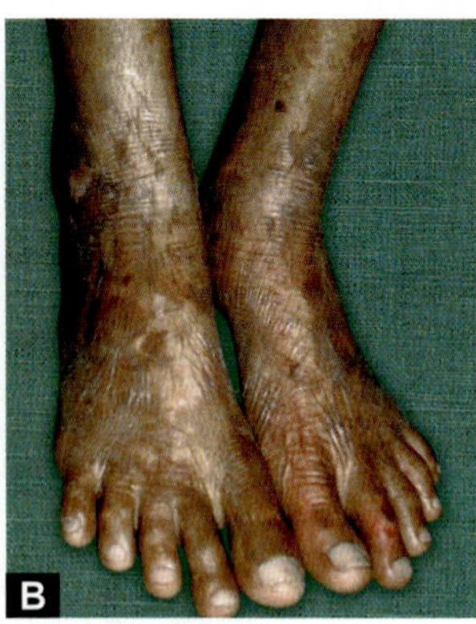


**FIG. 3:** Parchment-like skin over distal extremities in a patient with Rothmund–Thomson syndrome.

*Courtesy*: Dr Aparna Palit, Dr Arun C Inamadar, Department of Dermatology, Venereology and Leprosy, Shri BM Patil Medical College, Hospital and Research Center, BLDE University, Vijayapur, Karnataka.

## Rothmund-Thomson Syndrome

Rothmund-Thomson syndrome is rare and typically characterized with poikiloderma. It is also associated with increased risk of squamous cell carcinoma and osteosarcoma.

### Pathogenesis

Most cases are caused by *RECQL4* gene mutation. This gene synthesizes a human helicase called RecQ helicase and is located on 8q24.3. RTS is inherited as autosomal recessive disorder.

*Clinical features*: Rothmund–Thomson syndrome is characterized with poikiloderma, keratotic lesions, skeletal dysplasia, cataract, sparse hair, and increased risk of malignancy (squamous cell carcinoma and osteosarcoma). Patient may show recurrent diarrhea and vomiting.

Poikiloderma starts with inflammation at very early postnatal period (Fig. 2). There may be blisters. This is not photosensitivity-induced although distribution on face, dorsum of hands, feet, and other photoexposed areas may be involved. This stage may mimic sunburn or eczema. Covered areas like buttocks are also affected. Inflammation is followed by atrophy and telangiectasia (poikiloderma) (Fig. 3).

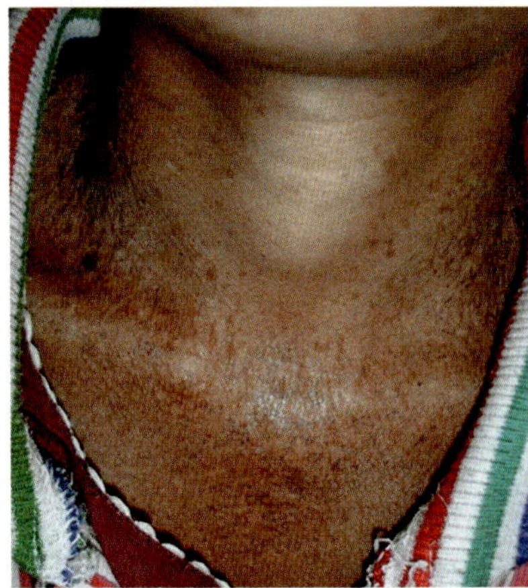

**FIG. 2:** Poikiloderma in a patient with Rothmund-Thomson syndrome.

*Courtesy*: Dr Aparna Palit, Dr Arun C Inamadar, Department of Dermatology, Venereology and Leprosy, Shri BM Patil Medical College, Hospital and Research Center, BLDE University, Vijayapur, Karnataka.

Warty keratotic lesions may be precancerous and involve acral areas and also knees.

This is one important cause of bilateral juvenile cataract.

Hairs are sparse and may involve eyebrows and eyelashes. There may be deformity of nails and teeth. Patients may also have hypogonadism.

Patients are often significantly short-statured. There is mid-facial hypoplasia like saddle nose deformity. A very classical and diagnostic skeletal deformity is absence or gross hypoplasia of thumb and radius. This is called "radial ray" defect.

Patients may die from cancers but overall mortality possibly is not higher.

### Diagnosis

Rothmund-Thomson syndrome may be confused with Kindler syndrome due to blistering at early life. Premature aging syndrome are also frequently mimicked. Both RTS and Bloom syndrome feature poikiloderma.

The RAPADILINO and Baller-Gerold syndrome are caused by mutation in same gene (*RECQL4*) and share many clinical features including radial ray defect but do not have poikiloderma.

### Treatment

This is essentially symptomatic. Retinoids may be used for keratoses.

## Cockayne Syndrome

Cockayne syndrome is a characterized by short stature, photosensitivity, and premature aging. There is impaired growth and development of head and nervous system. Unlike XP, there is no increased tendency for neoplasia.

## Pathogenesis

This rare disease has an autosomal recessive inheritance. CS develops from mutations in *ERCC8* gene (*CSA* gene, chromosome 5) and *ERCC6* gene (*CSB* gene, locus 10q11). These genes are involved in the DNA damage repair (DDR) mechanism, mainly in the pyrimidine pathway. DNA is constantly damaged be sun exposure, chemicals, and free radicals. CSA and *CSA* genes produce CSA and CSB proteins that are required for transcription-coupled NER of bulky UV-induced adducts. There might be some role of mitochondrial dysfunction in this.

It is important to note that the same genes are mutated in UVSS. The fact that these two conditions are not phenotypically similar, it is suggested that there might be some other mechanisms playing role in pathogenesis of CS and the following facts strongly support this.

Transcription-coupled repair defect in nucleus plays has been linked to photosensitivity and that in mitochondria is inducing premature aging. The latter phenotype is most possibly mediated through disturbances in ROS. POLG1 and POLG2 are essential for mtDNA replication. POLG1 inhibition is associated with premature aging. In CS, there is overexpression of HTRA3, a serine protease that selectively reduced POLG1 (DNA polymerase gamma) that might lead to premature aging.

### *Clinical Presentations*

Cockayne syndrome is rare and affects less than one in 2-2.5 per million newborns in the US.

Typical manifestations of CS are photosensitivity without lentigines or freckles (unless associated with XP), premature aging, and progressive neurological impairment involving central and peripheral nervous system. There may be calcification of basal ganglia.

Patient may have some typical appearance due to microcephaly, thin nose, "hollow" or sunken eyes, dwarfism, premature aging (progeroid) with wrinkled, aged pigmented skin, and loss of subcutaneous fat, unusually large ears, prognathism, dental malalignment, large hands and feet, long arms and legs, large joints with flexed deformity and kyphosis (Fig. 4).

Involvement of eyes and vision is significant. Patient may suffer from dry eyes, incomplete eyelid closure, cataract, optic atrophy, retinal degeneration, and blindness. There may also be hearing defect and hypogonadism (Box 3).

### *Diagnosis*

The diagnosis is essentially clinical. Genetic analysis may detect pyrimidine repair defect. CT scan of the brain may be done to detect any basal ganglia calcification.

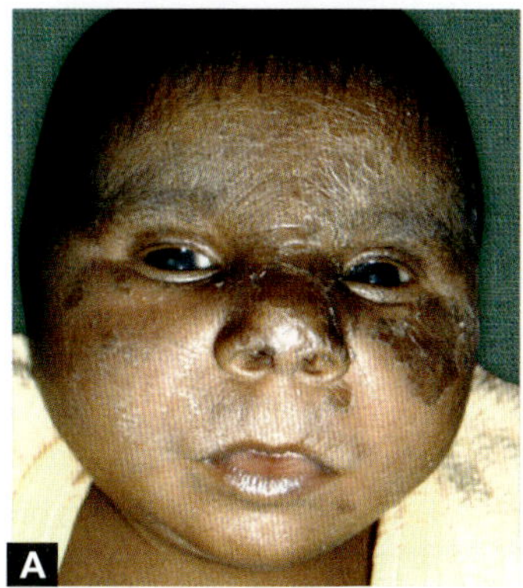


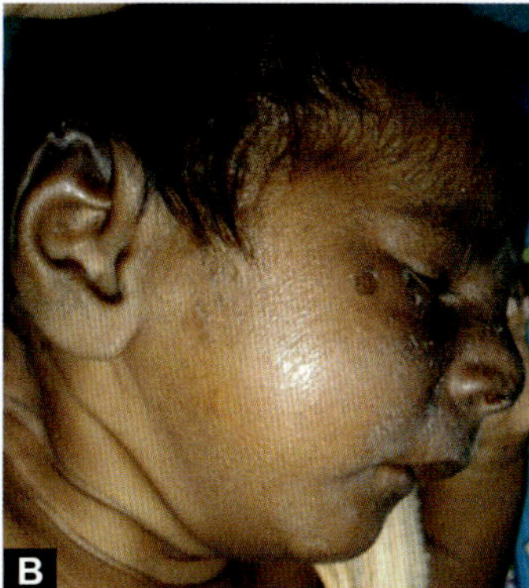


**FIG. 4:** Microcephaly, enophthalmos, photosensitivity and large pinna in an infant suggestive of Cockayne syndrome. The associated cataract in this patient indicates poor prognosis.

*Courtesy*: Dr Aparna Palit, Dr Arun C Inamadar, Department of Dermatology, Venereology and Leprosy, Shri BM Patil Medical College, Hospital and Research Center, BLDE University, Vijayapur, Karnataka.

**BOX 3 Classification of Cockayne syndrome**

**CS is classified into four subtypes**

- *Type I*: Manifests post infantile age. This consists of 25–30% of all cases. This may be fatal by 2nd decade (respiratory problems)
- *Type II*: Presents at birth. This is also known as cerebro-oculo-facio-skeletal (COFS) syndrome or Pena–Shokeir syndrome type II. This is most common type (70–75%) and has phenotypically identical withy type I other than age of onset. Death may occur by 6–7 years
- *Type III*: Manifests at childhood. This is the mildest one
- *Type IV*: Described recently. This fourth type has overlapping features of xeroderma pigmentosum and Cockayne syndrome (XP–CS). This type has features of XP-like widespread freckling and early skin cancers in addition to typical features of CS.

CS, Cockayne syndrome; XP, xeroderma pigmentosum.

### *Treatment*

Treatment is supportive. Genetic counseling and various rehabilitation therapies are helpful.

## UV-sensitive Syndrome

This is another rare photosensitivity syndrome that results from genetic defect involving same CS genes. Unlike XP, there is no higher chance of cancer and unlike CS; it does not have short stature and features of premature aging.

Features characteristic of photosensitivity like freckles, xerosis, pigmentation, and telangiectasia develop on sun-exposed skin (e.g., cheeks and nose) after repeated exposure.

### *Pathogenesis*

This is an autosomal recessive condition. Genetically, this is similar to CS and results from mutations in the *ERCC6* gene (*CSB* gene), the *ERCC8* gene (*CSA* gene), or the *UVSSA* gene (encoding UV stimulated scaffold protein A). Similar to CS, these patients also have defective repair of damaged DNA. There is defect in NER mediated through the deficiency in the subpathway called TC-NER or in short TCR. Additionally, cells are defective in TCR of cyclobutane pyrimidine dimers.

Despite these genetic similarities, they differ significantly in phenotypic expression. In UVSS, there is complete absence of CS proteins, whereas in CS, the genes produce severely truncated and malformed proteins. Possibly, complete absence of the proteins is less deleterious than presence of malformed CSB protein. This may explain the fact that UVSS lacks important features of CS like premature aging and neurological abnormalities. Unlike CS, mitochondrial involvement in UVSS has so far not been detected.

### *Clinical Presentation*

As described, UVSS is manifested by photosensitivity and freckles, normal growth, and life-span. It lacks other important features of CS like neurological abnormalities and premature aging. However, total number of cases is very few and the oldest known patient of UVSS is less than 50 years. Whether these will develop these features at an older age is yet not known.

## Werner Syndrome

This syndrome is characterized by premature aging with sclerodermatous skin changes and other features. This is a rare, autosomal recessive disorder.

### *Pathogenesis*

The primary defect lies in the mutation of *WRN/RECQL2* gene on chromosome 8, which codes for a DNA helicase. Due to defect, there is disarrayed DNA synthesis and spontaneous chromosome deletions and rearrangements.

### *Clinical Features*

There are sclerodermatous skin changes involving the face and extremities. Several signs of premature aging may be noted like wrinkled skin, sparse gray hair, beaked nose, etc. Overall, the patients present with a short stature and lean habitus. In many parts of body, subcutaneous calcification may be present. A group of patients may have increased risk of coronary atherosclerosis, DM, and malignancy (meningiomas, melanomas, carcinoma of thyroid.

### *Treatment*

There is no specific treatment; asymptomatic management forms the backbone of treatment. However, regular follow-up of these patients is required for early detection of malignancy and treatment of same.

## SUGGESTED READINGS


1. Aamann MD, Sorensen MM, Hvitby C, et al. Cockayne syndrome group B protein promotes mitochondrial DNA stability by supporting the DNA repair association with the mitochondrial membrane. FASEB J. 2010;24(7):2334-46.
2. Bradford PT, Goldstein AM, Tamura D, et al. Cancer and neurologic degeneration in xeroderma pigmentosum: long term follow-up characterises the role of DNA repair. J Med Genet. 2011;48:168-76.
3. Clausen T, Kaiser M, Huber R, et al. HTRA proteases: regulated proteolysis in protein quality control. Nat Rev Mol Cell Biol. 2011;12(3):152-62.
4. Cleaver JE, Lam ET, Revet I. Disorders of nucleotide excision repair: the genetic and molecular basis of heterogeneity. Nat Rev Genet. 2009;10(11):756-68.
5. Cleaver JE. Photosensitivity syndrome brings to light a new transcription-coupled DNA repair cofactor. Nat Genet. 2012;44(5):477-8.
6. DiGiovanna JJ, Kraemer KH. Shining a light on xeroderma pigmentosum. J Invest Dermatol. 2012;132(3 Pt 2):785-96.
7. Friedberg EC, Walker GC, Siede W, Wood RD (Eds). DNA Repair and Mutagenesis. Washington DC: American Society for Microbiology Press; 2005.
8. Friedberg EC, Walker GC, Siede W, Wood RD (Eds). DNA Repair and Mutagenesis. Washington DC: American Society for Microbiology Press; 1995.
9. German J. Bloom's syndrome. I. Genetical and clinical observations in the first twenty-seven patients. Am J Hum Genet. 1969;21(2):196-227.
10. Horibata K, Iwamoto Y, Kuraoka I, et al. Complete absence of Cockayne syndrome group B gene product gives rise to UV-sensitive syndrome but not Cockayne syndrome. Proc Natl Acad Sci U S A. 2004;101:15410-5.
11. Irvine AD, Mellerio JE. Genetics and genodermatoses. In: Burns T, Breathnach S, Cox N, Griffiths C (Eds). Rook's Textbook of Dermatology, 8th edition. United Kingdom: Wiley-Blackwell Publisher (P) Ltd; 2010. pp. 15.1-15.97.
12. Itoh T, Ono, T, Yamaizumi M. A new UV-sensitive syndrome not belonging to any complementation groups of xeroderma pigmentosum or Cockayne syndrome: siblings showing biochemical characteristics of Cockayne syndrome without typical clinical manifestations. Mutat Res. 1994,314:233-48.
13. Jaju PD, Ransohoff KJ, Tang JY, et al. Familial skin cancer syndromes: Increased risk of nonmelanotic skin cancers and extracutaneous tumors. J Am Acad Dermatol. 2016;74(3):437-51.
14. Kamileri I, Karakasilioti I, Garinis GA. Nucleotide excision repair: new tricks with old bricks. Trends Genet. 2012;28(11):566-73.
15. Keightley PD. Rates and fitness consequences of new mutations in humans. Genetics. 2012;190(2):295-304.
16. Lodish H, Berk A, Matsudaira P, et al. Molecular Biology of the Cell, 5th edition. New York, NY: WH Freeman; 2004.
17. Lyakhovich A, Graifer D, Stefanovie B, et al. Mitochondrial dysfunction in DDR-related cancer predisposition syndromes. Biochimica Biophysica Acta. 2016; 1865(2):184-9.
18. Maslov AY, Vijg J. Genome instability, cancer and aging. Biochim Biophys Acta. 2009;1790(10):963-9.
19. Nakazawa Y, Sasaki K, Mitsutake N, et al. Mutations in UVSSA cause UV-sensitive syndrome and impair RNA polymerase IIo processing in transcription-coupled nucleotide excision repair. Nat Genet. 2012;44(5):586-92.
20. Nance MA, Berry SA. Cockayne syndrome: review of 140 cases. Am J Med Genet. 1992;42(1):68-84.
21. O'Hagan HM, Mohammad HP, Baylin SB. Double strand breaks can initiate gene silencing and SIRT1-dependent onset of DNA methylation in an exogenous promoter CpG island. PLoS Genet. 2008;4(8):e1000155.
22. Schmitt MW, Prindle MJ, Loeb LA. Implications of genetic heterogeneity in cancer. Ann N Y Acad Sci. 2012;1267:110-6.

# 4 CHAPTER Primary Immunodeficiency Disorders

*Nilendu Sarma, Indrashis Podder*

## INTRODUCTION

Primary immunodeficiency disorders (PIDs) represent a heterogeneous group of disorders occurring due to genetic defects, where no secondary cause can be elicited and are characterized by the common feature of congenital immune system defects. Many of these disorders have prominent cutaneous manifestations, viz. eczematous or granulomatous dermatitis, and recurrent cutaneous infections. So for an astute dermatologist, skin often serves as a window for the diagnosis of these catastrophic disorders.

## CLASSIFICATION OF PRIMARY IMMUNODEFICIENCY DISORDERS

Classification of PID has been recently updated in 2013 by the International Union of Immunological Societies (IUIS) Expert Committee on Primary Immunodeficiency. This classification provides the most updated and complete list of all PIDs. Now, all the PIDs are classified into nine broad categories.

### Types of Primary Immunodeficiency Disorders

- Combined immunodeficiencies
- Combined immunodeficiencies with associated or syndromic features (Table 1)
- Predominantly antibody deficiencies
- Diseases of immune dysregulation
- Congenital defects of phagocyte number, function, or both
- Defects in innate immunity
- Autoinflammatory disorders
- Complement deficiencies
- Phenocopies of PID.

The ninth category is the newer addition to the older list. This entity, termed as—"Phenocopies of PID", although has phenotypic

**TABLE 1: Combined immune deficiencies with syndromic features**

| Disease | Inheritance pattern | Involved gene |
|---|---|---|
| • Congenital thrombocytopenia | | |
| ○ Wiskott–Aldrich syndrome (WAS) | XL | *WAS* |
| ○ WIP deficiency | AR | *WIPF1* |
| • DNA repair defects (diseases other than those mentioned in this table) | | |
| ○ Ataxia-telangiectasia | AR | *ATM* |
| ○ Nijmegen breakage syndrome | AR | *NBS1 (Nibrin)* |
| ○ Bloom syndrome | AR | *BLM; RecQ-like helicase* |
| ○ Immunodeficiency with centromeric instability and facial anomalies (ICF)—two different genetic defect with similar phenotypic presentation | AR | *DNMT3B (ICF1) or in ZBTB24 (ICF2)* |
| ○ *PMS2* deficiency | AR | *PMS2* |
| ○ *RNF168* deficiency | AR | *RNF168* |
| ○ *MCM4* deficiency | AR | *MCM4* |
| • Thymic defects with additional congenital anomalies | | |
| ○ DiGeorge anomaly | *De novo* defect in majority, some AD | Contiguous gene defects. Sometimes, heterozygous mutation in *TBX1* |

*Continued*

*Continued*

| Disease | Inheritance pattern | Involved gene |
|---|---|---|
| ○ CHARGE syndrome<br>Coloboma, heart anomaly, choanal atresia, retardation, genital and ear anomalies | *De novo* defect in majority, some AD | Two genetic defects—<br>*CHD7, SEMA3E, or unknown genes* |
| ○ Winged helix deficiency (nude) syndromic SCID | AR | *FOXN1* |
| • Immuno-osseous dysplasia | | |
| ○ Cartilage hair hypoplasia | AR | *RMRP (RNase MRP RNA)* |
| ○ Schimke syndrome | AR | *SMARCAL1* |
| • Hyper-IgE syndromes (HIESs) | | |
| ○ AD-HIES (Job's syndrome) | AD or *de-novo* defect | *STAT3* |
| ○ Comèl-Netherton syndrome | AR | *SPINK5* |
| ○ PGM3 deficiency | AR | *Mutations in phosphoglucomutase 3 (PGM3)* |
| • Dyskeratosis congenital (DKC) (many subtypes) | AR, AD, XL | *DKC1, NHP2, NOP10,*<br>*PCFT, RTEL1, TERC, etc.* |
| • Defects of vitamin B12 and folate metabolism (many subtypes) | | |
| ○ Anhidrotic ectodermal dysplasia with immunodeficiency (EDA-ID) | XL,<br>AD | *NEMO*<br>Gain-of-function mutation *in IKBA (NFKIAB)* |

WIP, WASP-interacting protein; AR, autosomal recessive; XL, X-linked; ATM: ataxia-telangiectasia mutated; AD, autosomal dominant; SCID, severe combined immunodeficiency.

*Source*: Modified and reproduced from Picard C, Al-Herz W, Bousfiha A, et al. Primary immunodeficiency diseases: an update on the classification from the International Union of Immunological Societies Expert Committee for Primary Immunodeficiency 2015. J Clin Immunol. 2015;35:696-726.

similarity to classical PID, does not occur due to germline mutations. Rather other acquired mechanisms like somatic mutations or autoimmune destruction of immunoprotective cells or cytokines can cause this.

## HYPER IMMUNOGLOBULIN E SYNDROME OR JOB SYNDROME OR BUCKLEY SYNDROME

This is a relatively rare condition, characterized by recurrent cutaneous and sinopulmonary infections, dermatitis from birth or early childhood, coarse facies, and excessively elevated levels of immunoglobulin E (IgE).

### Pathogenesis

This occurs due to dominant-negative heterozygous mutations in *STAT3* gene. Although most cases of Job syndrome are autosomal dominant, *de novo* defect has been reported from Turkey and Mexico. However, hyper IgE syndrome (HIES) may also occur due to mutations in *DOCK8* and *TYK2* genes.

Total numbers of circulating T as well as B cells are unchanged. However, Th-17 and T-follicular helper cells, switched and non-switched memory B-cells are reduced. B-cell activating factor level is increased, IgE level is high, and specific antibody production is diminished.

### Clinical Features

The disease usually manifests in the neonatal period with recurrent skin infections (mainly staphylococcal in origin) in the form of extensive impetigo and recurrent boils (particularly "cold abscesses"). Eczematous skin eruptions that may mimic atopic dermatitis are very typical of this disease. Recurrent sinopulmonary tract infections (*S. aureus* and sometimes *C. albicans*) and pneumatoceles (lung) are common. Coarse facial features like broad nasal bridge, thick doughy skin; wide, fleshy nasal tip, deep-set eyes, prominent forehead, and irregular jaws and cheeks are present. Other features are hyperextensible joints, osteopenia with fractures, scoliosis, dental abnormalities, and delay in shedding of primary teeth.

Autosomal recessive HIES (AR-HIES) does not present with skeletal or dental anomalies and lung pneumatoceles.

### Differential Diagnoses

Other immunodeficiency diseases presenting with recurrent skin or other infections and eczematous lesions should be ruled out (Box 1). It needs to be differentiated from Wiskott–Aldrich syndrome (lacks cold abscesses), Netherton syndrome (presence of hair abnormalities and ichthyosis linearis circumflexa), Omenn syndrome, DiGeorge syndrome, interleukin-1 receptor-associated kinase 4 (IRAK-4) deficiency (lacks eczematous dermatitis), and graft-versus-host disease (GVHD).

### Diagnosis

High degree of clinical suspicion is required. Classical clinical features along with laboratory investigations can diagnose this

**BOX 1 Primary immunodeficiency disorders with eczematous dermatitis**

- Hyper IgE syndrome
- Wiskott–Aldrich syndrome
- X-linked agammaglobulinemia
- Ataxia telangiectasia
- Chronic granulomatous disease
- Common variable immunodeficiency
- Severe combined immunodeficiency

condition. There are elevated levels of polyclonal IgE (mainly antistaphylococcal and anticandidal), high eosinophil count in peripheral blood and sputum, and lesional skin biopsy shows eosinophilic infiltration.

### Treatment

Supportive care is required, especially appropriate antibiotics, local wound care, and drainage of abscess. Surgical removal of pneumatoceles (if >6 months) may be necessary. Intravenous immunoglobulin (IVIg) and recombinant IFN-$\gamma$ may also be used.

## COMMON VARIABLE IMMUNODEFICIENCY

This is one of the most common causes of symptomatic primary immune deficiencies. This is a heterogeneous group of disorders characterized by deficiencies of immunoglobulins (IgG and IgA and some cases also IgM) with varying degrees of infective, autoimmune, and other complications.

Overall, this disease is very rare. Although the disease is congenital, due to its asymptomatic nature, diagnosis is typically delayed by many decades. There is no sexual predilection.

### Pathogenesis

Most cases are sporadic. Other cases are inherited as AR and some as dominant mode. Although it is a genetic disease, genetic defects are largely unknown. Mutations are detected in less than 10% of cases and have affected *CD19, CD20, CD21, CD81, BRAF, ICOS, TNFRSF13B*, and *TNFRSF13C*. *ICOS* gene regulates T-cell proliferation. Thus, it indicates intimate role of T-cells in immunoglobulin production.

### Clinical Features

Phenotypically, it can have diverse manifestations. Severity varies widely and regulates the time of first detection.

Recurrent infection mostly by bacteria and also by virus is very common and affects lungs, ear, and skin.

Infection with *Pneumococcus, Haemophilus influenzae, Streptococcus pneumoniae*, and *Staphylococcus aureus* is common. Infection with *Neisseria meningitidis, Pseudomonas aeruginosa,* and *Giardia lamblia* is also seen.

Other important and common manifestations are gastrointestinal inflammation leading to loss of villi, malabsorption, and diarrhea. Patients develop inflammatory bowel disease like ulcerative colitis and Crohn's disease. Nodular lymphoid hyperplasia develops in the gut.

Skin may develop granulomatous nodules. This may also be seen in some internal organs including liver. These show presence of non-caseating granuloma in histology. Lymphoid infiltration also present with lymphadenopathy and splenomegaly.

Although common variable immunodeficiency (CVID) is a disease of B-cell and immunoglobulin deficiency, paradoxical stimulation of B-cell and autoimmunity may develop. Autoimmune destruction of blood cells and rheumatoid arthritis is commonly observed. CVID is also characterized by increased risk of lymphoid malignancy (non-Hodgkin's lymphoma) and also of stomach, breast, bladder, and cervical epithelial cancers.

### Diagnosis

As most cases lack any known genetic defect, specific diseases presenting with similar clinical or laboratory abnormalities should be ruled out. This should be differentiated from agammaglobulinemia (XL or AR), hyper IgM syndrome (HIGM) that has low IgG, IgA, and IgE and may have slightly higher or even normal IgM, X-linked lymphoproliferative (XLP), and Wiskott-Aldrich syndrome.

There is low IgG and the level may be significantly low, even less than 100 mg/dL. IgA and IgM are also low. Lower capacity to raise immunoglobulins is also confirmed by antibody assay after vaccination (e.g., tetanus). Total B cell may be normal or low. Diagnosis is excluded in children below 4 years.

### Management

Management requires repeated courses of immunoglobulin (IVIg) throughout life. Antibiotics are frequently required to treat infections. TNF-$\alpha$ inhibitors may be used (recalcitrant noninfectious granulomas).

## X-LINKED AGAMMAGLOBULINEMIA OR BRUTON AGAMMAGLOBULINEMIA OR BRUTON–GITLIN SYNDROME

This is a relatively rare PID, where almost 90% of the cases show an X-linked recessive (XLR) inheritance; while the remaining 10% are transmitted in an AR fashion.

### Pathogenesis

This disorder occurs due to loss-of-function mutation of the *Bruton tyrosine kinase (BTK)* gene; thus resulting in the altered function and signaling of the pre-B-cell receptor. As a result, there is reduction in the total number of B-lymphocytes which leads to diminished quantities of all the immunoglobulins.

### Clinical Features

As a result of grossly diminished humoral immunity, recurrent bacterial infections with *Staphylococcus, Streptococcus, Pneumococcus, Haemophilus,* and *Pseudomonas* in the form of furuncles, cellulitis, boils, ecthyma gangrenosum, etc., begin in the first few years of life. Eczematous reactions can also occur. In some cases papular lesions and dermatomyositis like skin rash have been reported.

Recurrent systemic infections have also been reported, most notably in the form of pyogenic infections (mainly *Staphylococcal*), lower respiratory tract infections (LRTI), hepatitis B, viral meningoencephalitis, and joint space infections. There is an increased chance of lymphomas (~5%) in these patients.

### Diagnosis

This disorder must be differentiated from other similar disorders which present with eczematous skin eruptions like HIES, Bruton agammaglobulinemia, severe combined immunodeficiency (SCID), and ataxia-telangiectasia (Box 1). Prenatal diagnosis is possible by restriction fragment length polymorphism (RFLP) analysis of regions surrounding the *BTK* gene or direct gene analysis.

Laboratory investigations show diminished levels of B-lymphocytes and all the immunoglobulins.

### Treatment

Treatment of this condition is mostly symptomatic. Aggressive treatment of infections and antibody replacement by IVIg constitutes the cornerstone of management.

## WISKOTT–ALDRICH SYNDROME

Wiskott–Aldrich syndrome is a life-threatening primary immunodeficiency associated with a bleeding tendency, eczema, and recurrent pyogenic infection. However, this classic triad is seen in less than 30% cases.

Most cases have an XLR inheritance, boys more than girls; European population more than blacks and Asians.

### Pathogenesis

This syndrome occurs due to loss-of-function mutation of the WAS gene coding for the WAS protein (WASP). This leads to defective aggregation of actin filaments and abnormality of T-cell function. There is progressive loss of T-cell and reduced response to anti-CD3. There is diminished level of IgM associated in some cases with higher IgA and IgE. IgM antibody to polysaccharides is particularly decreased. There is reduced expression of CD21 and CD35. Recently, role of B cell intrinsic TLR7 signals has been implicated in WAS.

### Clinical Features

Predominant clinical presentation includes eczema that simulates atopic dermatitis, petechiae, ecchymoses of the skin and oral mucosa (due to thrombocytopenia), and recurrent bacterial, viral, and fungal infections of skin and systemic organs (Fig.1). Infection may be caused by all classes of microorganisms. Classically, there is thromobocytopenia with small platelets. IgA nephropathy is a known complication. Milder forms of WAS can manifest with isolated thrombocytopenia or neutropenia (both XL) Similar to other PIDs, autoimmune disease, and lymphoma is also seen. Platelet may be destroyed by autoimmunity (idiopathic thrombocytopenic purpura) increasing the bleeding risk.

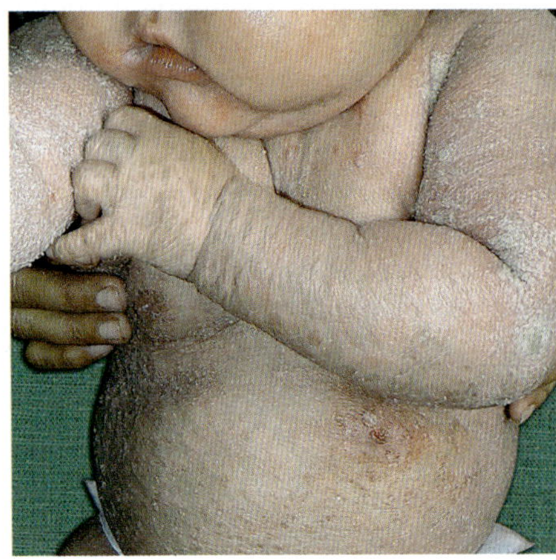

**FIG. 1:** Eczematous lesions, excoriation, and purpura in Wiskott-Aldrich syndrome.

### Diagnosis

As described, classical clinical triad is present in less number of cases. Evaluation of all other features is necessary. This condition has to be differentiated from other causes of primary immunodeficiency with eczematous dermatitis like HIES, Bruton agammaglobulinemia, SCID, and ataxia-telangiectasia (Box 1).

Laboratory investigations reveal persistent thrombocytopenia (platelet count < 80,000/cu.mm), low mean platelet volume (<5 fl), low IgM along with low IgD, and high IgA and IgE. Patients have defective antibody production capacity to polysaccharides or complex sugars. This can be confirmed in laboratory with poor antibody generation after vaccination with vaccines that contain polysaccharides or complex sugars such as *Streptococcus pneumoniae* vaccine.

### Treatment

Live vaccination is contraindicated. Hematopoietic stem cell transfusion is treatment of choice; IVIg may also be helpful. Platelet may be transfused before surgery or after massive hemorrhage. Currently, there is ongoing research regarding gene therapy with a lentivirus. Eltrombopag is a new drug shown to increase the platelet count. Splenectomy may be required in recalcitrant cases to prevent platelet destruction. Prior genetic counseling of prospective parents may prevent the occurrence of this disorder.

### Chronic Mucocutaneous Candidiasis

It is important to note that several PIDs may be characterized by chronic mucocutaneous candidiasis (CMC). It may be part of a complex clinical phenotype in some of these. In many other diseases, CMC may be the sole or the dominant clinical manifestations. This disorder is characterized by recurrent and progressive infections of the skin, nails, and mucosa with *Candida albicans*. Most cases are sporadic in nature; however autoimmune polyendocrinopathy-candidiasis–ectodermal dystrophy or dysplasia (APECED) and other familial forms may have AR inheritance. Onset in adult life may occur due to the presence of underlying thymoma.

### Pathogenesis

The primary pathological defect in this disorder is T-cell deficiency which may be specifically anticandidal. Recently, defective IL-17-mediated immunity, dominant-negative STAT3 deficiency, IL-12Rβ1 and IL-12p40 deficiencies have been detected. Reduced levels of natural killer cells (NK cells) and intercellular adhesion molecule-1 (ICAM-1) have also been reported. These immunological alteration leads to severe candidal infection of the integuments.

## Subtypes

There are several subtypes:

1. Familial chronic mucocutaneous candidiasis (CMC) (oral candidiasis > cutaneous; age <2 years)
2. Chronic localized candidiasis (Candida granuloma) (thick adherent crusts; face and scalp)
3. Candidiasis endocrinopathy syndrome (*AIRE* gene, hypoparathyroidism, hypoadrenocorticism)
4. Late-onset CMC (late childhood or early teenage)
5. Familial chronic nail candidiasis
6. CMC associated with keratitis (photophobia <2 years, alopecia, mucosal candidiasis)
7. CMC associated with other immunodeficiency disorders (SCID, HIGE, DiGeorge syndrome)
8. CMC associated with nonimmunologic conditions (KID syndrome, Acrodermatitis enteropathica, etc.).

## Clinical Features

Recurrent, persistent, and progressive Candidal infections of the skin, nails, and mucosa constitute the hallmark feature of this condition. Often there is diffuse and extensive oral involvement along with the presence of perlèche and lip fissures. The nails become thickened and dystrophic associated with paronychia (Figs 2 and 3). Cutaneous involvement leads to the development of hyperkeratotic, hornlike or granulomatous lesions.

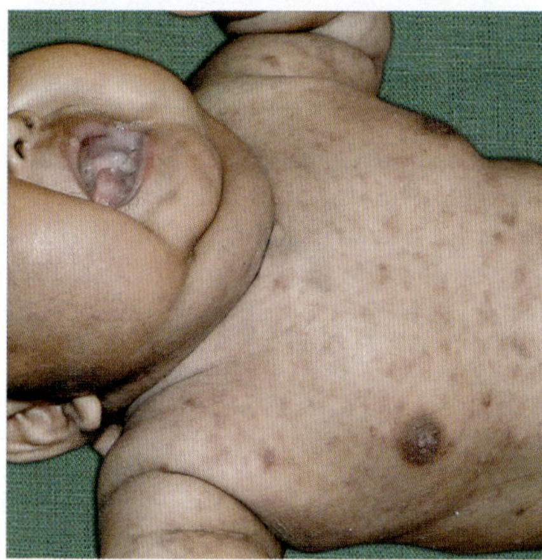

**FIG. 2:** Oral candidiasis and cutaneous erythematous papules in chronic mucocutaneous candidiasis.

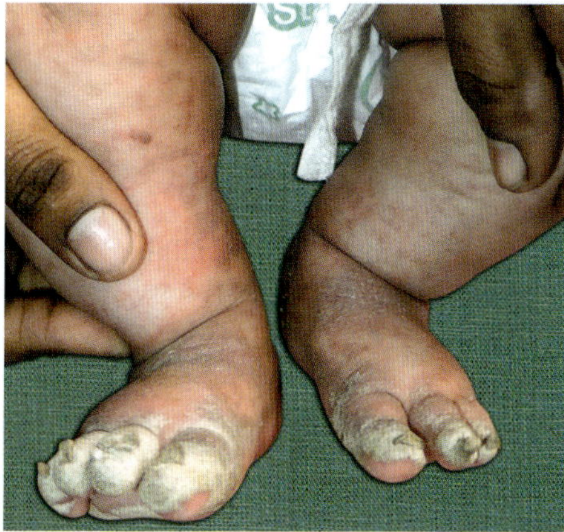

**FIG. 3:** Nail plate thickening and thick scaly plaques around nails in chronic mucocutaneous candidiasis.

## Differential Diagnosis

The most important differential diagnosis is the immune dysregulation, polyendocrinopathy, enteropathy, XLR (IPEX) syndrome. However in this condition eczematous dermatitis is present in addition to features of Candidal infection; thus helping us to rule out this disorder.

## Treatment

Systemic antifungal therapy with itraconazole, fluconazole, or ketoconazole is mandatory as topical medications are not effective. These drugs are usually given in higher dosage for prolonged duration; often courses need to be repeated. Hematopoietic stem cell therapy, fetal thymus grafts, and leukocyte infusion may be useful in persistent cases. There are few reports suggesting the use of oral Cimetidine as a successful immunomodulatory in these patients.

# ATAXIA–TELANGIECTASIA OR LOUIS–BAR SYNDROME

This disorder is characterized by oculocutaneous telangiectasias, progressive cerebellar ataxia, and selective immune deficiency often resulting in recurrent sinopulmonary infections. There is also increased sensitivity to ionizing radiation, which may predispose these patients to develop several malignancies (leukemias and lymphomas).

This is an AR disorder with occurrence of about 1 in 40,000 to 1 in 100,000. Carriers have an increased risk of breast carcinoma and hematologic malignancies. Death usually occurs in these patients due to neoplasia and ischemic heart disease.

## Pathogenesis

The primary defect is loss-of-function mutation of the *ATM* (ataxia-telangiectasia mutated) gene, which encodes a serine-threonine protease kinase; the latter playing an active role in the repair of DNA defect. So in these patients the repair system is defective, thus leading to increased occurrence of DNA double-stranded breaks. As a result there is cell cycle arrest and apoptosis of the cells of the immune system, thus resulting in diminished immunity. Ionizing radiation further aggravates the damage. Recently other genes have been implicated in addition to the *ATM* gene, viz. *MRE 11* and *NBS1* genes. The role of oxidative stress in the pathogenesis of this disease is under evaluation.

## Clinical Features

Progressive cerebellar ataxia is usually the first manifestation of this disease which usually becomes apparent when the child starts walking. There is swaying of the head and trunk along with choreoathetosis, dysarthria, and myoclonic jerks in some. However, this condition is suspected when the first evidence of oculocutaneous telangiectasias becomes evident around the age of 3–6 years. The telangiectasias first appear on the lateral and medial bulbar conjunctiva in the form of red, horizontal, and symmetrical streaks, subsequently involving the adjacent areas like the ears, neck, malar prominence, etc. Also 90% patients have progeric changes in the hair and skin most notably early greying of hair. Other cutaneous findings include viral infections (warts, molluscum), noninfectious granulomas (mainly on extremities), poikiloderma, eczematous eruptions, seborrheic dermatitis, keratosis pilaris, vitiligo, hirsutism, and acanthosis nigricans. Systemic bacterial and viral infection mainly in the form of chronic and recurrent sinopulmonary infection (80%) is an important feature. Enhanced susceptibility to radiation damage leads to the development of several malignancies like leukemia, lymphoma, colonic malignancy, etc.

### Diagnosis

This disorder has to be differentiated from Friedreich's ataxia (absence of ocular telangiectasia) and Bloom syndrome (absence of neurological abnormalities). This condition also needs to be differentiated from other causes of PID with eczematous dermatitis like HIES, Bruton agammaglobulinemia, SCID, and ataxia-telangiectasia (Box 1).

Laboratory investigations reveal reduced level of immunoglobulins (IgA, IgE, IgG2) and lymphopenia (70% cases) [mainly affecting the CD4+ cell line]. Elevated levels of α-fetoprotein, and carcinoembryonic antigen (CEA) have been demonstrated in some patients.

### Treatment

The treatment is mainly supportive in the form of antibiotics, IVIg, avoidance of sun exposure and sunscreens, and physical therapy (for neurological ds.). Aggressive screening is mandated for early detection of malignancy. However, if malignancy sets in, chemotherapy is essential, radiation, and radiomimetic agents like bleomycin should be avoided. Bone marrow transplant and levamisole therapy offer no added benefit.

## SEVERE COMBINED IMMUNODEFICIENCY OR GLANZMANN–RINIKER SYNDROME OR ALYMPHOCYTOSIS

Severe combined immunodeficiency (SCID) is the prototype disorder belonging to this group. This syndrome is characterized by recurrent infections, diarrhea, and failure to thrive within the first 3–6 months of life, due to defective humoral and cell-mediated immunity.

It is a relatively rare disease; occurring in 1:30,000–1:100,000 live births, boys more than girls. About 40% of the cases are XLR, while the remaining are AR. Almost 20% of the cases occur due to deficiency of the enzyme adenosine deaminase (ADA).

### Pathogenesis

Mutations in several genes have been implicated as the cause of this devastating syndrome, viz. ADA (most common), *IL2RG* (X-linked), *JAK3, IL7R, PTPRC*, etc. Recently another gene has been implicated called the *Artemis* gene in the pigs.

### Clinical Features

Widespread seborrheic dermatitis-like cutaneous eruption or morbilliform eruption constitute the major clinical presentation; especially in patients suffering from the Omenn variant. Recurrent bacterial (*Staphylococcus*) and fungal (Candidal) cutaneous infections are also very common due to the deranged immunity. Apart from these features, chronic diarrhea and failure to thrive within first few months, is seen in a group of these patients.

### Diagnosis

This condition has to be differentiated from other causes of immunodeficiency like HIV infection, GVHD, etc.

In laboratory investigations, we find low absolute lymphocyte count. Further detailed investigations reveal profound T-cell deficiency and diminished B lymphocyte and NK cell count. Distinct X-ray changes (cupping and flaring of costochondral joints) may be observed on the chest X-ray.

### Treatment

As this condition is genetic in nature, treatment is not much satisfactory. Human leukocyte antigen-identical hematopoietic stem cell transplantation is the most definitive form of therapy. Recently, enzyme replacement with polyethylene glycol-conjugated ADA and gene therapy are being tried in some centers. Apart from these modalities, early diagnosis and aggressive treatment of infections, barrier nursing, etc. are mandatory in these patients.

## CHRONIC GRANULOMATOUS DISEASE OR BRIDGES–GOOD SYNDROME OR QUIE SYNDROME

Chronic granulomatous disease (CGD) is a primary immunodeficiency disorder involving the phagocytic cells (neutrophils, monocytes, macrophages, and eosinophils), thus resulting in impaired killing of bacteria and fungi. The incidence of CGD is about 1 in 200,000 live births, 90% are boys; XLR more than AR inheritance.

### Pathogenesis

In CGD, there is a defect in the phagocyte NADPH oxidase. Recently five genes have been implicated, viz. *CYBA, NCF1, NCF2, CYBB,* and *NCF4* whose mutation may produce the defective NADPH oxidase. The defective NADPH oxidase system fails to generate superoxide ions, thus hampering the antimicrobial activity of phagocytes.

### Clinical Features

A variety of infections, e.g., lung (pneumonia), lymph nodes (lymphadenitis), liver (abscess), bone (osteomyelitis), and skin (abscesses or cellulitis) constitute the hallmark clinical feature of this condition. Colitis, which may be the solitary finding in some patients, has also been reported.

### Diagnosis

This condition should be differentiated from other related conditions like congenital neutropenia, cyclic neutropenia (recurrent oral ulceration and gingivitis), X-linked neutropenia, specific granule deficiency, and leukocyte adhesion deficiency.

Laboratory investigations reveal leukocytosis, elevated ESR, anemia, and diminished T-cells. There are two screening tests to detect this condition, viz. dihydrorhodamine (DHR) test and the nitroblue tetrazolium (NBT) test, the latter being used more widely. We may find cutaneous noninfective granulomas with histiocytic infiltrates on skin biopsy. Recently, use of flow cytometry has been advocated to detect the carrier state.

### Treatment

Gene therapy and hematopoietic stem cell transplantation are the only definitive forms of therapy. Aggressive treatment of infections must be pursued. Chronic prophylaxis with co-trimoxazole may be effective to prevent infections.

## COMPLEMENT DISORDERS

This group of disorders occurs as a result of deficiency of one or more components of the complement pathway, thus resulting in immunodeficiency. The most common disorders in this group are:

- C2 deficiency
- C1-esterase inhibitor deficiency
- C4-binding protein deficiency.

Amongst these disorders, C2 deficiency is the most common, with an incidence of about 1 in 20,000 live births.

### Pathogenesis

The basic defect lies in the HLA portion of chromosome 6 thus resulting in the defective synthesis of early complement components.

### Clinical Features

These disorders often mimic lupus erythematosus and angioedema clinically. Often, recurrent bacterial infections (especially capsulated organisms) occur. The lesions may occasionally become ulcerated.

### Diagnosis

This group of conditions has to be differentiated from lupus erythematosus (early and late), HIES, Leiner's disease, and Bruton agammaglobulinemia.

Laboratory investigations reveal deficiency of the complement factors.

### Treatment

Symptomatic treatment of infections is the cornerstone of management. Exogenous complement factors can also be administered.

## MISCELLANEOUS DISORDERS

A few of the disorders belong to the miscellaneous category; whose occurrence is extremely rare. Some of the important diseases are given below:

- Chédiak–Higashi syndrome, Griscelli syndrome (NK cell defect, abnormal neutrophils, recurrent infections, silvery streaks in the hair, and oculocutaneous albinism)
- Dyskeratosis congenita [cutaneous pigmentation, nail dystrophy, oral leukoplakia, malignancy, bone marrow failure, recurrent infections (bacterial), hypogammaglobulinemia, etc.]
- Anhidrotic ectodermal dysplasia (respiratory infections, hypohidrosis, elevated skin temperature, abnormal dentition, and typical facies)
- Papillon–Lefèvre syndrome [recurrent bacterial infections, impaired neutrophil function, PPKD (transgradiens), and dental anomalies].

## SUGGESTED READINGS


1. Frecha C, Toscano MG, Costa C, et al. Improved lentiviral vectors for Wiskott Aldrich syndrome gene therapy mimic endogenous expression profiles throughout haematopoiesis. Gene Ther. 2008;15:930-41.
2. Kapoor N, Raj R. Hematopoietic stem cell transplantation for primary immune deficiency disorders. Indian J Pediatr. 2016;83:450-4.
3. Kolhatkar NS, Scharping NE, Sullivan JM, et al. B-cell-intrinsic TLR7 signals promote depletion of the marginal zone in a murine model of Wiskott-Aldrich syndrome. Eur J Immunol. 2015;45:2773-9.
4. Ochs HD, Puck JM (Eds). Primary immunodeficiency diseases: a molecular and genetic approach. Oxford: Oxford University Press; 2013.
5. Picard C, Al-Herz W, Bousfiha A, et al. Primary immunodeficiency diseases: an update on the classification from the International Union of Immunological Societies Expert Committee for Primary Immunodeficiency 2015. J Clin Immunol. 2015;35:696-726.
6. Rezaei N, Aghamohammadi A. Hyper-IgE syndrome. JPGM. 2010;56:63-4.
7. Spickett GP, Schwarz T. Clinical immunology, Allergy and Photoimmunology. In: Burns T, Breathnach S, Cox N, Griffiths C (Eds). Rook's Textbook of Dermatology, 8th edition. United Kingdom: Wiley-Blackwell Publisher (P) Ltd; 2010. pp. 12-15.
8. Uzzan M, Ko HM, Mehandru S, et al. Gastrointestinal disorders associated with common variable immune deficiency (CVID) and chronic granulomatous disease (CGD). Curr Gastroenterol Rep. 2016;18:17.

5

CHAPTER

# Genodermatoses

Biju Vasudevan, Shilpa Garg, Shekhar Neema, Debdeep Mitra

## INTRODUCTION

Role of genetics may be important in the pathogenesis of large number of diseases. However, genetic makeup of an individual plays a predominant role in causation of some of these disorders.

Genodermatoses are a group of inherited skin disorders comprising of chromosomal, single gene, and polygenetic disorders. Transmission of these conditions may be autosomal dominant, recessive or X-linked (Table 1).

## CHROMOSOMAL DISORDERS

Chromosomal disorders may be due to qualitative or quantitative defect of either autosomes or sex chromosomes.

Many of these disorders have characteristic cutaneous manifestations that often play a crucial diagnostic role.

Salient features of chromosomal disorders are tabulated in table 2.

**TABLE 1: Classification overview of genodermatoses**

| Autosomal dominant | Autosomal recessive | X-linked dominant | X-linked recessive |
|---|---|---|---|
| • Neurofibromatosis<br>• Tuberous sclerosis<br>• Hereditary hemorrhagic telangiectasia (Osler–Weber–Rendu syndrome)<br>• Epidermolysis bullosa simplex | • Lamellar ichthyosis<br>• Ataxia-telangiectasia<br>• Albinism<br>• Autosomal recessive dystrophic epidermolysis bullosa | • Xeroderma pigmentosum | • X-linked ichthyosis<br>• Hypohidrotic ectodermal dysplasia |

**TABLE 2: Chromosomal disorders**

| Syndrome | Chromosomal defect | Salient noncutaneous features | Cutaneous features |
|---|---|---|---|
| ***Autosomal chromosome disorders*** | | | |
| Down syndrome | Trisomy 21 | Mongoloid slant of eyes, thick eyelids, sparse eyelashes, brushfield spots in iris, short stubby hands, simian palmar crease, mental retardation, and macroglossia | Xerosis, hypopigmented hairs, increased incidence of alopecia areata, onychomycosis, and pyoderma |
| Edward syndrome | Trisomy 18 | Severe mental retardation, low set ears, overlapping index and fifth fingers, and rocker bottom feet | Single palmar crease |
| Patau syndrome | Trisomy 13 | Microphthalmia, cleft palate or lip, low set ears, and death in infancy | Hyperconvex nails, cutis laxa of the neck |
| ***Sex chromosome disorders*** | | | |
| Turner syndrome | 45 XO | Growth failure, webbed neck, peripheral edema, broad chest, widely spaced nipples, wide carrying angle, low set ears, high-arched palate, and short fourth metacarpal and metatarsal | Cutis laxa, low posterior hairline, and keloidal tendency |
| Klinefelter syndrome | 47 XXY | Eunuchoid body proportions | Poorly developed secondary sexual characteristics, associations like systemic lupus erythematosus and incontinentia pigmenti |

## FAMILIAL MULTIPLE TUMOR SYNDROME

The most common of these disorders are neurofibromatoses and tuberous sclerosis. Less common disorders include Gardner's syndrome, Cowden's disease, multiple endocrine neoplasia type 1 (MEN 1), MEN 2, ataxia-telangiectasia, and Bloom syndrome.

### Neurofibromatoses

It is an autosomal dominant condition, though half of affected cases result from sporadic mutation. Variable expressivity of the gene determines the severity of disease in generations. The various forms of neurofibromatosis are classified in table 3.

#### Neurofibromatosis 1

It is the most common of the neurofibromatoses with incidence of approximately 1 in 3,000. It results from mutation or deletion of *neurofibromatosis 1 (NF1)* gene on chromosome 17 which codes for neurofibromin, a tumor suppressor gene.

##### *Clinical Features*

These patients may exhibit learning difficulties, endocrine disturbances like precocious puberty, acromegaly, Addison's disease, hyperparathyroidism and pheochromocytoma, urinary symptoms, and constipation. Skeletal complications like scoliosis, malignancies like malignant peripheral nerve sheath tumor, pheochromocytoma, and increased incidence of chronic myeloid leukemia and rhabdomyosarcoma may alter the course of the otherwise benign course of the disease.

##### *Diagnosis*

National Institutes of Health consensus criteria require two of the seven criteria for diagnosis of NF1 (Box 1).

##### *Treatment*

Treatment is symptomatic and mainly consists of removing any disfiguring lesions, looking actively for any complications, and genetic counseling.

#### Neurofibromatoses 2

It is relatively rare disorder with incidence of 1 in 40,000 characterized by vestibular schwannomas. Segmental neurofibromatosis is characterized by presence of café au lait macules and neurofibromas limited to one area of body.

**BOX 1 Criteria for diagnosis of neurofibromatosis 1**

- Six or more café au lait macules—more than 5 mm in prepubertal individuals and more than 15 mm in postpubertal individuals (Fig. 1)
- Two or more neurofibromas (Fig. 2) of any type or one plexiform neurofibroma
- Axillary or inguinal freckling
- Optic glioma
- Two or more Lisch nodules
- Sphenoid dysplasia or thinning of long bones with pseudoarthrosis
- First degree relative with NF1

NF1, neurofibromatosis 1.

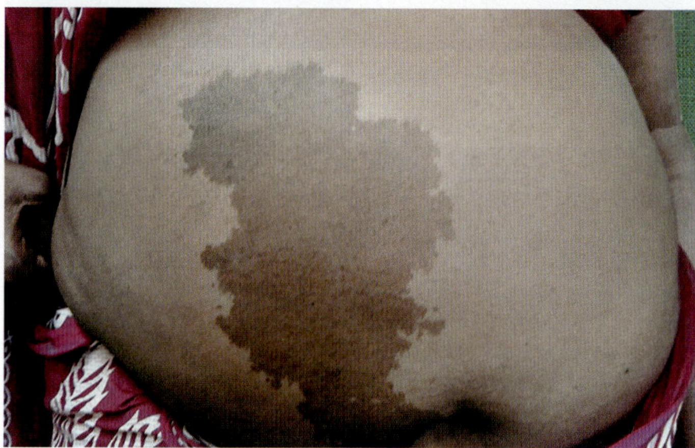

**FIG. 1:** Large café au lait macule.

*Courtesy*: Dr Sayantani Chakraborty, Assistant Professor, Department of Dermatology, RG Kar Medical College, West Bengal.

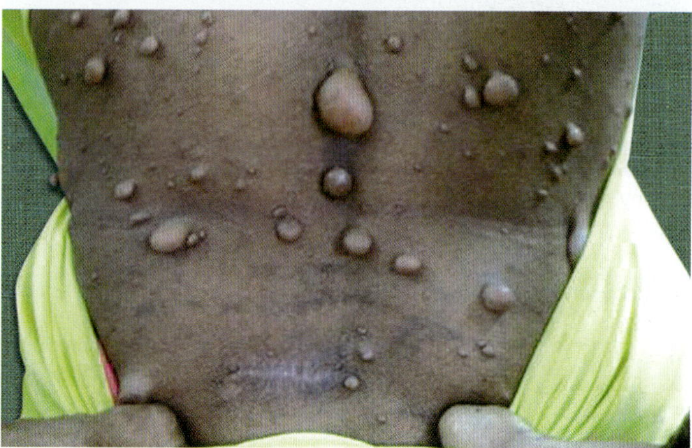

**FIG. 2:** Multiple neurofibromas.

**TABLE 3: Types of neurofibromatoses**

| Type | Inheritance pattern | Salient clinical features |
|---|---|---|
| Neurofibromatosis (NF1) | Autosomal dominant | Café au lait macules, neurofibromas, Lisch nodules, axillary freckling, bone and neurological alterations, and benign and malignant neoplasms |
| Acoustic (NF2) | Autosomal dominant | Bilateral acoustic neuromas, fewer café au lait macules, and neurofibromas |
| Mixed (NF3) | Autosomal dominant | Combination of features of NF1 and NF2 |
| Variant (NF4) | Unknown | Variations in café au lait macules, neurofibromas, CNS neoplasms, and Lisch nodules |
| Segmental (NF5) | Non-inheritable | Segmental neurofibromas and/or café au lait macules |
| Familial CLS (NF6) | Unknown | Familial café au lait macules |
| Late onset (NF7) | Unknown | Onset after third decade of life, neurofibromas, and few café au lait macules |
| Unspecified (NF8) | Unknown | Variable signs |

CLS, café au lait spots; CNS, central nervous system.

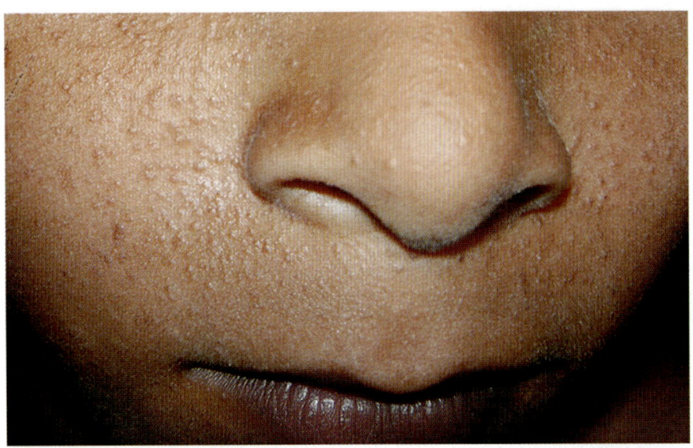

FIG. 3: Facial angiofibroma in tuberous sclerosis.

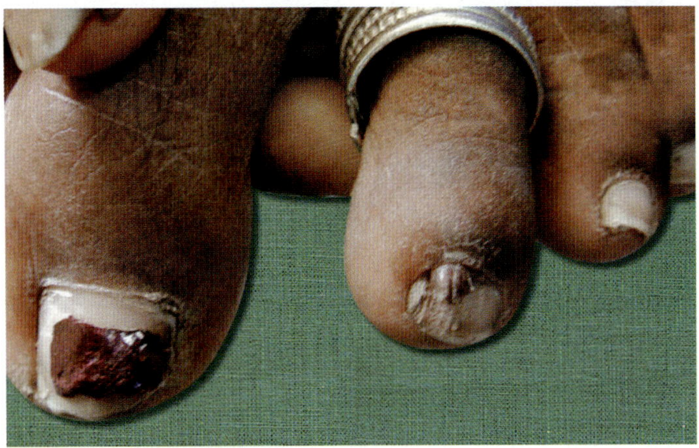

FIG. 4: Periungual fibroma in tuberous sclerosis.

## Tuberous Sclerosis

Tuberous sclerosis complex is an autosomal dominant syndrome with variable expressivity with an incidence of approximately 1 in 6,000 live births. Two-thirds of the cases are sporadic and one-third hereditary. It is caused by mutation in *TSC1* coding hamartin (chromosome 9) or *TSC2* coding tuberin (chromosome 17) gene.

### Clinical Features

The classical cutaneous features includes angiofibromas on face, dental enamel pits, periungual digital fibromas, shagreen patch, and forehead plaques. Gingival fibromas and ash leaf macules may also be present.

### Prognosis

It varies from a normal life expectancy to early death due to renal failure, seizures, hydrocephalus, arrhythmias, and respiratory failure.

### Diagnosis

Diagnostic criteria of tuberous sclerosis are listed in box 2.

### Treatment

Skin tumors can be removed surgically for cosmetic benefit. Carbon dioxide laser can be used for removal of skin tumors. Oral rapamycin is being tried for treatment of subependymal giant cell astrocytoma. There are successful reports of use of topical rapamycin for use of facial angiofibromas.

**TABLE 4: Enzyme deficiency diseases**

| Disease | Enzyme deficiency | Cutaneous features | Treatment |
|---|---|---|---|
| Phenylketonuria | Phenylalanine hydroxylase | Generalized hypopigmentation, blue eyes, blond hairs, mousy odor, atopic dermatitis, vomiting, and seizures | Low phenylalanine diet (250–550 mg/day) |
| Alkaptonuria | Homogentisic acid oxidase | Brown-to-black speckled skin discoloration, prominent over sun-exposed and sweat gland-rich areas, chromhidrosis, brownish discoloration of nails, sclera, and ear cartilage | Pain management, genetic counseling, avoiding high protein diet, and large amounts of dietary vitamin C |
| Tyrosinemia | Tyrosine amino transferases | Painful palmoplantar keratoderma (PPK), hyperhidrosis, painful corneal ulcers, and mental retardation | Low phenylalanine and tyrosine diet.<br>Oral retinoids—PPK |
| Biotinidase deficiency | Biotinidase | Seborrheic dermatitis, alopecia, and oral candidiasis | Vitamin B6: 10–40 mg/day |
| Holocarboxylase synthetase deficiency | Holocarboxylase synthetase | Seborrheic dermatitis | Vitamin B6: 10–40 mg/day |
| Hartnup disease | Increased tryptophan excretion | Pellagra-like dermatitis and photosensitivity | Oral nicotinamide 50–300 mg/day.<br>High protein diet |
| Homocystinuria | Cystathionine β-synthase | Marfanoid habitus, mental retardation, thin skin, sparse hairs, malar flush, and livedo reticularis | High dose<br>Vitamin B6: 150–300 mg/day |
| Prolidase deficiency | Prolidase | Chronic skin ulcers and recurrent skin infections | Skin ulcers: L-proline, glycine, vitamin C, and manganese |

Continued

*Continued*

| Disease | Enzyme deficiency | Cutaneous features | Treatment |
|---|---|---|---|
| Isovaleric acidemia | Isovaleryl-CoA dehydrogenase | Odor of sweaty feet, alopecia, and vomiting | Protein restricted diet, carnitine |
| Gout | Hypoxanthine guanine phosphoribosyl transferase (HGPRT) partial deficiency | Acute attacks of gout involving great toe, tophi over helix and antihelix | Acute—colchicines, nonsteroidal anti-inflammatory drugs.<br>Chronic—allopurinol |
| Lesch–Nyhan syndrome | Complete deficiency of HGPRT | Mental retardation, self-mutilation, e.g., biting of lower lip, features of gout | Allopurinol—features of gout.<br>Neurological—no effective treatment |

**BOX 2 Diagnostic criteria for tuberous sclerosis**

**Major**
- Facial angiofibroma (Fig. 3)
- Nontraumatic ungual or periungual fibroma (Fig. 4)
- Hypomelanotic macule (three or more)—ash–leaf macules
- Shagreen patch (connective tissue nevus)
- Multiple renal nodular hamartomas
- Cortical tuber
- Subependymal nodule
- Subependymal giant cell astrocytoma
- Cardiac rhabdomyoma
- Lymphangiomyomatosis
- Renal angiomyolipoma

**Minor**
- Dental pits
- Hamartomatous rectal polyp
- Bone cysts
- Cerebral white matter migration lines
- Gingival fibromas
- Non-renal hamartomas
- Retinal achromic patch
- Confetti skin lesions
- Multiple renal cysts

Definite—2 major or 1 major with 2 minor
Probable—1 major with 1 minor
Possible—1 major or 2 or more minor features

## GENETIC DISORDERS DUE TO ENZYME DEFICIENCIES

Inborn errors of amino acid metabolism are rare disorders and generally present with multiorgan dysfunction. Diseases of amino acid metabolism generally have an autosomal recessive inheritance. Most of these disorders present with mental retardation, failure to thrive or complaints like brittle hair or body odor (Table 4).

### Alkaptonuria

It is a rare (1 in 250,000) autosomal recessive disorder resulting from deficiency of enzyme homogentisic acid oxidase (HGO), the encoding gene being located on chromosome 3. Mutation, leads to inability to oxidize homogentisic acid, thereby resulting in accumulation of the same in various organs.

#### Clinical Features

- Dark color staining of diaper from urine is often the first sign. This occurs due to rapid oxidation of homogentisic acid when exposed to alkaline environment. Dark brown or black cerumen
- Chromhidrosis
- Scleral and ear cartilage pigmentation (Fig. 5)
- Arthropathy is the most disabling manifestation and presents during 3rd–4th decades. Hip, knee, shoulder joints, and spine are most commonly involved.

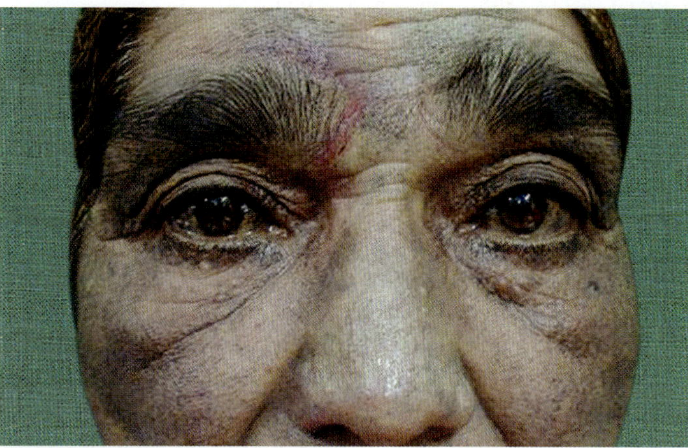

**FIG. 5:** Facial and scleral pigmentation in alkaptonuria.

**BOX 3 Laboratory diagnostic features of alkaptonuria**

- Darkening of urine on adding sodium hydroxide
- Detection of reducing substance in urine by Benedict's test and absence of glucose on oxidase test suggest the diagnosis
- Radiograph of spine—intervertebral disk calcification
- High performance liquid chromatography—quantification of homogentisic acid

#### Diagnosis of Alkaptonuria

The diagnostic features of alkaptonuria are listed in box 3.

#### Treatment

Management is only supportive like pain management, genetic counseling, avoiding high protein diet, and intake of large amounts of dietary vitamin C.

## POIKILODERMATOUS SYNDROMES

Poikiloderma means combination of—pigmentary changes, skin atrophy, and telangiectasia. The most common of these disorders are discussed briefly.

## Dyskeratosis Congenita

Also known as Zinsser–Engman–Cole syndrome, a rare disorder characterized by poikiloderma, nail dystrophy, leukoplakia, bone marrow failure, and predisposition to malignancies.

### Pathogenesis

It can have an X-linked recessive, autosomal dominant or autosomal recessive inheritance of which X-linked recessive form is the most common and therefore, 90% of the affected patients are males. The most common mutation identified in X-linked recessive dyskeratosis congenita (DKC) is in the dyskeratin gene, *DKC1*, located on the q28 region of X chromosome.

### Clinical Features

Dyskeratosis congenita presents with a triad of reticulate hyperpigmentation, mucosal leukoplakia, and dystrophic nails. The nails, often the earliest organ to get affected (about 5–13 years of age) present with longitudinal ridging, splitting, dystrophy with subsequent shedding, pterygium formation, recurrent episodes of suppurative paronychia, and onychogryposis. Skin pigmentation may develop along with the nail changes or 2–3 years thereafter. Grayish brown, fine lacy reticulate pigmentation is most prominently present on the neck and thighs, and may be admixed with hypopigmented macules. The skin is atrophic and may have numerous telangiectasias, giving a poikilodermatous appearance. Cicatricial alopecia and premature canities may be present. Lesions most frequently involve the oral mucosa, with small blisters and erosions which later develops into leukoplakia. Eye, gastrointestinal tract, and urogenital tract may also be involved resulting in stenosis. Bone marrow failure can be present in up to 93% of the patients. Myelodysplasia, Hodgkin disease, and acute myeloid leukemia have been reported. Because of the carcinoma and blood dyscrasia, the prognosis in patients with DKC is usually poor.

### Treatment

Patients are advised to avoid sun and cigarette smoking. Allogeneic bone marrow transplant can cure aplastic anemia. Hematological parameters can be improved with granulocyte colony stimulating factor. Other measures to treat bone marrow failure include transfusion of blood products, use of androgens like oxymetholone and erythropoietin. Use of retinoids may cause regression of leukoplakia, and hence can reduce the incidence of malignancy.

## Rothmund–Thomson Syndrome

### Pathogenesis

Rothmund–Thomson syndrome (RTS) is an autosomal recessive disease characterized by two types of compound heterozygous mutations in a DNA helicase gene *RECQL4*, present on chromosome 8q24.3. The RECQL4 protein is required for initiation of DNA replication and for efficient removal of ultraviolet light induced DNA damage. Depending on the presence or absence of mutations in *RECQL4*, RTS can be classified into two types. In RTS type 1, the gene defect is unidentified and patients have poikiloderma and juvenile cataract. In RTS type II, mutation in *RECQL4* is identified and patients present with typical poikiloderma and increased risk of osteosarcoma.

### Clinical Features

The skin is normal at birth. Earliest lesions are usually seen between 3 months and 6 months of age. Plaques of erythema with edema or diffuse transitory erythema develop on the face, neck, and trunk which are followed by atrophy, pigmentation, depigmentation, and telangiectasia present in varying combinations. The lesions resemble those seen in chronic radiodermatitis. Though photosensitivity may be seen in many cases, distribution of lesions may not be restricted to photoexposed areas, and poikilodermatous changes may develop without any preceding erythema. Severe photosensitivity leading to blister formation is more commonly seen during early childhood. Squamous cell carcinoma may develop in the keratotic lesions and in the surrounding atrophic skin. Hairs of the scalp, eyebrows, eyelashes, pubic and axillary region are often fine and sparse, and may be absent. Nails may be small and dystrophic or may be normal. Delayed physical development, proportionate small stature, slender delicate limbs, small hands and feet, and short fingers are noted. Small skull with bird-like facies with saddle nose may be seen. Patients usually have normal intelligence.

### Treatment

Sun protection is important. Patient should be under supervision for detection of malignancy. It is recommended to get a baseline radiograph of long bones by the age of 5 years as the underlying skeletal dysplasia can cause difficulty in differentiation from osteosarcoma. Retinoids are helpful for treating the skin changes and telangiectasia responds well to pulsed dye laser.

## Acrokeratotic Poikiloderma of Weary

### Pathogenesis

Also known as hereditary sclerosing poikiloderma, it is probably an autosomal dominant syndrome with incomplete penetrance generally most severe in males.

### Clinical Features

It presents with generalized poikiloderma that spares the face, scalp, and ears and is accentuated over the flexures. Other important findings are palmoplantar sclerosis, linear or reticular hyperkeratotic bands on flexural areas (like axillae, antecubital, and popliteal fossa), clubbing of fingers, Raynaud's phenomenon, and tissue calcinosis. Musculoskeletal (micrognathia, tendon contracture, bony abnormalities like maxillary bossing, mandibuloacral dysplasia), cardiovascular abnormalities, and progressive pulmonary fibrosis may also be associated.

## Kindler Syndrome

### Pathogenesis

It is an autosomal recessive disease. Loss-of-function mutations have been identified in the candidate gene *KIND1* that encodes the protein (kindlin1) on chromosome 20p12.3.

## Clinical Features

It is characterized by congenital acral blistering which is induced by trauma, photosensitivity, poikiloderma, atrophy of skin, and mucosal inflammation.[14] It shares features of inherited blistering skin disorders (dystrophic epidermolysis bullosa) and congenital poikilodermas (e.g. Rothmund-Thomson syndrome).

It presents in neonates and infants with skin fragility, blistering, and photosensitivity which improve through childhood. Progressive poikiloderma occurs later. Frequent acral blisters lead to sclerodermoid changes in the acral areas along with nail dystrophy and pseudosyndactyly of digits. Dental changes are prominent like periodontal disease and erosive gingivitis. Stenosis of esophagus, anus, urethra, and vagina may be present. Patients may be at increased risk for development of squamous cell carcinoma of skin and mucosa.

## Treatment

Avoidance of trauma, sun protection, and maintaining good oral hygiene are important. Mucosal strictures can be corrected by dilatation, although it is advised to avoid nonessential instrumentation in order to minimize worsening of stenosis.

# PREMATURE AGING SYNDROMES

Syndromes involving premature cutaneous aging present with characteristic skin changes like wrinkling, atrophy, canities, hair loss, loss of cutaneous fat, nail dystrophy, sclerosis, irregular pigmentation, poikiloderma, and skin ulceration.

## Classification of Various Premature Aging Syndromes

- *Defects in laminin A gene*:
  - Progeria (Hutchinson-Gilford syndrome)
  - Acrogeria (Gottron's syndrome)
  - Restrictive dermopathy
- *Defects in DNA repair*:
  - *Rec Q* gene associated:
    - Pangeria (Werner's syndrome): *WRN* gene defect
    - Bloom syndrome: *BLM* gene defect
    - Rothmund-Thomson syndrome: *RECQ4* gene defect
  - DNA nucleotide excision repair protein associated:
    - Cockayne syndrome
    - Xeroderma pigmentosum (Fig. 6)
    - Trichothiodystrophy
- *Other congenital progeroid syndromes*:
  - Neonatal pseudohydrocephalic progeroid syndrome (Wiedemann-Rautenstrauch syndrome)
  - Trisomy 21 (Down syndrome)
  - Ataxia-telangiectasia (Louis-Bar syndrome): ataxia-telangiectasia mutated gene mutation
  - Osteodysplastic geroderma
  - Wrinkly skin syndrome
  - Familial mandibuloacral dysplasia
  - Progeroid Ehlers-Danlos syndrome.

Among these disorders, progeria, acrogeria, and pangeria are the classical premature aging syndromes and they will be discussed in brief. Table 5 lists the main characteristics of these premature aging syndromes.

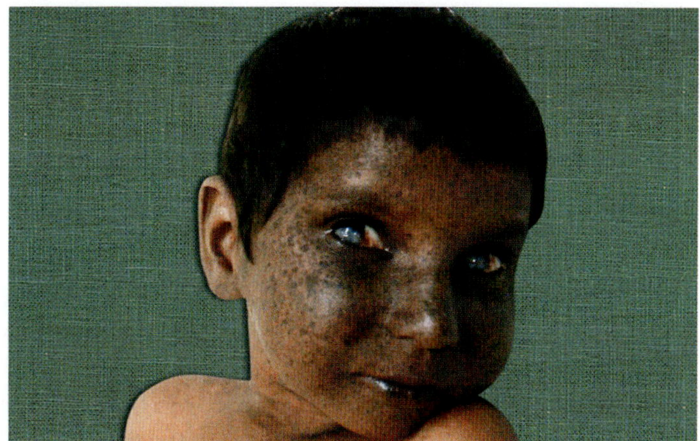

**FIG. 6:** Typical facies in a xeroderma pigmentosum child.

**TABLE 5: Characteristics of important premature aging syndromes**

| Features | Progeria | Pangeria | Acrogeria |
|---|---|---|---|
| Onset | Infancy | 3rd decade | Infancy |
| Death (decade) | 2nd | 5th/6th | Normal expectancy |
| ***Involvement*** | | | |
| Skin | + | + | + |
| Muscular | + | + | + |
| Skeletal | + | + | – |
| Photosensitivity | – | – | – |
| Visual impairment | – | + | – |
| Stunted growth | + | + | – |
| Mental deficiency | – | – | – |
| Cancer risk | – | + | – |

+, present; –, absent.

## Pangeria (Werner's Syndrome)

### *Pathogenesis*

Pangeria, also known as adult premature aging syndrome, is an inherited disorder mostly inherited as an autosomal recessive trait occurs due to mutation in *RecQ* type DNA helicase gene (*RECQL2* or *WRN* gene).

### *Clinical Features*

Graying of hair over the temples starts in the pubertal age groups and is the earliest manifestation of the syndrome. This may be associated with androgenic alopecia. Subsequently, signs of cutaneous atrophy and loss of subcutaneous fat starts appearing over the lower legs, feet, forearms, and hands. This leads to a tense, shining, and adherent appearance of the skin. Presents with bird-like facies, obese trunk and thin limbs, ankylosed joints, sclerodactyly, acral gangrene, and hoarseness of voice due to thinning of vocal cords and fixation of the epiglottis, mostly small stature and hypogonadal, with sparse or absent pubic and axillary hair. Diffuse or mottled pigmentation and telangiectasia on the limbs, face, and neck. Intelligence is usually normal. Insulin-dependent diabetes mellitus (in one-third), posterior subcapsular cataracts (in most) by the age of 30 years, and increased susceptibility to malignancies (especially fibrosarcoma) are also found. Skin cancers are rare, however squamous cell cancers can develop in long standing ulcers. Atherosclerosis is the leading cause of death along with malignancies by the age of 50–60 years.

**BOX 4 Clinical features of progeria**

- *A distinctive appearance*:
  - Narrowed face
  - Small lower jaw
  - Thin lips
  - Beaked nose
  - Head disproportionately large for face
  - Prominent eyes and incomplete closure of the eyelids
- Stunted growth, with below-average height and weight
- Alopecia, including eyelashes and eyebrows
- High-pitched voice
- Conspicuous veins
- Thinning, spotty, wrinkled skin
- Hardening and tightening of skin on trunk and extremities (similar to scleroderma)
- Delayed and abnormal dentition
- Stiff joints
- Hip dislocation
- Insulin resistance
- Hearing loss
- Loss of fat under the skin and loss of muscle mass
- Fragile bones
- Premature atherosclerosis

## Progeria (Hutchinson–Gilford syndrome)

This is a rare disorder characterized by retarded physical development and abnormal facies, skeletal abnormalities, and the onset in early childhood of scleroderma.

### *Pathogenesis*

This is caused by *lamin A* gene (*LMNA*) mutation resulting in reduced cell proliferation and altered DNA-damage responses.

### *Clinical Features*

Typical features are mentioned in box 4. Death usually occurs in the second decade as a result of severe and generalized atherosclerosis.

## Acrogeria (Gottron's Syndrome)

It is characterised by premature aging of the extremities.

### *Pathogenesis*

Most cases are sporadic, but cases with autosomal recessive and autosomal dominant inheritance have been reported. Mutation is detected in *COL3A1* gene (chromosome 2q31–q32). The same locus is affected in Ehlers–Danlos syndrome (IV).

### *Clinical Features*

Changes develop at or soon after birth. They have typical facies (Box 5). Some cases mimic variants of EDS-IV and have poor prognosis. Arterial fragility can lead to early onset arterial aneurysms and even death.

### *Diagnosis*

Skin biopsy from the affected areas commonly reveals epidermal atrophy, sparse appendages, thickened dermis, and subcutaneous fat replaced by hyalinized collagen. There is increase in glycosaminoglycans and abnormal elastic fibers.

### *Treatment*

Only symptomatic measures are available. The management of the recurrent, painful ulceration of the feet and legs is difficult, and amputation may be needed. Cataract surgery should be undertaken with special caution, for it is often complicated by severe degenerative changes of the cornea. Prenatal diagnostic tests are still being investigated and counseling of parents remains the cornerstone of treatment.

**BOX 5 Typical features of acrogeria**

- Dry, thin, transparent, and wrinkled skin over hands and feet
- Short stature
- Pinched facies, hollow cheek, owl-eye, beaked nose, thin lips, and micrognathism
- Lack of subcutaneous fat
- Easy bruising and arterial fragility
- Poikiloderma
- Atrophic or thickened nails

## Gorlin Syndrome

Gorlin syndrome, also known as Gorlin–Goltz syndrome or basal cell nevus syndrome, is a hereditary condition characterized by a wide range of developmental abnormalities and a predisposition to neoplasms. Incidence is 1 in 60,000 live births while 0.4% of patients with a basal cell carcinoma (BCC) are estimated to have Gorlin syndrome.

### *Genetics*

It is an autosomal dominant syndrome with complete penetrance and variable expressivity. It is related to mutation in *PTCH* tumor suppressor gene on chromosome 9. 35–50% of affected individuals are the result of new mutations.

### *Clinical Features*

It is characterized by the early onset development of multiple BCCs. Although this may develop at early childhood, typical age of onset is adolescence or early adulthood. Typical clinical features are odontogenic keratocysts of the jaw and palmar or plantar pits (Table 6).

Basal cell carcinomas may develop and are reported even in children of 3 or 4 years age. BCCs may vary in number (from a few to literally thousands) and range in size from 1 to 10 mm in diameter. They are most likely to appear on the sun-exposed parts of the body, but nonexposed areas may also be involved. After puberty, they become aggressive and invade locally. Evidence of metastastization has been rarely reported.

### *Diagnostic Criteria*

To make the diagnosis, either two major or one major and two minor criteria must be met (Box 6).

### *Differential Diagnosis*

Differential diagnosis includes Bazex syndrome (characterized by basal cell carcinoma associated with hypotrichosis, hypohidrosis, milia, and follicular atrophodermia), trichoepithelioma papulosum multiplex syndrome (Muir–Torre syndrome).

### *Investigations*

Genetic testing. X-ray of chest, skull, panoramic, cervical and thoracic spine, hands (for pseudocysts), and pelvic (female). Ovarian ultrasound (female) for ovarian fibroma and echocardiogram (children) for cardiac fibroma.

### *Management*

Keratocysts can be treated by surgical removal. Patients need to avoid excess sun exposure to prevent BCC formation.

**TABLE 6: Clinical features of Gorlin syndrome**

| Organ | Features |
|---|---|
| Skin | Cutaneous dyskeratosis, nodular or patch lesions, palmoplantar pits, multiple basal-cell carcinomas, benign dermal cysts, and multiple nevi |
| CNS | • *Ectopic calcification*: falx cerebri, tentorium cerebelli<br>• *Others*: meningioma, medulloblastoma, multiforme glioblastoma, moderate mental retardation, grand mal epilepsy, congenital hydrocephalus, and Huntington's chorea |
| Stoma | Odontogenic keratocysts, dental ectopy, heterotopy, impacted teeth, dental agenesis, malocclusion, cleft palate and lip, mandibular prognathism, high-arched palate, squamous-cell carcinoma, and other tumors |
| Eye | Cataract, coloboma, microphthalmia, chalazion, internal strabismus, exophthalmos, rotatory nystagmus, hypertelorism, and blindness |
| Muskulo-skeletal | Polyostotic bone cysts. Bifid, fused, splayed or missing ribs, bifid fused vertebra, scoliosis. Frontal, parietal, and temporal bossing. Polydactyly, syndactyly. Short fourth metacarpal and Sprengel shoulder |
| Genitouri-nary | Hypogonadism, cryptorchidism. Ovarian calcification, cysts, and fibroma |
| Ear | Otosclerosis, conductive hearing loss, and posteriorly angulated ears |
| Cardiac | Cardiac fibroma and absent internal carotid artery |
| Respiratory | Bronchogenic cysts and hyaline membrane disease |
| GI | Mesenteric cysts and gastric polyps |

CNS, central nervous system; GI, gastrointestinal.

**BOX 6 Criteria for diagnosis of Gorlin syndrome**

**Major criteria**
- *Basal cell carcinoma*: >2 or 1 under the age 20
- Odontogenic keratocysts
- *Palmar pits*: 3 or more
- Bilamellar calcification of the falx cerebri
- *Rib anomalies*: bifid rib, fused, splayed
- First degree relative with Gorlin syndrome

**Minor criteria**
- Macrocephaly
- Frontal bossing, cleft lip, or hypertelorism
- Sprengel deformity, pectus excavatum or pectus carinatum, syndactyly
- Bridging of the sella turcica, hemivertebrae, flame-shaped osseous radiolucencies
- Ovarian fibroma
- Medulloblastoma

Chemoprevention may be used to avoid skin lesions. Vitamin A analogs including isotretinoin may play an important role in preventing or slowing the development of new BCCs.

## Goltz Syndrome (Focal Dermal Hypoplasia)

This is an X-linked disorder, characterized by the classical cutaneous findings of linear or reticulate atrophic macules, fat herniation, and raspberry papillomas associated with multiple skeletal, ocular, and dental defects.

### *Pathogenesis*

This is caused by heterozygous mutation in the *PORCN* gene on chromosome Xp11.23. Defect in fibroblast growth leads to a dystrophic dermis and focal herniation of subcutaneous fat.

### *Clinical Features*

This is characterized by congenital streaks of very thin skin (dermal hypoplasia), yellowish-pink nodules of fat under the skin, areas where the top layers of skin are absent (cutis aplasia), small clusters of veins on the surface of the skin (telangiectasias), and streaks of slightly darker or lighter skin. Wart-like papillomas develop with age around the nostrils, lips, anus, and female genitalia and their presence in aerogastric tract can cause problems with swallowing, breathing, or sleeping. Hair on the scalp can be sparse and brittle or absent.

Systemic manifestations include skeletal changes like missing fingers or toes (oligodactyly), webbed or fused fingers or toes (syndactyly), and a deep split in the hands or feet with missing fingers or toes and fusion of the remaining digits (ectrodactyly). X-rays can show streaks of altered bone density, called osteopathia striata, ophthalmological manifestations like microphthalmia, absent or severely underdeveloped eyes (anophthalmia), and problems with the tear ducts and coloboma.

### *Treatment*

Focal dermal hypoplasia requires multispecialty care. The child usually leads a normal life with near normal intelligence. Papillomas can be removed by cryotherapy or cauterization, but may recur again. Proper genetic counseling, emphasizing the X-linked dominant inheritance, should be provided for the parents of affected offspring. Prenatal diagnosis is not possible, but ultrasonography can pick up some of the radiological abnormalities. Osteopathia striata may be present in 20% of gene carriers and they may show only noncutaneous defects associated with Goltz syndrome.

## Darier's Disease (Darier–White Disease)

Darier's disease (DD) was independently described by Darier and White in the year 1889. The disease has a worldwide distribution with a reported prevalence of 1 in 30,000–100,000. Men and women are equally affected. In 70% of the patients, the disease begins between 6 years and 20 years of age with the peak onset between 11 years and 15 years of age.

### *Pathogenesis*

*ATP2A2* is the defective gene in DD which is present on the chromosome region 12q23-24. The gene encodes a calcium pump sarco- or endoplasmic reticulum $Ca^{2+}$ adenosine triphosphatase (ATPase) isoform 2 (SERCA2), which transports $Ca^{2+}$ into the lumen of the endoplasmic reticulum from the cytosol. In DD there is breakdown of desmosomes with internalization of desmosomal components and the keratin filaments aggregate around the nucleus of the cell. This loss of adhesion between the cells triggers apoptosis which in turn forms the dyskeratotic cells (corps ronds and grains).

### *Histopathology*

Acantholysis and dyskeratosis are the prominent histological findings. Suprabasal lacunae present in the epidermis extend irregularly throughout the malpighian layer. "Corps ronds" are enlarged dyskeratotic cells having a dark staining nucleus and clear cytoplasm with a glistening ring-like membrane. These cells give rise to "grains" which are present in the upper epidermis as flattened parakeratotic small cells with shrunken cytoplasm. The epidermis overlying the acantholysis shows acanthosis, papillomatosis, and hyperkeratosis. Superficial dermis may show mild to moderate perivascular inflammatory infiltrate.

### Clinical Features

Darier's disease presents with firm, rough, dark papules which are greasy and distributed in the seborrheic areas of the face, trunk, scalp, ears, and lateral aspects of neck (Figs 7 and 8). Patient may complain of itching, pain, and malodor. Guttate leukoderma, scattered papules on the limbs, coalescing papillomatous masses or fissured warty plaques may all be present. In the flexures, the lesions may become vegetating and malodorous. The lesions show exacerbation with heat, sunlight, friction, and sweating. Characteristic nail changes include longitudinal red and/or white colored bands with a pathognomonic V-shaped nick at the free nail margin, brittle nails, painful longitudinal splits, fissuring, ridging, and wedge-shaped subungual hyperkeratosis. Palms and soles may exhibit minute pitting, punctate or filiform keratosis. Around 50–70% patients have presence of skin colored, flat topped papules involving the dorsum of hands and/or feet, resembling lesions of acrokeratosis verruciformis of Hopf. Oral lesions include painless white papules, white umbilicated or cobblestone papules, leukoplakia-like lesions, and gingival hypertrophy. The disease usually runs a chronic and relapsing course, though spontaneous remission is known to occur.

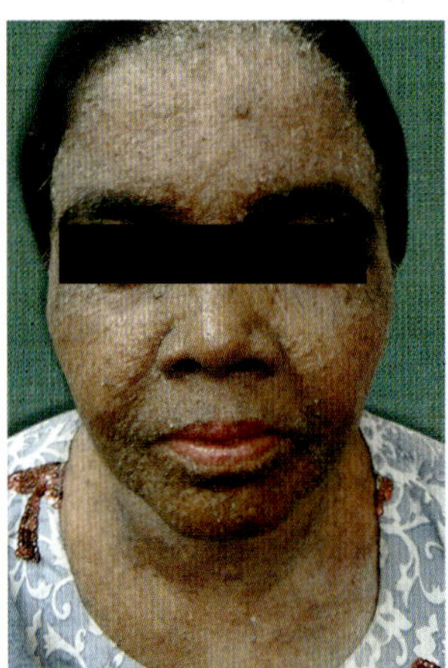

**FIG. 7:** Typical lesions of Darier's disease.

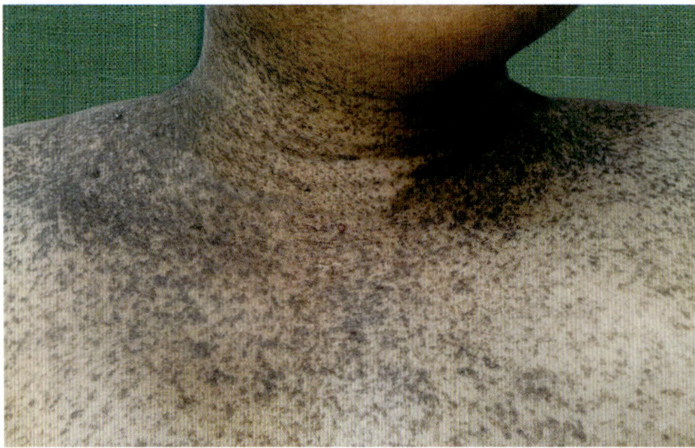

**FIG. 8:** Dirty papules on neck in Darier's disease.

### Types

- Predominantly vesiculobullous lesions
- Painful erosive variant
- Nipple hyperkeratosis
- Acral hemorrhagic lesions
- Segmental type
- Acantholytic dyskeratotic epidermal nevi–nevoid form of Darier's disease.

### Infectious Complications

The lesions of Darier's disease may get secondarily infected with bacteria, yeast or dermatophyte, herpes simplex, human papilloma virus, and poxvirus leading to formation of malodorous vegetating plaques. The increased frequency of infections in Darier's disease is most likely caused by epidermal barrier disruption. Kaposi's varicelliform eruption is common in patients with Darier's disease.

### Differential Diagnosis

- *Acrokeratosis verruciformis of Hopf*: This lacks acantholysis and dyskeratosis
- Acne
- Seborrheic dermatitis
- Discoid eczema—mimics the confluent lesions
- Hailey-Hailey disease—mimics clinically and histopathologically the flexural lesions of Darier's
- Acanthosis nigricans
- Dowling-Degos disease
- Confluent reticulate papillomatosis—this is characterized by presence of flat lesions mostly on the upper trunk.
- Follicular keratosis diseases
- Reticular erythematous mucinosis
- Prurigo pigmentosa.

### Treatment

Sunscreens, wearing lightweight clothes to prevent aggravation by heat, sweating, friction, and sun exposure is necessary. Keratolytics, emollients for scaling, and antimicrobial cleansers to prevent colonization with malodorous bacteria are also needed. Use of topical retinoids like tretinoin, isotretinoin, adapalene, and tazarotene are effective but can cause irritation, which can be managed with liberal application of emollients. Topical 5-fluorouracil, both 1% and 5% is found to be effective, however efficacy of calcipotriene is still not established in treatment of Darier's disease. Topical tacrolimus has also been used. Oral retinoids like acitretin (0.25–0.5 mg/kg/day) and isotretinoin (0.5 mg/kg/day) are used in severe disease. Severe inflammatory exacerbations, eczematization, and severe vulval disease and patients who fail to respond to oral retinoids respond well to cyclosporine. Surgical therapy, lasers, and photodynamic therapy may be effective in the treatment of focal recalcitrant lesions. Botulinum toxin has been used to decrease sweating in the recalcitrant flexural disease.

## Porokeratosis

It is a clonal disorder of keratinization manifesting as atrophic patches or plaques surrounded by distinctive cornoid lamella.

### Etiopathogenesis

Various risk factors are blamed namely genetic inheritance, ultraviolet radiation, and immunosuppression. Inherited or sporadic genetic defects are responsible for different forms of porokeratosis. Familial cases probably have an autosomal dominant inheritance pattern. Genetic mutations in the *SART3* and *MVK* genes have been found.

### Clinical Features

The variants of porokeratosis are:

- *Classic porokeratosis of Mibelli (PM)*: It is the second most common form of porokeratosis. It is seen in men more than women and first appears in childhood or young adulthood. Initially appearing as small, slightly pruritic lesion with central hypopigmentation, scaling and atrophy, and a raised hyperkeratotic ridged border, they slowly expand over a period of years. Classically, they are located on extremities, but can occur anywhere, including the palms, soles, genitalia (Fig. 9), or mucous membranes. Giant porokeratosis with lesions more than 10–20 cm may also occur
- *Disseminated superficial actinic porokeratosis (DSAP)*: It is the most common form of porokeratosis, and accounts for 50% of all cases. Annular macules with raised peripheral ridges, occurring predominantly on the extensor surfaces of arms and legs are characteristic with sparing of palms and soles (Fig. 10). Women in third and fourth decade with history of ultraviolet light exposure are more prone to develop this condition. Family history is contributory
- *Disseminated superficial porokeratosis (DSP)*: Very similar in morphology to DSAP, but occurs in a generalized distribution. Underlying immunosuppression is very likely
- *Linear porokeratosis*: Develop during infancy or early childhood and represents a segmental form of DSP. Unilateral reddish brown patches or linear keratotic papules and plaques distributed along Blaschko's lines are characteristic. There is a higher risk of malignant degeneration than other forms of porokeratosis
- Porokeratosis palmaris et plantaris disseminata (PPPD)
- Punctate porokeratosis (variant of PPPD)
- Porokeratosis ptychotropica (genital variant—localized to the groin or buttocks)
- Porokeratoma (porokeratotic acanthoma)

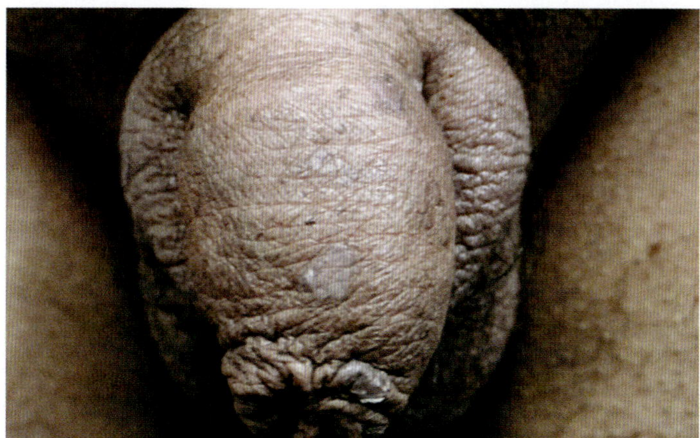

**FIG. 9:** Genital porokeratosis.

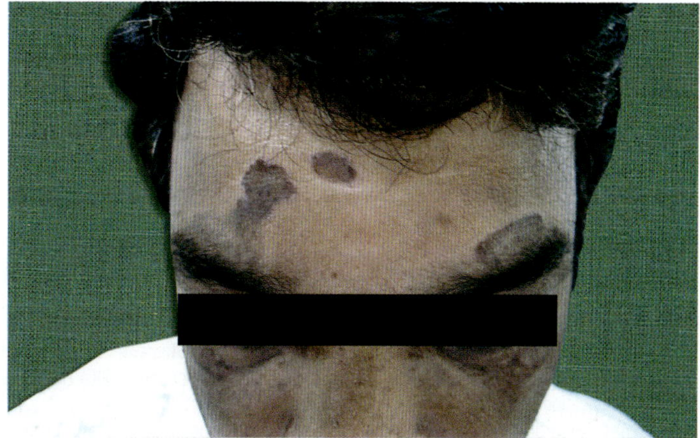

**FIG. 10:** Disseminated superficial actinic porokeratosis.

- *Porokeratotic adnexal ostial nevus (PAON)—two components*: Porokeratotic eccrine ostial and dermal duct nevus (PEODDN) and porokeratotic eccrine and hair follicle nevus (PEHFN)
- Pruritic papular porokeratosis.

Squamous cell carcinomas and rarely BCCs have been reported in all forms of porokeratosis. Large, long-standing, and linear lesions have the greatest risk of developing malignancy.

### Histopathology

The characteristic cornoid lamella consists of a thin column of tightly packed parakeratotic cells within a keratin-filled epidermal invagination. Within the parakeratotic column, the horny cells are homogeneous and have deeply basophilic pyknotic nuclei. Dyskeratotic cells are found beneath the parakeratotic column which does not have a granular layer. The papillary dermis beneath the cornoid lamella contains a moderately dense, lymphocytic infiltrate along with dilated capillaries.

### Treatment

Protection from sun, emollients, and observation for signs of malignancy are the cornerstones of therapy. Topical retinoids are the mainstay of topical therapy while others like 5-fluorouracil, calcipotriol, and imiquimod have also been found to be useful. Disseminated cases will benefit from oral retinoids which also can prevent development of malignancies. Destructive modalities like surgical excision, cryotherapy, and dermabrasion are advised for lesions which have become malignant. Lasers like pulsed dye, Q-Switched Nd:YAG, and Ruby are found to be beneficial in disseminated and linear variants.

## SUGGESTED READINGS


1. Bencini PL, Tarantino A, Grimalt R, et al. Prokeratosis and immunosuppression. Br J Dermatol. 1995;132:74-8.
2. Bornholdt D, Oeffner F, Konig A, et al. PORCN mutations in focal dermal hypoplasia: coping with lethality. Hum Mutat. 2009;30:E618-28.
3. Christopherson J, Geiger J-M, Danneskiol-Samsoe P, et al. A double-blind comparison of acitretin and etretinate in the treatment of Darier's disease. Acta Derm Venereol (Stockh), 1992;72:150-2.
4. Claudy AL, Gaudin OG, Granouillet R. Pox virus infection in Darier's disease. Clin Exp Dermatol. 1982;7:261-5.
5. Davidson HR, Connor JM. Dyskeratosis congenita. J Med Genet. 1988;25:843-6.

6. Fan W, Luo J. RecQ4 facilitates UV-induced DNA damage repair through interaction with nucleotide excision repair factor XPA. J Biol Chem. 2008;283:29037-44.
7. Fine JD, Eady RA, Bauer EA, et al. The classification of inherited epidermolysis bullosa (EB): report of the Third International Consensus Meeting on Diagnosis and Classification of EB. J Am Acad Dermatol. 2008;58:931-50.
8. Goltz RW, Peterson WC, Gorlin RJ, et al. Focal dermal hypoplasia. Arch Dermatol. 1962;86:708-17.
9. Grau Salvat C, Pont V, Cors JR, et al. Hereditary sclerosing poikiloderma of Weary: report of a new case. Br J Dermatol. 1999;140:366-8.
10. Heiss NS, Knight SW, Vulliamy TJ, et al. X-linked dyskeratosis congenita is caused by mutations in a highly conserved gene with putative nucleolar functions. Nat Genet. 1998;19:32-8.
11. Kitao S, Shimamoto A, Goto M, et al. Mutations in RECQL4 cause a subset of cases of Rothmund–Thomson syndrome. Nat Genet. 1999;22:82-4.
12. Knight S, Vulliamy T, Copplestone A, et al. Dyskeratosis Congenita (DC) Registry: identification of new features of DC. Br J Haematol. 1998;103:990-6.
13. Lai-Cheong JE, Tanaka A, Hawche G, et al. Kindler syndrome: a focal adhesion genodermatosis. Br J Dermatol. 2009;160:233-42.
14. Leow YH, Soon YH, Tham SN. A report of 31 cases of porokeratosis at the National Skin Centre. Ann Acad Med Singapore. 1996;25(6):837-41.
15. Liebermann S. Atrophoderma linearis maculosae papillomatosis congenitalis. Acta Dermatol Venereol. 1935;16:476-84.
16. Mansur AT, Elcioglu NH, Aydingoz IE, et al. Novel and recurrent KIND1 mutations in two patients with Kindler syndrome and severe mucosal involvement. Acta Derm Venereol. 2007;87:563-5.
17. Marks JG, Thor DE, Lowe RS. Darier's disease: an immunologic study. Arch Dermatol. 1978;114:1336-9.
18. Miyauchi Y, Daiho T, Yamasaki K, et al. Comprehensive analysis of expression and function of 51 sarco(endo)plasmic reticulum Ca2+-ATPase mutants associated with Darier disease. J Biol Chem. 2006;281:22882-95.
19. Munro CS. The phenotype of Darier's disease: penetrance and expressivity in adults and children. Br J Dermatol. 1992;127:126-30.
20. Murase J, Gilliam AC. Disseminated superficial actinic porokeratosis co-existing with linear and verrucous porokeratosis in an elderly woman: Update on the genetics and clinical expression of porokeratosis. J Am Acad Dermato. 2010;63(5):886-91.
21. Nobili B, Rossi G, De Stefano P, et al. Successful umbilical cord blood transplantation in a child with dyskeratosis congenita after a fludarabine-based reduced-intensity conditioning regimen. Br J Haematol. 2002;119:573-4.
22. Oster-Schmidt C. The treatment of Darier's disease with topical tazarotene. Br J Dermatol. 1999;141:603-4.
23. Otsuka F, Umebayashi Y, Watanabe S, et al. Porokeratosis large skin lesions are susceptible to skin cancer development: histological and cytological explanation for the susceptibility. J Cancer Res Clin Oncol. 1993;119:395-400.
24. Potozkin JR, Geronemus RG. Treatment of the poikilodermatous component of the Rothmund–Thomson syndrome with the flashlamp-pumped pulsed dye laser: a case report. Pediatr Dermatol. 1991;8:162-5.
25. Pritchard SL, Junker AK. Positive response to granulocyte-colony-stimulating factor in dyskeratosis congenita before matched unrelated bone marrow transplantation. Am J Pediatr Hematol Oncol. 1994;16:186-7.
26. Raychaudhury T, Valsamma DP. Giant porokeratosis. Indian J Dermatol Venereol Leprol. 2011;77:601.
27. Ringpfeil F, Raus A, DiGiovanna JJ, et al. Darier disease–novel mutations in ATP2A2 and genotype-phenotype correlation. Exp Dermatol. 2001;10:19-27.
28. Seishima M, Izumi T, Oyama Z, et al. Squamous cell carcinoma arising from lesions of porokeratosis palmaris et plantaris disseminata. Eur J Dermatol. 2000;10:478-80.
29. Shahidulla H, Humphreys F, Beveridge GW. Darier's disease: severe eczematisation successfully treated with cyclosporin. Br J Dermatol. 1994;131:713-6.
30. Shuttleworth D, Marks R. Congenital poikiloderma: treatment with etretinate. Br J Dermatol. 1988;118:729-30.
31. Siegel DH, Ashton GH, Penagos HG, et al. Loss of kindlin-1, a human homolog of the Caenorhabditis elegans actin–extracellular-matrix linker protein UNC-112, causes Kindler syndrome. Am J Hum Genet. 2003;73:174-87.
32. Siitonen HA, Sotkasiira J, Biervliet M, et al. The mutation spectrum in RECQL4 diseases. Eur J Hum Genet. 2009;17:151-8.
33. Stinco G, Governatori G, Mattighello P, et al. Multiple cutaneous neoplasms in a patient with Rothmund–Thomson syndrome: case report and published work review. J Dermatol. 2008;35:154-61.
34. Temple IK, MacDowall P, Baraister M, et al. Focal dermal hypoplasia (Goltz syndrome). J Med Genet. 1990;27:180-7.
35. Uitto J, Bauer EA, Santa-Cruz DJ, et al. Focal dermal hypoplasia: abnormal growth characteristics of skin fibroblasts in culture. J Invest Dermatol. 1980;765:170-5.
36. Weary PE, Hsu YT, Richardson DR, et al. Hereditary sclerosing poikiloderma. Report of two families with an unusual and distinctive genodermatosis. Arch Dermatol. 1969;100:413-22.

3

SECTION

# Environment and Skin

6

CHAPTER

# Environmental and Occupational Dermatoses

*Nilendu Sarma, Ishad Agarwal*

## INTRODUCTION

The human skin is a dynamic covering that ensheaths the framework of the human body. Being the largest human organ, it presents as an interface that interacts with the environment. Even though, the human beings have manipulated the environment to protect themselves from the various physical, chemical, and biological forces that it is composed of, there is still sometimes a deliberate or inadvertent exposure which could lead to injury of the skin. Environmental dermatoses are consequences of such interactions and result out of both the onslaught of environmental agents on skin and skin's reactions to them. Although, both macro-and micro environment affects the skin, the following discussion, would focus mainly upon the skin disorders due to physical agents such as heat, cold, water, chemicals, light and radiation, trauma, and certain environmental poisons.

## DERMATOSES DUE TO LIGHT

Dermatoses due to actinic injury or cutaneous reaction to light can be of following types:

- Acute and chronic normal effects of UV light
- Abnormal cutaneous effects of UV
- Immunologically mediated photodermatoses
- DNA defective repair mechanism disorders and inherited chromosomal disorders
- Photoaggravated disorders
- Chemical and drug-induced photosensitivity.

The terrestrial solar spectrum consists of wavelengths between 290 nm and 4,000 nm which contain the UV rays (UVR), visible rays and the infrared rays. The UVR has wavelength between 100 nm and 400 nm.

- UVC (100–290 nm)
- UVB (290–320 nm)
- UVA (320–400 nm), UVA1 (340–400 nm), UVA2 (320–340 nm)
- Visible light (400–700 nm)
- Infrared light (>700 nm).

## PHOTOBIOLOGICAL REACTIONS

The lights that fall on the surface of the skin are either reflected, refracted or absorbed. The depth of penetration of light is directly proportional to its wavelength. The photobiological reactions are mainly produced by the UVR and visible light and are due to interaction of light with the skin. Rays of smaller wavelength contain higher quantum of energy and hence their effects are more pronounced.

Sequence of photobiological reactions is as follows:

- Absorption of light by the chromophores in our skin like melanin, hemoglobin, amino acids, purines and pyrimidines, bilirubin
- Excitation of chromophores to singlet and triplet states
- Formation of photoproducts
- Initiation of biochemical response
- Cellular reactions.

## NORMAL RESPONSE OF SKIN TO SUN

### Tanning

Skin pigmentation produced as a result of sun exposure is a biphasic phenomenon that is mediated by both UVA and UVB lights. The tanning potential of the skin depends upon the Fitzpatrick skin types. The darker skin types tan more.

### Immediate Pigment Darkening

It is the protective response of skin to sun exposure. It is the darkening of skin that lasts for less than 2 hours. It is mainly due to UVA-induced photooxidation of the melanin content of the skin.

### Delayed Pigment Darkening

It is due to UVB and UVA rays both. The pigmentation lasts more than 24 hours. It appears at 72 hours and may last for weeks. The pathogenesis lies in increased number of melanin. It offers skin protection and increases the minimal erythema dose (MED) of the skin.

### Sunburn

The minimal amount of a particular wavelength of light capable of inducing erythema on an individual's skin is called the MED. Sunburn is the cutaneous response of skin to light above the MED. It is more pronounced in fair skinned individuals and characteristically there is erythema with or without blistering,

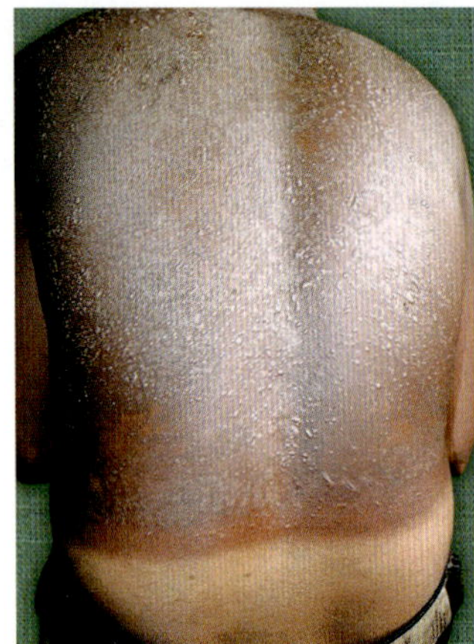

FIG. 1: Sunburn with intense erythema and vesicular eruptions.

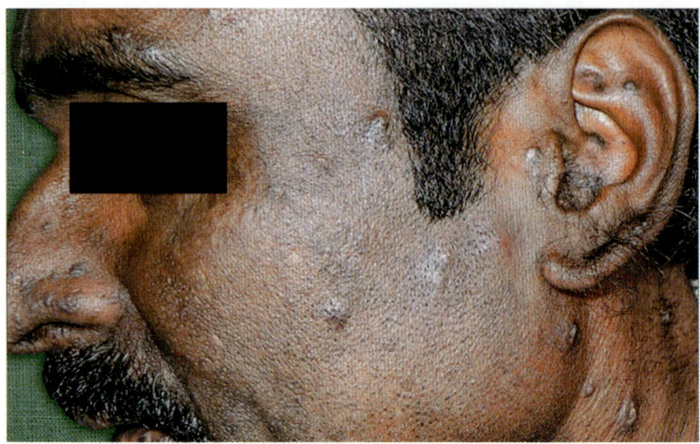

FIG. 2: Actinic prurigo.

pain and edema (Fig. 1). It is followed by desquamation and hyperpigmentation. It is seen more in higher altitudes.

### Treatment

Treatment of sunburn is supportive with pain management plus soothing topical emollients or corticosteroid lotions.

## PHOTOAGING

The characteristic changes of aging produced by chronic sun exposure is called photoaging or dermatoheliosis.

### Characteristic of Histological Changes

Photoaging is a dynamic process involving epidermis and dermis. Following histological changes are seen. Decreased content of collagen and basophilic degeneration of collagen with marked elastin content and elastosis. The fibroblasts are active. There is either increased or decreased melanocytes.

### Clinical Features

Photoaged skin is dry, lusterless, wrinkled, inelastic, and thick. There may be visible telangiectasias, comedones, deep furrows, freckles, and lentigines. Cutis rhomboidalis nuchae (sailor's or farmer's neck) is characteristic of long-term, chronic sun exposure and is seen in form of deep furrows over neck. Nodular elastoidosis with cysts and comedones occurs on the inferior periorbital and malar skin (Favre-Racouchot syndrome) on the forearms (actinic comedonal plaque) or helix of the ear. These lesions appear as thickened yellow plaques studded with comedones and keratinous cysts.

### Prevention

Strict usage of photoprotection, sunscreen, and moisturizers prevent aging.

## IMMUNOLOGICAL PHOTOMEDIATED DERMATOSES

This group of disorders contain:

- Polymorphous light eruptions (PMLEs)
- Chronic actinic dermatitis (CAD) and actinic reticuloid
- Hydroa vacciniforme
- Actinic prurigo (Fig. 2)
- Solar urticarial.

### Polymorphous Light Eruption

Polymorphous light eruption (PMLE) is the most common idiopathic photodermatoses induced by UVR. Some artificial light sources like welding arc and photocopy light may also induce polymorphic light eruption (PLE).

#### Pathogenesis

It is seen as a reaction to bright sunny light. It is a delayed type of hypersensitivity reaction to a light induced endogenous neoantigen which is yet to be characterized. UVB induces immunosuppression locally in normal individual. This is not seen in individual who are susceptible for PLE.

#### Clinical Features

The lesions of PMLE occur few minutes to hours after exposure to sun. Sometimes, it can develop after 1–3 days. It is seen more in early summer and progressively improves due to hardening effect of chronic sun exposure.

As the name suggests, the lesions are polymorphic. Classically they are grouped erythematous, papules, plaques, vesicles, rarely hemorrhagic, and even erythema multiforme like eruptions. This is seen over areas that are exposed but areas that are perennially exposed like dorsum of hands and face are spared. Commonly affected areas are extensor surface of forearms and arms, V-area of neck, and legs. Secondary eczematization may be seen but is rare. Rash remits in winter. Persistent rash even in winter and presence of eczematization should prompt meticulous search for alternate diagnosis.

There are some variants of PLE. Some young boys develop vesicular eruptions only on the helices of the ears in spring. This is known as juvenile spring eruptions.

Some individuals develop lichen nitidus-type lesions in exposed areas like V-area of neck. This is called photolichenoid PLE (Fig. 3). Some patients may have pruritus at exposed areas without any rash. This is called PLE sine eruption. Interestingly, one single individual persistently shows one particular type of PLE.

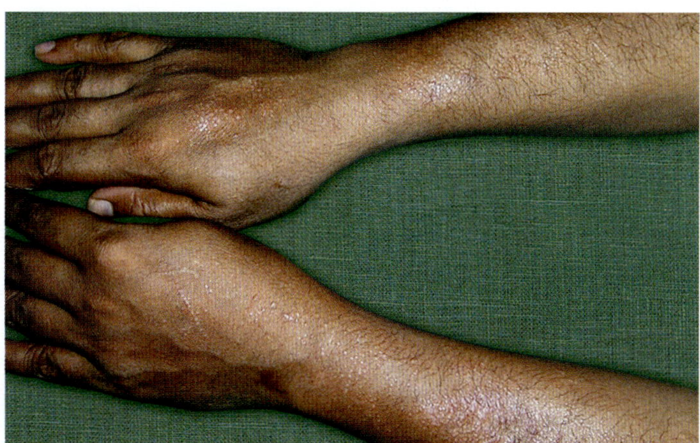

**FIG. 3:** Lichen nitidus-like polymorphous light eruption.

*Courtesy*: Dr Abhay Mani Martin, Senior Consultant and Head, Department of Dermatology, Baby Memorial Hospital, Kozhikode, Kerala.

### Diagnosis

In histopathology, dense perivascular lymphocyte collection is seen in upper and mid-dermis. Serum antinuclear antibodies (ANA) can help in differentiation from lupus erythematosus.

## Phototesting and Provocative Tests

Possibly, UVA is more important wavelength to induce PLE. Some smaller sections of patients are more sensitive to UVB or visible sunlight.

### Treatment

Strict photoprotection is advised to patients of PMLE. Physical protection, sunscreen should be used effectively. Sunscreen should be broad spectrum. Physical blockers effectively block UVA.

Desensitization is an important method of treatment. The principle of the therapy is to induce "hardening" by exposing the susceptible individual with suberythemal dose of UVB or UVA or PUVA. This is done 4–6 weeks prior to summer. People who are more sensitive to UVA are treated with UVB and vice versa. However, identification of sensitive spectrum has to be done with provocative test. If this is not available, selection of ray depends on availability, side effect profile and past treatment response. Flare-up of PLE is often induced during desensitization. It can be treated with topical corticosteroid.

Symptomatic treatment with antihistamines, topical corticosteroids may be given. In moderate cases hydroxychloroquine may be prescribed. In severe, unremitting cases systemic therapy like low dose azathioprine, ciclosporine, or thalidomide may be beneficial.

## Hydroa Vacciniforme

It is a more rare form of idiopathic photosensitivity which is seen in children. UVA is possibly more responsible than UVB in inducing hydroa vacciniforme (HV). Some cases are familial.

Early childhood (1–7 years) and a second peak at 12–16 years are commonly involved. Most cases that start in early childhood improve during adolescence. The lesions initially are recurrent painful, erythematous papules which occur symmetrically over face, hands, and buttocks. They develop into vesicles, bullae and crust and heal with varioliform scarring. These are often umbilicated. Some cases heal without scarring (hydroa aestivale). Common sites are cheeks, nose, ear, and dorsa of hands. Eyes are rarely affected and can lead to corneal scarring. Destructive changes in nose and ear are also seen occasionally. Management is generally similar to PLE.

## Chronic Actinic Dermatitis

Chronic actinic dermatitis (CAD) represents the end stage of progressive photosensitivity in some patients.

The basic components of chronic actinic dermatitis are:

- A persistent eczematous eruption of papules and vesicles in photoexposed distribution
- Histology consistent with features of eczema with or without lymphoma
- Reduction of MED in normal skin to UVB and sometimes to UVA.

### Pathogenesis

Chronic actinic dermatitis is caused and maintained by UVB, often UVA and sometimes visible light.

These patients often have exacerbated sensitivity to multiple contact allergens. The pathogenesis is similar to persistent allergic contact dermatitis with presence of CD8+ T-cells.

Following factors in host skin may predispose to development of CAD:

- Pre existing allergic contact dermatitis, frequently seen to sesquiterpene lactone, fragrances, and colophony may contribute. Chronic photostimulation and alteration of innate proteins by phototoxic agents exacerbate the disease
- Photoallergic contact dermatitis
- Drug-induced photosensitivity
- Endogenous eczema
- Immunosuppressive states.

### Clinical Features

This is seen mostly among older people (>50 years of age). Skin lesions occur primarily on chronically photoexposed skin which has borne the brunt of allergic contact dermatitis and other predisposing factors. They are edematous, scaly, thickened patches, and plaques that tend to be confluent. The sites such as retroauricular sulcus, between skin folds may be spared (Fig. 4). Appearance may mimick pseudolymphoma (actinic reticuloid) (Fig. 5). This is described as unremitting, lichenified, indurated, and plaques on photoexposed areas.

Some cases however show extensive involvement beyond exposed areas and even erythroderma can develop in few cases.

One subset of patients is called "persistent light reactors". In this, people retain light sensitivity even after the exposure to photosensitizing agent has ceased to occur.

### Diagnosis

Patch testing is very important. Widest possible allergens are to be used including compositae and sunscreen in addition to standard series. Photopatch test, if facilities are available, should also be attempted.

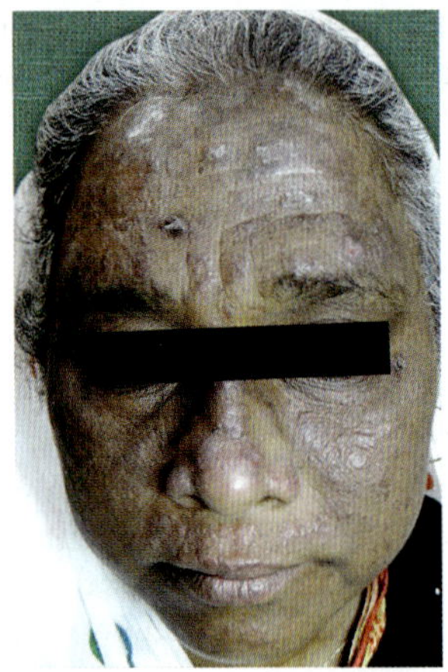

FIG. 4: Chronic actinic dermatitis with sparing of nasolabial furrow.

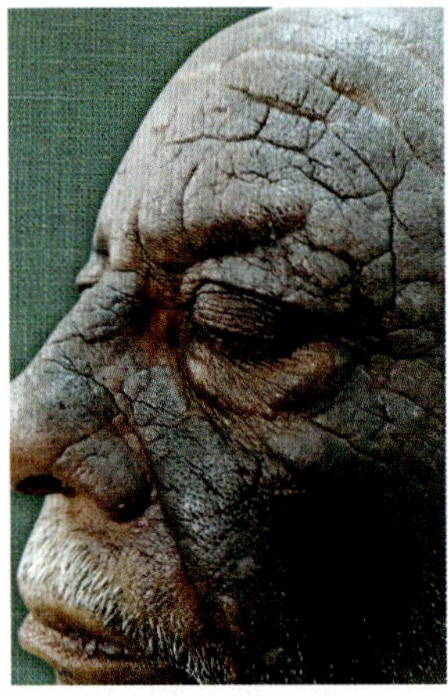

FIG. 5: Chronic actinic dermatitis progressing toward actinic reticuloid.
*Courtesy*: Dr Prerna, MO (Dermatologist), Dr B N Bose SD Hospital, Barrackpore, West Bengal.

Phototest—Although UVB is the most common spectrum, sensitivity frequently encroaches over longer wavelength of UVA and visible light. Positive test often shows a dermatitis response and this is highly diagnostic.

Histopathology shows presence of dermatitis. Some cases presenting with pseudolymphoma may have Sézary cells.

### Treatment

Photoprotection and avoidance form allergens are essential in all patients. Topical steroids are useful only in milder cases. Oral immunosuppressants, corticosteroids for initial control and azathioprine, cyclosporine, or mycophenolate mofetil for long-term control are given in resistant moderate to severe disease.

## PHOTOTOXIC AND PHOTOALLERGIC REACTIONS

Phototoxic reactions are direct cell injury resulting from a non-immunological reaction between the drug or metabolite and UVR, while photoallergic reactions are delayed type of hypersensitivity reactions between a photoproduct and UVR and consequent immune response that develops.

Phototoxic reactions usually can be distinguished from the photoallergic reactions by the sharp border and exclusive distribution over exposed areas (Fig. 6).

Agents that cause these reactions are mentioned in table 1.

Pathogenesis and important distinguishing clinical and histological features of these conditions are described in tables 2 and 3.

## DERMATOSES DUE TO HEAT

Thermoregulation is a complex process in which the cutaneous vasculature, lymphatics, and sweat glands play a vital role. Failure of body's ability to regulate its core temperature leads to a variety of skin related illnesses like heat exhaustion, heat stroke, heat cramps, and heat edema. However, in this chapter, we will discuss only the heat related illnesses that affect the skin.

### Miliaria

Miliaria is an eruption on skin caused due to blockage of the ducts of the eccrine sweat gland and resulting spillage of eccrine sweat in epidermis or dermis. It is produced in conditions which prevent dissipation of heat and moisture. Common precipitating factors are heat, humidity, fever, and some drugs like isotretinoin, doxycycline and bethanechol. Miliaria can be classified into various forms depending upon level of block

- *Miliaria crystallina (Sudamina)*: The site of blockage is the superficial stratum corneum. It is seen characterized by small,

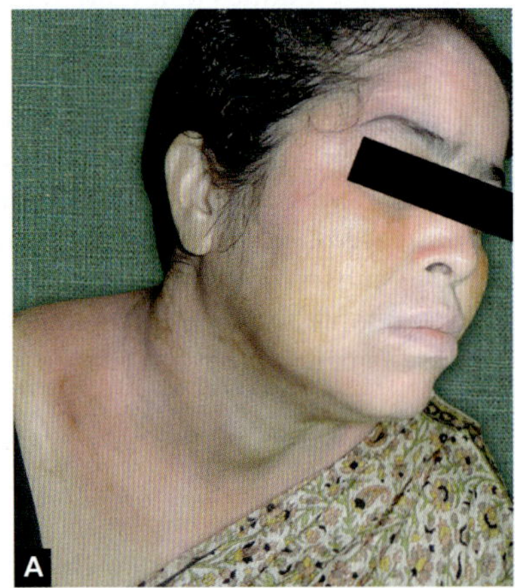

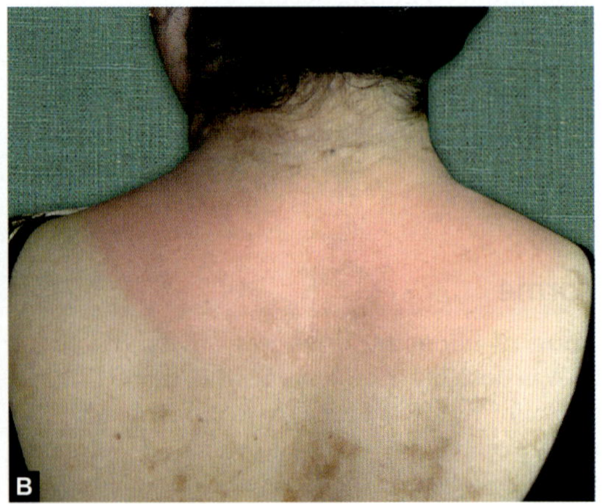

FIG. 6: Phototoxic reaction in a patient with vitiligo following oral psoralens intake and extended sun exposure.

**TABLE 1: Common causes of phototoxic and photoallergic reactions**

| | Phototoxic | Photoallergic |
|---|---|---|
| Topical agents | • Psoralen<br>• Tar | • Sunscreens<br>• Fragrances<br>• Antibacterials<br>• Plants of compositae family |
| Systemic agents | • Psoralens<br>• Nalidixic acid, doxycycline, and quinolones<br>• Fluorouracil, vinblastine<br>• Amitriptyline<br>• NSAIDs, phenothiazines, amiodarone, frusemide | • Griseofulvin<br>• Quinolones, sulfonamides<br>• NSAIDs, Ketoprofen, phenothiazine, thiazide |

NSAIDs, nonsteroidal anti-inflammatory drugs.

**TABLE 2: Pathogenesis of phototoxic and photoallergic reactions**

| Phototoxic reactions | Photoallergic reactions |
|---|---|
| Drug/antigen reaches the skin<br>↓<br>It absorbs light of a wavelength<br>↓<br>It gets excited to singlet and triplet state<br>↓<br>It returns to baseline and causes energy release and causes cell destruction | Drug/antigen gets converted into stable hapten by light<br>↓<br>This stable photo product binds to innate antigens<br>↓<br>Light alleviates this product into excited state<br>↓<br>This product causes type IV manifestations |

**TABLE 3: Clinical and histological features of phototoxic and photoallergic reactions**

| Phototoxic reactions | Photoallergic reactions |
|---|---|
| It requires large amount of drug | It requires less amount of drug |
| It occurs in a small span of time after exposure within minutes to hours | It occurs after a large delay of time after exposure and may even occur after the exposure has stopped |
| Skin lesions are acute, erythematous, blistering skin diseases with exaggerated sunburn like lesions which may heal with hyperpigmentation | Clinical features are chronic dermatitis like lesions. Lichenoid lesions, scaling may be seen in chronic lesions |
| Necrotic keratinocytes are seen in histology | Spongiotic dermatitis and lymphohistiocytic infiltrate are seen in histology |

superficial, clear vesicles which tend to rupture spontaneously and resolve after that. There is no inflammatory reaction

- *Miliaria rubra (Prickly heat)*: The lesions are produced due to blockage of the eccrine sweat duct at the level of stratum spinosum. Therefore, the spillage of sweat in epidermis produces erythema. The lesions are discrete, extremely pruritic papulovesicles which may be accompanied by tingling and burning. They may become confluent over a bed of erythema. Most commonly affected area are the antecubital fossa, inframammary folds under pendulous breasts, trunk, abdomen, popliteal fossa, and inguinal regions
- *Miliaria profunda (mammillaria)*: The lesions are small whitish papules which last for around 1 hour after the exposure of concentrated heat has ended. The blockage of sweat duct is at the level of dermo epidermal junction. It commonly occurs on trunk
- *Miliaria pustulosa*: The lesions consist of distinct superficial pustules which erupt on sites where sweat ducts have been destroyed due to a secondary pathology like contact dermatitis or lichen simplex chronicus. They may occur weeks after the initial pathology. Recurrent episodes may be a sign of salt loosing type 1 pseudohypoaldosteronism.

### Complications

The following complications may be seen:

- Secondary bacterial infections
- Tropical anhidrotic asthenia: It is a complication of widespread miliaria profunda in which destruction of sweat glands leads to anhidrosis and therefore heat exhaustion
- Widespread miliaria rubra in infants and small children may lead to thermoregulatory failures.

### Diagnosis and Treatment

Diagnosis is mainly clinical. Cornerstone of therapy is placing the patient in cool environment. Fans to circulate air may help. Topical anhydrous lanolin or hydrophobic lotion helps in sweat gland duct opening. Calamine liniment or lotion is also helpful.

## HEAT URTICARIA

Any condition that generates body heat like exercise, sweating, and hot showers or baths and occupational exposure to hot atmosphere can lead to development of wheals. This is also called cholinergic urticaria. This may be localized (localized heat urticaria). Urticaria that may be composed of very tiny eruptions develops 2–5 minutes which last for an hour.

### Kangri Ulcer

Kangri is a heated earthen pot kept inside a long coat by Kashmiri men to protect them from cold winters. Prolonged contact with heat, produces burns, scars and squamous cell carcinomas on skin where it comes in contact with the kangri.

Dermatoses of similar pathology influenced by cultural practices also occur in chutta smokers, kang cancers in China, turf cancers in Ireland and kairo cancer in Japan.

### Erythema ab Igne

Erythema ab igne (EAI) is a retiform cutaneous pattern caused by prolonged exposure to infrared rays which are not strong enough to cause a burn. Although, the incidence has decreased overtime due to rapid advancement of heating systems and cooking practices, it is still seen resulting due to changing cultural practices and application of heating devices such as hot water bottles. In India, it is still seen in women who cook over burning wood and fuel. Recently it has also been observed in people who use laptops for long periods of time.

## Clinical Features

Initially the lesions appear as painless, mottled, lace like blanchable erythema which subsides with residual hyperpigmentation. Telangiectasia, atrophy and scaling may also be seen in advanced cases. Rarely squamous cell carcinoma and Bowen's disease (BD) has been known to develop over lesions of EAI. Clinical hypothyroidism should be sought in older patients.

### Pathology

The basic pathology lies in dermal vascular network and histologically manifested initially by epidermal atrophy with loss of rete ridges, squamous atypia, dermal pigmentation, and vasodilatation. Focal hyperkeratosis and basophilic degeneration of connective tissue occurs later in the course of disease.

### Treatment

Treatment primarily consists of removing the source of heat. Topical 5-Fu or imiquimod cream may help to relieve BD developing over EAI. Depigmenting agents like hydroquinone, tretnoin may be used to reduce hyperpigmentation.

### Tropical Acne

Acne and acneiform lesions may occur in people living in hot and humid regions, predominantly because of blockage of pilosebaceous unit due to changes in corneocyte hydration.

# DERMATOSES DUE TO COLD

Exposure to cold causes injury to skin by one of the following mechanisms:

- Direct damage to tissue
- Response to skin to cold like cutaneous vasospasm

## Frostbite

Frostbite is a result of direct tissue freezing due to cold exposure. It is seen in people who are exposed to intense cold like army men, mountain climbers, and homeless men living in cold countries. Individuals who smoke or are diabetic, under treatment with beta-blockers might have higher risk.

## Pathogenesis and Clinical Features

The underlying pathogenesis in frostbite is a combination of tissue cooling, vascular insufficiency, and attack by inflammatory mediators. Severe cases may develop gangrene and even involving tendons, muscles, nerves, and bone. Following phases can be seen in the development of frostbite after cold exposure. The parts of body usually exposed are the extremities, fingers, toes, tip of nose and ears.

- *Phase 1*: This is the stage of cooling. Formation of extracellular ice (exposure at –2°C) or intracellular (–10°C ) and intravascular ice formation. This phase is clinically seen as woody hard extremity with loss of sensation and cold, blanched appearance. This is the first degree frostbite
- *Phase 2*: Stage of thawing and rewarming. In this stage, the tissue swell due to melting of ice resulting in edema. The blood vessels show vasodilation and the built of inflammatory mediators is released into tissues. Clinically the patient complains of intense pain and edema, hyperemia and blisters are seen. This is second degree of frostbite and it is due to a partial loss of the dermis
- *Phase 3*: This is the phase of extension of the injury. It is mainly due to thromboxane A2, platelet aggregation and leukocyte aggregation leading vascular compromise and furthering of the injury. Blisters may rupture at this stage. At this stage the skin may look mummified and blisters may be filled with hemorrhagic fluid. There is a full thickness loss of dermis. This is third degree of frostbite
- *Phase 4*: This is the stage of resolution. The injury may re-epithelize or it may lead to mummification of the tissues, necrosis, amputation of the limb. The vasomotor disturbances may perisist indefinitely. The tendons, bones, and muscles may be damaged and it is known as fourth degree of frostbite.

## Treatment

Fundamental therapeutic goals in frostbite are rapid rewarming, prevention of further cold exposure, and restoration of circulation. However, rubbing and using of heating pads, lamps, stove, or fireplace should be avoided as it can cause burn and further damage due to uneven rewarming. Moreover, if there is chance of refreezing before medical management starts, warming is avoided. Frostbite is a medical emergency and, if significant, it may require hospitalization. After the patient has been brought to a place where no refreezing can happen, rewarming is carried out with a water bath of temperature between 37°C and 39°C. If the patient is hypothermic, the core temperature should be raised before local rewarming. Wound care principles should be meticulously followed and surgical treatment should be sought wherever necessary.

# SKIN INJURY DUE TO NON FREEZING COLD EXPOSURE

Box 1 enlists most of the important and common conditions that occur due to exposure to cold that is above the freezing temperature. Some of these conditions have been discussed in greater details in other chapters. In the following discussion we will focus on chilblain, acrocyanosis, cutis marmorata, and livedo reticularis.

## Chilblain (Pernio)

Chilblain occurs due to abnormal vascular reaction to cold and occurs generally over extremities.

It is characterized by localized erythema and swelling of subcutaneous tissue.

**BOX 1 List of conditions due to non freezing cold exposure**

- Acrocyanosis
- Chilblain lupus
- Cold agglutinin disease
- Cold panniculitis
- Cold urticarial
- Cryofibrinogenemia
- Cryoglobulinemia
- Cutis marmorata
- Livedo reticularis
- Pernio
- Raynaud's phenomenon

### Pathogenesis and Precipitating Factors

It occurs due to sluggish blood flow and increased blood viscosity in superficial dermal vessels which are already under a vasospasm due to cold exposure. It is known to occur with cryofibrinogenemia, cold agglutinins, and cryoglobulinemia. It is also known to occur in lupus erythematosus, and leukemia.

### Clinical Features

The lesions of chilblain consist of localized, doughy, erythematous or violaceous swelling of extremities, mainly the dorsa of hands and fingers, proximal phalanges, ears, nose, heels 12–24 hours after exposure to cold (Fig. 7). The lesions are pruritic and patients complain of burning sensation. The lesions resolve within 2–3 weeks. However, blistering and ulceration may be seen in severe cases. In chronic pernio scarring may also occur.

### Treatment

Avoidance of cold exposure, protection from cold with proper clothing and warming is the mainstay of treatment, since the lesions resolve themselves. However in severe cases, medical management may be warranted with nifedepine, nicotinic acid, vitamin D3, calcium, and dipyridamole. Surgical management like sympathectomy may be done. Phototherapy and UV light has been reported to be efficacious.

## Acrocyanosis

Acrocyanosis is an uncommon condition affecting females predominantly, and is characterized by episodic violaceous discoloration of extremities after exposure to cold. It may also affect nose, ears, lips, and nipples. It is a temperature dependent disorder. The cyanosis increases with fall in temperature. The digits may show edema, especially after rewarming. Pain, if present, is a feature of severe disease known as remitting necrotizing acrocyanosis.

### Causes

This occurs mostly due to vasospasm. This may be primary without any reason or can be precipitated by emotional stress. It is also associated with cold agglutinin disease, postural tachycardia and may also occur as part of paraneoplastic acral vascular syndrome. It may also be seen in patients with anorexia nervosa, psychiatric, neurologic, autoimmune, infective, and after repeated injection of narcotics and inhalation of butyl nitrate.

### Treatment

Avoiding cold exposure, cessation of smoking, and management of any etiologic conditions especially emotional stress is key to management.

## Livedo

Livedo is characterized by transient or persistent, purple, blotchy, netlike appearance that reflects abnormality in the blood flow in cutaneous vasculature from various etiologies.

### Pathogenesis

Diminished blood flow to the feeding arteriole in the dermis, produces cyanosis at the anastomotic junction. It may be physiological, secondary to vascular, endocrine or a rheumatologic disease like lupus erythematosus, idiopathic or congenital. This is also known to be a complication of calciphylaxis.

### Etiology

This can be physiological or may represent some pathological condition.

Livedo has recently been classified into two forms, livedo reticularis (LR) and livedo racemosa.

Livedo reticularis is defined as livedo that is primary, affects younger people, appears as symmetric, uniform and most importantly it is temporary that improves spontaneously.

Livedo racemosa, on the other hand, is secondary to some pathological diseased conditions, asymmetric, nonuniform (frequently broken nets), and is generally persistent (Fig. 8). Antiphospholipid syndrome (APS) is the most common condition of livedo racemosa (Box 2).

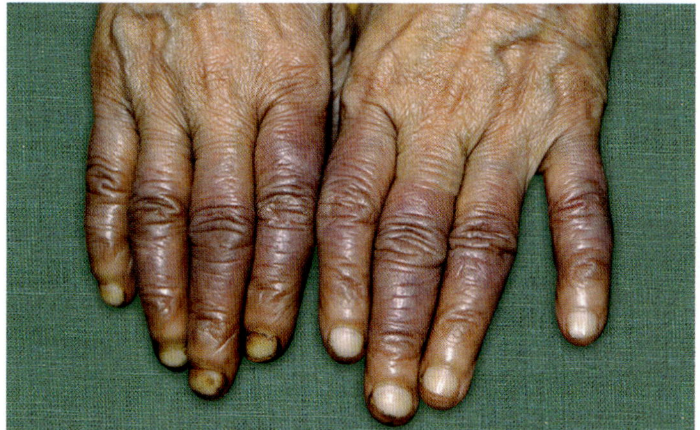

**FIG. 7:** Erythematous to violaceous patches in chilblain involving the dorsum of the fingers.

*Courtesy*: Dr Shekhar Neema, Assistant Professor, Department of Dermatology, Command Hospital, Kolkata, West Bengal.

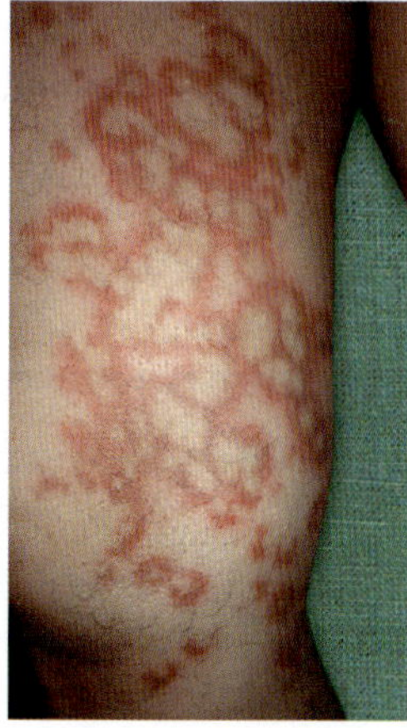

**FIG. 8:** Livedo racemosa in a middle-aged male suffering from lymphoma.

**BOX 2 Important causes of livedo racemosa**

- Sneddon's syndrome
- Livedoid vasculopathy
- Antiphospholipid syndrome
- Systemic lupus erythematosus
- Thromboangiitis obliterans
- Essential thrombocythemia
- Cryoglobulinemia, cryofibrinogenemia
- Polycythemia vera
- Polyarteritis nodosa
- Small and medium vessel vasculitis
- Cutaneous PAN
- Lymphoma

PAN, polyarteritis nodosa.

## Physiological Livedo Reticularis (Cutis Marmorata)

Livedo reticularis often represents a physiological manifestation to cold as seen in young females who develop LR in lower legs. Infants commonly show LR. This improves on warming.

Livedo reticularis may occur without any role of cold (primary LR). Amantadine is known to induce LR. There is a subset of LR that has been termed as idiopathic LR in which no precipitating factors are detected and are persistent. Possibly they actually reflect livedo racemosa and most have underlying APS or Sneddon's syndrome. Studies have shown that idiopathic LR is seen in 25% of migraine sufferers and is a marker for stroke in such patients.

## Congenital Livedo Reticularis or Cutis Marmorata Telangiectatica Congenital

It is a rare congenital presentation of red-purple vascular network on skin of a neonate in asymmetrical distribution over torso or limb, exacerbated by crying, and cold exposure. It resolves spontaneous by 2 years of age.

## Erythrocyanosis

Erythrocyanosis is persistent, dusky, erythema seen over areas where there is large amount of subcutaneous fat such as thighs, buttocks and lower legs of adolescent girls, obese boys and middle-aged women. It has been hypothesized that it is due to insulation of superficial dermal vessels from heat of underlying blood supply which renders it susceptible to cold injury. It may be associated with perniosis like lesions, telangiectasias, angiokeratoma, keratosis pilaris, and in later stages edema and fibrosis. Cold exposure prevention, calcium channel blockers, and vasodilators help.

## Cutaneous Injuries due to Water—Immersion Foot Syndromes

- *Trench feet*: This is a nonfreezing injury due to prolonged standing, immobilization and exposure to dampness, and cold water above freezing point. It was first seen in First World War in soldiers who had to stand in trenches filled with cold water for long time. The limbs become cold and numb initially, then they become edematous and painful and in severe cases there is blister formation, ulcer and gangrene. Treatment is conservative with analgesics, rest and surgical debridement where needed
- *Immersion foot*: This is a nonfreezing injury of skin due to immersion of foot in water for prolonged periods of time. It was described in sailors who were ship wrecked in the World War II (Table 4).

## Environmental Poisoning

### Arsenicosis

Arsenic (As) is a known carcinogen. Exposure to toxic level of arsenic can occur through drinking of contaminated ground water, and rarely through herbal medicines, occupational exposure or through other sources. Volcanic activity is the prime mechanism of arsenic intoxication of ground. Various anthropogenic activities like groundwater exploitation, use of fertilizers and pesticides, burning of coal, release from metal smelters can also contribute to this.

Arsenic intoxication of groundwater is reported from at least 35 countries with worst impact noticed in India and Bangladesh. Other affected countries are Cambodia, Myanmar, Nepal, and Vietnam.

Humans are exposed to groundwater arsenic while drinking the unsafe water. Additional routes of exposure are consumption of crops (e.g., rice) cultivated in affected fields.

#### *Clinical Features*

Arsenicosis manifests with two classical presentations called keratoses and pigmentary changes.

Palms and soles are classic site for keratoses but it may be seen on trunk. Typically, they appear as firm, spiny papules. Most are small (<1 cm) but may be bigger (Fig. 9). Palms and soles may be diffusely thickened. Dislodged keratoses present with depressed pits.

Both hyper and hypopigmention are seen, often simultaneously (Fig. 10). Well defined pigmentary changes are known as

**TABLE 4: Different temperature of the water and variations in clinical appearance of immersion foot**

| Variant (water temperature) | Time of exposure | Clinical features |
|---|---|---|
| Warm (15–32°C) | 1–3 days | Soddened, wrinkled skin, difficulty in walking |
| Tropical (21–32°C) | 3–7 days | Pruritus, edema, erythema, blisters, maceration, purpura, scaling, fever, lymphadenopathy |
| Cold (15–21°C ) | >7 days | There are three phases:<br>1. Prehyperemic: Cold, numb, edematous feet, with purpura, blisters, necrosis and nonpalpable pulse.<br>2. Hyperemic: Increase in vascularity leads to increased edema, erythema, cyanosis, blisters, vasomotor disturbances and higher risk of infections, myonecrosis, vasomotor changes<br>3. Posthyperemic: Blanching, cold sensitivity, hyperhidrosis, peripheral neuropathy and intermittent edema |

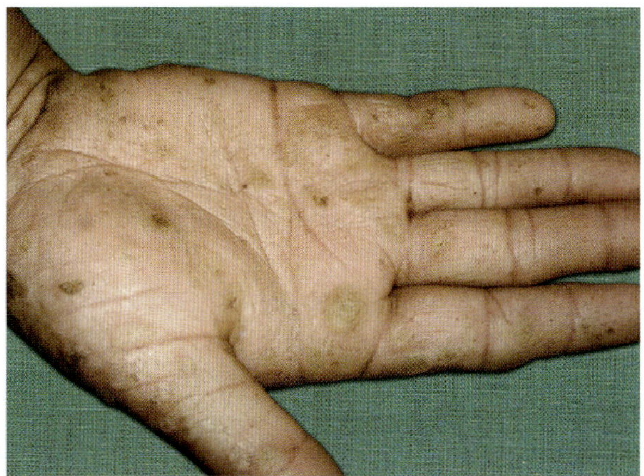

FIG. 9: Arsenical karatoses on palm.

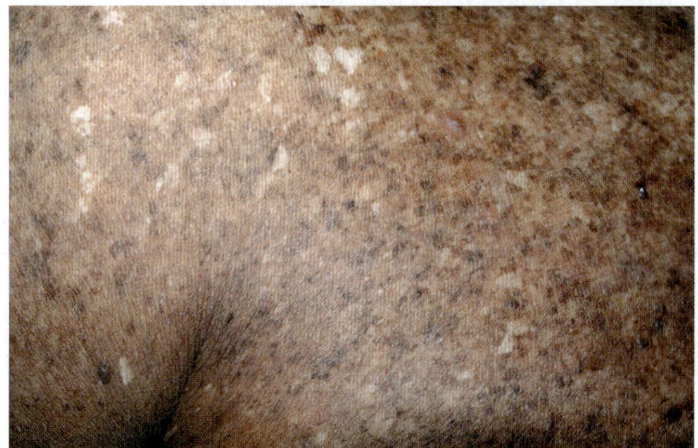

FIG. 10: Hypo and hyperpigmentation on chest in arsenicosis.

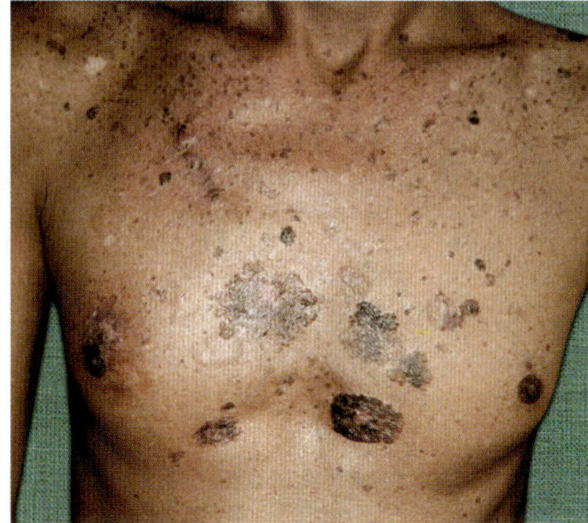

FIG. 11: Multiple Bowen's disease on chest in arsenicosis.

raindrop pigmentation. There may be diffuse hyperpigmentation of the trunk, palms, and soles.

Other manifestations are ulcer, transverse white bands in finger nails (Mee's lines).

Bowen's disease is very common in arsenicosis (Fig. 11). Frank malignancies like basal cell carcinoma, squamous cell carcinoma are also frequently noted.

## OCCUPATIONAL DERMATOSES

Occupational skin diseases are those skin conditions in which work-related exposure is a direct or major contributor in causation of the disease. They become significant because of loss of workdays and productivity. They account between 20% and 60% of all occupational diseases.

Plant dermatitis is very common in countries that depend on agriculture like India. Other very form of contact dermatitis (CD) that we see is household work-related CD seen in housewives due to detergents, soaps and vegetables. Other common forms of occupational contact dermatitis (OCD) are due to rapid industrialization and are seen in cashew nut workers, tea and coffee plantation workers, coconut climbers, farmers due to pesticides, mustard seeds, and animal husbandry employees.

Noxious agents that can cause occupational dermatoses are classified as:

- Mechanical—friction, pressure, vibration, mechanical disruption
- Chemical—elements and chemical compounds (organic, inorganic and proteins)
- Physical—heat, cold, radiation (UV and ionizing)
- Biological—organisms including viruses, bacteria, fungi, and parasites.

Different clinical presentations of occupations dermatitis is mentioned in box 3.

### Pigmentary Changes

Both hyper- and hypopigmentation may be seen in the spectrum of the pigmentary changes due to occupational diseases. Etiologic agents are mentioned in table 5.

**BOX 3 Important types of occupational dermatitis**

- Allergic and irritant dermatitis
- Chemical burn
- Contact urticaria
- Carcinogenesis
- Follicular diseases: Acne, folliculitis, chloracne
- Connective tissue disease: Systemic sclerosis (silica), pseudoscleroderma, vibration induced
- Pigmentary: Hyperpigmentation, hyopopigmentation
- Foreign body reactions
- Infections: Bacterial, fungal, viral, parasite

**TABLE 5: Etiologies of occupational pigmentation**

| Hyperpigmentation | Hypopigmentation (leukoderma) |
|---|---|
| • Physical agents such as heat and friction<br>• Foundry workers using a no-bake sand binder with an oil base<br>• Psoralens in fruits and vegetables<br>• Tars, mineral oils, halogenated hydrocarbons,<br>• Heavy metals, dyes, arsenic, and various pharmaceutical agents | • Chemical and thermal burns, ionizing radiation (X-ray induced radiodermatitis and necrosis), and blunt or repeated trauma to the skin<br>• Paratertiary butylphenol, paratertiary butylcatechol, monobenzyl ether of hydroquinone, hydroquinone and related compounds present in insecticides, paints, plastics and rubber, lubricating and motor oils, photographic chemicals, germicides and disinfectants, detergents and deodorants, and inks<br>• Phenolic/catecholic derivatives |

## Granulomatous Reactions

Occupational skin granulomas may be allergic, non-allergic or infectious in origin. Various causes of occupational granuloma have been mentioned in table 6.

## Occupational Acne (Acne Venenata)

Occupational acne is most commonly seen in workers exposed to insoluble cutting oils in the machine tool trade or in mechanics exposed to grease and lubricating oils. Bacteria present in the oils are not the cause.

The eruption may be mild, involving localized exposure, or covered areas of the body or severe, explosive and disseminated with involvement of almost every follicular orifice (Table 7).

## Occupational Connective Tissue Disorder Type Lesions

Pseduoscleroderma kind of lesions are known to occur in following:

- Vinyl chloride workers
- Occupational exposure to quartz
- Exposure occurs in the following industries and occupations: mining, stone industry, slate industry, foundry industry, fire-clay manufacture and processing, construction, rubber industry, ceramic and glass industries
- Bis (4-amino-3-methylcyclohexyl): Skin sclerosis, erythema, fatigue, myalgia, arthralgia methane—used in epoxy production
- Toxic oil syndrome
- Organic solvents.

## Occupational Carcinogenesis

Carcinogenesis in skin and other organs may develop due to exposure to carcinogenic substances while a person is engaged in a certain type of occupation (Table 8).

# MISCELLANEOUS OCCUPATIONAL DERMATOSES

Other miscellaneous occupational skin diseases are summarized in table 9.

**TABLE 6: Etiology of occupational granulomas**

| Allergic granulomas | Nonallergic granulomas | Infectious |
|---|---|---|
| Foreign body (non-allergic) granulomas follow inoculation or implantation of hard and sharp plant spines (thorns, cactus spikes), wooden splinters, hair (human hair in the case of barbers, and cow and sheep hair in animal tenders), or hard keratin animal parts into the skin | Powders, metals (lead, metallic mercury, beryllium, zirconium, chromium) and silica | Deep fungal or bacterial infections, or parasitic infestations |

**TABLE 7: Different types of occupational acne**

| Type of occupational acne | Description |
|---|---|
| Oil acne | Most common type of occupational acne. It is seen as erythematous papules and pustules on arms and legs and is sue to oil folliculitis |
| Coal tar or pitch acne | Coal tar, creosote, and pitch produce a comedonal type of acne with a predilection for exposed areas like the malar regions and typically around the eyes. The people involved usually have coal tar melanosis |
| Chloracne | It is one of the most sensitive indicators of systemic exposure to these toxic chemicals, occurring as trace contaminants during synthesis of industrial chemicals. It is very refractory and is characterized by follicular hyperkeratosis, noninflamed comedones and cysts caused by certain halogenated aromatic hydrocarbons. Chloracne can develop 2–4 weeks following initial chemical exposure. Excessive oiliness of the skin is followed by the appearance of multiple blackheads and straw-colored cysts on the cheeks (typically sparing the nose), retroauricular folds, axillae and groin region |
| Acne mechanica or sports-induced acne | It occurs in areas covered by protective gear in contact sports. It is caused by a combination of heat, pressure, occlusion, and friction. It can also be seen on dependent areas such as the back, secondary to friction in truck drivers |

**TABLE 8: Etiologies of occupational cancers**

| Occupational carcinogen | Occupation | Type of cancer |
|---|---|---|
| UV rays | Agriculturists, building workers | Bowen's disease, squamous cell carcinoma, basal cell carcinoma |
| Arsenic | • Manufacture of insecticide or herbicide<br>• Agricultural exposure to pesticide<br>• Smelting of copper, lead, zinc<br>• Mining of arsenic | Skin cancers, GIT cancer, bladder cancer |
| Benzidine, alpha- and beta-naphthylamine, magenta, auramine, 4-aminodipheny lether, and 4-nitrophenol | Rubber and dye workers | Bladder cancers |

*Continued*

*Continued*

| Occupational carcinogen | Occupation | Type of cancer |
|---|---|---|
| Polycyclic aromatic hydrocarbons (PAHs) such as benzo(a)pyrene, benzanthracene, benzo (b)fluoranthene, fuoranthene, and naphthalene | Tar and pitch workers, in aluminum production, coal gasification, coke production, iron and steel foundries, tar distillation, shale oil extraction, wood impregnation, roofing, road paving, carbon black production, carbon electrode production, chimney sweeping, and calcium carbide production | • Basal cell and squamous cell carcinomas and premalignant lesions.<br>• Tar keratoses (pitch warts) are precancerous, keratotic, epidermal tumors occurring years after exposure<br>• Pitch worker's cancer is carcinoma of the skin of the face or neck, arms and hands, or the scrotum, resulting from exposure to carcinogens in pitch |

GIT, gastrointestinal tract; UV, ultraviolet.

**TABLE 9: Miscellaneous occupational dermatoses**

| Sports injuries | | |
|---|---|---|
| **Injury** | **Clinical description** | **Sports** |
| Athelete's foot | Asymptomatic flesh-colored nodules located on the dorsal aspects of the feet, knees or knuckles that are caused by chronic pressure, friction or recurrent trauma by tight-fitting boots and sneakers | Surfing, boxing |
| Black heel | Black heel is a black discoloration on the posterior or posterolateral aspects of the heel caused by hemorrhage in a location where blood vessels are minimally protected by fatty tissue. It is due to frequent quick starts and stops | Tennis, basketball |
| Black palm | Black palm presents as grouped punctate hemorrhages in athletes who apply pressure to their hands | Tennis, weightlifting, gymnastics, golf |
| Golfer's nails | Seen in golfers who grip the club tightly and produce excessive pressure on the nail plate and underlying vascular bed causing splinter hemorrhages | Golf |
| Jogger's nipples | Painful eroded nipples that may bleed caused by repetitive friction of the nipples against a shirt due to running or other physical exercise | Running |
| Tennis toe | Painful subungual hemorrhages occurring on the first and second toe | Tennis |
| Turf toe | Acute tendonitis of the flexor and extensor tendons of the great toe | Football and hockey |
| Piezogenic pedal papules | Painful or asymptomatic, soft, skin-colored pressure induced papules probably caused by herniation of fat due to degeneration of dermal collagen present on the medial, posterior, and lateral aspects of the heels when standing and disappear when weight is taken off the foot | Long distance running |
| **Non eczematous occupational skin diseases** | | |
| **Disease** | **Occupation and agents** | |
| EM like lesions | Tropical woods and plants (e.g., poison ivy and primula); nickel and cobalt; proflavine and trinitrotoluene; epoxy resin, formaldehyde | |
| Purpuric lesions | Azo dyes, wood dust, N-isopropyl-n'-phenyl-1,4-phenylenediamine in rubber | |
| Lichenoid lesions | Epoxy resins. Color developers, methacrylic esters | |
| **Occupational diseases due to infectious agents** | | |
| **Organism/disease** | **Occupation** | |
| Anthrax | Butchers, meat handlers, food processing unit workers, tanners, carpet workers | |
| Cutaneous TB | Surgeons, morgue workers, pathologists, meat workers | |
| Swimming pool granuloma | Fishermen and swimming pool cleaners | |
| Brucellosis | Farmers, meat handlers, butchers | |
| Erysipeloid (fish-handler's disease) (Erysipelothrix rhusiopathiae) | Butchers, fishermen, farmers, poultry dressers | |
| Human papilloma virus | Butchers, slaughter house workers | |
| Orf (Parapox virus) | Veterinarians, farmers, shepherds | |
| Milker's nodules (Paravaccinia virus) | Dairy farmers, veterinarians | |

*Continued*

*Continued*

| Occupational diseases due to infectious agents | |
|---|---|
| **Organism/disease** | **Occupation** |
| Sporotrichosis (*Sporothrix schenckii*) | Farmers, forestry workers, outdoor inoculation through puncture occupation |
| Mycetoma (Fungi and actinomycetes) | Farmers, outdoor workers |
| Chromoblastomycosis | Agricultural and outdoor workers |
| Coccidioidomycosis | Farmers, construction workers |
| Scabies (*Sarcoptes scabiei*) | Medical personnel, care homeworkers |
| Swimmer's itch (*Schistosome cercaria*) | Skin divers, lifeguards, dockworkers |
| Lyme disease (*Borrelia burgdorferi*) | Outdoor workers, loggers, ranchers |

TB, tuberculosis.

## SUGGESTED READINGS


1. Brown PJ, Zirwas MJ, English JC 3rd. The purple digit: an algorithmic approach to diagnosis. Am J Clin Derm. 2010;11:103 16.
2. Chan CC, Chiu HC. Images in clinical medicine. Erythema ab igne. N Engl J Med. 2007;356(65):e8.
3. Doshi BR, Mahajan S, Kharkar V, et al. Granulomatous variant of giant centrifugal miliaria profunda. Pediatr dermatol. 2013;30(4):e48-51.
4. Elkeeb D, Elkeeb L, Maibach H. Photosensitivity: a current biological overview. Cutan Ocul Toxicol. 2012;31:263-72.
5. Gawkrodger DJ. Occupational skin cancers. Occup Med (Lond). 2004;54:458-63.
6. Gibbs MB, English JC 3rd, Zirwas MJ. Livedo reticularis: an update. J Am Acad Dermatol. 2005;52:1009-19.
7. Golant A, Nord RM, Paksima N, et al. Cold exposure injuries to the extremities. J Am Acad Orthop Surg. 2008;16:704-15.
8. Gupta G, man I, Kemmett D. Hydroa vacciniforme: a clinical and follow up study of 17 cases. J Am Acad Dermatol. 2000;42:208-13.
9. Huda M, Saha P. Pattern of dermatosis among pediatric patients attending a medical college hospital in northeastern region of India. Indian J Dermatol. 2009;49:189.
10. Iwatsuki K, Satoh M, Yamamoto T, et al. Pathogenic link between hydroa vacciniforme and Epstein–Barr virus-associated hematologic disorders. Arch Dermatol. 2006;142:587-95.
11. Kligman LH, Zheng P. An action spectrum for ultraviolet induced elastosis in hairless mice: Quantifications of elastosis by image analysis. Photochem Photobiol. 1991;53:237-42.
12. Koehler MM, Henninger CA. Orofacial and digital frostbite caused by inhalant abuse. Cutis. 2014;93:256-60.
13. Koh D, Goh CL. Skin disorders. In: Koh D, Seng CK, Jeyaratnam J (Eds). Textbook of Occupational Medicine Practice, 2nd edition. Singapore: World Scientific; 2001. pp. 111-44.
14. Kraemer M, Linden D, Berlit P. The spectrum of differential diagnosis in neurological patients with livedo reticularis and livedo racemosa. A literature review. J Neurol. 2005;252:1155-56.
15. Lakshmi C, Srinivas CR. Parthenium: A wide-angle view. Indian J Dermatol Venereol Leprol. 2007;73:296-306.
16. Lavker RM, Veres DA, Irwin CJ, et al. Quantitative assessment of cumulative damage from repetitive exposures to suberythemogenic doses of UVA in human skin. Photochem Photobiol. 1995;62:348-52.
17. Lehmann P. Diagnostic approach to photodermatoses. J Dtsch Dermatol Ges. 2006;4:965-75.
18. Levinbook WS, Mallett J, Grant-Kels JM. Laptop computer-associated erythema ab igne. Cutis 2007;80:319-20.
19. Ling TC, Gibbs NK, Rhodes LE. Treatment of polymorphic light eruption. Photodermatol Photoimmunol Photomed. 2003;19:217-27.
20. Magerl M, Borzova E, Gimenez-Arnau A, et al. The definition and diagnostic testing of physical and cholinergic urticarias--EAACI/GA2LEN/EDF/UNEV consensus panel recommendations. Allergy. 2009;64:1715-21.
21. McIntosh SE, Opacic M, Freer L, et al. Wilderness Medical Society practice guidelines for the prevention and treatment of frostbite: 2014 update. Wilderness Environ Med. 2014;25 (4 Suppl):S43-54.
22. Onoue S, Seto Y, Gandy G, et al. Drug-induced phototoxicity: an early in vitro dentification of phototoxic potential of new drug entities in drug discovery and development. Curr Drug Saf. 2009;4:123-36.
23. Sarma N. Arsenicosis- Indian Perspective. In: Ghosh S, Sarma N, De D Eds: Recent advances in Dermatology (Vol 3). Jaypee Brothers Medical Publishers (P) Ltd. New Delhi. 2014,134-153
24. Sarma N. Skin manifestations of chronic arsenicosis. In: States JC Ed. Arsenic: Exposure Sources, Health Risks, and Mechanisms of Toxicity. John Wiley and Sons, Inc. New Jersey. 2016,127-136.
25. Schornagel IJ, Knol EF, van Weelden H, et al. Diagnostic phototesting in PLE. Br J Dermatol 2005; 153:1234-6.
26. Shahi V, Wetter DA, Cappel JA, et al. Vasospasm is a consistent finding in pernio (chilblains) and a possible clue to pathogenesis. Dermatology. 2015;231:274-9.
27. Singh GK, Datta A, Grewal RS, et al. Pattern of chilblains in a high altitude region of Ladakh, India. Med J Armed Forces India. 2015;71:265-9.
28. Solak Y, Aksoy S, Kilickap S, et al. Acrocyanosis as a presenting symptom of Hodgkin lymphoma. Am J Hematol. 2006;81:151-2.
29. Williams J, Cahill J, Nixon R. Occupational autoeczematization or atopic eczema precipitated by occupational contact dermatitis? Contact Dermatitis. 2007;56:21-6.

# 4 SECTION Skin Disorders Through Ages

# 7 CHAPTER Neonatal Dermatoses

Nilendu Sarma, Tess McPherson

## INTRODUCTION

Skin in neonatal and pediatric ages behaves differently to the environmental agents and internal diseases than in an adult. In addition to its structural differences, its protective power, immunological reaction pattern, susceptibility to the infective and noninfective conditions that affect them have unique patterns that vary significantly with the adult skin. During the neonatal ages, there are many alterations that are absolutely normal. These can be confused as disease unless the physicians are aware of it. Many of the skin conditions that are typically seen in pediatric ages are described in other chapters. This chapter concisely describes some of the important skin conditions of the neonatal and pediatric population.

## SKIN CONDITIONS OF THE NEWBORN

### Transient Vascular Phenomena

Newborns show transient physiologic vascular reactions characterized by dilatation of cutaneous blood vessels. There are two conditions:

#### Cutis Marmorata

Cutis marmorata is characterized by a reticulated mottling symmetrically distributed all over the body when exposed to cold and disappears on exposure to warmth. This tendency persists for short periods but rarely may persist for long even early childhood (Fig. 1). Treatment is not necessary.

#### Harlequin Color Change

Affected infant shows erythema in one half of the body with sharp demarcation. Some physical activity like defecation or emotion of perineal stimulation may induce bradycardia and nonepileptic tonic seizure. This condition is known as paroxysmal extreme pain disorder (PEPD).

#### Etiology

This is considered to be immature hypothalamic center that controls the vascular tone of the peripheral blood vessels. This may be caused by brain injury. Prematurity and injury can be the etiology. PEPD is a caused by *SCN9A* mutation.

#### Clinical Manifestations

Harlequin color change (HCC) develops on 3$^{rd}$–4$^{th}$ day of life but may develop later during neonatal life. Erythema develops on the dependent part and on turning the baby on other side, position of erythema (and blanching) also shifts. Face, lips, tongue, and genitals are spared. HCC improves in neonatal period and PEPD may persist till late infancy. This persists for 30 seconds to 20 minutes. Transient nature of the condition differentiates from capillary malformations.

### Papulovesicular or Pustular Eruptions

Two conditions, erythema toxicum neonatorum (ETN) and transient pustular melanosis (TPM) present with papulovesicular and pustular eruptions. Both are noninfective and are seen in otherwise healthy neonates. If correctly diagnosed, these do not require extensive investigations and management is just supportive. However, there may be some infective conditions that may present with papulovesicular or pustular eruptions in the neonatal period (Box 1).

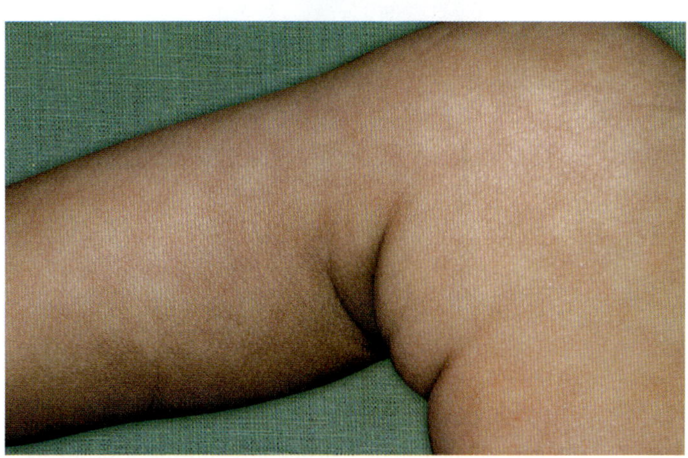

**FIG. 1:** Cutis marmorata in an infant.

**BOX 1 Infective etiology of neonatal papulovesicular or pustular rash**

- *Bacterial*: Group A or B *Streptococcus, Staphylococcus aureus, Listeria monocytogenes, Pseudomonas aeruginosa*
- *Congenital or neonatal candidiasis*
- Congenital syphilis
- *Viral*: Congenital cytomegalovirus, neonatal herpes simplex, congenital and neonatal varicella zoster

### Erythema Toxicum Neonatorum

This is possibly the most common transient skin eruptions in a healthy term baby (seen in 40–70% of normal baby).

Typically, it is very transient, develops on first 1–4 days of life and persists for 2–3 days. Erythematous macule that may form confluent patches with central tiny yellowish papule is the most common presentation. Pustules, with surrounding erythema are also seen in lesser number of cases. It often has a "flea-bitten" look. The most common site is back, arm, thighs, and face. It spares the palms and soles (Fig. 2).

Cytology shows many eosinophils. Histology shows edema and eosinophils (and neutrophils). Peripheral eosinophilia is also detected in some cases.

Management: No treatment is necessary.

### Transient Pustular Melanosis

Overall, this is less common (5% of black, 1% of white newborn). This is present at birth. This is characterized by flaccid vesiculopustular eruptions (1.5–3 mm in diameter) without any surrounding erythema (Fig. 3). All parts of the body including palms and soles are affected. Common sites are neck, nape, chin, upper chest, lower back, and buttocks. Pustules heal with distinct and collarette scale. They also leave pigmented macule. Pigmented macules are typically seen simultaneously. ETN and TPM are frequently present together.
Treatment is not required.

## Neonatal Erythroderma

Generalized erythema (with or without scaling) as seen in adults may also be seen in neonates but is rare than adults. The conditions that result in neonatal erythroderma are different than in adults and are mentioned in box 2. However, the prognosis is poor similar to adults. The prognosis is dependent on the conditions that precipitates this and also on the complications of erythroderma itself.

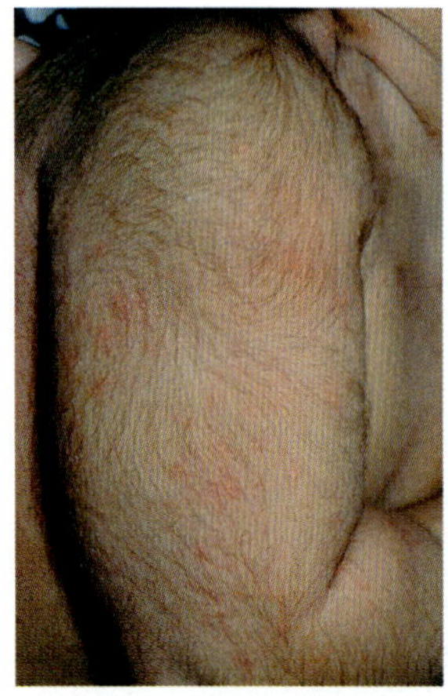

**FIG. 2:** Confluent erythematous patches in erythema toxicum neonatorum.

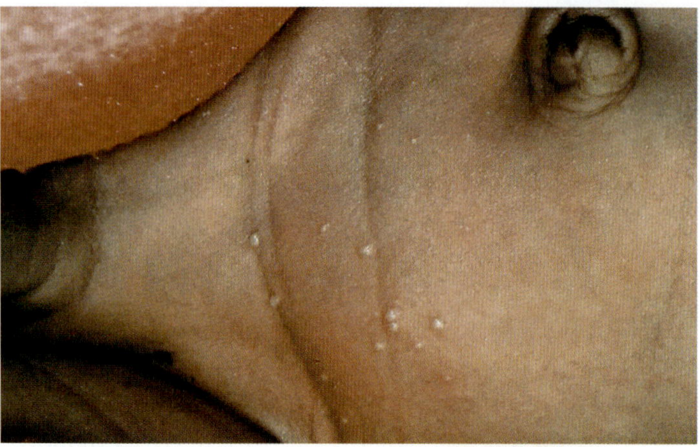

**FIG. 3:** Pustular eruptions in transient neonatal pustular melanosis.

**BOX 2 Causes of neonatal erythroderma**

**Transient dermatoses**
- Erythema toxicum neonatorum

**Dermatoses**
- Seborrheic dermatitis
- Atopic dermatitis
- Psoriasis
- Pityriasis rubra pilaris
- Diffuse cutaneous mastocytosis
- Ichthyosis (NBIE, BIE)
- Syndromic ichthyosis (Chanarin–Dorfman syndrome, Conradi–Hünermann–Happle syndrome), trichothiodystrophy with ichthyosis
- Netherton syndrome
- Ectodermal dysplasia

**Infections**
- Scabies
- Congenital syphilis
- Staphylococcal scalded skin syndrome (SSSS)
- Congenital and neonatal candidiasis

**Drug induced**
- SJS and TEN
- Red man syndrome

**Immunological disorders**
- Omenn syndrome(familial reticuloendotheliosis with eosinophilia)
- Graft versus host disease (GVHD)
- Severe combined immunodeficiency (SCID) and other primary immunodeficiency
- Hypogammaglobulinemia

**Metabolic error**
- Sjogren–Larsson syndrome
- Hydroxy carboxylase synthetase deficiency
- Gaucher disease type 2
- Amino acid metabolism disorders
- Cystic fibrosis
- Essential fatty acid deficiency
- Disorders of biotin metabolism

**Mastocytosis**
- Diffuse cutaneous mastocytosis

NBIE, nonbullous ichthyosiform erythroderma; BIE, bullous ichthyosiform erythroderma; SJS, Stevens–Johnson syndrome; TEN, toxic epidermal necrolysis.

### Clinical Manifestations

Primary skin diseases are the most common etiology of infantile erythroderma. In most of these skin diseases, diagnosis is primarily clinical.

Seborrheic dermatitis is generally less pruritic, and is characterized by more sharply demarcated, erythematous with yellowish hue, greasy scaly patches, most severe on scalp and folds (Fig. 4). Not uncommonly, it can lead to generalized erythematous lesions (Fig. 5).

Atopic dermatitis is rare before 2-3 months of life and is pruritic. Psoriasis may occasionally manifest as neonatal erythroderma with extensive psoriasiform scaling (Fig. 6). More commonly, it starts few months after birth. Initial disease is frequently a localized disease like napkin psoriasis.

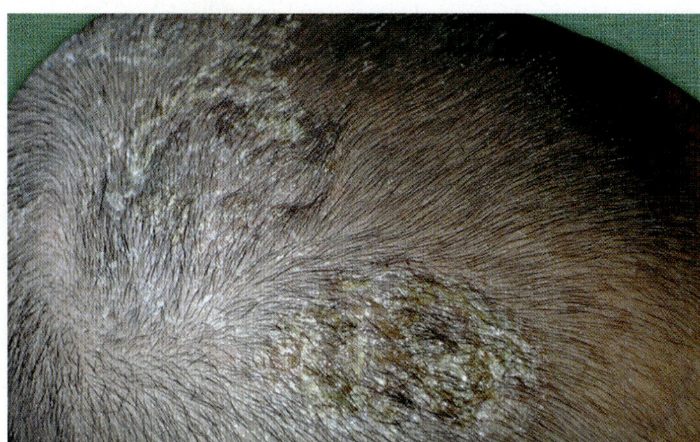

**FIG. 4:** Scaly greasy lesions of seborrhea capitis.

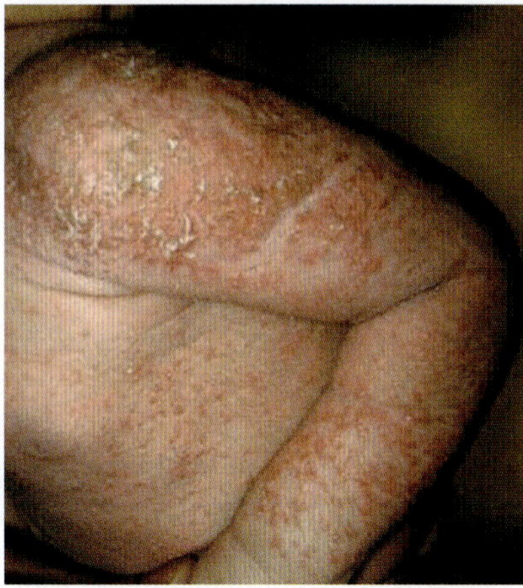

**FIG. 5:** Generalized erythematous scaly patches from seborrheic dermatitis.

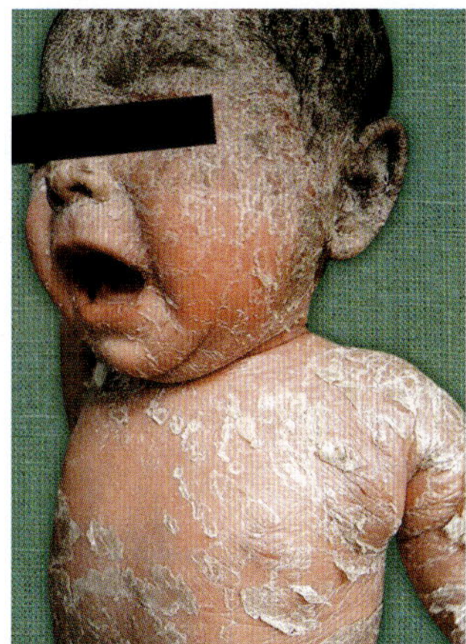

**FIG. 6:** Psoriatic erythroderma that started at 2 months of age.

Netherton syndrome (NS) may be mimicked but is also generally rare in neonatal age. NS is caused by mutation in *SPINK5* gene and is characterized by typical polycyclic serpiginous double-edged scaly patches called ichthyosis linearis circumflexa (ILC). Other typical features are trichorrhexis invaginata (bamboo hair), hypotrichosis, and elevated serum IgE. However, hair abnormalities may not develop until childhood and IgE can also be normal in neonatal period. There is profound skin barrier dysfunction leading to high chance of hypernatremic dehydration and failure to thrive. Patient may improve from erythroderma with age. Signs of atopy usually develop later in life.

Collodion membrane appears as waxy coating of entire body surfaces of the newborn. Soon, this sheds off and underlying erythroderma manifests (Fig. 7). Most such cases ultimately develop autosomal recessive congenital ichthyosis (ARCI). Two major subtypes of ARCI are lamellar ichthyosis (LI) and congenital ichthyosiform erythroderma (CIE), usually present at birth with collodion baby. Rare causes of collodion membrane are some metabolic disorders like Neu-Laxova syndrome, Conradi-Hünermann-Happle syndrome, and even ectodermal dysplasias. LI has darker and thicker scales than CIE and can cause significant morbidity due to ectropion, eclabium, and digital autoamputation (Figs 8 and 9).

Bullous congenital ichthyosiform erythroderma generally manifests with severe blistering and may subsequently develop palmoplantar hyperkeratosis. It is not always possible to

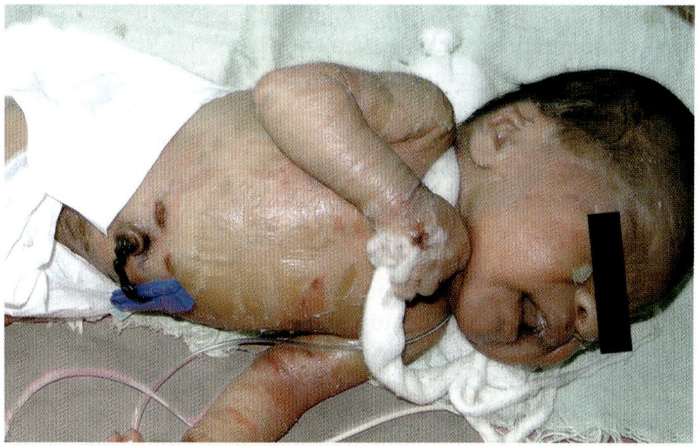

**FIG. 7:** Shedding of collodion membrane leaving erythroderma in a neonate.

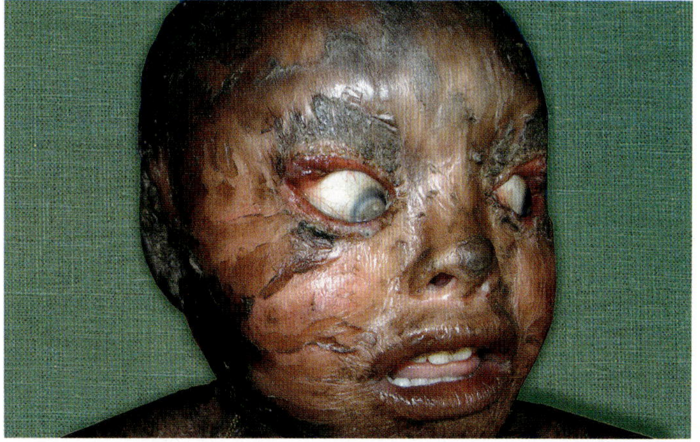

**FIG. 8:** Thick scaling, ectropion, and corneal opacity in lamellar ichthyosis.

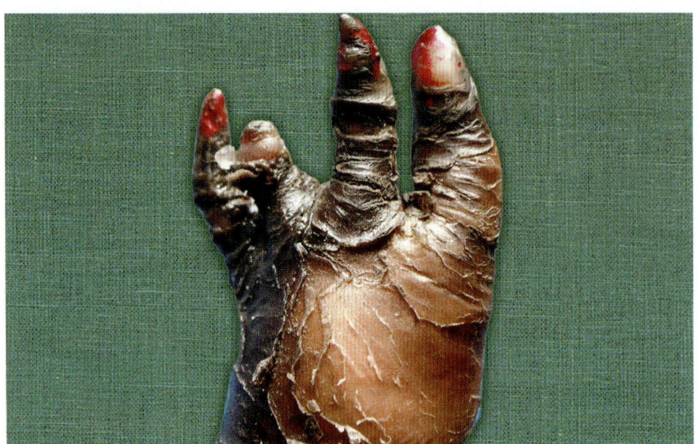

FIG. 9: Digital autoamputation in lamellar ichthyosis.

differentiate idiopathic ichthyosis from the syndromic ichthyosis. Presence of other signs and investigations are required for proper diagnosis.

Harlequin ichthyosis (HI) is the most severe form and fatal autosomal recessive congenital erythrodermic ichthyosis. This is caused by mutation in *ABCA12* gene. The appearance is very distinctive. The neonate, often premature is coated with thick keratotic scale, firmly adherent over the entire body. Soon after birth, this coat ruptures and forms deep fissures. This appearance mimics Harlequin's costume. Tight skin over the body leads to formation of ectropion, eclabium, ainhum (and thus autoamputation of digits), and difficulty in feeding as well as respiration. Corneal damage occurs due to inability to close the eyes. After this is shed off, erythroderma manifests. HI may be associated with other abnormality or may present with complications of poor respiration and feeding, secondary infection, hypoglycemia, and renal failure. This is fatal in about half of the cases. Cases that survive may mimic ARCI.

Chanarin–Dorfman syndrome, also known as neutral lipid storage disorder, is caused by mutation in *ABDH5* gene. Manifestation is usually similar to nonbullous ichthyosiform erythroderma or erythrokeratodermia variabilis (EKV). Other signs are impaired sweating, palmoplantar keratosis, and rhomboid lichenification of nuchal skin. Systemic signs are myopathy, sensorineural deafness, cataract, and growth retardation. Lipid vacuoles are found in the granulocytes and monocytes in the peripheral blood smear and also in keratinocytes.

Conradi–Hunnermann–Happle syndrome, caused by X-linked dominant mutation in *EBP* gene (emopamil binding protein), is also known as chondrodysplasia punctata type 2. This typically presents with ichthyosiform erythroderma in females (fatal in males). Scaly ichthyotic plaques may develop along Blaschko's lines. Other features are sparse eyebrow, patchy cicatricial alopecia, follicular atrophoderma, frontal bossing, hearing defect, sectorial cataract (mosaicism), mental retardation, and asymmetric facial appearance, and musculoskeletal defect leading asymmetrical growth. Most of these develop much late. Punctuate or stippled epiphysial calcification is a very important sign.

Trichothiodystrophy with ichthyosis is characterized by brittle hair that under polarized hair microscopy shows presence of alternate light and dark band. Other hair changes like trichoschisis and trichorrhexis nodosa are also detected. There may be photosensitivity.

Ectodermal dysplasia (AEC syndrome) may present with neonatal erythroderma.

Diffuse cutaneous mastocytosis has features like urticaria, flushing, thickened skin, diarrhea, and anaphylaxis. Systemic involvement should be ruled out. Serum tryptase level is high.

Congenital cutaneous candidiasis occurs due to infection of the fetus during pregnancy from candidal chorioamnionitis. Neonatal candidiasis occurs due to infection to the neonate during vaginal delivery. Affected neonate presents with extensive erythematous maculopapular eruption, pustules or even bullous eruptions. Placenta shows whitish lesions. Napkin area and oral mucosa is spared (affected in neonatal candidiasis).

### Diagnosis

Clinical evaluation is most vital. Investigations should be directed to identify the etiology.

### Management

Erythroderma per se is a life-threatening condition in most. Basic life support is of vital importance. (see chapter on Dermatologic Emergency for a detailed description).

High risk of hypothermia, fluid loss and hypovolemia, hyponatremia, hypoproteinemia, and higher risk of infection necessitates special management strategy. Management in isolation is required, preferably in intensive care unit with high humidity. Multidisciplinary action is always required. Regulation of fluid, electrolyte, and temperature should be carefully monitored. Prevention of infection is of utmost importance. Specific management and drug treatment depends on the exact cause of the condition.

## Subcutaneous Fat Necrosis

Subcutaneous nodules that are freely mobile and not fixed to underlying tissue are present over buttocks and back and usually spare face and anterior trunk. Sometimes, these may be present extensively. This is supposed to be developed from trauma or ischemia during delivery. Usual time of onset is around 6 weeks following birth in a full-term baby. They generally heal within 6 months. However, some of these may calcify, rupture, and atrophy may occur rarely. Hypercalcemia is a possible yet rare systemic complication.

### Pathogenesis

Pathogenesis is not known. Local trauma during delivery, deficiency of brown fat, elevated prostaglandin E, and hypercalcemia are possible; etiology; perinatal asphyxia, and difficult labor may be the predisposing factors.

### Pathology

Fat necrosis, calcification, refractile crystals, and occasional giant cells are typical findings.

### Treatment

Prognosis is good. Systemic complications need to be addressed.

## Sclerema Neonatorum

In contrast to subcutaneous fat necrosis, sclerema neonatorum (SN) is seen in very sick neonates. Tightening of skin and underlying tissues appear as diffuse hardening. This starts over buttocks, thighs, and legs and then involves entire body (Figs 10 and 11). Characteristically palms, soles, and genitals are spared. Complications like respiratory difficulty and flexion deformity are seen. It may be fatal in some cases.

### Pathogenesis

Any forms of serious illness like sepsis, prematurity, hypoxia, hypothermia, metabolic acidosis, glucose and electrolyte imbalance, neurological, and cardiopulmonary disease may lead to SN.

### Treatment

Management of systemic condition is the only option.

# IMPORTANT CONGENITAL DEVELOPMENTAL ANOMALY

## Median Raphe Cyst and Canal

Cystic lesion may be seen in the midline, anywhere from penile tip to anus. Distal penis is most common location. Sometimes they are longer and called median raphe canal (Fig. 12). They are developed from genital folds and are benign in nature. Surgical treatment is curative.

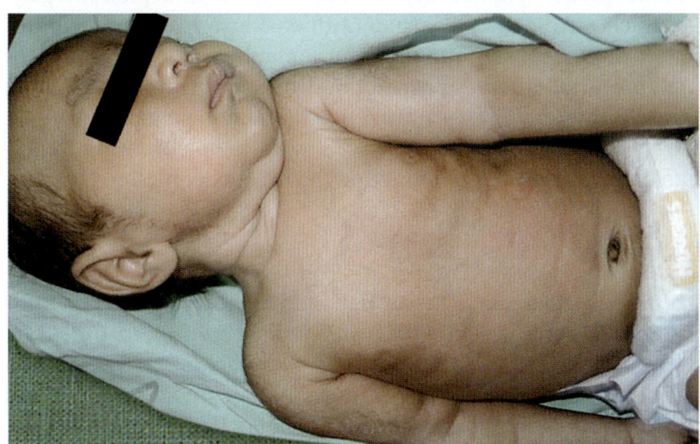

FIG. 10: Smooth shiny waxy appearance and stiff generalized skin in sclerema neonatorum.

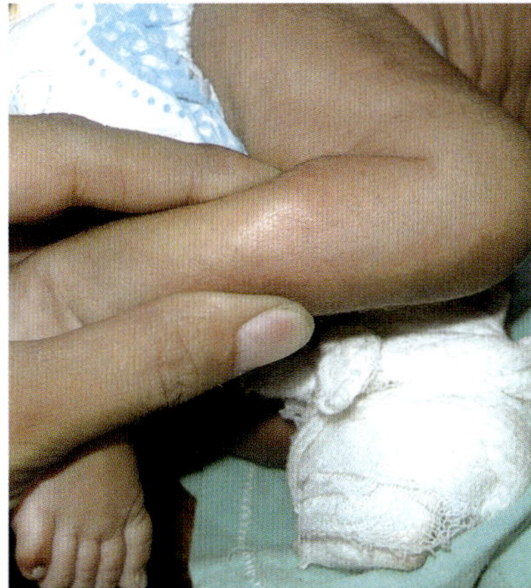

FIG. 11: Induration of skin frequently starts in the legs in sclerema neonatorum.

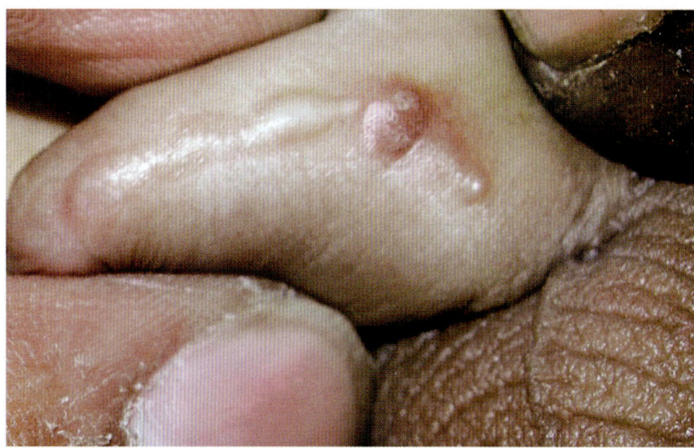

FIG. 12: Median raphe canal.

## Aplasia Cutis Congenita

Aplasia cutis congenita (ACC) manifests with absence of skin involving single or multiple areas. By definition, they are present at the time of birth.

### Pathogenesis

This could be a genetic condition, many autosomal dominant cases have been described. However, aplasia developing due to intrauterine events like amniotic bands, trauma, viral infections, and drugs (methimazole) may be difficult to differentiate. Frieden have classified nine subtypes of ACC.

### Clinical Features

This may be single (most common) or multiple, small (1–3 cm) or large, may have associated other developmental anomaly and systemic abnormalities or as isolated condition (commoner). Lesions over trunk and limbs are generally large (Fig. 13). Affected areas are covered with thin scar-like tissue. Involvement of deeper structures like bone and meninges are also seen. Larger lesions may be associated with ulcers that also eventually heal with scar.

## Staphylococcal Scalded Skin Syndrome

Staphylococcal scalded skin syndrome (SSSS) is induced by exfoliative or epidermolytic toxins (ET-A and ET-B) released by Staphylococci that form an infected focus of pharynx, nose, or other areas. Blisters in SSSS are not infectious.

Widespread flaccid blisters develop rapidly within 1–2 days following scarlatiniform erythematous eruptions that show a typical flexural accentuation (Figs 4, 14, and 15). The affected infant or child is irritable, febrile, and has significant skin tenderness. Blisters rupture easily leaving denuded areas. Mortality is low in children but may be significantly higher in adults. There are no intraoral lesions as this area lacks granular cell layer. However, conjunctivitis and lip crusting are present.

Differential at early stages are toxic shock syndrome (TSS), scarlet fever and later, when blisters are present, it mimics toxic epidermal necrolysis (TEN). Other bullous diseases that

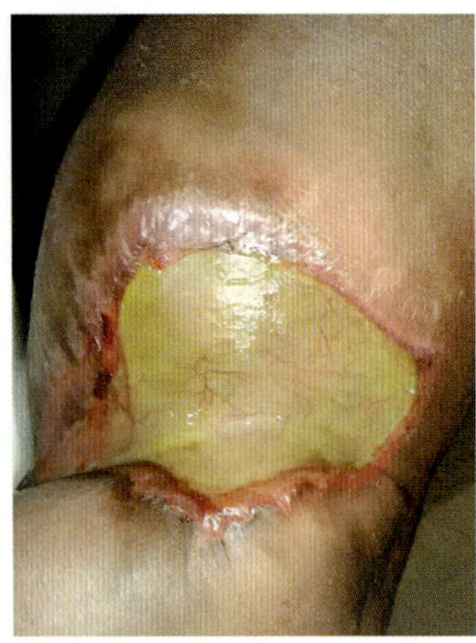

**FIG. 13:** Large aplasia cutis on trunk.
*Courtesy*: Dr Sayantani Chakraborty, Assistant Professor, Department of Dermatology, RG Kar Medical College, West Bengal.

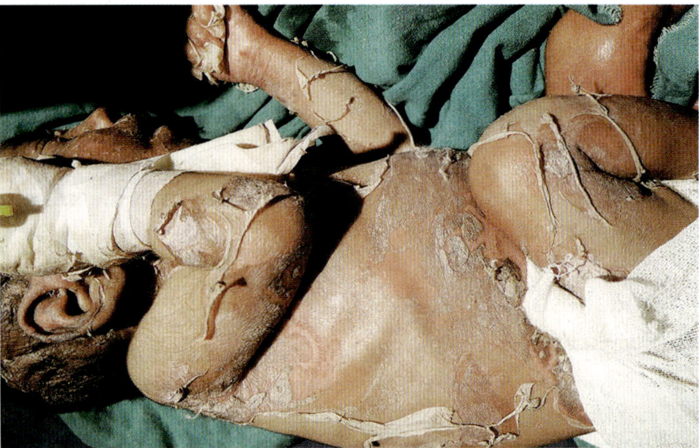

**FIG. 14:** Generalized superficial blisters in Staphylococcal scalded skin syndrome.

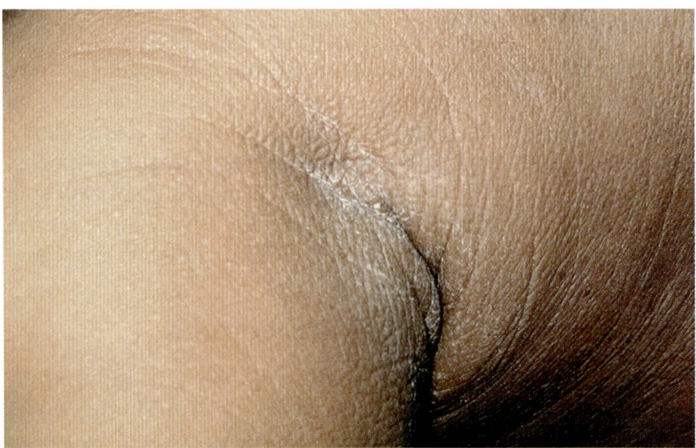

**FIG. 15:** Scarlatiniform eruptions with flexural accentuation preceding Staphylococcal scalded skin syndrome.

may develop at neonatal ages or early in life like epidermolysis bullosa (EB) are also mimicked. Differentiation from TEN is very important. EB is a genetic disease and thus history of consanguinity and involvement of other family members have to be sought.

Urgent management with intravenous (IV) antibiotics (penicillinase-resistant penicillin) is required.

## CONGENITAL AND NEONATAL INFECTIONS

### Congenital Rubella Syndrome

Congenital rubella syndrome (CRS) occurs in a fetus born to a mother who contacts rubella infection during first 16 weeks of pregnancy. Chance of fetal infection is highest during first 8–12 weeks when it can affect the fetus in 80% of the cases. Pathogenesis of its fetopathic effects is mediated through endothelial damage, cytolysis, and inhibition of cellular mitosis.

Maternal infection during pregnancy frequently goes unnoticed. It manifests with fever, upper respiratory symptoms, mild maculopapular rash, lymphadenopathy (suboccipital and posterior auricular mostly), and conjunctivitis.

#### Clinical Manifestations

Characteristic cutaneous manifestations are generalized blue-red infiltrative nodules present at birth or develop within first 2 days of life (blueberry muffin lesion). Blueberry muffin lesions represent extramedullary hematopoiesis and this may be seen in many conditions other than CRS (Box 3).

Other types of cutaneous eruptions are smaller purpuric lesions, nonspecific maculopapular lesions, reticulate erythema of face and extremities, pigmentation, and urticaria.

Classic triad of CRS is congenital cataract, deafness, and cardiac defect. Other features are growth and mental retardation, microcephaly, pigmentary retinopathy, hepatosplenomegaly, jaundice, cardiac defects (patent ductus arteriosus and pulmonary artery stenosis), radioluscent metaphyseal lesion, diabetes mellitus and other endocrinopathies, and thrombocytopenia. Disease may manifest at birth or gradually develop with time. Rarely, progressive encephalitis may develop. Immune deficiencies (hypogammaglobulinemia) have also been seen.

#### Diagnosis

Council of State and Territorial Epidemiologists (CSTE) published case definition of rubella and defined confirmed, probable, and suspected case of CRS. Confirmed case of CRS has been defined as presence of one or more of the clinical symptoms in the infant and laboratory evidence of congenital rubella infection. Laboratory evidence of rubella infections are:

- Isolation of rubella virus
- Rubella-specific IgM antibody
- Higher and persistent level of rubella antibody that is not due to passive transfer from mother (as suggested by the following—rubella titer that does not drop two-fold per month)
- Polymerase chain reaction (PCR)-positive specimen.

**BOX 3** **Causes of blueberry muffin lesion**

- Infection
  - Rubella
  - Toxoplasmosis
  - Cytomegalovirus enterovirus
  - Parvovirus B19
- Erythroblastosis fetalis
- Neoplasia
  - Neuroblastoma
  - Leukemia
  - Histiocytosis

Fetal infection is suggested by presence of IgM antibody, IgG seroconversion, or a more than or equal to 4-fold rise. Virus isolation is done through culture and/or reverse transcriptase-PCR/RT-PCR from throat (preferred) sample, respiratory secretion, urine, cerebrospinal fluid (CSF), blood, and amniotic fluid. IgM antibody against rubella in the child is also diagnostic.

### Management

Rubella is a vaccine preventable disease. When infection occurs to the mother in early pregnancy, abortion is suggested. Management of affected child is only supportive. Role of IVIg to prevent infection in the fetus (when pregnant mother is infected) is not confirmed and can be attempted when the mother refuses termination of pregnancy.

## Congenital Cytomegalovirus Infection

Congenital cytomegalovirus (CMV) is the largest and very complex member of the human herpesvirus family. CMV infection is common and this is a common cause for mental retardation and the nonhereditary cause of sensorineural hearing loss. Many cases are asymptomatic. Infection to the fetus occurs through transplacental spread from infected mother, exposure during vaginal delivery, or through breast milk.

### Etiology

This is common in poor socioeconomic groups and in developing countries. CMV is present in urine, saliva, cervicovaginal secretions, semen, breast milk, tears, and blood products. It can spread easily in crowded living condition through contact with these materials.

### Clinical Manifestations

Only about 10% of cases manifest (symptomatic congenital CMV disease). Sensorineural hearing loss, often bilateral and progressive, starts frequently after infancy (median 18 months) and is seen in asymptomatic cases also.

Symptomatic congenital CMV disease presents with striking features that is characterized by sensorineural hearing loss, growth restriction, prematurity, microcephaly, jaundice, low platelet count and petechiae, hepatosplenomegaly, chorioretinitis, motor defects, pneumonitis, and dental defects. Congenital CMV infection causes multiorgan involvement like hepatosplenomegaly, eye involvement (chorioretinitis, strabismus and optic atrophy), and central nervous system (CNS) defects. Intracerebral calcification is common.

Infection occurring late in pregnancy can cause pneumonia, hepatosplenomegaly, hepatitis, thrombocytopenia, sepsis-like syndrome, and atypical lymphocytosis.

### Diagnosis

Viral detection through culture or PCR.

### Management

Mostly supportive. Ganciclovir given parenterally may prevent hearing deterioration and improve developmental outcomes, but its use remains restricted to infants with severe symptomatic neonatal CNS disease. Oral formulation of ganciclovir called valganciclovir has also been tried. Other drugs that can be used are cidofovir, foscarnet, and fomivirsen.

## Toxoplasma Infection

### Etiology

The sexual stage of the organism is in cat's intestine. Humans get the systemic infection through ingestions of the contaminated food (oocysts present in cat's feces). Foods like vegetables, fruits, water, or infected milk are the frequent source of infection. Undercooked seafood, poultry, and livestock also transmit the infection.

Once within the body, the cyst ruptures and spreads through lymphatics and blood. Infection is transmitted to the fetus during fresh infection or from latent infection in the mother.

### Clinical Manifestations

Infection to the fetus at an early trimester induces more serious disease than when it occurs late. The classic triad is chorioretinitis, hydrocephalus, and intracranial calcifications. However this can be seen in some other conditions also. Severe neonatal disease can cause abortion, retarded development, bilateral chorioamnionitis, hepatosplenomegaly, jaundice, lymphadenopathy (a very common finding), eosinophilia, bleeding, and skin rash. The organism has high affinity for CNS causing retarded higher function, macro, or microcephaly, hydrocephalus or other structural defect, encephalitis, seizure, and impaired psycho-behavioral development. It can also commonly cause visual and auditory inflammatory disorders, and cardiovascular abnormalities.

Toxoplasma infection can lead to chronic inflammatory and autoimmune disorders like antiphospholipid syndrome, autoimmune thyroid diseases, systemic sclerosis, rheumatoid arthritis, systemic sclerosis, and inflammatory bowel disease (Crohn's disease and ulcerative colitis).

Disease may manifest few weeks postpartum or even later in life with neurological signs and retinochoroiditis. Some cases may have subclinical disease. Cases may go undiagnosed and manifest later with complications.

### Diagnosis

Diagnosis of maternal infection is very important to prevent infection to the fetus. Elevated IgM antibody or a rising IgG titer is highly suggestive. Sabin–Feldman dye test is the "international gold standard" test, relatively sensitive and specific but not readily available.

Amniotic fluid examination (20–24 weeks) can be done to check the fetal infection status. Congenital toxoplasmosis can be diagnosed with serology (ELISA) and PCR (from blood, CSF, amniotic fluid, bronchoalveolar lavage fluid). RT-PCR for DNA in amniotic fluid is highly sensitive (98%) and specific (100%).

Anti-toxoplasma IgA and IgE antibodies are highly sensitive (less specific), even more than IgM antibody for congenital toxoplasmosis.

Serum alpha fetoprotein is an important marker to indicate fetal death as well as systemic diseases affected by diseases.

CT scan of brain in CNS toxoplasmosis shows bilateral, ring-enhancing lesions, typically multiple in number. MRI is a more definitive method of diagnosis.

### Management

A combination approach is always preferred using at least two drugs from sulfasalazine, pyrimethamine, sulfadiazine, atovaquone, and clindamycin. These can be used even when fetal infection is suspected. Pyrimethamine is always used. Folinic acid is used to avoid bone marrow suppression. Glucose-6-phosphate dehydrogenase level should be checked before using pyrimethamine and sulfadiazine.

Pyrimethamine is started first (2 mg/kg/day for 2 days followed by 1 mg/kg/day; maximum 25 mg) along with leucovorin (10 mg, 3 times/week). Sulfadiazine (50 mg/kg/twice daily; maximum 4 g) is given after neonatal jaundice improves. After 6 months, pyrimethamine is given on alternate days for another 6 months. Sulfadiazine and leucovorin are continued at the same dose.

Spiramycin monotherapy is effective as preventive monotherapy in early pregnancy before fetal exposure. However, it is less active in later pregnancy and when fetal infection is suspected.

Other drugs that have been used (without any definite or proven efficacy) are azithromycin, clarithromycin, dapsone, and co-trimoxazole. Combination of atovaquone and Diclazuril has been effectively used in pregnant women.

Systemic steroids are used when vision is threatened (for active chorioretinitis) or if CSF protein is more than 1 g/dL.

## Congenital Varicella Syndrome and Neonatal Varicella

Congenital varicella syndrome (CVS) is rare. This occurs when pregnant mother contracts primary varicella infection before 20–24 weeks of pregnancy with highest chance during 12–20 weeks. As most of these defects seen in CVS are dermatomal, it is postulated that the intrauterine herpes zoster is the basis of CVS and not the primary fetal varicella infection. Very short latency in developing intrauterine varicella zoster may be due to defect in cell-mediated immunity in the fetus. Maternal chicken pox in later pregnancy may lead to neonatal varicella or zoster.

### Clinical Manifestations

Affected child shows presence of dermatomal distribution of vesicles or scar and in severe cases, cutis aplasia. Noncutaneous features of this condition are low birth weight, developmental delay, eye defects like microphthalmia, cataract, chorioretinitis, and neurological defects like mental retardation, seizure, and encephalomyelitis, unilateral limb shortening gastrointestinal abnormalities.

### Diagnosis

Diagnostic criteria proposed by Alkalay et al. is mentioned below:

- Maternal varicella during pregnancy
- Dermatomal distribution of skin lesions and/or neurologic defects, eye disease, and limb hypoplasia
- Proof of intrauterine varicella zoster virus infection as confirmed through the following:
  - Viral DNA in the infant
  - Presence of specific IgM
  - Persistent IgG even after 7 months of age
  - Zoster during early infancy.

### Management

Overall, the chance of fetal involvement is rare. So termination of pregnancy when a mother contracts varicella during pregnancy is not advisable. Vaccination of all woman planning pregnancy and who never had varicella infection may offer benefit. When a woman is vaccinated with Oka strain (a live vaccine), pregnancy should be delayed for at least 1 month.

When the mother is exposed to chicken pox, she should be treated with varicella zoster immune globulin within 96 hours. Duration of protection lasts for about 3 weeks.

Varicella zoster immune globulin was recommended for neonates in the following situations:

- *Exposure from mother*: Mother had chicken pox up to and including 5 days before delivery or up to 2 days after delivery
- Exposure from other source: Exposed to varicella during neonatal period when mother was susceptible
- Less than 28 weeks age of gestation
- Infant weighing less than 1000 g at birth who are exposed to Varicella regardless of maternal history (because they may not have acquired maternal antibodies).

Acyclovir crosses placenta. Increase risk for malformations with acyclovir is not reported. Rather, its use in pregnant woman as postexposure prophylaxis is possibly beneficial for the child. However, definitive evidence to suggest treatment of pregnant woman with acyclovir to prevent fetal infection or embryopathy is lacking. Oral acyclovir is ideally given on seventh day of exposure to the mother to prevent secondary viremia.

Role of prophylactic use of acyclovir in neonate to prevent neonatal varicella is not known. In active action of the neonate, treatment with acyclovir (60 mg/kg/day for 2–3 weeks) is indicated.

## Neonatal Herpes Infection

Neonatal herpes infection is infection of the neonate from the infected mother during vaginal delivery, through ascending infection or acquired from other people after birth. Herpes simplex virus type 2 is a commoner etiology and has a poorer prognosis than herpes simplex virus type 1. Transplacental infection causes congenital herpes infection that is more severe leading to chorioretinitis, microphthalmia, and microcephaly. Neonatal herpes can occasionally also occur from transplacental spread of infection.

### Clinical Manifestations

Disease generally manifests within first 2 weeks or sometimes delayed for another 2–3 weeks.

Neonatal herpes can be of varying severity ranging from localized to disseminated disease. Skin involvement is common but not universal and may sometimes be even absent in disseminated disease. Neurological involvement is common but may also be absent in disseminated disease.

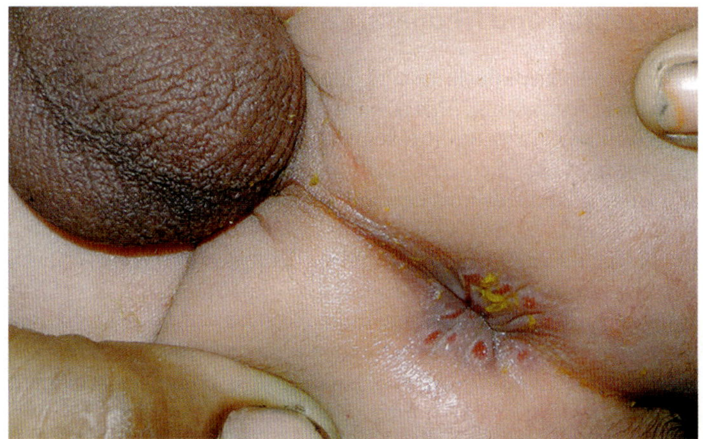

FIG. 16: Neonatal herpes simplex of the perianal area.

Localized disease can have isolated neurological disease without skin or other organ involvement or skin, eye and mouth (SEM) involvement without any other organ involvement. Disseminated infection means involvement of multiple organs (not necessarily skin or CNS in all cases) leading to hepatitis, pneumonitis, disseminated intravascular coagulation, encephalitis, lethargy, hypotonia, and seizures.

Characteristic skin lesions of neonatal herpes are erythematous macules, grouped or zosteriform vesicles, scattered and few to generalized vesiculopustular eruptions (Fig. 16). Ulcers may eventually develop in some lesions mimicking diseases like EB. Keratitis is a very typical eye finding in neonatal herpes infection.

## Diagnosis

Clinical presentation is helpful especially when vesicular lesions are present. Disseminated disease without skin involvement may be difficult to diagnose. Isolated CSF lymphocytic pleocytosis, thrombocytopenia, and hepatitis may be the indicator of the condition.

Laboratory investigations are done for confirmation. These are Tzanck smear from the vesicle base (less sensitive and specific), direct fluorescent antibody of lesions scraping (highly sensitive and specific), and viral culture (most specific and gold standard) from various tissues (vesicle fluid, CSF, urine, blood, eyes).

## Management

Progressive worsening of disease that initially appears milder is not rare. Disease presenting as localized skin vesicles, if untreated may turn to more serious disease within 7–10 days. Mortality is very high in untreated disseminated disease (>80%) and in CNS disease (about 50%). Long term sequels may develop in untreated cases. Proper treatment significantly reduces mortality and complications.

Intravenous acyclovir is the drug of choice with dose of 15–30mg/ kg/day (higher doses may be better) for 2 weeks for milder or skin involvement.

For disseminated or neurological involvement, 60 mg/kg/day (three divided doses), IV for 3 weeks is used. In CNS involvement, this should be followed by continuous therapy for next 6 months with oral acyclovir with 300 mg/m$^2$.

# Congenital Syphilis

This is caused by *Treponema pallidum*, a spirochete. Infection from mother to intrauterine fetus occurs after 16 weeks of gestations. Infection in fetus can cause still birth, hydrops fetalis, or preterm delivery. Manifestation in the fetus occurs due to direct infection by the organism as well as immunological reactions in the fetus. Many factors control the extent and severity of fetal involvement such as—timing (temporal relation) of infection and pregnancy, stage of disease, and promptness in diagnosis and management. This risk of fetal involvement may reach up to 100% depending upon these parameters.

## Clinical Manifestations

About two-thirds of cases are asymptomatic at birth. Traditionally, neonatal syphilis is classified in two stages—early congenital syphilis (that develop within first 2 years of life) and late congenital syphilis (develop after 2 years). Late lesions develop due to immunological reactions in the child and are noninfectious. Stigmata of early disease that persists beyond 2 years of life also represent late disease. Late lesions may appear due to absence of or incomplete treatment at early stage.

Early disease results directly from the infection, so these lesions are infections. These can be equated with the secondary stage of adult syphilis.

### Early Congenital Syphilis

Manifestation of disease usually takes first few weeks (about 4 weeks) of life unless it is very severe when it may be apparent at birth indicating a poorer prognosis.

Fever, rhinitis, skin eruptions, and hepatosplenomegaly are three major features.

Rhinitis (snuffles) or ulceration of nasal mucosa extending in severe cases to cartilage is generally the earliest manifestation. It develops during 2–6 weeks of life.

Wide range of skin manifestations may occur.

Bullous lesions on palms or soles and weeping mucous patches at the mucocutaneous junctions are considered (highly specific). Deep mucosal erosion affecting oral mucocutaneous area may leave circumoral scar (rhagades).

Skin lesions similar to secondary syphilis appear. Erythematous papulosquamous eruptions, mostly on plasma and soles similar to secondary syphilis appear and it leaves coppery pigmentation. Condylomata lata (moist, soft and flat papules) develops mostly over anogenital, perinasal, and angle of mouth. Erythema multiforme like lesions and pustular eruptions are reported.

Palms and soles may also feature induration and fissuring. Exfoliation of larger scales from entire body is also noted. Umbilical cord may show presence of nonexudative spiral zones of red or blue and white discoloration (necrotizing funisitis). Acute bacterial infection of the cord leads to exudative inflammation.

This leads to multiorgan involvement. It can cause hepatosplenomegaly, ascitis, generalized lymphadenopathy (enlarged epitrochlear node is highly suggestive), jaundice, anemia, leukocytosis, thrombocytopenia, edema, osteochondritis involving mostly the long bones, and diffuse periostitis leading to new bone formation outside cortex (onion peel appearance). Severe periostitis of the epiphysial area may lead to fracture and painful movement of limbs (pseudoparalysis of Parrot). Few cases show neurological involvement (meningitis, choroiditis, seizures, mental retardation, or complication like hydrocephalus).

### *Late Congenital Syphilis*

Distinctive signs are noted in permanent teeth like notched permanent central incisor with tapered end (Hutchinson's teeth). This looks like screwdriver. Crowed, poorly developed cusps in first molar appear as mulberry (mulberry molar). It is rapidly lost (so not seen in adult life). Hutchison's triad is very specific (Hutchinson's teeth, interstitial keratitis, and eighth nerve palsy) rarely seen as eighth nerve palsy. Maxilla maldevelopment results in "bulldog" facies.

Other signs are frontal bossing (due to gross periostitis and new bone formation on frontal bone leading to overhanging forehead), gumma (may be ulcerated), saber shin, rhagades, saddle nose, and paroxysmal cold hemoglobinuria. Thickening of inner third of unilateral clavicle (Higoumenaki's sign) is also seen but not specific.

Neurosyphilis is usually asymptomatic. Patient may develop juvenile paresis and tabes. Progressive sensorineural deafness or blindness is due to optic atrophy, recurrent interstitial keratitis and scarring.

### Diagnosis

Affected newborn has a peculiar dirty look owing to presence of jaundice, anemia, edema, and other skin changes. Many of the cutaneous changes are very specific and highly diagnostic.

Nontreponemal serological tests (quantitative, VDRL, RPR) should be done in neonate and titer measured successively. Specific treponemal tests (FTA-ABS, MHA-TP) should also be done. There are few facts that should be remembered while evaluating serology in neonates. Maternal transfer of antibody (that persists in infant till 4–6 months) may give false positive result. Infection (in mother or fetus) may give false negative result. A rising titer, value higher than mother and persistent antibody after 6 months is diagnostic.

Confirmation can be done with dark ground microscopy of swab from umbilical cord, condyloma latum or mucous patches.

### Treatment

Immediate treatment with parenteral crystalline penicillin G (1–1.5 lac units/kg/day, IV, in two divided dose for first 7 days of life and then four times daily for next 3 days). Involvement of CNS requires 2–3 lac units/kg/day IV in 4 divided doses for 14 days.

## Neonatal Listeriosis

Listeriosis is an uncommon yet serious foodborne disease. This is caused by *Listeria monocytogenes* (LM), a gram-positive bacterium. Infection spreads through contaminated foods like milk, meat, fish, and vegetables. Infection may be transmitted to intrauterine fetus from mother transplacentally or rarely through ascending infection. It generally causes mild, febrile gastroenteritis in healthy individual. People with impaired immunity or high risk population like pregnant women and neonates are primarily affected who may develop more severe illness like sepsis, meningitis, or encephalitis that can lead to persistent consequences. Death may also occur. It can cause abortions, stillbirths, preterm birth, and neonatal listeriosis.

## Congenital and Neonatal Candidiasis

Congenital candidiasis occurs during pregnancy from chorioamnitis in the mother. This is exceedingly rare possibly because of high number of intrauterine fetal death as well as underdiagnosis in healthy baby. Preterm labor is also common. Any form of intrauterine devices and cervical cerclage (in mother) as well as very low birth weight (<1500 g) are known risk factor.

Neonatal infection by Candida can occur during vaginal delivery from mother or from other persons. Very low birth weight, prolonged hospitalization with use of central venous catheters, urinary catheter, and parenteral alimentation are risk factors. *Candida albicans* is the most common organism for both conditions. Two forms are recognized, superficial, and disseminated. Extensive cutaneous vesicles and pustules are noticed in disseminated form and oral mucosa and napkin-area are involved in superficial form (Figs 17 and 18).

### Clinical Manifestations

Neonate with congenital candidiasis presents with extensive erythematous maculopapular eruption, pustules, or even bullous eruptions. Placenta shows whitish lesions (white placenta-red baby). Napkin area and oral mucosa is spared (affected in neonatal candidiasis). Systemic involvement like pulmonary infection can also occur. Skin involvement is not always detected.

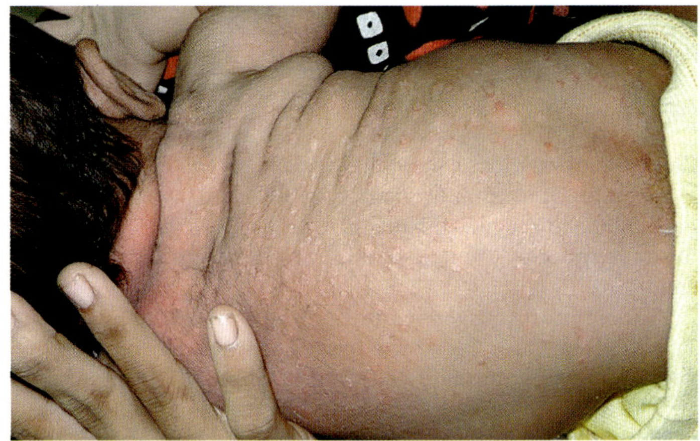

**FIG. 17:** Extensive neonatal candidiasis.

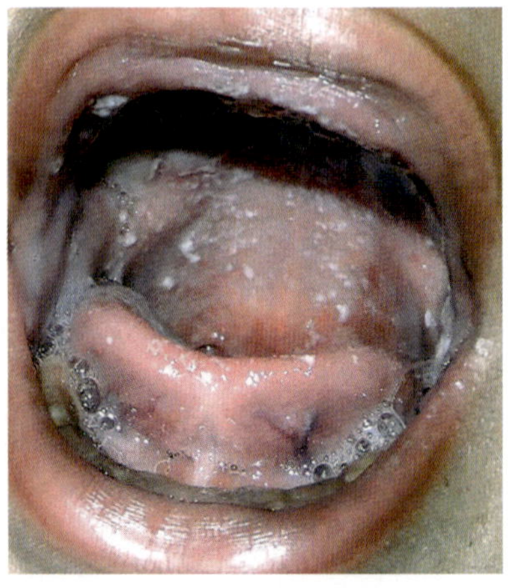

**FIG. 18:** Oral candidiasis in a 1-month-old baby.

Severe cases of neonatal candidiasis may present with signs of sepsis. In disseminated infections, in addition to skin and mucosa (diaper rash, thrush) other organs like CNS, kidney, heart, eyes, bones, and joints may be affected.

## Diagnosis

This should be differentiated from LM infection, impetigo, neonatal varicella, and neonatal herpes virus infection.

Diagnosis of the condition is done with microscopical examination and culture from skin lesions. Blood culture can detect systemic infection. Culture should also be done in suspected disseminated infection from other body fluids like urine and CSF. Systemic examination should include examination of eyes, heart, kidney, and bones.

## Treatment

Full-term healthy baby with only cutaneous disease may not require treatment. Systemic involvement and signs of sepsis may warrant systemic antifungal therapy with fluconazole or amphotericin B (gold standard).

# SUGGESTED READINGS


1. Ahn KH, Park YJ, Hong SC, et al. Congenital varicella syndrome: A systematic review. J Obstet Gynaecol. 2016;36(5):563-6.
2. Alkalay AL, Pomerance JJ, Rimoin DL. Fetal varicella syndrome. J Pediatr. 1987; 111:320-3.
3. D McIntosh, D Isaacs. Varicella zoster virus infection in pregnancy. Arch Dis Child. 1993;68(1 Spec No):1-2.
4. Grose C. Varicella infection during pregnancy. Herpes. 1999;6:33-7.
5. McLean H, Redd S, Abernathy E, et al. VPD surveillance manual, fifth edition, 2012. Available from https://www.cdc.gov/vaccines/pubs/surv-manual/chpt14-rubella.pdf. [Accessed April 2018].
6. Moss WJ, Griffin DE. Measles. Lancet. 2012;379:153-64.
7. Ratanajamit C, Vinther Skriver M, Jepsen P, et al. Adverse pregnancy outcome in women exposed to acyclovir during pregnancy: a population-based observational study. Scand J Infect Dis. 2003;35:225-9.
8. Stone KM, Reiff-Eldridge R, White AD, et al. Pregnancy outcomes following systemic prenatal acyclovir exposure: Conclusions from the international acyclovir pregnancy registry, 1984-1999. Birth Defects Res A Clin Mol Teratol. 2004;70(4):201-7.
9. Tan MP, Koren G. Chickenpox in pregnancy: revisited. Reprod Toxicol. 2006;21: 410-20.
10. Yazigi A, De Pecoulas AE, Vauloup-Fellous C, et al. Fetal and neonatal abnormalities due to congenital rubella syndrome: a review of literature. J Matern Fetal Neonatal Med. 2017;30(3):274-8.

# 8
# CHAPTER Geriatric Skin Disease

*Joyeeta Chowdhury*

## INTRODUCTION

Aging in humans refers to a multidimensional process of physical, psychological, and social change. Senescence is the state or process of aging.

Skin is the most superficial body organ and plays an important role in protecting the body from environmental damage and in forming social relations. Skin changes are among the most visible signs of aging (Box 1).

Skin aging is a complex process combined with intrinsic and extrinsic factors like environmental factors, genetic makeup, nutrition, and other factors. Intrinsic or chronological skin aging results from the passage of time and is influenced by genetic factors. Extrinsic skin aging is mainly determined by UV irradiation, and this is also known as photoaging. Both cause dermal matrix alterations that mostly contribute to the formation of wrinkles, laxity, and fragility of aged skin. Although the typical appearance of photoaged and chronologically aged human skin can be readily distinguished, recent evidence indicates that chronologically aged and UV-irradiated skin share important molecular features including altered signal transduction pathways that promote matrix-metalloproteinase (MMP) expression, decreased procollagen synthesis, and connective tissue damage. UV irradiation accelerates the chronological aging process in human skin.

**BOX 1 Chronological aging skin changes**

- Skin
  - Skin is thin and inelastic
  - Xerosis
  - Uneven pigmentation
  - Lentigines
  - Idiopathic guttate hypopigmentation
  - Facial lines
  - Baggy eyelids and jawline
  - Solar elastosis
  - Yellowish sallow complexion
  - Open and closed comedones and cysts (Favre-Racouchot syndrome) (Fig. 1)
  - Seborrheic keratosis (Fig. 2)
  - Telangiectasia
  - Cherry angioma
  - Senile purpura
- Hair
  - Graying of hair
  - Thinning
  - Male and female pattern alopecia
  - Coarse facial hairs in women
- Nails
  - Dull and brittle
  - Yellow and coarse
  - Longitudinal ridges

## CONTRIBUTING FACTORS

Skin aging is the result of several factors such as intense physical and psychological stress, alcohol intake, poor nutrition, overeating, environmental pollution, and UV exposure.

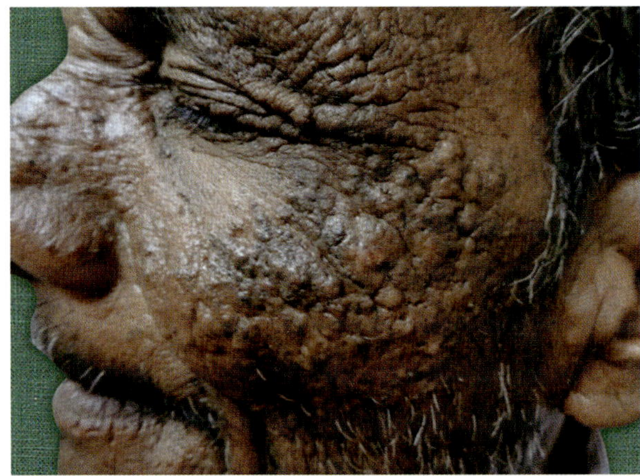

**FIG. 1:** Solar elastosis and multiple senile comedones.

*Courtesy*: Dr Aprana Palit, Dr Arun C Inamadar, Department of Dermatology, Venereology and Leprosy, Shri B.M. Patil Medical College, Hospital & Research Center, BLDE University, Vijayapur, Karnataka.

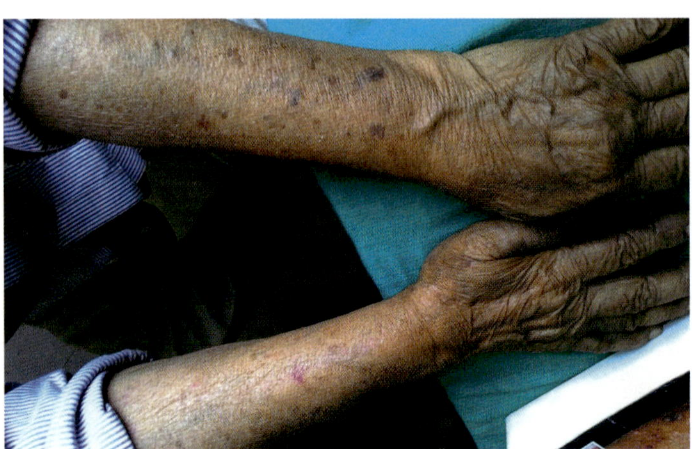

**FIG. 2:** Seborrheic keratosis.

### Intrinsic Factors

- *Genetics*: Cellular aging or "replicative senescence" is due to DNA damage induced by factors such as UV radiation, toxins, or age-related deterioration. A hallmark of replicative senescence is the shortening of telomeres
- *Hormones*: With aging, there is a decline in the level of sex hormones (estrogen, testosterone, and dehydroepiandrosterone sulfate) and growth hormone

  This is significantly seen in women after menopause when estrogen levels decline. Estrogen binds to receptors on skin cells, activating gene expression that modulates skin cell renewal.
- *Oxidative stress*: Skin being the barrier faces UV radiation and environmental pollution. These exposures induce the production of highly volatile molecules called free radicals. Chronic free radical assault leads to the appearance of uneven, blotchy pigmentation, and subverts the structural framework of the skin, giving rise to wrinkles and sagging skin. Free radicals also arise from internal, metabolic reactions like glycation from elevated blood sugar. Oxidative stress plays a central role in initiating and driving events that cause skin aging at the cellular level

  Oxidative stress causes collagen degeneration, damages DNA, and promotes the release of proinflammatory mediators (cytokines), which trigger the generation of inflammatory skin diseases.
- *Elevated blood sugar levels and glycation-glucose-driven intrinsic aging*: Sugar molecules attach themselves to the amino groups of tissue proteins such as collagen to form advanced glycation end products (AGEs). AGE molecules undergo extensive cross-linking collagen proteins leading to their breakage. Glycation reactions are promoted by oxidative stress and lead to the production of reactive oxygen species in the skin. Glycation directly increases the release of MMP-1, which preferentially breaks down collagen.

### Extrinsic Factors

- *Ultraviolet radiation and "photoaging"*: One of the most important extrinsic factors in accelerated skin aging is solar ultraviolet radiation (UVR)

  Chronic sun exposure damages the dermal connective tissue and alters normal skin metabolism. In addition to depressing immunity, and stimulating oxidative stress and inflammation, UV radiation increases the production of MMPs, enzymes that degrade collagen. Collagen damage is a major contributor to the loss of skin suppleness and structure that occurs with advancing age.

  The major targets of UV irradiation in the skin are the surface epidermal layers UVA radiation induces oxidative stress that stimulates post-UV inflammation and hyperpigmentation. UVB radiation damages DNA and epidermal keratinocytes.
- *Others*: Tobacco and pollution also cause premature aging.

## HISTOPATHOLOGICAL CHANGES

### Epidermis

- The thickness of epidermis decreases with age. The rete ridges also flatten, cell turnover rate is decreased
- The permeability of the skin also changes with age and become more permeable to chemical substances
- The corneocytic transit time increases, the water binding capacity of the stratum corneum is reduced
- The number of melanocytes decreases, but increase in size thus leading to irregular pigmentation, freckles. Langerhans cells decline in number.

### Dermis

The visible change of skin aging like wrinkling is mostly due to dermal changes. The dermal thickness reduces by almost 20%.

Grossly the collagen bundles become fragmented and disoriented and elastin fibers become progressively reduced. There is loss of collagens I and III in the papillary dermis with an associated increase in MMPs.

But in photoaging, paradoxically, there is increase in fibers that take up elastin stains. The dermal thickness decreases and the collagen per unit area of unexposed skin decreases with age. The number of mast cells, mononuclear cells, and neutrophils increase. The fibroblasts show a stellate phenotype and, ultrastructurally, a highly activated endoplasmic reticulum that reflects increased biosynthetic activity.

Mechanical effects also contribute to decreased collagen synthesis especially in the photoaged dermis.

The blood vessels of the dermis become more fragile. This leads to bruising, bleeding under the skin (often called senile purpura), cherry angiomas, and similar conditions.

- *Nerves*: There is no structural variation but there is decreased sensory perception and increase in threshold for pain
- *The subcutaneous fat layer*: This thins, reducing its normal insulation and padding. Thus, there is easy injury and hypothermia
- *Sebaceous gland*: The secretory activity declines with age. This occurs earlier in women
- *Eccrine glands*: Sweating declines in old age due to reduction in the number of glands and secretion.

## CHANGES IN NAILS AND HAIR

Decrease in growth and increase in brittleness. Ingrown toenails may be more common. Black hair turns to gray with age. The follicles of gray hairs have a few melanocytes but the cytoplasm may contain large vacuoles and the melanosomes may be only lightly melanized. The follicles of fully white hairs may completely lack melanocytes. Androgenetic alopecia is seen in both sexes. Scalp hair becomes sparse and there is tendency of terminal hairs to change to vellous hair.

## PHOTOAGING

Severity of photoaging has been classified as below:

- *Mild—early photoaging*: No wrinkles, mild pigment changes, no keratosis, and minimal wrinkles
- *Moderate—early-to-moderate photoaging*: Wrinkles in motion, early brown spots visible, keratosis palpable but not visible, parallel smile lines begin to appear
- *Advanced—advanced photoaging*: Wrinkles at rest, obvious discolorations, visible capillaries (telangiectasias), and visible keratosis

**BOX 2 Skin diseases commonly found in elderly**

- Pruritus without skin lesions: Etiology that need to be ruled out are:
  - Anemia
  - Thyroid disease
  - Malignancy especially lymphomas
  - Polycythemia vera
  - Liver or renal pruritus
- Dermatitis
  - Eczema craquele
  - Allergic contact dermatitis
  - Irritant contact dermatitis
  - Seborrheic dermatitis
  - Nummular eczema
  - Atopic dermatitis
- Bullous diseases: Bullous pemphigoid, paraneoplastic pemphigus, cutaneous malignancies (seborrheic keratoses, basal cell carcinoma, and melanoma)
- Cutaneous infections
  - Bacterial: Staphylococcal folliculitis, necrotizing fasciitis
  - Viral: Herpes zoster with postherpetic neuralgia
  - Fungal: Onychomycosis and candidiasis
  - Others: Scabies
- Miscellaneous
  - Ecchymosis
  - Nutritional
  - Adverse drug reactions
  - Leg ulcers

- *Severe—Severe photoaging*: Only wrinkles, yellow-gray skin color, prior skin malignancies, wrinkles throughout—no normal skin—Roughening.

  There are certain skin diseases commonly found in elderly as mentioned below (Box 2).
- *Eczema*: Aged skin is dry and asteatotic dermatitis is frequently associated with it. This is due to decrease in water holding capacity of the skin and decrease in the natural skin oils. Atopic dermatitis flares up due to dry skin
- *Psoriasis*: Peak of onset of psoriasis is in later life, between the ages of 55 and 60 years. Flexural psoriasis is a particular problem in the elderly patient
- *Senile pruritus*: It is one of the most common old age skin problem. It may be due to dryness, atopy or may be due to underlying disorders like diabetes, hypothyroidism, malignancies, adverse drug reaction, and infestations. Senile pruritus is a nonspecific pruritus in old age and happens due to:
  - Decreased lipid content of skin
  - Decreased sweat and sebum production
  - Impaired barrier function of skin
  - Xerosis.

Whenever elderly patients present with chronic pruritus, senile pruritus needs to be differentiated from other specific etiologies as mentioned earlier. Clinically, it manifests as dry skin sometimes with excoriation marks and ecchymosis. Regular use of emollients can provide some relief.

## Infections

Common infections in old ages are:

- *Bacterial*: Staphylococcal folliculitis is common in elderly. Cellulitis, erysipelas, necrotizing fasciitis, and pseudomonal cellulitis is found more often in elderly than young. These may be precipitated by underlying diabetes
- *Viral*: There is increase in incidence of herpes zoster (Fig. 3). Postherpetic neuralgia is also much more common in elderly people
- *Fungal*: Onychomycosis, tinea pedis, and mucocutaneous candidiasis are frequently found
- *Parasitic*: Scabies flares up due to decrease immunity. There is increase chance of crusted scabies in the debilated.

## Ulcers

*Leg ulcers*: Most are caused by venous hypertension but arterial disease becomes increasingly important with advancing years. Poor wound healing in elderly people, perhaps associated with other illnesses and poor nutrition may also have a role in the perpetuation of some ulcers.

*Decubitus ulcers*: Due to decrease mobility, bed-ridden conditions, and poor wound healing.

## Neoplasms

Most skin tumors are more common in elderly people:

- *Benign, tumors*—seborrheic keratoses, senile lentigines and skin tags dysplastic-actinic keratoses, and Bowen's disease
- *Malignant*—basal cell carcinoma (Fig. 4), squamous cell carcinoma, melanoma, and Merkel cell carcinoma
- *Others*: *Bullous pemphigoid*—common above 60 years. Due to flattening of rete ridges and increase in circulating autoantibodies. Adverse drug reactions are common due to multiple medications.

  Skin changes due to vitamin deficiencies like angular cheilitis and glossitis is also common.
- *Senile purpura*: It is also known as Batman purpura. It results from increased fragility of blood vessels and decreased dermal tissue. It occurs due to both chronic and photoaging. There is appearance of purplish ecchymotic patches especially on the extensor surface of limbs (Fig. 5). History of preceding trauma is absent or minimal. The color gradually changes to brown due to hemosiderin pigment and resolves slowly over months. Drugs like corticosteroids and anticoagulants may

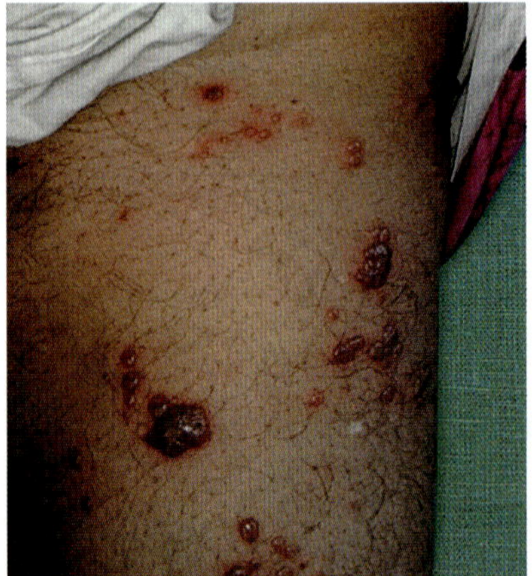

**FIG. 3:** Herpes zoster in aged patient.

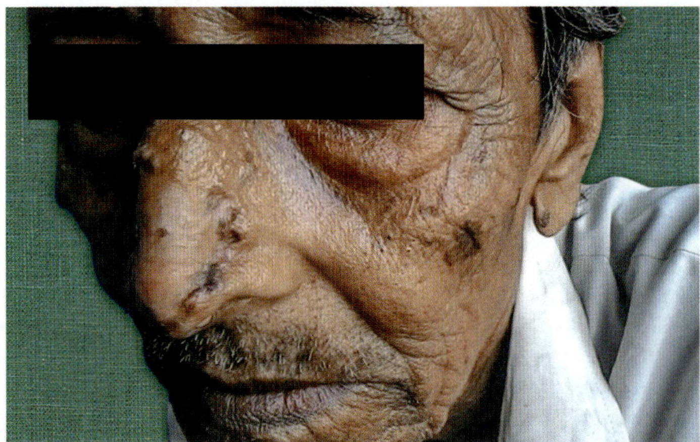

**FIG. 4:** Basal cell carcinoma over nose.

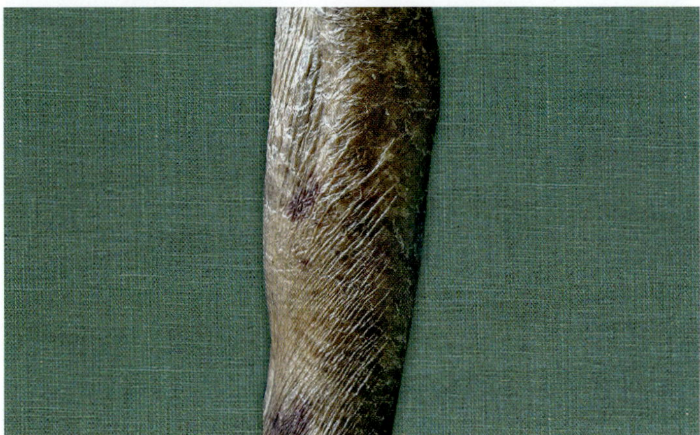

**FIG. 5:** Senile purpura with xerosis.

aggravate the condition. Histology shows thinned epidermis, decreased collagen tissue in dermis with extravasated red blood cells. The condition requires no treatment. Sunscreens and protective clothing is beneficial.

## SUGGESTED READINGS


1. Antonicelli F, Bellon G, Debelle L, et al. Elastin-elastases and inflamm-aging. Curr Top Dev Biol. 2007;79:99-155.
2. Ashcroft GS, Horan MA, Ferguson MW. The effects of ageing on cutaneous wound healing in mammals. J Anat. 1995;187:1-26.
3. Chahal HS, Drake WM. The endocrine system and aging. J Pathol. 2007;211(2):173-80.
4. Commo S, Gaillard O, Bernard BA. Human hair greying is linked to a specific depletion of hair follicle melanocytes affecting both the bulb and the outer rootsheath. Br J Dermatol. 2004;150:435-43.
5. Fisher GJ, Kang S, Varani J, et al. Mechanisms of photoaging and chronological skin aging. Arch Dermatol. 2002;138(11):1462-70.
6. Harvell JD, Maibach HI. Percutaneous absorption and inflammation in aged skin: a review. J Am Acad Dermatol. 1994;31:1015-21.
7. Kimberlin DW, Whitley RJ. Varicella-zoster vaccine for the prevention of herpes zoster. N Engl J Med. 2007;356:1338-43.
8. Kumar P, Barton SP, Marks R. Tissue measurements in senile sebaceous gland hyperplasia. Br J Dermatol. 1988;118:397-402.
9. Marks R. Measurement of biological ageing in human epidermis. Br J Dermatol. 1981;104:627-33.
10. Ma W, Wlaschek M, Tantcheva-Poor I, et al. Chronological ageing and photoageing of the fibroblasts and the dermal connective tissue. Clin Exp Dermatol. 2001;26:592-9.
11. Moloney MC, Grace P. Understanding the underlying causes of chronic leg ulceration. J Wound Care. 2004;13:215-8.
12. Norman RA, Blanco PM. Papulosquamous diseases in the elderly. Dermatol Ther. 2003;16:231-42.
13. Rabe JH, Mamelak AJ, McElgunn PJ, et al. Photoaging: mechanisms and repair. J Am Acad Dermatol. 2006;55:1-19.
14. Silver AF, Montagna W, Karacan I. The effect of age on human eccrine sweating. In: Montagna W (Ed). Advances in Biology of Skin, vol. 6. Aging. Oxford: Pergamon; 1965. pp. 129-50.
15. Van Boekel MA. The role of glycation in aging and diabetes mellitus. Mol Biol Rep. 1991;15:57-64.
16. Verdier-Sévrain S. Effect of estrogens on skin aging and the potential role of selective estrogen receptor modulators. Climacteric. 2007;10(4):289-97.

5 SECTION

# Pruritus and Eczematous Disorders

9 CHAPTER

# Eczema and Pruritus

*Tarang Goyal, Nadia Zakir, Vijay Zawar*

## ECZEMA

## INTRODUCTION

Eczema (or dermatitis) may manifest as any combination of pruritus, scaling, erythema, thickening or lichenification of the skin, hyperpigmentation, oozing or chronic resistant dermatitis. The usual progression of a skin disease involves an underlying trigger that causes primary lesions such as papules, pustules, and vesicles.

Eczemas are classified as exogenous or endogenous (Table 1).

- *Endogenous eczema*: Here the process originates within the body itself
- *Exogenous eczema*: It is triggered by external factors.

## PHYTODERMATITIS AND PHYTOPHOTODERMATITIS

Contact dermatitis due to plants or their products is quite common (Table 2). Phototoxic eruption (phytophotodermatitis) is very common amongst gardeners, florists, farmers, and people living in rural areas. Plants can cause allergic, irritant, and phototoxic dermatitis.

- *Acute stage*: Erythema, edema, vesicles, and bullae. Patterns may be seen in some cases as poison ivy. A diffuse, patchy eruption may occur as a result of indirect exposure to extracts. Dermatitis starts on exposed areas as face, extensor of extremities and spread later to involve axillae, groins, ankles, waist, and feet
- *Chronic stage*: Lichenification, fissuring of finger tips, and hyperpigmentation may be seen.

**TABLE 1: Classification of eczemas**

| Exogenous causes | Endogenous causes |
|---|---|
| • Irritant contact dermatitis<br>• Allergic contact dermatitis<br>• Photo contact dermatitis<br>• Infective dermatitis<br>• Eczematous dermatophytosis<br>• Dermatophytid | • Atopic dermatitis<br>• Seborrheic dermatitis<br>• Nummular eczema<br>• Asteotic eczema<br>• Pityriasis amiantacea<br>• Stasis dermatitis<br>• Pityriasis alba<br>• Juvenile plantar dermatitis<br>• Pompholyx |

### Diagnosis

Patch tests and photopatch test with active ingredients or standard concentration of plant extracts should be used. Tests with saw dust are done dry as well as wet. In cases of primula and poison ivy, these tests are not advisable due to risk of aggravation or sensitization.

## INFECTIVE DERMATITIS

Skin infection may secondarily induce eczematization. This is caused by the microorganisms or their products. This is known as infective dermatitis (ID). Secondary infection may also occur in any eczematous skin lesion. This is known as infected eczema. The distinction between infective and infected eczema is difficult (Table 3). This condition seems to occur particularly in patients

**TABLE 2: Common sensitizing plants**

| Family | Common name |
|---|---|
| Anacardiaceae<br>• *Rhus radicans*<br>• *Mangifera indica*<br>• *Anarcardium occidentale* | <br>• Poison ivy<br>• Mango<br>• Cashew |
| Compositae<br>• *Chrysanthemum*<br>• *Parthenium* | <br>• Mums<br>• Feverfew |
| Liliaceae<br>• *Tulipa* | <br>Tulip |
| Primulaceae | Primula |
| Amaryllidaceae | Narcissus, daffodil |
| **Vegetables** | |
| *Alliceae* | Chive, onion, garlic |
| *Compositae* | Chicory, endive, artichoke, lettuce |
| *Cruciferae* | Horseradish, brussel sprout, cabbage |
| *Liliaceae* | Asparagus |
| *Umbelliferae* | Celery, parsnip, carrot, parsley |

**TABLE 3: Infected eczema versus infective eczema**

| Infective eczema | Infected eczema |
|---|---|
| • Usually presents as an area of advancing erythema, sometimes with micro vesicles<br>• Seen predominantly around discharging wounds or ulcers, or moist skin lesions of other types<br>• Primary source can be boiled or discharging sinus or a wound<br>• The area involved is usually in contiguity of primary focus<br>• Infection may be bacterial, viral, or fungal<br>• Rapid response to antimicrobial therapy<br>• For example, ID may develop secondary to otitis media, tinea pedis, infected scabies, or pediculosis. | • Erythema with exudation and crusting<br>• Margin is characteristically sharply defined. There may be small pustules and fissures in the advancing edge<br>• Infection may be bacterial, viral, or fungal<br>• Rapid response to antimicrobial therapy |

ID, infective dermatitis.

with poor standards of hygiene. Hyperhidrosis and heavy footwear may act as important predisposing factors.

## SEBORRHEIC DERMATITIS

Seborrheic dermatitis (SD) is a common papulosquamous disorder and involves different age groups. It is found in areas with high sebaceous gland concentration and larger body folds. It was first described by Unna who also suspected *Malassezia furfur* (Pityrosporum ovale) as the causative factor. However, etiology is uncertain and possibly is multifactorial (Box 1).

### Clinical Features

Two peaks may be seen—infantile and adult

- *Infantile form*: This is common in first 3 months. This is mostly self-limiting. Initially scales are mild and greasy, found on the vertex, extending later to involve entire scalp. Inflammation and oozing leads to crusting and yellowish brown adherent scale called "cradle cap" (Fig. 1). Lesions also found on face, neck, retroauricular folds, trunk, proximal extremities, axillae, and inguinal folds (Fig. 2). Superimposed candidal infection may also be found

**BOX 1 Probable etiologies of seborrheic dermatitis**

- *Malassezia furfur* (Pityrosporum ovale)
- Higher surface lipid levels of triglycerides and cholesterol
- Abnormal immune response to *Malassezia* leading to increased IL-10 and decreased IFN-γ and IL-2
- Low humidity, cold temperature; early spring
- *Drugs*: Griseofulvin, lithium, chlorpromazine, phenothiazines, stanozolol, psoralen, cimetidine, gold, methyldopa, buspirone, arsenic, haloperidol, etc.
- *Neurotransmitter abnormality disorders*: Parkinson's, Alzheimer's, epilepsy, CVA, trigeminal nerve injury, poliomyelitis

IFN-γ, interferon-gamma; IL, interleukin; CVA, cardiovascular accidents.

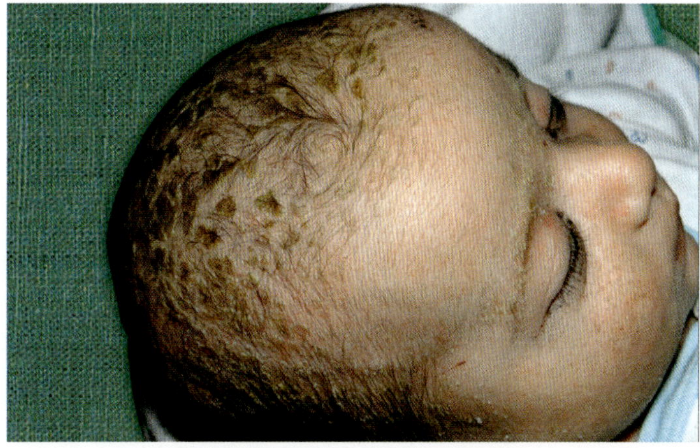

**FIG. 1:** Cradle cap in an infant showing yellowish brown adherent scales.

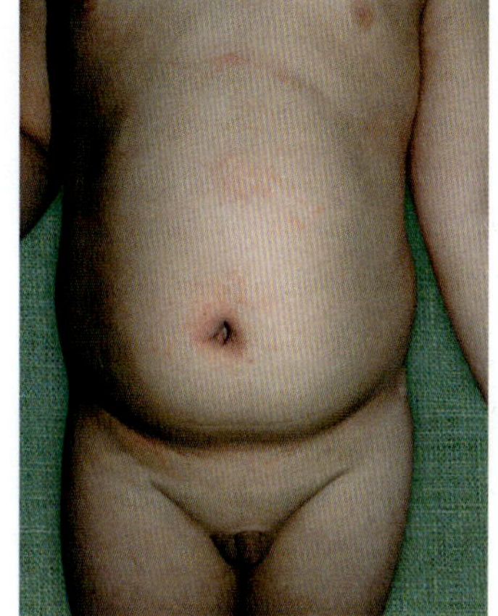

**FIG. 2:** Seborrheic dermatitis involving the trunk (presternal and periumblical regions).

- *Adult form*: Another peak is seen at 40 years of age, more commonly in males. Flaky greasy white scaling is seen symmetrically on face, affecting the forehead, medial eyebrows, upper eyelids, nasolabial folds, retroauricular areas, occiput, and neck. Typical bran-like scale is seen (Figs 3 and 4). The lesions on the chest assume a petaloid form; inguinal and other body folds can have an intertrigo-like appearance

Severity of seborrheic dermatitis may depend on various factors (Box 2).

- *Differential diagnosis*: Infantile SD has to be differentiated from other conditions such as atopic dermatitis, candidiasis, psoriasis, other eczematous disorders including immunodeficiency syndromes like Wiskot-Aldrich syndrome, and Langerhans cell histiocytosis. Adult form of SD should be differentiated from atopic dermatitis, psoriasis, pityriasis rosea, and pityrosporum folliculitis (Fig. 5).

### Histopathology

In acute stage, folliculocentric scale, orthokeratosis, and focal parakeratosis with neutrophils, mild focal spongiosis, and sparse superficial perivascular infiltrate are found. In subacute stage, mild psoriasiform hyperplasia is seen. Numerous yeast cells may also be found and in chronic stage, superficial dilatation of capillaries with pronounced psoriasiform hyperplasia is found. Diagnosis is essentially clinical.

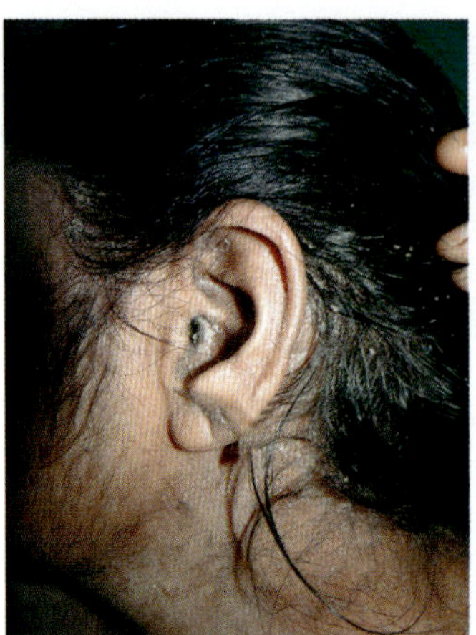

**FIG. 3:** Seborrheic dermatitis of the scalp involving the external ear.

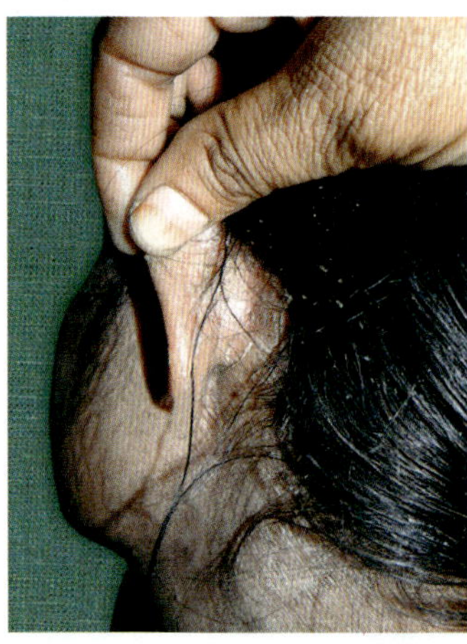

**FIG. 4:** Seborrheic dermatitis involving the retroauricular fold.

**BOX 2 Conditions associated with more incidence/increased severity of seborrheic dermatitis (SD)**

- HIV/AIDS
- Parkinson's disease
- Premature infants
- Congestive heart failure patients
- Alcoholic patients
- Obesity disorders

HIV, human immunodeficiency virus; AIDS, acquired immune deficiency syndrome.

## Treatment

It is commonly treated with antifungal creams, shampoo or as stay on product (ketoconazole, oxiconazole, and climbazole).

- Selenium sulfide 2.25% has been in use for long time
- If there is significant inflammation, mild to moderate steroid lotions or shampoo or coal tar is used. Tacrolimus, pimecrolimus can also be used. Topical steroid (lotion) may be used if there is prominent inflammation. If scaling is gross, keratolytic like salicylic acid may be used in the form of a lotion or shampoo. Oral drugs like ketoconazole, fluconazole, and itraconazole may be used in severe cases.

# PITYRIASIS AMIANTACEA

This is also known as asbestos scalp, tinea asbestina, and keratosis follicularis amiantacea. It was first described by Alibert in 1832.

Localized or diffuse massive silvery scales appear on scalp along with inflammation. Hairs are matted due to the scaling.

Proposed etiologies are psoriasis, seborrheic dermatitis, atopic dermatitis, pemphigus disorders, lichen planus, and Darrier's disease (Fig. 6).

## Histopathology

Spongiosis, mild exocytosis of lymphocytes and acanthosis, hyper- and parakeratosis surrounding the hair shafts are seen.

## Treatment

It occurs at any age and is resistant to treatment. Mineral/vegetable oils, e.g., olive oil followed by shampoos can be used to remove scales. Some cases may require oral antibiotics or oral antifungals.

# NUMMULAR ECZEMA

The term "nummular" is derived from Latin *"nummulum"*= "coin shape" of lesions, is a form of eczema that presents with coin-shaped lesions. This is also called as discoid eczema and microbial eczema.

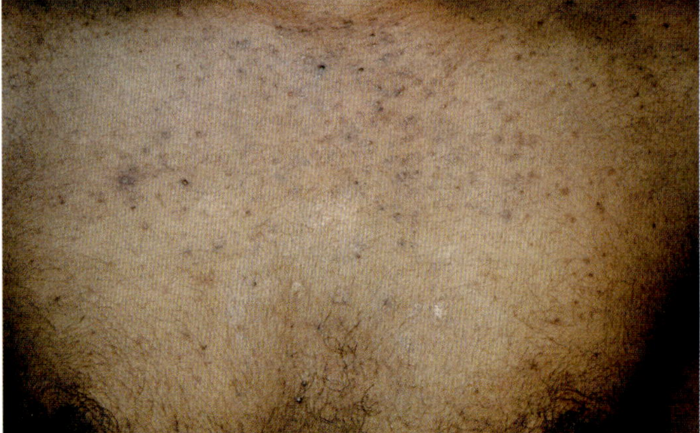

**FIG. 5:** Pityrosporum folliculitis.

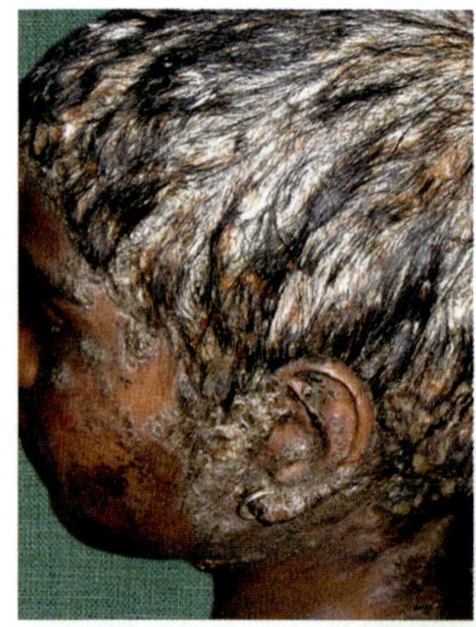

**FIG. 6:** Thick adherent asbestos like scales of pityriasis amiantacea.

| BOX 3 | Disease with coin-shaped eczematous lesions |
|---|---|
| • Nummular eczema | • Asteotic eczema |
| • Atopic annular lesions | • Stasis dermatitis |

## Pathogenesis

Whether this is a specific entity is uncertain. Similar type of coin-shaped lesions may be noted in some other disorders (Box 3). Hydration of skin, atopy, internal hidden focus of infection, environmental allergens as house dust mite, and *Candida albicans* are proposed to have some etiological relation. Drugs as gold, mercury amalgam, and isotretinoin are also implicated. Patients having hepatitis C virus infection, treatment with interferon α-2b and ribavarin combination therapy may induce generalized lesions.

## Clinical Features

It is seen as chronic, persistent, single or multiple well-demarcated round or oval erythematous plaques which may be dry, scaly or vesicular, and oozing. Pinpoint oozing or crusted vesicles are characteristic (Fig. 7). Variable degree of pruritus is seen.

It is predominantly a disease of adults. Peak incidence is seen in 50–60 years of age, males are affected more than females. Extremities, lower legs are commonly affected in males and forearms in females.

Oid-Oid disease is a name given to a therapy resistant variant, also called as Sulzberger-Garbe syndrome.

## Treatment

This is similar to other common eczemas.

# ASTEATOTIC ECZEMA

This is also known as winter eczema, winter itch, eczema craquelè, and dessication dermatitis.

## Etiology

Dry and excessive cold weather, use of soaps, surfactants or even water in excess, marasmus, hemodialysis, and atopic dermatitis are known to cause this condition.

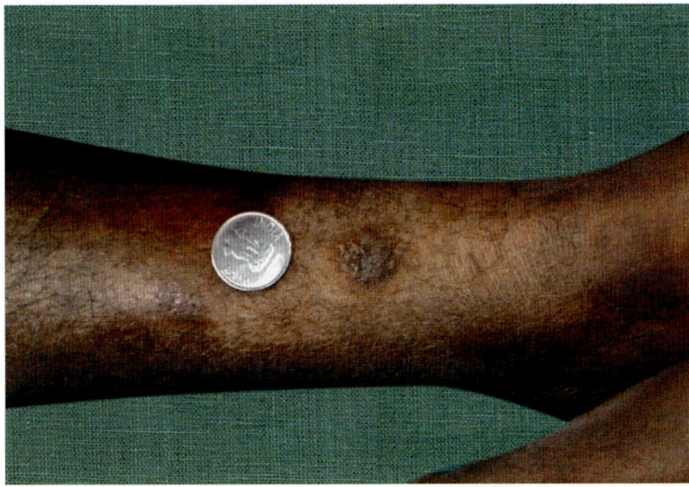

FIG. 7: Coin shaped lesions of nummular eczema.

## Clinical Features

Skin may appear to have dry and dull with fine powdery bran-like scales that progresses to develop criss-cross pattern of dry skin with superficial cracks and fissures (crazy paving; eczema craquelè) with erythema (Fig. 8). Eczematous changes like oozing, crusting, excoriations, and lichenification may develop.

## Pathogenesis

There is decrease of intercellular lipids and altered ratio of esterified fatty acids to ceramides. There is decreased synthesis of natural moisturizing factor.

## Differential Diagnosis

Stasis dermatitis, allergic contact dermatitis, atopic dermatitis.

## Treatment

Hydration of skin with use of topical corticosteroids is helpful. Use of urea, ceramide, or lactic acid containing emollients is beneficial. Antibiotics must be given in secondarily infected cases.

# STASIS DERMATITIS

- *Syn*: Gravitational dermatitis, varicose eczema, and congestion eczema
- The term stasis dermatitis was first used by Pillsbury.

## Pathogenesis

Chronic venous insufficiency and microangiopathy leading to chronic inflammation are responsible for stasis dermatitis. Typically lesions occur in the medial supramalleolar regions where microangiopathy is most intense. Scratching and sensitization secondary to various topical products induce eczematous changes (stasis dermatitis).

## Clinical Features

- *Early sign*: Pitting edema of medial shin and calf region proximal to the ankle. Spotty hemosiderin deposits may be seen later due to stasis purpura

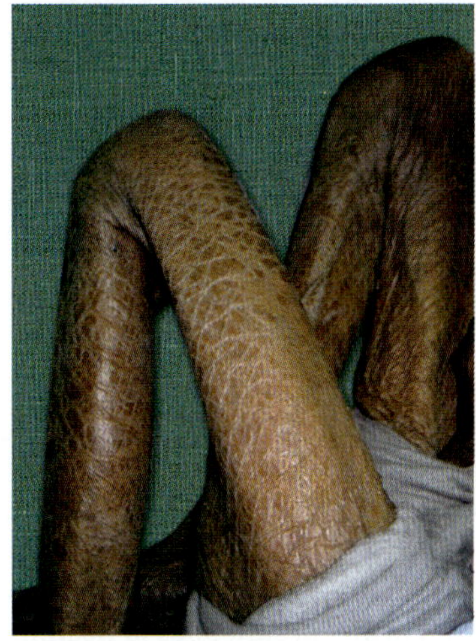

FIG. 8: Crazy paving pattern of asteatotic eczema.

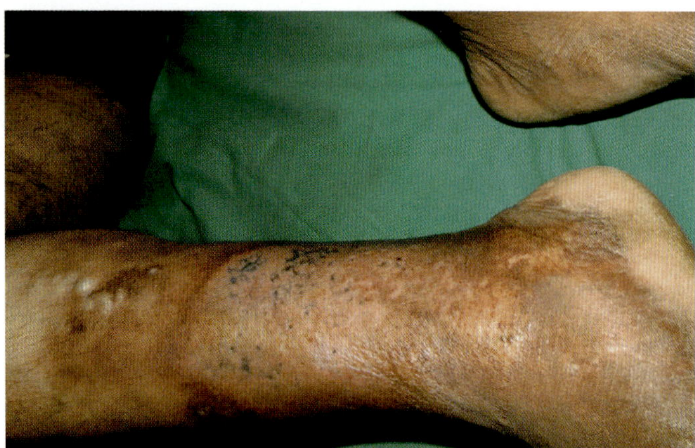

FIG. 9: Stasis dermtitis showing atrophie blanche, hemosiderin pigmentation with varicose veins.

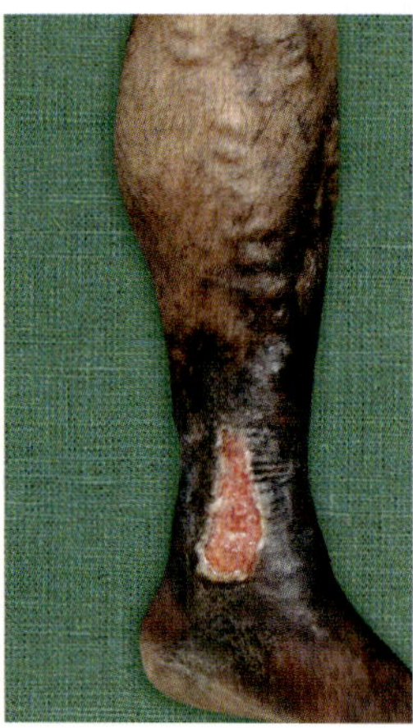

FIG. 10: Venous ulcer with lipodermatosclerosis giving the leg an inverted bottle apperance.

- *Later sequelae*: Ascending edema covering distal one-third calf, inflammation, and subfascial edema appears. Next, the skin, subcutaneous adipose tissue and deep facia become adherent to appear as stiffness of the skin called chronic lipodermatosclerosis. A firm circular cuff formed seems to strangle the distal calf, giving the appearance of "Inverted Wine Bottle". The skin may show porcelain white atrophic spots called atrophie blanche, hemosiderin pigmentation, and venous ulcers (Fig. 9).

Stasis dermatitis appears as erythema, scaling, episodes of vesiculation, and lichenification. There may be eventually formation of ulcers (Fig. 10).

### Differential Diagnoses

Irritant contact dermatitis, contact dermatitis, nummulae eczema, psoriasis, or even mycosis fungoides.

### Treatment

Venous incompetence has to be treated properly. Use of compression stockings, lifestyle modification, postural changes as well as avoidance of long-standing is necessary. In some selected cases surgical approach may be considered. Use of emollients and sometimes topical corticosteroids are used. Topical application of any product has to be minimized.

## PITYRIASIS ALBA

It is a disorder of children and young adults characterized by erythematous faint hypopigmented ill-defined patches. Pityriasis-scaly; alba-white.

### Clinical Features

Face is the most common site. Upper arms, neck, or shoulders or even legs uncommonly are affected. This manifests as rounded, oval or irregular hypopigmented mildly erythematous patches having fine lamellar or branny scales with ill-defined margins (Fig. 11). Usually 4–20 lesions are present. Less commonly, hyperpigmented variety is seen.

### Treatment

Pityriasis alba resolves spontaneously. Tacrolimus ointment, pimecrolimus cream, low-potency topical steroids as hydrocortisone, desonide may be used in cases with erythema and pruritus. Psoralen plus ultraviolet A (PUVA) or PUVAsol may be used for the hypopigmentation.

## JUVENILE PLANTAR DERMATOSIS

It occurs primarily in children with atopic diathesis. It mainly affects kids above 3 years of age, occurs more in winter and has a male predominance. Also called atopic winter feet or forefoot dermatitis.

### Pathogenesis

Atopy, occlusive shoes, and friction are known as precipitating factors.

### Clinical Features

*Sites*: Balls of feet and toe pads, distal feet.

Symmetrical, well-defined, shiny, and glazed erythematous dry skin develops on the distal sole especially balls of feet and toe pads. Cracks and fissures may also be present in more severe cases (Fig. 12).

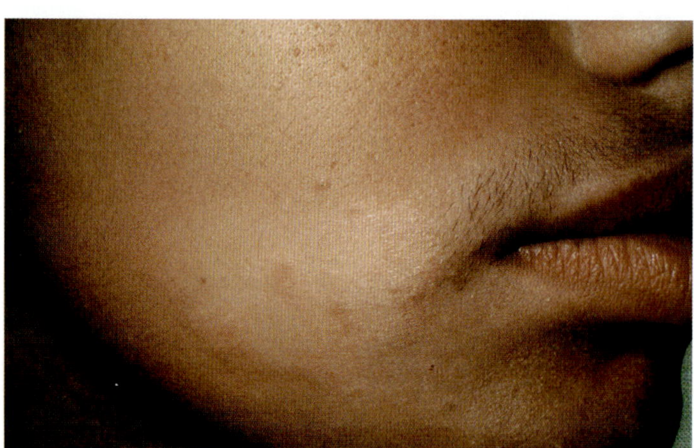

FIG. 11: Pityriasis alba.

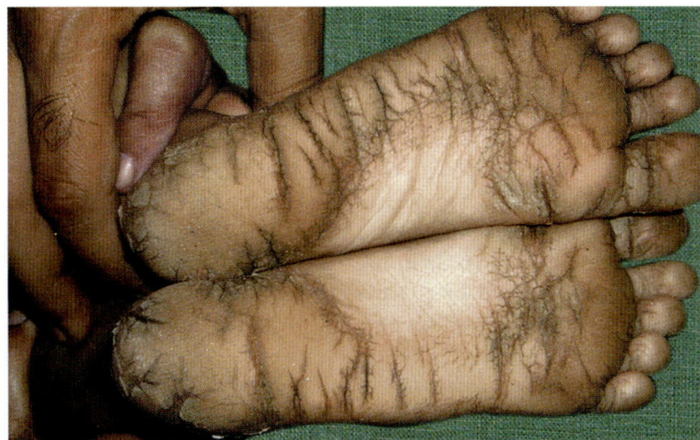

FIG. 12: Juvenile planter dermatoses showing severe fissuring with relative sparing of the instep.

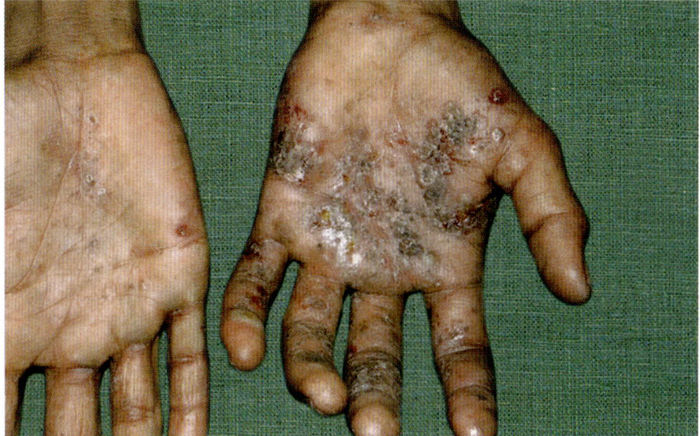

FIG. 13: Dyshidrotic eczema showing multiple deep seated vesicles with crusting and oozing.

### Differential Diagnosis

Tinea pedis, allergic contact dermatitis, psoriasis, and irritant contact dermatitis may mimick this.

### Treatment

Avoidance of impermeable socks and shoes, and rest are same on the pattern of allergic contact dermatitis.

## DYSHIDROTIC ECZEMA

Syn: Pompholyx, acute, and recurrent vesicular hand dermatitis.

It is chronic relapsing palmoplantar eczematous dermatitis characterized by pruritic vesicles and bullae.

### Pathogenesis

This is unknown. Late stage atopic dermatitis, hyperhidrosis, acute or subacute allergic contact dermatitis may manifest as pompholyx.

### Clinical Features

Symmetrical deep seated vesicles and bullae develop on palms, lateral and medial fingers, and soles. The size of vesicles vary from pin point (tapioca-like when grouped), to larger clear fluid filled bullae (Fig. 13). Lesions are usually itchy.

### Differential Diagnosis

Tinea manuum and pedis, pustular psoriasis, erythema multiforme, fixed drug eruption, allergic contact dermatitis, and infantile acropustulosis.

### Treatment

Topical corticosteroids is usually the first line therapy. Topical calcineurin inhibitors, PUVA therapy, and UVB therapy have all been tried. Systemic corticosteroids are used in acute severe cases.

## LOCALIZED NEURODERMATITIS

This is also known as lichen simplex chronicus. Lesions are lichenified or excoriated, usually unilateral and limited to a single patch. Nape of neck, wrists, anterior lower legs, ankles, ears, or anal area are commonly affected. Predominantly follicular pattern is also seen.

### Pathogenesis

It starts as a small patch of dermatitis. Persistent itch aggravates the condition (itch-scratch-itch) without any role of allergies. There is no familial predisposition or seasonal variation. Female preponderance is present.

Stress acts as an aggravating factor. Neurodermatitis may be secondary to atopic eczema, contact dermatitis, or any other dermatosis like lichen planus, psoriasis, or insect bite.

### Treatment

It includes complete avoidance of scratching, occlusive steroid dressings, emollients, and sedating antihistaminics. Intralesional steroid injection can be given for chronic and bigger lesion.
Stress management and/or medication is often necessary.

## PRURIGO NODULARIS

Prurigo nodularis is a chronic pruritic skin condition characterized by intense itchy papules or nodules. Hyde and Montgomery first described prurigo nodularis in 1909. Also known as nodular prurigo, Hyde's disease, picker's nodules, nodular lichen simplex chronicus, and nodular neurodermatitis circumscripta.

### Pathogenesis

This is unknown. It is known to be induced by intense picking and scratching, leading to the formation of lumps or nodules. Calcitonin gene-related peptide and substance P immunoreactive nerves are markedly increased in number and activity in the skin of patients with prurigo nodularis as compared to normal skin. But whether this represents a causative etiology or arises as a result of chronic scratching and skin irritation is not known. Emotional stress seems to be a contributory factor. It can also commence as a reaction after an insect bite or another form of dermatitis. Prurigo nodularis has also been reported to be associated with internal diseases including iron deficiency anemia, chronic renal failure, celiac diseases, HIV infection, etc. It has also been speculated that widespread prurigo nodularis may also follow sensitization of the spinal nerves and that the nodules appear because of scratching.

## Clinical Features

It can occur at all ages, but mainly at 20–60 years of age. Both sexes are equally affected. This appears as discrete, symmetrical, firm nodule, measuring 1–3 cm in diameter, firm to hard on palpation, often with raised warty surface and sometimes with excoriation. Pruritus is usually severe. Prurigo nodularis often affects the extensor aspects of the body. Lesions may vary in number from few to more than hundred. The disease runs a long and chronic course. This runs a chronic course with persistence and recurrence of lesions.

## Diagnosis

Skin biopsy and histopathology is useful to confirm the diagnosis. Under the microscope, the changes resemble those of lichen simplex, but the hyperkeratosis is greater and the downward projection of epidermis is so marked so as to suggest pseudoepitheliomatous hyperplasia. There is dense dermal infiltrate and neural and vascular hyperplasia.

- Direct immunofluorescence is often negative
- Patch testing can diagnose allergic contact dermatitis (ACD)
- Investigations to rule out systemic diseases are necessary.

## Differential Diagnosis

- Perforating disease
- Hypertrophic lichen planus
- Pemphigoid nodularis
- Lichen simplex chronicus
- Actinic prurigo
- Multiple keratoacanthomas
- Nodular scabies
- Dermatitis herpetiformis
- Knuckle pads
- Actinic keratosis
- Milker's nodules
- Squamous cell carcinoma
- Cutaneous T-cell lymphoma
- Lymphocytoma cutis.

## Treatment

Emollients, ultrapotent topical steroids creams, applied under occlusion to enhance the effect, coal tar ointment as steroid alternative, calcipotriol ointment, and capsaicin cream are used. In resistant cases, intralesional corticosteroids injections or cryotherapy may be used. Oral antihistaminics and tricyclic antidepressants (amitriptyline or doxepin) are used for pruritus.

In resistant cases, other options may be tried. These are phototherapy (both broad and narrow band UVB and PUVA), oral corticosteroids, methotrexate, gabapentin, thalidomide, cyclosporine, azathioprine, systemic retinoids such as acitretin and isotretinoin.

## REGIONAL DERMATITIS

- *Eyelids*: It is the most common type of the allergic contact dermatitis. Eyelids react readily to the direct application of allergens in cosmetics (mascara), medications, airborne allergens (pollens, dust, hair sprays, and hair dyes), and to allergens carried by the fingers such as nail polish. Edema of the eyelids may be the sole manifestation of airborne dermatitis
- *Lips and perioral area*: It is manifested by dryness, flaking, and most common cause is use of lipsticks. Perioral dermatitis is a relatively common condition, often due to excessive use of a topical fluorinated corticosteroid. Lipsticks, lip pomades, sun screens, toothpaste, tooth powders, mouth washes, and cigarette can cause dermatitis. Foods like pineapple, orange, lemon, carrot, and raw mango can cause such eruptions. Nail polishes, and nail hardeners in nail biters and thumb suckers, nickel, and nickel objects held in the mouth, pins, hair pins, and keys are common causes
- *Neck*: Common causes of contact dermatitis of the neck are cosmetics, shaving lotions and acne medications, metal chains and necklaces, usually containing nickel, and perfumes are common allergen. Sun light may aggravate
- *Face*: Face is mostly affected by direct application of cosmetic or medications. Fingers may also cause allergic contact dermatitis due to indirect spread of allergens. Contact dermatitis of adjacent areas as scalp, e.g., use of a hair dye can also cause reaction. The eyelids are usually the first area of the face to be affected. In men, a common cause is shaving lotion, while in teenagers, cosmetics are often responsible for a low-grade chronic dermatitis
- *Conjunctiva*: Ophthalmic preparations, medications. Products used for cleansing or preserving contact lenses, eye washes, hair sprays, pomades, bleach, shampoos, dyes, and rinses
- *Genitals*: In both sexes the genitals show pronounced edema and pruritus upon exposure to allergens. The sensitizing agent may be carried to the area by the fingers
- *Vulvitis*: Feminine hygiene products, cleansers, topical medications, deodorants, permicides, sexual partner, perfumed or colored toilet paper, sanitary napkins, tightly fitting underwear, pantyhose, or metallic clips or zippers in persons allergic to nickel, poison ivy, nail polish (allergen transmitted by fingers)
- *Balanitis*: Condoms (rubber), powders, lubricants, topical medications for treatment of genital lesions or parasitic infections (pediculosis). Toilet preparations (soaps, lotions), hygienic products, powders, and lubricants or other preparations used by the sexual partner
- *Dermatitis of hands and forearms*: Approximately two-thirds of all cases of contact dermatitis affect the hands. Although the dermatitis is primarily due to irritants, the eruption may spread to the forearms, face, and other body areas. The primary affected site also has diagnostic importance, e.g., liquids usually first affect the interdigital spaces. Contact dermatitis in housewives often begins under wedding ring. Most cases of irritant dermatitis begin on the dorsal aspect of the hands even if the contact is with the palms.

The forearms are often affected as an extension of the dermatitis of the hands. In workers who wear protective gloves the dermatitis often begins at the level of the upper border of the gloves. The anticubital spaces are often the site for airborne agents
- *Perianal dermatitis*: Suppositories used for hemorrhoids contain sensitizers such as benzocaine or dibucaine and frequently cause a perianal dermatitis.
  Neomycin or triple combinations containing salicylates may also cause a dermatitis. Irritation from feces, especially in cases of diarrhea, is a common cause of dermatitis
- *Thigh and lower legs*: Clothes, underwear, objects carried in the pockets such as keys and coins are often causes of dermatitis. Stasis dermatitis is an important cause of lower leg dermatitis.

# PRURITUS

## INTRODUCTION

Pruritus is defined as the unpleasant cutaneous sensation that elicits the desire to scratch. This is a common clinical sign in many diseases, and in conditions that are not inherently pruritic, it is often present because of secondary infections or as a result of production of inflammatory mediators. As dermatitis becomes chronic, acute signs of inflammation subside and primary lesions become obscured by signs of chronic inflammation. Resolution of dermatitis requires identification of the underlying cause and treatment of secondary infections or other complications.
Pruritus may be:
- Localized
- Generalized
- Paroxysmal
- Unremitting.

## ETIOLOGY

There are numerous causes of pruritus (Box 4).

**BOX 4 Causes of pruritus**

- *Infection and infestation*: Scabies, pediculosis, insect bites, folliculitis, impetigo, viral exanthema like chicken pox, measles, etc., tinea
- *Eczematous disorders*: Atopic dermatitis, papular urticaria, seborrheic dermatitis, allergic contact dermatitis, irritant contact dermatitis, lichen simplex chronicus, stasis dermatitis, xerotic dermatitis, air-borne contact dermatitis, chronic actinic dermatitis, prurigo simplex, prurigo nodularis, etc.
- *Inflammatory disorder*: Psoriasis, parapsoriasis, PRP, lichen planus, urticaria, mastocytosis, eosinophilic folliculitis, polymorphous light eruption
- *Bullous diseases*: Bullous pemphigoid, dermatitis herpetiformis, pemphigus foliaceus, pemphigus vulgaris, Darier, Hailey–Hailey, etc.
- *Genetic*: Inflammatory linear verrucous epidermal nevus (ILVEN), incontinentia pigmenti
- *Neoplastic*: Cutaneous T-cell lymphoma
- *Others*: Scars, keloids, cutaneous amyloidosis, aquagenic pruritus

*Pruritus in Systemic conditions*
- *Renal*: Chronic renal failure, dialysis associated pruritus
- *Hepatogenic*: Cholestatic jaundice, primary biliary cirrhosis
- *Hematological*: Polycythemia vera, iron deficiency anemia, Hodgkin's and Non-Hodgkin's lymphoma
- *Endocrine*: Diabetes, hypothyroidism, hyperthyroidism
- Pruritus in pregnancy
- Neurogenic pruritus
- Pruritus in HIV

HIV, human immunodeficiency virus; PRP, platelet rich plasma.

## PATHOPHYSIOLOGY

The absence of itching in areas insensitive to pain and in persons with congenital absence of cutaneous pain sensation has given a better understanding toward neurophysiology of pruritus. Histamin is the most powerful mediator of pruritus. However, there are many other mediators (Box 5).

**BOX 5 Mediators of pruritus**

| *Primary mediators* | *Secondary mediators* |
|---|---|
| • Histamine | • Prostaglandin E1,2 |
| • Tryptase | • Substance P |
| • Cathepsin S | • μ-Opioid receptor antagonist |
| • Interleukin-31 | • Nerve growth factor |
| | • Interleukin-2 |

The use of microneurography (insertion of fine glass electrodes into C fibers) has led to identification of exceptionally slow conducting neurons which are 10–15% of total number of C fibers. These respond to both pruritogenic and thermal stimuli. Increasing the temperature leads to lowering of threshold of these fibers, due to which the patient complaints of increased itch in patients with increased temperatures.

### Itch Pathway

Stimulated C fibers → ipsilateral dorsal root ganglion → synapse with itch-specific sensory neurons → neurons cross over → ascend in lateral spinothalamic tract → somatosensory cortex of postcentral gyrus → activation of both angular cingulated cortex and supplemental motor area.

## INVESTIGATIONS

Box 6 shows outline of investigations in pruritus.

## CENTRAL NERVOUS SYSTEM PRURITUS

It is also called as neurogenic itching, occurs due to cerebral stroke, tumor, abscess, multiple sclerosis or can be idiopathic. It is characterized by intense episodes of uncontrollable itching.

## UREMIC PRURITUS

Chronic renal failure patients with uremia exhibit pruritus. Patients who are on maintenance hemodialysis, the incidence is higher. The itching intensity increases immediately after dialysis treatment which has been postulated to be due to accumulation of pruritogenic metabolites to the products from dialysis equipment.
The following may be the causes of uremic pruritus:
- Xerosis
- Secondary hyperparathyroidism
- Abnormal mast cell proliferation
- Abnormal cutaneous innervations
- Increased histamine levels.

**BOX 6 Outline of investigations in a case of pruritus**

*Initial screening*
- Complete blood count with differential leukocyte count
- Liver and renal profile
- Hepatitis C screening
- Thyroid panel
- Urine analysis
- Stool examination
- HIV screening
- Chest X-ray
- Routine skin biopsy

*Advanced screening*
- Skin biopsy for mast cells and immunofluorescence
- Serum protein electrophoresis
- Ferritin levels
- Desired tests to rule out malignancy as CT scan or MRI
- 5-hydroxyindoleacetic acid in urine

HIV, human immunodeficiency virus; CT, computed tomography; MRI, magnetic resonance imaging.

### Management

- Modification of dialysis to ensure adequate solute clearance
- Topical emollients with high water content to be used for 4 weeks
- Tacrolimus 0.03% and 0.1%
- Gamma-linoleic ointment
- Topical local anesthetic as pramoxine.
- Oral gabapentin (300 mg three times a week for 4 weeks or 100 mg three times a week) and pregabalin (25 mg three times a week)
- Naltrexone 50 mg daily
- Ultraviolet B (UVB) therapy

## HEPATOGENIC PRURITUS

It is common in patients with cholestasis associated hepatitis and almost 50% patients present with itching as the initial symptom. There has been no linkage found between the levels of bile salt and intensity of pruritus, but lowering of bile salts definitely leads to lessening of pruritus.

### Management

- *Cholestyramine (4 g one to three times daily)*: First-line therapy.
- *Others*: Rifampicin (300–450 mg daily) (contraindicated in patients with advanced liver disease with elevated bilirubin levels), opiate antagonists as naltrexone, and SSRTIs as sertraline can be used cautiously. Danazol, a synthetic androgen, has been used in primary biliary cirrhosis, urticaria, and idiopathic pruritus.

  Recently MARS (molecular adsorbent recirculating system) an extracorporeal hemofiltration system has been used successfully.

  Recently, nalfurafine, TRK-820 (μ-Opioid receptor antagonist) has shown efficacy in cholestatic and renal pruritus patients.

## PRURITUS ASSOCIATED WITH HEMATOLOGIC DISEASES

Polycythemia vera, Hodgkin's disease and iron deficiency anemia have been found to be associated with severe pruritus.

In Hodgkin's disease the itching occurs at night time and in legs. Generally pruritus precedes manifested disease by months or years.

### Management

- Cyproheptadine
- Pizotifen (0.5 mg three times daily)
- Interferon α-2b plus UVA therapy
- Iron replacement
- Aprepitant (neurokinin 1 receptor antagonist) is used as antiemetic in oncology patient (e.g., in Sézary syndrome or Erlotinib-induced pruritus patients).

## AQUAGENIC PRURITUS

Polycythemia rubra vera and other myeloproliferative disorders are associated with aquagenic pruritus which starts 1–5 minutes after water contact and may persist up to 2 hours or more.

## NOTALGIA PARESTHETICA

It is a type of sensory neuropathy in T2–T6 division and is associated with localized pruritus on back. Degenerative changes of spine have been thought to be the causative factor in this type of pruritus.

## BRACHIORADIAL PRURITUS

It is associated with intense pruritus along with the distribution of brachioradial nerve on the lateral forearm, solar dermapathy has been implicated as the cause.

## SCALP DYESTHESIA

Mostly seen in women with stress as a precipitating factor, mild erythema may be seen.

## HIV-ASSOCIATED PRURITUS

It may be the presenting sign of AIDS. With advancing disease there is a switch from Th1 to Th2 cytokine profile and an associated immune dysregulation. Basophils and mast cells exhibit degranulation and peripheral neuropathy may aggravate the problem.

## SUGGESTED READINGS


1. Bowers AG. Phytophotodermatitis. Am J Contact Dermat. 1999;10:89-93.
2. Gupta AK, Versteeg SG. Topical treatment of facial seborrheic dermatitis: A systematic review. Am J Clin Dermatol. 2017;18:193-213.
3. Inui S. Nalfurafine hydrochloride to treat pruritus: a review. Clin Cosmet Investig Dermatol. 2015;8:249-55.
4. Mettang T. Uremic itch management. Curr Probl Dermatol. 2016;50:133-41.
5. Miazek N, Michalek I, Pawlowska-Kisiel M, et al. Pityriasis alba--common disease, enigmatic Entity: up-to-date Review of the literature. Pediatr Dermatol. 2015;32:786-91.
6. Nishizawa A. Dyshidrotic eczema and Its relationship to Metal Allergy. Curr Probl Dermatol. 2016;51:80-5.
7. Pereira MP, Ständer S. Chronic pruritus: Current and emerging treatment options. Drugs. 2017.
8. Pongcharoen P, Fleischer AB Jr. An evidence-based review of systemic treatments for itch. Eur J Pain. 2016;20:24-31.
9. Rowe B, Yosipovitch G. Paraneoplastic itch management. Curr Probl Dermatol. 2016;50:149-54.
10. Sasseville D. Clinical patterns of phytodermatitis. Dermatol Clin. 2009;27:299-308.
11. Wollina U. Pompholyx: a review of clinical features, differential diagnosis, and management. Am J Clin Dermatol. 2010;11:305-14.

# 10 CHAPTER Atopic Eczema

Attila S Antal, Thomas Ruzicka

## INTRODUCTION

The term atopy (greek 'atopos'; out of place) is defined as hypersensitivity to everyday influences which is characteristic for atopic disorders. Atopic hypersensitivity contains immunoglobulin E (IgE)-mediated reactions as well as intolerance to mechanical, physical, and chemical impacts. Often, but not mandatory atopic eczema (AE) occurs simultaneously or delayed together with allergic rhinoconjunctivitis and/or allergic asthma, whereas the "atopic march" typically starts with AE of infancy.

There is an obvious genetic background as the risk of a child to develop an atopic disorder with no family history is around 15%; if both parents suffer from atopy-associated diseases, the incidence rises up to 60–80%.

Atopic eczema can resolve until adolescence in most of the cases however, hypersensitivity of the skin and the airways remains for the lifetime. The commonness of the disease and its particular early onset turns atopic dermatitis (AD) into a special endeavor in dermatology.

## ETIOLOGY

Patients suffering from AE reveal a barrier dysfunction of the skin (genetics) which leads to higher transepidermal water loss with consecutive xerosis cutis. Dry skin results in pruritus, which in turn causes scratch trauma with further barrier defects. Mechanical trauma induces the production of proinflammatory cytokines and chemokines recruiting inflammatory cells to the skin. In the context of constitutional barrier deficiency, consecutive advantaged penetration of irritants and allergens can foster the sensitization to environmental products. Under these inflammatory conditions, epidermal keratinocytes preferentially produce cytokines, supporting a Th2-type differentiation. In turn, Th2-associated cytokines reduce the production of antimicrobial peptides (AMPs) in keratinocytes and facilitate bacterial colonization.

After the acute exudative stage, AE develops into a chronic, squamous, and lichenified, Th1-dominated eczema. Effector cytokines of Th1 and Th2 cells determinate the histological and clinical picture of AE. With their induction of characteristic chemokine signatures they support the recruitment of eosinophils, T-cells, dendritic cells, and mast cells and the activation of epithelial and stromal cells which react via enhanced keratin production and fibrotic remodeling. Eventually, emotional stress and atopic skin inflammation can modulate the pruritus threshold or can directly cause itch which leads into a vicious circle resulting in the AE phenotype.

## GENETICS

Twin sample studies demonstrated impressively the role of genetic factors in the development of AE. The concordance rate among monozygotic twins (0.72–0.77) is significantly higher compared to heterozygotic twins (0.15–0.23). The importance of inherited factors is furthermore supported through the fact that a positive family history is the strongest risk factor for the occurrence of AE in lifetime. Numerous epidermal structural genes as well as key elements of the immune system have been identified in the past playing a crucial role in the development of the clinical picture of AE. A mutation on chromosome 1q21 in the *profilaggrin–filaggrin* gene is probably crucial factor in the pathogenesis.

Further genetic factors are known to be found in the *SPINK5* gene which encodes for the serine protease inhibitor—LEKTI. Complete loss-of-function results in Netherton syndrome and interestingly polymorphisms are found in AE patients abundantly often. In addition continuing investigations revealed that besides genetic deficiencies in barrier function, polymorphisms in tight junction-associated *Claudin*-1 gene lead to reduced protein levels of Claudin-1 and 3. These observations indicate that defects in the stratum corneum and tight junctions compromise the barrier function of AE patients.

Besides the epidermal differentiation complex further candidate genes were identified in the past on 1q23, 5q23, 5q31, 11q13m 11q22, 16p12, and 17q11 associated with an AE phenotype. Genes in these regions encode for proteins with crucial functions in the immune system [IL-4, IL-5, IL-13, GM-CSF, CCL5 (RANTES), IL-4R, IL-18 or FcεR1].

## EPIDERMAL BARRIER

Xerosis cutis is a characteristic feature of AE. It is caused via an elevated transepidermal water loss. Following mechanisms are assumed to be responsible:

- Dysregulation of ceramide constitution reduces barrier function and water-binding capacity
- Elevation of the skin pH level results in an activation of serine proteases which in turn inhibit, via the PAR2 receptor, the secretion of lamellar bodies into the stratum corneum and directly initiates inflammatory reactions

- The defect or reduction of filaggrin leads to a diminished hydration of the stratum corneum
- Epidermal barrier dysfunctions result in increased penetration of allergens into the skin resulting in allergic sensitization.

## INFLAMMATION NETWORK

In AE, epidermal keratinocytes produce thymic stromal lymphopoietin (TSLP), IL-25, and IL-33, a group of cytokines responsible for the differentiation of naïve CD4+-T-cells toward a Th2 phenotype. Recent investigations demonstrated that a dysfunction of the epidermal barrier induces the production of TSLP and IL-25 reduces the production of filaggrin. Therefore, the barrier dysfunction directly seems to promote the differentiation of IL-4, IL-5, and IL-13 producing Th2 cells.

The Th2-associated cytokines IL-4 and IL-13 instruct B cells to abundantly produce IgE, in addition IL-5 enhances the survival of eosinophils resulting in frequently observed elevated systemic eosinophil counts of AE patients.

## INNATE IMMUNITY

A severe colonization by *Staphylococcus aureus* is observed on lesional and nonlesional skin of AE patients. During the last years, it has been shown that AE patients revealed significantly lower levels of AMPs in the epidermis. Th2 cytokines, such as IL-4 and 13 downregulate AMPs. These findings together with the observations of reduced levels of human beta-defensin-2 and 3, cathelicidin LL-37, and dermicidin could explain the high susceptibility to bacterial infections.

### Pruritus and Neurogenic Inflammation

Emotional stress is an important trigger of atopic skin inflammation. Although the precise mechanisms of neuroendocrine and neuroimmunologic mechanisms are not unraveled yet it could be shown the nerve endings produce abundantly higher levels of substance P which mediates itch and inflammation.

Another recently discovered factor seems to be the cytokine IL-31 which is abundantly expressed in Th2 cells of AE patients. Transgenic mice overexpressing IL-31 through a lymphocyte-specific promoter showed severe pruritus and an AE phenotype, furthermore IL-31-challenged mice showed severe pruritus. Therefore IL-31 seems to represent a cytokine directly mediating itch from T-cells to the nervous system.

## CLINICAL PRESENTATION

The morphology of eczema in the acute stage can be characterized by poorly circumscribed erythema, edematous swelling, infiltrate, seropapules, intraepidermal vesicles, erosions, and crusts; in a later or chronic stage lichenification, excoriation, and nodules dominate. Xerosis cutis is a defining feature of atopic skin inflammation and due to the increased cholinergic response to scratches there is a so called white dermographism. Depending on the age of the patient, the clinical presentation of AD can differ enormously:

- *Atopic dermatitis of infancy*: The mainly affected areas in infancy are the scalp, cheeks, extensor aspects of the extremities, and trunk (Fig. 1). The lesions usually occur after the age of 3 months and are characterized by erythema, papules, vesicles, oozing, excoriations, and formation of crusts
- *Atopic dermatitis of childhood and adolescence*: The predilection areas tend to shift in toddlers and older children to the flexures of the elbows and knees, as well as wrists and ankles (Fig. 2)
- *Atopic dermatitis of adulthood*: In adulthood, the face is more often affected together with the head and neck region (head-neck-shoulder-dermatitis) (Fig. 3)
- *Special manifestations*: The following types of eczema can occur solitarily or in combination with other forms. Capillitium—an increased pityriasis simplex capillitii can occur due to sebostasis. Depending on severity and degree of inflammation hair loss can occur
- *Eyelids*: Isolated AE of the eyelids can be found due to exposure to allergens or irritants (Fig. 4)
- *Earlobes*: Rhagades often can be found in the earlobe region.
- *Lips*: Preferentially in the colder time of year, patients suffer from cheilitis sicca with pruritus and burning sensations (Fig. 5)
- *Hands and feet*: Common manifestations of AE are dry fingertips (pulpitis sicca) with a tendency to extension to the paronychium with the complication of severe forms of onychodystrophy. On the palms and plantar region dyshidrotic eczema can occur on the margins of the fingers and feet with itching vesicles.

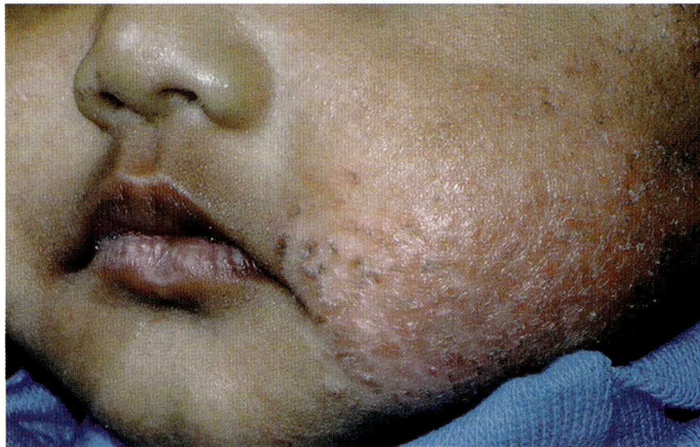

**FIG. 1:** Typical eczematous patches on cheeks in infantile atopic dermatitis.

*Courtesy*: Dr Nilendu Sarma, Associate Professor and Head, Department of Dermatology, Dr BC Roy Post Graduate Institute of Pediatric Sciences, West Bengal.

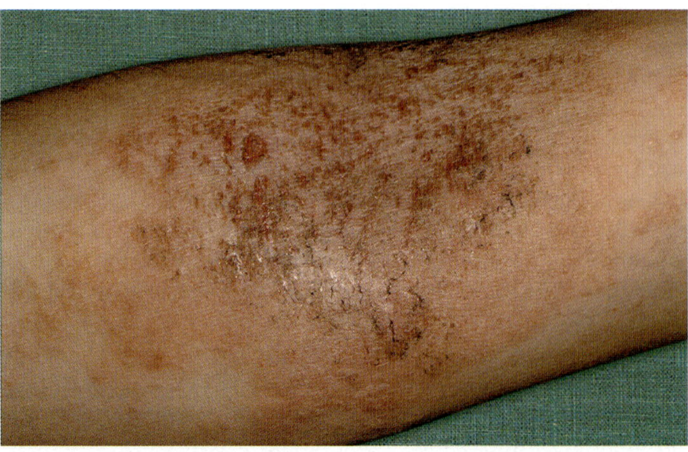

**FIG. 2:** Exudative flexural eczema.

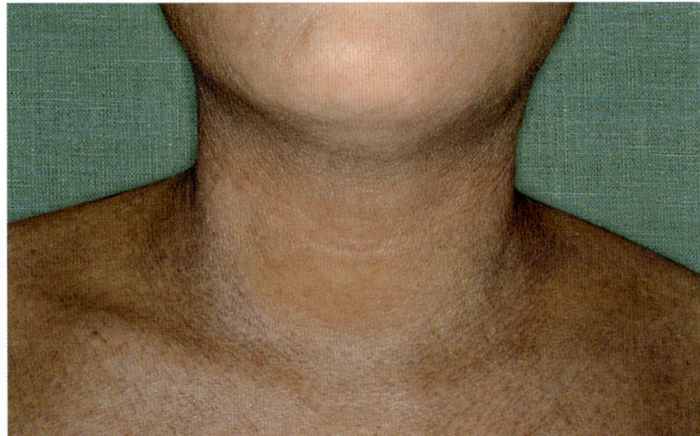

FIG. 3: Atopic eczema in adulthood.

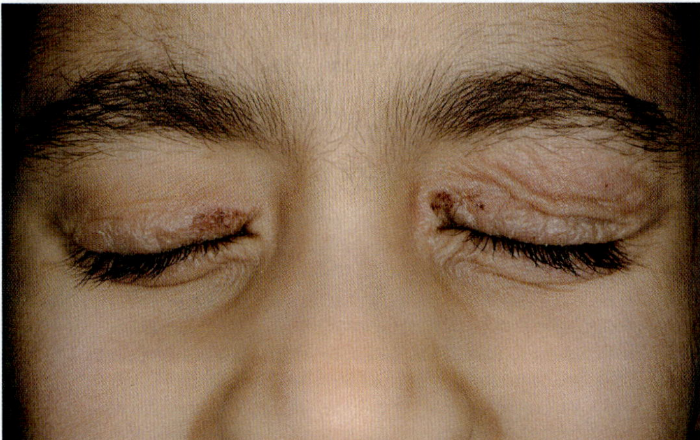

FIG. 4: Eczema of the eyelids.

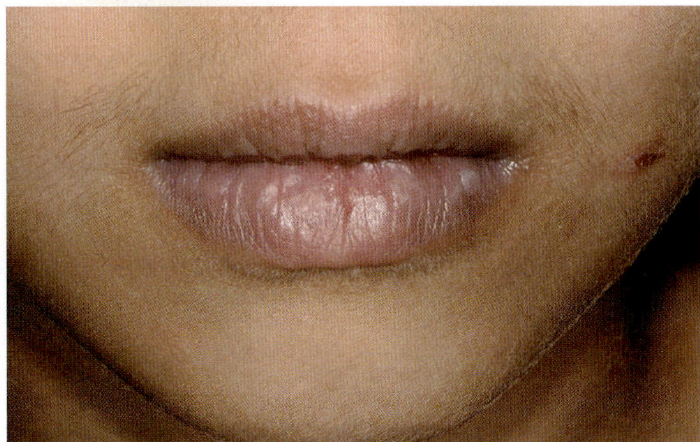

FIG. 5: Cheilitis sicca.

## HISTOLOGY

The histomorphology of AE resembles the clinical bandwidth of eczema. In the acute phase, the alterations can be very subtle with mild spongiosis, up to spongiotic blisters and orthokeratosis. In the dermis a superficial perivascular lymphohistiocytic infiltrate with eosinophils can be observed. Later stages are characterized by acanthosis with mild parakeratosis and reduced spongiosis. The inflammatory infiltrate is dominated by $CD4^+$ lymphocytes.

## DIFFERENTIAL DIAGNOSES

In infancy, seborrheic eczema, nummular eczema, and psoriasis can resemble AE. Eczematous stages of mycosis fungoides or Sézary syndrome as well as ichthyosis and psoriasis should be excluded in adolescents and adults. Furthermore scabies as a commonly occurring infection has to be differentiated from AE.

## TRIGGER FACTORS

- *Physical factors*: Physical impacts, especially if the interaction occurs intensively, long-lasting or repeatedly such as—UV exposure, irritating cloth, wool, occlusive clothing, severe sweating, soaps, and alcoholic detergents or cold and dry climate
- Immunoglobulin E-mediated reactions with delayed-type reactions. The allergen administration can occur directly through the skin or systemically via ingestion—house dust mite allergen, pollen, animal fur, and molds
- Contact urticaria and consecutive protein contact dermatitis with animal proteins such as crustacean, fish, and meat or aeroallergens. Systemically through ingestion of inhalable allergens or food
- Pseudoallergic reactions or intolerance reactions to biogenic amines such as citrus fruits
- Neurovegetative factors: Stress and psychiatric disorders
- Localized infections with *Malassezia* species and staphylococcal infections
- Systemic infections such as streptococcal, staphylococcal or HIV infection.

## COMPLICATIONS

### Bacterial Secondary Infection

Impetiginization with yellow crusts caused by *Staphylococcus aureus* is a frequently observed complication in children.

### Viral Secondary Infection

Eczema herpeticum can be observed after infection with herpes simplex virus on a preexisting eczema. Up to 3 mm in diameter measuring vesicles disrupt and leave hemorrhagic erosions. Fever, malaise, and lymph node swelling usually can be found.

Eczema molluscatum caused by molluscum contagiosum can be found in children and resolves in general spontaneously.

## DIAGNOSTIC APPROACH

Hanifin and Rajka developed the most widely used diagnostic criteria for AD which were later revised by the American Academy of Dermatology (Box 1). Several scoring systems exist to score the severity of eczema where if the most common ones are SCORAD and EASI.

### Anamnesis

Seasonal fluctuation should be inquired as well as hormonal factors such as pregnancy or menses. Especially psychological pressure, occupation, leisure activities, or contact to animals could be of interest. Hypersensitivity to food or aeroallergens must be evaluated.

**BOX 1 Diagnostic criteria according to Hanifin and Rajka. Three major and three minor criteria are mandatory**

**Major criteria**
- Pruritus
- Typical morphology
- Chronic relapsing course
- Atopy in family history

**Minor criteria**
- Sebostasis, Ichthyosis
- Type I sensitizations
- Elevated total IgE level
- Early onset of disease
- Hand- and foot eczema
- Mammillary eczema
- Cheilitis
- Relapsing conjunctivitis
- Keratoconus
- Anterior subcapsular cataract
- Periorbital dark circles
- Pruritus when sweating
- Pityriasis alba
- Keratosis follicularis
- White dermographism

## Allergy Diagnostics

Due to multiple sensitizations to allergens of AE patients, the correct identification of relevant substances becomes a diagnostic endeavor. To avoid unnecessary restrictions for the patient a distinct identification is inevitable.

Laboratory investigations should include total IgE and eosinophil cationic protein levels. Determination of specific IgE is even more important as it can give useful hints for disease-relevant allergens.

Skin testing requires areas of unaffected skin. To evaluate type-I sensitizations, prick testing should be chosen. Furthermore, epicutaneous testing is recommended to exclude relevant contact allergies.

## THERAPY

Main objectives of the therapy are to minimize the degree of the skin alterations and to reduce the number and intensity of flares.

- *Basic therapy*: The headstone of AE therapy is the use of emollients to avoid dryness of the skin and to maintain the skin barrier. The therapy must be performed constantly and repeatedly. In general, greasy formulations are recommended for very dry conditions whereas creams and lotions with higher water content should be left for mild eczemas. To elevate the water-binding capacity of the skin, urea containing preparations in a concentration of 3–5% should be applied several times a day

  The choice of the preparation depends on the patient's preferences.
- *Topical anti-inflammatory treatment*: The anti-inflammatory treatment of choice is glucocorticoids for moderate to severe AD. In the acute and lichenified phase of dermatitis, halogenated glucocorticoids of classes III or IV should be applied, after initial improvement the therapy can be reduced to glucocorticoids of classes I or II. Modern, non-atrophogenic substances should be preferred such as methylprednisolone aceponate, prednicarbate, or mometasone furoate.

  Calcineurin inhibitors, such as tacrolimus and pimecrolimus turned out to be an effective and beneficial supplement to glucocorticoids especially, when chronic causes prohibit a long-term use of glucocorticoids. Proactive treatment is an effective concept to reduce the risk of relapsing flares. After the last exacerbation is under control, two to three times a week glucocorticoids or calcineurin inhibitors will be applied to the sites likely to become active. Because the overall quantity of glucocorticoid is smaller than that used under a reactive strategy this regime should be advocated.
- *Phototherapy*: UV light has beneficial effects on widespread eczema although the long-term side effects limit its use especially for children. UVB-311 nm is proven to alleviate pruritus and UVA-1 can be beneficial for some patients in the acute phase of eczema
- *Systemic therapy*: While the new generation of non-sedative antihistamines (ebastine, desloratadine, fexofenadine, levocetirizine, mizolastine, and rupatadine) have minor effects on itch, the sedative side effect of older antihistamines such as clemastine, dimetindene, hydroxyzine or doxylamine can help the patient at night to find sleep
- *Anti-inflammatory systemic therapy*: In severe cases short-term tapered treatment with prednisolone 0.5–1 mg/kg body weight is beneficial; in children this procedure should be well-considered. Therapy refractory cases needing a long-term systemic treatment can be treated with cyclosporine in a dosage of 2.5 mg/kg body weight. To avoid the risk of long-term adverse effects the therapy should be discontinued after 2 years.

## SUGGESTED READINGS


1. Bieber T, Kraft S, Jürgens M, et al. New insights in the structure and biology of the high affinity receptor for IgE (Fc epsilon RI) on human epidermal Langerhans cells. J Dermatol Sci. 1996;13(1):71-5.
2. De Benedetto A, Kubo A, Beck LA, et al. Skin barrier disruption: a requirement for allergen sensitization? J Invest Dermatol. 2012;132(3 Pt 2):949-63.
3. De Benedetto A, Rafaels NM, McGirt LY, et al. Tight junction defects in patients with atopic dermatitis. J Allergy Clin Immunol. 2011;127(3):773-86.
4. Hanifin JM, Cooper KD, Ho VC, et al. Guidelines of care for atopic dermatitis, developed in accordance with the American Academy of Dermatology (AAD)/American Academy of Dermatology Association "Administrative Regulations for Evidence-Based Clinical Practice Guidelines". J Am Acad Dermatol. 2004;50(3): 391-404.
5. Hanifin JM, Thurston M, Omoto M, et al. The eczema area and severity index (EASI): assessment of reliability in atopic dermatitis. EASI Evaluator Group. Exp Dermatol. 2001;10(1):11-8.
6. Homey B, Steinhoff M, Ruzicka T, et al. Cytokines and chemokines orchestrate atopic skin inflammation. J Allergy Clin Immunol. 2006;118(1):178-89.
7. Irvine AD, McLean WHI, Leung DYM. Filaggrin mutations associated with skin and allergic diseases. New Engl J Medicine. 2011;365:1315-27.
8. Ong PY, Ohtake T, Brandt C, et al. Endogenous antimicrobial peptides and skin infections in atopic dermatitis. N Engl J Med. 2002;347(15):1151-60.
9. Palmer CN, Irvine AD, Terron-Kwiatkowski A, et al. Common loss-of-function variants of the epidermal barrier protein filaggrin are a major predisposing factor for atopic dermatitis. Nat Genet. 2006;38:441-6.
10. Ring J, Alomar A, Bieber T, et al. Guidelines for treatment of atopic eczema (atopic dermatitis) Part II. J Eur Acad Dermatol Venereol. 2012;26(9):1176-93.
11. Ruëff F, Bergmann KC, Brockow K, et al. Skin tests for diagnostics of allergic immediate-type reactions. Guideline of the German Society for Allergology and Clinical Immunology. Pneumologie. 2011;65(8):484-95.
12. Schultz Larsen FV, Holm NV, et al. Atopic dermatitis in a population based twin series. Concordance rates and heritability estimation. Acta Derm Venereol Suppl (Stockh). 1985;114:159.
13. Sonkoly E, Muller A, Lauerma AI, et al. IL-31: a new link between T cells and pruritus in atopic skin inflammation. J Allergy Clin Immunol. 2006;117(2):411-7.
14. Soumelis V, Reche PA, Kanzler H, et al. Human epithelial cells trigger dendritic cell mediated allergic inflammation by producing TSLP. Nat Immunol. 2002;3(7):673-80.
15. Spergel JM. From atopic dermatitis to asthma: the atopic march. Ann Allergy Asthma Immunol. 2010;105(2):99-106.
16. Severity scoring of atopic dermatitis: the SCORAD index. Consensus report of the European Task Force on Atopic Dermatitis. Dermatology. 1993;186(1):23-31.
17. Weidinger S, Illig T, Baurecht H, et al. Loss-of-function variations within the filaggrin gene predispose for atopic dermatitis with allergic sensitizations. J Allergy Clin Immunol. 2006;118(1):214-9.
18. Wollenberg A, Bieber T. Proactive therapy of atopic dermatitis--an emerging concept. Allergy. 2009;64(2):276-8.

# 11 CHAPTER Allergic Contact Dermatitis

*Nilendu Sarma*

## INTRODUCTION

Jadassohn first described allergic contact dermatitis (ACD) in 1895. An ACD is a delayed type of induced sensitivity (allergy) resulting from cutaneous contact with a specific allergen to which the patient has developed a specific sensitivity. Approximately 3,000 chemicals are well documented as specific causes of allergic contact dermatitis.

## PATHOGENESIS

Allergic contact dermatitis is a type IV hypersensitivity reaction, mediated through T-cells. The prerequisite for ACD is contact with a low molecular weight substance (<500 D) commonly known as hapten. Hapten then binds to the proteins (Box 1).

This complex is recognized by the dendritic antigen presenting cells like epidermal Langerhans cell or dermal dendritic cells. They form a complex and stimulate various costimulatory molecules and cytokines. This complex migrates to regional lymph node and is presented to the naïve T-cells in the lymph node. Hapten specific major histocompatibility complex (MHC) class I and/or MHC class II restricted T-cells are differentiate. Mostly, Th1 and Th17 subset of T-cells are differentiated.

This entire process is called sensitization phase of contact hypersensitivity (CHS).

Any subsequent exposure results in stimulation of "effector phase" of CHS. This arm of CHS is lesser explored in comparison to sensitization phase.

$CD8^+$ T-cells play significant role in effector pathways. $CD4^+$ T-cells play a suppressive role to control the tissue damage in this phase. A multitude of cytokines are known to be secreted that control the entire process. Recently, interleukin (IL)-9 has also been identified to have regulatory role through allergen-specific Th1-lymphocyte responses and stimulating IL-4 production.

Toll-like receptors (TLRs) are an important molecule in human that play great role in the innate immune system where they identify the pathogens though their molecular patterns. They have at least 11 members. TLRs are expressed on local immune cells in the skin like dendritic cells, important immune cells like macrophages, granulocytes, natural killer cells, and T-cells, and nonimmune cells, such as fibroblasts and epithelial cells.

These TLRs play important role in both allergic and irritant dermatitis, especially the elicitation phase.

Following exposure to infective or noninfective molecules, arrays of immunological alterations takes plays. This is characterized by expression of many transcription factors, synthesis of genes, and release of high number of cytokines. Toll like receptors are shown to be actively involved with these steps. Studies suggested significant role of TLRs in the elicitation phase of both ACD and irritant contact dermatitis (ICD) and relatively less role in sensitization phase.

Penetration of hapten is enhanced with defective barrier function of epidermis. Filaggrin is a protein that has important role in skin barrier. Loss of function mutation in filaggrin gene is significantly associated with atopic dermatitis (AD). Possibly, there is well-known genetic association with contact dermatitis also. However, it is unclear whether this risk is mediated through simultaneously present AD.

An important hypothesis regarding CHS is that ACD is rather more a natural phenomenon. Thus, people not developing ACD are protected by specific subset of $CD4^+$ T-cells that secret IL-10.

Inherent risk for ACD is genetically controlled. Different steps of sensitization and elicitations are controlled by different genetic loci. These steps are often specific for different chemicals.

Epidermal enzyme N-acetyltransferases (NATs) is required for during the sensitization phase for some antigens. Genetic polymorphism for of this enzyme thus regulates risk of ACD. This association is complicated. Rapid acetylating NAT1 is found to have a lower risk of paraphenylenediamine (PPD) sensitization. Chromate sensitization among cement workers has been linked to mutation in the genes for tumor necrosis factor (at position 308).

Why some individuals are more susceptible to develop ACD while others are not given the same level of exposed environment can possibly be explained by the genetic susceptibility.

**BOX 1 Haptens**

- Haptens are low-molecular weight molecule that are antigenic and induce sensitization after binding to skin protein
- Substances that need metabolic activation in skin to form a hapten are called prohapten. Metabolic activation makes them capable of biding to skin protein
- Substances that are activated outside our body form a hapten which are called prehapten

## ETIOLOGY

Although there can be large numbers of allergens leading to development of ACD, most common substances are fragrances, metals (nickel and cobalt), rubber, hair dye (p-phenylenediamine), textiles, preservatives used in cosmetics, moisturizers, and topical medications. In various reports, most commonly elicited allergens are nickel and fragrances.

## PREDISPOSING FACTORS

Any predisposing skin inflammatory condition increases the chance of ACD. The list includes irritant dermatitis, leg ulcer (especially stasis ulcer), and possibly AD. Thus, many cases of ACD are preceded by and associated with ICD.

Atopic dermatitis is also now known to increase chance for ACD. However, these two diseases have different immunological alterations. This results in different presentation of some of the observed effects of ACD.

Old age is a risk factor for sensitization but elicitation and induction of ACD is less efficient in old age.

Higher prevalence among females may be due to higher exposure rate as well as hormonal influence. Fragrance allergy is more common among males. Darker skin color (not race) races have higher skin barrier leading to lower risk of ACD than white people.

Allergic contact dermatitis is one of the most common dermatoses among occupational dermatoses, although irritant dermatitis is commoner.

## CLINICAL PRESENTATION

Allergic contact dermatitis occurs more at least twice as frequently in women than men. Prevalence of ACD among children is rising. It presents with erythema, papules, vesicles, and other features of dermatitis or eczema (Figs 1 and 2).

Pigmentation or depigmentation may follow when eczematous lesions heal (Fig. 3). Pigmentary alterations or other noneczematous presentation may also develop as primary manifestation (Fig. 4).

Presentation may vary based on the locations and etiologic agents.

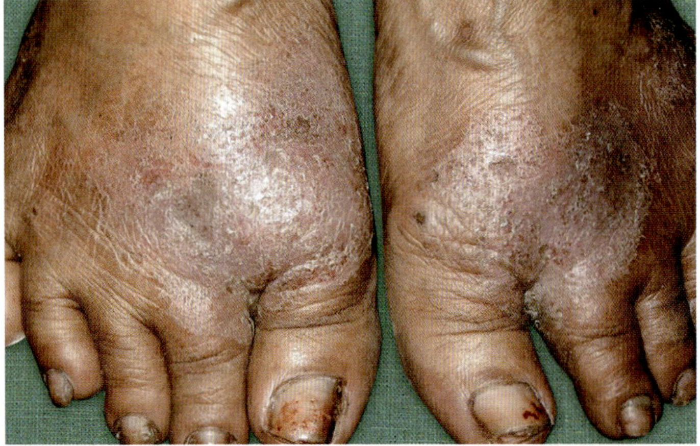

**FIG. 1:** Eczematous lesions due to allergic contact dermatitis to footwear.

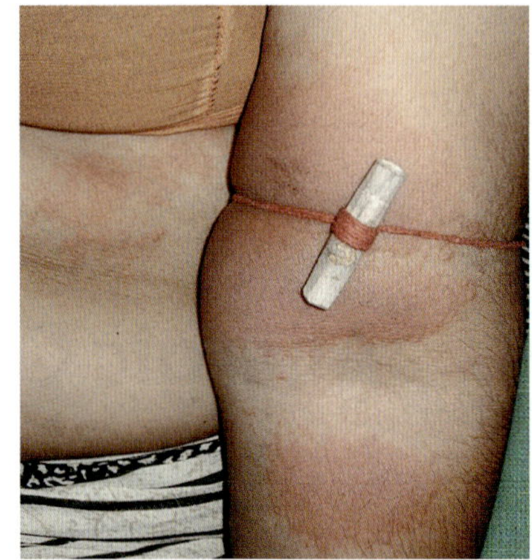

**FIG. 2:** Allergic contact dermatitis to azo dye present in red colored cord.

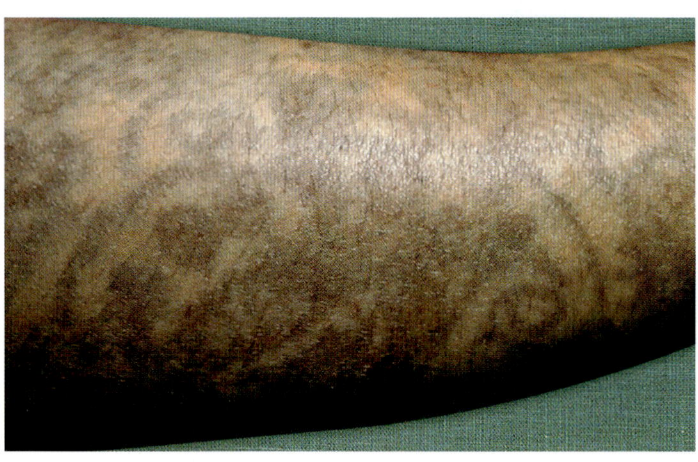

**FIG. 3:** Postinflammatory hyperpigmentation following allergic contact dermatitis to henna.

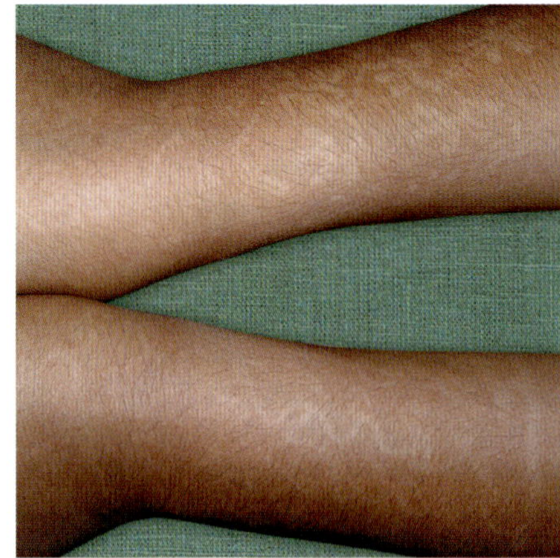

**FIG. 4:** Chemical leukoderma developing following henna application.

### Regional Dermatitis

#### Eyelid and Periorbital Areas

Eyelid is considered to be one of the top body locations affected by ACD along with face and hands. On the other hand, ACD is the most common cause (about 81%) of all cases of eyelid dermatitis. Eyelid has a thinner skin. Rubbing causes damage of eyelid skin

**TABLE 1: Common allergens in eyelid and periorbital areas**

| Source | Allergenic substances |
|---|---|
| Airborne allergens | Plant allergens, weed pollens |
| **Cosmetics** | |
| Fragrances | Fragrance mix, Balsam of Peru |
| Eyeliners, mascara, eye shadow | Shellac, black iron oxide |
| Preservative in eye cosmetics | Paraben, phenyl mercuric acetate (antimicrobial), imidazolidinyl urea (formaldehyde releaser used as antimicrobial), quaternium-15 (formaldehyde releaser used as antimicrobial), and ditertiarybutyl hydroquinone (antioxidant) |
| Nail products like acrylic nails, polishes, hardeners, repair agents, and wraps | Tosylamide, formaldehyde resin, and acyrlates |
| **Eye medications** | |
| Preservatives and antibiotics | Neomycin sulfate, benzalkonium (preservative), thimerosal 10% (preservative), phenyl mercuric acetate, chlorobutanol, chlorhexidine |

leading to enhanced penetration of chemicals. Both allergic and irritant dermatitis are common in eyelids. Irritant dermatitis is also common in eyelids. Personal care products and cosmetics (used for eyelid or other areas like face, scalp, and body) account for most of cases of eyelid ACD. Apart from primarily eye care products, airborne allergens, and any substances used on scalp, face, and hands can cause ACD of eyelid even when site of primary contact may not show any signs of allergy. Other causes that can have a similar presentation are seborrheic dermatitis, AD, irritant dermatitis, and sometimes psoriasis (Table 1).

Ophthalmic solutions are less common cause of periobital dermatitis as found in North American study. This area is more commonly sensitized by nickel and fragrances.

## Face and Lips

Allergic contact dermatitis on face is almost always bilateral. The exception being ACD from nail cosmetics that occurs unilaterally. Allergic contact dermatitis may develop on lips due to cosmetics, lipsticks, food preservatives, and tooth pastes (Fig. 5).

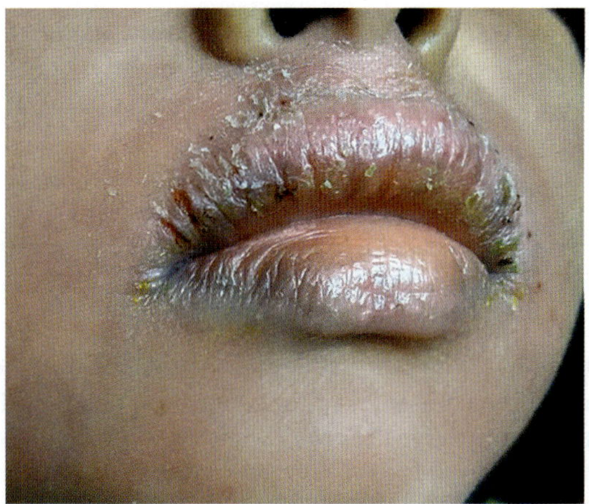

**FIG. 5:** Allergic contact dermatitis on lips due to contact allergy to preservatives.

## Ear

Mild degree of ACD from shampoo and hair dye may primarily or exclusively affect the ear helix. Allergic contact dermatitis may involve other parts of ear depending on the source of allergy. Allergy may develop from ear preparations containing neomycin, framycetin, gentamicin, sulfonamide, benzocaine (local anesthetic), parabens, and topical corticosteroids. Prior infection of the external ear or trauma from habitual insertion of objects may precipitate or aggravate the condition. Other sources of allergy are ear ring, hearing aid, and metals from spectacle.

## Neck

Common causes are metals from chains. Allergic contact dermatitis may also develop from cosmetics. "Fiddler's neck" develops from contact with violin.

## Genitals

Allergic contact dermatitis may involve male and female genital areas like vulva, scrotum, and penis. Deodorant sprays may cause allergy in vulva from the preservatives and antibacterial agents. Spermicides containing hexylresorcinol, nonoxyl, phenylmercuric acetate, and borate can cause allergy. Occasionally, nail cosmetics, including wet nail polish, textiles (dyes, resins), and medications can also cause allergy in vulva. Irritant dermatitis may develop from spermicides as well as soaps. Allergy from rubber condom in sensitive individuals may develop in both males and females. Moreover, allergy from substances used by the female partners (spermicides, hygienic sprays, or medications) may affect male partners.

# DIAGNOSIS

Clinical suspicion is of prime importance. Mostly, ACD presents with dermatitis or eczema. However, noneczematous presentations are also not uncommonly encountered.

Site of primary contact with the substance that cause allergic reaction may not develop allergy.

It is interesting to know that many times, sites away from the primary exposure develop allergy. Thus, substances used on head or hair causes allergy on face, nail cosmetics leading to allergy on face or eyelids. This is called ectopic ACD.

Allergic contact dermatitis has to be differentiated from many other common conditions (Box 2).

## Patch Test

Patch test is scientific method to identify the cause of allergic contact dermatitis. Despite many difficulty and limitations, this is considered the gold standard method for etiological diagnosis of ACD.

**BOX 2 Differential diagnosis of allergic contact dermatitis**

- Atopic dermatitis
- Irritant contact dermatitis
- Dyshidrotic dermatitis
- Seborrheic dermatitis
- Psoriasis
- Pruritic conditions with nonspecific eruptions
- Dermatitis herpetiformis
- Rare forms of eczema like mycosis fungoides

**BOX 3 Grading of patch test reactions**

| | |
|---|---|
| ? | Faint erythema, nonpalpable. Doubtful reaction |
| + | Nonvesicular, erythema, slight infiltration (edema) or few micro-papules. Weak reaction |
| ++ | Vesicles, erythema, papules, infiltration. Strong reaction |
| +++ | Bulla. Very strong reaction |
| NR | Negative reaction |
| IR | Irritant reaction |
| NT | Not tested |

## Principles and Method

List of allergens are applied to back inside a closed chamber (Finn chamber) on the back and kept in contact for 48 hours. The area is read after another 24–48 hours. Allergens to which individual is already sensitized, will show allergic reactions (positive test). The principal is simple and straightforward. If someone has contact allergy to some substance, the same allergen, when applied for sufficient period on other areas of body like back should also show signs of sensitization.

Patch testing is advocated when allergic contact dermatitis is suspected and also in any other cases of eczema that is resistant to standard treatment. Another important indication is any type of skin and mucosal eruptions, including delayed drug eruptions where delayed-type hypersensitivity is suspected.

Patch test should be postponed in any individual suffering from active dermatitis of severe degree or generalized nature undergoing an immunosuppressive treatment and test site either showing active dermatitis, recently treated with topical corticosteroids within last 7 days, or undergone ultraviolet ray exposure.

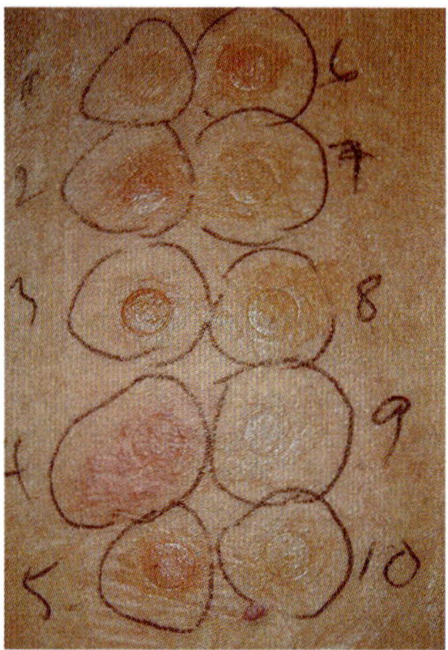

FIG. 6: Positive reaction to nickel.

## Interpretation of Patch Test

Interpretation of patch test is based on severity of reaction that is classified into few grades (Box 3).

### *Irritant Reaction*

An irritant reaction (IR) has as "glazed" appearance. A reaction present mostly over the edge is also indicative of IR. Other features that suggest IR are follicular papules and pustules. More severe IR may appear as burn like area or even necrosis. Features that suggest IR is sharply localized area of reaction that heals faster than allergic reaction. Allergic reaction, on the other hand, when strong, can spread beyond the margin of patch test chamber, shows progressively stronger reaction on second visit (72/96 h) than first visit (48 h) and heals slowly (Figs 6 and 7). Distinction is difficult or even impossible when the reaction is milder.

Equivocal reaction or weak reaction: This is not sure what does a weak reaction that presents as erythema with or without slight edematous appearance indicate. This may represent either allergy or irritant reaction.

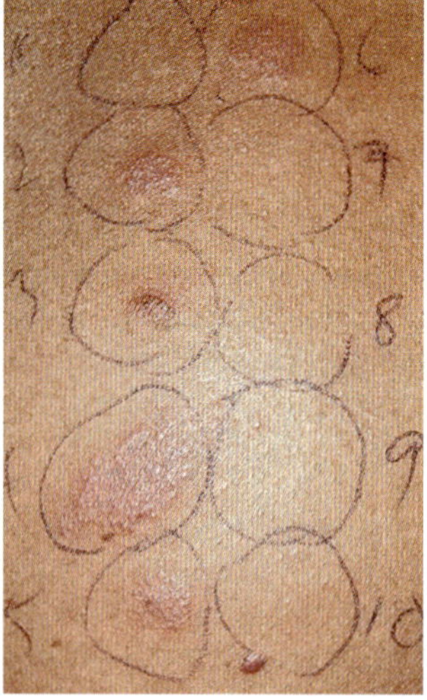

FIG. 7: Stronger reaction to nickel and new positive reactions to few other allergens.

### *Relevance*

A positive test reaction has less importance unless the relevance of such reaction to practical life can be elicited. Positive reaction may indicate a past sensitization and may not be related to present dermatitis. A positive reaction is said to be relevant when this allergen is found to be the cause of present dermatitis (as primary or aggravating factor for the present dermatitis). Assessment of relevance is the most difficult job in diagnostic evaluation of ACD. Detailed clinical history, use test, and work-site visit to understand the exposure status is often required to assess the relevance.

### *Cause*

Many substances can cause both allergy and irritation depending upon the concentration of it and the hyper-irritability of the skin. Cleaning the area of patch testing with soaps or solvents increases the chance of irritant reaction. Presence of active eczematous disease elsewhere and use of a nonstandard allergen.

## Modification of Standard Methods

### Photopatch Test

When photocontact dermatitis is suspected, photopatch test is done with the standard photoallergen series. Patches are applied in duplicate. One set is irradiated with ultraviolet A light, 5 J/cm$^2$ after 48 hours (or 24 h). Reading is taken simultaneously on both sides at 72–96 hours. A positive reaction at exposed side and not on unexposed side reflects positive photoallergy.

This method is applied to check allergy from any substances present in a finished product. Another use of open test is to detect the contact urticaria.

In open test, the substance is applied directly on the skin (e.g., retroauricular area in suspected contact urticaria) and reading is done at 15–30 minutes after application.

There are many modification and variation of open test. If the pen test is negative and immediate reactions are excluded, the test area is covered with tape and thus open test is converted into closed test. This is called semi-open test.

Sometimes, the substance (usually cosmetics) is directly applied on the antecubital fossa, twice daily for 7 days over an area of 3 cm diameter. This is called "repeated open application test (ROAT)" or "use test."

The major reason why open test is used instead of standard closed patch test is nonavailability of suspected allergens in standard concentration. When a finished product is used for patch testing when standard concentration of the allergens are unknown and not available, open test is a recommended method before closed patch is done.

Open test generally does not show IR. This is another advantage of open test over closed test.

## Problems Associated with Patch Test

### False Negative Test

- Patch test, although reproduces a situation that is very close to real life, cannot be the same. Sweating, damaged skin, pre-existing skin condition, and repeated exposure of variable duration are all important factors that controls sensitization in real life
- Nonavailability of allergen
- Very high or very low concentration of allergen. If high, there may be an IR and if low, there may a false negative reaction
- Faulty method or improper fixation of patch
- Prolonged topical corticosteroid used at the site of patch test may result in a negative test.

### Ways to Minimize False Negative Test

- In case of negative reaction, if the suspicion is high, then a final reading should be done on 7$^{th}$ day. There are some allergens that can show a delayed positive reaction
- In some cases, ultraviolet rays play important role in inducing contact dermatitis. Photopatch test should be done in such cases instead of standard patch test that may result in a negative test.

#### *Anaphylaxis*

Anaphylactic reaction from patch test material is very rare. Penicillin, neomycin, gentamicin, and natural rubber are reported to cause anaphylactic reaction. This is considered similar to stage-3 contact urticaria syndrome.

#### *Angry Back Syndrome or Excited Skin Syndrome*

A strongly positive reaction to some allergen can lead to false positive reaction to other allergens. This often happens if patch test is done when the patient has active eczema at some areas. These false positive reactions are generally not seen when they are tested sequentially or tested at different site away from the allergen that showed a strong reaction.

# MANAGEMENT

Diagnosis of allergen by patch test is the only scientific approach to management of ACD. This should be attempted in all cases. However, this is not possible in many situations. Patch testing with unknown allergens is difficult and may not be safe.

Avoidance of allergens is the most crucial step. For occupational ACD, workplace visit by the specially trained personnel may be of great value. Avoidance of exposure to allergens can be attempted with using gloves during work, barrier creams, and substitution of job are important primary steps that can minimize the damage and necessity for use of strong medications. Not all these are feasible in all cases. Using gloves may not be practical in all working atmosphere. Barrier creams are not highly effective or recommended. But stringent avoidance policy remains the mainstay in the management of allergic contact dermatitis.

Based on severity, topical corticosteroid is generally the first line therapy. Ample use of moisturizers is also helpful in restoring the skin barrier defect. When this fails, other drugs can be used. An oral retinoids called alitretinoin is reported to be highly effective in chronic hand eczema. Topical Grenz rays, ultraviolet B, psoralen, and ultraviolet A are also found to be of benefit in chronic hand eczema. In acute and extensive cases, systemic corticosteroid can be used for short course.

In nickel allergic cases, nickel elimination diet has been shown to be useful.

# SPECIAL FORMS OF ALLERGIC CONTACT DERMATITIS

## Systemic Contact Type Dermatitis

This is a special type of contact dermatitis where systemic exposure of a substance, to which the individual has developed sensitization from previous exposure, leads to extensive eruptions of various patterns. Systemic exposure may occur through oral or other mucosal route, inhalation, and injection.

### Etiology

Many allergens are present in substances that are available for cutaneous contact (cosmetics, topical drugs, and occupational exposure) as well as in substances that can be taken orally (drugs, foods) or other routes. These allergens can cause systemic contact type dermatitis (SCTD). Nickel, chromate, and cobalt are common allergen causing dyshidrotic eruptions (Box 4).

**BOX 4 Important causes of systemic contact dermatitis**

- *Metals*: Mercury, nickel, gold
- *Fragrances*: Balsam of Peru
- *Formaldehyde*: Preservative in textiles, cosmetics, detergents, instant coffee
- Plants and herbal products: Compositae and Anacardiaceae
- *Medications*: Neomycin, gentamicin antibacterials, corticosteroids, and aminophylline
- *Others*: Aspartame (artificial sweetener)

**BOX 5 Clinical manifestations of systemic contact type dermatitis**

- Dyshidrotic hand eczema
- Eczematous rash
- Predominantly flexural, and generalized maculopapular rash
- Erythema multiforme like rash
- Vasculitic eruptions
- Urticaria and anaphylaxis
- Flare up of previously positive patch test site
- Systemic manifestations

## Clinical Presentations

Clinical manifestations can be varied (Box 5). In some cases, there may be systemic manifestations like nausea, vomiting, headache, and fever. Symmetrical drug-related intertriginous and flexural exanthema, also known as Baboon's syndrome (a term that is better avoided), is possibly a manifestation of SCTD. Although this is shown to be precipitated by systemic exposure to some drugs, now it is known that previous topical sensitization may not be important in most of the cases. Known etiologies are penicillin V, amoxicillin, erythromycin, aminophylline, nickel, and mercury.

## Diagnosis

Patch testing with the suspected allergen is generally positive and confirmatory. In patients with drug induced skin rash including eczematous rash, erythema multiforme (EM)-like rash, vasculitic or maculopapular rashes, patch test can be done after 6–12 weeks after complete healing of rashes. Patch testing is preferable in such cases than more risky oral provocation test. Patch testing with any new substances should be initially done with open test followed by standard patch test.

Positive patch test for some drugs like penicillin excludes its systemic use. In many cases of true penicillin allergy, patch test is positive even when intracutanoeus test is negative.

# Primary Endogenous Contact Eczema

This is reverse of SCTD. Here allergens, mostly drugs, are sensitized through systemic exposure. When these substances were subsequently applied topically, develop localized eczema.

# Noneczematous Presentation of Allergic Contact Dermatitis

Contact dermatitis can present without eczema, the classical manifestation. Noneczematous manifestations can be of many types (Box 6).

**BOX 6 Noneczematous allergic contact dermatitis**

- Pigmented CD
- Contact leukoderma
- Lichenoid CD
- Erythema multiforme-like CD
- Purpuric CD
- Acneiform CD
- Pustular CD
- Dyshidrotic CD
- Granuloma gluteale infantum
- Granulomatous CD (as seen in tattoos)
- Lymphomatoid CD
- Primarily dermal involvement (to metal or hydroquinone)
- Scleroderma like CD (due to organic solvents)
- Edematous CD (e.g., PPD)

CD, contact dermatitis; PPD, paraphenylenediamine.

## Erythema Multiforme-like Contact Dermatitis

This is one of the most common noneczematous CDs. Common allergens are exotic woods and plants, medicaments, and ethylenediamine.

Topical medications like sulfonamide, promethazine, neomycin, topical nonsteroid anti-inflammatory drugs like phenylbutazone, and topical corticosteroids, budesonide, and metals like nickel and cobalt are known induce EM-like CD. Erythema multiforme-like lesions are preceded by eczematous lesions at contact site. Post-sensitization and possibly due to systemic exposure, EM-like rash develops with wider distribution.

## Pigmented Contact Dermatitis

People with darker skin types are at higher risk. White people generally develop eczematous eruptions. Common site of pigmentation is forehead, temporal, and zygomatic areas of face. Other areas like lips and axilla thighs are also commonly affected.

There may or may not be any preceding inflammatory phase and pigmentation generally develops without any signs of dermatitis. Face is the commonest area where pigmentation can develop following ACD. Photocontact dermatitis is a common cause of pigmented CD. In Japan, Riehl's melanosis is used almost synonymously with pigmented CD (Fig. 8).

This is possibly a form of idiosyncratic reaction with definite role of genetic susceptibility.

Allergen induced inflammation stimulates the enzymatic activity of melanocytes leading pigmentation.

Initial cases of pigmented CD were from optical whitener (Tinopal CH 3566) that was used in washing powders. There was an epidemic of pigmented CD from azo dye Naphthol AS used in textile. Other azo dyes like Brilliant Lake Red R and Sudan-1 are reported to induce this. Kumkum (bindi, used in India) is a special source of pigmented CD in India. Kumkum contains azo dyes.

Nowadays, commonly implicated allergens are fragrances like hydroxycitronella, benzyle salicylates, and jasmine. Other causes are para-tertiary butylphenol resin (leather), bactericides, and chromates.

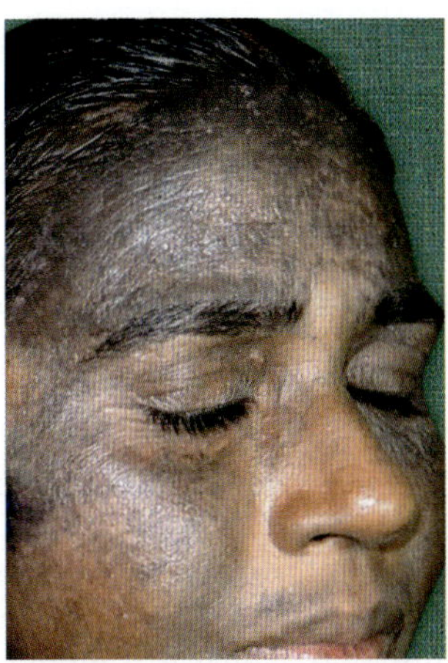

FIG. 8: Pigmented contact dermatitis involving forehead and sides of face.

### Diagnosis

Suspected allergens can be detected with patch test, photopatch test, use test, and ROAT.

### Management

Removal of allergens is most important step.

## Chemical Leukoderma

Chemical leukoderma (CL) occurs due to repeated contact with some chemicals. This is also known as occupational leukoderma, occupational vitiligo, and contact leukoderma.

### Etiology

Chemical leukoderma occurs from commonly used substances like rubber, plastic, resin, adhesives, detergent, alta, bindi, deodorants, and hair dye, as well as from industrial substances of like tar and tar products, industrial oils, and printing ink. Chemical leukoderma is reported from polyvinyl chloride (stethoscope ear piece) and cinnamic aldehyde (toothpaste) (Box 7).

### Etiopathogenesis

Melanocytes are possibly destroyed. Melanogenesis might be blocked from yet unknown mechanism. Due to their structural similarity with tyrosinase, catechols and phenols can destroy the melanocytes. Free radical formation, apoptosis, and monobenzyl ether of hydroquinone induces necrosis are proposed mechanism.

**BOX 7 Agents causing chemical leukoderma**

- Derivatives of phenols and catechols, monobenzylether of hydroquinone: Para-tertiary butyl phenol, para-tertiary butyl phenol formaldehyde, para-tertiary octyl phenol, para-tertiary butyl catechol, para-tertiary amylphenol
- Sulfhydryls, mercurials, arsenics, cinnamic aldehyde, p-phenylenediamine
- Drugs like chloroquine and fluphenazine, eserine and thiotepa (otic preparation), azelaic acid, corticosteroids, imatinib mesylate, hydroquinone, azo dyes (present in alta, lipsticks, lipliner, eyeliners, etc.)
- Skin brightening cosmetics: Rhododendrol, raspberry ketone, hydroquinone monomethyl ether, p-hydroxyphenylacetamide

Increased expression of heat shock protein and tumor necrosis factor-related apoptosis-inducing ligand on the dendritic cells have been detected.

It should be understood that CL can result from both ACD and ICD.

### Clinical Presentations

Depigmented or hypopigmented macules develop after repeated contact with allergen. Shape and distribution often indicate the contact with the suspected allergen (Fig. 4). However, CL may develop at areas away from the contact of allergen. Visible inflammation is often absent in contrast to postinflammatory leukoderma.

Clinically, differentiation from postinflammatory leukoderma or vitiligo is difficult. There are suggestions that this may actually represent a subtype of vitiligo.

### Diagnosis

Patch test should be performed. Result is, however, often negative or may take long time to become positive. Repeated open application test may be a better alternative. Test site may develop depigmentation that may be hazardous.

### Management

Contact with suspected substances should be avoided. Topical corticosteroid, calcineurin inhibitor, phototherapy, photochemotherapy, and 308 nm excimer laser therapy have been used.

## Contact Urticaria

Contact urticaria can be of two types—immunologic and non-immunologic.

### Nonimmunologic Contact Urticaria

Contact with some substances stimulates direct mast cells release leading to nonimmunologic contact urticaria (NICU) that usually develops within 45 minutes after first exposure. Urticaria is associated with sensations like tingling and itching. Cinnamic acid, cinnamic aldehyde, sorbic acid, and benzoic acids are common agents. This is more common than immunologic contact urticaria (ICU). This is a local reaction and systemic manifestations are generally not seen. Urticaria develops on intact skin but it depends on concentration of the substances. High concentration is generally required to develop urticaria (Box 8).

### Immunologic Contact Urticaria

Common agent causing ICU is latex protein present in natural rubber latex (NRL). Food proteins, generally uncooked can cause ICU. Drugs (antibiotics), preservatives, fragrances, animal dander, and human semen are reported to induce ICU. Immunologic contact urticaria is more common in damaged skin and in atopics.

### Combined Nonimmunologic Contact Urticaria and Immunologic Contact Urticaria

Some agents may induce both allergic and nonallergic contact urticaria. Nonimmunologic contact urticarial develop first time. Immunologic contact urticarial manifest with subsequent exposure. This is seen with some arthropod bite (Box 9).

Four stages of contact urticaria have been described in box 10.

**BOX 8 Agents causing nonimmunologic contact urticarial**

- Cinnamic acid
- Cinnamic aldehyde
- Sorbic acid
- Benzoic acids
- Preservatives
- Fragrances present in food or cosmetics (shampoo, mouthwash, and chewing gum)

**BOX 9 Agents causing immunologic contact urticaria**

- Natural rubber latex
- *Foods*: Milk protein (casein), egg white, potato, sea foods (fish), chicken, lamb, beef, peach skin, and banana (often cross reaction with natural rubber latex allergy)
- *Drugs*: Neomycin, bacitracin, chloramphenicol, chlorhexidine, diphencyclopropenone, dinitrochlorobenzene, topical vitamin E
- Preservatives, vehicles, and other associated ingredients like paraben, benzyl alcohol, polyethylene glycol
- *Metals*: Nickel
- Formaldehyde

**BOX 10 Stages of contact urticaria**

- Localized reaction (redness and swelling) with nonspecific symptoms (burning, itching, tingling)
- Generalized reaction
- Extracutaneous symptoms (rhinoconjunctivitis, oropharyngeal, and gastrointestinal dysfunction)
- Anaphylactic shock

### *Clinical Presentation*

Urticaria develops within 30–45 minutes after exposure. Immunologic contact urticarial requires past exposure. Some individuals may develop dermatitis that may be clinically indistinguishable from ACD especially when involves classic sites of ACD like hands. Both ICU and NICU may manifest with eczema preceded by urticaria. As mentioned, NICU is localized disease. In contrast, ICU may, in some cases be more severe with systemic involvement and even develop anaphylaxis. This dermatitis is not mediated through delayed hypersensitivity, so patch test is negative.

### *Diagnosis*

Immediate patch test/contact test is positive. There may many reasons for a negative test. Testing may result in anaphylaxis. Thus, it should be done with complete arrangement to manage such reaction. Patch test in NICU should be done only in intact skin. Chance of patch test positive reaction in ICU increases when it is done in previously affected skin or even in eczematous skin or with a scratch test. When ICU is suspected in eczema (e.g., hand eczema), scratch patch test or immediate patch test with suspected raw and whole foods may be required.

### *Treatment*

Antihistamines are effective in both ICU and NICU. Nonsteroidal anti-inflammatory drugs are a drugs (topical and systemic) can inhibit NICU.

## Lichenoid Contact Dermatitis

Lichen planus-like eruptions may develop on skin and mucous membrane. This is relatively rare. Common allergens are paraphenylenediamine, nickel, epoxy resins, aminoglycoside antibiotics, and methacrylic acid esters. The source of PPD is various color developers like Kodak CD2, Kodak CD3 (used in film processing industry). Hair dye is another source of PPD. Resins used in dental material can cause oral mucosal lesions.

Diagnosis can be done with patch testing that develops mostly eczematous eruptions and sometimes lichenoid lesions.

## Lymphomatoid Contact Dermatitis

Lymphomatoid CD or pseudolymphomatous CD is a rare entity. The first case of lymphomatoid CD was from phosphorus sesquisulfide from match box and it was reported in 1976 by Orbaneja et al. Many of the cases in Europe were due a chemical named dimethyl fumarate, which is a mould inhibitor used in leather furniture. This is why the distribution involved typically hips and legs and its description as "toxic sofa" dermatitis. Other known allergen causing this form of CD are rubber chemicals, dyes, metals (nickel, gold sodium thiosulfate, and cobalt naphthenate), preservatives, and isopropylamino diphenylamine.

Typical distribution includes pelvis, hips, and lower legs that mimics the bathing trunk distribution of mycosis fungoides (MF). These is a male predominance. This polyclonal T-cell disorder shares many clinical and histological features that closely simulate classical MF.

Unlike all other cases of CD, this is primarily limited to adult and older population (average ages of 57–80 years) further making the differential diagnosis difficult.

Diagnosis is difficult in many cases even histology as subbasal band like lymphocytic infiltration and intraepidermal mononuclear cells simulating Pautrier's microabscess are noted in epidermis. Spongiosis in the epidermis, when present is helpful.

## SUGGESTED READINGS


1. Antico A, Soana R. Chronic allergic-like dermatopathies in nickel sensitive patients. Results of dietary restrictions and challenge with nickel salts. Allergy Asthma Proc. 1999;20:235-42.
2. Blömeke B, Brans R, Coenraads PJ, et al. Para-phenylenediamine and allergic sensitization: Risk modification by N-acetyltransferase 1 and 2 genotypes. Br J Dermatol. 2009;161:1130-5.
3. Bonamonte D, Foti C, Vestita M, et al. Noneczematous contact dermatitis. ISRN Allergy. 2013;2013:361746.
4. Bourke J, Coulson I, English J. Guidelines for the management of contact dermatitis: An update. Br J Dermatol. 2009;160:946-54.
5. Brasch J, Becker DT, Aberer W et al. S1-guidelines of the German Contact Allergy Group (DKG) of the German Dermatology Society (DDG), the Information Network of Dermatological Clinics (IVDK), the German Society for Allergology and Clinical Immunology (DGAKI), the Working Group for Occupational and Environmental Dermatology (ABD) of the DDG, the Medical Association of German Allergologists (AeDA), the Professional Association of German Dermatologists (BVDD) and the DDG. Allergo J Int. 2014;23:126-38.
6. Cavani A, Nasorri F, Prezzi C, et al. Human CD4þ T lymphocytes with remarkable regulatory functions on dendritic cells and nickel-specific Th1 immune responses. J Invest Dermatol. 2000;14:295-302
7. Bangert C, Friedl J, Stary G, et al. Immunopathologic features of allergic contact dermatitis in humans: Participation of plasmacytoid dendritic cells in the pathogenesis of the disease? J Invest Dermatol. 2003;121:1409-18.
8. de Jongh CM, Khrenova L, Verberk MM, et al. Loss-of-function polymorphisms in the filaggrin gene are associated with an increased susceptibility to chronic irritant contact dermatitis: A case-control study. Br J Dermatol. 2008;159:621-7.
9. Guin JD. Eyelid dermatitis: A report of 215 patients. Contact Dermatitis. 2004; 50:87-90.

10. Johansen JD, Aalto-Korte K, Agner T, et al. European Society of Contact Dermatitis guideline for diagnostic patch testing—recommendations on best practice. Contact Dermatitis. 2015;73:195-221.
11. Liu J, Harberts E, Tammaro A, et al. IL-9 regulates allergen-specific Th1 responses in allergic contact dermatitis. J Invest Dermatol. 2014;134:1903-11.
12. Kawai T, Akira S. Toll-like receptor and their crosstalk with other innate receptors in infection and immunity. Immunity. 2011;34:637-50.
13. Kezic S, O'Regan GM, Yau N, et al. Levels of filaggrin degradation products are influenced by both filaggrin genotype and atopic dermatitis severity. Allergy. 2011;66:934-40.
14. Krob HA, Fleischer AB Jr, D'Agostino R Jr, et al. Prevalence and relevance of contact dermatitis allergens: A meta-analysis of 15 years of published T.R.U.E. test data. J Am Acad Dermatol. 2004;51:349-53.
15. Maibach HI, Johnson HL. Contact urticaria syndrome: Contact urticaria to diethyltoluamide (immediate-type hypersensitivity). Arch Dermatol. 1975;111: 726-30.
16. Orbaneja JG, Diez LI, Lozano JL, et al. Lymphomatoid contact dermatitis: A syndrome produced by epicutaneous hypersensitivity with clinical features and a histopathologic picture similar to that of mycosis fungoides. Contact Dermatitis. 1976;2:139-43.
17. Peiser M, Tralau T, Heidler J, et al. Allergic contact dermatitis: Epidemiology, molecular mechanisms, in vitro methods and regulatory aspects. Current knowledge assembled at an international workshop at BfR, Germany. Cell Mol Life Sci. 2012;69:763-81.
18. Rai R, Shenoy MM, Viswanath V, et al. Contact sensitivity in patients with venous leg ulcer: A multi-centric Indian study. Int Wound J. 2018;1-5.
19. Reed JT, Ghadially R, Elias PM. Skin type, but neither race nor gender, influence epidermal permeability barrier function. Arch Dermatol. 1995;131: 1134-8.
20. Sarma N, Ghosh S. Clinico-allergological pattern of allergic contact dermatitis among 70 Indian children. Indian J Dermatol Venereol Leprol. 2010;76:38-44.
21. Sarma N, Samson JF. Chemical leukoderma. In: Majid I, ed. IADVL Recent advances in dermatology. Jaypee Brothers Medical Publishers (P) Ltd. New Delhi. 2016, 206-210.
22. Sarma N, Samson JF. Pigmented contact dermatitis. In: Majid I, ed. IADVL Recent advances in dermatology. Jaypee Brothers Medical Publishers (P) Ltd. New Delhi. 2016, 238-240.
23. Sarma N. Late reaction, persistent reaction and doubtful allergic reaction: the problems of interpretation. Indian J Dermatol. 2009;54(1):56-8.
24. Knackstedt TJ, Zug KA. T cell lymphomatoid contact dermatitis: A challenging case and review of the literature. Contact Dermatitis. 2014;72:65-74.
25. Usatine RP, Riojas M. Diagnosis and management of contact dermatitis. Am Fam Physician. 2010;82:249-55.
26. Wang BJ, Shiao JS, Chen CJ, et al. Tumour necrotizing factor-a promoter and GST-T1 genotype predict skin allergy to chromate in cement workers in Taiwan. Contact Dermat. 2007;57(5):309-15.
27. Warshaw EM, Belsito DV, Taylor JS, et al. North American Contact Dermatitis Group patch test results: 2009 to 2010. Dermatitis. 2013;24:50-9.
28. Wilson LD, Hinds GA, Yu JB. Age, race, sex, stage, and incidence of cutaneous lymphoma. Clin Lymphoma Myeloma Leuk. 2012:12:291-6.

# 12 CHAPTER Irritant Dermatitis

*Nilendu Sarma*

## INTRODUCTION

Irritant contact dermatitis (ICD) also known as irritant reaction (IR) is nonimmunological damage of the skin and occurs due to direct contact with some irritant substances. Unlike allergic contact dermatitis (ACD), there is no role of any form of sensitization and T-cells. Important differences between allergic and irritant dermatitis is given in table 1. Irritant dermatitis often predisposes enhanced sensitization leading to increased chances of allergic contact dermatitis.

## PATHOGENESIS

In contrast to ACD that is immunologically mediated, there is no sensitization phase in ICD. Recent knowledge on the pathogenesis of contact dermatitis however indicates that there might be significant overlap in the pathogenic mechanism between ICD and ACD. Many, if not most of the substances, can induce both allergic and irritant dermatitis. Immunological mechanisms are possibly important in ICD also. IR results in damage of the epidermal barrier and keratinocytes, and subsequent release of cytokines, upregulation of adhesion molecules. Tumor necrosis factor (TNF)-$\alpha$ is now shown to play an important role.

Damage in the skin from ICD depends on strength of irritant, duration of contact, frequency of exposure, pre-existing condition of the skin, and associated conditions that also damage the skin barrier. There are some diseases where there is impaired skin barrier function like atopic dermatitis. These can aggravate or increase the chance of ICD.

Filaggrin is an important component in epidermis that provides structural barrier capacity to the skin. Filaggrin polymorphism results in functional deficiency of filaggrin and such defect is found in various diseases like ichthyosis vulgaris, atopic dermatitis, and irritant dermatitis.

Irritant contact dermatitis thus depends on both the agents and endogenous factor. Sex, age, atopy, and barrier defect are endogenous factors. Wet work and occupational exposure are important exogenous factors. Important irritants are mentioned in box 1.

## PREDISPOSING ENVIRONMENTS OF IRRITANT CONTACT DERMATITIS

Irritant contact dermatitis is seen in both household work and occupational fields. Housewives are prone to develop hand eczema in the hands. ICD is the most common etiology of occupational skin disease as well. Overall, occupational skin disease shares the top position with few others in occupational diseases having been present in about 30% of all cases in industrialized countries. Occupational exposures that have high risk of development of ICD are found among kitchen workers and food handlers, bakers, bar tenders, hairdressers, metalworkers, construction workers, people exposed to repeated hand washing or wet works like housewives and maids, nurses, and fishermen.

**TABLE 1: Differences between allergic and irritant dermatitis**

| | Allergic contact dermatitis | Irritant contact dermatitis |
|---|---|---|
| Pathogenesis | T-cell mediated delayed hypersensitivity reaction | Primarily nonimmunological reactions. Its direct damage from the irritant effect of the agent. Thus, it depends on the strength of the irritants |
| Symptoms | Itching is primary | Burning, pain primary |
| Morphology | Eczematous, vesicular | Broad spectrum, erythema, dry, fissured lesions in milder cases and necrosis in acute severe cases |
| Contact area and disease spread | Often spreads outside contact area | Restricted to the contact area |
| Gap between exposure and lesion | Clinical manifestation usually requires more than one exposure. Prolonged first contact may lead to sensitization and manifestation form a single contact | No sensitization required. So, strong irritant can lead to manifestation from first contact. Milder irritant may take more than one exposure |

**BOX 1 Important irritants**

- Water/wet work
- Soaps and detergents
- Temperature variation and low humidity
- Acids and alkalis
- Biocide/fungicide
    - Isothiazolinone, chlorothalonil
- Plastics and resins
    - Epoxy, phenolic, and acrylic monomers
    - Amine catalysts
    - Styrene, benzoyl peroxide
- Metal salts
    - Nickel, chromium, cobalt, platinum, arsenic
- Metal working fluids
- Degreasing agents
- Solvents
    - Alcohol solvents
    - *Aliphatic*: Petrol/gasoline, diesel, petroleum spirit, white spirit, and kerosene
    - *Aromatic*: Benzene, toluene, xylene, naphthalene, and styrene
    - *Halogenated*: Chloroform, trichloroethylene, methylchloride, and ethylene dichloride
    - *Miscellaneous*: Water, alcohols, ketones, glycols, and turpentine.
- Plants
    - Irritant hairs of the plant
    - Unsaturated lactones (protoanemonin)
    - Latex (especially cactus plant)
    - Enzyme [pineapple juice, Mucunain (Mucuna pruriens/itch plant)]
    - Oxalic acid (present in dieffenbachias, philodendrons, agaves, and daffodil plants)
    - Phytophotodermatitis: Psoralens (meadow grass, apiaceae plants like celery, carrot, parsnip, fennel and Rutaceae plants/citrus fruits).
- Dusts/friction and mechanical trauma
- Sodium lauryl sulfate

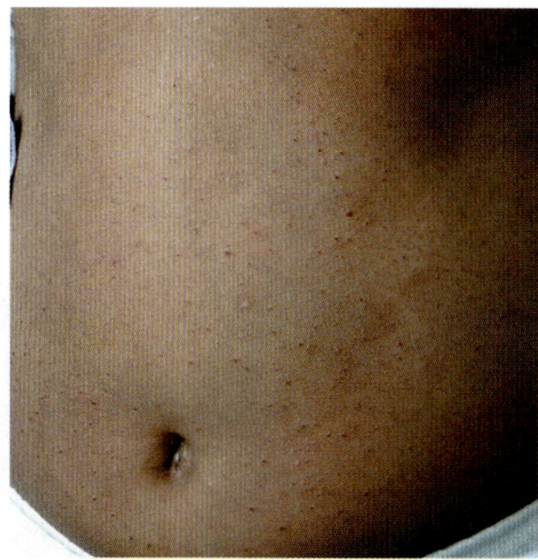

**FIG. 1:** Irritant dermatitis due to mustard oil massage.

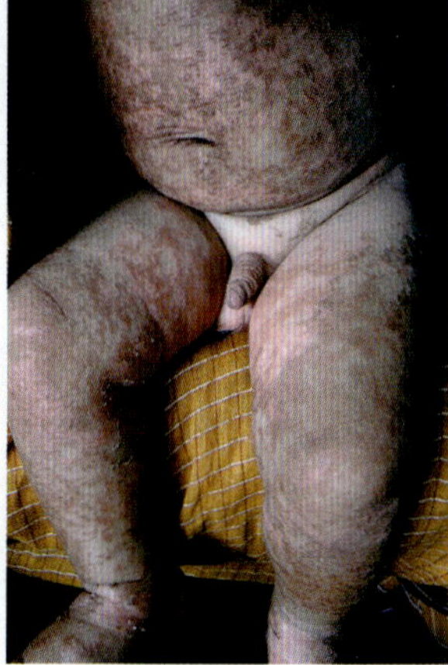

**FIG. 2:** Irritant reaction due to antiseptics containing chlorhexidine and cetrimide.

## CLINICAL PRESENTATION

Common presentations of ICD are erythema, edema, scaling, glazed appearance, dryness, fissuring, and blistering. Presentations vary according to the irritant potential of the irritants, type and duration of exposure (see classification). Chronic low-grade reaction may appear indistinguishable from ACD. Common ICD include hand dermatitis, saliva dermatitis, and napkin dermatitis.

Mustard oil massage in the children, a common practice in Indian subcontinent frequently leads to irritant dermatitis and it often presents with follicular lesions (Fig. 1). Some antiseptic solutions are also known to commonly induce IR (Fig. 2).

## CLASSIFICATION

Irritant contact dermatitis has been subdivided into the following clinical subtypes:

- *Subjective irritancy*: This is a subjective sensation of stinging and smarting without any objective signs. The sensation of irritancy appears immediately after the contact with some cosmetics or sunscreen. This is seen in some people as an idiosyncratic reaction
- *Acute irritant contact dermatitis (ICD)*: This occurs after single (or few exposures happened in very short interval). This occurs when strength of the substance is high enough to induce reaction after single exposure. Common examples are strong acids and alkalis and solvents like ethylene oxide, carbon disulfide, and mustine. This presents as erythema, edema, and more severe acute reaction from strong corrosive substances may lead to formation of blister and even ulcer (Figs 3 and 4)
- *Chronic or cumulative irritant contact dermatitis (CICD)*: This is the most common presentation. Exposure to weaker irritants occurring repeatedly at some interval can lead to CICD. Each exposure causes some damage to the epidermis. Re-exposure before the skin heals completely results in more damage. Disruption of epidermal barrier occurs progressively in a step-wise manner. At some point, ICD manifests clinically. Hand is the most common site affected. Dorsum of hand and finger webs is most common sites. Housewives are very commonly affected with hand dermatitis and ICD is the most common etiology of hand dermatitis among the housewives (Figs 5 and 6).

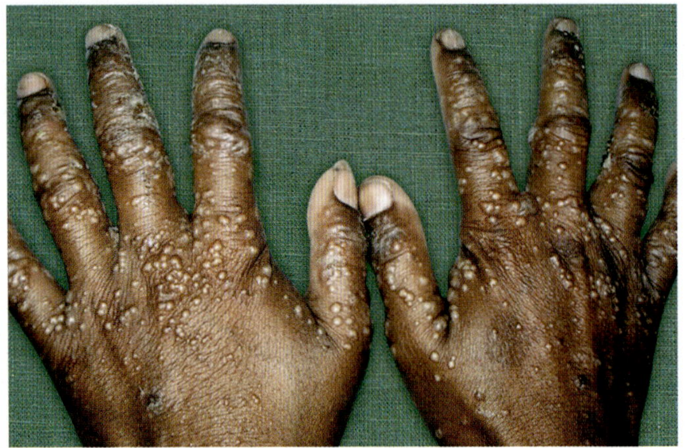

FIG. 3: Acute blistering due to irritant dermatitis.

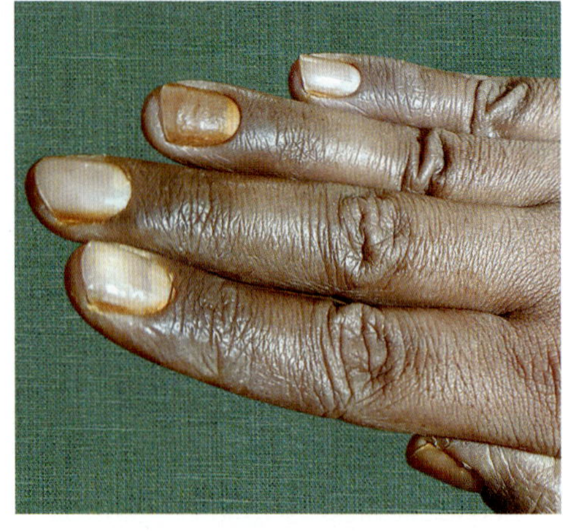

FIG. 6: Chronic irritant dermatitis on the dorsum of finger.

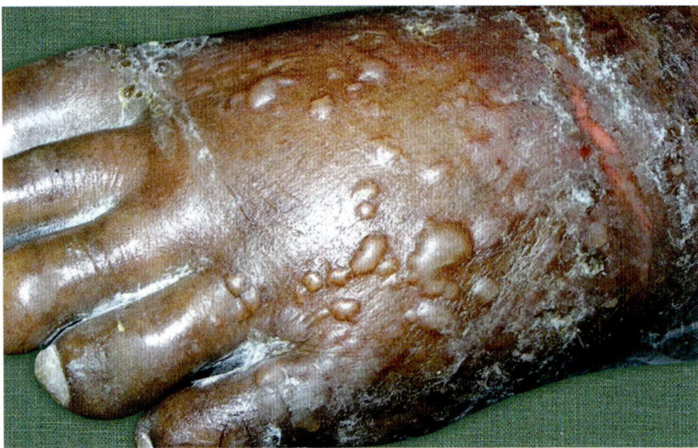

FIG. 4: Irritant contact dermatitis (ICD) due to strong caustic chemical contact.

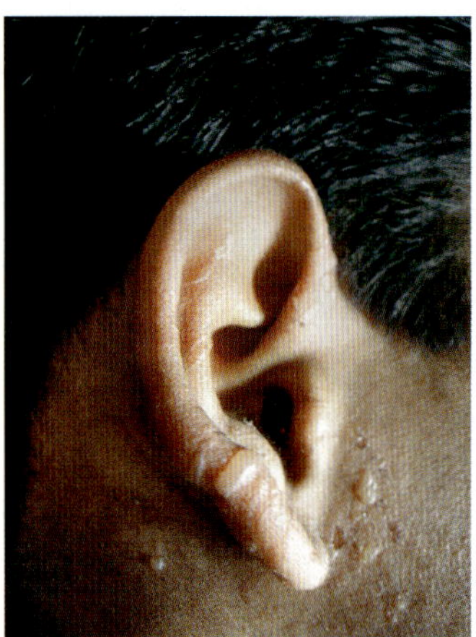

FIG. 7: Blistering phytophotodermatitis.

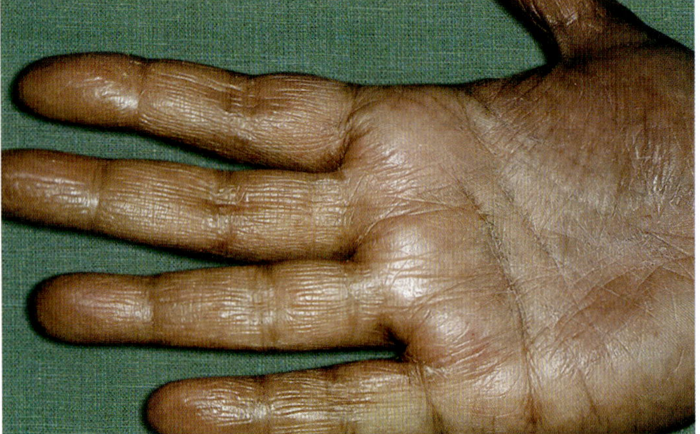

FIG. 5: Glazed appearance on the palmar aspect in chronic irritant dermatitis.

## PHYTOPHOTODERMATITIS

This is caused by psoralens, a furocoumarin present in plants and subsequent sun exposure. UV light with wavelength higher than 320 nm (UVA). Contact with plants or plant product containing psoralens and subsequent exposure to sunlight leads to, usually after 48 hours, development of burning sensation, erythema, edema, and in sometimes blister. Hyperpigmentation without any other form preceding skin changes has also been noted (Fig. 7).

Pseudo-phytophotodermatitis is a condition where dermatitis develops not due to plants but plant arthropods or chemicals and biocides applied to the plants.

### Diagnosis

Dermatitis in ICD is generally limited to the exposed site and there may be a well-defined cut-off margin. This is in contrast to ACD where lesion extends from the contact area and with continuous exposure this may spread much beyond the exposed site.

Irritant contact dermatitis commonly develops on dorsum of hands, finger webs and ACD on the palmar aspect. ICD classically shows erythema, glazed appearance, dryness, fissuring whereas ACD and endogenous eczema manifest with vesicular eruptions. But this is not followed as a rule. It should be remembered that common sites like hand, face, eyelids or some other exposed areas are susceptible to develop ACD, ICD and even endogenous eczema. Thus, meticulous identification and exclusion has to be employed in all cases. Patch test can be done to rule out presence of associated ACD.

Patch testing is an important tool that can rule out ACD. As mentioned earlier, clinical differentiation from ACD is not always possible and both may be associated in many cases. In fact presence of ICD increases the chance of developing ACD. Recently, an *invivo* noninvasive technique called high-definition optical coherence tomography (HD-OCT) that is a real-time three-dimensional imaging technique with cellular resolution has been shown to be useful in differentiating ICD and ACD.

### Treatment

Avoidance from the irritants is most important step. Application of emollients, moisturizers, and topical steroid are primary treatment to help restore the skin damage and to reduce skin inflammation. Non-soap detergents should also be used. More severe cases that are resistant to primary treatment may require other drugs like topical PUVA, azathioprine, and cyclosporin.

A very important step to reduce occupational ICD is to reduce exposure to strong irritants. Education, proper training, use of gloves and other measures, decreasing contact time, use of less damaging substances, shifting to other departments or profession can be rewarding.

## SOME IMPORTANT SUBSTANCES CAUSING ALLERGIC CONTACT DERMATITIS AND IRRITANT CONTACT DERMATITIS

### Metals

Nickel, cobalt, and chromium are the most commonly encountered metal allergens in clinical practice with the former being more common than latter. Nickel is often found to be the most common allergen among general population as found in some.

Females are more commonly affected than males because of increased exposure from jewellery, ear, and body-piercing habits. Nickel exposure can also occur from various foods like soy, chocolate, nuts, green beans, peas, and canned foods, cocoa, beans. Orthodontic appliances also release nickel.

Chromium (CrVI) is present in cement at very high concentration in many countries. Workers exposed to cement like construction workers manifest chromium allergy. European Union (EU) has regulated its use in cement since 2005. It has drastically reduced allergy to this among the workers. Many other countries including India however still have no such system. Other source of CrVI is shoe and other leather goods.

Presence of nickel and also cobalt can be identified with the use of spot test.

### Rubber Materials

Natural rubber is obtained from plants, Hevea brasiliensis being the largest plant source of rubber in the world. This plant is mostly cultivated in Southeast Asia. To prevent coagulation that turns liquid rubber into solid form, ammonia, thiurams, or other preservatives like sodium pentachlorophenate are added at the source point.

Natural rubber latex (NRL) is used to produce items like surgical gloves and condoms. Natural rubber is also processed into a dry form that is used to make tires.

Rubber is also made artificially (synthetic rubber) worldwide. Chemically there are various forms of synthetic rubbers depending upon the chemical composition of the polymer like polyisoprene rubber, butadiene rubber, neoprene, silicone rubber, and chloroprene rubber.

Synthesis of rubber requires various steps of treatment. Untreated rubber has poor strength and elasticity. Vulcanization or curing is a process of cross-linking of polymer chains. This makes the rubber elastic. This requires addition of additives like sulfur and lead. To speed up the process of vulcanization, some additives called accelerator are added like thiurams, carbamates, mercaptobenzothiazole, thiourea, and benzothiazole sulfenamide. Oxidation makes the rubber brittle with time. Antioxidants are used to prevent this. Commonly used antioxidants are paraphenylenediamine, cinnamates, phenols (butylated hydroxytoluene), and carbamates. In addition to these, there are many other additives used those act as plasticizers, and retarders.

Natural rubber latex causes type-1 immediate hypersensitivity from after contact with the latex protein. Atopics and poor quality rubbers increase the risk. The powder used in gloves (cornstarch powder) absorbs the latex protein and increase the chance of allergy. They also increase the risk of inhalation. Mucosal exposure can lead to more severe attack. Contact urticaria is the most common manifestation. More severe cases may develop anaphylaxis. Repeated exposure may lead to eczematous presentation mimicking allergic contact dermatitis.

Diagnosis can be confirmed by anti-latex IgE RAST. Contact with NRL (with increasing duration) can detect allergy but is risky as it may lead to anaphylaxis.

Allergic contact dermatitis to synthetic rubber additives is far more common than immediate hypersensitivity from NRL. Mercaptobenzothiazole is one of the most common rubber allergens. Footwear is a common source of rubber allergy.

### Plastics and Related Substances

Plastics are also called polymer. Smaller molecules called monomers are joined to form a long chain polymers or plastics. This process is called polymerization or "curing". Plastic is a rare cause of allergy. Common cause of allergy from plastic material is presence of incompletely cured substances, setting agents or diluting agents. Common types of plastics are cellulose ester plastics (commonly found in pens, spectacle frame, tooth brush), epoxy resin (present in tennis racket, surface coating paints, adhesives), formaldehyde resin, phenol formaldehyde resin, p-tert butylphenol formaldehyde resin, polyurethanes, acrylic plastics and polyethylene.

Plastics can cause ACD and ICD. P-tertbutylphenol is known to cause depigmentation.

### Preservatives

Preservatives are used in personal care products including cosmetics, medicines, home care products as well as in many substances that are used only in specific occupation. Thus, allergy to preservatives is seen in large number and in wide spectrum of population. Preservatives are added to prevent contamination and early decay.

Formaldehyde is a very commonly used preservative and allergy to this is very common. However, this can also lead to irritant dermatitis.

**BOX 2 Nonformaldehyde releasing preservatives**

- Chloroxylenol
- Iodopropynyl butylcarbamate
- Methylchloroisothiazolinone/methylisothiazolinone (MCI/MI)
- Parabens
- Phenoxyethanol
- Thimerosal

Its role as a disinfectant is an added advantage. Formaldehyde is used in instant coffee, cod fish, mushrooms, smoked ham, liquid soaps, hand-washes and dish-washes, detergents, shampoos, and deodorants. Metalworking fluid is an important source of fomaldehyde exposure. This is also found in chemicals used in paints, lithoprinting materials, photographic developers, papers and paper products (newspaper, paper-back cover, and tissue paper), root canal disinfectant. Products like shampoos are often rinsed, so, hair dressers more commonly show allergy than common individuals.

Apart from direct use of formaldehyde, there are many preservatives that release formaldehyde. These are called formaldehyde-releasing preservatives (FRPs). Commonly used FRPs are quaternium-15, diazolidinyl urea, imidazolidinyl urea, DMDM hydantoin, 2-bromo 2-nitropropane-1,3 diol, and sodium hydroxymethylglycinate (used as an additive to hair care products for straightening or softening). Avoiding formaldehyde (or FRP) can be a challenging task due to its omnipresence in various products.

There are many nonformaldehyde preservatives also that can also cause ACD (Box 2).

## Fragrances

Fragrances are one of the most common allergens. These are present in cosmetics, day care products and also in pharmaceutical products and foods. At least 2,500 fragrance substances are known to exist. More than 100 substances may be present in a single cosmetic product.

Balsam of Peru is an important fragrance material and allergy to this is very common. Other common allergens are cinnamyl alcohol, cinnamic aldehyde, eugenol, isoeugenol, citronellol, and coumarin. Fragrances can also induce irritant dermatitis.

A new allergen called hydroxyisohexyl 3-cyclohexene carboxaldehyde (HICC), used in deodorants, is being more frequently reported to cause allergy nowadays.

Common clinical patterns are eczematous rash, photoallergic and phototoxic reactions, pigmented contact dermatitis, and contact urticaria. Common sites of involvement are face, hands, neck, axilla, and venous stasis site.

## Textiles

Textile fibers or fabrics are rare causes of allergic or irritant dermatitis. Generally the additives are sources of allergic rash. Formaldehyde resins are commonly used in textiles. This makes the fabrics wrinkle-resistant. Formaldehyde is a common cause of ACD. Dyes are next most common cause of ACD in textiles. Paraphenylenediamine, azo and anthraquinone based dyes [e.g., disperse blue 106, 124, disperse yellow (DY) 3; disperse orange (DO) 1 and 3 and disperse red (DR) 1 and 17] are known to induce ACD. Allergens also known to be present in textiles are chrome, cobalt, latex and rubber accelerators. Metal buttons (nickel), fasteners, elastic materials used in clothing can also commonly induce ACD.

Dermatitis due to ACD from allergens form textiles has a specific distribution pattern that follows the prolonged contact with the tightly fitted clothes. Thus, posterior neck, upper back, flexural areas or folds, waist, buttocks, scrotum or vulva are affected with sparing of vaults of folds.

Fabrics that are heavy, and stiff, wrinkle-free/resistant, colorfast and stain-resistant have higher concentration of formaldehyde resin. These are not safe for who have developed sensitivity to formaldehyde. Soft, easily wrinkled fabrics are considered safe.

Patch test is necessary to confirm a case of formaldehyde allergy. Strength of reaction may be very weak and delayed.

## Hair Dye

Hair dye is a commonly used material. Thus allergy to the components is also very common. Principal allergen is p-phenylenediamine (PPD) which is an extreme sensitizer. But there are other sensitizers like toluene-2,5-diamine (PTD), p-aminophenol, m-aminophenol, and resorcinol. There is cross reaction with antioxidant isopropylphenyl p-phenylenediamine (IPPD) also.

Due to cross reactivity, patchy testing with PPD can identify many cases of allergy to these molecules but definitely not all. Possibly there are many other allergens. However, these are not studied well.

Common presentations are eczematous rash on face, eyelid, ear, scalp, and other body areas. Acute and severe reaction can be associated with significant angioedema. Involvement of face may be more prominent than scalp. Hair dressers may develop allergy over hands.

## Solvents

Solvents are substances that are used to dissolve or make other substances thinner. This is used in lacquers, varnishes, paints, resin, rubber, glue, and cement. They are also used to extract fats, waxes, and oils.

When comes in contact with skin, they dissolve the natural skin lipid making it dry. Repeated exposure leads to fissuring and chronic dermatitis. ICD is a more common reaction to solvents. Occupational contact with solvents can occur mostly from the practice of using the available solvents as hand cleaning substance by the workers.

## Metalworking Fluids

Metalworking fluids (MWFs) are liquids used during cutting of metals to reduce friction and for faster conduction of heat. These can be neat oils (insoluble oil), soluble oil, and aqueous fluids (synthetic and semisynthetic). The last ones are used most commonly. To prevent rancidity (caused by growth of organisms), biocides are added. Other additives and associated substances in cutting oils are fragrances, emulsifiers, antioxidants and metals (cobalt, nickel, and chromate).

Exposure to these oils may cause oil acne, folliculitis, hyperpigmentation, eczema (allergic or irritant), leukoderma, phototoxic reaction and pigmentation. Irritant dermatitis is possibly more common than allergic dermatitis.

Complete protection of the workers from the MWFs is extremely difficult due to many practical problems. Severe reactions may require shifting of job.

## Plants

Many plants can induce ACD. Some can also induce ICD or urticaria. Different parts of plants are implicated in induction of skin rash like leaf, fruits, seed cover, or the roots.

Poison ivy, poison oak, myroxylon balsamum (Balsam of Peru), pinus palustris (colophony), Gingko, ragweed, pyrethrum (sesquiterpene lactone), chrysanthemum (sesquiterpene lactone), onion, garlic and primrose plants are known for their ability to sensitize. ICD can occur from the thiocyanates present in the bulb of garlic plant.

# SUGGESTED READINGS

1. Boone MA, Jemec GB, Marmol VD. Differentiating allergic and irritant contact dermatitis by high-definition optical coherence tomography: a pilot study. Arch Dermatol Res. 2015;307:11-22.
2. Bourke J, Coulson I, English J. Guidelines for care of contact dermatitis. Br J Dermatol. 2001;145:877-85.
3. Carlson RM, Smith MC, Nedorost ST. Diagnosis and Treatment of Dermatitis Due to Formaldehyde Resins in Clothing. Dermatitis. 2004;15(4):169-75.
4. Diepgen TL, Coenraads PJ. The epidemiology of occupational contact dermatitis. In: Kanerva L, Elsner P, Wahlberg JE, Maibach HI (Eds). Handbook of Occupational Dermatology. Berlin: Springer; 2000. pp. 3-16.
5. Douglas JD. Allergic Contact Dermatitis: Topical Preservatives, Part-I. Dermatology Nursing © 2010.
6. English JS. Current concepts of irritant contact dermatitis. Occup Environ Med. 2004;61:722-6.
7. Fonacier L, Bernstein DI, Pacheco K, et al. Contact Dermatitis: A Practice Parameter—Update 2015. J Allergy Clin Immunol Pract. 2015;3:S1-S39.
8. Geier J, Krautheim A, Uter W, et al. Occupational contact allergy in the building trade in Germany: influence of preventive measures and changing exposure. Int Arch Occup Environ Health. 2011;84(4):403-11.
9. Malten KE. Thoughts on irritant contact dermatitis. Contact Dermatitis. 1981;7:435-8.
10. Mathias CG. Prevention of occupational contact dermatitis. J Am Acad Dermatol. 1990;23:742-8.
11. Meding B, Swanbeck G. Prevalence of hand eczema in an industrial city. Br J Dermatol. 1987;116:627-34.

# 6 SECTION Urticaria, Mastocytosis and Flushing Disorders

# 13 CHAPTER Urticaria, Angioedema and Urticarial Syndromes

Sanjay Ghosh, Saurav Kundu

## INTRODUCTION

Urticaria, hive or wheal is a circumscribed, erythematous or white, nonpitting swelling of the integument, usually pruritic plaque that that resolves completely within hours or days.

Angioedema is characterized by sudden marked swelling of the lower dermis and subcutis, pain rather than itching and frequent involvement of the mucous membrane and resolution that is slower than wheals.

## URTICARIA

A wheal comprises of three typical features—a central swelling of variable size, almost invariably surrounded by a reflex erythema, associated itching or sometimes burning sensation and a fleeting nature with the skin returning to its normal appearance usually within 1–24 hours.

### Epidemiology

Around 15–20% of people have urticaria at least once during their lifetime. There is no age bar for urticaria or angioedema, although urticaria is mostly seen after adolescence. The highest incidence of urticaria is seen in young adults. Exact epidemiology of chronic urticaria in India is not known. Worldwide, it occurs in 0.1–3% of the population. Women are twice commonly affected compared to men.

### Etiopathogenesis

On the basis of etiopathogenesis, urticaria can be histaminergic (i.e., mediated by histamine) or nonhistaminergic.

#### Histaminergic Urticaria

Mast cell is the key effector cell of acute and chronic urticaria. Studies using conventional histochemical stains show mast cell predominance in urticarial leisons. Among the mediators released during mast cells degranulation, histamine, and leukotrienes (LTC4, D4, E4) appear to be most important. Roles of heparin and tryptase remain unclear. Histamine is mainly responsible for the wheals and itch whereas flare is mediated by substance P.

LTC4, D4 and E4 play an important role in nonselective nonsteroidal anti-inflammatory drug (NSAID)-induced urticaria which result in diversion of arachidonic acid metabolism from prostaglandin E2 (PGE2) to leukotrienes. The reduced PGE2 level has a permissive effect on immunological mast cell degranulation. That is not seen with selective cyclooxygenase-2 (COX-2) inhibitors.

Cells that play important role in the late phase of urticaria have been discussed in table 1.

#### Nonhistaminergic (Not Mediated by Mast Cell) Urticaria

Stimulation of Hageman factor XII activates the intrinsic coagulation system, generation of plasmin, and production of bradykinin. There is a complex interconnecting system of feedback loops involving the C1-esterase inhibitor which has an inhibitory influence on the complement, kallikrein, coagulation, and fibrinolytic system. The bradykinin, which is generated by the action of kallikrein on kininogen, appears to be the primary mediator of hereditary angioedema. The angiotensin-converting enzyme inhibitors (ACEIs) result in accumulation of kinin and lead to angioedema without wheals.

Immunological stimuli of mast cell degranulation may be:

- *Allergen*: By cross linking of high affinity immunoglobulin E (IgE) receptor
- *Functional autoantibody*: Presence of anti FcεRI and anti IgE
- *Complement induced*: C5a acts as a stimulus for mast cell histamine release
- Direct mast cell liberators: Drugs such as opiates and polymyxin B.

The lower threshold for urticaria in some persons is due to enhanced ability of mast cells to release mediators. This, in

**TABLE 1: Cells with released mediators responsible for late phase of urticaria**

| Cells | Released mediators |
|---|---|
| Eosinophils | Eosinophil cationic protein, major basic protein |
| Basophil | Histamine and leukotrienes |
| PMNs | No specific role |
| T helper lymphocytes | IL3, TNF-α |

IL, interleukin; TNF, tumor necrosis factor; PMNs, polymorphonuclear neutrophils.

turn, is due to presence of functional autoantibodies, dietary pseudoallergens, stress, viral infection, drugs, and other unknown intrinsic factors.

## Scoring of Urticaria

Several scoring systems have been proposed but the most widely used scoring system is urticaria activity score (UAS7) as the scoring is done for 7 days (Table 2).

## Classification

Urticaria has been classified into acute and chronic urticaria based on the duration of each attack. Urticaria has also been classified based on the etiology (Box 1).

## Clinical Features

### Acute Urticaria

Acute urticaria is characterized by spontaneous appearance of wheal and angioedema which lasts less than 6 week. The prevalence of acute urticaria is higher in people with atopic disease. It is characterized by discrete scattered wheals size usually larger than 1 cm (Fig. 1). Urticaria may be associated with systemic symptoms like shortness of breath, dizziness, headache, nausea, and diarrhea.

Most common triggering factors of acute urticaria are acute viral upper respiratory tract infection (most common in children), foods and food additives (most common in children) and drugs, mainly penicillin and NSAIDS (IgE-mediated). However, acute urticaria is self-limited in more than 99% patients and hence extensive diagnostic tests are not recommended.

**TABLE 2: The urticaria activity score (UAS7) for assessing disease activity in chronic spontaneous urticaria (CSU)**

| Score | Wheals | Pruritus |
|---|---|---|
| 0 | None | None |
| 1 | Mild (<20 wheals/24 h) | Mild (not troublesome) |
| 2 | Moderate (21–50 wheals/24 h) | Moderate (troublesome but not disturbing daily activities/sleep) |
| 3 | Intense (>50 wheals/24 h or large confluent areas of wheals) | Intense (troublesome with daily activity and sleep disturbance) |

**BOX 1 Classification of urticaria based on etiology**

- Spontaneous
  - Acute spontaneous urticaria
  - Chronic spontaneous urticaria
- Inducible
  - Symptomatic dermographism
  - Delayed pressure urticaria
  - Cold contact urticaria
  - Solar urticaria
  - Heat urticaria
  - Vibratory angioedema
  - Cholinergic urticaria
  - Contact urticaria
  - Aquagenic urticaria

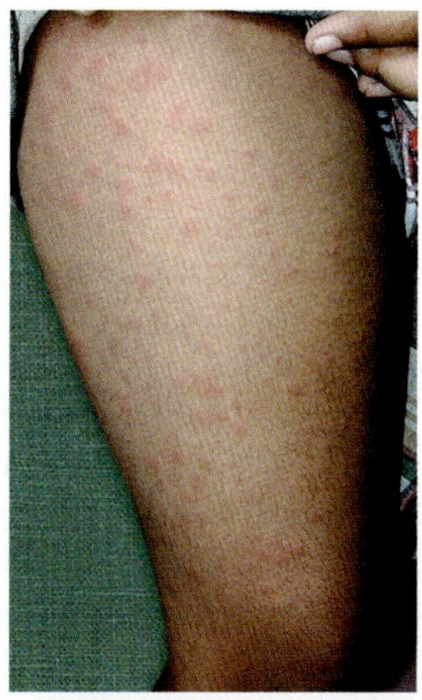

**FIG. 1:** Blanching, erythematous plaques of acute urticaria.

*Courtesy*: Dr Nilendu Sarma, Associate Professor and Head, Department of Dermatology, Dr BC Roy Post Graduate Institute of Pediatric Sciences, West Bengal.

**BOX 2 Triggering factors of chronic urticaria**

- *Autoreactivity*: Due to anti-IgE or anti-IgE receptor antibody
- *Infective*: Bacterial infections such as *Helicobacter pylori*, viral infections such as Hepatitis A and B and parasitic infections include *Toxocara canis, Giardia lamblia,* and *Blastocystis hominis.*
- *Due to intolerance*: Food pseudoallergens such as food colorants, taste intensifiers.
- *Miscellaneous*: Chronic inflammatory process such as gastritis, reflux esophagitis, and chronic cholecystitis.

### Chronic Urticaria

This is defined as sudden appearance of wheals and/or angioedema daily or almost daily for at least 6 weeks (the duration is taken arbitrarily).

The mean duration of chronic urticaria is 4 years ranging from few months to few decades with 50% of chronic urticaria patients showing spontaneous remission within the first 10 years of disease. Symptoms are usually episodic with symptom-free period ranging from few days to few months.

Various triggering factors of urticaria are suggested in box 2.

### Some Important Subtypes of Urticaria

#### *Chronic Autoimmune Urticaria*

These patients have complement activating against the high affinity IgE receptor FcεRI or less commonly against IgE itself. Demonstration of serum antithyroid antibodies is suggestive. Autologous serum skin test (ASST) positivity indicates the presence of autoreactivity.

#### *Physical Urticaria*

Urticaria is triggered by physical stimuli such as pressure, cold heat, and friction. They occur most frequently in person between 17 years and 40 years of age. May occur as a single entity or may coexist with chronic spontaneous urticaria (CSU).

Symptomatic dermographism: Most common form of physical urticaria where patients complain of itching but the lesions are polymorphic varying from linear (most common) or oblong shape to patchy papular erythema which can all occur simultaneously. The triggering factor may be pressure of clothing and jewelry. Mucosal involvement does not occur, but vulvar swelling after sexual intercourse has been reported. There is no association with systemic disease, atopy, food allergy, or autoimmunity.

The duration is maximum up to 1 hour and disease intensifies in the evening. Delayed dermographism is delayed pressure urticaria (DPU) like response to frictional stimulus.

### Delayed pressure Urticaria

A sustained pressure stimulus when applied to the skin produces a whealing response which appear between 30 minutes and 6 hours. This variety of urticaria is usually nonresponsive to antihistamine. Triggering factors include tight clothing, tight shoes, seat belt, carry bags, walking, and jogging. DPU may be associated rarely with arthralgia.

Lesions are generally deeper than those of ordinary urticaria involving subcutaneous tissues. Histology shows more pronounced infiltrate than other form of urticaria. The lesion can be reproduced by pressure. When a 15 lb weight suspended from forearm for 15 minutes, lesions are produced within 30 minutes to 6 hours.

### Heat and Cold Urticaria

Heat urticaria is a very rare disorder. But, cold urticaria is relatively more common with prevalence of 0.5% in general population with highest prevalence in young adults.

Types of cold urticaria:

- Positive cold stimulation test
  - Primary cold urticaria
  - Secondary cold urticaria—infection, drugs, cryoglobulinemia, vasculitis
- Negative cold stimulation test
  - Delayed cold urticaria
  - Cold dependent dermographism
  - Acquired and familial cold urticaria
  - Cold-induced cholinergic urticaria.

Most important cell in pathogenesis of cold urticaria is mast cells, which get activated on cooling below threshold. But, the mechanism of heat urticaria is unclear.

Heat and cold urticaria can be elicited by:

- Environmental exposure
- Food
- Handling objects
- Aquatic exposure.

Major symptoms are immediate development of wheals and or angioedema which are typically nonpseudopodic and may be localized or generalized. Exposure of cold to upper aerodigestive tract may lead to swelling of lips, tongue, pharynx or larynx and even lead to syncope.

It may be dangerous when attacks occur during aquatic activities as it may lead to drowning. It carries a poor prognosis and tolerance induction may be tried.

### Solar Urticaria

Wheals develop between 5 minutes and 10 minutes of exposure to visible light or ultraviolet light and last for few hours. Covered body areas are more prone to develop this. Age between second and fourth decade and females are more commonly affected and this may be seasonal (spring and autumn). Symptoms such as headache, nausea, wheezing, and dyspnea may be associated. Histamine plays an important role. Eosinophils and neutrophils also play an important part.

This may be associated with atopy, polymorphic light eruption, chronic actinic dermatitis, systemic lupus erythematosus, and other physical urticaria.

### Cholinergic Urticaria

Cholinergic urticaria is characterized by small, short-lived wheals with disproportionately large surrounding flare occurring after a rise in the core temperature. It is common in young adults.

Other cutaneous disorders precipitated by alteration in the core temperature:

- Cholinergic pruritus
- Exercise-induced anaphylaxis
- Persisting cholinergic erythema
- Cold-induced cholinergic urticaria
- Cholinergic dermographism
- Localized heat urticaria.

Triggering factors include exercise, eating hot or spicy food, exposure to high temperature, and hot showers.

Pathogenesis: Apart from mast cell degranulation, role of acetylcholine released from local sympathetic nerve ending has been speculated.

Lesions usually develop within 15–20 minutes of exposure to stimulus and last up to 1 hour. Lesions are most often focused in upper trunk and proximal extremities and may be associated with systemic symptoms such as dizziness, flushing, headache, abdominal pain, nausea, diarrhea, breathlessness, and syncope.

### Exercise-induced Anaphylaxis

It is a rare entity and is triggered by physical exertion only and not by other cause which induces increase in core temperature. This distinguishes it from cholinergic urticaria. In some case, foodstuff such as wheat, shellfish, apples, peaches, or drugs such as aspirin may enhance the attack. Mast cell degranulation plays an important role during attack. Systemic features such as flushing, nausea, diarrhea, headache, and vertigo may occur.

### Contact Urticaria

It is defined as the wheals that appear following contact of substances with the skin. This may be of two types:

- Immunologic contact urticaria or allergic contact urticarial (IgE mediated)
- Nonimmunologic contact urticaria.

*Immunologic contact urticaria*: Common inducers of immunologic contact urticaria are animal products like hair, blood, gelatin, plant products mainly latex, and other foods such as banana, tomatoes, onion, garlic, dairy product, fish, honey, medications like phenothiazine, pyrazolone, benzocaine, and also the epoxies and acrylic.

*Nonimmunologic contact urticaria*: Common triggering factors of nonimmunologic contact urticaria are plants—stinging nettle (contains toxin in their leaves), animal—caterpillars, jellyfish, mosquito, ants, fleas, and direct histamine liberators—spices (mustard, cinnamon), fragrance (cinnamon aldehyde).

The lesions are localized to the site of contact. Hand is most often involved in food handler whereas perioral erythema and swellings are very common in children with atopy.

### Urticarial Vasculitis

This clinicopathologic entity is characterized by:

- Urticarial papules and plaques lasting longer than 24 hours

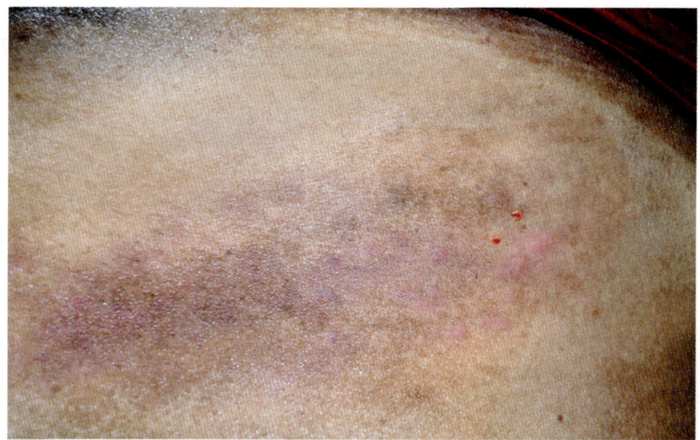

FIG. 2: Urticarial plaque leaving pigmented patch in urticarial vasculitis.
*Courtesy*: Dr Nilendu Sarma, Associate Professor and Head, Department of Dermatology, Dr BC Roy Post Graduate Institute of Pediatric Sciences, West Bengal.

- Resolving with faint purpura or residual hyperpigmentation (Fig. 2)
- Histologically characterized by presence of leukocytoclastic vasculitis around capillaries and postcapillary venules with or without fibrinoid necrosis.

Triggering factors include autoimmune connective tissue disease, hepatitis A and B, paraproteinemias, inflammatory bowel disease, and idiopathic.

Types include normocomplementemic and hypocomplementemic. Hypocomplementemic variety is associated with systemic manifestations.

This has to be differentiated from other vasculitis like leukocytoclastic vasculitis, and also from papular urticaria, polymorphic light reaction, maculopapular exanthems, urticaria pigmentosa, and erythema multiforme.

This is diagnosed by biopsy, direct immunofluorescence, and investigation to identify the triggers and complications.

## Histology

Histologically, wheals are characterized by edema of upper and mid dermis with dilatation of postcapillary venules whereas in angioedema, mainly lower dermis and subcutis are affected. There is a mixed cellular infiltrate of both acute and chronic inflammatory cells. More neutrophils and eosinophils predominate in lesions over 12 hours than below 4 hours in biopsies of CSU. Evidence of leukocytoclasia and red cell extravasation is found in urticarial vasculitis.

## Diagnosis of Urticaria

Because of the heterogeneity of the disease, initial evaluation should start with detailed history and routine physical examination.

Identification of some primary or etiological factors is of prime importance in management and prognosis. Apart from physical mode of precipitation, other causative factors like drugs, foods, infection, and internal disease need to be identified.

Infection is a common cause of urticaria. Infectious cause should be considered in urticaria associated with ear, nose, and throat infections. *Anisakis* simplex, a sea fish nematode is frequently associated with urticarial in population who consume uncooked sea fish. Other infections associated with urticaria are *Helicobacter pylori, Streptococcus spp., Staphylococcus spp., Giardia,* and hepatitis.

Examination of lesion is important to rule out signs of vasculitis. Presence of angioedema is an important finding. Ruling out malignancies is warranted only if patient's history is suggestive.

Invasive and costly investigations are to be strongly discouraged. Specific laboratory test and provocation test should be performed if there are suggestive features in history (Table 3).

Currently, the only available test to screen for autoantibodies is ASST, which is a nonspecific test that evaluates the presence of histamine releasing factor. It is a very simple, quick test which consists of intradermal injection of patient's own serum with a 0.4 mm needle into the volar aspect of forearm. Positive control with histamine and negative control with 0.9% saline is also injected 3–5 cm apart. The reading is taken 30 minutes later and the diameter of the wheal at the test site is measured. Positive reading means diameter at the test site should be at least 1.5 mm larger than the negative control.

Basophils of patients with chronic urticaria are hyporesponsive to polyclonal anti-IgE (Basophil histamine release test).

Other blood tests such as antinuclear antibody test can also be considered if history points at this. Elevated serum D-dimer level is seen in few patients of CSU.

For most types of physical urticaria, no validated tools for provocation testing exist with few exceptions.

In cold urticaria, a Peltier element-based provocation device is available (Temp test). Besides determining the threshold levels for whealing, the system can also be used for treatment monitoring. For symptomatic dermographism and DPU, dermographometers have been developed which can reproduce similar lesions. Ergometer provocation in cholinergic urticaria has produced demonstrable results. Finally, contact urticaria should be demonstrated with cutaneous provocation tests, for example, prick tests.

### Test for Food-elicited Urticaria Diet

Conduction of pseudoallergen low diet can provide information on the presence of chronic urticaria due to food intolerance. Patient should be informed that at least 3 weeks adherence is necessary and effect may not be seen until 10–14 days. Intake of antihistamines and glucocorticoids must be reduced to minimum (Table 4).

### Prick Test

This test is performed in cases of suspected contact urticaria. In this test, a small drop of allergen is applied to the skin of forearm and then the skin is pricked with a lancet without breaking the skin. Histamine solution and normal saline are used as positive and negative control, respectively. Results are read after 15 minutes. The largest diameter and the diameter perpendicular to it is measured for the test and the positive and negative controls.

To calculate the value, the sum of largest and perpendicular diameter is divided by 2. Positive reaction means more than half the size of histamine wheal provided the negative control shows no reaction.

**TABLE 3: Recommended diagnostic tests in urticaria (From EAACI/GA²LEN/EDF/WAO 2013 guideline)**

| Types | Subtypes | Routine diagnostic tests | Extended diagnostic tests (if history suggests) |
|---|---|---|---|
| Spontaneous urticaria | a) Acute spontaneous urticaria | None | None |
| | b) Chronic spontaneous urticaria | Differential blood count, ESR, CRP, mission of suspected drugs | Tests for infectious disease, functional autoantibodies, thyroid hormones and autoantibodies, pseudoallergen free diet, tryptase assay, ASST, lesional skin biopsy |
| Inducible urticaria | a) Cold urticaria | Cold provocation test | Differential blood count, ESR, CRP, cryoproteins, and infectious disease detection |
| | b) Delayed pressure urticaria | Pressure test | None |
| | c) Heat urticaria | Heat provocation test | None |
| | d) Solar urticaria | Ultraviolet and visible light threshold test | Rule out other photodermatosis |
| | e) Symptomatic dermographism | Test for dermographism | Differential count, ESR, CRP |
| | f) Vibratory angioedema | Test with vortex | None |
| | g) Aquagenic urticaria | Wet clothes at body temperature for 20 minutes | None |
| | h) Cholinergic urticaria | Exercise and hot bath provocation | None |
| | i) Contact urticaria | Prick test | None |

ESR, erythrocyte sedimentation rate; CRP, C-reactive protein; ASST, autologous serum skin test.

**TABLE 4: Foods allowed and forbidden to test food-elicited urticaria diet**

| | Foods allowed | Foods forbidden |
|---|---|---|
| Basic foods | Additive-free bread, potatoes, rice, unprocessed cereals, flour | Cake, biscuit, potato chips |
| Fats | Butter, plant oils | Margarine, mayonnaise |
| Milk products | Fresh milk, natural yoghurt, cream without stabilizers | All others |
| Animal food | Fresh meat | Sea food, seasoned meat, eggs |
| Vegetables | Except those forbidden | Peas, mushroom, tomatoes, spinach, olives |
| Fruits | None | All including dried fruits |
| Herbs and spices | Salt and onion | All including garlic and herbs |
| Sweets and beverages | Sugar, honey, coffee, black tea | All sweets including chewing gum, beer, wine, spirits |

## Management of Urticaria

### Identification and Elimination or Avoidance of the Triggers or Stimulus

This step is vital. For DPU and symptomatic dermographism, emphasis is to be placed in reducing the contact area, e.g., broadening the shapes of handbag can be beneficial. Similarly, in cold urticaria, impact of cold wind and cold water needs to be emphasized. In solar urticaria, identification of the wavelength and its avoidance is to be emphasized. However, in most patients, the threshold of physical triggers is low and total avoidance of symptoms is impossible, e.g., mild exercise can trigger cholinergic urticaria or loose fitting clothing can develop wheals of dermographism.

### Eradication of Infectious Agent and Treatment of Inflammatory Process

Chronic spontaneous urticaria is often reported to be associated with infection of the gastrointestinal tract with *H. pylori* and infestation with bowel parasites although meta-analysis shows low-level evidence.

### Reduction of Functional Autoantibodies

Reduction of functional autoantibodies by plasmapheresis has been shown to have temporary benefit in severely affected patients.

### Dietary Management

Dietary pseudoallergens found in food additives can both elicit and aggravate CSU. Avoidance of the relevant allergen must be maintained for minimum 3 weeks before beneficial effects are observed. It is highly recommended that avoidance of a particular food item should be based on double blind oral provocation test or a clear history.

### Inducing Tolerance

It can be useful in cold urticaria, cholinergic urticaria, and solar urticaria. But, the tolerance induction is only short lasting, requiring daily exposure.

### Pharmacological Treatment

The treatment of urticaria is mainly aimed to reduce the effect of mast cell and release of its mediators such as histamine, platelet-activating factor, and leukotrienes. Patient should be properly counseled regarding continuous use of H1 histamines instead of as and when needed basis. Being inverse agonist and helping in stabilizing the histamine in inactive form, these drugs reduces further attack with continuous use.

Newer generation antihistamines are often preferred because of the lower adverse effects and lesser drug interactions.

### Other Therapeutic Options

Omalizumab (anti-IgE) has been shown to be very effective in CSU in double-blind, placebo controlled trial and has been effective as a third-line agent. It has very good safety profile and good efficacy. Only cost is prohibitive.

Cyclosporin A has been recommended for patients with severe disease refractory to any dose of antihistamine and it has been confirmed by double-blind, placebo-controlled trial.

Leukotriene receptor antagonist of which montelukast is best used have a low-level evidence and worth trying in aspirin and food additive-intolerant persons and in ASST-positive patients.

Systemic corticosteroids are recommended for patients only in short course (maximum 10 days) in urticarial as a third-line drug. But, long-term use is strictly discouraged.

Before changing to alternative therapy, it is recommended to wait for 1–4 weeks to allow the drug to show full effectiveness. It is recommended to follow up the patients every 3–6 months for continuing on alternative treatment.

Other therapies, which have low level of evidence in treatment of CSU, are dapsone, sulfasalazine, methotrexate, intravenous immunoglobulin, plasmapheresis, interferon and ultraviolet B. Proper trials are lacking for the above-mentioned agents.

Therapies which are formally proposed but lacked a double-blind, placebo-controlled trial include tranexamic acid for CSU, nifedipine in symptomatic dermographism, and colchicine and indomethacin in DPU.

### Treatment in Children

It is strongly recommended that second-generation antihistamines are to be used in children as first-line agent in urticaria as they have a high safety profile than the first generation antihistamines. Even updosing (weight adjusted) is recommended in children similar to adults. Cetirizine, desloratadine, fexofenadine, levocetirizine, and loratadine have been well studied and their long-term safety has been well established in children.

### In Pregnancy and Lactation

No report of birth defect has been reported in women receiving modern second-generation antihistamines but most of the studies suggest the use of loratadine, desloratadine, cetirizine and levocetirizine was safe during pregnancy. Use of second-generation antihistamines is advised in nursing mother as infants occasionally develop sedation from old first-generation antihistamines. If at all first-generation drugs are to be used chlorpheniramine and diphenhydramine have the highest safety profile.

## ANGIOEDEMA

It is defined as transient localized swellings of the deep dermis, and subcutaneous and submucosal tissues. It may or may not be associated with wheals (Table 5).

### Drugs causing Angioedema

- *Nonsteroidal anti-inflammatory drugs*: Aspirin, diclofenac, indomethacin, and ibuprofen are potent COX-1 inhibitors and have higher propensity to cause angioedema than paracetamol and pyrazolones
- *Angiotensin-converting enzyme inhibitors*: Enalapril and ramipril usually during first month of therapy.

### Hereditary Angioedema

This is an autosomal dominant disorder and is caused by mutation in C1-inhibitor gene on chromosome. This is mainly of two type:

- *Type 1*: Most common (85%), decreased level of C1-inhibitor about 35–50% of normal
- *Type 2*: Functional inactivity of C1-inhibitor but levels normal or elevated.

A third type called estrogen-dependent angioedema but C1-inhibitor levels are normal.

### Acquired Angioedema

C1-inhibitor deficiency associated with monoclonal gammopathy of unknown significance (MGUS) and other B cell malignancies, is caused due to:

- C1-inhibitor consumption by complement activators
- C1-inhibitor depletion by autoantibodies.

**TABLE 5: Classification of angioedema**

| Angioedema without wheals | Angioedema with wheals |
|---|---|
| • Idiopathic (40%)<br>• Allergic<br>• Drug induced (e.g., NSAID)<br>• C1 deficiency<br>• Hereditary (Type 1, 2, 3)<br>• Acquired<br>• Angioedema with eosinophilia<br>  ○ Gleich syndrome-Episodic angioedema with weight gain<br>  ○ Nonepisodic angioedema<br>• Angioedema due to physical triggers<br>  ○ Vibratory angioedema<br>  ○ Exercise-induced angioedema | Similar to urticaria in terms of assessment and management |

NSAID, nonsteroidal anti-inflammatory drug.

## Mediators of Angioedema

Angioedema can be mediated by:
- *Histamine*: Idiopathic, allergic
- *Bradykinin*: Hereditary angioedema, ACEI induced.

## Clinical Features

Presentation depends on the tissue affected:
- *Subcutaneous tissue*: Nonpitting, nonpruritic, affects hand, feet, genitalia
- *Intestinal*: Abdominal pain, watery diarrhea
- *Laryngeal*: Dyspnea, dysphoria, dysphagia.

Hereditary angioedema manifests usually in children or adolescent and is often triggered by trauma, stress, and infection. This may be preceded by prodromal symptoms such as headache, paresthesia, and flu-like symptoms (Fig. 3).

Angiotensin-converting enzyme inhibitor-induced angioedema usually shows a site of predilection involving lower face, tongue, and larynx. Triggers include trauma, bee string, and hemodialysis. Persons predisposed to develop this subtype include:
- Caribbean origin
- Hereditary angioedema
- ACEI associated cough.

## Differential Diagnosis

- Acute contact dermatitis
- Cellulitis
- Melkersson–Rosenthal syndrome
- Cheilitis granulomatosa.

## Investigations

All patients with recurrent angioedema should undergo screening for C4 level and, if low, for qualitative and quantitative assay of C1-inhibitor.

Elevated eosinophil (>1,500/mm$^3$) count should point toward Gleich syndrome.

## Treatment

Hereditary angioedema: Acute attacks managed by C1-inhibitor concentrate and fresh frozen plasma.
Acute attack is managed by:
- Intramuscular epinephrine injection
- Parenteral antihistamine and steroid
- Intravenous immunoglobulin in Gleich syndrome.

## Symptomatic Management

- Close monitoring in intensive care unit
- Endotracheal intubation or tracheostomy.

## Prophylaxis

- Low-dose attenuated androgens such as danazol or stanozolol
- Antifibrinolytic agents: Aminocaproic acid, tranexamic acid
- Avoidance of triggering drugs.

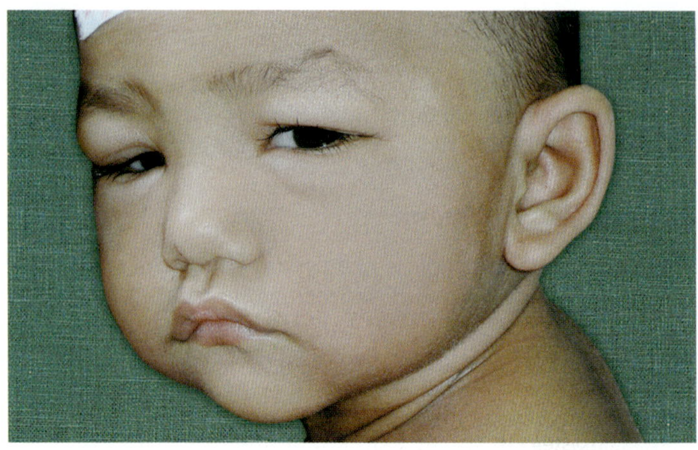

**FIG. 3:** Hereditary angioedema in a child

*Courtesy*: Dr Nilendu Sarma, Associate Professor and Head, Department of Dermatology, Dr BC Roy Post Graduate Institute of Pediatric Sciences, West Bengal.

## Newer Drugs in Management of Hereditary Angioedema

- Kallikrein inhibitor (DX 88)
- Icatibant (bradykinin B2 receptor antagonist)
- Recombinant C1-inhibitor.

# URTICARIAL SYNDROMES

Urticarial syndromes are of two types:
- Familial
- Nonfamilial.

## Familial Urticaria

These groups of diseases are associated with urticarial lesions in presence of positive family history, neonatal onset, systemic involvement, periodic fever, amyloidosis, and neutrophilic predominance in histopathology (Table 6).

Usually lesions are non-pruritic and non-responsive to conventional treatment.

### Treatment

Interleukin-1 antagonist such as Anakinra has been shown to be beneficial in cryopyrin-associated periodic syndrome, hyperimmunoglobulin D syndrome (HIDS) and familial mediterranean fever (FMF). Etanercept has been found beneficial in tumor necrosis factor receptor-associated periodic syndrome (TRAPS). Colchicine has found useful in FMF and TRAPS. Bone marrow transplantation has shown promise in HIDS. Corticosteroids have been tried in TRAPS and HIDS with some benefit.

## Nonfamilial Autoinflammatory Diseases

This group presents with neutrophilic urticaria of unknown etiology. They are usually acquired or polygenic in inheritance. Two diseases are described in this category (Table 7).

**TABLE 6: Familial urticarial syndrome**

| Disease | Mode of inheritance | Skin manifestation | Systemic manifestation | Genes responsible | Diagnostic tests |
|---|---|---|---|---|---|
| 1. Cryopyrin associated periodic syndrome (CAPS)—3 subtypes | AD | – | – | *CIAS1* gene product Cryopyrin | – |
| a) Familial cold-induced autoinflammatory syndrome | – | Cold-induced atypical urticarial eruption | Fever, arthralgia. Attacks are almost regular. | Same as above | CRP, ESR, genetic testing |
| b) Muckle–Wells syndrome | – | Atypical urticarial eruption | Fever, arthralgia. Attacks are almost regular | Same as above | CRP, ESR, serum amyloid A, urinalysis, creatinine level, genetic testing |
| c) Neonatal onset multisystem inflammatory disease | – | Atypical urticarial eruption | Fever, arthralgia, sensorineural deafness, renal amyloidosis. Attacks are almost regular | Same as above | CRP, ESR, urinalysis, creatinine level, neurologic evaluation, genetic testing |
| 2. Familial Mediterranean fever | AR | Erysipelas like erythema at acral sites, atypical urticarial lesions, nonspecific purpuric lesions | Fever, peritonitis, pleuritis, arthritis, renal amyloidosis, meningitis. Variable period between 2 attacks | *MEFV* gene product pyrin | CRP, ESR, WBC count, serum amyloid A, urinalysis, creatinine level, genetic testing |
| 3. Tumor necrosis factor receptor associated periodic syndrome (TRAPS) | AD | Migratory erythematous papules and plaques overlying areas of myalgia, nonspecific purpuric lesions | Fever, abdominal pain, pleurisy. Average duration of attack 21 days. Number of episodes per year is 6 on an average | *TNFRSF1A* gene product tumor necrosis factor receptor 1 | CRP, ESR, serum amyloid A, genetic testing |
| 4. Hyper IgD syndrome (HIDS) | AR | Intermittent morbilliform rash | Arthralgia, abdominal pain, lymphadenopathy. Average duration of attack 1–2 days. Number of episodes per year is 6 | *MVK* gene product mevalonate kinase | CRP, ESR, serum IgD level, urine mevalonate level, genetic testing |

ESR, erythrocyte sedimentation rate; CRP, C-reactive protein; WBC, white blood cell; IgD, immunoglobulin D; AR, autosomal recessive; AD, autosomal dominant.

**TABLE 7: Nonfamilial urticarial syndrome**

| Disease | Skin manifestation | Systemic manifestation | Diagnostic tests | Treatment |
|---|---|---|---|---|
| Still's disease | Evanescent erythematous eruption, PG like, rheumatoid nodule like lesions | Seronegative arthritis, hepatosplenomegaly, lymphadenopathy, CNS manifestations, ocular disease | CRP, ESR, RA factor, ANF | Methotrexate, hydroxychloroquine, leflunomide, TNF blockade |
| Schnitzler's disease | Painful urticaria | Fever, monoclonal IgM gammopathy, bone pain, arthralgia, hepatosplenomegaly, lymphadenopathy | CBC, serum protein electrophoresis | Corticosteroids, cyclosporine A, thalidomide, anakinra |

CRP, C-reactive protein; ESR, erythrocyte sedimentation rate; CBC, complete blood count; TNF, tumor necrosis factor; IgM, immunoglobulin M; CNS, central nervous system; ANF, atrial natriuretic factor; PG, pyoderma gangrenosum; RA, rheumatoid arthritis.

## SUGGESTED READINGS


1. Asero R, Tedeschi A. Usefulness of a short course of oral prednisolone in antihistamine resistant chronic urticaria: a retrospective analysis. J Investig Allergol Clin Immunol. 2010;20:386-90.
2. Belkhir R, Moulonguet-Doleris L, Hachulla E, et al. Treatment of familial Mediterranean fever with anakinra. Ann Intern Med. 2007;146:825-6.
3. Bowen T, Cicardi M, Farkas H, et al. Canadian 2003 international consensus algorithm for the diagnosis, therapy, and management of hereditary angioedema. J Allergy Clin Immunol. 2004;114(3):629-37.
4. Church MK, Maurer M, Simons FE, et al. Risk of first–generation H1 antihistamines: a GA²LEN position paper. Allergy. 2010;65:459-66.
5. Davis AE III. The pathophysiology of hereditary angioedema. Clin Immunol. 2005;114(1):3-9.
6. Konstantinou GN, Asero R, Maurer M, et al. The following protocol is recommended by an EACCI/GA²LEN task force. Allergy. 2009;64(9):1256-68.
7. Mager M, Borzova E, Gimenez-Arnau A, et al. The definition and diagnostic testing of physical and cholinergic urticaria-EAACI/GA²LEN/EDF/UNEV consensus panel recommendations. Allergy. 2009;64:1715-21.
8. Mitzel-Kaoukhov H, Staubach P, Muller-Brenne T. Effect of high dose intravenous immunoglobulin treatment in therapy resistant chronic spontaneous urticaria. Ann Allergy Asthma Immunol. 2010;104:253-8.
9. Neven B, Valayannopoulos V, Quartier P, et al. Allogenic bone marrow transplantation in mevalonic aciduria. NEJM. 2007;356:2700-3.
10. Staevska M, Popov TA, Kralimarkova T, et al. The effectiveness of levocetirizine and desloratidine in up to 4 times conventional doses in difficult to treat urticaria. J Allergy Clin Immunol. 2010;125:676-82.
11. Zingale LC, Castelli R, Zanichelli A, et al. Acquired deficiency of the inhibitor of the first complement component: presentation, diagnosis, course and conventional management. Immunol Allergy Clin North Am. 2006;26(4):669-90.
12. Zuberbier T, Aberer W, Asero R, et al. The EAACI/GA²LEN/EDF/WAO Guideline for the definition, classification, diagnosis and management of urticaria: the 2013 revision and update. Allergy. 2014;69(7):868-87.
13. Zuberbier T, Asero R, Bindslev-Jensen C, et al. EAACI/GA²LEN/EDF/WAO guideline: definition, classification and diagnosis of urticaria. Allergy. 2009;64:1420-6.
14. ZurawBL. Novel therapies for hereditary angioedema. Immunol Allergy Clin North Am. 2006;26(4):691-708.

# 14 CHAPTER Mast Cell and Mast Cell Activation Disorders

*Nilendu Sarma*

## INTRODUCTION

Mast cell, also called mastocyte, an important cell for defence, is basically a granulocyte that is derived from bone marrow myeloid stem cell. Its granules contain various biologically important secretory molecules like histamine and heparin (Box 1). Previously, it was thought to be a cell very similar to basophil, they are actually different cell and are derived from different hematopoietic lineages.

Mast cells originate from myeloid progenitor cells expressing the CD34 molecule in the bone marrow and are released in the immature form. Once they settle in the tissue, they are matured. T lymphocyte-derived interleukin-3 have role in its maturation.

Mast cell is distributed over many tissues like skin, lymph nodes, digestive and urinary tracts, and respiratory tract.

Mast cell plays important role in allergy. This is the key cell involved in anaphylaxis. Its other important roles are innate immune defence system and tolerance, wound healing, angiogenesis, immune tolerance, and blood-brain barrier function.

**BOX 1 Mediators of mast cells**

**Preformed mediators**
- Tryptase
- Histamine
- Serotonin
- Heparin

**Newly formed**
- Eicosanoids like thromboxane, prostaglandin D2, and leukotriene C4

**Cytokines and chemokines**
- Eosinophil chemotactic factor

## MANIFESTATIONS OF MAST CELL ACTIVATION

Whatever be the etiology and mechanism, the final result is release of mediators. The mediators affect many organs of the body and the symptoms depend on the organs affected.

Typical manifestations are:
- Urticaria, angioedema, flushing (skin)
- Nausea, vomiting, diarrhea, pain, bloating (gastrointestinal)
- Hypotension, unconsciousness, tachycardia (cardiovascular)
- Wheezing (respiratory)
- Conjunctival injection, nasal stuffiness (nose and eye)
- Headache, paresthesias, cognitive dysfunction (neurological)
- Anaphylaxis.

These symptoms may be precipitated spontaneously or after some precipitating events like heat, cold, stress, trauma, medications, insect stings, and foods.

## PHYSIOLOGICAL MAST CELL ACTIVATION

Mast cells express a high affinity receptor (FcεRI) on its surface. This binds to the Fc region of immunoglobulin E (IgE) antibody. Mast cells thus are coated with IgE. When antigen (allergens) bind to the IgE, mast cells are activated and release histamine and other mediators. There are other mechanisms (non-IgE mediated) as well that can stimulate the mast cells to release the mediators. These are physical injury, pathogen-associated molecular pattern receptors (for pathogens), and complement mediated mechanisms.

KIT is a transmembrane receptor. This is encoded by the proto-oncogene *c-Kit*. Point mutation (D816V) in *c-Kit* results in gain of function of the KIT resulting in spontaneous mast cell activation without IgE or other receptors. This occurs in mastocytosis.

## DISORDERS OF MAST CELL ACTIVATION

Mastocytosis, as discussed in next section, is the well-recognized mast cell activation disorders. However, activation of mast cell has a much wider spectrum than just mastocytosis. Common to all these conditions are the clinical manifestations of urticaria, flushing, abdominal pain, diarrhea, vomiting, and other features as mentioned above. Mast cell activation may be functional hyperactivity without any significant increase in mast cell number either in bone marrow or peripheral blood (mast cell hyperplasia) or there may increase in number of hyperactive mast cells.

Mast cell activation may be seen in following situations:
- Monoclonal proliferation of mast cell—as seen in mastocytosis, chronic eosinophilic leukemia and monoclonal mast cell activation syndrome
- Mast cell activation secondary to stimulation form other conditions like allergic disease (IgE or non-IgE mediated as in drugs, hormones), various infections and infestations of some chronic inflammatory or neoplastic disorders, chronic autoimmune urticarial, and physical urticarial
- Idiopathic mast cell degranulation. This is seen in case of idiopathic urticaria, angioedema, anaphylaxis, and in mast cell activation syndrome (MCAS).

## Monoclonal Mast Cell Activation Syndrome

This is now considered one important condition under clonal mast cell activation disorders. Since the diagnostic criteria of mastocytosis have been defined, condition that have features of clonal mast cell activation yet not fulfilling the criteria for mastocytosis are grouped under this entity.

Signs that indicate clonal mast cell activation are aberrant mast cell morphology, CD25 expression, and/or presence of the *c-Kit* D816V point mutation. These are all the minor criteria of mastocytosis. Monoclonal mast cell activation syndrome features one or two of these and lack the major criteria of mastocytosis that is defined as cluster of abnormal mast cell, each cluster being formed by more than 15 cells. Bone marrow may have increased number of aberrant mast cell but that does not reach up to classical mastocytosis level, serum tryptase levels may be slightly elevated, *c-Kit* mutation, if detectable, is limited bone marrow only.

This typically manifest with recurrent intermittent signs of mast cell degranulation like urticarial, angioedema and flushing, light-headedness and abdominal cramping, nausea and diarrhea, or in severe cases, life-threatening hypotension and unconsciousness. The episodes may last for a few minutes to several hours. Usually, these symptoms starts without any identifiable triggers but some cases may develop this after hymenoptera stings and exercise. This indicates that the condition also increases sensitivity to this IgE mediated pathway.

There is less information whether these conditions will ultimately transform to mastocytosis.

## Mast Cell Activation Syndrome

This is a yet ill-defined entity but requirement for such a condition is felt necessary as many of the patients presenting with symptoms of mast cell degranulation do not have presence of increased mast cell population. Thus, MCAS is considered an idiopathic state of mast cell hyper-responsiveness or increased function without any increase in mast cell number. This is considered an idiopathic condition. Common to all mast cell activation disorders, symptoms are due to mast cell degranulation. As mentioned, diagnosis requires involvement of more than two organs.

Diagnostic criteria of MCAS has been recently proposed by Akin et al. The proposed diagnostic criteria are:

1. Episodic clinical symptoms in two or more systems (skin, gastrointestinal, cardiovascular, respiratory, and naso-ocular)
2. Response to antihistamines, antileukotriene medications, and cromolyn sodium
3. Laboratory confirmation of increased mast cell release
4. Primary and secondary mast cell activation disorders ruled out.

Three mandatory criteria (out of the 4) have been included to ensure that only conditions of mast cell abnormality are included as, occasionally, some nonmast cell disorders might present with similar symptoms.

Baseline serum tryptase levels more than 15 ng has been considered as a satisfactory criterion for laboratory confirmation of mast cell activation. Increase serum tryptase level during symptomatic period should be repeated once more to confirm mast cell activation. Total serum tryptase is mentioned as the preferred method than 24-hour urine histamine metabolites, or 11-beta-prostaglandin F2. Laboratory evaluation of mast cell release has made stringent to avoid picking-up any non mast cell condition.

## SUGGESTED READINGS


1. Akin C, Valent P, Metcalfe DD. Mast cell activation syndrome: Proposed diagnostic criteria: Towards a global classification for mast cell disorders. J Allergy Clin Immunol. 2010;126(6):1099-104.
2. Frieri M. Mast Cell Activation Syndrome. Clin Rev Allergy Immunol. 2015 May 6. [Epub ahead of print].
3. Moon TC, Befus AD, Kulka M. Mast cell mediators: Their differential release and the secretory pathways involved. Front Immunol. 2014;5:569.
4. Valent P, Akin C, Escribano L, et al. Standards and standardization in mastocytosis: Consensus statement on diagnostics, treatment recommendations and response criteria. Eur J Clin Invest. 2007;37:435-53.

# 15 CHAPTER Mastocytosis

Sayantani Chakraborty, Nilendu Sarma

## INTRODUCTION

Mastocytosis are a heterogeneous group of disorders characterized by abnormal growth and accumulation of mast cells (MCs) in one or more organ systems. Skin is the most common organ to be affected but other organs like bone marrow and gastrointestinal (GI) tract may be affected too. It results from a clonal, neoplastic proliferation of morphologically and immunophenotypically abnormal MCs that accumulate in one or more organ systems.

The first description of mastocytosis was made by Nettleship and Tay in 1869 and Sézary coined the term mastocytosis.

The clinical presentation of the disease is spectral ranging from skin-limited disease [(cutaneous mastocytosis (CM)], particularly in pediatric cases where the majority have disease-onset within the first 2 years of life with spontaneous regression in most of the cases. While in adults, it presents mostly as systemic disease with extracutaneous involvement [systemic mastocytosis (SM)] that may be associated with multiorgan dysfunction/failure and shortened survival.

## PATHOGENESIS

Mastocytosis is frequently associated with somatic gain of function point mutations within KIT (D816V). KIT (CD117) is a type III receptor with intrinsic tyrosine kinase activity expressed by MC, melanocytes, hematopoietic progenitor cells, and interstitial cells of Cajal in the GI tract. It is functionally relevant for normal MC development, hematopoiesis, gametogenesis, melanogenesis, and regulation of slow gastric waves.

Mast cells retain high levels of cell surface KIT expression and the interaction with the KIT ligand with stem cell factor (SCF) plays a key role in regulating MC proliferation, maturation, adhesion, chemotaxis, and survival. Somatic mutations that leads to gain of function of KIT tyrosine kinase, particularly the D816V mutation is associated with SM. While childhood type is mostly associated with germ-line or acquired activating KIT mutations.

Rare germline KIT mutations that target the transmembrane domain and that are associated with familial mastocytosis include F522C and A533D.

Mast cells are multipotent effector cells of the immune system that produce histamine, tryptase, chymase, carboxypeptidase A, heparin, chondroitin sulfate glycosaminoglycans, prostaglandin D2, leukotrienes (LTC4, LTD4, LTE4), vascular endothelial growth factor, platelet-activating factor, multifunctional cytokines [tumor necrosis factor (TNF)-α, TNF-β, SCF, interleukin (IL)-1, IL-2, IL-3, IL-4, IL-5, IL-6, IL-9, IL-10, IL-13, granulocyte-macrophage colony stimulating factor (GM-CSF)], and chemokines (IL-8, monocyte chemotactic protein-1, macrophage inflammatory protein-1α). These mediators are responsible for a wide variety of clinical symptoms in patients affected by mastocytosis.

### Extent of the Involvement

Mastocytosis is an unusual clonal disease of bone marrow-derived hematopoietic progenitor cells, which manifests with a broad spectrum of clinical and morphological appearances.

Cutaneous mastocytosis is defined by increased numbers of skin MCs in the absence of the involvement of extracutaneous tissues. SM is characterized by proliferation and accumulation of MCs in at least one extracutaneous organ. Bone marrow is considered the most frequently affected internal organ. Thus, evaluation of bone marrow has been the backbone in all further classification and diagnosis of SM.

## CLINICAL FEATURES

Mastocytosis is a spectral form of disease. Lesions may range from mere presentation of a cutaneous sign, localized skin lesions to widespread systemic involvement.

Clinical presentation of mastocytosis ranges in a spectrum from good-prognosis forms, such as CM, indolent systemic mastocytosis (ISM), and extracutaneous mastocytoma to poor-prognosis, advanced forms like aggressive systemic mastocytosis (ASM), SM associated with clonal hematological non-MCs lineage diseases (SM-AHNMD), mast cells leukemia (MCL), and mast cell sarcoma.

Childhood onset mastocytosis usually consists of skin disease characterized by a benign and self-limiting course. Children having MC disease present with urticaria pigmentosa/maculopapular type, diffuse cutaneous mastocytosis (DCM) and solitary mastocytoma of the skin.

Mastocytoma present as a solitary nodular or plaque lesion, which resolves spontaneously with age. This is seen in children and appears at very early age (Fig. 1).

Urticaria pigmentosa is a form of CM and is characterized by small, brown macules and papules. The plaque form consists of

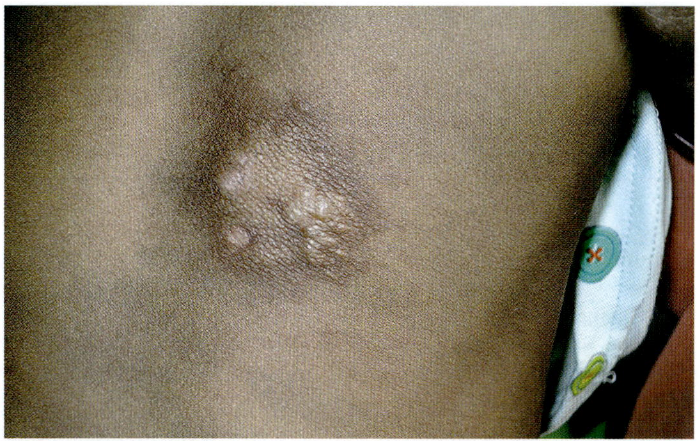

**FIG. 1:** Solitary mastocytoma developing urticarial rash after rubbing (Darier sign).

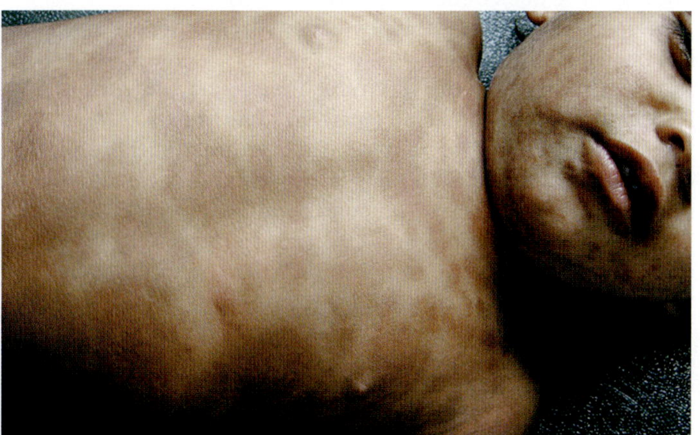

**FIG. 2:** Generalized brown patches of urticarial pigmentosa.

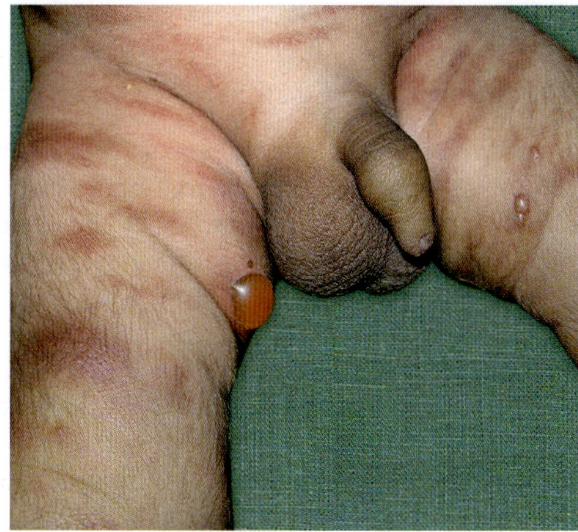

**FIG. 3:** Bullous lesion in mastocytosis.

slightly tanned or brown, flat or slightly elevated plaques up to several centimeters in diameter and usually occurs in infancy and early childhood. These usually resolve spontaneously (Fig. 2).

Diffuse cutaneous mastocytosis is the most severe form of CM, and is characterized by infiltration of MCs involving almost the entire skin. Diffuse cutaneous mastocytosis usually occurs at birth or in early infancy. Widespread hemorrhagic blisters may be the first clinical presentation of DCM.

Bullous lesions are commonly seen in childhood mastocytosis (Fig. 3).

In DCM, a diffuse thickening and leather grain appearance of the skin in found as the child grows up. There are four different forms of DCM like large hemorrhagic bullous, infiltrative small vesicular, and pseudoxanthomatous and pachydermic forms.

Systemic mastocytosis often occur in DCM. Diffuse cutaneous mastocytosis cases associated with MCs infiltration of the liver, spleen, lymph nodes and bone marrow, chronic diarrhea, malnutrition, and myeloproliferative disorders have been described. Otherwise the incidence of SM is rare in children. Some cases of SM associated with acute myelomonocytic leukemia and acute myeloid leukemia may occur in children.

Mechanical irritation of skin lesions leads to release of MCs mediators, and thus to reddening and urticarial swelling. This reaction is known as Darier's sign and is pathognomonic for all forms of CM.

Telangiectasia macularis eruptiva perstans is a rare subtype of CM and is often less adequately discussed in current classification system. Mast cell number in the skin is very less in comparison to other types. Thus, it does not urticate on rubbing and lesions are very small and macular with faint erythematous telangiectatic component. This tends to be very persistent.

Systemic mastocytosis frequently present with intermittent symptoms of mediator release. Patients commonly complain of flushing, itching, blistering, diarrhea, abdominal cramping and pain, vomiting, peptic symptoms, hypotensive episodes with vascular collapse, anaphylaxis, headache, and bone pain. Urticaria, angioedema, sneezing, rhinorrhea, and wheezing are commonly present. Indolent systemic mastocytosis is usually associated with skin involvement and a benign course. Aggressive systemic mastocytosis is characterized by life-threatening impaired organ function due to MCs. In MCL, bone marrow aspirate smears show >20% MCs. Associated cutaneous disease, if present, serves as important diagnostic clue.

## DIAGNOSIS

Diagnosis of mastocytosis requires many considerations. The purpose of diagnosis is not fulfilled unless it leads to fruitful management planning. Precisely, the approach to diagnosis should be directed to diagnose mastocytosis, identify cases of SM, and classify them into various subtypes. Each subtype has different prognosis and management strategies.

World Health Organization (WHO) has classified mastocytosis into seven subtypes (Box 1). Among them, the first one is CM and the rest are SM. Diagnosis of CM depends largely on clinical presentation, presence of Darier's sign, and findings on skin biopsy.

World Health Organization has also proposed diagnostic criteria for diagnosis of SM (Box 2). Classification of individual SM types sometimes requires in depth analysis of multiple laboratory parameters, criteria defined for disease burden (B-findings) and disease aggressiveness (C-findings) (Box 3).

All cases of CM should be evaluated to rule out SM. There are some basic principles in this regard:

1. All cases of CM should be clinically evaluated for presence of systemic signs and symptoms of SM
2. Adults with CM have high chance of SM. So, all adult cases should be thoroughly investigated as per standard protocol
3. Children with CM have very less chance of SM except for DCM. So they should be investigated only with specific indications.

**BOX 1 World Health Organization classification of mastocytosis**

1. Cutaneous mastocytosis
2. Indolent systemic mastocytosis
   a. Isolated bone marrow mastocytosis
   b. Smouldering systemic mastocytosis
3. Systemic mastocytosis with associated clonal hematologic non-mast cell lineage disease
4. Aggressive systemic mastocytosis
5. Mast cell leukemia
6. Mast cell sarcoma
7. Extracutaneous mastocytoma

**BOX 2 World Health Organization diagnostic criteria for systemic mastocytosis**

**Major criterion**

- Multifocal dense infiltrates of mast cells (>15 in aggregate) in tryptase stained biopsy sections of the bone marrow or of another extracutaneous organ

**Minor criterion**

- In biopsy of bone marrow or other extracutaneous organ(s), more than 25% of the mast cells show abnormal morphology (that is, are atypical mast cell type I or are spindle shaped) in multifocal lesions in histological examination
- Detection of a point mutation at codon 816 in the KIT receptor gene. This may be found in bone marrow, blood, or other internal organ
- KIT positive mast cells in bone marrow, blood, or other internal organs are found to express CD2 and/or CD25
- Serum total tryptase level persistently more than 20 ng/mL*

*This criterion cannot be used if the patient has a clonal non-mast cell associated hematological disorder.

**BOX 3 B and C findings (World Health Organization)**

*B findings*:

- Infiltration grade of mast cells in bone marrow >30% on histology and serum total tryptase levels >200 ng/mL
- Hypercellular bone marrow with loss of fat cells, discrete signs of dysmyelopoiesis without substantial cytopenias or WHO criteria for myelodysplastic syndrome or myeloproliferative disorder
- Hepatomegaly, splenomegaly, or lymphadenopathy without impaired organ function

*C findings (reflect impaired organ function because of infiltration of mast cells)*:

- One or more cytopenia(s), but no obvious non-mast cell hematopoietic malignancy
- Hepatomegaly with ascites and impaired liver function
- Palpable splenomegaly with hypersplenism
- Malabsorption with hypoalbuminemia and weight loss
- Large osteolytic lesions and/or severe osteoporosis causing pathological fractures

As per WHO criteria, bone marrow examination plays the pivotal role in the diagnosis of SM. The presence of multifocal dense aggregates of MCs in bone-marrow has been categorized as major criterion of SM by the WHO diagnostic system. The presence of one major and one minor criteria or three minor criteria constitute the diagnosis of SM.

**BOX 4 Diagnosis of mastocytosis in skin**

- Skin exanthema of cutaneous mastocytosis (major criteria)
- Lesional skin biopsy shows monomorphic, tryptase positive mast cell in cluster (>15/cluster) or scattered (>20 cells/high power field)
- Skin biopsy shows KIT mutation at 816 codon

Bone marrow MC smear (<20% vs. ≥20%) examination is the foundation in the subdivision of SM into two major subtypes as proposed by Valent et al. Subtype with ≥20% MC in the bone marrow has been further divided into two subtypes based on the MC count in the peripheral blood smear. These are aleukemic MCL (<10% MC) and MCL (≥10% MC).

Subtypes with <20% MC in the bone marrow need to be evaluated for any evidence of SM-AHNMD. If no such evidence is found, then there may be three subtypes—ISM (no B and no C findings), SSM (B findings), and ASM (C findings). B and C findings have been defined by WHO (Box 3).

Recently, another subtypes called "well-differentiated SM" has been described.

Mast cell sarcoma is very rare. There is no evidence of SM. Neoplastic MCs are detected focally in some organs.

As diagnosis of SM requires specific criteria, there will be cases that might have highly suggestive features but lack required major or minor criteria. Two such conditions require mention. Patients with CM who meet criteria for SM only partially (no major criteria, only one or two minor criteria) are often designated as "mastocytosis in skin" (Box 4).

With time, many of these cases may turn to typical SM. Cases without any cutaneous manifestations and having similar partial SM criteria, if have signs of clonal MC proliferation (D816V), are often diagnosed as MMAS (See chapter on 'Mast Cell and Mast Cell Activation Disorders').

## Laboratory Diagnosis

### Cytological Evaluation

Mast cells in the bone marrow are also assessed for the cytological atypicality. Bone marrow MCs are recommended as the best for KIT mutation analysis and evaluation of CD25 expression. Subtyping of SM (e.g., SSM, ASM) also depend on assessment of atypical MC number in the bone marrow.

#### *Serum Tryptase*

Serum tryptase level is another important noninvasive marker. As mentioned earlier, this serves as the most important marker to decide bone marrow examination in children presenting with CM. However, there may be persistent (>24 h) rise in serum tryptase above 20 ng/mL, which may be raised in other myeloid malignancies. The serum tryptase level is also important in evaluating the disease state because it is an indicator of the total body burden of MCs, and it correlates closely with the disease course and is considered a marker of disease severity. Decline in tryptase levels is associated with improvement of these symptoms.

### Histopathology

Histopathology from lesional skin reveals increased number of MCs in all the layers of skin. There is increased pigment in the epidermis. Mast cell infiltrates are predominantly found around blood vessels and skin appendages in the papillary dermis. The

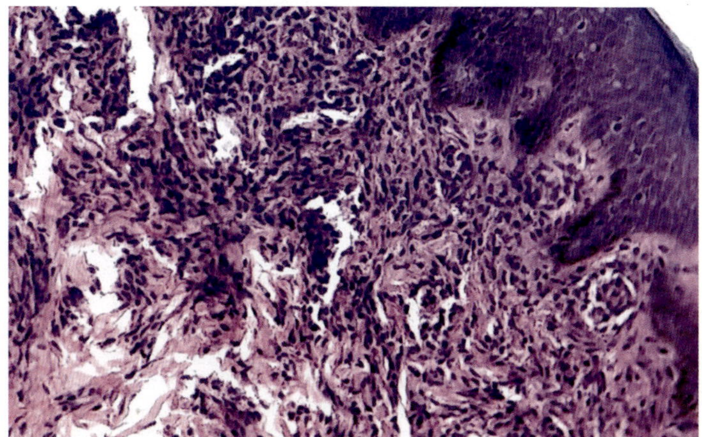

**FIG. 4:** Abundant round to oval basophilic mast cells in papillary dermis in mastocytosis (100x, H&E stain).

MCs are usually oval or spindle-shaped and have granules that stain metachromatically with toluidine blue Giemsa and Astra blue stains are also useful. Cytoplasma is abundant with distinct margin (Fig. 4).

### Immunohistochemistry

Immunohistochemical study with tryptase and anti-KIT (CD117) in lesional skin and bone marrow is helpful. Clonal proliferation is assessed with atypical morphology and immunoreactivity for CD2 and/or CD25. KIT mutations (*KIT D816V*) in highly purified bone marrow MCs and other hematopoietic cells with the use of sensitive diagnostic methods like multi-parametric flow cytometry can also detect clonality.

Immunophenotypical positivity for anti-CD25 is considered one of the most sensitive parameters, typically expressed on the neoplastic MCs. Therefore, some recommend this as the marker of choice. In advanced SM bone marrow, MCs often display lower levels of CD2 compared with ISM, and show strong expression of CD30 (Ki-1 antigen).

## TREATMENT

Treatment in CM is mostly symptomatic as none of the currently available therapeutic measures induces permanent involution of cutaneous or visceral lesions. Patients are advised to avoid agents that precipitate mediator release, such as aspirin, nonsteroidal anti-inflammatory drugs, codeine, morphine, alcohol, quinine, opiates, gallamine, procaine, radiographic dyes, dextran, polymyxin B, scopolamine, and D-tubocurarine, heat, friction, etc.

Histamine type 1 ($H_1$) receptor antagonists or combined $H_1$ and $H_2$ receptor antagonists are often helpful in controlling many of the symptoms associated with mastocytosis. The second-generation antihistaminics are more advantageous as they have longer half-lives and are more receptor specific. Addition of an $H_2$ antihistaminics may be helpful as they act synergistically.

Mast cell stabilizers like, oral cromolyn sodium and ketotifen may be helpful in stabilizing the MC related symptoms like pruritus, whealing, and flushing, as well as systemic symptoms such as diarrhea, abdominal pain, bone pain, and disorders of cognitive function.

Topical class 1 topical corticosteroids or intralesional corticosteroids may be helpful in treating the cutaneous lesions. Systemic corticosteroids may be helpful in reducing systemic and GI symptoms. Some people have also used systemic corticosteroids with cyclosporine which is helpful in relieving in cutaneous and GI symptoms.

Psoralens plus ultraviolet A therapy given four times a week can help control the pruritus and cutaneous whealing in patients with mastocytosis. They only provide symptomatic relief but do not have any action on disease progression by only reducing MC histamine content. This is more helpful in alleviating the cutaneous symptoms associated with telangiectasia macularis eruptiva perstans.

Interferon-α is helpful in treating aggressive form of the disease. Interferon-α (with or without corticosteroids) can control dermatological, hematological, GI, skeletal, and mediator-release symptoms.

Though with limited success, chemotherapeutic agents are used in the treatment of SM. Intravenous cladribine (2-chlorodeoxyadenosine) was reported to be effective in eliminating skin lesions and reducing the number of bone marrow MCs remarkably in a patient with advanced systemic disease. It has broad therapeutic activity and helpful in debulking disease.

Local radiation therapy may be helpful in reducing the bone pain.

Imatinib mesylate is a tyrosine kinase inhibitor which has variable response in halting the disease progression as per reports. Though it is said to be less useful in the patients having D816V mutation, there is one successful case report from 2008 described treatment of progressive c-*kit* mutation CM with imatinib, halting disease symptoms and progression and improving the length of disease course.

Imatinib is approved by the Food and Drug Administration for use in patients with aggressive SM with organ dysfunction without D816V c-*kit* mutation or unknown c-*kit* mutation status.

The other newer tyrosine kinase inhibitor which may be effective in treating systemic or severe MC disease are dasatinib, masitinib, nilotinib, and sunitinib.

Patients with mastocytosis should be equipped with emergency equipment like epinephrine self-injector and get trained about the use of it. Patients with recurrent episodes of vascular collapse may be prophylactically placed on $H_1$ and $H_2$ antihistamines to lessen the severity of attacks.

## SUGGESTED READINGS


1. Akin C, Fumo G, Yavuz AS, et al. A novel form of mastocytosis associated with a transmembrane c-kit mutation and response to imatinib. Blood. 2004; 103: 3222-5.
2. Bains SN, Hsieh FH. Current approaches to the diagnosis and treatment of systemic mastocytosis. Ann Allergy Asthma Immunol. 2010;104(1):1-10; quiz 10-2, 41.
3. Castells M, Metcalfe DD, Escribano L. Diagnosis and treatment of cutaneous mastocytosis in children. Am J Clin Dermatol. 2011;12:259-70.
4. Escribano L, Akin C, Castells M, et al. Current options in the treatment of mast cell mediator-related symptoms in mastocytosis. Allergy. 2006;5:61-77.
5. Escribano L, Alvarez-Twose I, Sanchez-Munoz L, et al. Prognosis in adult indolent systemic mastocytosis: A long-term study of the Spanish Network on mastocytosis in a series of 145 patients. J Allergy Clin Immunol. 2009;124:514-21.
6. Garcia-Montero AC, Jara-Acevedo M, Teodosio C, et al. KIT mutation in mast cells and other bone marrow hematopoietic cell lineages in systemic mast cell disorders: A prospective study of the Spanish Network on Mastocytosis (REMA) in a series of 113 patients. Blood. 2006;108:2366-72.

7. Hoffmann KM, Moser A, Lohse P, et al. Successful treatment of progressive cutaneous mastocytosis with imatinib in a 2-year-old boy carrying a somatic KIT mutation. Blood. 2008;112(5):1655-7.
8. Horny HP, Akin C, Metcalfe DD, et al. Mastocytosis (Mast cell disease). In: Swerdlow SH, Campo E, Harris NL, editors. World Health Organization (WHO) classification of tumors: pathology and genetics. In: Tumours of haematopoietic and lymphoid tissues Lyon: IARC Press, 2008, pp. 54-63.
9. Kar R, Rao S, Pati HP. Systemic mastocytosis with acute myelomonocytic leukemia: A case report. Indian J Hematol Blood Transfus. 2008;24:182-5.
10. Kleewein K, Lang R, Diem A, et al. Diffuse cutaneous mastocytosis masquerading as epidermolysis bullosa. Pediatr Dermatol. 2011;28:720-5.
11. Kurosawa M, Amano H, Kanbe N, et al. Response to cyclosporin and low dose methylprednisone in aggressive systemic mastocytosis. J Allergy Clin Immunol. 1999;103:S412-20.
12. Lange M, Niedoszytko M, Nedoszytko B, et al. Diffuse cutaneus mastocytosis: Analysis of 10 cases and a brief review of the literature. J Eur Acad Dermatol Venereol. 2012;26:1565-71.
13. Mamadeo KM, Wolgast L, McMahon C, et al. Systemic mastocytosis in a child with t(8;21) acute myeloid leukemia. Pediatr Blood Cancer. 2011;57:684-7.
14. Morgado JM, Sanchez-Munoz L, Teodosio CG, et al. Immunophenotyping in systemic mastocytosis diagnosis: CD25 positive alone is more informative than the CD25 and/or CD2. Mod Pathol. 2012;25:516-21.
15. Niedoszytko M, de Monchy J, van Doormaal JJ, et al. Mastocytosis and insect venom allergy: Diagnosis, safety, and efficacy of venom immunotherapy. Allergy. 2009;64:1237-45.
16. Quintas-Cardama A, Jain N, Verstovsek S. Advances and controversies in the diagnosis, pathogenesis, and treatment of systemic mastocytosis. Cancer. 2011;117:5439-49.
17. Srivastava N, Chand S, Singh S. Pseudoxanthomatous mastocytosis. Int J Dermatol. 2008;47:50-1.
18. Tang X, Boxer M, Drummond A, et al. A germline mutation in KIT in familial diffuse cutaneous mastocytosis. J Med Genet. 2004;41:e88.
19. Teferi A, Li CY, Butterfield JH, et al. Treatment of systemic mast cell disease with cladribine. N Engl J Med. 2001;344:307-8.
20. Valent P, Akin C, Arock M, et al. Definitions, criteria and global classification of mast cell disorders with special reference to mast cell activation syndromes: A consensus proposal. Int Arch Allergy Immunol. 2012;157:215-25.
21. Valent P, Akin C, Escribano L, et al. Standards and standardization in mastocytosis: consensus statements on diagnostics, treatment recommendations and response criteria. Eur J Clin Invest. 2007;37:435-53.
22. Valent P, Sotlar K, Horny HP. Aberrant expression of CD30 in aggressive systemic mastocytosis and mast cell leukemia: A differential diagnosis to consider in aggressive hematopoietic CD30-positive neoplasms. Leuk Lymph. 2011;52:740-4.
23. Verstovsec S. Advanced systemic mastocytosis: The impact of KIT mutations in diagnosis, treatment, and progression. Eur J Hematol. 2012;90:89-98.

# 16 CHAPTER Figurate Erythema

Sayantani Chakraborty, Nilendu Sarma

## INTRODUCTION

Erythemas are change in color of the skin due to vasodilatation which may be venous or arterial in origin. They may arise from both papillary dermis and reticular dermis. Depending upon the etiology, they may be transient or persistent and they may be divided into regional, diffuse, reticulated and figurate.

Figurate erythemas are a group of distinct conditions characterized by annular, arciform or polycyclic lesions often mimicking a large group of other annular and polycyclic lesions. They have different underlying causes and may often be idiopathic. The triggering factors are often systemic ranging from infections, malignancies both hematological and solid organs, allergies, drugs, connective tissue diseases, etc. They are often confused with other dermatological entities, most commonly urticaria, mastocytosis, granuloma annulare, etc. Hence, it is very important to perform a detailed workup of the cases to find out the underlying causes responsible for the conditions as they sometimes serve as important indicators to underlying more serious disorders.

The common morphological types of annular erythemas are as:

- Erythema annulare centrifugum (EAC)
- Erythema gyratum repens
- Erythema marginatum
- Necrolytic migratory erythema
- Erythema migrans
- Annular erythema of infancy.

## ERYTHEMA ANNULARE CENTRIFUGUM

Erythema annulare centrifugum is an inflammatory skin disease. The ambiguity embraced at all aspects of this condition starting from clinical description to etiology and thence management. Important clinical parameters playing role in creating this confusion are its pruritic versus nonpruritic nature, scaling versus nonscaling surface, just erythema, or palpable margin and so on. Over the years, our knowledge has advanced and the spectrum of clinical manifestations has expanded to incorporate all these.

The list of conditions that have been suggested to have etiological relationship is ever expanding. Infections, drugs, foods, connective tissue disease, and even numerous malignant conditions have been reportedly implicated as its etiology, in addition to a large group of patients in whom none of these are detected.

Despite these numerous unknown facets, this is considered as an important dermatological entity, common in prevalence and distinctly different from paraneoplatic figurate erythema or figurate erythema due to infection (e.g., erythema marginatum, erythema chronicum migrans, lupus, lymphoma or pseudolymphoma).

Thus, EAC is a condition that has figurate shape, flat or elevated, and scaly or non-scaly margin, is gradually progressive, and may be pruritic or nonpruritic. It can result from numerous etiologies, many of which can also result in non-EAC annular lesions of specific nature. Generally, EAC is often the preferred diagnosis when the condition fulfils the clinical descriptions of the conditions and all other similar-appearing specific entities are ruled out.

### Pathogenesis

This is considered to be an allergic or hypersensitive reaction to diverse etiologic factors (Box 1).

**BOX 1 Etiologies of erythema annulare centrifugum**

**Infection**

- *Bacteria*: *Escherichia coli*, streptococci, *Mycobacterium tuberculosis*, and *Borrelia*
- *Fungi*: Dermatophytes, *Malassezia furfur*, *Candida albicans*, and blue cheese *Penicillium*
- *Parasites*: *Ascaris lumbricoides*, and *Phthirus pubis* infestation
- *Viruses*: Epstein–Barr virus, molluscum contagiosum

**Drugs**

- Finasteride, chloroquine, hydroxychloroquine, and rituximab

*Neoplasia*

- Hodgkin disease, non-Hodgkin's disease, acute myelogenous leukemia (AML), chronic lymphocytic leukemia, squamous cell carcinoma, non-small cell lung cancer, multiple myeloma, prostate adenocarcinoma, breast cancer, and malignant histiocytosis

**Foods**

- Blue cheese, and tomatoes

**Systemic conditions**

- Recurrent acute appendicitis, cholestatic liver disease, and Graves' disease
- Menstruation, hypereosinophilic syndrome, Sjögren syndrome, and sarcoidosis
- Osteoarthritis, stress, and pregnancy

Possible etiologic agents are many. Mechanism of this reaction is unknown. It has been postulated that there are some role of type IV hypersensitivity, type 1 T helper (Th1) dependent pathway, tumor necrosis factor-alpha, interleukin-2, and other proinflammatory cytokines and vasoactive peptides.

Erythema annulare centrifugum manifesting as paraneoplastic disorder is rare but has been reported with lymphoproliferative malignancies, specifically lymphoma and leukemia. Paraneoplastic erythema annulare centrifugum eruption (PEACE) is thought to be a result of cytokine or other tumor-associated factors.

Recently, it has been proposed that EAC represents another manifestation of *Borrelia* infection that causes erythema migrans.

Spongiotic changes in the superficial variety indicate allergic mechanisms like id eruption. Deep variety has many histological alterations that suggest some close relation with lupus erythematosus. Rarely, EAC can be familial.

## Clinical Features

This starts with a small erythematous papular eruption expanding centrifugally and eventually developing central clearing. They may appear annular, polycyclic, or incomplete arcs. It progresses faster (few mm in a day) than erythema gyratum repens that progresses relatively slower (in months) (Fig. 1).

Central part of the lesions becomes clear without any atrophy except occasional case. Some cases may show a trailing scale at the inner side of a progressive margin. However, postinflammatory hyperpigmentation may develop. In the deep type of EAC, there is an indurated and apparent border, without desquamation and the lesion rarely itches.

There is a predilection for the trunk, buttocks, thighs and the legs but, upper extremities and the face are also affected. The palms and the soles are usually spared.

There is no age and sex predilection.

## Histopathology

Two histological types of EAC are found to exist, deep and superficial. Original description (Jean Darier in 1916) of EAC was of deep type. The subdivision is based on the level at which inflammatory infiltrate and other changes are detected. Characteristic changes in superficial variety are perivascular lymphocytic infiltrate with occasional eosinophils, spongiosis and papillary edema. Superficial type shows presence of parakeratosis that clinically is represented with scaling.

Deep infiltration, on the other hand, manifests with a palpable margin. Histologically, there is a sleeve-like arrangement of the superficial and deep lymphocytic infiltrate. Other changes are melanophages, with occasional dermal-epidermal junction vacuolation and individual necrotic keratinocytes. Many of the changes are similar to lupus erythematous.

## Diagnosis

Erythema annulare centrifugum has to be differentiated from all other annular erythematous lesions (Table 1).

History of progression and clinical examination is important. Underlying disorders should be ruled out with extensive investigations. Routine laboratory tests, hemogram, Mantoux

**TABLE 1: Figurate lesions**

| Uncertain etiology | Specific entities |
|---|---|
| Erythema annulare centrifugum | Erythema chronicum migrans (*Borrelia burgdorferi* infection) |
| Familial annular erythema (FAE) | Paraneoplastic |
| Eosinophilic annular erythema | Erythema gyratum repens |
| Annular erythema of infancy (AEI) | Necrolytic migratory erythema |
| Neutrophilic figurate erythema (variant of AEI) | • Sweet's syndrome<br>• Lupus erythematous (LE)—neonatal LE, subacute LE<br>• Erythema marginatum<br>• Pseudolymphoma<br>• Superficial fungal infection (Tinea)<br>• Mycoses fungoides<br>• Granuloma annulare (Fig. 2)<br>• Urticaria (Fig. 3)<br>• Migratory keratoderma<br>• Resolving erythema nodosum<br>• Nonvesicular stage of bullous pemphigoid<br>• Psoriasis<br>• Erythema multiforme |

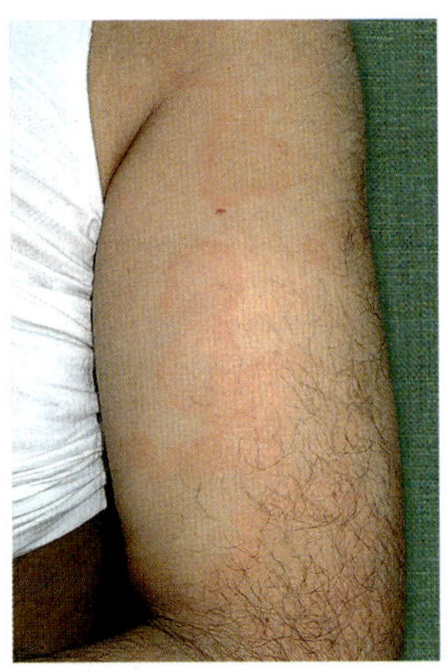

**FIG. 1:** Erythema annulare centrifugum in an adult.

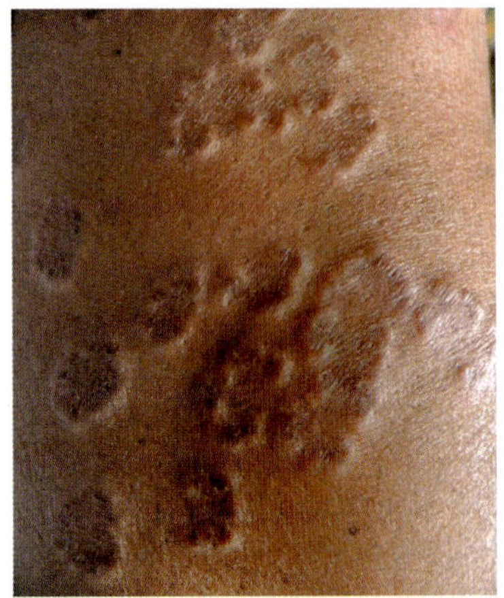

**FIG. 2:** Figurate lesions due to granuloma annulare.

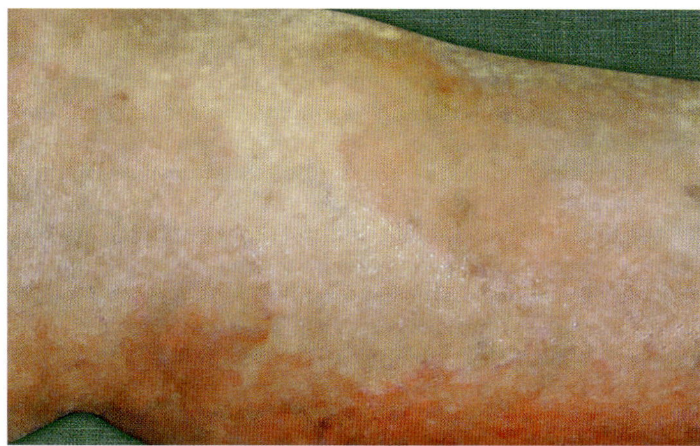

FIG. 3: Figurate lesion in urticarial vasculitis.

test, scraping for fungal elements, urine analysis, serum antinuclear antibody should be done. Skin biopsy is indicated in order to rule out other mimicking conditions.

## Treatment

The course is usually self-limiting in uncomplicated cases. Topical or systemic corticosteroids may help in remission but this is temporary and recurrence may happen on withdrawal of the drug. Resolution of the underlying condition may often help in clearing of the lesions. Several other drugs are also used in isolated cases like topical tacrolimus, topical calcipotriol, oral metronidazole, subcutaneous etanercept, subcutaneous interferon-α, etc.

# ERYTHEMA GYRATUM REPENS

Erythema gyratum repens was first reported in 1952 by Gammel in a woman with breast carcinoma.

Erythema gyratum repens represents an immune reaction in which there is a cross-reaction between tumor antigens and cutaneous antigens. Direct immunofluorescence (DIF)-demonstrated deposits of immunoglobulin G (IgG) and C3 in the basement membrane zone of the skin. In cases associated with malignancy, similar deposits were seen in the associated neoplasm.

There is an underlying malignancy in about 80% of the cases of erythema gyratum repens. The most frequently seen malignancies are lung, breast and esophagus cancers, and on rare occasion with hematological malignancy like in blast crisis of chronic myeloid leukemia.

Apart from malignancy, tuberculosis, CREST (calcinosis, Raynaud phenomenon, esophageal dysmotility, sclerodactyly, and telangiectasia) syndrome, drug hypersensitivity, hypereosinophilic syndrome, systemic lupus erythematosus, and pregnancy have also been reported.

Clinically, the rash is characterized by serpiginous erythematous bands with a wood grain appearance and a scaling edge which spreads centrifugally on the trunk and extremities sparing hands, feet, and face. Pruritus may be debilitating. The diagnosis is based upon its characteristic clinical pattern. Erythema gyratum repens is a rare condition that has been considered to be an obligate paraneoplastic syndrome.

The lesions spread fast and are associated with desquamation and pruritus.

Erythema gyratum repens is seen primarily in adults.

## Diagnosis

It should be differentiated from tinea imbricate, vasculitis, lupus erythematosus, pemphigoid, annular psoriasis, etc.

Histologic features are nonspecific and include hyperkeratosis, focal parakeratosis, moderate patchy spongiosis and a mild, perivascular lymphohistiocytic infiltrate. In some cases, eosinophils, and melanophages are seen in the dermis.

## Treatment

Treatment of erythema gyratum repens should be directed to the underlying condition.

Antihistamines may be used for intense pruritus.

## Erythema Marginatum

It is a sign seen in about 20% of patients with acute rheumatic fever. It is seen more commonly in children than in adult as acute rheumatic fever is higher in children than in adults. The peak age of onset is between 5 years and 15 years.

The lesions of erythema marginatum begin as erythematous macules that spread peripherally. Fully-developed lesions are annular erythematous plaques without much scaling. The lesions are migrating in nature and are usually asymptomatic. New groups of lesions appear mostly during bouts of fever and are mostly noticeable during afternoon. The most common locations are the trunk, axillae, and proximal extremities. It is one of the major Jones' criteria, along with carditis, migratory polyarthritis, chorea, and subcutaneous nodules and is thought to be a response to streptococcal antigens. It usually precedes joint inflammation and often occurs during episodes of carditis.

Erythema marginatum-like lesions may also present in absence of rheumatic fever like in drug induced (Sorafenib). It has been associated with a unique presentation of erythema marginatum with hemorrhagic lesions.

Skin biopsy shows an interstitial and perivascular infiltrate composed predominantly of neutrophils without vasculitis. There can be extravasation of erythrocytes in the later stages.

Lesions often resolve spontaneously and are unaffected by treatment of the primary condition.

# ERYTHEMA CHRONICUM MIGRANS

Lyme's borreliosis is associated with a unique type of migrating erythema. This condition is caused by infection with *Borrelia burgdorferi* sensu lato, *Borrelia afzelii* or *Borrelia garinii*. The primary infection at the site of tick bite is a solitary flat or elevated lesion mildly inflammatory. However, hemorrhagic or urticated lesions in the beginning may also be found. Lesions of *B. burgdorferi* are usually more inflammatory. It gradually expands in target like concentric ring-like pattern. Nonannular lesions may be more common in infections caused by *B. afzelii*. The lesion expands slowly over a period of weeks to a median size of about 15 cm with central clearing. There may be hemorrhagic lesions too. Malaise, flu-like symptoms, and lymphadenopathy are common in this stage of disease. Within one to few weeks, additional, usually multiple, annular plaques may develop in most of the patients. These lesions may resemble EAC.

Borrelial lymphocytoma is another accompanying feature during this stage of the disease which manifests as small plaques, usually on the earlobe, nose, areola, scrotum, or over bony prominences.

If left untreated, this may progress to a more chronic stage known as acrodermatitis chronica atrophicans.

Histology of early localized or disseminated stage erythema migrans shows a superficial perivascular lymphocytic infiltrate rich in plasma cells, and which may extend more deeply around vessels or appendages. *Borrelia*-specific IgG antibody may be considered to be diagnostic.

Treatment is recommended with doxycycline 100 mg BD for 2–3 weeks.

## NECROLYTIC MIGRATORY ERYTHEMA

This type of figurate erythema is seen in pancreatic neuroendocrine tumors (PNETs), especially glucagonoma as paraneoplastic manifestation. It is called glucagonoma syndrome in such cases. Glucagon or its metabolites are thought to be responsible.

Rarely, it may be associated other neoplastic disorders like myelodysplastic syndrome, hepatocellular carcinoma, bronchial carcinoma, and jejunal adenocarcinoma.

Association with non-neoplastic diseases like chronic pancreatitis, chronic hepatitis, zinc and essential fatty acid deficiency, is also seen. In such circumstances, it is known as pseudoglucogonoma syndrome.

This appears as erythematous scaly lesions with centrifugal growth.

The lesions show regression once the tumor is debulked and/or with reduction in glucagon levels. Recurrence of symptoms is a sensitive indicator of recurrence of the tumor.

## ANNULAR ERYTHEMA OF INFANCY

Annular erythema of infancy presents as figurate erythema clinically similar to EAC in the infantile age group. This is a vaguely defined entity, often overlapping with differentiating entities like neonatal lupus erythematous and fungal infections. Intestinal colonization with *Candida* and Epstein–Barr virus infection were reported in some affected cases. There may be face presentation of neonatal lupus erythematous with positive antibodies. Some types where there is central atrophy are named erythema gyratum repens and atrophicans transiens, are also described. Lichenoid and lymphomatoid annular erythema may represent a varied set of presentation. Persistent annular erythema of infancy has been described with intestinal candidal colonization.

Histopathology resemble with EAC. Neutrophilic figurate erythema of infancy is a distinct term that has been attributed to patients with lesions having neutrophilic predominance.

Annular erythema of infancy is a benign disease in most cases unassociated with other conditions. It is usually self-limiting over a few months, even though a chronic course may rarely occur.

## SUGGESTED READINGS


1. Cardoso Filho Fde A, Feitosa RG, Fechine CO, et al. Glucagonoma syndrome associated with necrolytic migratory erythema. Rev Assoc Med Bras. 2015;61(3):203-6.
2. Carvalho SM, Dalben I, Corrente JE, et al. Rheumatic fever presentation: A case series report. Rev Bras Reumatol. 2012;52(2):241-6.
3. De La Torre-Lugo EM, Sanchez JL. Erythema gyratum repens. J Am Acad Dermatol. 2011;64:e89-90.
4. Durani BK, Andrassy K, Hartschuh W. Neutrophilic dermatosis with an erythema gyratum repens-like pattern in systemic lupus erythematosus. Acta Derm Venerol. 2005;85:455-6.
5. Eubanks LE, McBurney E, Reed R. Erythema gyratum repens. Am J Med Sci. 2001;321:302-5.
6. Feder HM Jr, Abeles M, Bernstein M, et al. Diagnosis, treatment and prognosis of erythema migrans and Lyme Arthritis. Clin Dermatol. 2006;24(6):509-20.
7. Gore M, Winters ME. Erythema Gyratum Repens: A rare Paraneoplastic Rash. West J Emerg Med. 2011;12(4):556-8.
8. Kiyohara T, Kumakiri M, Kobayashi H, et al. Erythema gyratum repens accompanied by essential thrombocythemia, followed by a blastic crisis. Acta Derm Venereol. 2003;83:133-4.
9. Morita A, Sakakibara N, Tsuji T. Erythema gyratum repens associated with hypereosinophilic syndrome. J Dermatol. 1994;21:612-4.
10. Mu EW, Sanchez M, Mir A, et al. Paraneoplastic erythema annulare centrifugum eruption (PEACE). Dermatol Online J. 2015;21(12).
11. Nadelman RB. Erythema migrans. Infect Dis Clin North Am. 2015;29(2):211-39.
12. Patrizi A, Savoia F, Varotti E, et al. Neutrophilic figurate erythema of infancy. Pediatr Dermatol. 2008;25(2):255-60.
13. Rübsam K, Flaig MJ, Ruzicka T, et al. Erythema marginatum hemorrhagicum: a unique cutaneous side effect of sorafenib. J Am Acad Dermatol. 2011;64(6):1194-6.
14. Stachowitz S, Abeck D, Schmidt T, et al. Persistant annular erythema of infancy. Clin Exp Dermatol. 2000;25(5):404-5.
15. Weyers W, Diaz-Cascajo C, Weyers I. Erythema annulare centrifugum: results of clinicopathologic study of 73 patients. Am J Dermatopathol. 2003;25:451-62.

# 17 CHAPTER Autoinflammatory Syndromes

*Nilendu Sarma, Sayantani Chakraborty*

## INTRODUCTION

Autoinflammatory syndromes are characterized by spontaneous, abnormal activation of innate immunity leading to spontaneous inflammation in the absence of any pathogenic role of autoantibodies or autoreactive T lymphocytes. Clinically, these manifest as recurrent episodes of fever, skin rashes, inflammation of serous membranes, eyes, joints, lymph nodes, gastrointestinal tract, and nervous system and high risk of secondary amyloidosis in the long run.

The majority of the syndromes are inherited as Mendelian traits with strong influence of environmental factors in some types. Thus, involvement of first- or second-degree family members is generally found. Genes are related to inflammatory activation pathway, especially activation of interleukin-1β (IL-1β). Genetic defects of most of the autoinflammatory syndromes have been identified (Table 1).

Many new conditions are being identified and the list is getting bigger day by day. Very recently, a new disease caused by high-penetrance heterozygous germline mutations in *TNFAIP3*, which encodes the nuclear factor-kappa B (NF-κB) regulatory protein A20, has been identified among six unrelated families with early-onset systemic inflammation. This disorder resembles Behçet's disease.

However, genetic defect is yet to be identified for some other common autoinflammatory syndromes like periodic fever, aphthous stomatitis, pharyngitis, and adenitis (PFAPA) syndrome, congenital dyserythropoietic anemia, some neutrophilic dermatoses and Still's disease.Diseases included under the umbrella of autoinflammatory syndrome are constantly increasing. Atopic dermatitis, psoriasis, vitiligo, alopecia, rosacea, and diabetes are also considered to be autoinflammatory syndromes.

Commonly, autoinflammatory syndromes are classified in the following subtypes:

- Monogenic periodic fever syndromes
  - Familial Mediterranean fever (FMF)
  - Tumor necrosis factor receptor-associated periodic syndrome (TRAPS)
  - Mevalonate kinase deficiency (MKD).
- Cryopyrin-associated periodic syndromes (CAPSs)
  - Muckle-Wells syndrome (MWS)
  - Familial cold autoinflammatory syndrome (FCAS)
  - *NLRP12*-associated autoinflammatory disorder (*NLRP12AD*)
  - Chronic infantile neurological, cutaneous, and articular (CINCA) syndrome.
- Autoinflammatory pyogenic disorders
  - Pyogenic arthritis, pyoderma gangrenosum and cystic acne (PAPA) syndrome
  - Deficiency of the IL-1 receptor antagonist (DIRA)
  - Majeed syndrome (MS).
- Autoinflammatory granulomatous disorders
  - Blau syndrome (BS)
  - Early-onset sarcoidosis (EOS).

During attacks, levels of acute phase reactants are high. After the attack, the level becomes little lower but remains persistently higher than normal.

Some of the conditions have specific laboratory abnormality. Mevalonic acid can be detected in urine during attack in patients with hyper immunoglobulin D (IgD) syndrome.

Histopathology is of limited value.

Genetic studies to identify the gene defect can be confirmatory but are less sensitive and not available in all setup.

## FAMILIAL MEDITERRANEAN FEVER

Familial Mediterranean fever is transmitted by autosomal recessive inheritance. Mutation of *MEFV* gene that encodes pyrin leads to decreased production of pyrin permits apoptotic speck protein-induced (apoptosis-associated speck-like protein with a caspase recruitment domain) IL-1 processing and inflammation that is most possibly initiated after a minor serosal injury.

Clinically, it is characterized by recurrent acute fever, arthritis, polyserositis, and erythema that typically resemble erysipelas. There are three phenotypes of this condition:

- Phenotype 1: Recurrent inflammatory episodes, each lasting about 12–72 hours, frequently manifested with fever and abdominal pain are triggered by events like stress, physical exercise, or infections. Sometimes arthralgia and myalgia are also found. Nonspecific symptoms like lack of appetite, malaise, and irritability may precede the episodes.

  Erysipelas-like lesions of about 10 cm in diameter appear during the episode and persist for short period (usually 12–48 hours). Legs, hip, knee and dorsum of feet are commonly affected.

**TABLE 1: Autoinflammatory syndromes and the identified genetic defects**

| Conditions | Genetic defect |
|---|---|
| **Inflammasome mediated** | |
| Autoinflammation and PLCγ2-associated antibody deficiency and immune dysregulation (APLAID) | *PLCG2* |
| Familial cold autoinflammatory syndrome 1 (FCAS1) | *CIAS1* (*PYPAF1* or *NALP3*) |
| Familial Mediterranean fever | *MEFV* |
| Mevalonate kinase deficiency (hyper-IgD syndrome) | *MVK* |
| Muckle-Wells syndrome | *CIAS1* (also called *PYPAF1* or *NALP3*) |
| Neonatal-onset multisystem inflammatory disease (NOMID) or chronic infantile neurological, cutaneous, and articular (CINCA) syndrome | *CIAS1 (PYPAF1* or *NALP3)* |
| NLRC4-related macrophage activation syndrome (NLRC4-MAS)/FCAS4 | *NLRC4* |
| PLCγ2-associated antibody deficiency and immune dysregulation (PLAID)/FACS3 | *PLCG2* |
| **Noninflammasome mediated** | |
| ADAM17 deletion | *ADAM17* |
| Blau syndrome | *NOD2* (also called *CARD15*) |
| CARD14-mediated psoriasis (CAMPS) | *CARD14* |
| Chronic atypical neutrophilic dermatosis with lipodystrophy (CANDLE) | *PSMB8* |
| Cherubism (diseases of the bones) | *SH3BP2* |
| Chronic recurrent multifocal osteomyelitis and congenital dyserythropoietic anemia (Majeed syndrome) | *LPIN2* |
| Copa defect | *COPA* |
| Deficiency of the interleukin-1 receptor antagonist (DIRA) | *IL-1RN* |
| Deficiency of the IL-36 receptor antagonist (DITRA) | *IL-36RN* |
| HOIL1 deficiency functional defect | *HOIL1* |
| Pyogenic sterile arthritis, pyoderma gangrenosum and acne (PAPA) syndrome | *PSTPIP1* |
| SLC29A3 mutation | *SLC29A3* |
| Tumor necrosis factor receptor-associated periodic syndrome (TRAPS) | *TNFRSF1* |

Modified and reproduced from Picard C, Al-Herz W, Bousfiha A, et al. Primary immunodeficiency diseases: an update on the classification from the International Union of Immunological Societies Expert Committee for Primary Immunodeficiency 2015. J Clin Immunol. 2015;35:696-726.

- Phenotype 2: Some of the FMF patients may present with proteinuria or kidney failure due to amyloidosis.
- Phenotype 3: These patients have mutations (homozygous or heterozygous) in the *MEFV* gene.

Inflammatory markers are raised in blood [e.g., erythrosedimentation rate (ESR), C-reactive protein (CRP), serum amyloid A (SAA), neutrophil leukocytosis, thrombocytosis].

Colchicine is frequently used to prevent the acute episodes and also to prevent secondary complications of amyloidosis. IL-1 inhibitors (anakinra, rilonacept) and anti-TNF-α agents (etanercept, infliximab, adalimumab) have also been used, especially in resistant cases.

## TUMOR NECROSIS FACTOR RECEPTOR-ASSOCIATED PERIODIC SYNDROME

This is an autosomal dominant condition associated with mutation in the *TNFRSF1A* gene (TNF receptor). This mutation results in increased TNF inflammatory signaling. There is dysregulation in the secretion of IL-1 and IL-6. This may even result in oxidative damage and production of mitochondrial-free radicals.

### Clinical Presentation

The syndrome is characterized by inflammatory attacks of variable intensity and duration comprising of fever episodes accompanied more or less constantly by sterile peritonitis with abdominal pain, diarrhea or constipation, nausea, and vomiting.

Arthritis, arthralgia, and musculoskeletal pain are characteristics of this condition. Mono-ocular and/or bilateral periorbital edema is hallmark sign of the disease. This may be associated with periorbital pain and conjunctivitis.

Different kinds of skin rashes are described. These include a migratory macular erythema, edematous dermal plaques, serpiginous or annular lesions, purpuric lesions. Rash may be painful. Histologically, there is presence of perivascular lymphocytic and monocytic infiltrates.

During acute episodes, there is acute rise in ESR, CRP, and SAA. There may be marked increase in neutrophils, haptoglobin, fibrinogen, and platelets.

Proteinuria may be an important marker of kidney damage.

Genetic tests determining mutation in the TNFRSF1A are indispensible for cases suspicious of TRAPS.

### Treatment

High doses of nonsteroidal anti-inflammatory drugs (NSAIDs) and corticosteroids may prove useful during acute phases.

Colchicine and immunomodulating or immunosuppressant agents have also been proven to have very little efficacy in TRAPS.

Etanercept has been proven to be useful in reducing the intensity and duration of acute attacks, although in some cases.

Treatment with anti-IL-1 agents, also has been proven to be particularly efficacious in preventing attacks and inducing a rapid and long-lasting remission of the disease, as well as in the prevention and even regression of amyloidosis.

Recently, the IL-6 receptor antagonist tocilizumab has been used in etanercept- and anakinra-resistant patients with good results.

## MEVALONATE KINASE DEFICIENCY/HYPER-IGD SYNDROME

This is transmitted as an autosomal recessive disease and is caused by mutations in the *MVK* gene. Inflammatory reactions are mediated through IL-1β.

Proinflammatory isoprenoids are overproduced along with reduced synthesis of cholesterol. Mevalonic acid is increased in plasma and urine.

Attacks are more common in childhood and adolescence. This is characterized by recurrent fever (above 38.5°C), mouth ulcers, abdominal pain, vomiting, and/or diarrhea and headache. Cervical or sometimes generalized lymphadenopathy is present.

A nonspecific maculopapular rash, mostly affecting palms and soles are often noted. Urticaria, erythema nodosum, and purpura are less commonly seen.

Acute phase reactants are elevated during attacks. Serum IgD is often high (even above 100 IU/mL). Serum IgA may also be elevated.

Elevated urinary mevalonic acid during acute febrile flares may aid in diagnosis. Genetic testing may be done to confirm the diagnosis.

During acute attacks, NSAIDs and corticosteroids may be helpful. Simvastatin may be efficacious in reducing the duration of acute episodes by reducing production of mevalonic acid by blocking the enzyme 3-hydroxy-3-methylglutaryl coenzyme A reductase. Anti-IL1 and anti-TNF-alpha may be helpful in resistant cases.

## CRYOPYRIN-ASSOCIATED PERIODIC SYNDROME

Cryopyrin-associated periodic syndromes are a group of autoinflammatory diseases caused by mutations in the *NLRP3* gene (also called *CIAS1* or *PYPAF*) encoding for cryopyrin. *NLRP3* stands for NOD-like receptor family pyrin domain 3. All are transmitted by autosomal dominant inheritance.

Cryopyrin is a crucial inflammasome protein that have role in leukocyte apoptosis and NF-κB signaling and IL-1 processing. Mutation leads to constitutive activation of the NLRP3 inflammasome

There are three known forms of CAPS:
1. Familial cold autoinflammatory syndrome
2. Muckle-Wells syndrome
3. Chronic infantile neurological, cutaneous, and articular syndrome.

Clinically, these patients manifest with recurrent fever attacks associated with other multiple inflammatory symptoms. Many of these patients tend to develop secondary amyloidosis, kidney, and neurological disorder.

The FCAS generally appears during the first few months of life and is characterized by brief recurrent inflammatory episodes, usually triggered by generalized exposition to low temperatures or sudden changes in temperature. Symptoms include fever, urticaria-like rash that responds poorly to antihistamines. Besides, there may be conjunctivitis, headache, arthralgia, arthritis, and fatigue. FCAS generally does not progress to amyloidosis.

Muckle-Wells syndrome generally presents very early in life or during childhood. Presentation may be recurrent episodic or even chronic. Common manifestations are neurosensorial deafness, episcleritis, and secondary amyloidosis.

The CINCA syndrome manifests during the first weeks of life and is the most severe form.

Eyes and central nervous system are frequently affected and manifest with papilledema, uveitis, optic nerve atrophy, blindness, mental retardation, chronic aseptic meningitis, cerebral atrophy, and increased intracranial pressure. Sometimes, a form of deforming osteoarthropathy of the large joints and hypertrophy of growth plates is seen.

Renal involvement may occur due to amyloidosis. Nonpruritic urticaria-like skin rash is noted.

### Treatment

Interleukin antagonist anakinra may often help in improving neurological symptoms. Other IL-antagonists which may be useful are rilonacept and canakinumab.

## BLAU SYNDROME/GRANULOMATOUS AUTOINFLAMMATORY DISEASES

Blau syndrome is an autosomal dominant granulomatous inflammatory disease caused by mutations in the region encoding for the nucleotide-binding domain region of the *NOD2/CARD15* gene with subsequent dysregulation of the inflammatory response and formation of noncaseous granulomas.

The protein NOD2 is mainly expressed in monocytes and plays a crucial role in the clearance of bacteria, particularly, *Mycobacterium tuberculosis*, as it is capable of interacting with peptidoglycan and activating the NF-κB signal route.

Early-onset sarcoidosis and BS are possibly the two variants of the same disorder with same genetic defect. EOS is considered by some as sporadic BS.

Disease manifests in childhood. It affects joints, skin, and eyes. Systemic manifestations include recurrent (or persistent) fever, granulomatous arteritis, cranial nerve neuropathies, and hearing loss. This commonly presents with symmetrical polyarthritis of small and medium sized joints often leading to ankylosis. Photophobia, blurred vision, recurrent bilateral anterior uveitis or bilateral granulomatous panuveitis are major problem of this condition.

Symmetrical, dark red maculorpapular or nodular eruptions, lichenoid-like lesions, those may heal with scarring are seen on the trunk and limbs. Noncaseating granulomas with giant cells are found with the skin eruptions.

Early-onset sarcoidosis, a multiorgan sporadic disease characterized by onset in the first 4 years of life, joint, skin, eye, lymph node involvement, and recurrent fevers, with possible abdominal or central nervous system involvement. Histologically, presence of noncaseous epithelioid granulomas is observed in the involved tissues. Pulmonary parenchyma, involved in more than 90% of patients with adult sarcoidosis, is usually spared in EOS.

There is no established therapy. In the acute phases, high doses of corticosteroids may be utilized but with variable success. The use of anti-TNF-α and anti-IL-1 biological agents also seems encouraging.

## HEREDITARY PYOGENIC DISORDERS

Three disorders, namely PAPA syndrome (pyogenic arthritis, pyoderma gangrenosum and acne), MS and DIRA are often grouped together due to the similarity in their clinical presentation with presence of sterile abscesses that mainly affect the skin, joints, and bones.

The PAPA syndrome appears in early childhood and is characterized by joint involvement, manifested with severe self-limiting pyogenic arthritis. In terms of skin involvement, the appearance of pyoderma gangrenosum and nodular-cystic acne is described in early childhood.

It is an autosomal dominant disease caused by mutations in the *PSTPIP1* gene. This encodes for CD2-binding protein 1 (*CD2BP1*), involved in the proper assembly of the cytoskeleton, which normally inhibits pyrin-mediated inflammatory signals and the activation of caspase-1.

## MAJEED SYNDROME

Majeed syndrome is a rare autosomal recessive disease caused by homozygous mutations in the *LPIN2* gene (Table 1) that encodes for lipin 2. This manifests during early childhood.

Recurrent febrile attacks along with multifocal sterile osteomyelitis, dyserythropoietic anemia are seen. Skin manifestation includes chronic diffuse neutrophilic dermatoses.

The DIRA is another rare autosomal recessive disease caused by missense mutations in the *IL1RN* gene that encodes for the IL-1 receptor antagonist. It is manifested during the first few weeks of life, generally with multifocal osteomyelitis, periostitis, skin pustules, neonatal sepsis, hepatosplenomegaly and even multiorgan failure.

## PFAPA SYNDROME

The acronym stands for periodic fever, aphthous stomatitis, pharyngitis, and adenitis. Familial cases have been found. No genetic defect has been detected so far. A recent study has shown that this is unlikely to be a monogenic disease. None of the known genes that are involved in other autoinflammatory syndromes are involved. They proposed oligogenic or a complex inheritance multiple genes or nongenetic factors to be involved in this condition.

Clinically, this manifests in childhood age (before 5 years age) with periodic (every 2–6 weeks) high fever (>39°C that last for 3–6 days). Oral aphthae on the labial mucosa, tender enlargement of cervical lymphadenopathy, follicular exudative tonsillitis are the most common features that are usually present either single or in combination.

This possibly represents the most frequent cause of periodic fever of unknown origin in childhood. Disease generally improves by adolescence with only occasional cases persist in adulthood.

Other features are headache, malaise, arthritis, nausea, and vomiting. Overall general condition and growth remains normal. Genital ulcer has been reported.

This has to be differentiated from Behçet's disease. Diagnosis is clinical and depends on exclusion of other similar diseases. Treatment is done with oral prednisolone and cimetidine. Tonsillectomy has been advocated by some.

## DIAGNOSTIC APPROACH

Diagnosis is essentially clinical. Details history and clinical examination during the attack are important. Cutaneous as well as systemic manifestations should be evaluated properly.

Unexplained recurrent fever is a sine qua non feature of all autoinflammatory syndromes. The number, frequency and gap between each attack and age of onset are important parameters. Chronic infections like tuberculosis (TB), systemic lupus erythematosus (SLE), vasculitis, malignancy like leukemia and lymphoma have to be ruled out. Age is an important criterion for diagnosis. Frequently, therapeutic challenge with drugs like steroids, antibiotics, tonsillectomy, colchicine, and IL-1 inhibitors assists in diagnosis.

Recurrent constitutional symptoms, as well as specific tissue inflammation involving joint and skin symptoms are also important manifestations of these conditions. Now, with expanding knowledge from translational research, various conditions with diverse clinical manifestations have been incorporated into the spectrum of autoinflammatory disease.

## TREATMENT

Traditional anti-inflammatory drugs like systemic corticosteroids are generally not effective in most autoinflammatory disorders except in some specific indications. Prednisolone is the main drug used during acute attacks in hyper-IgD syndrome. Anakinra is also highly effective. Immunosuppressive drugs like methotrexate and cyclosporine are used in some specific disorders like Balu syndrome.

- *Nonsteroidal anti-inflammatory drugs*: They are very useful in many autoinflammatory diseases. Indomethacin works significantly well in chronic recurrent multifocal osteomyelitis (CRMO).

Following drugs are used in autoinflammatory disorders:

- *Colchicine*: Useful in most (not all) cases of FMF
- Anti-TNF: Etanercept has been used successfully in some cases of TRAPS
- *Interleukin-1 receptor antagonist*: IL-1 is involved in the pathogenesis of CAPS [FCAS, MWS, and neonatal-onset multisystem inflammatory disease (NOMID)] and *NLRP3* (*CIAS1*) gene is involved in these
- *Anakinra*: Short half-life requiring daily injections
- *Rilonacept, canakinumab, and gevokizumab*: All these drugs are found to be effective in these conditions. Some cases required higher dosage of anakinra. Daily or twice daily injection of anakinra was a disadvantageous. Moreover, this injection is painful. Rilonacept and canakinumab are also effective and are now the Food and Drug Administration (FDA)-approved for these indications.

Interleukin-1 antagonists have now been used for conditions other than CAPS like colchicine-resistant FMF, hyper-IgD syndrome, etanercept-resistant TRAPS, BS, pyogenic arthritis, pyoderma gangrenosum, and acne, Schnitzler syndrome, systemic-onset juvenile idiopathic arthritis (SoJIA), adult-onset Still's disease and for chronic gout-associated joint pain.

### Other Drugs

- Hypolipidemic drugs: Simvastatin
- Kinase-blocking small molecules
- Rituximab
- Glyburide
- Anticytokines
- Peroxisome proliferator-activated receptor agonists
- Micro-RNAs
- Histone deacetylase inhibitors.

## SUGGESTED READINGS


1. Abramovits W, Oquendo M. Introduction to autoinflammatory syndromes and diseases. Dermatol Clin. 2013;31:363-85.
2. Aksentijevich I, Galon J, Soares M, et al. The tumor-necrosis-factor receptor-associated periodic syndrome: new mutations in TNFRSF1A, ancestral origins, genotype-phenotype studies, and evidence for further genetic heterogeneity of periodic fevers. Am J Hum Genet. 2001;69(2):301-14.
3. Almeida de Jesus A, Goldbach-Mansky R. Monogenic autoinflammatory disease: concept and clinical manifestations. Clin Immunol. 2013;147(3):155-74.
4. Altunoğlu A, Erten Ş, Canoz MB, et al. Phenotype 2 familial Mediterranean fever: evaluation of 22 case series and review of the literature on phenotype 2 FMF. Ren Fail. 2013;35(2):226-30.
5. Brizi MG, Galeazzi M, Lucherini OM, et al. Successful treatment of tumor necrosis factor receptor-associated periodic syndrome with canakinumab. Ann Inter Med. 2012;156(12):907-8.
6. Cantarini L, Capecchi PL, Lucherini OM, et al. Familial Mediterranean fever diagnosed in an elderly patient. Clin Exp Rheumatol. 2010;28(4):S91.
7. Cantarini L, Lucherini OM, Muscari I, et al. Tumour necrosis factor receptor-associated periodic syndrome (TRAPS): state of the art and future perspectives. Autoimmunity Reviews. 2012;12(1):38-43.
8. Cattalini M, Soliani M, Rigante D, et al. Basic characteristics of adults with periodic fever, aphthous stomatitis, pharyngitis, and adenopathy syndrome in comparison with the typical pediatric expression of disease. Mediators Inflamm. 2015;2015:570418.
9. Chae JJ, Wood G, Richard K, et al. The familial Mediterranean fever protein, pyrin, is cleaved by caspase-1 and activates NF-κB through its N-terminal fragment. Blood. 2008;112(5):1794-803.
10. Cush JJ. Autoinflammatory syndromes. Dermatol Clin. 2013;31:471-80.
11. Di Gioia SA, Bedoni N, von Scheven-Gête A, et al. Analysis of the genetic basis of periodic fever with aphthous stomatitis, pharyngitis, and cervical adenitis (PFAPA) syndrome. Sci Rep. 2015;5:10200.
12. Femiano F, Lanza A, Buonaiuto C, et al. Oral aphthous-like lesions, PFAPA syndrome: a review. J Oral Pathol Med. 2008;37:319-23.
13. Gattorno M, Pelagatti MA, Meini A, et al. Persistent efficacy of anakinra in patients with tumor necrosis factor receptor-associated periodic syndrome. Arthritis Rheum. 2008;58(5):1516-20.
14. Hill SC, Namde M, Dwyer A, et al. Arthropathy of neonatal onset multisystem inflammatory disease (NOMID/CINCA). Pediatric Radiology. 2007;37(2):145-52.
15. Hoffman HM. Therapy of autoinflammatory syndromes. J Allergy Clin Immunol. 2009;124:1129-40.
16. Martinon F, Petrilli V, Mayor A, et al. Gout-associated uric acid crystals activate the NALP3 inflammasome. Nature. 2006;440:237-41.
17. Masters SL, Simon A, Aksentijevich I, et al. Horror autoinflammaticus: the molecular pathophysiology of autoinflammatory disease (*). Annu Rev Immunol. 2009;27:621-68.
18. Miettunen PM, Wei X, Kaura D, et al. Dramatic pain relief and resolution of bone inflammation following pamidronate in 9 pediatric patients with persistent chronic recurrent multifocal osteomyelitis (CRMO). Pediatr Rheumatol Online J. 2009;7:2.
19. Miyamae T. Cryopyrin-associated periodic syndromes: diagnosis and management. Paediatr Drugs. 2012;14(2):109-17.
20. Ozturk MA, Kanbay M, Kasapoglu B, et al. Therapeutic approach to familial Mediterranean fever: a review update. Clin Exp Rheumatol. 2011;29(4):S77-86.
21. Picard C, Al-Herz W, Bousfiha A, et al. Primary immunodeficiency diseases: an update on the classification from the International Union of Immunological Societies Expert Committee for Primary Immunodeficiency 2015. J Clin Immunol. 2015;35:696-726.
22. Radakovic S, Holzer G, Tanew A. Erysipelas-like erythema as a cutaneous sign of familial Mediterranean fever: a case report and review of the histopathologic findings. J Am Acad Dermatol. 2013;68(2):e61-3.
23. Rigante D. The fresco of autoinflammatory diseases from the pediatric perspective. Autoimmunity Reviews. 2012;11:348-56.

# 7 SECTION Acne, Rosacea and Related Disorders

# 18 CHAPTER Acne

Rajeev Sharma, Abhijit Saha

## INTRODUCTION

Acne vulgaris is a multifactorial, chronic inflammatory disorder of pilosebaceous unit primarily affecting the adolescents. It is clinically characterized by pleomorphic nature with comedone being the most unique and pathognomonic feature, others are papules, pustules, and nodules. Though the course may be self-limiting, the potentially life-long sequelae may lead to huge economic and psychological burden.

## EPIDEMIOLOGY

Around 79–95% of the adolescent population in Western countries is affected. Though traditionally considered as a disease of youth, adult acne is not uncommon and is reported in 12.5% of female and 3% of males beyond 45 years of age. Other studies have reported acne in 28–61% of school children in the age group 10–12 years; 79–95% in the age group 16–18 years; and even in children in the age group 4–7 years. One Indian study reported affection of 50.6% of boys and 38.13% of girls in the age group 12–17 years with acne.

## PATHOGENESIS

Acne is a chronic inflammatory disease of sebaceous follicle (large sebaceous gland with a small, rudimentary hair follicle) located on face, chest, shoulder, and back.

In nutshell, the pathogenesis of acne can be illustrated by the following interrelated events: Androgenic influence on sebocytes and keratinocytes leads to seborrhea and sebaceous hyperplasia and altered follicular keratinization and accumulation of desquamated keratinocytes respectively which in turn creates a favorable follicular milieu for *P. acne* leading to proliferation of the bacteria and consequent inflammation. This inflammation again upregulates sebum production y and influences follicular keratinization by elaboration of LT-B4 and IL-1 respectively.

- *Altered follicular keratinization*: The primary change is the altered pattern of follicular keratinization which starts with hyperproliferation of infundibular epithelium. This leads to production of excess, altered keratin with increased cohesiveness. Accumulation of these abnormally desquamated keratinocytes in the follicular ostium forms keratin plug and thus heralding the process of comedogenesis
- Proposed factors implicated in keratinocyte hyperproliferation:
  - Decreased sebaceous linoleic acid
  - Androgenic stimulation via 5α-reductase activity
  - Increased interleukin (IL)-1α activity.
- *Seborrhea and sebaceous gland hyperplasia*: The severity of acne directly correlates with rate of sebum excretion. Triglyceride of sebum is broken down by *Propionibacterium* acnes to free fatty acids which in turn favor further bacterial colonization in follicle and incite inflammation
- *Acne and androgen*: Androgens increase in sebum production and enhance follicular hyperkeratosis. Conditions of hyperandrogenism have been found to be associated with seborrhea and severe acne. Acne-prone skin exhibits higher androgen receptor density and higher 5α-reductase activity than uninvolved skin
- *Bacterial colonization and inflammation*: The immunological events involved in pathogenesis of acne are led by perifollicular accumulation of CD4+ cells which elaborate interleukin-1 (IL-1). *Propionibacterium acnes* triggers innate immunity and activates a cytoplasmic complex of protein called inflammasome and through this secretes various inflammatory mediators, the principal mediator of which is IL-1, a strong proinflammatory cytokine, activation of toll-like receptors, and induction of matrix metalloproteinases (MMPs). *Propionibacterium acnes* stimulates several MMPs that are involved in tissue destruction and induce scar formation. Delayed, persistent, and more specific inflammatory responses lead to scarring in predisposed individuals.

## CLINICAL FEATURES

The primary site of affection is the face with involvement in around 99% cases; other less commonly affected areas are back (60%), chest (15%), and shoulders. Distribution of acne varies according to the age group as in case of neonatal acne, it involves the whole face including eyelids, whereas preadolescent acne usually predominates over the forehead and adult acne is largely restricted to jaw areas.

Although polymorphic, one type of lesion may predominate in a single case. The microcomedo is the primary and precursor lesion of acne and it evolves to open and closed comedone and

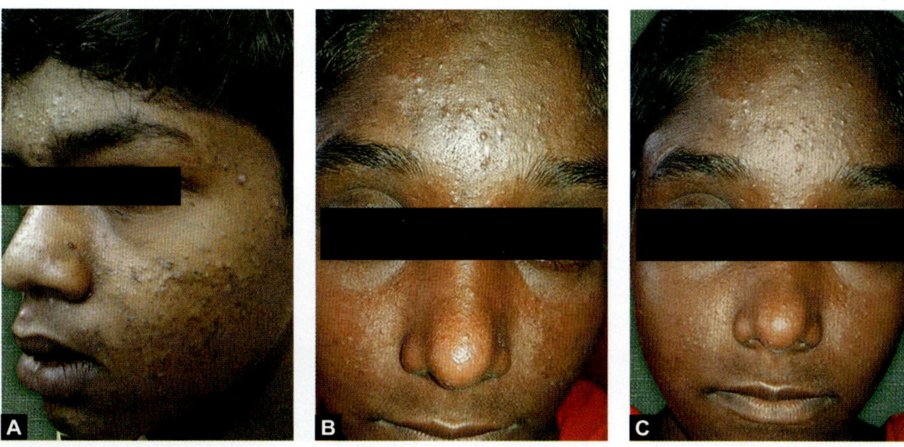


FIG. 1: Preadolescent acne with mostly comedonal lesions.

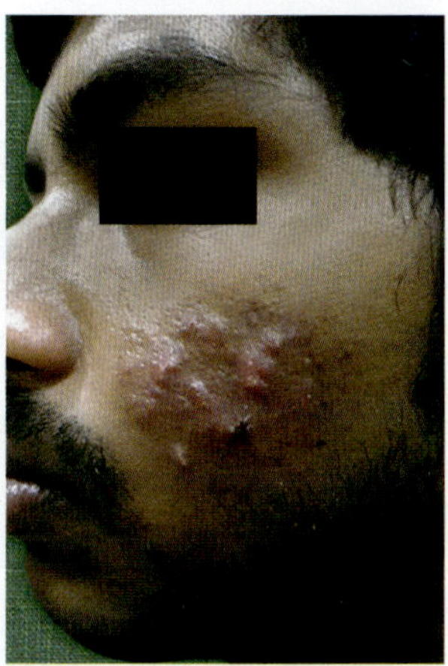

FIG. 2: Inflammatory acne.

further into inflammatory lesions like papules and nodules. Preadolescent acne is largely comedonal (Fig. 1). Open comedo or blackhead represents flat or slightly elevated papule with dilated central opening filled with keratin. The black color may be due to oxidation of melanin and presence of certain lipids in sebum or due to interference in light transmission through compact keratin. Other types of comedones are macrocomedones (3–4 mm), sandpaper comedones, submarine comedones, missed comedones, nevoid comedones, and drug-induced comedones.

The inflammatory lesions vary from small papules to pustules and large, tender nodules (Fig. 2). Sometimes, the nodules become fluctuant and are erroneously termed as cysts. The term nodulocystic acne has been replaced by a newer nosology, severe nodular acne. At times, the inflammation may be so pronounced that it may lead to formation of coalescent indurated or fluctuant plaques with sinus tract and serosanguineous or purulent discharge.

Scarring, the most bothersome complication of acne, may follow inflammatory and even noninflammatory lesions. It may be of atrophic type, hypertrophic type, or mixed acne scar. Atrophic scar are of several types—ice pick scar (narrow, deep scar that taper to a point in the dermis), boxcar (wide sharply demarcated), rolling scar (shallow, wide scar with an undulating appearance), perifollicular elastolysis, and macular scar (Fig. 3). Hypertrophic scar which are less common can be classified into keloid, papular scar, and perifollicular fibrosis. Scarring also shows tropism like atrophic scars are usually encountered in face while keloidal changes are seen in jaw line and trunk.

## Grading of Acne Severity

There are inherent difficulties in objectively measuring acne. European Dermatology Forum uses the following classification:
- Comedonal acne
- Mild to moderate papulopustular acne
- Severe papulopustular acne, moderate nodular acne
- Severe nodular acne, conglobate acne.

There are other classifications of grading like:
- Grade I: Comedonal with occasional papule (Fig. 4)
- Grade II: Comedones, many papules and few pustules (Fig. 5)
- Grade III: Predominantly pustules, nodules, and abscesses
- Grade IV: Cysts or abscesses with scarring.

### Adult Acne

Adolescent acne persisting beyond the age of 25 years is called persistent adult acne whereas acne appearing for the first time after the age of 25 years is called as late-onset adult acne. The prevalence of persistent acne is much higher than that of late-onset one. In persistent acne, patients have lesions on most of the days and may experience a premenstrual flare. Late-onset acne can be further subdivided into inflammatory acne with premenstrual flare which occurs around the chin and perioral area, and sporadic acne which occurs suddenly in adult life without any distinguishing features.

The classical presentation of adult acne has been described as inflammatory papulopustular lesions in the mandibular and chin area (Fig. 6). Another variant called comedonal postadolescent acne, in which inflammatory lesions are sparse but large prominent cyst-like comedones are homogeneously distributed on the whole face with a relative absence on the lower third of the face and the jaw line. This variant is common in smokers.

Hormones, colonization by resistant bacteria, the use of cosmetics, drugs, and chronic stress have been thought to play possible role in the pathogenesis.

### Acne Variants

Acne presents with wide range of clinical subtypes, some of them having acute fulminant course with systemic involvement.

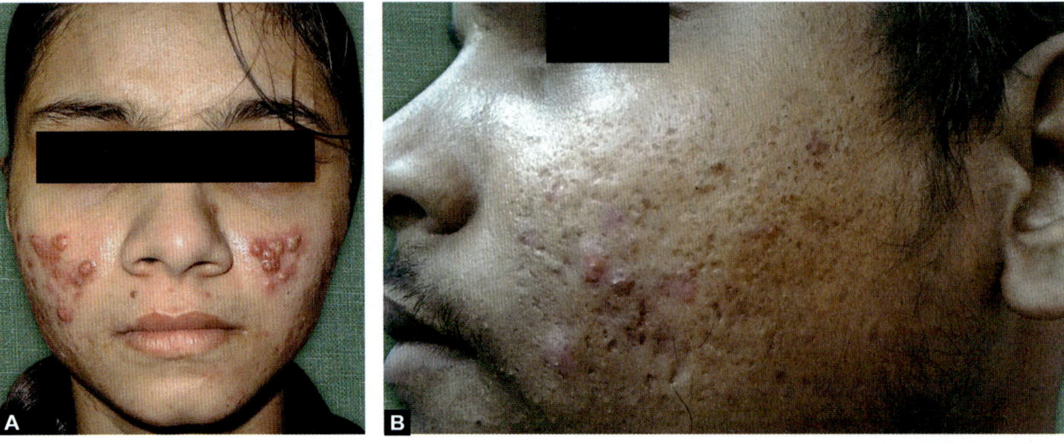

**FIG. 3:** **A,** Inflammatory acne with pustules, nodules and marked surrounding erythema; **B,** Nodular acne with different types of scars (rolling, ice-pick, boxcar).

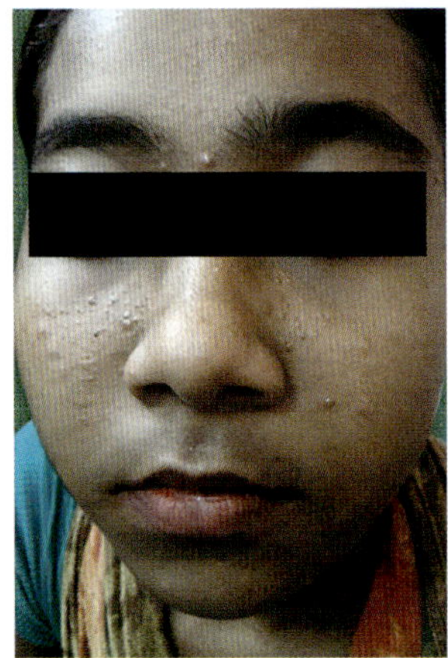

**FIG. 4:** Grade I: Comedonal with occasional papule.

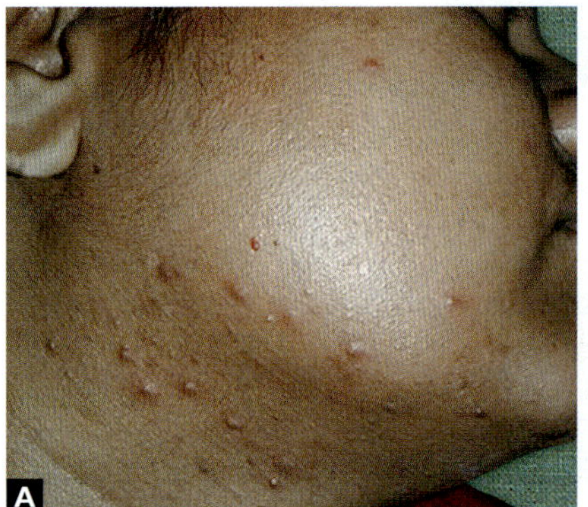

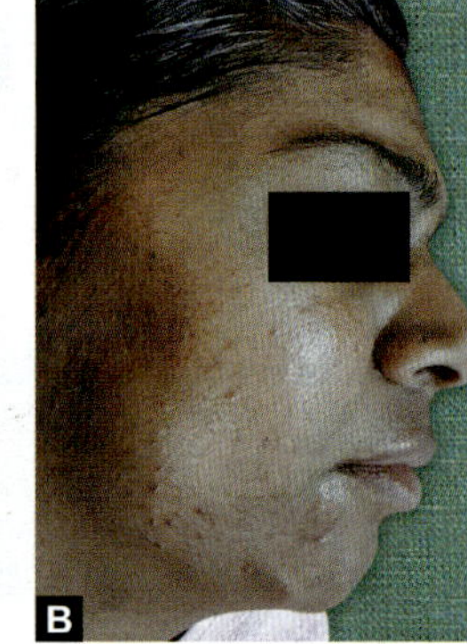

**FIG. 6:** Adult acne with typical distribution over the mandibular area.

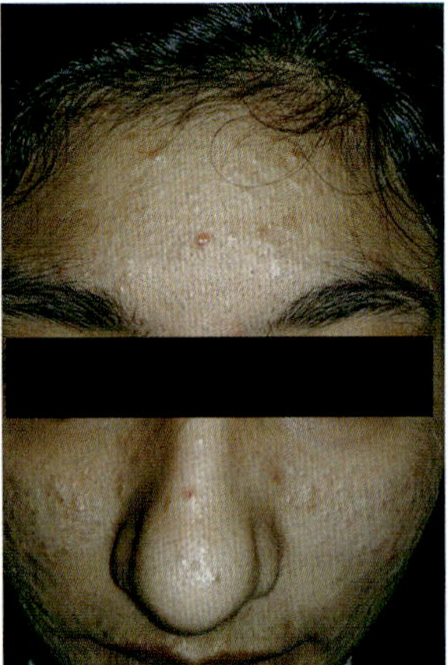

**FIG. 5:** Grade II: Comedones, many papules and few pustules.

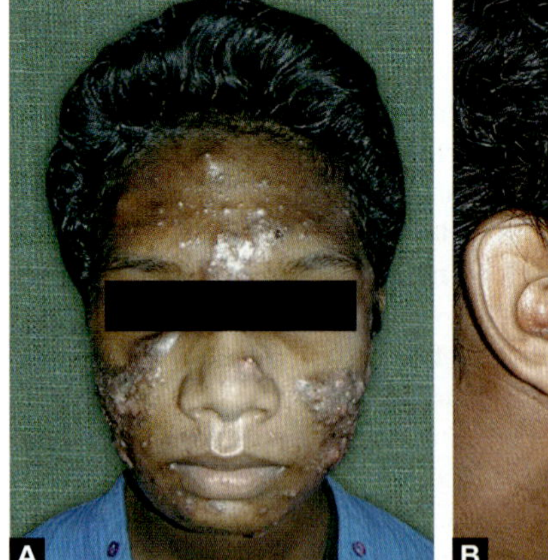

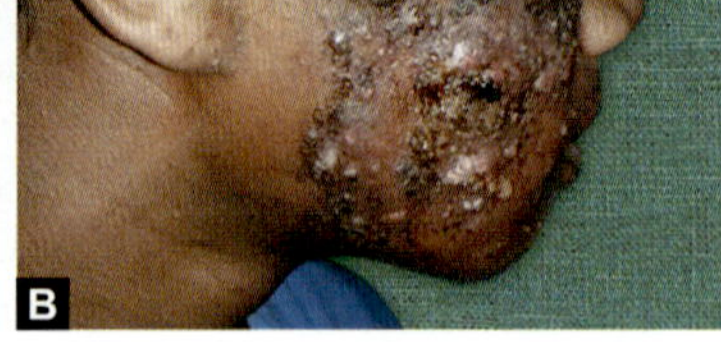

**FIG. 7:** **A,** Acne conglobata grouped inflammatory nodules, cysts, and large abscesses with discharging sinus; **B,** Acne conglobata: Close-up view.

- *Neonatal acne*: Not an infrequent finding, seen in around 20% of healthy newborns. Appears by 2 weeks of age and resolves spontaneously by 3 months. Due to absence of comedones, thought to be a variant of neonatal cephalic pustulosis
- *Infantile acne*: Appears by 3–6 months. Though comedones are the primary finding, inflammatory lesions, and even scarring are not unusual. If severe, evaluations for adrenal and gonadal tumors are warranted
- *Acne conglobata*: Clinically characterized by multiporous comedones, grouped inflammatory nodules, cysts, and large abscesses with interconnecting sinus tracts (Fig. 7) involving mainly posterior neck and back
- *Acne fulminans*: This most severe form of nodular acne is characterized by explosive onset of acutely suppurative, tender, and friable plaques with hemorrhagic crusts in association with variable systemic manifestations. This is a

disease of teenage males. There is preferential involvement of chest and back with characteristic sparing of face. Systemic involvement in the form of fever, polyarthralgia, myalgia, hepatosplenomegaly, and bone pain make this variant of acne a medical emergency. Erythema nodosum is an occasional accompaniment. The acute inflammatory flare is managed with systemic glucocorticoids in conjunction with systemic antibiotics followed by isotretinoin

- *SAPHO syndrome*: It is characterized by osteoarticular and dermatological symptoms. The acronym stands for synovitis, acne (acne conglobata/fulminans), pustulosis on the skin, often psoriatic, mainly on the palm and soles, and hyperostosis and osteitis
- *PAPA syndrome*: This is an auto-inflammatory syndrome due to mutation of CD2 binding protein and is characterized by Pyogenic Arthritis, Pyoderma gangrenosum, and Acne
- *Acne mechanica*: This comedonal acne variant results from repeated mechanical and frictional obstruction of pilosebaceous unit
- *Acne excoriée*: This is disease of young female. It is typified by comedones and papules with extensive neurotic excoriations resulting in crusted erosions with scar. Usually associated with underlying psychiatric component in the forms of depression, obsessive disorders, anxiety, etc.
- *Acne with solid facial edema*: Also known as Morbihan disease is a disfiguring variant of acne characterized by woody induration of mid-third of face due to soft tissue swelling. The course is fluctuating, but spontaneous resolution does not occur. Can be successfully treated with isotretinoin alone or in combination with ketotifen
- *Acne-associated syndromes*: Acne accompanied by hirsutism, irregular menstrual cycle, deepening of voice, increased libido, therapy-resistant acne, late-onset acne, in presence of premenstrual flare, stress aggravated acne, and cutaneous signs of hyperinsulinemia like acanthosis nigricans or skin tags may indicate necessity for hormonal assessment. The most common endocrinopathies associated with acne are polycystic ovarian syndrome (PCOS) and its subset hyperandrogenism and insulin resistance- acanthosis nigricans (HAIR-AN)—hyperandrogenism (HA), insulin resistance (IN), and acanthosis nigricans (AN), congenital adrenal hyperplasia, nonclassical adrenal hyperplasia, etc.
  - Polycystic ovarian syndrome accounts for 95% of hyperandrogenemia in women and affects around 6% of the female population. It is an amalgamation of endocrine abnormalities arising from generalized dysregulation of steroidogenesis, with or without ovarian cyst formation. Presence of at least two out of three findings—oligoovulation or anovulation manifesting as oligomenorrhea or amenorrhea, clinical or biochemical evidence of androgen excess, and polycystic ovaries on ultrasound confirms the diagnosis of PCOS (Rotterdam criteria for PCOS) (Fig. 8)
  - Nonclassical adrenal hyperplasia—predominantly reflects features of androgen excess rather than adrenal insufficiency. The patients usually present with hirsutism, acne vulgaris, alopecia areata, anovulation, and infertility
  - HAIR-AN syndrome (hyperandrogenism-HA, insulin resistance-IR and acanthosis nigricans-AN)—It is thought to be a subset of PCOS. Occasionally found to be accompanied by some autoimmune diseases such as Hashimoto thyroiditis, Grave's disease, and vitiligo. In younger women, hyperandrogenism manifests as seborrhea, acne vulgaris, hirsutism, menstrual irregularities, androgenetic alopecia, clitoromegaly, and changes in muscle mass
  - SAHA syndrome (seborrhea, acne, hirsutism, and androgenetic alopecia)—Generally occurs in young to middle-aged women due to elevated blood levels of androgens or an increased androgen-driven peripheral response of the pilosebaceous unit with normal circulating androgen levels. This syndrome may be frequently associated with AN, when the acronym SAHA-AN may be used.

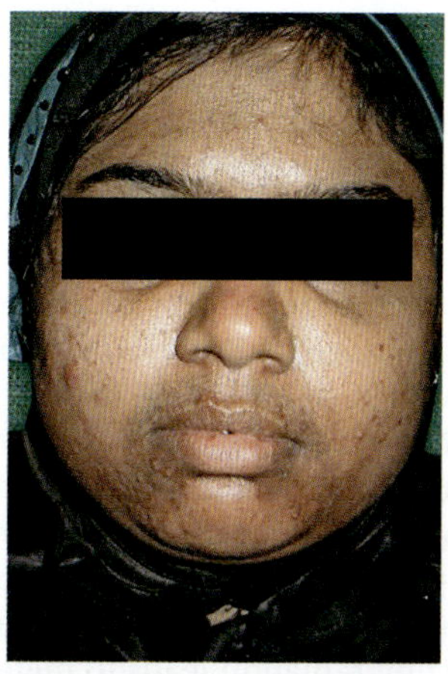

**FIG. 8:** Polycystic ovary syndrome with late onset acne, hirsutism, obesity, and acanthosis nigricans.

## Acneiform Eruption

A group of dermatoses which morphologically resembles acne vulgaris but is of different etiology and is differentiated from the latter by the following features:

- Monomorphic lesion
- Not necessarily confined to the usual sites of acne vulgaris
- Sudden onset
- Lack of comedones
- Different age of presentation.

These are follicular reactions presenting with inflammatory papules and pustules.

Causes of acneiform eruption:

- *Drug-induced acne*: Often accompanied by signs of systemic drug toxicities like fever, malaise, etc. Offending drugs are:
  - Corticosteroids
  - Anabolic steroids
  - *Antiepileptic*: Carbamazepine, phenytoin, gabapentin, topiramate, etc.
  - *Psychopharmacologic drugs*: Lithium, sertraline, pimozide, amitriptyline, etc.
  - *Antitubecular*: Isoniazid, rifampicin, and pyrazinamide
  - *Antineoplastic*: Dactinomycin, pentostatin, etc.
  - *Antiviral*: Ritonavir, ganciclovir, etc.
  - *Immunosuppressive*: Cyclosporine
  - *Halogens*: Potassium iodide
  - *Vitamins*: B1, B6, B12
  - *Epidermal growth factor receptor inhibitors*: Gefitinib, cetuximab, etc.

  - *Miscellaneous*: Psoralen plus ultraviolet A (PUVA), cabergoline, thiouracil, disulfiram, isosorbide mononitrate, etc.
- *Gram-negative folliculitis*: It is usually seen in patients with pre-existing acne following long-term treatment with oral antibiotics especially tetracyclines and are of two types—papulopustular lesions around nose or deep seated nodules
- *Occupational acne*: Acneiform eruptions may occur following occupational exposure to various industrial chemicals such as fumes generated in the manufacture of chlorine or its byproducts (chloracne), cutting and lubricating oils, and tar derivatives. The lesions tend to be more common in covered parts of the body and are characterized by large comedones, inflammatory papules, pustules, nodules, and true cysts
- *Radiation acne*: It may follow either ionizing radiation or UV radiation. Ionizing radiation leads to metaplasia of follicular infundibulum and thus resulting in keratotic plugs
- *Tropical acne*: These are folliculitis resulting from extreme heat of tropical climates or occupational environment. Typically involves trunk and buttocks and clinically resembles acne conglobata
- *Acne aestivalis*: Also referred to this as Mallorca acne, since it occurred in many Scandinavians after they had been on a sunny vacation in Mallorca, are clinically characterized by monomorphic papular lesions
- *Acne necrotica*: Uncommon, papulopustular follicular eruption that eventually leaves depressed superficial scars resembling small pox scars
- *Apert syndrome*: This autosomal dominant disorder, also known as acrocephalosyndactyly is characterized by disfiguring synostoses of bones of the hands, feet, vertebral bodies, and cranium and is associated with diffuse follicle-based acneiform papules
- *Pseudoacne of nasal crease*: Acneiform papules developing over the transverse, linear groove across the middle of nose (nasal crease) along with milia.

## LABORATORY TESTS

The tests are not generally indicated unless hyperandrogenism is suspected. In majority of the patients, serum androgens are within normal range.

## DIFFERENTIAL DIAGNOSIS

Clinically acne vulgaris mimics a vast majority of dermatoses, but by the age of onset, lesional morphology, and distribution, we can narrow down the options (Table 1).

## COMPLICATIONS

All types of acne lesions resolve with some form of sequelae (Fig. 9). Transient erythema is almost inevitable. This may persist for long time. Postinflammatory hyperpigmentation and scarring are commonly noted. Depression, anxiety, and decreased quality of life are also not uncommon.

## TREATMENT (TABLE 2)

### Topical Therapy

Topical therapy is indicated in mild to moderate acne alone or in combination and in maintenance therapy.

- *Benzoyl peroxide*: It is an effective topical agent and is available in different formulation and concentrations (2.5–10%).

**TABLE 1: Differential diagnosis of acne**

| **Neonatal acne** | |
|---|---|
| Sebaceous hyperplasia | Transient yellowish papules over cheeks, nasal bridge, forehead |
| Milia | Small, pearly white or yellow, non-inflammatory papules |
| Miliaria rubra | Red inflammatory papules due to overheating or bundling of neonates |
| Candidal infection | Inflammatory papules and pustules are diffusely distributed |
| **Comedonal acne: Closed** | |
| Milia | Primary milia are small, superficial keratin cysts concentrated especially in periorbital region. Secondary milia follow blistering dermatoses |
| Sebaceous hyperplasia | Seen in adults. Lobulated, yellowish papules over forehead and cheeks |
| • Appendageal tumors<br>  ○ Syringoma<br>  ○ Trichoepithelioma<br>  ○ Trichodiscomas<br>  ○ Eruptive vellus hair cyst<br>  ○ Steatocystoma multiplex | • Typically noninflammatory<br>• Typical distribution<br>• Occasional systemic association |
| **Open comedone** | |
| Favre-Racouchot syndrome | • Appears in middle to late adulthood<br>• Interspersed within areas of solar elastosis<br>• Typically distributed in temporal and periorbital areas |
| Nevus comedonicus | • Presents at birth or during childhood<br>• Grouped or linear comedones often along the Blaschko's line |
| Trichostasis spinulosa | Multiple vellus hairs arising from dilated follicular orifice, most commonly located on nose |
| Dilated pore of Winer | Solitary enlarged comedone, seen in elderly individual |
| Contact acne | Discussed in the section of occupational acne |
| **Inflammatory acne** | |
| Rosacea | • Later age of onset<br>• Lack of comedones<br>• Typically involves convexities of face<br>• Telangiectasia and flushing |
| Perioral dermatitis | • Typical distribution: perioral and periorbital<br>• Presence of microvesicles and micropustules<br>• Lack of comedones<br>• Rebound after discontinuation of potent topical steroids |

*Continued*

*Continued*

| Inflammatory acne | |
|---|---|
| **Folliculitis** | |
| • Gram-negative<br>• Other bacterial<br>• Eosinophilic (associated with HIV infection)<br>• Pityrosporum<br>• Demodex<br>• Candidal<br>• Molluscum<br>• Lack of comedones<br>• Monomorphic lesion<br>• Particular distribution | |
| Pseudofolliculitis barbae and acne keloidalis nuchae | Occur primarily in black or in men of African descent |
| Lupus miliaris disseminatus faciei | • Discrete red-brown papules<br>• Predilection for the periorbital region<br>• Positive diascopy<br>• Granuloma with caseation necrosis on histopathology |
| Kertaosis pilaris | • Early age of onset<br>• Autosomal dominant inheritance<br>• Association with atopic dermatitis and ichthyosis |

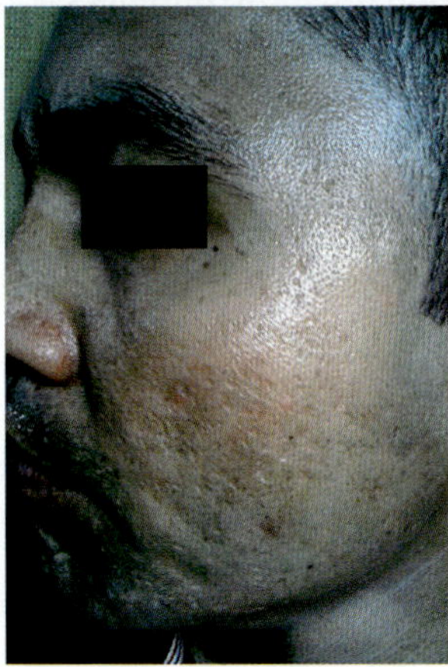

**FIG. 9:** Sequelae of acne: Postinflammatory hyperpigmentation, erythema and scar.

The drug has a bactericidal, anti-inflammatory, comedolytic, and keratolytic properties, and is indicated in mild to moderate acne. The major limitation is dryness and irritation which can be addressed by choosing proper formulation and concentration

- *Topical retinoids*: Topical retinoids should be used as first line therapy in mild to moderate inflammatory acne and is also preferred agent for maintenance therapy. Retinoids are the only agents which address all the four key steps of acne pathogenesis. Topical retinoids target the abnormal follicular proliferation and reduce follicular plugging and thus formation of microcomedones. Enhanced efficacy can be achieved if combined with benzoyl peroxide or other topical antibiotics as topical retinoids act synergistically by enhancing the penetration of coadministered drug.

  Currently available topical retinoids are tretinoin, adapalene, tazarotene, isotretinoin, metretinide, retinaldehyde, and β-retinoyl glucuronide.
- *Topical antibiotics*: They act by inhibiting *P. acne* and reduce inflammation.

  Clindamycin and erythromycin are frequently used. Newer topical antibiotics like nadifloxacin, azithromycin, and clarithromycin are also used.

  To avoid emergence of bacterial resistance and cross resistance, topicals should not be used as monotherapy. Combination of topical tretinoin and benzoyl peroxide found to be superior to monotherapy. A combination of topical retinoid and topical antimicrobial is more effective in reducing both inflammatory and noninflammatory acne lesions than either agent used alone.
- *Salicylic acid*: It has been used for many years in acne as a comedolytic and anti-inflammatory agent, but is less potent than topical retinoid
- *Azelaic acid*: It is a naturally occurring dicarboxylic acid available as 10–20% topical cream and has been shown to be effective in inflammatory and comedonal acne. In addition it helps in reducing post-inflammatory hyperpigmentation
- *Other drugs*: Picolinic acid gel 10% and dapsone gel 5%.

## Systemic Therapy

- *Oral antibiotics*: These are indicated in moderate to severe inflammatory acne not responding to topical therapies. They act by suppressing the growth of *P. acnes* and thereby reducing production of inflammatory cytokines. Some of these also possess intrinsic anti-inflammatory effects. Commonly used agents are tetracycline (500 mg–1 g/day) and its derivatives doxycycline (50–200 mg/day), minocycline ((50–200 mg/day), lymecycline (150–300 mg/day), erythromycin (500 mg–1 g/day); cotrimoxazole, trimethoprim, and azithromycin (500 mg thrice weekly). Among these, doxycycline and minocycline are found to be superior.

  Most common side effect is gastrointestinal upset. Photosensitivity is seen with doxycycline, whereas pigmentation of skin, mucosa, and nails are reported with the use of minocycline. Serious adverse effects like autoimmune hepatitis, serum sickness like reaction and systemic lupus erythematosus occur rarely with minocycline. Another complication with long-term antibiotic therapy is gram-negative folliculitis.

  An ensuing problem with oral antibiotics is emergence of resistance, most commonly seen with erythromycin. This can be avoided by optimizing antibiotic therapy; by avoiding monotherapy, encouraging combination therapy (with topical benzoyl peroxide or topical retinoids as per need), and limiting the duration of therapy. If retreatment is required same antibiotic should be repeated and benzoyl peroxide can be used during the interim period.
- *Hormonal therapy*: It is best indicated in females in adult onset acne. Because of the potential risk associated with hormonal therapy, prior consultation with gynecologist is recommended
  - *Oral contraceptives*: In most of the formulations, estrogen is combined with a progestin to minimize the risk of endometrial cancer. The currently approved preparation are norgestimate with ethinyl estradiol (35 μg), ethinyl

**TABLE 2: Treatment algorithm of acne vulgaris**

| | Mild | | Moderate | | Severe |
|---|---|---|---|---|---|
| | Comedonal | Papular/pustular | Papular/pustular | Nodular | Conglobata/ fulminans |
| First line therapy | Topical retinoid | Topical retinoid + topical antibiotic | Oral antibiotic + Topical retinoids+/-BPO | Oral antibiotics +Topical retinoids +/- BPO | Oral isotretinoin oral corticosteroids may be added (especially in case of acne fulminans) |
| Others | • Azelaic acid<br>• Salicylic acid<br>• BPO (low strength of recommendation) | • Azelaic acid<br>• Salicylic acid<br>• BPO<br>• Systemic antibiotic | Oral antibiotic+ topical retinoids with Azelaic acid | Azelaic acid in place of BPO | • Dapsone<br>• High dose oral antibiotic + topical retinoid + BPO |
| Surgical options | Comedo extraction | – | Comedo extraction | Comedo extraction<br>IL steroid | IL steroid |

BPO, benzoyl peroxide; OCP, oral contraceptives; IL, intralesional.

estradiol with norethindrone, and ethinyl estradiol (20 µg)-rospirenone combination

- *Spironolactone*: It acts primarily as a steroidal androgen receptor blocker. In doses 50–100 mg twice daily it has been shown to reduce sebum production and improve acne. It may cause hyperkalemia, menstrual irregularities, breast tenderness, and feminization of male fetus
- *Cyproterone acetate*: It is the first androgen receptor blocking agent to be well-studied and found to be effective in females with acne. Higher doses have been found to be more effective than lower dose. It is also combined (2 mg) with ethinyl estradiol (35 or 50 µg) as an oral contraceptive formulation
- *Flutamide*: It is useful in acne when given in females with hirsuitism. It has been used in doses of 250 mg twice a day for 6 months in combination with oral contraceptives for the treatment of acne. Fatal hepatitis is a serious side effect and warrants monitoring of liver function test. And in view of feminization of male fetus, pregnancy is contraindicated during therapy hence concomitant oral contraceptive pill use is beneficial
- *Gonadotropin releasing hormone (GnRH) analogs*: Gonadotropin releasing hormone analogs inhibit ovarian androgen production by blocking the cyclical release of luteinizing hormone and follicle-stimulating hormone from the pituitary. However, there are no published studies using GnRH analogs for acne alone and their use is limited by their high cost and menopausal symptoms including bone loss on their long-term use
- *Insulin sensitizer*: Metformin is used, especially in acne in association with PCOS, HAIR-AN syndrome, obese patients, or biochemical evidence of hyperinsulinemia. It is usually given in a dose of 500 mg once a day to twice a day doses to up to 2,000 mg/day
- *Isotretinoin*: This is indicated in severe, recalcitrant nodular acne, acne with physical and psychological scarring, and acne unresponsive to conventional therapies. The approved dose is 0.5–2 mg/kg/day, which is usually given for 20 weeks or up to a total cumulative dose of 120–150 mg/kg. Recent trends are low-dose long-term isotretinoin regimens and use of micronized formulations (0.4 mg/kg)
- *Low dose isotretinoin*: The lower dose isotretinoin (0.25–0.5 mg/kg/day for 24 weeks) offers a good balance between efficacy and dose-related side effects. The low dose isotretinoin can be given in any regimen (daily, alternate day or intermittent) for duration of around 6–7 months.

Side effects of isotretinoin include those of musculoskeletal, mucocutaneous, and ophthalmic systems, as well as headache and central nervous system effects. Most of the side effects are temporary. Oral isotretinoin is a potential teratogen. Therefore, a pregnancy prevention program (initially SMART, now iPLEDGE) has been implemented in the United States ensuring compulsory registration of all female patients receiving isotretinoin.

Female patients are advised to use at least one but ideally two methods of contraception for 1 month before starting treatment, including a barrier method, and to continue to use effective contraception throughout the treatment period and for at least 1 month after cessation of treatment. Ideally, hormonal contraception is recommended along with the barrier method; either the combined contraceptive pill or injectable or implantable hormonal aids should be used. Progesterone only pills are generally avoided as this may act adversely on the severity of acne.

All female patients of childbearing potential should have a medically supervised pregnancy test from blood or urine just before starting therapy, monthly pregnancy tests throughout therapy and the last test 5 weeks after stopping course of therapy. This can be done by measurement of human chorionic gonadotropin in blood or in urine using a urine test with minimum sensitivity of 25 mIU/mL. In patients with irregular menses, the timing of this pregnancy test should reflect the sexual activity of the patient and be undertaken at least 3 weeks after the patient last had unprotected sexual intercourse.

## Physical Treatment

### Lesional Therapy

- *Comedone extraction*: Both open and closed comedones can be removed mechanically with comedone extractor
- *Aspiration and intralesional injection*: Intralesional triamcinolone acetonide (2–5 mg/mL) alone can also dramatically improve the deep nodular lesions

- Phototherapy
- Visible light: These act via photodestruction of *P. acnes*. Blue light (peak at 415 nm), and mixed blue and red light (peak at 415 and 660 nm) have been used
- Photodynamic therapy: Found to be effective but further studies are recommended to substantiate the efficacy and safety.

### Physical Treatment of Scars

Acne and diet: Consumption of high milk and hyperglycemic diets possibly exacerbates acne by increasing the insulin/insulin-like growth factor 1 signaling.

## CONCLUSION

There is a major step forward in the understanding of acne over the last few years. It is hoped that the newer insight into the pathogenesis will help to design further targeted therapy in future. Still we cannot deny the economical and psychosocial burden of this ubiquitous disease. Clinical management should integrate psychological intervention to improve the quality of life of acne sufferers.

## SUGGESTED READINGS


1. Aktan S, Ozmen E, Sanli B. Anxiety, depression, and nature of acne vulgaris in adolescents. Int J Dermatol. 2000;39:354-7.
2. Amichai B, Shemar A, Grunwald MH. Low-dose isotretinoinin the treatment of acne vulgaris. J Am Acad Dermatol. 2006;54:644-6.
3. Bardazzi F, Savoia F, Parente G, et al. Azithromycin, a new therapeutic strategy for acne in adolscents. Dermatol Online J. 2007;13:4.
4. Betti R, Bencini PL, Lodi A, et al. Incidence of polycystic ovaries in patients with late-onset or persistent acne: hormonal reports. Dermatologica. 1990;181(2):109-11.
5. Capitano B, Sinagra JL, Bordignon V, et al. Underestimated clinical features of postadolescent acne. J Am Acad Dermatol. 2010;63:782-8.
6. Chen HC, Smith SJ, Tow B, et al. Leptin modulates the effects of acyl CoA: diacylglycerol acyltransferase deficiency on murine fur and sebaceous glands. J Clin Invest. 2002;109:175-81.
7. Cordain L, Lindeberg S, Hurtado M, et al. Acne vulgaris: A disease of western civilization. Arch Dermatol. 2002;138:1584-90.
8. Cordain L. Implications for the role of diet in acne. Semin Cutan Med Surg. 2005;24:84-91.
9. Cunliffe WJ, Gollnick HP. Acne: Diagnosis and management. London: Martin Dunitz; 2001. pp. 49-103.
10. Cunliffe WJ, Goulden V. Phototherapy and acne vulgaris. Br J Dermatol. 2000;142:855-6.
11. Danby FW. Acne and milk, the diet myth, and beyond. J Am Acad Dermatol. 2005;52:360-2.
12. Del Rosso JQ. Combination topical therapy in the treatment of acne. Cutis. 2006;78:5-12.
13. Del Rosso JQ. New topical therapies for the treatment of acne vulgaris. Cutis. 2007;80:400-10.
14. Deplewski D, Rosenfield RL. Role of hormones in pilosebaceous unit development. Endocrine Rev. 2000;21:363-92.
15. Dhir R, Gehi NP, Agarwal R, More YE. Oral isotretinoin is aseffective as a combination of oral isotretinoin and topical antiacneagents in nodulocystic acne. Indian J Dermatol Venereol Leprol. 2008;74:187.
16. Elman M, Lebzelter J. Light therapy in the treatment of acne vulgaris. Dermatol Surg. 2004;30:139-46.
17. Elmer KB, George RM. HAIR-AN syndrome: a multisystem challenge. Am Fam Physician. 2001;63(12):2385-90.
18. Fried RG, Wechsler A. Psychological problems in the acne patient. Dermatol Ther. 2006;19:237-40.
19. Fulton JE Jr, Plewig G, Kligman AM. Effects of chocolate on acne vulgaris. JAMA. 1969;210:2071-4.
20. Goodfield MJ, Cox NH, Broswer A, et al. Advice on the safe introduction and continued use ofisotretinoin in acne in the U.K. 2010. British J Dermatol. 2010;162:1172-9.
21. Goodman G. Post acne scarring: a review. J Cosmet Laser Ther. 2003;5:77-95.
22. Goulden V, Clark S, Cunliffe W. Post-adolescent acne: A review of clinical features. Br J Dermatol. 1997;136:66-70.
23. Goulden V, Stables GI, Cunliffe WJ. Prevalence of facial acne in adults. J Am Acad Dermatol. 1999;41:577-80.
24. Handojo I. The combined use of topical benzoyl peroxide and tretinoin in the treatment of acne vulgaris. Int J Dermatol. 1979;18:489-96.
25. Harrison PV. A comparison of doxycycline and minocycline in the treatment of acne vulgaris. Clin Exp Dermatol. 2003;139:459-64.
26. Heffernan MP, Nelsoa MM, Anadkat MJ. A pilot study of the safety and efficacy of picolinic acid gel in the treatment of acne vulgaris. Br J Dermatol. 2007;136:548-52.
27. Henkel V, Moehrenschlager M, Hegerl U, et al. Screening for depression in adult acne vulgaris patients: Tools for the dermatologist. J Cosmet Dermatol. 2002;1:202-7.
28. Holland DB, Jeremy AH, Roberts SG, et al. Inflammation in acne scarring: A comparison of the responses in lesions from patients prone and not prone to scar. Br J Dermatol. 2004;150:72-81.
29. Huber J, Walch K. Treating acne with oral contraceptives use of lower doses. Contraception. 2006;73:23-9.
30. Ingham E, Eady EA, Goodwin CE, et al. Pro-inflammatory levels of interlukin 1 alpha-like bioactivity are present in the majority of open comedones in acne vulgaris. J Invest Dermatol. 1992;98:895-901.
31. Itoh Y, Ninomiya Y, Tajima S, et al. Photodynamic therapy of acne vulgaris with topical delta-aminolaevulinic acid and incoherent light in Japanese patients. Br J Dermatol. 2001;144:575-9.
32. Jacob CI, Dover JS, Kaminer MS. Acne scarring: A classification system and review of treatment options. J Am Acad Dermatol. 2001;45:109-17.
33. Jain S. Topical tretinoin or adapalene in acne vulgaris: An overview. J Dermatol Treat. 2004;15:200-7.
34. Jemec GB, Jemec B. Acne: Treatment of scar. Clin Dermatol. 2004;22:434-8.
35. Jeremy AH, Holland DB, Roberts SG, et al. Inflammatory events are involved in acne lesion initiation. J Invest Dermatol. 2003;121:20-7.
36. Kapetanovic R, Cavaillon JM. Early events in innate immunity in the recognition of microbial pathogens. Expert Opin Biol Ther. 2007;7:907-18.
37. Khunger N, Kumar C. A clinico-epidemiological study of adult acne: Is it different from adolescent acne? Indian J Dermatol Venereol Leprol. 2012;78:335-41.
38. Kim J, Ochoa MT, Kruzik SR, et al. Activation of toll-like recptor 2 in acne triggers inflammatory cytokine responses. J Immunol. 2002;169:1535-41.
39. Krautheim A, Gollnick H. Acne: topical treatment. Clin Dermatol. 2004;22:398-407.
40. Kubba R, Bajaj AK, Thappa DM, et al. Acne in India: guidelines for management - IAA consensus document. Indian J Dermatol Venereol Leprol. 2009;75 Suppl 1:1-62.
41. Lee JW, Yoo KH, Park KY, et al. Effectiveness of conventional, low-dose and intermittent oral isotretinoin in the treatment of acne: a randomized, controlled comparative study. Br J Dermatol. 2011;164:1369-75.
42. Levine RM, Rasmussen JE. Intralesional corticostaeroids in the treatment of nodulo-cystic acne. Arch Dermatol. 1983;119:480-1.
43. Leyden JJ, Shalita A, Thiboutot D, et al. Topical tretinoin in inflammatory acne: A retrospective, investigator-blinded, vehicle-controlled, photographic assessment. Clin Ther. 2005;27:216-24.
44. Muhlemann MF, Carter GD, Cream JJ, et al. Oral spironolactone: an effective treatment for acne vulgaris in women. Br J Dermatol. 1986;115:227-32.
45. Nast A, Dreno B, Bettoli V, et al. European evidence-based (S3) guidelines for the treatment of acne. J Eur Acad Dermatol Venereol. 2012;26:1-29.
46. Orfanos CE, Adler YD, Zouboulis CC. The SAHA syndrome. Horm Res. 2000;54(5-6):251-8.
47. Pandey SS. Epidemiology of acne vulgaris. Indian J Dermatol. 1983;28:109-10.
48. Papageorgiou P, Katsambas A, Chu A. Phototherapy with blue (415 nm) and red (660nm) light in the treatment of acne vulgaris. Br J Dermatol. 2000;142:973-8.
49. Parsad D, Pandhi R, Nagpal R, et al. Azithromyin monthly pulse vs daily doxycyline in the treatment of acne vulgaris. J Dermatol. 2001;28:1-4.
50. Polenghi MM, Zizak S, Molinari E. Emotions and acne. Dermatol Psychosomatics. 2002;3:20-5.

51. Poli F, Dreno B, Verschoore M. An epidemiological study of acne in female adults: Results of a survey conducted in France. J Eur Acad Dermatol Venereol. 2001;15:541-5.
52. Rotterdam ESHRE\ASRM sponsored PCOS Consensus Workshop Group. Revised 2003 consensus on diagnostic criteria and long term health risk related to polycystic ovary syndrome. Hum Reprod. 2004;19:41-7.
53. Sardana K, Garg VK. Efficacy of low-dose isotretinoin in acne vulgaris. Indian J Dermatol Venereol Leprol. 2010;76:7-13.
54. Shaw JC, White LE. Persistent acne in adult women. Arch Dermatol. 2001;137: 1252-3.
55. Sheth R, Poonevala V. Isotretinoin: an Indian experience. Indian J Dermatol Venereol Leprol. 2001;67:180-2.
56. Simpson NB, Cunliffe WJ. Disorders of the sebaceous glands. In: Burns T, Breathnach S, Cox N, Griffiths C (Eds). Rook's Textbook Of Dermatology, 7th edition. Oxford: Blackwell Science; 2004. pp. 43.28-43.34.
57. Singhi MK, Ghiya BC, Dhabhai RK. Comparison of oral azithromycin pulse with daily doxycycline in the treatment of acne vulgaris. Indian J Dermatol Venereol Leprol. 2003;69:274-6.
58. Smith RN, Mann NJ, Braue A, et al. The effect of a high-protein, low glycemic-load diet versus a conventional, high glycemic-load diet on biochemical parameters associated with acne vulgaris: A randomized, investigator marked, controlled trial. J Am Acad Dermatol. 2007;57:247-56.
59. Thiboutot DM, Knaggs H, Gilliand K, et al. Activity of type 1 5-$\alpha$-reductase and 17-$\beta$-hydroxysteroid dehydrogenase in the infrainfundibulum of subjects with and without acne vulgaris. Dermatology. 1998;196:38-42.
60. Thorneycroft IH, Gollnick H, Schellschmidt I. Superiority of combined contraceptive containing drospirenone to a triphasic preparation containing norgestimate in acne treatment. Cutis. 2004;74:123-30.
61. Tutakne MA, Chari KV. Acne, rosacea and perioral dermatitis. In: Valia RG, Valia AR (Eds). IADVL Textbook and Atlas of Dermatology, 2nd edition. Mumbai: Bhalani Publishing House; 2003. pp. 689-710.
62. Williams C, Layton AM. Persistent acne in women. Implications for the patient and for therapy. Am J Clin Dermatol. 2006;7:281-90.
63. Wolfe JE. An update of recent clinical trials examining adapalene and acne. J Eur Acad Venereol. 2001;15:23-9.
64. Yagyu H, Kitamine T, Osuga J, et al. Absence of ACAT-1 attenuates atherosclerosis but causes dry eye and cutaneous xanthomatosis in mice with congenital hyperlipidemia. J Biol Chem. 2000;275:21324-30.
65. Yang DJ, Quan LT, Hsu S. Topical antibacterial agents. In: Wolverton SE (Ed). Comprehensive Dermatologic Drug Therapy, 2nd edition. Philadelphia: Saunders Elsevier; 2007. pp. 525-46.
66. Yazici K, Baz K, Yazici AE, et al. Disease-specific quality of life is associated with anxiety and depression in patients with acne. J Eur Acad Dermatol Venereol. 2004;18:435-9.
67. Zaenglein AL, Graber EM, Thiboutot DM. Acne vulgaris and acneiform eruptions. In: Wolff K, Goldsmith LA, Katz SI, Gilchrest BA (Eds). Fitzpatrick's Dermatology In General Medicine, 7th edition. McGraw Hill; 2003. pp. 690-703.
68. Zheng Y, Eilertsen KJ, Ge L, et al. Scd1 is expressed in sebaceous glands and is disrupted in the asebia mouse. Nat Genet. 1999;23:268-70.

# 19 CHAPTER Rosacea and Perioral Dermatitis

*Abhijit Saha, Rajeev Sharma*

## ROSACEA

Rosacea is a chronic inflammatory facial dermatosis predominantly affecting the convexities of face and manifesting with flushing, persistent erythema, and telangiectasia. The chronic course is punctuated by episodes of "flares" with development of additional features like edema, papules, and pustules.

### Epidemiology

This is a common dermatosis especially in fair skinned individuals with an estimated overall prevalence of 0.5–10%. It has been called as the "Curse of Celts" because of its increased prevalence in Celtics and Northern Europeans. Though females outnumber males (M:F = 3:1), phymatous changes are almost exclusive to men. Usual age of onset is in between 30 years and 50 years. However, children, adolescents, and young adults may also be affected and in them it usually coexists with acne.

### Pathogenesis

The exact pathogenesis is still an enigma and a number of hypothesis and theories have been documented including mechanistic explanations that explain the clinical presentations of defined clinical subtypes. There is a complex interplay of several intrinsic and extrinsic factors like genetic predisposition, impaired epidermal barrier function, vascular abnormalities, dermal matrix degeneration, environmental factors, and microorganisms.

- *Neurogenic dysregulation*: Some receptors have been detected in the sensory nerve endings (four vanilloid receptors and one ankyrin receptor) that get stimulated and contribute to rosacea and manifest with flushing and burning.
- *Defective barrier function and increased transepidermal water loss (TEWL)*: There is defective regulation of innate immunity of skin, the pathogenesis of which is not understood. There is elevated expression of cathelicidin, antimicrobial peptides (AMPs), and a serine protease called kallikrein 5. There is also elevated toll-like receptor 2, and matrix metalloproteinases (MMPs). LL-37 peptide form of cathelicidin, in addition to proteolytically processed forms of LL-37, have been found in significantly different amounts in rosacea patients compared with healthy individuals. LL-37 is expressed by polymorphonuclear leukocytes and lymphocytes. LL-37 interacts with endothelial cells and stimulates angiogenesis both *in vitro* and *in vivo*. It also modulates the expression of vascular endothelial growth factor (VEGF)
- Ultraviolet (UV) light radiation—stimulates kallikrein 5 cathelicidin inflammatory cascade through reactive oxygen species (ROS) and toll-like receptor 2.

Microbial organisms may play role through different known and unknown mechanisms. *Demodex folliculorum, Staphylococcus epidermidis, Helicobacter pylori,* and *Bacillus oleronius* have been implicated (Flowchart 1).

### Triggers of Rosacea

- Hot and cold temperature
- Sunlight
- Wind
- Hot drinks
- Exercise
- Spicy food
- Alcohol
- Emotions
- Cosmetics
- Topical irritants
- Drugs.

### Classification and Clinical Features

Despite its apparent high incidence, the nosology of rosacea is not well established; therefore, the National Rosacea Society (NRS) assembled a committee to develop a standard classification system based on morphologic characteristics. This classification system describes the primary features of rosacea and defines four subtypes and one variant. Evolution from one subtype to another may or may not occur. This NRS classification also incorporated a provisional grading system—mild, moderate, and severe forms. Rosacea can be diagnosed by some characteristic features which typify the disease entity like—typical affection of the convexities of the central face along with presence of one or more primary features like flushing, nontransient erythema typically sparing periorbital areas, papules and pustules, and telangiectasia. Diagnosis is also aided by the presence of secondary features of burning

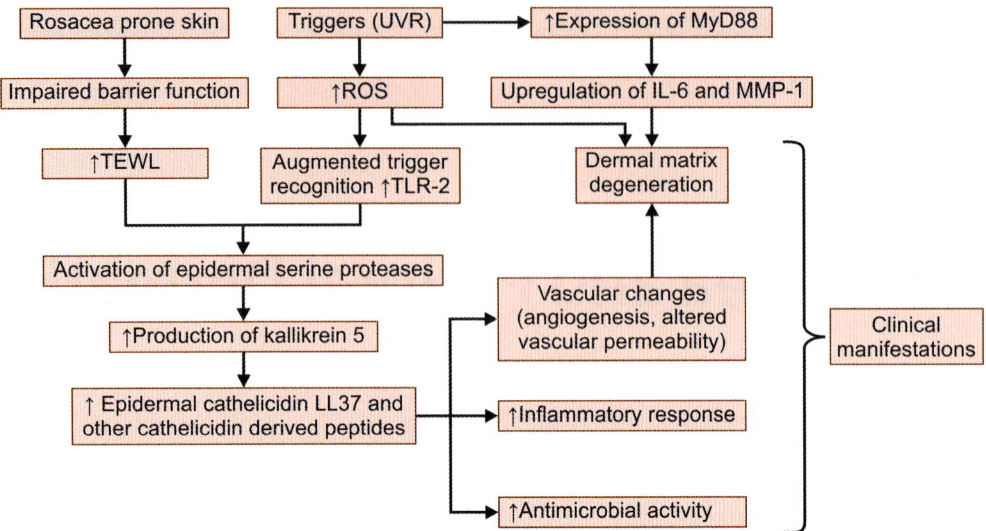


UVR, ultraviolet radiation; MyD88, myeloid differentiation factor; ROS, reactive oxygen species; TEWL, transepidermal water loss; TLR, toll-like receptor; MMP, matrix metalloproteinase.

**FLOWCHART 1:** Schematic representation of the pathogenesis of rosacea.

or stinging, dry appearance, and edema, which at times may become severe enough to form solid facial edema. Edema may accompany or follow prolonged facial erythema or flushing. Ocular involvement, phymatous changes, and peripheral location are some of the others secondary changes.

## Subtypes

The aforementioned primary and secondary features often occur simultaneously. The subtypes as described by the NRS (2002), include few signs sufficient to diagnose a specific subtype and features of more than one subtype may be found in a single patient.

- *Erythematotelangiectatic*: Characterized by flushing and persistent central facial erythema with or without telangiectasia. Central facial edema, stinging and burning sensations, and roughness or scaling may also be reported
- *Papulopustular*: Persistent central facial erythema with transient, central facial papules, or pustules or both. Papule and pustules may also develop periorificially. This variant is differentiated from acne by the absence of comedone (Fig. 1)
- *Phymatous*: Characteristic findings are thickening of skin, irregular surface, nodularities, and enlargement of the affected area. May occur on the nose (rhinophyma), (Fig. 2) chin (gnathophyma), forehead (metophyma), eyelids (blepharophyma), or ears (otophyma)
- *Ocular*: Blepharitis is the most common form of presentation, other being conjunctivitis, scleritis and rosacea keratitis, and corneal ulceration, which may lead to visual loss. The common manifestations are foreign body sensation, burning or stinging, dryness, itching, photophobia, and blurring of vision, telangiectases of the conjunctiva and lid margin, or lid and periocular erythema. Multiple chalazia result from meibomian gland dysfunction. Ocular rosacea usually accompanies cutaneous lesions but it may precede the development of cutaneous lesions or may appear thereafter (Fig. 3).

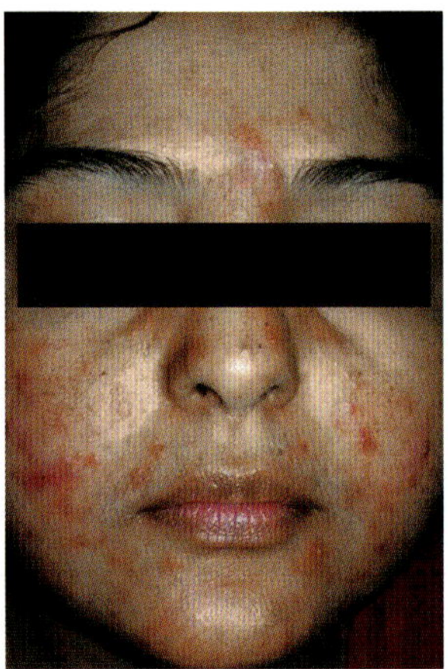

**FIG. 1:** Typical papulopustular lesions in rosacea.

*Courtesy*: Dr Brijesh Nair, Consultant Dermatologist, Military Hospital, Jaipur, Rajasthan.

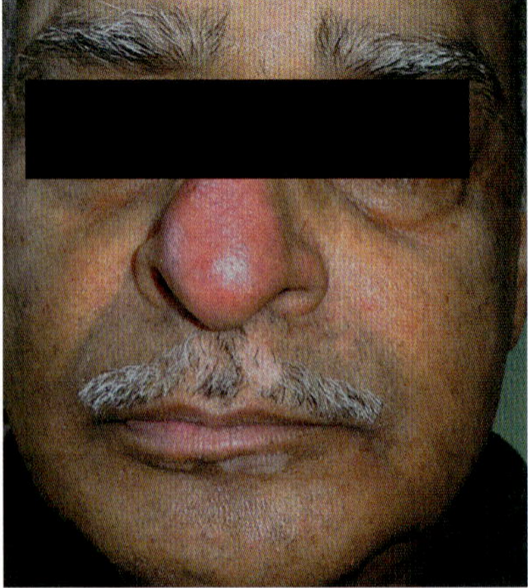

**FIG. 2:** Early rhinophymatous changes in rosacea.

*Courtesy*: Dr Nilendu Sarma, Associate Professor and Head, Department of Dermatology, Dr BC Roy Post Graduate Institute of Pediatric Sciences, West Bengal.

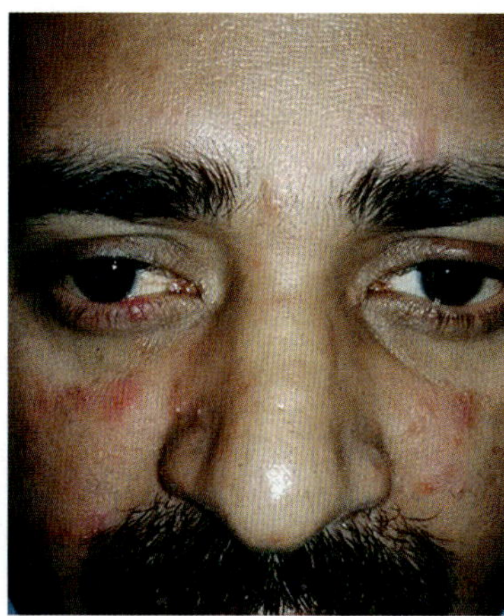

FIG. 3: Eye changes along with facial lesions in rosacea.
*Courtesy*: Dr Brijesh Nair, Consultant Dermatologist, Military Hospital, Jaipur, Rajasthan.

## Variant of Rosacea

The only variant is granulomatous rosacea. It is characterized by noninflammatory, hard, brown, yellow, or red monomorphic papules or nodules with preferential involvement of cheeks, and periorificial facial skin. Diascopy reveals apple jelly nodule and granuloma on histopathology.

Rosacea though a solely dermatological disorder usually without any known systemic associations and complications; it has a negative impact on quality of life through stigmatizing feelings and anxiety of patients. Recently, it has been found to be associated with increased risk for cardiovascular disease. It is becoming an increasing health problem in elderly population of western countries (Table 1).

## Treatment

Rosacea is a difficult to treat condition. One important aspect of management is avoidance triggers. The classical approach of therapy is based on the type of presentation.

### General Measures

- Use of broad spectrum sunscreen, preferably physical block
- Avoidance of triggers
- Avoidance of irritants (soaps, alcoholic cleansers, tinctures and astringents, abrasives, and peeling agents)
- Use of gentle and soap free cleanser
- Protective, gentle emollient to reduce the discomfort like burning and stinging
- Cosmetic coverage of erythema and telangiectasia with light green or yellow tinted foundation
- Circular massage to improve the edema of central face.

### Topical Therapy

- *Metronidazole*: Metronidazole, a synthetic nitroimidazole-derivative with antibacterial and antiprotozoal properties, is a major topical therapy for rosacea. It works as an oxygen scavenger, thereby decreasing ROS and inhibiting neutrophils. It is available in 0.75% aqueous gel (MetroGel) or 1% cream and is applied once or twice daily. It is effective

**TABLE 1: Differential diagnosis of rosacea**

| | |
|---|---|
| **Systemic causes:** | |
| • Polycythemia vera<br>• Connective-tissue diseases (systemic lupus erythematosus and dermatomyositis)<br>• Carcinoid syndrome<br>• Neurologic causes | Only flushing. No other primary or secondary features |
| **Drugs (mainly vasodilators) and food additives:** | |
| • Calcium channel blockers<br>• Niacin<br>• Cholinergic drugs<br>• Amyl and butyl nitrites<br>• Bromocriptine<br>• Tamoxifen<br>• Systemic steroids<br>• Cyclosporine | Only flushing |
| **Dermatological causes:** | |
| Acne vulgaris | • Early age of onset<br>• Presence of comedones<br>• Not limited to convexities of face<br>• Telangiectasia and flushing are usually absent |
| Perioral dermatitis | • Typical distribution; perioral and occasionally periorbital<br>• Presence of microvesicles and micropustules<br>• Absence of central facial erythema<br>• Rebound after discontinuation of potent topical steroids |
| Steroid-induced acneiform eruption | Monomorphic lesions |
| Rosacea fulminans | • Classically seen in young females<br>• Abrupt onset of confluent papules, pustules, and coalescent nodules with draining sinuses on a background of diffuse erythema<br>• Typically involving chin, cheeks, and forehead |
| Seborrheic dermatitis | • Eczematous changes<br>• Distributed mainly over perinasal areas, nasolabial folds, retro auricular groove, and extrafacial sites |
| Photodermatitis | • Seasonal<br>• Photo distributed areas |
| Chronic photodamage | • Affects periphery of the face, neck, upper chest, and postauricular area<br>• Additional feature: Dyspigmentation<br>• Submental sparing |
| Haber's syndrome | • Genodermatosis<br>• Persistent facial erythema and telangiectases<br>• Follicular and verrucous papules, and atrophic pitted scars<br>• Xerosis |

against inflammatory papular and pustular rosacea but does not alter erythema, telangiectasia, or flushing. The main side effect is burning or stinging.

- *Azelaic acid*: 15% azelaic acid gel another US Food and Drug Administration (US FDA) approved topical therapy for rosacea, is as effective as topical metronidazole. Probably the anti-inflammatory activity of azelaic acid accounts for a substantial proportion of the therapeutic effect. Azelaic acid reduces ROS, inhibits kallikrein 5 and increases serine protease activity.
- *Sodium sulfacetamide or 10 % sulfur*: It is better tolerated as a cleanser formulation.

Other topical agents used for rosacea include benzoyl peroxide, clindamycin, erythromycin, topical calcineurin inhibitors, and topical retinoids. Topical antibiotics act via anti-inflammatory effect rather than antibacterial. Tetracyclines and erythromycin reduce leucocyte migration and phagocytosis. Imidazoles are increasingly used for treatment of rosacea. The mechanism of action may be anti-inflammatory or immunosuppressive rather than bactericidal. Imidazoles seem to have low toxicity and are well tolerated by patients with sensitive skin. Benzoyl peroxide improves the papule and pustules of rosacea but it is better to avoid in sensitive patients. Topical retinoid is another option for maintenance therapy. With long-term use tretinoin promotes connective tissue remodeling and minimizes dermal inflammation. Recently, topical ivermectin 1% has been evaluated in two randomized, double-blind, and controlled studies for 12 weeks. It acts as a ligand of farnesoid X receptor, which seems to decrease the density of *Demodex* mites in rosacea skin.

### Systemic Therapy

Rosacea generally responds well to oral antibiotics. Tetracycline hydrochloride (HCl), oxytetracycline, doxycycline, and minocycline are preferred antibiotics. They act via anti-inflammatory effect (inhibit chemotaxis, MMPs, and protein kinase C) and thereby improve the inflammatory papulopustular lesions of rosacea. Treatment is started with a higher dose and once acute flare is controlled doses are lowered down. Doses of 250–500 mg tetracycline HCl or oxytetracycline, or 50 mg minocycline or doxycycline, per day are generally sufficient. Unnecessary long-term use of antibiotics should be discouraged.

Isotretinoin is exceptionally effective and is of particular importance in all forms of severe or therapy resistant rosacea. It is also indicated in early phymas. The dose required for control of rosacea varies. Refractory cases usually respond well to a dose of 0.5–1 mg/kg/day. Low-dose isotretinoin is much better and safer. 0.1–0.2 mg/kg per day is usually effective in severe rosacea, though clearing may take longer.

Other oral agents used are macrolides, metronidazole, antiandrogens [oral contraceptive pill and spironolactone], beta-blockers, clonidine, naloxone, and selective serotonin reuptake inhibitors.

Azithromycin has found to be effective in both ocular and cutaneous rosacea. 1.5% ophthalmic solution of azithromycin is efficacious in ocular rosacea in children. During pregnancy, acute rosacea flare-ups may occur. Fuentelsaz et al. described a pregnant woman with rosacea fulminans who was successfully treated after a 3-month tapering course of azithromycin.

Combination of topical and systemic therapy provides better and faster results in initiation therapy but topical treatment is preferred for maintenance.

### Laser and Light Therapy

All previously mentioned medical treatments fail to improve erythema. Diffuse central facial erythema of rosacea is often chronically present, even in patients who are not experiencing acute flare-ups. Erythema with telangiectasias may improve by laser or intense pulsed light therapies.

### Treatment of Phyma

Early phyma is treated with oral isotretinoin. In advanced cases, surgical interventions such as tangential excision, dermabrasion, electrocautery, radiofrequency electrosurgery, and laser ablation are undertaken.

### Ocular Rosacea

Ocular rosacea has a significant impact on quality of life. The treatment of ocular rosacea is based on systemic anti-inflammatory drug therapy, topical therapy with artificial tears, and eyelid hygiene, 10% sodium sulfacetamide eye ointment. Once-daily low dose (40 mg) doxycycline is a safe and effective treatment. 0.05% cyclosporine. A ophthalmic emulsion has been shown to be effective in ocular rosacea. A recent alternative to systemic low-dose tetracyclines is topical azithromycin eye drops. The alpha-1-selective inhibitor oxymetazoline has been used off-label as 0.05% solution in some cases.

## PERIORAL DERMATITIS

Perioral dermatitis (POD) is a distinctive disorder first described in 1957 and is characterized by discrete papules and pustules in a periorificial distribution primarily around the mouth with a narrow zone of sparing around the vermillion border of lips. Initially described in young females, but is also seen in children. Granulomatous POD, a subset of POD is exclusively a disease of children and shows granuloma on histopathology. It was first reported in the French literature in 1970 by Gianotti et al.

### Epidemiology

It is a common dermatosis with increasing trend. POD in adults predominantly affects women, but in children there is no gender predilection. The granulomatous form is reported in prepubertal age group. This subset is more common in dark skinned (Afro-Caribbean, African American, and Asian).

### Etiology and Pathogenesis

The precise etiopathogenesis is still unknown; however, the long-term use of fluorinated topical steroids for minor skin alterations of the face often precedes the manifestation of POD. Though the disease is prevalent in young women, hormonal influence is not established. Several microbiological agents (candida, demodex, and fusiform bacteria) were thought to be implicated in the pathogenesis but their exact role was not proved. Allergic contacts with fluorides of toothpaste and dentifrices have also been reported. External physical factors like UV radiation, heat may exacerbate it. While external factors are often implicated, periorificial dermatitis may actually result from epidermal barrier dysfunction. A combination of external factors and intrinsic factors such as atopy predispose individuals to develop periorificial dermatitis.

## Clinical Features

Subjective symptoms of stinging or burning may be there, but itching is absent. Often, long-term use of topical steroids for minor or even undiagnosed skin conditions precedes the development of POD.

The primary skin lesions are discrete or grouped, tiny papules, vesicles, and pustules on an erythematous base distributed symmetrically around the perioral, perinasal, and periorbital areas. The lesion may be unilateral. Distinctive feature is sparing of 5 mm clear zone around the vermillion border (Figs 4 and 5).

Perioral dermatitis is more appropriately termed as periorificial dermatitis. A recent study found that 70% of pediatric patients with periorificial dermatitis had perioral, 43% perinasal, and 25% periocular involvement. Other studies reported up to 100% perioral involvement, 57% perinasal, and 25% periocular involvement.

Childhood granulomatous periorificial dermatitis characterized by monomorphous, dome-shaped, skin-colored to yellowish-brown papules with occasional overlying scale affecting the perioral, and periocular and perinasal areas predominantly. Extra-facial involvement affecting the neck, trunk, extremities, and genitalia has been reported. It is benign self-limiting condition and heals without any sequelae, but healing with atrophic scarring has been reported.

## Diagnosis

*Histopathology*: Spongiotic changes in the outer root sheath of hair follicles. Childhood granulomatous periorificial dermatitis shows upper dermal noncaseating granulomas with predilection for follicle and perifollicular dermis and mixed infiltrate of lymphocytes, histiocytes with occasional epidermal changes such as hyperkeratosis, acanthosis, and spongiosis.

## Differential Diagnosis

The differential diagnosis of POD is shown in table 2.

## Prognosis and Clinical Course

Benign self-limited disorder with fluctuating course recurs on treatment with topical steroids. With proper treatment it resolves with minimal recurrence.

**FIG. 4:** Perioral dermatitis.
*Courtesy*: Dr Nilendu Sarma, Associate Professor and Head, Department of Dermatology, Dr BC Roy Post Graduate Institute of Pediatric Sciences, West Bengal.

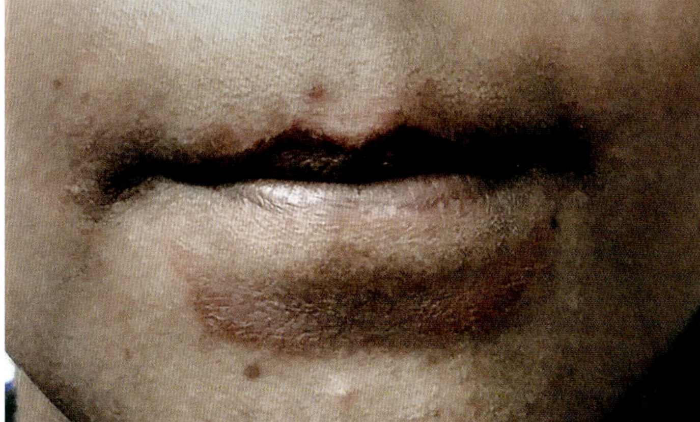

**FIG. 5:** Perioral dermatitis with classical sparing area.
*Courtesy*: Dr Sayantani Chakraborty, Assistant Professor Department of Dermatology, RG Kar Medical College, West Bengal.

**TABLE 2: Differential diagnosis of perioral dermatitis**

| POD | |
|---|---|
| Rosacea | • Involvement of convexities of face<br>• Persistent erythema<br>• Telangiectasia |
| Seborrheic dermatitis | • Concentrated around nasolabial folds<br>• Scaling |
| Allergic contact dermatitis | History of contact with allergens |
| Lip licking cheilitis | • Common in children<br>• Scaling<br>• Well demarcated |
| Acne vulgaris | • Presence of comedones<br>• Other sites of involvement |
| Gram negative folliculitis | • History of long-term antibiotic use<br>• Predominance of pustules |
| Demodex folliculitis | Immunocompromised host |
| **Granulomatous periorificial dermatitis** | |
| Granulomatous rosacea | • Persistent erythema and flushing<br>• Telangiectasia<br>• Edema |
| Sarcoidosis | • Rare in children<br>• Associated systemic involvement |
| Lupus miliaris disseminates faciei | • Adult onset<br>• Chronic course<br>• Predilection for central face and periorbital area<br>• Heals with depressed scar |
| Blau syndrome | • Skin lesions of varying morphology<br>• Synovial cysts<br>• Uveitis<br>• Arthritis |

## Treatment

Discontinuation of topical corticosteroids should be done. In case of potent fluorinated steroid, initial substitution with low potent hydrocortisone cream may reduce the flare. Patient education and counseling form important aspect of management.

In mild cases, as well as in most children and pregnant women, individualized topical therapy is generally recommended. Antimicrobial agents like metronidazole, erythromycin, and clindamycin are administered in a nongreasy base (e.g., gel, lotion, and cream). Topical calcineurin inhibitors have been used successfully. Other topical medicines tried with variable responses are azelaic acid, sulfur-based preparations, and adapalene.

In severe forms of POD, systemic treatment with antibiotics is required. The drugs of choice are tetracycline, doxycycline, and minocycline for a period of around 8–10 weeks. In unresponsive and granulomatous forms, oral isotretinoin may be considered. Oral erythromycin can be used in pediatric patients with more severe or refractory involvement.

Photodynamic therapy has been reported to be helpful although large studies have not yet been performed.

## SUGGESTED READINGS


1. Bhatia ND, Del Rosso JQ. Optimal management of papulopustular rosacea: rationale for combination therapy. J Drugs Dermatol. 2012;11(7):838-44.
2. Böhm D, Schwanitz P, Stock Gissendanner S, et al. Symptom severity and psychological sequelae in rosacea: Results of a survey. Psychol Health Med. 2014;19(5):586-91.
3. Coda AB, Hata T, Miller J, et al. Cathelicidin, kallikrein 5, and serine protease activity is inhibited during treatment of rosacea with azelaic acid 15% gel. J Am Acad Dermatol. 2013;69(4):570-7.
4. Cox ES, Shannon AB. Papular facial eruption in an African American adolescent-quiz case. Arch Dermatol 2006;142(6):775-80.
5. Culp B, Scheinfeld N. Rosacea: A Review. P T. 2009;34(1):38-45
6. Darlenski R, Kazandjieva J, Tsankov N, et al. Acute irritant threshold correlates with barrier function, skin hydration and contact hypersensitivity in atopic dermatitis and rosacea. Exp Dermatol. 2013;22(11):752-3.
7. Del Rosso JQ. Update on rosacea pathogenesis and correlation with medical therapeutic agents. Cutis. 2006;78(2):97-100.
8. Doan S, Gabison E, Chiambaretta F, et al. Efficacy of azithromycin 1.5% eye drops in childhood ocular rosacea with phlyctenular blepharokeratoconjunctivitis. J Ophthalmic Inflamm Infect. 2013;3:38.
9. Duman N, Ersoy Evans S, Atakan N: Rosacea and cardiovascular risk factors: a case control study. J Eur Acad Dermatol Venereol. 2014;28(9):1165-9.
10. Fuentelsaz V, Ara M, Corredera C, et al. Rosacea fulminans in pregnancy: successful treatment with azithromycin. Clin Exp Dermatol. 2011;36(6):674-6.
11. Generali JA, Cada DJ. Oxymetazoline (topical): rosacea. Hosp Pharm. 2013;48(7): 558-9.
12. Hall CS, Reichenberg J. Evidence based review of perioral dermatitis therapy. G Ital Dermatol Venereol. 2010;145(4):433-44.
13. Holmes AD. Potential role of microorganisms in the pathogenesis of rosacea. J Am Acad Dermatol. 2013;69(6):1025-32.
14. Hussain W, Daly BM. Granulomatous periorificial dermatitis in an 11-year-old boy: dramatic response to tacrolimus. J Eur Acad Dermatol Venereol. 2007;21(1):137-9.
15. Jansen T. Azelaic acid as a new treatment for perioral dermatitis: results from an open study. Br J Dermatol. 2004;151(4):933-4.
16. Ljubojevic S, Lipozencic J, Turcic P. Perioral dermatitis. Acta Dermatovenerol Croat. 2008;16(2):96-100.
17. Mantelli F, Di Zazzo A, Sacchetti M, et al. Topical azithromycin as a novel treatment for ocular rosacea. Ocul Immunol Inflamm. 2013;21(5):371-7.
18. Marks JG, Miller JJ. Rosacea. Principles of Dermatology, 4th edition. Philadelphia: Elsevier/Saunders; 2006.
19. Meyer-Hoffert U, Schröder J: Epidermal proteases in the pathogenesis of rosacea. J Investig Dermatol Symp Proc. 2011;15(1):16-23.
20. Narayanan S, Hünerbein A, Getie M, et al. Scavenging properties of metronidazole on free oxygen radicals in a skin lipid model system. J Pharm Pharmacol. 2007;59(8):1125-30.
21. Oppel T, Pavicic T, Kamann S, et al. Pimecrolimus cream (1%) efficacy in perioral dermatitis - results of a randomized, double-blind, vehicle-controlled study in 40 patients. J Eur Acad Dermatol Venereol. 2007;21(9):1175-80.
22. Pelle MT. Rosacea. In: Wolff K, Goldsmith LA, Katz SI, Gilchrist BA, Paller AS, Leffell DJ (Eds). Fitzpatrick's Dermatology in General medicine, 7th edition. New York: McGraw-Hill; 2008. pp. 703-9.
23. Richey DF, Hopson B. Photodynamic therapy for perioral dermatitis. J Drugs Dermatol. 2006;5(2 Suppl):12-6.
24. Ríos-Yuil JM, Mercadillo-Perez P. Evaluation of Demodex folliculorum as a Risk Factor for the Diagnosis of Rosacea In Skin Biopsies. Mexico's General Hospital (1975-2010). Indian J Dermatol. 2013;58(2):157.
25. Schechter BA, Katz RS, Friedman LS. Efficacy of topical cyclosporine for the treatment of ocular rosacea. Adv Ther. 2009; 26(6):651-9.
26. Scheinfeld N: A review of deferasirox, bortezomib, dasatinib, and cyclosporine eye drops: possible uses and known side effects in cutaneous medicine. J Drugs Dermatol. 2007;6(3):352-5.
27. Scheinfeld NS. Rosacea. Skinmed. 2006;5:191-4.
28. Smith JR, Lanier VB, Braziel RM, et al. Expression of vascular endothelial growth factor and its receptors in rosacea. Br J Ophthalmol. 2007;91(2):226-9.
29. Sobolewska B, Doycheva D, Deuter C, et al. Treatment of ocular rosacea with once-daily lowdose doxycycline. Cornea. 2014;33(3):257-60.
30. Stein L, Kircik L, Fowler J, et al. Efficacy and safety of ivermectin 1% cream in treatment of papulo-pustular rosacea: results of two randomized, double-blind, vehicle controlled pivotal studies. J Drugs Dermatol. 2014;13(3):316-23.
31. Voegeli R, Rawlings AV, Doppler S, et al. Increased basal transepidermal water loss leads to elevation of some but not all stratum corneum serine proteases. Int J Cosmet Sci. 2008,30(6):435-42.
32. Wilkin J, Dahl M, Detmer M, et al. Standard classification of rosacea: Report of the National Rosacea Society Expert Committee on the Classification and Staging of Rosacea. J Am Acad Dermatol. 2002;46(4):584-7.
33. Yamasaki K, Gallo RL. The molecular pathology of rosacea. J Dermatol Sci. 2009;55(2):77-81.
34. Yamasaki K, Kanada K, Macleod DT, et al. TLR2 expression is increased in rosacea and stimulates enhanced serine protease production by keratinocytes. J Invest Dermatol. 2011;131(3):688-97.
35. Yücel A, Yilmaz M. Rosacea Ön Tanılı Hastalarda Demodex folliculorum ve Demodex brevis Yaygınlığının Araştırılması. Turkiye Parazitol Derg. 2013;37:195-8.

# 20 CHAPTER

# Hidradenitis Suppurativa

*Nilendu Sarma, Abhijit Saha*

## INTRODUCTION

Hidradenitis suppurativa (HS) is characterized by chronic painful, deep-seated, inflamed lesions with mucopurulent discharge, sinus formation and scarring of the apocrine gland-bearing areas.

## HISTORY

It was named by Verneuli in 1854. Owing to its distribution, it was considered a disorder of the apocrine glands. Later, Brunsting discovered the basic alteration as altered keratinization of the terminal hair follicle. It was included into the follicular occlusion triad by Pillsbury. Plewig named it acne inversa.

## EPIDEMIOLOGY

Overall prevalence among general population is about 1%. It generally begins after puberty. Onset after menopause is rare. It shows female predilection with a female to male ratio as high as 2-5:1.

## PATHOGENESIS

Pathogenesis of HS is not explained. Infection, genetic predisposition, and comorbidities and many environmental factors are all important in this. Hyperkeratosis of terminal follicular epithelium is affected initially with secondary involvement of apocrine glands. It begins with follicular plugging due to follicular hyperkeratosis that obstructs the apocrine gland ducts and leads to perifolliculitis. This is followed by rupture of the follicular epithelium that results in inflammation and all its complications like rupture of the overlying skin, fibrosis and sinus tract formation. Primary factor contributing to development of HS could also be inflammation. This leads to follicular occlusion.

Role of infection as the primary factors is not proven. Lymph nodes are generally not also enlarged. Coagulase-negative *Staphylococcus* (*Staphylococcus epidermidis*) is repeatedly discussed as an important etiology. These are commensal in skin. Possibly, they induce inflammation. Various gram-negative organisms and anerobic organisms also contribute to the HS phenotype. Presence of biofilm is considered one important mechanism of persistent infection and resistance to antibiotics and frequent relapse. Presence of *Staphylococcus aureus* and *Streptococcus pyogenes* is very rare and possibly reflect secondary infection.

Genetic factor is another very important factor. There is an autosomal dominant inherited form of HS with mutation in the gamma-secretase genes *NCSTN, PSENEN*, and *PSEN1* resulting in an extensive disease with early age of onset.

Comorbidities that are frequently associated with HS include obesity, metabolic syndrome inflammatory bowel disease especially perianal Crohn's disease, follicular occlusion triad, polycystic ovarian syndrome, pyoderma gangrenosum, nephrotic syndrome, amyloidosis, pityriasis rubra pilaris, acanthosis nigricans, steatocystoma multiplex, and Dowling-Degos disease, rheumatological conditions like spondyloarthropathies and SAPHO syndrome (synovitis, acne, pustulosis, hyperostosis and osteitis).

Despite the apparent strong clinical influence of androgens like age of occurrence, postpartum and premenstrual flare, most patients have normal hormonal profile. Additionally, apocrine glands are not androgen sensitive.

## CLINICAL FEATURES

This is a chronic disease with variable course. It involves apocrine gland-bearing areas with a predilection for the intertriginous regions. The axillary and inguinoperineal, perineum, gluteal area, and inframammary (in women) regions are commonly affected. Other zones less commonly affected are areola of the breast, scalp, zygomatic and malar areas of the face, nape of the neck, the external auditory meatus, and eyelids. Disease generally starts after puberty.

The disease starts with inflammatory, painful nodules, and sterile abscesses followed by tissue fibrosis. Over time, sinus tracts and fistulas develop bridging individual lesions. Hypertrophic scarring can often be seen. This is accompanied by chronic discharge. Sinuses have been reported to involve deeper tissues including muscle, fascia, urethra, and bowel (Fig. 1).

Multiple open comedones and double-ended comedones or bridged comedones are the tell-tale signs of HS; and may frequently progress to multiple abscesses and sinus tract formations. Pain is a major symptom and characteristic of pain is variable. This is a chronic disease with recurrence of the same process in an adjacent area or in different areas of predilection.

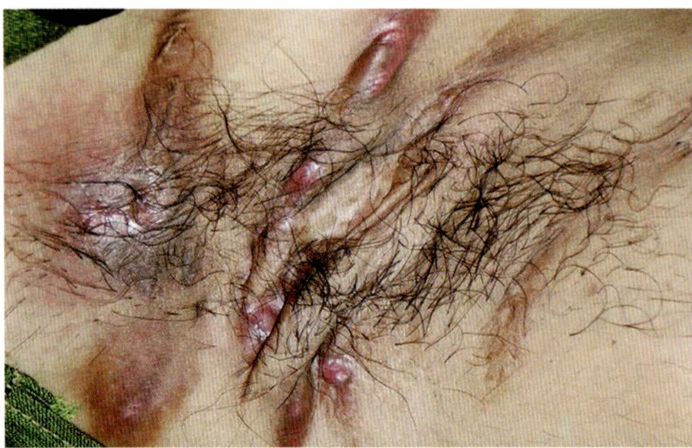

FIG. 1: Nodules, discharging sinus and scarring in axilla in hidradinitis suppurativa.

The disease has significant negative impact on quality of life with pain being one of the major contributing factors. Depression and stigmatization are associated mainly with anogenital lesions.

## CLASSIFICATION AND SCORING

Based on severity, HS has been classified into three stages by Hurley:

- *Stage I*: Single lesion without sinus tract formation. This is most common
- *Stage II*: More than one lesion or area, with limited tunneling
- *Stage III*: Multiple lesions, with more extensive sinus tracts and scarring.

Sartorius scale assists in assessment treatment response.

Recently, Physician Global Assessment and Patient Global Assessment have become useful tools to evaluate patient severity as well as responses to therapy. "Hidradenitis suppurativa score" (HSS) includes risk factors like smoking and obesity.

## DIAGNOSIS

Diagnosis is primarily clinical. Following three features are helpful in diagnosis:

- Typical lesions deep-seated nodules and/or fibrosis
- Typical localizations--genitoanal and axillary region, often symmetrical
- Typical relapsing course and chronicity.

### Laboratory Studies

Patients with acute lesions may have an elevated erythrocyte sedimentation rate, elevated white blood cell count (occasionally), a low serum iron level, and serum protein abnormalities on electrophoresis.

## HISTOPATHOLOGY

Typically, it demonstrates follicular hyperkeratosis and mixed cellular infiltrate in the lower half of the dermis and subcutis. Occasionally, foreign body giant cells may be detected.

Active lesions may show abscess and sinus tract may be visible and extensive fibrosis with destruction of appendageal structures in chronic cases.

## DIFFERENTIAL DIAGNOSIS

- Crohn's disease (intestinal Crohn's disease is usually associated)
- Staphylococcal infection
- Simple abscess (generally single lesion)
- Nodular acne
- Tuberculosis
- Leprosy
- Furunculosis
- Actinomycosis
- Lymphogranuloma venereum
- Lymphadenitis
- Donovanosis
- Epidermoid or dermoid cyst
- Pilonidal sinus.

## COMPLICATIONS

- Local:
  - Scarring
  - Infection
  - Anal, urethral or rectal stricture
  - Urethral fistula
  - Secondary lymphedema (scrotal or vulvar)
  - Lymphangioma circumscriptum of the vulva
  - *Squamous cell carcinoma*: This tends to be more aggressive with early metastatic spread and a devastating mortality rate.
- Systemic:
  - Septicemia
  - Anemia
  - Hypoproteinemia
  - Nephritic syndrome
  - Arthopathies
  - Polyarthritis
  - Dactylitis
  - Synovitis, acne, pustulosis, hyperostosis, and osteitis (SAPHO) syndrome
  - Secondary amyloidosis with multi-organ involvement
  - Interstitial keratitis.

## TREATMENT

A variety of therapeutic options are available, including preventive, medical, surgical, and psychological strategies with variable outcomes. Treatment is directed towards disease manifestations and stage of the disease.

*General or preventive measures*: Mild disease can be handled with these measures:

- Pain management
- Weight reduction
- Avoidance of prolonged exposure to heat and humidity
- Avoidance of shaving, if irritation occurs
- Avoidance of tight, synthetic clothing near affected area
- Stress management
- Topical antiseptics and antibacterial soap
- Warm compresses, warm baths, and hydrotherapy
- Non-narcotic analgesics
- Cessation of cigarette smoking.

## Medical Therapy

The only effective topical antibiotic is clindamycin.

Antistaphylococcal agents are advocated for axillary disease, and more broad-spectrum coverage is required for perineal disease. Dicloxacillin, erythromycin, tetracycline, minocycline, and cephalosporins have been used with variable success. Duration of therapy is adjusted depending on the course of the disease.

Many studies have used combination of antibiotics like rifampicin and clindamycin, rifampicin, moxifloxacin, and metronidazole. Isoniazid has not shown to be of any benefit.

Parenteral antibiotics can be used in severe cases. Ertapenem (IV) and ceftriaxone (IV) was reported to be effective as was combination of linezolid and meropenem.

Oral contraceptive agents that contain a high estrogen-to-progesterone ratio and low androgenicity of progesterone, cyproterone acetate in combination with ethinyl estradiol and other contraceptives have shown variable efficacy. Finasteride and cyproterone acetate have been found to be effective in some studies.

Oral retinoids initially thought to be a promising treatment option because of its action on follicular keratinization, demonstrated modest therapeutic benefit. Isotretinoin is of limited value. Pretreatment with isotretinoin at a dosage of 0.5–1.0 mg per kg daily for a few months before surgery has been recommended to reduce the inflammatory components. Acitretin is of proven efficacy. Alitretinoin has also showed significant benefit. It has shorter half-life and is useful in females.

Other drugs used are biologics like adalimumab, ustekinumab, infliximab, systemic corticosteroids, azathioprine, cyclosporine, dapsone, and methotrexate. Etanercept was not found to be of much benefit.

Intralesional corticosteroid works rapidly. But, presence of cellulitis has to be ruled out. Systemic steroid has also been used for short duration with good result.

Dapsone has shown only mild-to-moderate efficacy.

Colchicine, metformin, zinc gluconate, intravenous immunoglobulin, botulinum toxin injection, and oral tacrolimus have been used but more evidence is necessary. Cyclosporine is not very safe to be used.

## Surgery

It is the cornerstone for acute abscess pain relief and for treatment of advanced disease. For early, limited disease that presents with a fluctuant abscess, incision, and drainage may be a good first option. In mild-to-moderate acne inversa (Hurley grade I and II), surgery with primary closure is a treatment option whereas in more advanced disease, extensive surgery with second intention healing is the gold standard. Relapse is frequent even after successful treatment with antibiotics and other drugs. Surgical debridement is possibly required to remove the biofilm that is considered as the source of infection.

Carbon dioxide laser has also been used for excision.

## Other Treatment Modalities

Initial studies with neodymium-doped yttrium aluminum garnet laser have shown promising results. Intense pulsed light, photodynamic therapy, blue light therapy, radiotherapy, and cryotherapy have also been used.

## SUGGESTED READINGS


1. Amankwah Y, Haefner H. Vulvar edema. Dermatol Clin. 2010;28:765-77.
2. Bettoli V, Join-Lambert O, Nassif A. Antibiotic treatment of hidradinitis suppurativa. Dermatol Clin. 2016;34:81-9.
3. Blanco R, González-Vela MC, González-López MA, et al. Interstitial keratitis secondary to severe hidradenitis suppurativa responding to adalimumab. Cornea. 2012;31:206.
4. Bong JL, Shalders K, Saihan E. Treatment of persistent painful nodules of hidradenitis suppurativa with cryotherapy. Clin Exp Dermatol. 2003;28:241-4.
5. Canoui-Poitrine F, Revuz JE, Wolkenstein P, et al. Clinical characteristics of a series of 302 French patients with hidradenitis suppurativa, with an analysis of factors associated with disease severity. J Am Acad Dermatol. 2009;61:51-7.
6. Danby FW, Margesson LJ. Hidradenitis suppurativa. Dermatol Clin. 2010;28:779-93.
7. Fioravanti A, Lauraflori M, Guidelli GM, et al. Dactylitis as a first manifestation of arthritis associated with hidradenitis suppurativa. Indian J Dermatol Venereol Leprol. 2011;77:74-6.
8. Girouard SD, Falk RH, Rennke HG, et al. Hidradenitis suppurativa resulting in systemic amyloid A amyloidosis: A case report and review of the literature. Dermatol Online J. 2012;18:2.
9. Highton L, Chan WY, Khawa N, et al. Treatment of hidradenitis suppurativa with intense pulsed light: A prospective study. Plast Recosntr Surg. 2011;128:459-65.
10. Hurley HJ. Axillary hyperhidrosis, apocrine bromhidrosis, hidradenitis suppurativa and familial benign pemphigus surgical approach. In: Roenigk RK, Roenigk HH (Eds). New York: Dermatologic Surgery Marcel Dekker; 1989. pp. 729-39.
11. Losanoff JE, Sochaki P, Khoury N, et al. Squamous cell carcinoma complicating chronic suppurative hidradenitis. Am Surg. 2011;77:1449-53.
12. Miller IM, Ellervik C, Vinding GR, et al. Association of metabolic syndrome and hidradenitis suppurativa. JAMA Dermatol. 2014;150(12):1273-80.
13. Pagliarello C, Paradisi A. The perils of a defective medical communication: Fatal neglected squamous cell carcinoma arising in perineal hidradenitis suppurativa. Case Rep Dermatol. 2011;3:5-7.
14. Passeron T, Khemis A, Ortonne JP. Pulsed dye laser-mediated photodynamic therapy for acne inversa is not successful: A pilot study on four cases. J Dermatolog Treat. 2009;20:297-8.
15. Schweiger ES, Riddle CC, Aires DJ. Treatment of hidradenitis uppurativa by photodynamic therapy with aminolevulinic acid: Preliminary results. J Drugs Dermatol. 2011;10:381-6.
16. Sims SM, McLean FW, Davis JD, et al. Vulvar lymphangioma circumscriptum: A report of 3 cases, 2 associated with vulvar carcinoma and 1 with hidradenitis suppurativa. J Low Genit Tract Dis. 2010;14:234-7.
17. Van Rappard DC, Mooij JE, Baeten DL, et al. New onset polyarthritis during successful treatment of hidradenitis suppurativa with infliximab. Br J Dermatol. 2011;165:194-8.
18. von der Werth JM, Jemec GB. Morbidity in patients with hidradenitis suppurativa. Br J Dermatol. 2001;144(4):809-13.
19. Xu LY, Wright DR, Mahmoud BH, et al. Histopathologic study of hidradenitis suppurativa following long-pulsed 1064-nm Nd: YAG laser treatment. Arch Dermatol. 2011;147:21-8.
20. Yazdanyar S, Jemec GB. Hidradenitis suppurativa: A review of cause and treatment. Curr Opin Infect Dis. 2011;24:118-23.
21. Yu CC, Cook MG. Hidradenitis suppurativa: a disease of follicular epithelium, rather than apocrine glands. Br J Dermatol. 1990;122(6):763-9.

# 8 SECTION Blistering Disorders of Skin

# 21 CHAPTER Genetic Bullous Diseases

*Vesarat Wessagowit*

## INTRODUCTION

Genetic bullous diseases are a group of inherited bullous disorders characterized by skin fragility and blistering often induced by minor trauma. Phenotypes in most of these conditions are frank blisters but sometimes can appear as crusted plaques in the flexural areas, generalized verrucous plaques or prematurely aged skin. The onset is usually from birth but can be as late as third decade of life. Clinical recognition, investigations, and history taking are important in making the correct diagnosis and lead to proper management.

## PATHOGENESIS

Skin is the body's largest organ which keeps the internal organs from mechanical, physical or microbial noxae.

Integrity of the skin is maintained through cohesion between the keratinocytes (through keratinocyte cell-cell adhesion) themselves as well as that between the keratinocytes, the basement membrane (through hemidesmosomal structures) and the dermis. Defects of any of these cohesions, whether inherited or acquired, lead to skin fragility (Fig. 1).

Tonofibrils are fibrillar structural proteins composed of with tonofilaments which converge at desmosomes and hemidesmosomes (Fig. 1). They are composed of keratin-1 and 10 and reside in keratinocytes. Keratin-1 and 10, coexpressed in terminally differentiated epidermis, are specific markers for terminal differentiation in mammalian epidermis. Defects of these proteins result in epidermolytic ichthyosis [Online Mendelian Inheritance in Man (OMIM) accession number 113800].

Calcium homeostasis is important in the keratinocyte adhesion and differentiation, with an increasing epidermal gradient in the normal skin, from the basal layer to the superficial layers. Defects in intracellular calcium transport result in two different inherited skin fragility disorders. Abnormal sarco/endoplasmic reticulum calcium adenosine triphosphatase 2 (SERCA2) endoplasmic reticulum calcium transport results in Darier-White disease (OMIM 124200), whereas defective human secretory pathway $Ca^{2+}$-ATPase 1 (hSPCA1) Golgi apparatus calcium transport gives rise to benign chronic pemphigus (OMIM 169600).

The dermal-epidermal junction of the skin is tightly anchored by hemidesmosomal complex, an electron-dense structure at the base of basal keratinocytes. They are composed of multiple structural proteins.

The heterotypic keratins 5 and 14 are coexpressed in the basal layer of the epidermis. These cytoskeletal proteins, together with plectin, are linked with hemidesmosomal protein bullous pemphigoid antigen 1 (BPAG1). The $\alpha6\beta4$ integrins and type XVII collagen help to anchor basal cells to the dermis via adhesion to type VII collagen in anchoring fibrils.

Focal contacts link the basement membrane with the epithelial cortical actin network. Kindlin, talin, vinculin, integrin $\alpha3\beta1$ and type XIII collagen are localized to the focal contacts.

Defects in these structures result in inherited bullous skin diseases, such as epidermolysis bullosa simplex (EBS; OMIM 131800, 131900), EBS with muscle dystrophy (OMIM 226670), junctional epidermolysis bullosa, Herlitz type (OMIM 226700), junctional epidermolysis bullosa, non-Herlitz type (OMIM 226650), epidermolysis bullosa junctional is with pyloric atresia (OMIM 226730), autosomal recessive epidermolysis bullosa dystrophica (OMIM 226600) and Kindler syndrome (OMIM 173650).

## EPIDERMOLYTIC ICHTHYOSIS

Epidermolytic ichthyosis is an autosomal dominant condition with a prevalence of 1 case per 200,000–300,000 population, with 50% *de novo* mutations in probands.

Phenotypically patients present with erythema and widespread formation of epidermal blisters developing at birth, hence the name bullous congenital ichthyosiform erythroderma. Later in life, bullosis is replaced by progressive hyperkeratosis with or without palmoplantar keratoderma also known as epidermolytic hyperkeratosis.

Epidermolytic ichthyosis is classified on clinical ground into two groups and six different subtypes (Table 1). The ichthyosis can be generalized with accentuation over flexures and overlying joints, typically described as corrugated cardboard-like (Fig. 2). NPS-1 subtype (hystrix) has characteristic porcupine-like spiny papules (Fig. 3). Mosaic epidermolytic ichthyosis has lesions limited to Blaschko's lines (Fig. 4). Patients usually have a characteristic pungent odor, caused by superinfection from mixed flora.

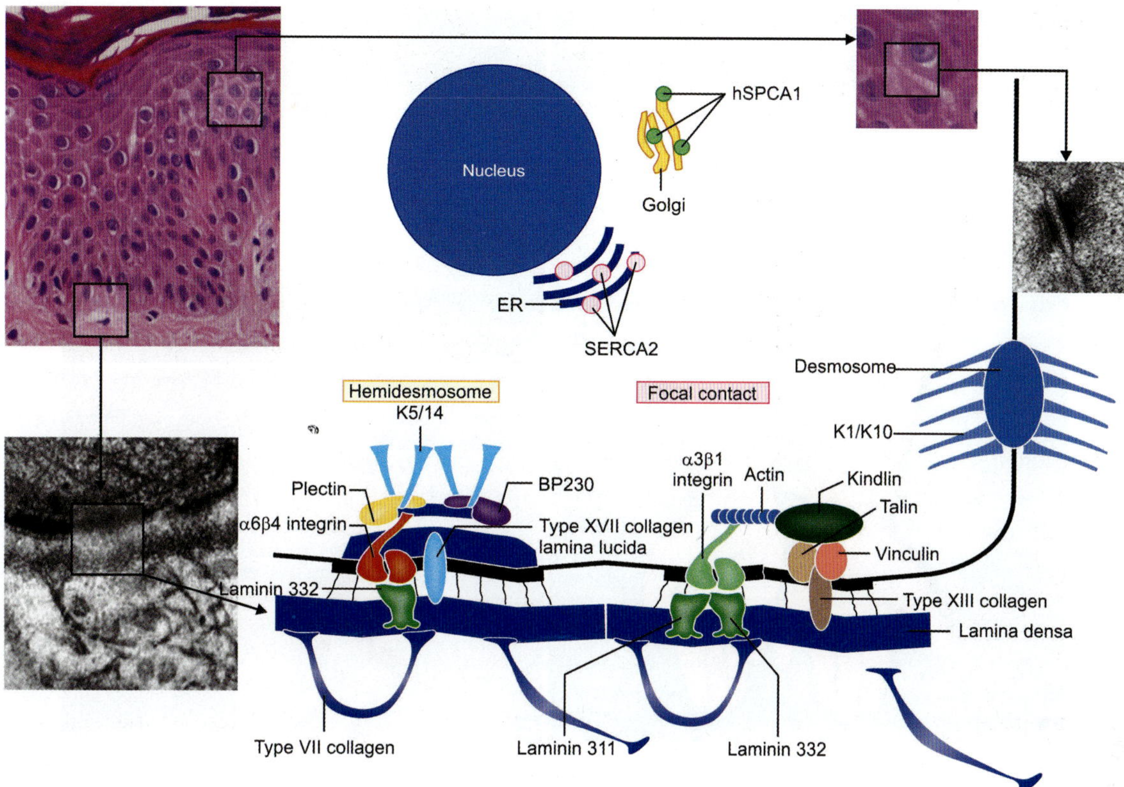


ER, endoplasmic reticulum; SERCA2, sarco/endoplasmic reticulum calcium adenosine triphosphatase 2.

**FIG. 1:** Schematic diagram of the components of the skin involved in the pathogenesis of genetic bullous diseases. Integrity of the skin is maintained by cohesion between neighboring keratinocytes via desmosomal cell-cell adhesion and between the overlying epidermis and the dermis underneath through the hemidesmosomal complex. The tonofibrils, composed of heterotypic keratin 1/10, attach themselves to desmosomes. Intracellular calcium homeostasis is important in cellular function and the defects in either calcium pumps, namely, sarcoplasmic/endoplasmic reticulum $Ca^{2+}$-ATPase 2 (SERCA2) in endoplasmic reticulum or human secretory pathway $Ca^{2+}$-ATPase 1 (hSPCA1) in the Golgi apparatus, can result in skin fragility. At the hemidesmosomal complex, intermediate filaments containing keratin 5/14 together with plectin are linked with BP230 protein. The α6β4 integrin and type XVII collagen help to anchor basal cells to the dermis via adhesion to type VII collagen in anchoring fibrils. Kindlin is a key regulatory component of cell–extracellular matrix junctions, such as focal adhesions. Alteration of these proteins can result in inherited bullous disorders. Not drawn to scale.

**TABLE 1: Subtypes of epidermolytic ichthyosis, classified by palm-sole involvement and the mutated genes**

| Phenotype | NPS-1 | NPS-2 | NPS-3 | PS-1 | PS-2 | PS-3 |
|---|---|---|---|---|---|---|
| PPK | Absent | | | Present | | |
| Palm/sole surface | Normal | | Hyperlinear | Smooth | | Cerebriform |
| Digital contracture | No | | | | Yes | No |
| Scales | Hystrix | Brown | Flat, white | Mild | White scales to peel | Tan |
| Distribution | Generalized | | | Localized | Generalized | |
| Erythroderma | – | | + | – | + | – |
| Blistering | + | | | Localized | + | Neonatal |
| Mutations | *KRT10* | | | *KRT1* | | |

NPS, Nonpalm-sole; PS, palm-sole.

## Differential Diagnosis (Box 1)

During the neonatal period, the phenotype is similar to other blistering conditions as shown in box 1.

## Diagnosis

Histopathology of epidermolytic ichthyosis is distinctive and called epidermolytic hyperkeratosis (Fig. 2C). Findings include marked hyperkeratosis, a thick granular layer, coarse keratohyaline granules, and vacuolar degeneration of the upper epidermis.

In general, patients with palmoplantar keratoderma have mutations in *KRT1* and patients without palm-sole hyperkeratosis have mutations in *KRT10*, except patients with exclusive palmoplantar involvement (the so-called Vörner type) who have mutations in *KRT9*.

## Management

Treatment is symptomatic and focuses on hydration, lubrication, keratolysis, and treatment of superficial skin infections. Epidermolytic ichthyosis tends to improve with increasing age.

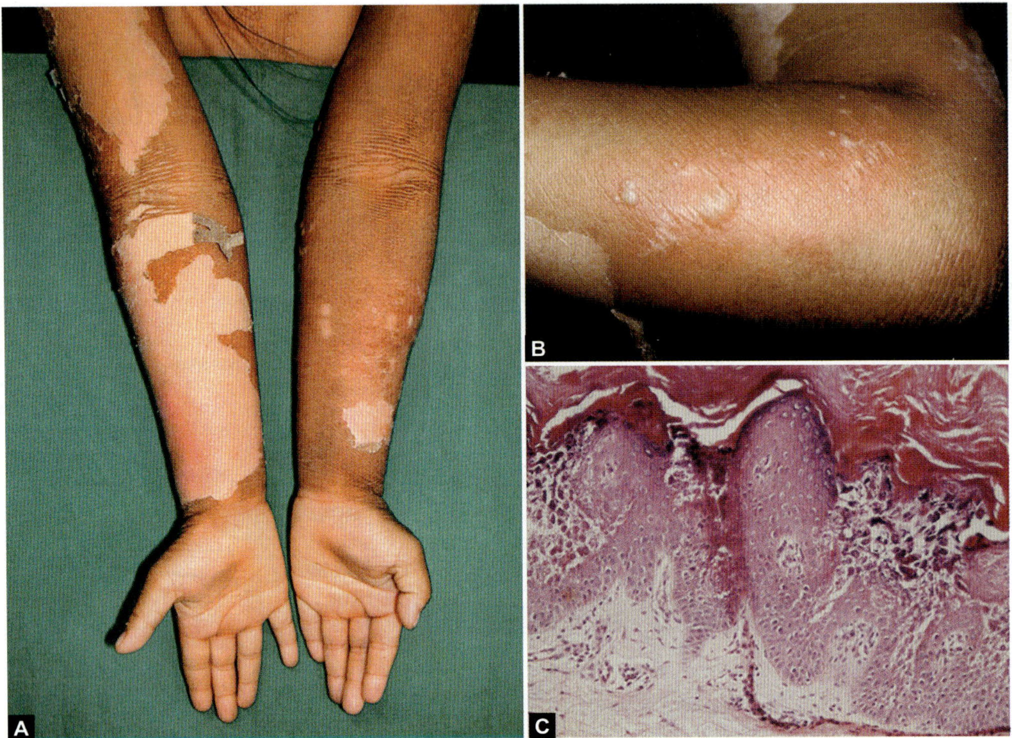


**FIG. 2:** Epidermolytic ichthyosis. **A,** Diffuse hyperkeratosis with flexural accentuation in the "corrugated cardboard" appearance of skin folds. The scales can be peeled off leaving normal skin underneath; **B,** Blister formation in the forearm; **C,** Epidermolytic hyperkeratosis histology showing markedly thickened stratum corneum and characteristic vacuolar degeneration and hypergranulosis of the stratum granulosum and stratum spinosum.

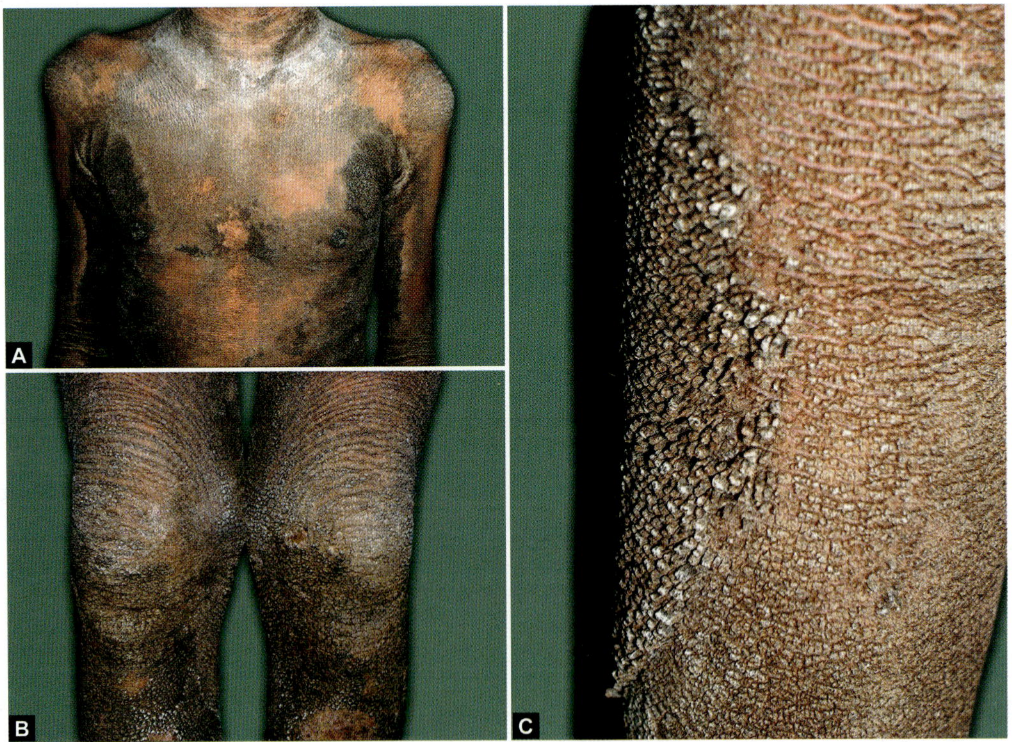


**FIG. 3:** Epidermolytic ichthyosis, hystrix type. Diffuse, porcupine-like spiny papules involving the entire body sparing the face. **A,** Trunk; **B,** Knees; **C,** Close-up picture showing massive hyperkeratosis with prominent spiky scales.

Patients with extensive skin involvement can have a dramatic respond to oral acitretin but dose increment should be gradual as it can paradoxically enhance blistering. Acitretin is teratogenic and should not be used with cyclines, methotrexate, or vitamin A and its derivatives. Re-esterification to longer half-life etretinate occurs thus alcohol consumption is discouraged. For females in childbearing age, two different methods of contraception should be used for 2 years after discontinuation of acitretin.

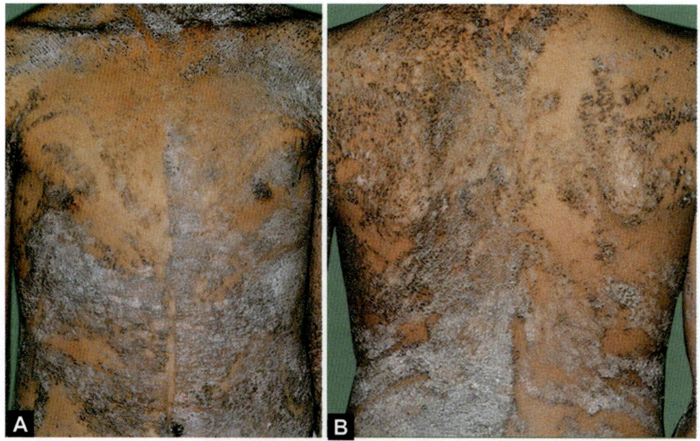

**FIG. 4:** Epidermolytich ichthyosis, mosaic type. Thick, hyperpigmented hyperkeratotic lesions arranged along Blaschko's line. **A,** Chest; **B,** Back.

| BOX 1 | Differential diagnosis of epidermolytic ichthyosis |
|---|---|
| *Early, generalized vesicles* | *Late, hyperkeratotic lesions* |
| • Epidermolysis bullosa<br>• Staphylococcal scalded skin syndrome<br>• Bullous pemphigoid | • Other ichthyoses<br>• Pityriasis rubra pilaris |

Progestin-only contraceptives and minipills are not acceptable because of failure possibility.

## DARIER–WHITE DISEASE

Darier–White disease is a rare, late-onset autosomal dominant condition with a variable prevalence depending on the country, from 1 case per 36,000 in England to 1 in 100,000 in Denmark. Spontaneous mutations are frequently seen.

The onset of disease is usually around puberty. Patients present with greasy, skin-colored to brown keratotic papules, which may be isolated or may form relatively large, crusted, and confluent plaques (Fig. 5). The sites of predilection are the seborrheic areas of the face and trunk, upper chest, and back. Other areas frequently involved include the forehead, ears, scalp, sides of the neck, groins, perianal area, and axillae. The skin lesions can become very thick in the body folds with secondary bacterial infection. The disease is chronic with exacerbations throughout life. Precipitating factors include heat, sweat, sunlight, friction, and infections. Eczema herpeticum can complicate pre-existing lesions. Localized lesions in Blaschkoid distribution are also found.

Nail changes are specific for this condition. These include alternating red and white longitudinal stripes and nail fragility, resulting in V-shaped nicking at the free margin (Fig. 6).

Other characteristic findings in Darier–White disease patients include pits/punctated keratoses on palms and soles (Fig. 5), and cobblestone white papules on the hard palate (Fig. 6). Sometimes discrete, flat skin-colored papules similar to acrokeratosis verruciformis of Hopf are seen on dorsal aspect of hands and feet (Fig. 6).

Neurological and psychiatric disorders have been reported in patients with Darier disease.

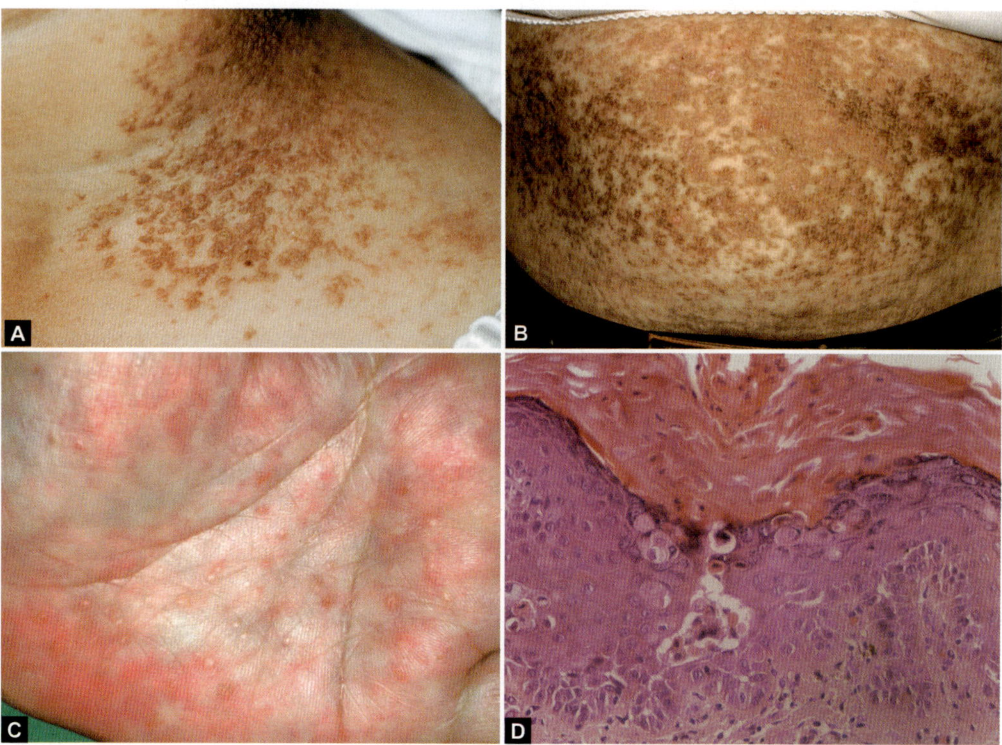

**FIG. 5:** Darier's disease. **A,** Greasy, skin-colored to brown keratotic papules on side of neck; **B,** Relatively large, crusted, and confluent plaques on the abdomen; **C,** Punctated keratosis on the palm; **D,** Histology shows hyperkeratosis and suprabasal clefts containing acantholytic cells and dyskeratotic cells in the stratum spinosum (corps ronds) and upper layers (grains).

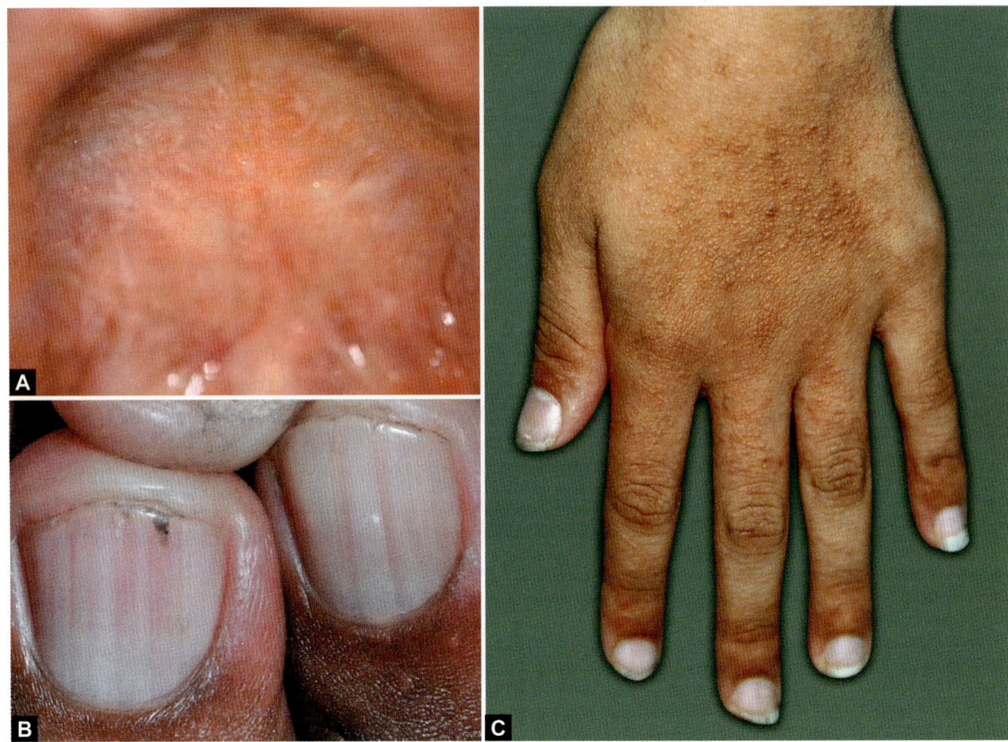

FIG. 6: Darier–White disease. **A,** Cobblestone papules on the hard palate; **B,** Alternate white and red bands and V-shaped nicking at the free margin of nails; **C,** Discrete, flat skin-colored papules on dorsal hand.

**BOX 2 Differential diagnosis of Darier–White disease**

*Limited seborrheic lesions*
- Seborrheic dermatitis

*Acral lesions*
- Verruca plana

*Nail changes*
- Lichen planus

*Erosive lesions*
- Benign chronic pemphigus
- Pemphigus vulgaris
- Candidal intertrigo

*Vegetative lesions*
- Pemphigus vegetans

## Differential Diagnosis

Lesions can be variable and resemble many different conditions (Box 2).

**BOX 3 Management for Darier–White disease**

*Avoiding precipitating factors*
- Sunscreens, heat and sweat avoidance, loose-fitting, cotton clothing

*Treat superimposed infections*
- Bacterial—topical/systemic
- Viral especially herpes—oral antivirals

*Topical treatment*
- Emollients
- Corticosteroids
- Retinoids—irritation is a common side effect

*Systemic treatment*
- Acitretin—can be very effective but relapse is common when the drug is discontinued

## Diagnosis

Histological examination shows hyperkeratosis, focal dyskeratosis associated with suprabasal acantholysis leading to suprabasal clefts (Fig. 5).

Heterozygous mutations in *ATP2A2*, coding for SERCA2 protein, are found in the patients.

## Management

There is no specific treatment for this condition (Box 3). Acitretin is effective but should be titrated from the smallest dosage (10 mg/day) as cutaneous side effects are common.

# BENIGN CHRONIC PEMPHIGUS (HAILEY–HAILEY DISEASE)

Hailey-Hailey disease is a rare, autosomal dominant condition with the prevalence of 1 in 50,000 population. The disease onset is later than Darier-White disease, usually in adulthood.

Phenotypically lesions are very similar to Darier-White disease, albeit limited only to the sites of friction and flexures (neck, axillae, submammary region, groin, and perineum) (Fig. 7). Lesions can be malodorous and painful.

## Differential Diagnosis

Hailey-Hailey lesions are found mainly in the intertriginous regions thus differential diagnosis includes diseases confined to the flexures (Box 4).

## Diagnosis

Histopathology shows similar features to Darier-White disease but acantholysis is widespread, giving the appearance of a "dilapidated brick wall" with mild dyskeratosis (Fig. 7).

Heterozygous mutations in *ATP2C1*, coding for human secretory pathway $Ca^{2+}/Mn^{2+}$ ATPase 1 (hSPCA1) protein, are found in the patients.

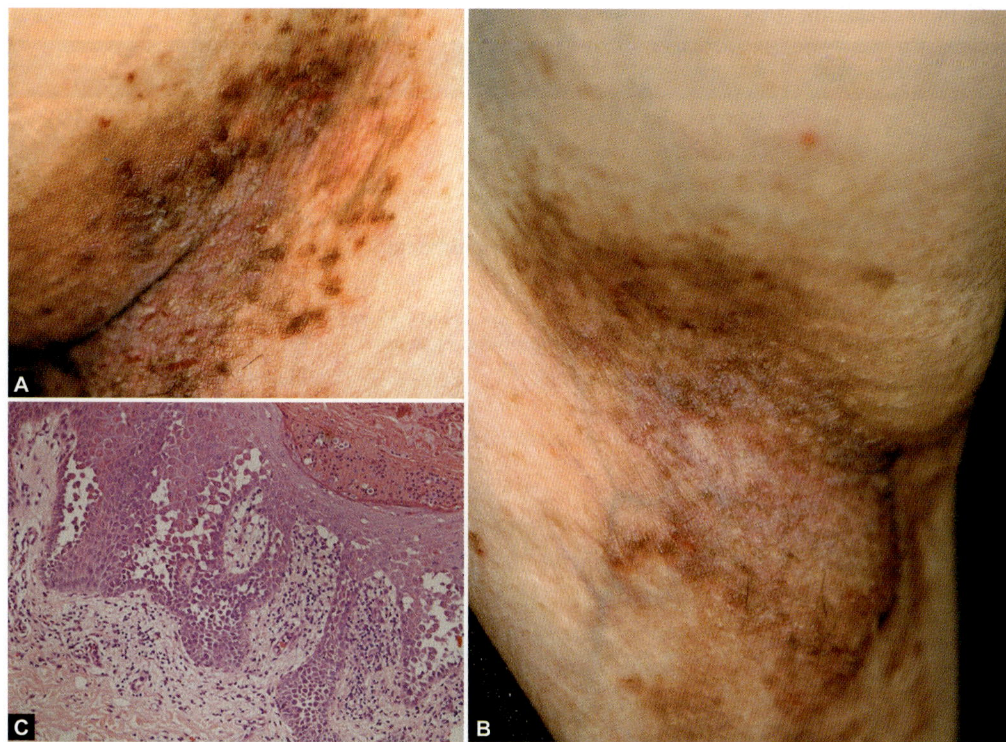


FIG. 7: Hailey–Hailey disease. Hypertrophic and macerated plaques with painful fissures at **A,** submammary; **B,** axilla; **C,** histology shows hyperkeratosis and widespread acantholysis of keratinocytes with the appearance of a "dilapidated brick wall". Dyskeratosis is mild.

**BOX 4 Differential diagnosis of Hailey–Hailey disease**

- Darier-White disease
- Candidosis
- Intertrigo
- Pemphigus

**BOX 5 Treatment of Hailey–Hailey disease**

*Avoiding precipitating factors*
- Heat and friction avoidance

*Treat superimposed infections*
- Bacterial—topical/systemic

*Topical treatment*
- Emollients
- Corticosteroids
- Calcipotriol
- Tacrolimus
- Gentamicin

*Surgery*
- $CO_2$ laser ablation—can result in long-lasting remission (Fig. 8)

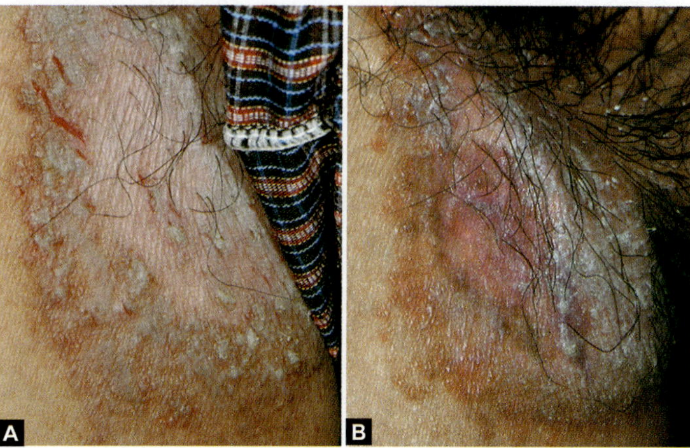


FIG. 8: Treatment of Hailey–Hailey disease with $CO_2$ laser vaporization. **A,** Preoperative photograph of the right crural area; **B,** $CO_2$ laser ablation of the outer half results in clearing of the lesion.

## Management

There is no specific treatment for this condition (Box 5).

# EPIDERMOLYSIS BULLOSA

Epidermolysis bullosa (EB) is a group of inherited diseases characterized by trauma-induced blister formation of the skin and/or mucosae. Moreover, wound healing is usually defective, leading to excessive granulation tissue formation, chronic ulcers, and carcinoma. The phenotypes of EB differ according to the underlying heritable molecular defects. EB can be transmitted by autosomal dominant or recessive pattern of inheritance. In the United States, the incidence of EB between 1986 and 1990 was 19.6 per 1 million live births.

Epidermolysis bullosa is subdivided according to the level of separation into four groups from the most superficial (intraepidermal) to the deepest (sublamina densa) and the mixed type (Table 2).

1. *Epidermolysis bullosa simplex (EBS)*: Blisters in EB simplex are the most superficial amongst all EB types, being intraepidermal. This group of EB is the most common, with incidence 10.8 per 1 million live births.
   Epidermolysis bullosa simplex is further classified into two subtypes: (1) suprabasal EBS and (2) basal EBS.
   The level of separation in the superbasal group is very superficial, resulting in milder phenotypes in general apart from the fatal autosomal recessive acantholytic EBS. Clinical appearances vary from mere superficial peeling in acral peeling skin syndrome to skin fragility syndromes.

**TABLE 2: Epidermolysis bullosa classification**

| Level of skin cleavage | Major EB type | Major EB subtypes | Phenotype | Targeted proteins (genes) |
|---|---|---|---|---|
| Intraepidermal | EBS | Suprabasal EBS | Acral peeling skin syndrome | Transglutaminase 5 (*TGM5*) |
| | | | Skin fragility syndromes | |
| | | | • Desmoplakin deficiency<br>○ EBS-desmoplakin<br>○ Skin fragility-woolly hair syndrome | Desmoplakin (*DSP*) |
| | | | • Plakoglobin deficiency<br>○ EBS-plakoglobin<br>○ Skin fragility-plakoglobin deficiency | Plakoglobin (*JUP*) |
| | | | • Plakophilin deficiency<br>○ EBS-plakophilin<br>○ Skin fragility-ectodermal dysplasia syndrome | Plakophilin 1 (*PKP1*) |
| | | | Acantholytic EBS | Desmoplakin/plakoglobin (*DSP/JUP*) |
| | | | EBS, superficialis | Unknown |
| | | Basal EBS | EBS, localized | K5/K14 (*KRT5/KRT14*) |
| | | | EBS, generalized, severe | |
| | | | EBS, generalized intermediate | |
| | | | EBS, with mottled pigmentation | K5 (*KRT5*) |
| | | | EBS, migratory circinate | |
| | | | EBS, autosomal recessive K14 | K14 (*KRT14*) |
| | | | EBS with muscular dystrophy | Plectin (*PLEC*) |
| | | | EBS with pyloric atresia | Plectin/α6β4 integrin (*PLEC/ITGA6/ITGB4*) |
| | | | EBS Ogna | Plectin (*PLEC*) |
| | | | EBS, autosomal recessive—BP230 deficiency | BPAG1 (*DST*) |
| | | | EBS, autosomal recessive—exophilin 5 deficiency | Exophilin 5 (*EXPH5*) |
| Intralamina lucida | JEB | JEB, generalized | JEB, generalized severe | Laminin-332 (*LAMA3/LAMB3/LAMC2*) |
| | | | JEB, generalized intermediate | Laminin-332/type XVII collagen (*LAMA3/LAMB3/LAMC2/COL17A1*) |
| | | | JEB with pyloric atresia | α6β4 integrin (*ITGA6/ITGB4*) |
| | | | JEB, late onset | Type XVII collagen (*COL17A1*) |
| | | | JEB with respiratory and renal involvement | α3 integrin (*ITGA3*) |
| | | JEB, localized | JEB, localized | Type XVII collagen/α6β4 integrin/laminin-332 (*COL17A1/ITGB4/LAMA3/LAMB3/LAMC2*) |
| | | | JEB, inversa | Laminin-332 (*LAMA3/LAMB3/LAMC2*) |
| | | | JEB, Laryngo-onychocutaneous syndrome | Laminin-332 (*LAMA3*) |
| Sublamina densa | DEB | DDEB | DDEB, generalized | Type VII collagen (*COL7A1*) |
| | | | DDEB, acral | |
| | | | DDEB, pretibial | |
| | | | DDEB, pruriginosa | |
| | | | DDEB, nail only | |
| | | | DDEB, bullous dermolysis of the newborn | |
| | | RDEB | RDEB, generalized severe | |
| | | | RDEB, generalized intermediate | |
| | | | RDEB, inversa | |
| | | | RDEB, localized | |
| | | | RDEB, pretibial | |
| | | | RDEB, pruriginosa | |
| | | | RDEB, centripetalis | |
| | | | RDEB, bullous dermolysis of the newborn | |
| Mixed | Kindler syndrome | – | Kindler syndrome | Kindlin-1 (*FERMT1*) |

EBS, epidermolysis bullosa simplex; JEB, junctional epidermolysis bullosa; DEB, dystrophic epidermolysis bullosa; DDEB, dominant dystrophic epidermolysis bullosa; RDEB, recessive dystrophic epidermolysis bullosa.

Epidermolysis bullosa simplex, localized (Weber–Cockayne) is the most common form, often presents during infancy and childhood but occasionally in early adulthood on the feet during sports/military activities. Blisters are limited only to the traumatic areas, particularly the hands and feet and healed with postinflammatory hyperpigmentation (Fig. 9).

Epidermolysis bullosa simplex, generalized intermediate (Koebner) is more extensive than EBS, localized, with lesions at the hands, feet, and extremities and the onset is usually from birth. Thickened soles are seen during late childhood.

Epidermolysis bullosa simplex, generalized severe (Dowling-Meara/herpetiformis) is the severest amongst the basal EBS, with generalized extensive blisters present at birth. Mucosal involvement is common. Later, during childhood, spontaneous herpetiform lesions appear on trunk and proximal proximities. Nail dystrophy and diffuse palmoplantar keratoderma are also seen.

Other rare forms of EBS with distinctive phenotypes include EBS Ogna, described solely in Norway with acral blisters and onychogryphosis of great toenails; acral peeling skin syndrome with painless peeling of skin on hands and feet (Fig. 9); EBS with muscular dystrophy and EBS with pyloric atresia.

For EBS—autosomal recessive with BP320/exophilin 5 deficiency, the blisters are limited and mild (Fig. 9).

2. *Junctional EB (JEB)*: These autosomal recessive EB are divided into the generalized and localized junctional groups. As separation occurs intralamina lucida, blisters heal with scars. The incidence of JEB is 2.0 per 1 million live births.

   Junctional EB, generalized severe (Herlitz) is the severest type with high mortality within the first year of life. Extensive periorificial granulation tissue typically occurs on the face later during infancy (Fig. 10). Nails and teeth are involved, as well as all mucosae leading to failure to thrive.

   Junctional EB, generalized intermediate (non-Herlitz) can have similar but milder phenotype to JEB, generalized severe. Oral erosions are limited and extracutaneous involvement is rare.

   Junctional EB with pyloric atresia is similar to EBS with pyloric atresia but with nail and tooth involvement and blisters healed with scars (Fig. 11).

   Junctional EB with respiratory and renal involvement patients have mild blisters with very severe interstitial lung disease with nephrotic syndrome.

   Junctional EB, localized and inversa are very rare with limited blistering. JEB, laryngo-onychocutaneous syndrome is seen in Pakistani patients with hoarseness of voice, nail dystrophy and crusted, granulation tissue on the face without any blisters.

3. *Dystrophic EB (DEB)*: It is characterized by scars and milia formation as the plane of separation is the deepest. It is subclassified into dominant DEB (DDEB) and recessive DEB (RDEB). The incidence of DDEB and RDEB are 2.9 and 2.0 per 1 million live births, respectively.

   Dominant DEB, generalized (Cockayne–Touraine) patients have blisters, hypertrophic scars and milia limited to traumatic areas, such as elbows and knees, sacrum and acral areas (Fig. 12). Nail dystrophy is commonly seen but oral mucosae are usually spared.

   Dominant DEB can be limited to the pretibial area. These lesions can be extremely pruritic leading to trauma-induced pruritic nodules and linear lesions (Fig. 13).

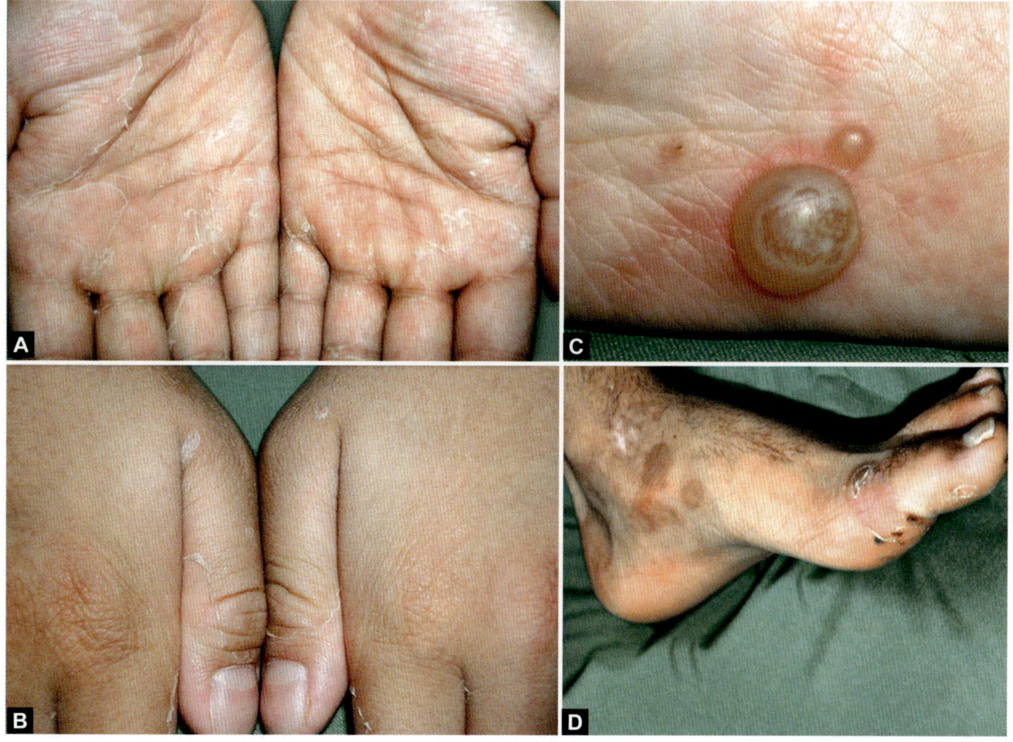

**FIG. 9:** Epidermolysis bullosa simplex (EBS). **A** and **B,** Acral peeling skin syndrome with lesions on palmar and dorsal sides of both hands. Lesions can be easily peeled off without discomfort; **C,** EBS, localized form. Blisters on the sole after mechanical injury; **D,** Autosomal recessive EBS with exophilin 5 deficiency*. Mild blister formation on the left foot.

**Courtesy*: John McGrath, Professor of Molecular Dermatology, St John's Institute of Dermatology, UK.

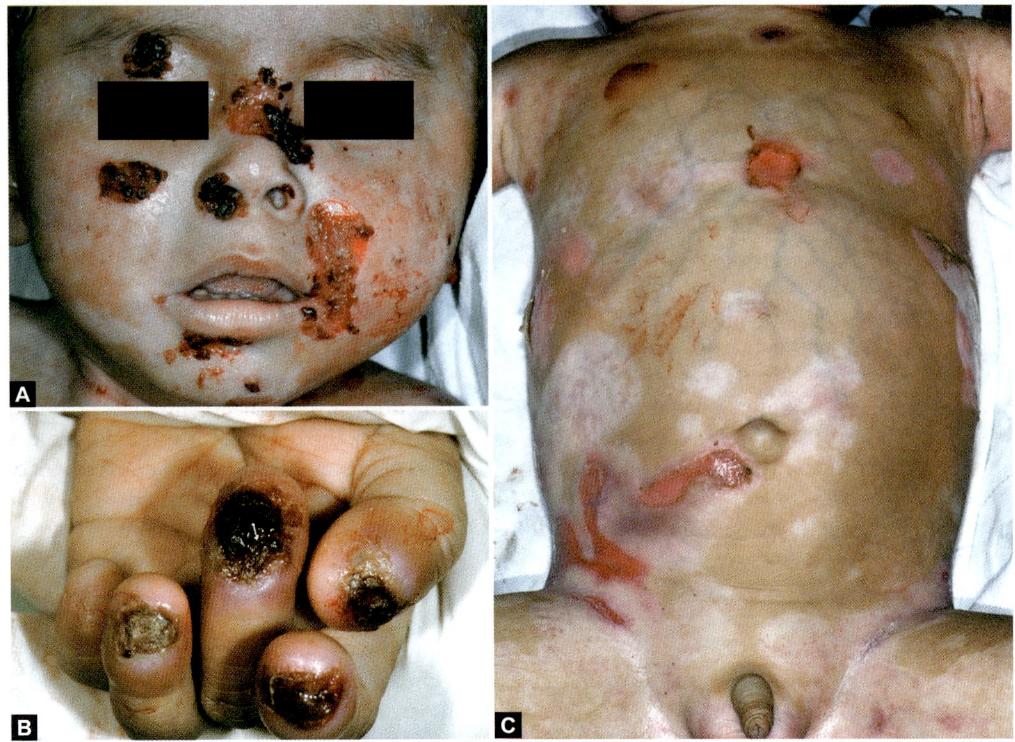

**FIG. 10:** Junctional epidermolysis bullosa, generalized severe type. Generalized blister formation-granulation tissue formation on **A,** Face; **B,** Fingernails; **C,** Blisters and ulcers on the trunk are seen.

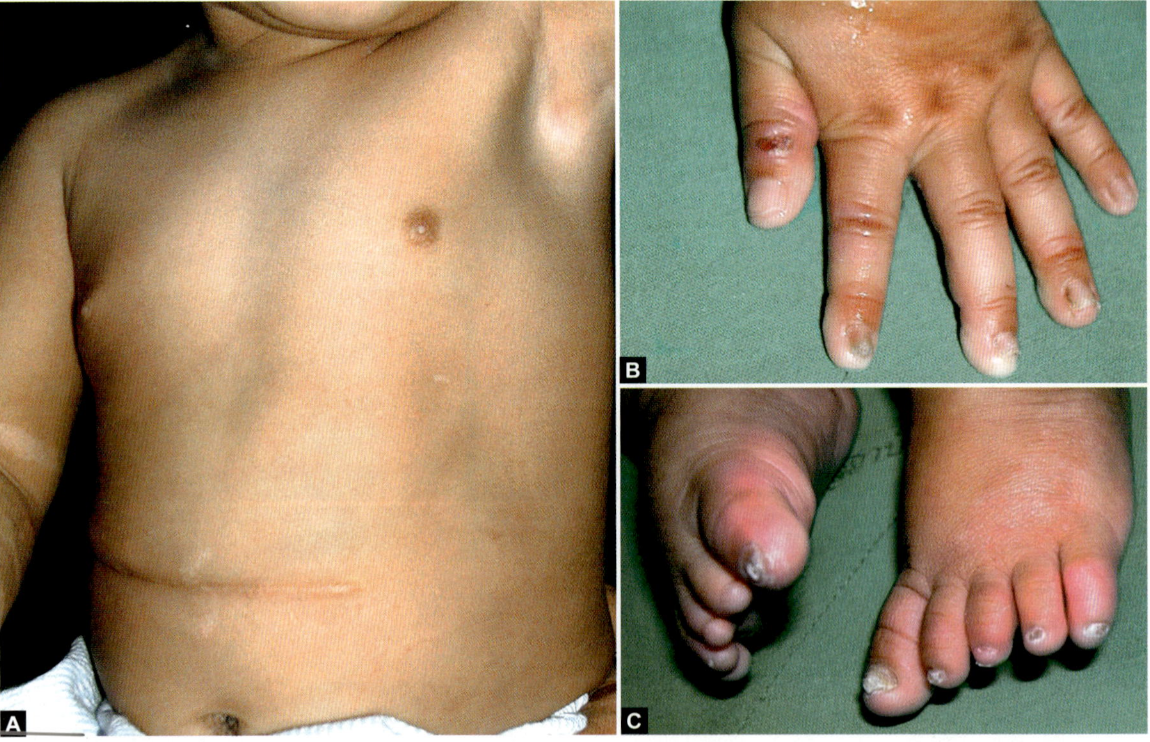

**FIG. 11:** Junctional epidermolysis bullosa with pyloric atresia. **A,** Surgical scar to relieve pyloric atresia; **B,** Blisters and nail dystrophy on the hand; **C,** Nail dystrophy both feet.

Dominant DEB, bullous dermolysis of the newborn is a limited form of DDEB with complete remission within the age of one. Antigen mapping with antibodies to type XVII collagen shows granular basilar keratinocyte perinuclear intracytoplasmic and dermal-epidermal staining.

Recessive DEB, generalized severe patients present with extensive blister formation from birth (Figs 14 and 15).

Scarring of the hands and feet lead to fusion of the digits called "mitten" deformity (Fig. 15). Periorificial granulation tissue typical of JEB, generalized severe is not seen. Congenital

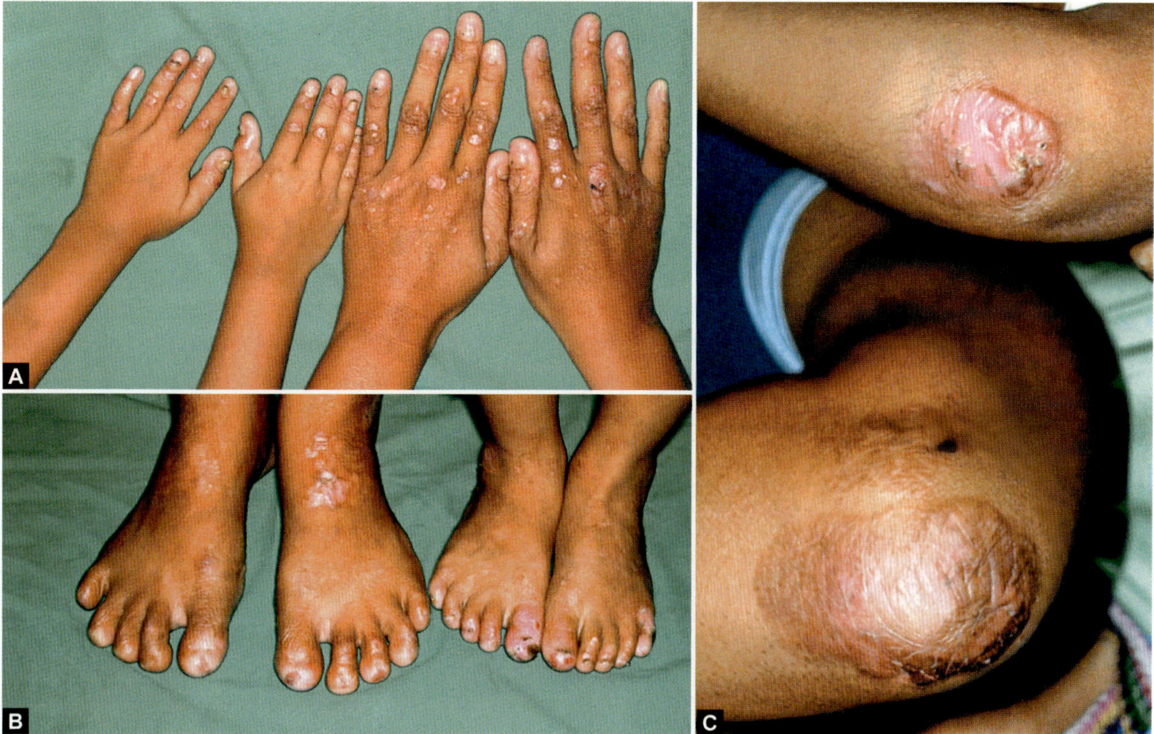


FIG. 12: Dominant dystrophic epidermolysis bullosa, generalized type. Hypertrophic scars, milia and nail dystrophy on **A,** Dorsal hands; **B,** Dorsal feet,;and **C,** Elbows in the mother and her daughter.

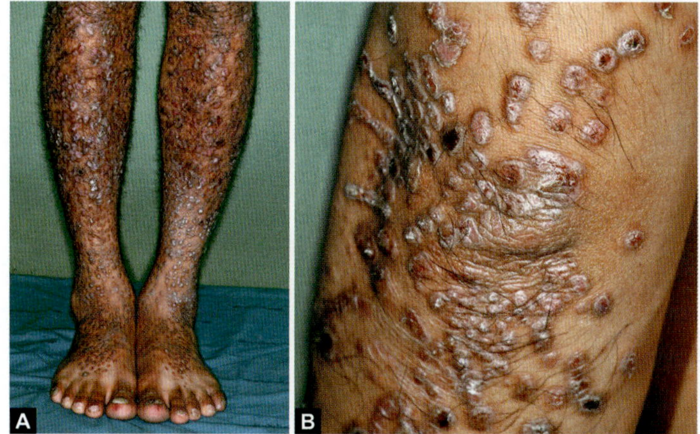


FIG. 13: Dominant dystrophic epidermolysis bullosa, pruriginosa type. Numerous hyperkeratotic, excoriated papules on **A,** Shins; **B,** Elbow. Many lesions are confluent into bizarre linear formation.

absence of the skin (aplasia cutis congenita/Bart's syndrome) is commonly found. Mucosal involvement is extensive, leading to oral ulcers, esophageal and laryngeal stricture, poor intake and anemia. Patients typically have failure to thrive. Squamous cell carcinoma (SCC) developed in chronic, unhealed ulcers is usually fatal.

Depending on the types of mutations, RDEB can have milder phenotypes not distinguishable from DDEB on clinical ground alone (Fig. 16).

4. *Kindler syndrome*: Kindler syndrome is a rare autosomal recessive condition. The prevalence is not known. Patients present with blistering and photosensitivity during infancy/childhood. Recurrent blister formation occurs primarily on trauma-prone areas of hands and feet, which may prompt an incorrect diagnosis of EB. Poikiloderma in sunexposed skin appears gradually and become more prominent as the patient ages, mimicking premature aging (Fig. 17). Periodontitis is commonly seen. Other less common features include palmar pits, punctate palmoplantar keratoderma, finger and toe webs, and nail dystrophy.

## Differential Diagnosis

The only unifying characteristic of EB is blister formation, thus the main differential diagnosis is acquired vesiculobullous diseases (Box 6).

## Laboratory Diagnosis

Investigations are very important in the management strategy (Flowchart 1) but in resource-poor setup it is always better to have a strong clinical suspicion as one has to rely on purely clinical manifestation. Routine light microscopy, direct immunofluorescence (DIF) and indirect immunofluorescence can be helpful in excluding other conditions such as autoimmune bullous dermatosis. Antigenic mapping using monoclonal antibodies against various basement membrane zone antigens is very helpful in establishing the correct diagnosis in autosomal recessive cases with null mutations on both alleles as the staining will be greatly diminished or negative (Fig. 18). Transmission electron microscopy can show typical structural alteration specific to each type of EB (Fig. 18).

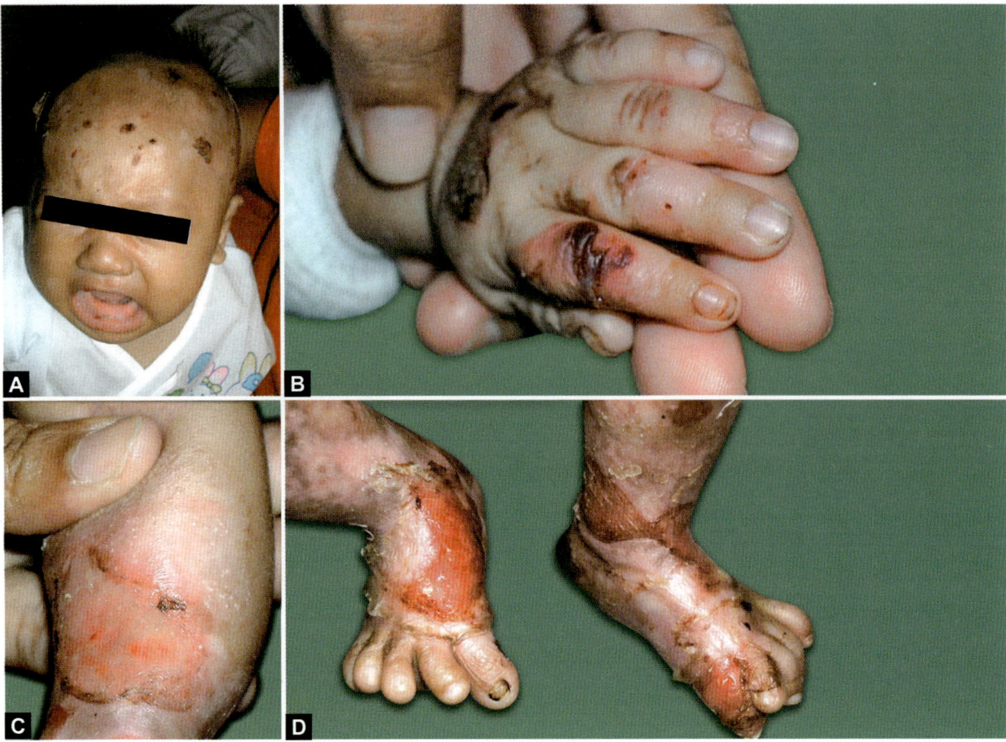


**FIG. 14:** Recessive dystrophic epidermolysis bullosa, generalized severe type. Generalized blisters can be seen on the **A,** Face; **B,** Hand; **C,** Healed with milia on the shin. Congenital absence of skin is seen around the **D,** ankles. Excessive granulation tissue formation is not found.

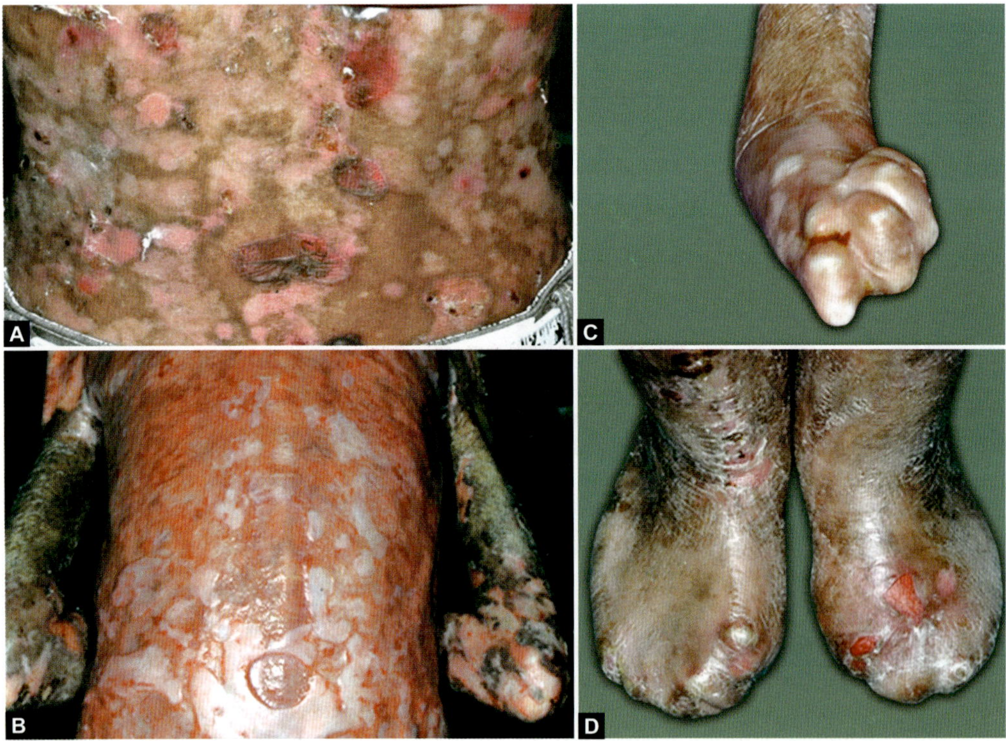


**FIG. 15:** Recessive dystrophic epidermolysis bullosa, generalized severe type. Extensive blisters and denuded skin on **A,** Abdomen; **B,** back with scarring; **C** and **D,** contraction of digits and toes leading to "mitten" deformity of the hands and feet.

## Molecular Diagnosis

Deoxyribonucleic acid (DNA) mutation detection can identify the specific genetic mutation in probands and relatives (Fig. 19). The choice of genes to investigate is guided by clinical information and laboratory findings (Table 2).

Knowledge in prevalence of different mutation types, genes and population hotspot mutations is important in mutation detection, e.g., in generalized severe JEB mutations in *LAMB3* are much more common than either *LAMA3* or *LAMC2*, hence it is more economical to start mutation screening with *LAMB3* sequencing (Table 3).

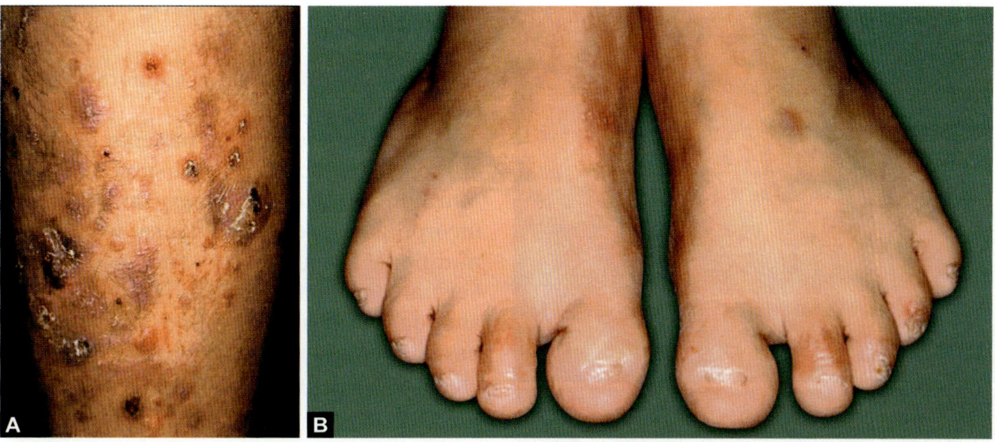

**FIG. 16:** Recessive dystrophic epidermolysis bullosa, generalized intermediate type. **A,** Blisters, crusting and scars are seen mainly on the shin of this 8-year-old boy; **B,** Nail dystrophy is also seen.

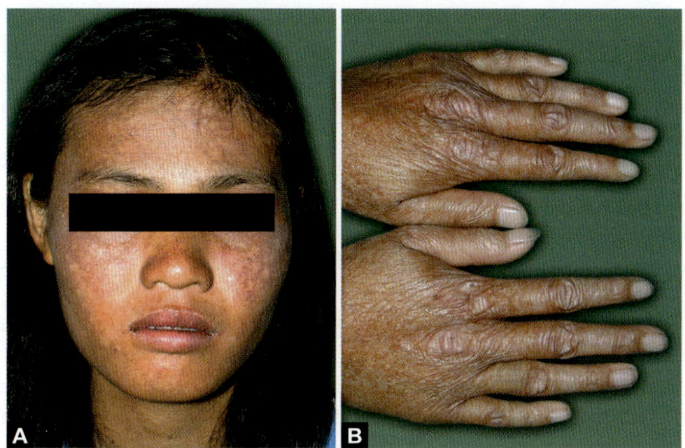

**FIG. 17:** Kindler syndrome. **A,** Poikiloderma is seen on the face of this 15-year-old girl; **B,** Skin on back of hands of this same girl is photodamaged and atrophic, with the appearance of premature photoaging.

**BOX 6 Differential diagnosis of epidermolysis bullosa (EB)**

*Differential diagnosis of EB*
- Bullous pemphigoid
- Epidermolysis bullosa acquisita
- Friction blisters
- Dyshidrotic eczema
- Dermatitis herpetiformis
- Bullous lupus erythematosus
- Thermal burns

*Differential diagnosis of dominant DEB (DDEB), pretibial/pruriginosa*
- Prurigo nodularis

*Differential diagnosis of Kindler syndrome*
- Infancy—EB
- Later—defective DNA repair syndromes, e.g., Bloom syndrome, Cockayne syndrome, xeroderma pigmentosum, and Rothmund-Thomson syndrome

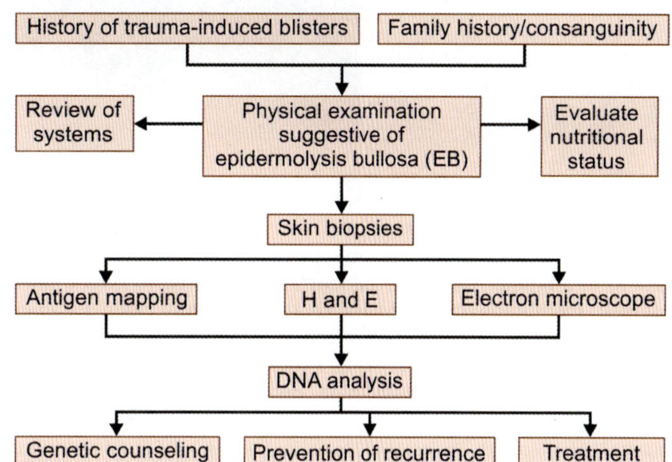


**FLOWCHART 1:** Approach to epidermolysis bullosa (EB) patients. When seeing a patient with EB, detailed history of blisters and family history are important. Physical examination can lead to the correct diagnosis if characteristic features are present. In severe patients, nutritional status should be evaluated as failure to thrive is commonly seen in this group. Antigenic mapping with specific monoclonal antibodies against basement membrane zone antigens is very helpful in establishing a correct diagnosis. Routine histology and electron microscope can also be helpful in certain cases. Molecular diagnosis is important for determining prognosis, genetic counseling, prevention of recurrence and treatment.

Splicing mutations in *PKP1* is found in 50% of cases, thus changes which potentially lead to cryptic splicing should be analyzed carefully (Table 3).

Certain mutations are frequently seen in a specific population and mutation screening for hotspots can be cost effective, e.g., *LAMB3* R365X in European population.

However, sequencing can be very expensive, especially when clinical and investigative data are not informative or the panel of gene screening is big. Indeed, standard capillary sequencing techniques fail to find mutations in 15% of EB cases.

Next generation sequencing, which can screen the whole exome or genome, has been shown to help in such instances and the technology is getting more affordable.

*In vitro* fertilization coupled with preimplantation genetic diagnosis/haplotyping is now used successfully in many countries to prevent recurrence in successive pregnancies.

Current classification of EB, the so-called "onion ring" approach, takes into account sequentially the major EB subtype, mode of inheritance, phenotype, antigen mapping findings, and mutation(s) in the proband as can be elucidated. For example, RDEB, generalized severe, type VII collagen absent, *COL7A1* +/+ c.5797C >G, p.R1933X.

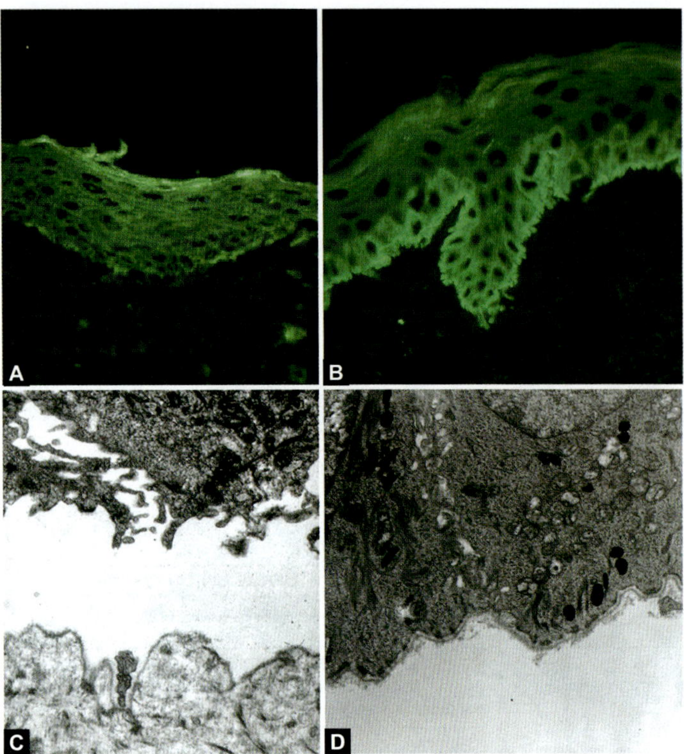


**FIG. 18:** Laboratory investigations in epidermolysis bullosa. **A,** Immunofluorescence antigenic mapping shows markedly reduced staining in a Kindler syndrome patient*; **B,** compared to bright, linear basement membrane zone and basal keratinocyte anti-kindlin-1 staining in normal control*. Transmission electron microscopy of the dermal-epidermal junction shows; **C,** lamina lucida separation in junctional epidermolysis bullosa; **D,** sublamina densa separation in recessive dystrophic epidermolysis bullosa.

**Courtesy*: John McGrath, Professor of Molecular Dermatology, St John's Institute of Dermatology, UK.

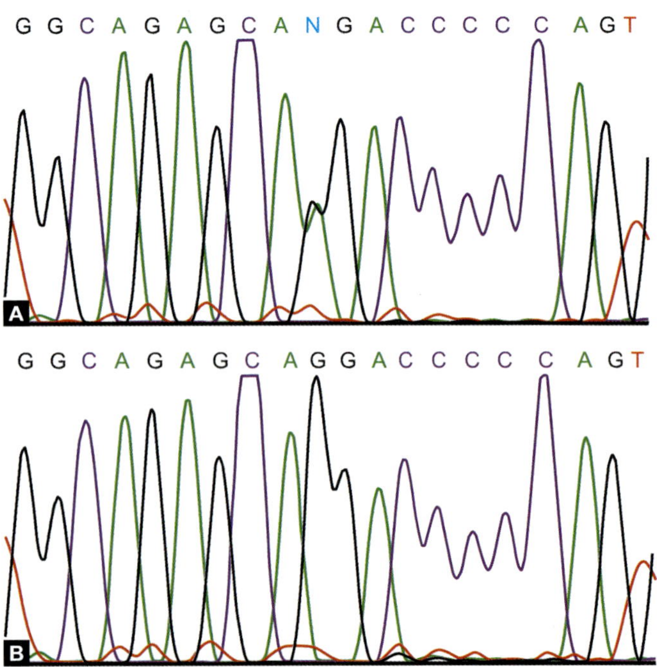


**FIG. 19:** Mutation detection using capillary sequencing. **A,** An electropherogram shows a heterozygous missense mutation in *COL7A1* gene, which changes amino acid glycine to arginine; **B,** normal control sequence.

## Treatment

Treatment of EB is mainly supportive, as underlying mutations cannot be corrected.

Caring for severe EB patients requires a multidisciplinary approach, including general surgery, chest medicine, dentistry, nutrition and dermatology, amongst other. Optimal care incorporates trauma avoidance, wound care, infection control, nutritional requirement and gastrointestinal management. Several specific treatment options like drugs (doxycycline, aminoglycosides), cell-based therapy, gene therapy, protein-based therapy, etc. have emerged which are showing some effectivity in the treatment of this group of disorders (Table 4).

### Supportive Care

Wound care is one of the most important aspects of EB management. Blisters occur in all types of EB following minor trauma. They can expand quite readily, thus lancing is recommended. A sterile hypodermic needle should pass through the blister roof at the lowest point parallel to the skin to create and entry and exit holes so that exudates can be removed. Blister roof should not be removed.

For denuded areas, antiseptic wound soak followed by topical antimicrobial application and semiocclusive nonadhesive dressing can reduce the risk of local infection.

Different types of EB need different approach (Table 5 and Flowchart 1).

Severe EB patients may have low resistance to bacterial infection due to malnutrition.

*Staphylococcus aureus* and *Streptococcus pyogenes* are the most common pathogens but *Pseudomonas aeruginosa* infection can occur. In generalized severe JEB, sepsis can be a frequent cause of death.

Squamous cell carcinoma can develop in nonhealing areas. Surveillance of such areas is very important in RDEB patients as metastasis is commonly seen.

Heat avoidance can reduce new blister formation in EBS.

Esophageal constriction, oral ulcers, tooth decay, and chronic gastrointestinal bleeding lead to impaired nutritional status. Maintaining food intake is thus very important. Gastrostomy tube insertion can improve nutrition in EB patients with poor oral intake.

Aminoglycoside was capable to induce *premature termination codon* (PTC)-read through and restore functional protein in EB caused by nonsense mutations. As gentamicin has severe side effects such as nephrotoxicity and ototoxicity, its use in patients should be based on mutation analysis information, as this PTC-read through relies heavily on the nature of the surrounding nucleotides and the stop codons themselves, the best being UGA (Table 2).

Corrective gene therapy technologies, such as short inhibitory ribonucleic acids (siRNAs) and spliceosome-mediated RNA trans-splicing (SMarT), are the most promising approaches that enable inhibition of expression of the mutant alleles without affecting wild-type gene expression. This SMarT technique has been used *in vitro* to rectify the plectin gene, collagen XVIII and keratin 14 gene in EB patients and hence is considered as a promising therapy of several autosomal dominant blistering genodermatoses because it clears the mutation while increases normal allele expression.

**TABLE 3: Prevalence of published gene lesions in genes related to genetic bullous diseases. From the human gene mutation database (http://hgmd.cf.ac.uk). In bracket = percentage**

| Gene | Missense/ nonsense | Splicing | Regulatory | Small deletions | Small insertions | Small indels | Gross deletions | Gross insertions/ duplication | Complex rearrange- ments | Repeat variations |
|---|---|---|---|---|---|---|---|---|---|---|
| *KRT1* | 33 (73.33) | 4 (8.89) | 0 | 4 (8.89) | 1 (2.22) | 1 (2.22) | 1 (2.22) | 0 | 1 (2.22) | 0 |
| *KRT10* | 25 (65.79) | 5 (13.16) | 0 | 3 (7.89) | 2 (5.26) | 3 (7.89) | 0 | 0 | 0 | 0 |
| *ATP2A2* | 99 (58.93) | 14 (8.33) | 2 (1.19) | 35 (20.83) | 14 (8.33) | 0 | 1 (0.59) | 2 (1.19) | 1 (0.59) | 0 |
| *ATP2C1* | 55 (43.65) | 21 (16.67) | 0 | 33 (26.19) | 9 (7.14) | 1 (0.79) | 4 (3.17) | 0 | 3 (2.38) | 0 |
| *TGM5* | 3 (100) | 0 | 0 | 0 | 0 | 0 | 0 | 0 | 0 | 0 |
| *DSP* | 49 (70) | 5 (7.14) | 0 | 10 (14.28) | 3 (4.28) | 2 (2.85) | 0 | 1 (1.43) | 0 | 0 |
| *JUP* | 8 (72.73) | 1 (9.09) | 0 | 1 (9.09) | 1 (9.09) | 0 | 0 | 0 | 0 | 0 |
| *PKP1* | 3 (25) | 6 (50) | 0 | 1(8.33) | 0 | 1 (8.33) | 0 | 1 (8.33) | 0 | 0 |
| *KRT5* | 91 (85.85) | 5 (4.72) | 0 | 7 (6.60) | 1 (0.94) | 2 (1.89) | 0 | 0 | 0 | 0 |
| *KRT14* | 70 (78.65) | 3 (3.37) | 0 | 11 (12.36) | 1 (1.12) | 1 (1.12) | 0 | 2 (2.25) | 1 (1.12) | 0 |
| *PLEC* | 26 (48.15) | 2 (3.70) | 0 | 12 (22.22) | 8 (14.81) | 0 | 3 (5.56) | 3 (5.56) | 0 | 0 |
| *ITGA6* | 2 (40) | 1 (20) | 0 | 2 (40) | 0 | 0 | 0 | 0 | 0 | 0 |
| *ITGB4* | 30 (43.48) | 9 (13.04) | 0 | 23 (33.33) | 4 (5.79) | 1 (1.45) | 2 (2.89) | 0 | 0 | 0 |
| *DST* | 1 (50) | 0 | 0 | 0 | 0 | 0 | 0 | 0 | 1 (50) | 0 |
| *EXPH5* | 1 (33.33) | 0 | 0 | 0 | 0 | 2 (66.67) | 0 | 0 | 0 | 0 |
| *LAMA3* | 17 (47.22) | 6 (16.67) | 0 | 10 (27.78) | 3 (8.33) | 0 | 0 | 0 | 0 | 0 |
| *LAMB3* | 36 (42.86) | 14 (16.67) | 0 | 22 (26.19) | 8 (9.52) | 1 (1.19) | 1 (1.19) | 2 (2.38) | 0 | 0 |
| *LAMC2* | 13 (37.14) | 5 (14.28) | 0 | 12 (34.28) | 1 (2.86) | 3 (8.57) | 0 | 1 (2.86) | 0 | 0 |
| *COL17A1* | 28 (34.56) | 14 (17.28) | 0 | 23 (28.39) | 14 (17.28) | 0 | 1 (1.23) | 1 (1.23) | 0 | 0 |
| *ITGA3* | 1 (33.33) | 1 (33.33) | 0 | 0 | 0 | 1 (33.33) | 0 | 0 | 0 | 0 |
| *COL7A1* | 325 (54.35) | 102 (17.05) | 1 (0.17) | 101 (16.89) | 47 (7.86) | 11 (1.84) | 9 (1.51) | 1 (0.17) | 1 (0.17) | 0 |

**TABLE 4: Mode of action for different therapeutic options**

| Therapy | Mode of action |
|---|---|
| Doxycycline | Small molecule-based approach: downregulates matrix metalloproteinase, reduces inflammation and bulla formation in epidermolysis bullosa simplex (EBS) |
| Aminoglyco-sides | Induce premature termination codon (PTC)-read through and restore functional protein in EB |
| Isothiocyanate sulforaphane | Induce keratin 16 and 17 that are complementary to K14 |
| Gene therapy | Short inhibitory RNAs (siRNAs), spliceosome-mediated RNA trans-splicing (SMarT) inhibition of expression of the mutant alleles without affecting wild-type gene expression |
| Protein replacement therapy | Protein replacement by normal functional protein like collagen VII in recessive dystrophic epidermolysis bullosa (RDEB) |
| Cell-based therapy | Allogeneic bone marrow transplantation, induced pluripotent stem cells (iPSCs) and revertant mosaicism therapies |
| Nanotechnol-ogy | To deliver therapeutic molecules like siRNA genes, etc. |

Emerging therapies, such as protein therapy and stem cell therapy, have all shown promise for severe RDEB patients.

**TABLE 5: Approach to wound care for epidermolysis bullosa (EB)**

| EB types | Special wound care |
|---|---|
| Epidermolysis bullosa simplex (EBS) | Avoid occlusive dressing—can lead to overheating, sweating, and further friction-induced blistering |
| Epidermolysis bullosa simplex Dowling-Meara (EBS-DM) | Thin layer of paraffin preferred—any dressings have the potential to induce blisters around the wound |
| Junctional epidermolysis bullosa (JEB) | Avoid mesh dressing as granulation tissue can grow through; use of superpotent corticosteroid can reduce hypergranulation and promote healing |
| Dystrophic epidermolysis bullosa (DEB) | Nonadhesive dressing allowing exudates to pass through; treat infections and itchiness |

Protein replacement has been shown to restore function in many genetic diseases, such as Fabry disease. As patients with severe RDEB lack type VII collagen, administration of the deficient protein should ameliorate skin fragility. Indeed, topical, lesional and intravenous applications of recombinant type VII collagen were shown to restore anchoring fibril formation and dermal-epidermal adherence in mouse models. However, introduction of an exogenous protein into patients could potentially cause autoantibody formation. Indeed, patients with RDEB were shown

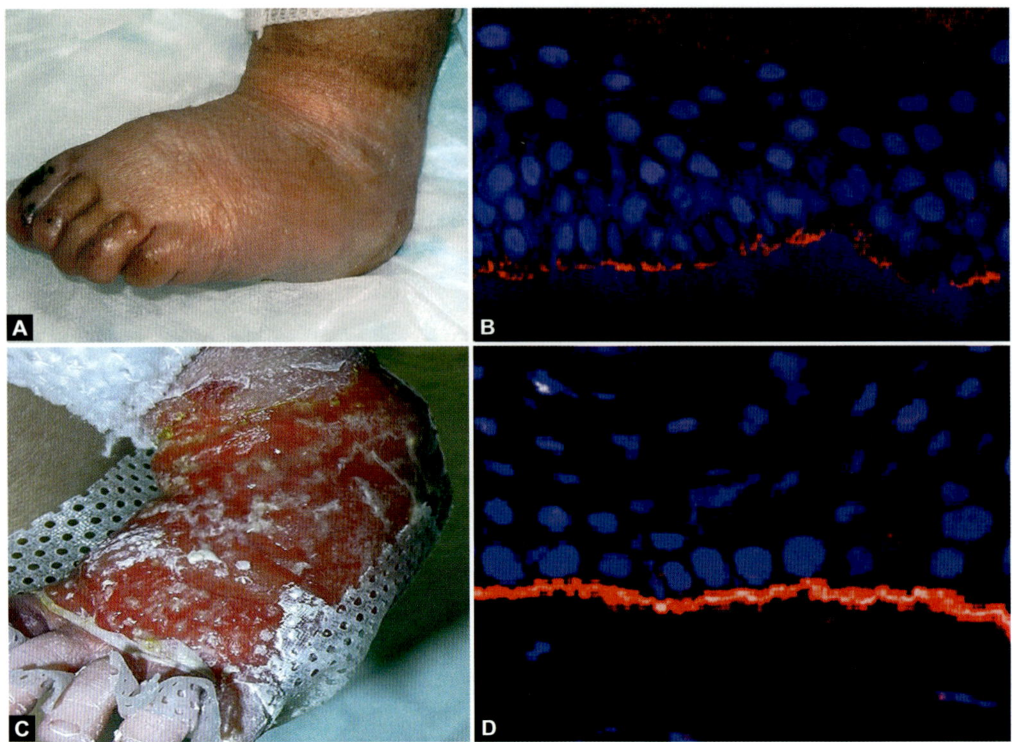


FIG. 20: Myeloablation and whole bone marrow transplantation in an 8-month-old child with severe generalized recessive DEB (RDEB). **A,** Left foot before treatment, showing extensively denuded skin; **B,** Same foot, 100 days after bone marrow transplantation, showing excellent healing; **C,** Antigen mapping of the patient's skin revealing reduced staining of type VII collagen; **D,** Much stronger, linear anti-type VII collagen staining 100 days after bone marrow transplantation.

*Courtesy*: Jakub Tolar, Professor and Director, Stem cell Institute, Division of Blood and Marrow Transplantation, Department of Pediatrics, University of Minnesota.

to have circulating autoantibodies against type VII collagen and type XVII collagen arisen *de novo*. The pathogenic role of these antibodies has so far not been demonstrated. Currently there are no trials of type VII collagen protein replacement on humans.

Many different cell types have propensity to be used for treatment in RDEB.

Allogeneic fibroblast injections directly into the wounds were shown to upregulate the patient's own *COL7A1* alleles, probably through the expression of cytokines, such as heparin-binding EGF-like growth factor.

The *COL7A1* expression was shown to last many months after one single injection into the patients' wounds, but eventually treatments have to be repeated.

Treatment of RDEB using stem cells has shown promise in laboratories and is making impact in patients' lives. Human cord blood-derived unrestricted somatic stem cells have been shown to accelerate wound healing when injected intradermally in a mouse model and, when administered intrahepatically, has been demonstrated to improve blistering phenotype.

Several centers around the world are studying the therapeutic benefits of allogeneic bone marrow stem cell transplantation in patients with RDEB, the rational being that bone marrow-derived cells can be guided into becoming skin cells, given the right microenvironment. Indeed, bone marrow transplant after myeloablation in RDEB patients was shown to improve wound healing and reduce new blister formation, although fatality is around 25% (Fig. 20).

Improved conditioning, nonmyeloablative regimen has resulted in the survival of all allogeneic marrow recipients. Although markedly improved, the skin and mucosal lesions have not become entirely normal. A specific subgroup of bone marrow-derived mesenchymal stem cells which is PDGFRα+ was shown to migrate specifically to injured skin in a mouse model. Transplantation of these cells into type VII collagen-null mice has been shown to ameliorate the blistering phenotype. Whether selective transplantation could reduce complications and improve effectiveness in patients remains to be seen.

Revertant mosaicism is commonly seen in patients with recessive EB. Using these autologous cells to treat RDEB patients could potentially remove all problems associated with allogeneic transplantation. Keratinocytes cultured from reverted patches can be transformed to inducible pluripotent stem cells (iPSCs), which can be dedifferentiated into skin cells. Clinical trials are eagerly anticipated.

## SUGGESTED READINGS


1. Burge SM, Wilkinson JD. Darier-White disease: a review of the clinical features in 163 patients. J Am Acad Dermatol. 1992;27(1):40-50.
2. Burge SM. Hailey-Hailey disease: the clinical features, response to treatment and prognosis. Br J Dermatol. 1992;126(3):275-82.
3. Chan YM, Yu QC, Fine JD, et al. The genetic basis of Weber-Cockayne epidermolysis bullosa simplex. Proc Natl Acad Sci U S A. 1993;90(15):7414-8.
4. Chen MA, Bonifas JM, Matsumura K, et al. A novel three-nucleotide deletion in the helix 2B region of keratin 14 in epidermolysis bullosa simplex: delta E375. Hum Mol Genet. 1993;2(11):1971-2.
5. Christiano AM, Greenspan DS, Hoffman GG, et al. A missense mutation in type VII collagen in two affected siblings with recessive dystrophic epidermolysis bullosa. Nat Genet. 1993;4(1):62-6.
6. Denyer J, Pillay E. Best practice guidelines for skin and wound care in epidermolysis bullosa—International Consensus. Wounds International, DEBRA. 2012. pp. 1-41.

7. Fine JD, Bruckner-Tuderman L, Eady RA, et al. Inherited epidermolysis bullosa: updated recommendations on diagnosis and classification. J Am Acad Dermatol. 2014;70(6):1103-26.
8. Fine JD, Johnson LB, Suchindran C, et al. The epidemiology of inherited EB: findings within American, Canadian and European study populations. In: Fine JD, Bauer EA, McGuire J, Moshell A (Eds). Epidermolysis Bullosa: Clinical, Epidemiologic, and Laboratory Advances, and the Findings of the National Epidermolysis Bullosa Registry. Baltimore: Johns Hopkins University Press; 1999. pp. 101-13.
9. Floquet C, Hatin I, Rousset JP, et al. Statistical analysis of readthrough levels for nonsense mutations in mammalian cells reveals a major determinant of response to gentamicin. PLoS Genet. 2012;8(3):e1002608.
10. Germain DP, Charrow J, Desnick RJ, et al. Ten-year outcome of enzyme replacement therapy with agalsidase beta in patients with Fabry disease. J Med Genet. 2015;52(5):353-8.
11. Happle R, van de Kerkhof PC, Traupe H. Retinoids in disorders of keratinization: their use in adults. Dermatologica. 1987;175 Suppl 1:107-24.
12. Hu Z, Bonifas JM, Beech J, et al. Mutations in ATP2C1, encoding a calcium pump, cause Hailey-Hailey disease. Nat Genet. 2000;24(1):61-5.
13. Iinuma S, Aikawa E, Tamai K, et al. Transplanted bone marrow-derived circulating PDGFRalpha+ cells restore type VII collagen in recessive dystrophic epidermolysis bullosa mouse skin graft. J Immunol. 2015;194(4):1996-2003.
14. Inoue M, Tamai K, Shimizu H, et al. A homozygous missense mutation in the cytoplasmic tail of beta4 integrin, G931D, that disrupts hemidesmosome assembly and underlies non-Herlitz junctional epidermolysis bullosa without pyloric atresia? J Invest Dermatol. 2000;114(5):1061-4.
15. Itoh M, Kiuru M, Cairo MS, et al. Generation of keratinocytes from normal and recessive dystrophic epidermolysis bullosa-induced pluripotent stem cells. Proc Natl Acad Sci U S A. 2011;108(21):8797-802.
16. Jobard F, Bouadjar B, Caux F, et al. Identification of mutations in a new gene encoding a FERM family protein with a pleckstrin homology domain in Kindler syndrome. Hum Mol Genet. 2003;12(8):925-35.
17. Liao Y, Itoh M, Yang A, et al. Human cord blood-derived unrestricted somatic stem cells promote wound healing and have therapeutic potential for patients with recessive dystrophic epidermolysis bullosa. Cell Transplant. 2014;23(3):303-17.
18. Liao Y, Ivanova L, Zhu H, et al. Rescue of the mucocutaneous manifestations by human cord blood derived nonhematopoietic stem cells in a mouse model of recessive dystrophic epidermolysis bullosa. Stem Cells. 2015;33(6):1807-17.
19. Liu L, Mellerio JE, Martinez AE, et al. Mutations in EXPH5 result in autosomal recessive inherited skin fragility. Br J Dermatol. 2014;170(1):196-9.
20. McGrath JA, Gatalica B, Christiano AM, et al. Mutations in the 180-kD bullous pemphigoid antigen (BPAG2), a hemidesmosomal transmembrane collagen (COL17A1), in generalized atrophic benign epidermolysis bullosa. Nat Genet. 1995;11(1):83-6.
21. Munro CS. The phenotype of Darier's disease: penetrance and expressivity in adults and children. Br J Dermatol. 1992;127(2):126-30.
22. Nagy N, Almaani N, Tanaka A, et al. HB-EGF induces COL7A1 expression in keratinocytes and fibroblasts: possible mechanism underlying allogeneic fibroblast therapy in recessive dystrophic epidermolysis Bullosa. J Invest Dermatol. 2011;131(8):1771-4.
23. Nakano A, Chao SC, Pulkkinen L, et al. Laminin 5 mutations in junctional epidermolysis bullosa: molecular basis of Herlitz vs. non-Herlitz phenotypes. Hum Genet. 2002;110(1):41-51.
24. Oji V, Tadini G, Akiyama M, et al. Revised nomenclature and classification of inherited ichthyoses: results of the First Ichthyosis Consensus Conference in Soreze 2009. J Am Acad Dermatol. 2010;63(4):607-41.
25. Pulkkinen L, Christiano AM, Airenne T, et al. Mutations in the gamma 2 chain gene (LAMC2) of kalinin/laminin 5 in the junctional forms of epidermolysis bullosa. Nat Genet. 1994;6(3):293-7.
26. Pulkkinen L, Meneguzzi G, McGrath JA, et al. Predominance of the recurrent mutation R635X in the LAMB3 gene in European patients with Herlitz junctional epidermolysis bullosa has implications for mutation detection strategy. J Invest Dermatol. 1997;109(2):232-7.
27. Reis A, Hennies HC, Langbein L, et al. Keratin 9 gene mutations in epidermolytic palmoplantar keratoderma (EPPK). Nat Genet. 1994;6(2):174-9.
28. Rothnagel JA, Dominey AM, Dempsey LD, et al. Mutations in the rod domains of keratins 1 and 10 in epidermolytic hyperkeratosis. Science. 1992;257(5073):1128-30.
29. Ruzzi L, Gagnoux-Palacios L, Pinola M, et al. A homozygous mutation in the integrin alpha6 gene in junctional epidermolysis bullosa with pyloric atresia. J Clin Invest. 1997;99(12):2826-31.
30. Sakuntabhai A, Burge S, Monk S, et al. Spectrum of novel ATP2A2 mutations in patients with Darier's disease. Hum Mol Genet. 1999;8(9):1611-9.
31. Siegel DH, Ashton GH, Penagos HG, et al. Loss of kindlin-1, a human homolog of the Caenorhabditis elegans actin-extracellular-matrix linker protein UNC-112, causes Kindler syndrome. Am J Hum Genet. 2003;73(1):174-87.
32. Simpson CL, Patel DM, Green KJ. Deconstructing the skin: cytoarchitectural determinants of epidermal morphogenesis. Nat Rev Mol Cell Biol. 2011;12(9):565-80.
33. Smith FJ, Eady RA, Leigh IM, et al. Plectin deficiency results in muscular dystrophy with epidermolysis bullosa. Nat Genet. 1996;13(4):450-7.
34. Szigeti R, Kellermayer R. Autosomal-dominant calcium ATPase disorders. J Invest Dermatol. 2006;126(11):2370-6.
35. Takeichi T, Liu L, Fong K, et al. Whole-exome sequencing improves mutation detection in a diagnostic epidermolysis bullosa laboratory. Br J Dermatol. 2015;172(1):94-100.
36. Tampoia M, Bonamonte D, Filoni A, et al. Prevalence of specific anti-skin autoantibodies in a cohort of patients with inherited epidermolysis bullosa. Orphanet J Rare Dis. 2013;8:132.
37. Tolar J, Wagner JE. Allogeneic blood and bone marrow cells for the treatment of severe epidermolysis bullosa: repair of the extracellular matrix. Lancet. 2013;382(9899):1214-23.
38. Vidal F, Aberdam D, Miquel C, et al. Integrin beta 4 mutations associated with junctional epidermolysis bullosa with pyloric atresia. Nat Genet. 1995;10(2):229-34.
39. Vidal F, Baudoin C, Miquel C, et al. Cloning of the laminin alpha 3 chain gene (LAMA3) and identification of a homozygous deletion in a patient with Herlitz junctional epidermolysis bullosa. Genomics. 1995;30(2):273-80.
40. Wagner JE, Ishida-Yamamoto A, McGrath JA, et al. Bone marrow transplantation for recessive dystrophic epidermolysis bullosa. N Engl J Med. 2010;363(7):629-39.
41. Wang X, Ghasri P, Amir M, et al. Topical application of recombinant type VII collagen incorporates into the dermal-epidermal junction and promotes wound closure. Mol Ther. 2013;21(7):1335-44.
42. Wessagowit V, McGrath JA. Clinical and molecular significance of splice site mutations in the plakophilin 1 gene in patients with ectodermal dysplasia-skin fragility syndrome. Acta Derm Venereol. 2005;85(5):386-8.
43. Wong T, Gammon L, Liu L, et al. Potential of fibroblast cell therapy for recessive dystrophic epidermolysis bullosa. J Invest Dermatol. 2008;128(9):2179-89.
44. Woodley DT, Wang X, Amir M, et al. Intravenously injected recombinant human type VII collagen homes to skin wounds and restores skin integrity of dystrophic epidermolysis bullosa. J Invest Dermatol. 2013;133(7):1910-3.

# 22 CHAPTER Autoimmune Blistering Diseases

*Anuradha Jindal, Raghavendra Rao*

## INTRODUCTION

Autoimmune blistering diseases (AIBDs) are a heterogeneous group of conditions characterized by presence of autoantibodies against the distinct adhesion molecules of epidermis or dermoepidermal junction. Common unifying feature of AIBD are the presence of blisters in the skin with or without mucosal involvement. Based on the level of blister formation, they are broadly classified into intraepidermal or subepidermal AIBD (Table 1).

## PEMPHIGUS

"Pemphix" (Greek word) means to bubble or blister. Pemphigus is the prototype of intraepidermal AIBD. It is potentially a life-threatening disease that results from the damage to adhesive molecules in the epidermis, namely "desmoglein".

**TABLE 1: Classification of autoimmune blistering diseases**

| | Condition | Target antigen |
|---|---|---|
| Intraepidermal AIBD | Pemphigus vulgaris | Dsg1 and Dsg3 |
| | Pemphigus foliaceus | Dsg1 |
| | Immunoglobulin A pemphigus | Dsc3 |
| | Paraneoplastic pemphigus | Dsg1, Dsg3, BP180, envoplakin, periplakin |
| Subepidermal immunobullous diseases (SIBDs) | Bullous pemphigoid | BP230 and BP180 |
| | Pemphigoid gestationis | BP180 |
| | Mucous membrane pemphigoid | • BP180<br>• α6β4 integrin<br>• Laminin332 (Laminin 5) |
| | Linear IgA disease | LABD 97 and LAD-1 |
| | Epidermolysis bullosa aquisita | Type VII collagen |
| | Dermatitis herpetiformis | Epidermal TG3 |
| | Laminin γ-1 pemphigoid (p-200 pemphigoid) | Laminin γ-1 |

Dsg, desmoglein; TG3, transglutaminase 3; Dsc, desmocollin; AIBD, autoimmune blistering disease.

### Epidemiology

The incidence of pemphigus is approximately 0.68–1 per 100,000 population. Pemphigus vulgaris (PV) is the most common variant of pemphigus with an incidence of 0.1–0.5 per 100,000 population. PV accounts for 70% of all pemphigus in many Asian countries, including India. Those with Jewish ancestry seem to, have a particularly high incidence. PV is most common in middle age though it can occur at any age. It seems to affect both sexes equally.

### Pathogenesis

The etiology of pemphigus is not clear. PV is strongly associated with the human leukocyte antigen (HLA) serotypes HLA-DR4 and HLA-DR6. A close interaction between genetic and external factors may lead to disease initiation. Various environmental and pharmacologic factors have been implicated in the pathogenesis of pemphigus, including medications, pesticides, malignancy, ultraviolet radiation, and stress. Foods containing an allium, phenol, thiol, or urushiol group have also been reported to trigger pemphigus.

The autoantibodies in PV target the desmosomal cadherin molecule namely, desmoglein 3 (Dsg3) and desmoglein 1 (Dsg1). Acetylcholine receptors on keratinocytes may also be the potential target antigens in PV.

### Clinical Features

Depending on the level of intraepidermal split, five main types of pemphigus have been recognized; PV, pemphigus foliaceus (PF), paraneoplastic pemphigus (PNP), immunoglobulin A (IgA) pemphigus, and drug-induced pemphigus.

### Pemphigus Vulgaris

Pemphigus vulgaris typically presents initially with painful oral erosions. They are usually seen on the buccal mucosa bilaterally; in about two-third of patients, it might be the only manifestation of the disease and is often misdiagnosed as aphthous ulcers. Though oral mucosa is commonly affected, erosions may sometimes be seen on the lining epithelium of conjunctiva, nasal, larynx, esophagus, urethra, vulva, and cervix. Subsequently, over a latent

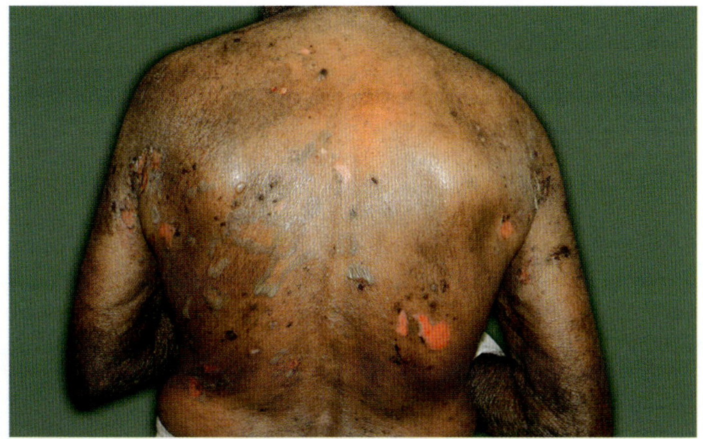

FIG. 1: Flaccid blisters and erosions on the back in pemphigus vulgaris.

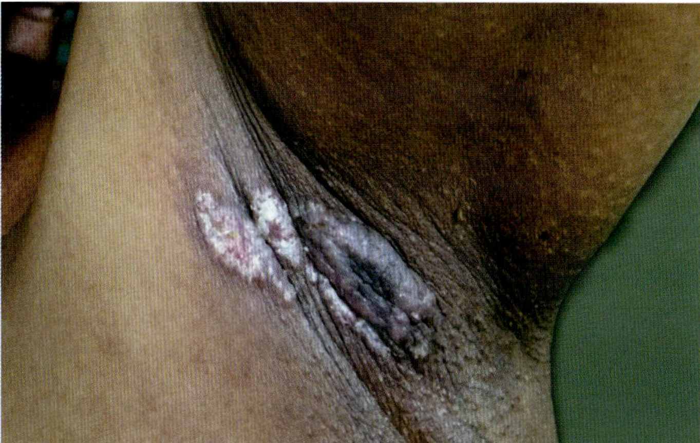

FIG. 2: Vegetative plaque on the left axilla in pemphigus vegetans.

**TABLE 2: Signs in autoimmune blistering diseases**

| Sign | Description |
|---|---|
| Direct Nikolsky sign | • Lateral digital shearing pressure using thumb or finger pad of index finger on the bony prominence causes dislodgment of upper epidermis from the lower epidermis<br>• Indicates disease severity; first sign to disappear when the patient responds to treatment |
| Marginal Nikolsky sign<br>*Synonym*: Indirect Nikolsky sign I | Elicitation close to existing lesion; may persist for longer time |
| Nikolsky's phenomenon | Development of blister instead of erosion |
| Wet Nikolsky sign | Base of erosion has a moist, glistening appearance. It indicates disease activity |
| Dry Nikolsky sign | Base of erosion is dry; indicate re-epithelialization beneath the blister |
| Pear sign in pemphigus | It is described by Sheklakov. Fresh blisters are more or less tense but the older blisters become flaccid and resemble a rubber sack filled with fluid and acquire a pear shape |
| • Asboe–Hansen sign<br>Syn: Bulla spreading sign<br>• Lutz sign<br>• Indirect Nikolsky sign II | Margin of the bulla is marked by a pen. Then a gentle unidirectional pressure is applied to the center of the blister. This leads to the peripheral extension of the bullae. It is seen in both pemphigus and subepidermal immunobullous disease (SIBD). In pemphigus, the extension has an angulated border while in SIBD like BP, it has as regular border |
| Sheklakov's sign (false- Nikolsky sign) | Perifocal subepidermal separation (as indicated by presence of minute bleeding spots). It is seen in BP, DH, and PG. |
| Pseudo-Nikolsky's sign | Can be elicited only over the lesional (erythematous) skin<br>• Seen in TEN/SJS<br>• Due to necrosis and not due to acantholysis |

SJS, Stevens–Johnson syndrome; TEN, toxic epidermal necrolysis; BP, bullous pemphigoid; DH, dermatitis herpetiformis; PG, pemphigoid gestationis.

period ranging from few weeks to months, affected patients will develop flaccid blisters and erosions involving the trunk, face, scalp, and proximal limbs (Fig. 1). Erosions often shows tendency to spread peripherally in the absence of treatment. Nikolsky's and bulla spreading sign (Table 2) are positive in majority of patients with active disease. Pemphigus vegetans (Fig. 2) is a variant of PV that is characterized by "heaped up" vegetating lesions especially on the intertriginous areas.

## Differential Diagnosis

When patients presents with only oral lesions, herpes, oral lichen planus, severe aphthae, and mucous membrane pemphigoid (MMP) should be considered in the differential diagnosis. Other AIBDs and severe cutaneous drug reactions (such as Stevens-Johnson syndrome, toxic epidermal necrolysis, erythema multiforme) should be ruled out in patients who presents with mucocutaneous disease.

## Diagnosis

Biopsy for routine histopathological examination should preferably be taken from the untreated, fresh blister. The histological hallmark of pemphigus is "acantholysis" (loss of cohesion between the keratinocytes) leading to intraepidermal cleft. More specifically, PV is characterized by suprabasal cleavage; basal keratinocytes are separated from each other but still attached to the dermoepidermal junction, gives a "rows of tombstone" appearance. An inflammatory infiltrate composed of variable amounts of neutrophils, eosinophils, and lymphocytes may be present.

Direct immunofluorescence (DIF) from the perilesional skin is the gold standard in confirming the diagnosis of pemphigus and is virtually positive in all patients with active disease. It shows intercellular staining of epidermis with immunoglobulin G (IgG) +/- C3 giving a "fish-net" or "chicken-wire" appearance (Fig. 3). Circulating autoantibodies can be detected by indirect

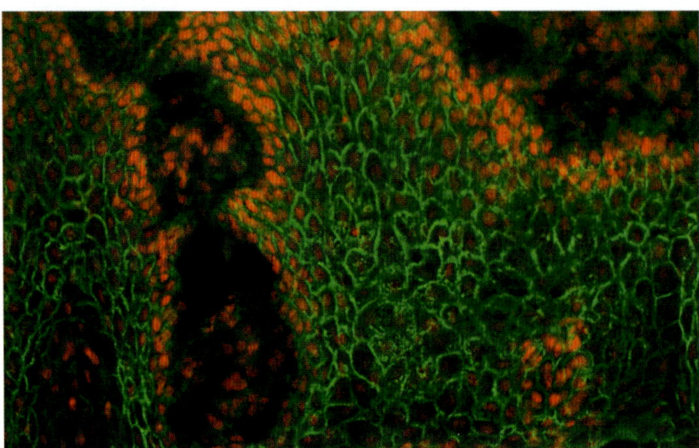

**FIG. 3:** Intercellular staining of epidermis with immunoglobulin G (FITC, x20) in pemphigus vulgaris.

**TABLE 3: Ideal substrate for indirect immunofluorescence**

| Condition | Substrate |
|---|---|
| Pemphigus vulgaris | Monkey esophagus |
| Pemphigus foliaceus | Normal human skin (NHS) |
| Paraneoplastic pemphigus | Rat bladder |
| SIBD | Salt-split NHS |

SIBD, subepidermal immunobullous diseases.

**TABLE 4: Summary of principle of tests directed against the detection of antibodies**

| Test | Principle |
|---|---|
| DIF | • Ideal site of biopsy is perilesional skin<br>• Transported to the laboratory in Michel's medium<br>• Frozen section of skin biopsy taken using cryostat and are stained with FITC-labeled antibodies with specificities against IgG, IgM, IgA, C3, and FB<br>• Examined under fluorescence microscopy |
| IIF | • Two-step procedure<br>• Serum of patient is diluted in serial titer with PBS<br>• It is then incubated with frozen section of suitable substrate (NHS, MO, salt-split skin)<br>• Step 2 is similar to DIF and frozen sections are then stained with FITC-labeled IgG (occasionally with IgA)<br>• Examined under fluorescence microscope |
| ELISA | • Serum of patients at recommended dilution is incubated in the well of an appropriate ELISA system (for example, desmoglein ELISA for pemphigus)<br>• ELISA plate wells are precoated with recombinant antigen<br>• Antigen–antibody reaction can be detected by the color changes; intensity corresponds to the amount of circulating antibodies |

FITC, fluorescein isothiocyanate; PBS, phosphate buffer saline; ELISA, enzyme-linked immunosorbent assay; IG, immunoglobulin; IIF, indirect immunofluorescence; NHS, normal human skin; MO, monkey esophagus; DIF, direct immunofluorescence.

immunofluorescence (IIF). Sensitivity of IIF is generally lower (around 90% in PV) and depends upon the substrate used (Table 3). Studies have shown that IIF titer generally correlates with the disease activity and is, therefore, used to monitor the disease activity.

In recent years, recombinant and cell-derived forms of the target antigens have been applied in the development of sensitive and specific enzyme-linked immunosorbent assays (ELISAs) for the detection of circulating autoantibodies. ELISA system is useful both for confirmation of diagnosis and for monitoring of disease activity. In pemphigus, patients suffering from only mucosal lesion will have antibodies against Dsg3 only, while patients with mucocutaneous disease will have antibodies against both Dsg1 and Dsg3 (Table 4).

## Pemphigus Foliaceus

Pemphigus foliaceus is considered traditionally as the superficial type of pemphigus.

### Pathogenesis

In PF, autoantibodies target Dsg1 which is strongly expressed in the upper epidermis. This explains the subcorneal location of blisters in this condition. Most of the patients with PF do not have mucosal involvement.

### Clinical Features

Primary lesions of PF are flaccid, superficial vesicles and bullae of the skin that tends to rupture easily due to their location in the subcorneal plane. These patients rather present with erosions, scaling and crusting on an erythematous background. Lesions are often seen on seborrheic areas of the body, i.e., scalp, face, chest and back (Fig. 4). Occasionally, erythema, scaling may be generalized leading to exfoliative dermatitis.

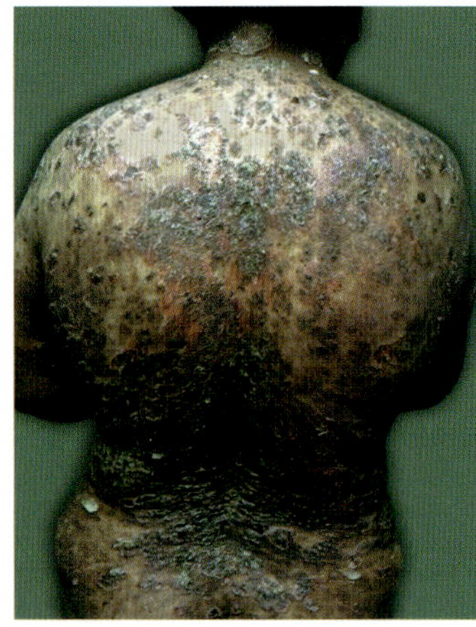

**FIG. 4:** Extensive scaling and crusting over the trunk in pemphigus foliaceus.

### Differential Diagnosis

Differential diagnosis of PF includes seborrheic dermatitis, bullous impetigo, IgA pemphigus, pemphigus herpetiformis, drug eruption, subcorneal pustular dermatosis (SPD), and lupus erythematosus (LE).

### Diagnosis

Histopathology shows subcorneal blister and helps to distinguish it from PV. There are variable amounts of acantholytic keratinocytes, neutrophils, and fibrin within the blisters. Dyskeratotic cells are present within the epidermis. DIF findings are similar to PV and shows intercellular staining of epidermis with IgG with or without C3. The staining with IgG may be more intense in upper epidermis reflecting the abundance of Dsg1 in the superficial epidermis.

## Pemphigus Erythematosus (Senear–Usher Syndrome)

Pemphigus erythematosus (PE) is a rare, localized variant of PF which shows immunological coexistence of two autoimmune conditions, i.e., PE and LE.

### Clinical Features

Patients with PE presents with erythematous scaly or crusted plaques in the malar region (resembling LE) and other seborrheic areas. Lesions on the trunk are similar to PF and occur in a localized or generalized distribution. Oral mucosa is usually spared.

### Diagnosis

Direct immunofluorescence (DIF) shows intercellular deposition of IgG and C3 in a fish net-like pattern on the cell surface of keratinocytes (similar to pemphigus); in addition, there will be granular basement membrane zone (BMZ) staining with these immunoreactants, similar to LE. Antinuclear antibodies (ANA) may also be found in the serum of these patients.

## Paraneoplastic Pemphigus

Anhalt et al. in 1990 first reported and proposed criteria for the diagnosis of PNP (Box 1).

### Pathogenesis

The exact mechanisms by which neoplasia induces PNP are incompletely understood. Circulating antibodies are directed against both desmoglein and plakin family of proteins in the patients with PNP.

### Clinical Features

It is characterized by recalcitrant mucosal erosions and a polymorphous skin rash (lichenoid, erythema multiforme-like or pemphigus-like) which occur in the setting of underlying malignancy (usually lymphoproliferative). PNP is characterized by multiple internal organ involvement (lungs, thyroid, kidney, smooth muscle) and is, therefore, sometimes referred as paraneoplastic autoimmune multiorgan syndrome (PAMS).

**BOX 1 Criteria for the diagnosis of paraneoplastic pemphigus (Anhalt's criteria)**

- Painful mucosal ulcerations and a polymorphous skin eruption in the context of occult neoplasm
- Vacuolar interface change, keratinocytes necrosis and intraepidermal acantholysis
- Deposition of immunoglobulin G and C3 in the intercellular spaces, and granular-linear complement deposition along the epidermal basement membrane zone
- Serum antibodies that bind not only to cell surfaces of skin and mucosa in a pattern typical of pemphigus vulgaris, but also to simple, columnar, and transitional epithelia
- Serum antibodies that recognize epidermal antigens of 250, 230, 210, and 190 kDa

### Diagnosis

Histopathology of PNP shows considerable variability and depends on the phenotypic presentation. Hence, it may show suprabasal clefting, dyskeratotic keratinocytes, basal cell vacuolization or interface dermatitis like histological findings. Immunofluorescence is considered as one of the main diagnostic criteria for PNP. The pattern of fluorescence at the BMZ is similar to bullous pemphigoid (BP). Antibodies in PNP bind to the desmosomes of both simple as well as transitional epithelia. Hence, IIF using rat bladder as a substrate confirms the diagnosis of PNP, and it has a sensitivity and specificity of 86% and 98%, respectively. PNP targets multiple antigens; of these, ELISA system for the detection of antibodies against envoplakin (N terminus) is commercially available.

## Immunoglobulin A Pemphigus

It is an uncommon variant of pemphigus in which IgA rather than IgG is deposited in the intercellular space of epidermis. There are two distinct types of IgA pemphigus: (1) SPD type; and (2) intraepidermal neutrophilic (IEN) type.

### Pathogenesis

Though the exact target antigen of IgA pemphigus is not known, antibodies against desmocollin 1 have been detected in patients with SPD type of IgA pemphigus.

### Clinical Features

Patients with both types of IgA pemphigus clinically present with flaccid vesicles or pustules on erythematous or normal skin. Lesions are seen predominantly in the axillae and groin but sometimes trunk and the proximal extremities may be involved. The pustules tend to coalesce to form an annular or circinate pattern with crusts in the center, so called "sunflower-like" pattern. Oral mucosa is usually spared in IEN type of IgA pemphigus.

### Differential Diagnosis

Differential diagnosis of IgA pemphigus includes SPD, PF, and pustular psoriasis.

### Diagnosis

Immunoglobulin A pemphigus is characterized by minimal acantholysis. There will be infiltration of epidermis with neutrophils. In SPD type of IgA pemphigus, pustules are located subcorneally in the upper epidermis, whereas in IEN type, pustules are seen either in the suprabasal plane or throughout the epidermis.

Direct immunofluorescence microscopy helps to confirm the diagnosis; it shows intercellular IgA staining in the epidermis.

**TABLE 5: Drugs causing autoimmune blistering diseases**

| Condition | Drugs |
|---|---|
| Pemphigus | D-penicillamine, captopril, and rifampin |
| Linear IgA disease | Vancomycin, penicillin, cephalosporins, captopril, and nonsteroidal anti-inflammatory drugs (diclofenac, naproxen) |

## Drug-induced Pemphigus

Drugs may exacerbate or induce pemphigus. Both thiol and non-thiol drugs have been associated with pemphigus.

### Etiopathogenesis

Pemphigus can be induced by a variety of drugs (Table 5); D-penicillamine and angiotensin-converting enzyme (ACE) inhibitors are the most often culprits. Drugs with sulfhydryl (-SH) group may directly interact with the -SH group of desmoglein or bind to them creating a new epitope. Non-SH group may alter the function of B-cell activity leading to autoantibody production. The time interval between the initiation of medication and the onset of disease ranges from 8 to 12 months.

### Clinical Features

Drug-induced pemphigus is usually PF or PE; occasionally, it can have PV-like presentation with oral involvement.

### Diagnosis

Histopathologically, eosinophils in the dermis characterize the early stages of drug-induced pemphigus. DIF and ELISA findings are similar to other types of pemphigus and depend on the phenotypic presentation.

## Other Unusual Variants

Pemphigus herpetiformis is an uncommon variant of pemphigus characterized by intensely pruritic, vesicular eruption. These vesicles show a tendency for grouping and are distributed in the predilection site for dermatitis herpetiformis (DH). DIF is the same as the classic forms of pemphigus—intercellular deposits of IgG and C3 in the epidermis. Endemic PF (fogo selvagem) is more common in South American countries, especially central Brazil. It is usually seen in outdoor workers and affects young men. Distribution of disease corresponds to the distribution of black fly. Though clinical and immunological profile is identical to PF, patients experience burning pain in the affected areas.

## Treatment of Pemphigus

Goal of treatment in pemphigus is to achieve complete clinical as well as immunological remission. Treatment plan is outlined in flowchart 1.

Therapy should be initiated with systemic corticosteroids (prednisolone 1 mg/kg/day). This should be continued till the disease is consolidated (defined as the time at which there is cessation of new lesions in conjunction with the healing of pre-existing lesions). Dose of steroids may be increased if the patient continues to develop new lesions (up to a maximum of 2 mg/day).

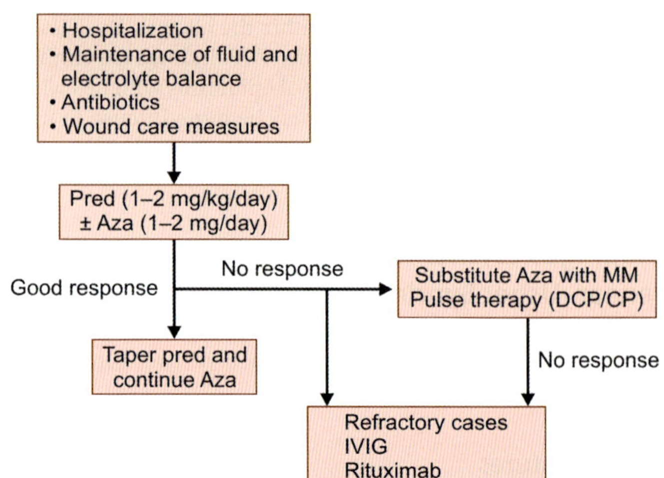


Pred, prednisolone; Aza, azathioprine; MM, mycophenolate mofetil; DCP, dexamethasone-cyclophosphamide pulse; CP, cyclophosphamide; IVIG, intravenous immunoglobulin; PV, pemphigus vulgaris; PF, pemphigus foliaceus.

**FLOWCHART 1:** Treatment outline of pemphigus.

Once the disease is controlled, dose of steroids should be tapered to minimize the side effects of long-term steroid therapy. Once the patient achieves the clinical remission, further tapering of steroids should be based on the immunological activity of the disease as measured by IIF or ELISA (Dsg 1 and 3).

Many patients develop the relapse of their disease when the steroid dose is being tapered off. Hence, the experts in the field of pemphigus now recommend immunosuppressive agents as the first-line treatment of pemphigus along with steroids so that the total cumulative dose of steroids is reduced. Immunosuppressive agents that are commonly recommended are azathioprine (1–2 mg/kg), mycophenolate mofetil (2–3 gm/day) or cyclophosphamide pulse therapy (500 mg intravenously). Since these agents are associated with potential toxicity, baseline investigations should be done in all patients before instituting the therapy with immunosuppressive agents, which needs to be repeated periodically (Box 2).

### Dexamethasone—Cyclophosphamide Pulse

Pulse therapy means the administration of large (supra-pharmacologic) doses of drugs in an intermittent manner to enhance the therapeutic effect and reduce the side effects. Dexamethasone-cyclophosphamide pulse (DCP) consists of four phases:

- *Phase I*: It comprises of administering 100 mg dexamethasone dissolved in 500 mL of 5% glucose as a slow intravenous drip over 2 hours repeated on three consecutive days. On the second day, the patient is also given 500 mg cyclophosphamide in the same drip. This constitutes one cycle of DCP. Such DCP cycles are repeated at exactly 28-day intervals counted from the first day of the pulse. In between the DCPs, the patient receives only 50 mg/day of oral cyclophosphamide. Once the skin and the mucous membrane lesions heal completely, the patient is considered to have entered phase II
- *Phase II*: The patient remains in clinical remission and receives nine more DCPs along with 50 mg cyclophosphamide orally per day
- *Phase III*: DCP therapy is withdrawn and only oral cyclophosphamide 50 mg is given daily for 9 months

**BOX 2 Monitoring guidelines for steroids and immunosuppressive drugs**

*Monitoring guidelines for long-term steroid therapy*

Baseline
- TB screening: Tuberculin skin test, chest X-ray
- Biochemistry test: FBS, triglycerides, potassium level
- Hepatitis B surafce antigen and hepatitis C viral study

Follow-up

At 1 month, repeat every 3–4 months
- Fasting and postprandial sugars, triglycerides, potassium levels

In case of long-term steroid administration, early morning cortisol levels [to check for hypothalamus pituitary adrenal axis (HPA axis) suppression]

*Monitoring guidelines of azathioprine*
- Baseline
  - Pregnancy test (in women of childbearing potential)
  - Complete blood count including platelets
  - Liver and renal function test
  - Urine analysis
  - Tuberculin test
- Special test - TPMT* levels
- Follow-up (every 2 weeks for first 2 months, then every 2–3 months)
  - CBC
  - AST and ALT
  - TPMT <6.3 U/mL: Do not give azathioprine
  - TPMT between 6.3 and 15 U/mL: 1 mg/kg
  - TPMT between 15.1 and 26.4 U/mL: 2–2.5 mg/kg

*Monitoring guidelines for mycophenolate mofetil*
- Baseline
  - Complete blood count with platelets
  - Liver and renal function test
  - Hepatitis B and C panel
  - Tuberculin test
  - Pregnancy test
- Follow-up
  - Complete blood count, including platelet
  - Serum creatinine
  - Liver function tests

*Monitoring guidelines for cyclophosphamide*
- Baseline
  - Complete blood counts with platelets
  - Liver and renal function test
  - Urinalysis
  - Pregnancy test
- Follow-up
  - Complete blood counts weekly for 2–3 months, then biweekly for 2–3 months, then every month
  - Urinalysis weekly for 2–3 months, then biweekly for 2–3 months, then every month
  - Liver function test: Monthly for first 3–6 months, quarterly then

* Thiopurine methyltransferase (TPMT) levels

TPMT, thiopurine methyltransferase; AST, aspartate aminotransferase; ALT, alanine aminotransferase; FBS, fasting blood sugar.

**TABLE 6: Rituximab dosage schedule**

| Protocol | Dose |
|---|---|
| Rheumatoid arthritis | 1000 mg (or 500 mg) on day 1 and day 15 |
| Lymphoma | 375 mg/m$^2$ weekly for 4 weeks |
| Repeat the cycle after 6–9 months (if necessary) | |

- *Phase IV*: After this, the treatment for pemphigus is withdrawn completely and the patient is followed up for the next 10 years to look for any relapse.

Dexamethasone-cyclophosphamide pulse therapy is reserved for patients who fail to respond to augmented dose of steroid (1.5–2 mg/kg of prednisolone) therapy.

Rituximab is a chimeric murine-human monoclonal antibody to CD20 which induces depletion of B cells *in vivo*. CD20 is a B-cell-specific antigen expressed on the surface of B lymphocytes throughout the differentiation phase from the pre-B-cell to the mature B-cell stage. Rituximab's cytotoxicity is mediated by three mechanisms including antibody-dependent cellular cytotoxicity, complement-mediated lysis, and direct disruption of signaling pathways and triggering of apoptosis. At present, rituximab is quite expensive drug and is usually reserved for patients with recalcitrant disease (Table 6).

Extensive and widespread PF should be treated in the same way as that of PV. Localized disease can be controlled by potent topical steroids or dapsone. Dapsone is also the drug of choice for IgA pemphigus. Treatment of PNP is more difficult and should be directed against the underlying tumor along with the specific pemphigus therapy. Cessation of inciting drug along with dapsone therapy is found to be beneficial in drug-induced pemphigus.

## PEMPHIGOID

Pemphigoid is derived from the Greek word meaning "form of blister" (pemphix, blister; edios, form). Pemphigoid group of diseases comprises of BP, pemphigoid gestationis (PG), MMP, and linear IgA bullous disease (LAD).

### Bullous Pemphigoid

Bullous pemphigoid is the prototype of subepidermal immunobullous diseases (SIBD) in which autoantibodies are produced against distinct components of BMZ.

#### Epidemiology

Bullous pemphigoid is the most common AIBD in the western world. The incidence of BP is estimated to be between 4.5 and 14 new cases per million per year. BP typically affects people aged 70 years and older. The risk of patients developing BP in patients older than 90 years appears to be 300-fold higher than for those aged 60 years.

#### Pathogenesis

The exact etiology of BP is not known. Two antigenic target in BP are hemidesmosomal proteins namely BP230 and BP180 (also known as collagen XVII). BP230 (BPAg1) is a hemidesmosomal protein, located in the basal keratinocytes, while BP180 (BPAg2) is a transmembranous molecule. Autoantibody in majority of patients with BP recognizes an epitope located in the amino-terminal of noncollagenous domain of BP180 (NC16A).

Numerous triggers have been implicated in the disease onset of BP patients, including trauma, burns, radiotherapy, ultraviolet (UV) radiation, and a variety of drugs (especially spironolactone, phenothiazines with aliphatic side chains).

## Clinical Features

The diagnosis of BP should be considered in all elderly patients who presents with a generalized pruritic eruption with widespread blister formation. Blisters are tense, 1–3 cm in diameter and are seen on the background of normal or urticarial base. Lesions are distributed predominantly over the trunk, abdomen, and proximal extremities (Fig. 5). Vegetating plaques may be present in intertriginous areas. Mucosal involvement is seen in about 30% of the patients; painful erosions and rarely intact bullae may be seen involving the oral cavity, eyes, nose, pharynx, esophagus, and anogenital area (Table 7).

## Differential Diagnosis

Bullous pemphigoid has to be differentiated from other SIBD. Prebullous eruption may mimic urticaria, DH, scabies, or dermatitis.

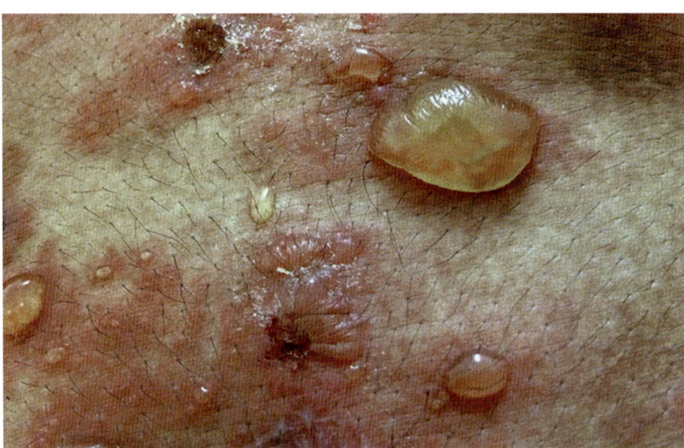

**FIG. 5:** Tense blisters on an erythematous base in bullous pemphigoid.

**TABLE 7: Atypical forms of bullous pemphigoid**

| Variants | Description |
|---|---|
| Pemphigoid vegetans | Vegetative plaques in the intertriginous area |
| Pemphigoid nodularis | Prurigo nodularis-like lesions |
| Vesicular pemphigoid | DH-like presentation with smaller, grouped vesicles |
| Lichen planus pemphigoides | Coexistence of LP and BP |
| Localized BP | Pretibial/vulvar/peristomal/umbilical |
| Dyshidrosiform pemphigoid | Deep-seated vesicles in the palms and soles |

DH, dermatitis herpetiformis; LP, lichen planus; BP, bullous pemphigoid.

## Diagnosis

Routine histopathology of an early intact vesicle typically reveals a subepidermal cleavage with a superficial dermal inflammatory infiltrate typically rich in eosinophils. DIF of the perilesional skin shows linear deposition of C3 and IgG along the BMZ (Fig. 6). IIF is less sensitive than DIF; sensitivity of IIF can be increased by using salt-split normal human skin ("indirect salt-split study"). It typically shows linear staining of IgG on the epidermal side of the split ("roof pattern") or occasionally a combined "roof" and "floor" pattern (Fig. 7).

The ELISA using recombinant BP180 and BP230 is now available commercially and is used for the detection of circulating antibodies; antibodies against BP180 seems to correlate with the disease activity.

## Treatment

Oral prednisolone (0.5–1 mg/kg/day) is the mainstay of treatment; disease control is usually achieved within 1–2 weeks. Other agents (Box 3) that have been used includes tetracycline with nicotinamide, dapsone, immunosuppressive agents like mycophenolate, azathioprine, cyclophosphamide, methotrexate, and cyclosporine A. Intravenous immunoglobulin (IVIG) and rituximab are reserved for severe, refractory disease.

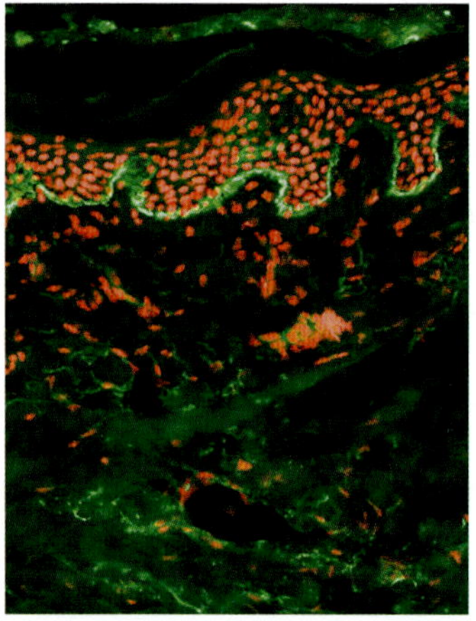

**FIG. 6:** Linear staining of basement membrane zone with C3 (FITC, x20).

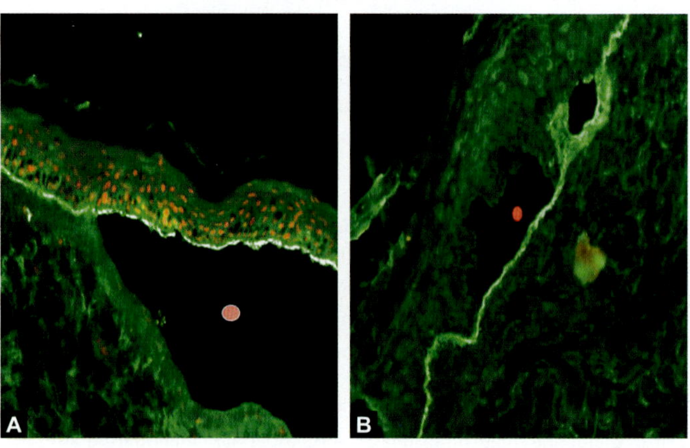


**FIG. 7:** Linear basement membrane zone band: **A,** on the epidermal side ("roof pattern") of the split (as indicated by red circle) with immunoglobulin G in bullous pemphigoid; **B,** on the dermal side of the split ("floor pattern") in epidermolysis bullosa acquisita (FITC, x20).

**BOX 3 Treatment of bullous pemphigoid**

*First-line of management*
- Limited skin involvement: Potent topical steroids
- Extensive skin involvement: Oral steroids (prednisolone 0.5–1 mg/kg)

*Alternative treatment options*
- Tetracycline with nicotinamide
- Dapsone
- Azathioprine
- Cyclophosphamide
- Mycophenolate mofetil

*Refractory cases*
- Intravenous immunoglobulin
- Rituximab

## Mucous Membrane Pemphigoid

Mucous membrane pemphigoid (MMP), known previously as cicatricial pemphigoid is a unique SIBD characterized by involvement of the mucous membrane predominantly and tendency for scarring.

### Epidemiology

Mucous membrane pemphigoid is the second most common SIBD after BP, with an annual incidence of 1 per million in central Europe. It is primarily a disease of elderly and is more common in females as compared to males.

### Etiopathogenesis

The disease is more common in people with HLA-DR4 and DQw7. BP180 is the target antigen in majority of patients. However, in contrast to BP, the antibodies target the carboxy terminus of BP180, which is present in the lower end of BP180 near lamina densa. Apart from this, few patients with MMP show antibodies against diverse proteins such as laminin 332, integrin ($\alpha 6\beta 4$) and type VII collagen.

### Clinical Features

The disease typically begins in the mouth with blisters and erosions often involving the gingiva ("desquamative gingivitis"), buccal mucosa, palate, inner surface of the lips, and the tongue. Lesions almost always heal without scar formation.

Eyes are frequently affected and may sometimes be the only site of involvement. It starts as unilateral nonspecific conjunctivitis that gradually involves the other eye. Conjuctival inflammation and erosions that scar, cause symblepharon, ankyloblepharon, entropion, trichiasis, corneal damage, and neovascularization. Evaluation by an experienced ophthalmologist is critical to differentiate MMP from other ocular problems. Rarely, patients may have involvement of nasopharyngeal, esophageal and genital mucosal lesions. About 30% of MMP patients will have cutaneous involvement which is seen predominantly on the head and neck region. It presents as erythematous plaque which becomes the site for recurrent blister formation. These lesions may heal with atrophic scarring. It must be differentiated from Brunsting–Perry disease, in which mucosa is spared and antibodies are directed against type VII collagen.

### Diagnosis

Histopathology is quite similar to BP and shows subepithelial blisters admixed with mixed inflammatory infiltrate comprising of plasma cells and lymphohistiocytes. Older lesion may show predominant fibrosis. DIF shows linear deposition of IgG, IgA and C3 along the BMZ. IIF on salt-split skin may show mixed pattern (roof, floor or combined) reflecting the antigenic heterogenicity.

### Treatment

Treatment of MMP depends upon the extent and severity of the disease. Oral disease may respond to topical steroids. Systemic drugs are necessary for severe ocular or other mucosal disease. Dapsone is often used as the first-line agent; best immunosuppressive agent for MMP is cyclophosphamide. A multidisciplinary approach is ideal for these patients with severe mucosal disease.

## Pemphigoid Gestationis

Pemphigoid gestationis (PG), formerly known as herpes gestationis, is a rare SIBD of pregnancy and the peripartum period. The incidence of PG is very low, estimated at approximately 1 case per 50,000 pregnancies.

### Pathogenesis

The major target antigen in PG is BP180 similar to BP. Hence, DIF findings are similar to BP and shows linear BMZ band with C3. ELISA would typically reveal circulating IgG antibodies against BP180, in particular against the NC16A domain of BP180.

There is an increased risk of prematurity and small-for-gestational-age babies. Newborns may rarely be born with transient blisters which resolve in few days.

### Clinical Features

The disease presents usually in the third or sometimes in the second trimester of pregnancy. It is more common in multigravida women, and can invariably recur in their subsequent pregnancies. If it recurs, it often presents early in the pregnancy. There are also reports of this disease occurring in women with trophoblastic tumors, hydatidiform mole, or choriocarcinoma. The patient initially presents with pruritic urticarial papules and annular plaques, followed by vesicles and bullae. The most common site of the eruption is abdomen (especially, periumbilical area in 90% of patients) and thighs.

### Treatment

Potent topical steroids are used as the first-line treatment. The disease in most patients will be adequately controlled with potent or highly potent topical corticosteroids in combination with H1-receptor antagonists. Oral prednisolone can be added at an initial dose of 0.25–0.5 mg/kg/day day in patients who have extensive blisters. IVIG and rituximab have been used in the postpartum period to control disease flares.

## Linear Immunoglobulin A Disease

Linear IgA disease (LAD) is an acquired SIBD, characterized immunopathologically by linear deposition of IgA along the

BMZ. The disease affects both children and adults; although there are some differences in their clinical presentations, there is considerable overlap with shared immunopathology and immunogenetics.

## Epidemiology

Linear IgA disease is a rare disorder with an incidence of 0.5 per 1 million population in Western Europe; however, it may be more common in Asian countries, including Indian subcontinent. It has a bimodal onset; one peak is seen during the childhood (previously known as chronic bullous disease of childhood or CBDC) and the second peak occurs in adults after 60 years of age.

## Pathogenesis

Evidence suggests genetic susceptibility to this disease with an increased incidence of HLA-B8, HLA-DR3, and HLADQW2. Autoantibodies in LAD are directed against these cleaved ectodomains of BP180 molecule, i.e., LAD-1 and LABD-97. Certain triggering factors may play a crucial role in the initiation of disease in genetically predisposed individuals; these include drugs, malignancy and vaccination.

## Clinical Features

- *LAD (childhood)*: It is a disease of preschool children with mean age of onset at 4.5 years (range 6 months to 10 years). The classic primary lesions of LAD are clear or hemorrhagic blisters developing on normal or erythematous skin. Blisters are often arranged in annular fashion around the central crust giving a "strings of pearl" appearance (Fig. 8). The periorificial region of face and perineal area are commonly affected with occasional involvement of lower abdomen, vulva, thighs, and buttocks. Mucosal involvement may be seen in 80% of LAD patients, but it is usually less severe in childhood LAD when compared to adult LAD. Affected patients may present with oral erosions, nasal bleeding, and conjunctivitis
- *LAD (adults)*: Clinical presentation of adult onset of LAD is similar to BP. Tense blisters are seen on an erythematous skin; this may be associated with variable degree of pruritus and burning sensation. Lesions are seen predominantly on the trunk; the face, scalp, and the extremities may be involved as well. The distinctive "string of pearls" appearance of blisters is less common in adults
- *Drug-induced* LAD: LAD is probably the most common autoimmune blistering condition precipitated by drugs (Table 5). Though it may have a similar presentation as that of classic disease, occasionally it may present as erythema multiforme-like, toxic epidermal necrolysis like or morbilliform rash without blistering.

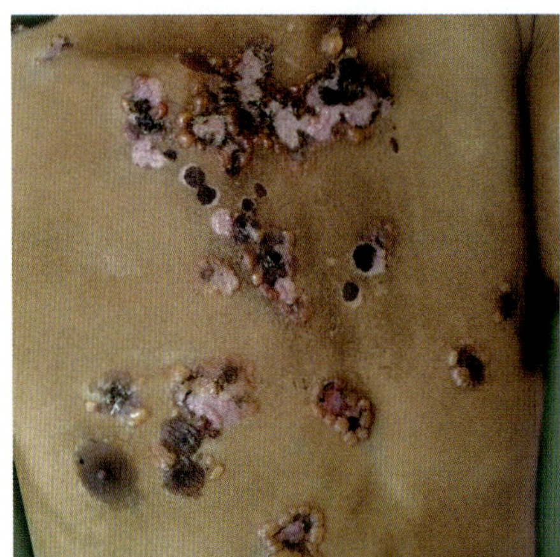

FIG. 8: Tense vesicles in an annular configuration showing "string of pearls" appearance in linear immunoglobulin A.

## Differential Diagnosis

In children, LAD is usually mistaken for bullous impetigo, but the history of frequent relapses raises the possibility of LAD. Hereditary epidermolysis bullosa (EB) is often present at birth and is also differentiated from LAD by the family history. Childhood BP may resemble LAD. In adults, it is most often confused with BP and DH.

## Diagnosis

Histology is characterized by a subepidermal blister with primarily neutrophilic infiltrate in the papillary dermis, although mononuclear cells and occasional eosinophils are also seen. DIF of perilesional skin shows linear staining of BMZ with IgA. Occasionally, other classes of immunoglobulin deposition, especially IgG, may be present along the BMZ and may lead to diagnostic confusion. This type of "dual" staining of IgA and IgG has been reported in children and is known as "mixed immunobullous disease of childhood". Circulating IgA autoantibodies can be detected by IIF in both children (75% of cases) and adults (30% of cases). Indirect salt-split study shows "roof pattern" in majority of patients, with few patients showing combined pattern.

## Treatment

Most cases of LAD respond well to dapsone or sulfapyridine. Widespread involvement may require oral steroids along with dapsone to control the initial disease activity. Other drugs that have been used with success include erythromycin, colchicine, mycophenolate mofetil, and IVIG.

# DERMATITIS HERPETIFORMIS

Dermatitis herpetiformis, also known as Duhring Brocq disease, is a chronic, recurrent, pruritic, papulovesicular disease. Another hallmark of DH is the presence of gluten-sensitive enteropathy.

## Epidemiology

Dermatitis herpetiformis is a relatively rare disease; it is more prevalent in Scandinavian and Eastern European countries and uncommon in African-Americans or Asians. Mean age of onset of DH is in the fourth decade and is more common among men.

## Pathogenesis

Dermatitis herpetiformis is usually seen in persons with HLA-DQ2 and HLA-DQ8. All patients with DH have gluten-sensitive enteropathy and observe worsening of their condition after taking gluten-rich diet, just as in celiac disease (CD). Dermatitis herpetiformis may be considered as the skin manifestation of CD. Granular IgA deposits are seen in the dermal papilla and circulating IgA anti-endomysium antibodies can be demonstrated in the affected patients. The anti-endomysium antibodies are directed against the tissue transglutaminase (TG2) which is homogeneous to epidermal transglutaminase (TG3). Binding of antibodies to TG3 might stimulate complement system by alternate pathway leading to neutrophil chemotaxis.

## Clinical Features

Dermatitis herpetiformis is a polymorphous skin disease characterized by 1–3 mm large papules, papulovesicles, crusted erosions, and excoriations typically distributed over extensor aspect of elbows and knees, buttocks, shoulders, midline of back, and scapula in decreasing order of frequency. Affected patients will experience severe itching, which can precede the development of skin lesions. Gastrointestinal symptoms, such as steatorrhea (20–30%) and symptoms similar to CD (<10%) may be present.

## Diagnosis

Striking histopathologic change is the presence of papillary tip microabscess comprising of collection of neutrophils and subepidermal blister. DIF characteristically shows granular deposition of IgA on top of the dermal papillae and sometimes along the dermal-epidermal junction. Circulating antibodies against tissue transglutaminase (anti-TTG), antiepidermal transglutaminase (anti-ETG) and deamidated antigliadin may be detected is some patients.

## Treatment

Dapsone (50–150 mg/day) is the drug of choice. It dramatically improves the pruritus within few hours in the affected patients. A strict, gluten-free diet should be advised to DH patients.

# EPIDERMOLYSIS BULLOSA ACQUISITA

Epidermolysis bullosa acquisita (EBA) is an SIBD disorder characterized by the presence of autoantibodies of IgG class and less often by IgA class against type VII collagen (COL7), a major component of anchoring fibrils.

## Epidemiology

The incidence of EBA is estimated to be between 0.2 and 0.5 new cases per million per year. No gender or racial predilection has been reported. EBA is usually seen in adults with a mean age of onset at 50 years; few cases have been reported in children as well.

## Pathogenesis

Autoantibodies in EBA are directed against type VII collagen (COL7), a major component of anchoring fibrils, located in the lamina densa and sublamina densa region. In majority of patients with EBA, autoantibodies target epitopes within the NC1 region of the protein.

## Clinical Features

Clinically, four phenotypic variants of EBA have been described:
- Classical or mechanobullous variant
- Inflammatory
- Brunsting–Perry disease
- MMP-like.

### Classical (Mechanobullous) EBA

It comprises majority of the cases of EBA; clinically, it is characterized by skin fragility and appearance of tense vesicles, and bullae on the normal skin ("noninflammatory blisters"). These blisters have a tendency to heal with scarring and milia formation. Lesions develop over the trauma-prone surfaces, such as the extensor aspect of the limbs (elbows, knees, dorsal aspect of the hands, toes, and ankles). Scarring alopecia and nail dystrophy, even leading to acquired anonychia, may be seen in severe cases. Mucous membrane involvement is rare in classical variant.

### Inflammatory EBA

Clinically this form of EBA is indistinguishable from BP; widespread tense blisters on erythematous skin are seen over the trunk, body folds, and the extremities (Fig. 9).

### Brunsting—Perry Disease

This is characterized by localized blistering or erythematous plaques involving the head and neck region, which heals with atrophic scarring. Mucous membrane is spared.

### Mucous Membrane Pemphigoid-like

This variant of EBA resembles MMP with predominant mucosal lesions. Ocular involvement results in conjunctival inflammation and fibrosis leading to ankyloblepharon and blindness.

## Differential Diagnosis

Epidermolysis bullosa acquisita may be confused with hereditary form of EB, BP, LAD, MMP, porphyria and bullous systemic LE.

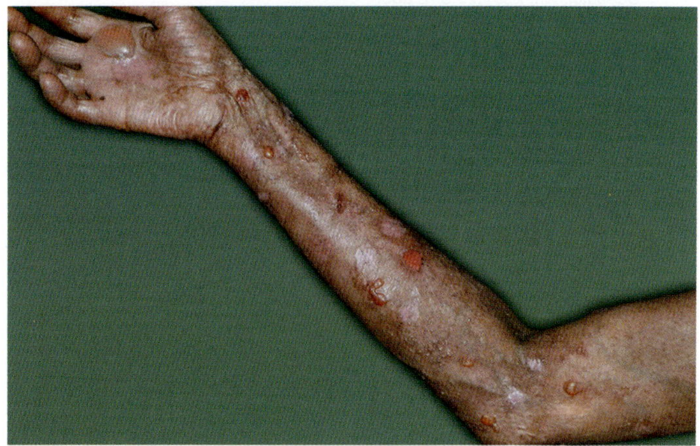

FIG. 9: Tense bullae and milia over upper limb in epidermolysis bullosa acquisita.

**TABLE 8: Salt-split study**

| | |
|---|---|
| Exclusive 'roof' pattern | BP, LAD, MMP, PG |
| Exclusive 'floor' pattern | EBA, MMP (Laminin 332), Laminin γ-1 pemphigoid, bullous systemic lupus erythematosus |
| Combined pattern | BP, LAD, MMP |

BP, bullous pemphigoid; LAD, linear IgA bullous disease; MMP, mucous membrane pemphigoid; PG, pemphigoid gestationis; EBA, epidermolysis bullosa acquisita.

## Diagnosis

Histopathology shows a non- or pauci-inflammatory subepidermal blister in classic EBA. In the inflammatory form, there is neutrophil-rich infiltrate with variable number of eosinophils. DIF demonstrates linear deposition of IgG and less commonly C3, along the BMZ. Deposits of multiple conjugates (IgM, IgA, or properdin) at the BMZ is also more frequently seen in the setting of EBA compared to BP. IIF is either negative or positive in low titer in classic form of the disease. On salt-split skin, antibodies bind to the dermal side ["floor pattern" (Fig. 7)] in contrast to "roof" pattern seen in BP (Table 8).

## Treatment

Treatment of EBA is similar to other AIBD and includes systemic corticosteroids with or without immunosuppressive agents. In general, EBA is more resistant to treatment and may require higher dose of steroids and immunosuppressive drugs than BP.

# LAMININ γ1 PEMPHIGOID (P-200 PEMPHIGOID)

This is newly described subepidermal autoimmune disease in which autoantibodies are directed against laminin γ1, present at the interface between lamina lucida and lamina densa. Clinically, it is indistinguishable from BP. DIF features are similar to BP; IIF on salt-split skin, however, shows a dermal binding ("floor") pattern resembling EBA.

# SUGGESTED READINGS


1. Amann PM, Megahed M. Pemphigus erythematosus. Hautarzt. 2012;63:365-7.
2. Baroni A, Lanza A, Cirillo N, et al. Vesicular and bullous disorders: pemphigus. Dermatol Clin. 2007;25:597-603.
3. Bastuji-Garin S, Joly P, Lemordant P, et al. Risk factors for bullous pemphigoid in the elderly: a prospective case-control study. J Invest Dermatol. 2011;131:637-43.
4. Bonciani D, Verdelli A, Bonciolini V, et al. Dermatitis herpetiformis: from the genetics to the development of skin lesions. Clin Dev Immunol. 2012;239:691.
5. Caux F. Diagnosis and clinical features of epidermolysis bullosa acquisita. Dermatol Clin. 2011;29:485-91.
6. Cheng SW, Kobayashi M, Kinoshita-Kuroda K, et al. Monitoring disease activity in pemphigus with enzyme-linked immunosorbent assay using recombinant desmogleins 1 and 3. Br J Dermatol. 2002;147:261-5.
7. Chhabra S, Minz RW, Saikia B. Immunofluorescence in dermatology. Indian J Dermatol Venereol Leprol. 2012;78:677-91.
8. Clarindo MV, Possebon AT, Soligo EM, et al. Dermatitis herpetiformis: pathophysiology, clinical presentation, diagnosis and treatment. An Bras Dermatol. 2014;89:865-77.
9. Di Zenzo G, Della Torre R, Zambruno G, et al. Bullous pemphigoid: from the clinic to the bench. Clin Dermatol. 2012;30:3-16.
10. Eming R, Hertl M. Autoimmune bullous disorders. Clinc Chem Lab Med. 2006;44:144-9.
11. Frew JW, Murrell DF. Paraneoplastic pemphigus (paraneoplastic autoimmune multiorgan syndrome): clinical presentations and pathogenesis. Dermatol Clin. 2011;29:419-25.
12. Groves RW. Pemphigus: a brief review. Clin Med. 2009;9:371-5.
13. Intong LRA, Murrell DF. Pemphigoid Gestationis: Pathogenesis and Clinical Features. Dermatol Clin. 2011;29:447-52.
14. Junkins-Hopkins JM. Dermatitis herpetiformis: pearls and pitfalls in diagnosis and management. J Am Acad Dermatol. 2010;63:526-8.
15. Khandpur S, Verma P. Bullous pemphigoid. Indian J Dermatol Venereol Leprol. 2011;77:450-5.
16. Kourosh AS, Yancey KB Pathogenesis of mucous membrane pemphigoid. Dermatol Clin. 2011;29:479-84.
17. Monsh B, Groth S, Richter L, et al. A long-term study of a patient with anti-p200 pemphigoid: correlation of autoantibody levels with disease activity and an example of epitope spreading. Br J Dermatol. 2012;167:1179-83.
18. Pohla-Gubo G, Hintner H. Direct and indirect immunofluorescence for the diagnosis of bullous autoimmune diseases. Dermatol Clin. 2011;29:365-72.
19. Porro AM, Caetano Lde V, Maehara Lde S, et al. Non-classical forms of pemphigus: pemphigus herpetiformis, IgA pemphigus, paraneoplastic pemphigus and IgG/IgA pemphigus. An Bras Dermatol. 2014;89:96-106.
20. Rashid KA, Stern JN, Ahmed AR. Identification of an epitope within human integrin alpha 6 subunit for the binding of autoantibody and its role in basement membrane separation in oral pemphigoid. J Immunol. 2006;176:1968-77.
21. Sinha AA. The Genetics of Pemphigus. Dermatol Clin. 2011;29:381-91.
22. Sitaru C, Mihai S, Otto C, et al. Induction of dermalepidermal separation in mice by passive transfer of antibodies specific to type VII collagen. J Clin Invest. 2005;115:870-8.
23. Venning VA. Linear IgA disease: clinical presentation, diagnosis, and pathogenesis. Immunol Allergy Clin North Am. 2012;32:245-53.
24. Venugopal SS, Murrell DF. Diagnosis and clinical features of pemphigus vulgaris. Dermatol Clin. 2011;29:373-80.

# 9 SECTION Pigmentation Disorders

# 23 CHAPTER Nevomelanocytic Nevi

*Nilendu Sarma, Sayantani Chakraborty*

## INTRODUCTION

Nevi are circumscribed, fixed, non-neoplastic cutaneous or mucosal lesions. They occur due to mosaicism. In contrast to epidermal and vascular nevi, melanocytic or nevomelanocytic nevi may have some malignant potential. Melanocytic nevi may be congenital and acquired, atypical, or dysplastic.

Based on onset time, nevomelanocytic nevi is classified into two subtypes—congenital and acquired.

## CONGENITAL MELANOCYTIC NEVI

Congenital melanocytic nevi (CMN) appears at birth. Development may be delayed, within 2 years of life (nevus tardive).

It is characterized by a homogenous color that may darken with age. Variegated color, rough verrucous, or cerebriform surface with papules, and rugosity may indicate benign neurotization of the nevus, but may also be the signs of malignant alteration (Fig. 1).

This is classified based on its size

- Small (<1.5 cm)
- Medium (between 1.5 and 19.9 cm)
- Large or giant (≥20 cm).

Giant variety is also known as bathing trunk nevus, garment nevus, giant hairy nevus, giant pigmented nevus, and nevus pigmentosus and pilosus.

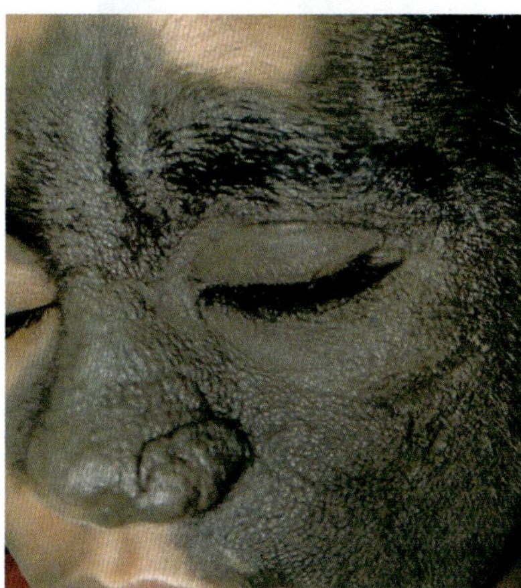

**FIG. 1:** Large congenital melanocytic nevi with rugose surface.

There may be conspicuous sparing of areola, or penis.

The risk of melanoma increases with size of nevi. Risk is very low in small CMN. Presence over trunk, presence of many satellite nevi and giant CMN are considered risk factors. Giant CMN has higher risk of malignancy (51.6% compared to general population).

### Histopathology

Nevus cells are present in the subcutaneous tissue and lower two thirds of the dermis. Cells show "Indian files," or "cords of cells" pattern where single cell extends between the collagen bundles of the reticular dermis. Distributed in and around appendages (hair follicles, sebaceous glands, eccrine apparatus), capillaries, nerves, and arrector pili are typical of CMN.

### Management

Early surgical excision with reconstruction is generally advocated.

## ACQUIRED MELANOCYTIC NEVUS

Acquired melanocytic nevi (AMN) are uncommon. They generally appear after 6 months. Incidence after 3rd decade is very less. Epidermal melanocytes may proliferate along the dermoepidermal junction (junctional nevus) and then migrates to the dermis by the "dropping off" phenomenon (theory of Abtropfung or dropping off of nevus cells by Unna, 1883) maintaining the junctional activity (compound nevus). Junctional activity may gradually diminish and it becomes purely intradermal (dermal nevus). At junctional stage, they are flat. With more intradermal infiltration of nevi, they turn to raised lesions with less intense color and even skin colored papule (Fig. 2).

Acquired melanocytic nevus may be familial. Sun exposure is considered an important risk factor. They are seen in Noonan's syndrome and Turner's syndrome.

Risk of melanoma in AMN is low and prophylactic removal of these lesions is not mandatory. Total number of nevi and presence of atypical nevi are independent risk factors for the development of malignancy.

Nevi on the nail matrix/nail bed leads to formation of a longitudinal brown stripe on under surface of the nail plate. This may mimic melanoma of nail bed. Melanoma is characterized by

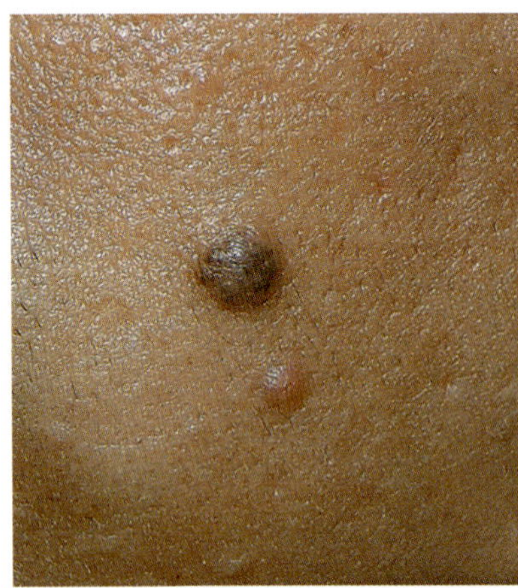

FIG. 2: Dermal mole with gradually fading pigmentation.

variable color, wide proximal diameter due to rapid growth, and extension of the proximal end beyond the proximal nail fold.

## DYSPLASTIC AND ATYPICAL NEVI

Dysplastic nevi (presence of histopathological dysplasia) have higher risk for development of multiple myeloma. They can be sporadic and familial.

Atypical nevus is mainly a clinical description based on the presence of various atypical features of melanoma. They should not be used interchangeably. Clinical atypical features and histological dysplasia may not correlate. Although, melanoma may develop without preceding atypical or dysplastic nevi, their presence increases the risk.

Atypical nevi appear much later, usually around puberty. They may involute with age, but more commonly, they continue to appear throughout the life. They are called atypical because they have features of melanoma (ABCD rule) like asymmetry, border irregularity, color variation, and diameter >6 mm. Tucker described the following clinical features for atypical nevi:

- ≥5 mm in size
- Complete or partially flat surface.

And, two of the following three features:

1. Variable pigmentation
2. Irregular and asymmetrical outline
3. Indistinct borders.

Dermatoscopic examination has become an important tool in evaluation of atypicality and risk of melanoma. Eccentric peripheral hyperpigmentation has been particularly mentioned as rare but highly atypical feature with higher chance of melanoma. Other dermatoscopic features like presence of light brown structure, less area, and central homogeneous pattern with peripheral reticulated network or dots that indicated active growth state are described as markers of higher chance of melanoma. All suspected lesions should be excised for histological confirmation.

In the original description by Clark et al., dysplastic nevus was described to have four main features:

1. Atypical melanocytic hyperplasia
2. Melanocytes with cytological features characteristic of malignant melanocytes
3. Mesenchymal changes in the papillary dermis (eosinophilic fibroplasia)
4. Lymphocytic infiltrate.

Subsequent modifications to these criteria have been done by other groups like the University of Pennsylvania, World Health Organization, the European Organization for Research and Treatment of Cancer, and Duke University.

Definition of dysplastic nevus syndrome (B-K mole syndrome, atypical mole syndrome, and familial atypical multiple-mole melanoma/FAMMM syndrome) is proposed by National Institute of Health Consensus Conference. The criteria are:

- Occurrence of melanoma in one $1^{st}/2^{nd}$ degree relative
- Large number of nevi (often >50), some of which are clinically atypical
- Nevi with certain distinct histopathological features.

## SPECKLED LENTIGINOUS NEVI

Speckled lentiginous nevus (SLN) is possibly a subtype of congenital melanocytic nevus. Developmental defect of the neural crest derived melanoblast possibly results in SLN. This is generally present at birth and appears as café au lait macule. Full development with speckled macules and papules takes more time.

### Clinical Features

There is a diffuse background pigmentation over which there are tiny darker lentigine-like pigmented macules or even papules. Speckled lentiginous nevus may be oval, block-like, zosteriform, or linear. Distribution is along the lines of Blaschko. Darker maculopapular spots are usually distributed evenly (Fig. 3).

This may be a feature of speckled lentiginous nevi syndrome, FACES (facial features, anorexia, cachexia, and eye and skin anomalies) syndrome, Ebstein syndrome, phacomatosis pigmentovascularis (PPV), and phacomatosis pigmentokeratotica (PPK). Speckles of SLN are macular in PPV and papular in PPK. Speckled lentiginous nevus syndrome is characterized by SLN, ipsilateral sensory and/or motor neuropathy, and spinal muscular atrophy or hypertrophy.

In PPK, nevus spilus is associated with an organoid nevus with sebaceous differentiation. Presence of SLN in PPV and PPK is explainable by a mechanism called "twin spotting."

### Histological Features

Histologically, nevus cells are present as nest in the speckled area. They may be distributed in various patterns like lentigines,

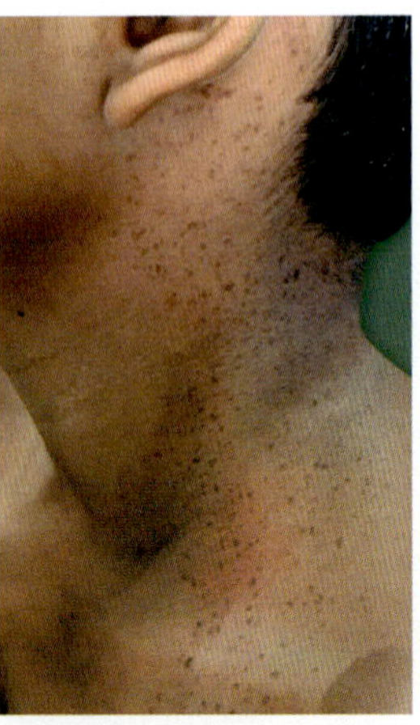

FIG. 3: Speckled lentiginous nevus in a segmental pattern along with a café au lait macule.

junctional, compound or dermal nevi, blue nevi, or even Spitz nevi and features may change with time. When many SLN are present, few may lack background and some may lack pigmentation. Nevus cells that are diagnostic of the condition may be detected even in normally pigmented background areas.

## Differential Diagnosis

This has to be differentiated from agminated lentiginosis and agminated Spitz nevi. These lack background hyperpigmentation.

## Treatment

Lasers like Q-switched ruby, neodymium-doped yttrium aluminum garnet, or alexandrite laser may be used for specked area. Background pigmentation is relatively resistant and may even recur.

# PHACOMATOSIS PIGMENTOVASCULARIS

Phacomatosis pigmentovascularis was described by Ota, Kawanura, and Ito in 1947. There is coexistence of a pigmented nevus and a cutaneous vascular malformation. Nevus flammeus is present in all types of PPV. Phacomatosis pigmentovascularis has been classified into four types on the basis of the type of pigmented nevus (Table 1) (Fig. 4). Phacomatosis pigmentovascularis with only skin manifestation is classified as subtype "a", and those having additional systemic manifestations are classified as subtype "b". Systemic involvement determines the prognosis. A fifth type characterized by cutis marmorata telangiectatica congenita, dermal melanocytosis (with or without nevus spilus) is described.

**TABLE 1: Types of phacomatosis pigmentovascularis**

| | |
|---|---|
| Type I | Nevus flammeus, nevus depigmentosus, and verrucous epidermal nevus |
| Type II | Nevus flammeus, dermal melanocytosis (nevus of Ota/nevus of Ito/aberrant Mongolian spots) with or without nevus anemicus |
| Type III | Nevus flammeus and nevus spilus with or without nevus anemicus |
| Type IV | Nevus flammeus, dermal melanocytosis (nevus of Ota/nevus of Ito/aberrant Mongolian spots), nevus spilus with or without nevus anemicus |

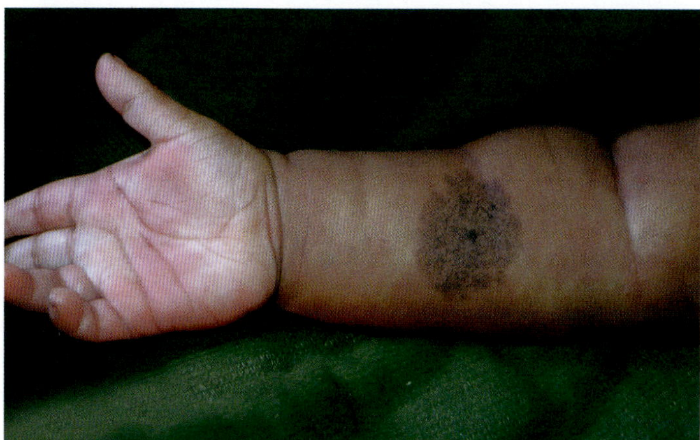

**FIG. 4:** Phacomatosis pigmentovascularis in a child showing presence of nevus flammeaus and nevus spilus.

## Pathogenesis

Simultaneous involvement of melanocytic and vascular abnormality is hypothesized to result from "twin spotting" or didymosis.

## Differential Diagnosis

Sturge-Weber syndrome (nevus flammeus, intracranial and visceral angioma, and seizure), and Klippel-Trenaunay syndrome (nevus flammeus, lymphangioma and/or limb hemihypertrophy).

# SPITZ NEVI

This is a rare type of benign melanocytic lesion. This is seen mostly in children below 14 years of age, but rarely may appear in adults.

In older people, clinical and histopathological differentiation from malignant lesions may be difficult and evaluation should be done very cautiously. For this reason, terms like "atypical Spitz nevus" or "Spitzoid tumor of uncertain biological potential" are sometimes used.

Typically, Spitz nevi appear as single pinkish, erythematous, or dark pigmented or nonpigmented asymptomatic small nodular or dome shaped lesions that grows fast to reach about 1 cm in diameter. Thereafter, growth ceases and it remains stationary for years. Common sites are face, cheeks, and legs. It usually spares palms, soles, and mucous membranes.

Occasionally, it may be multiple, in cluster, eruptive wide spread, larger, and may have atypical symptoms like bleeding and itching.

It mimics melanoma, juvenile xanthogranuloma, pyogenic granuloma, or malignant melanoma.

In dermoscopy, uniform rounded structures with prominent blood vessels is noted. Pigmented streaks may appear as radially with a "starburst pattern". It may also appear structureless or show presence of globular pigmentation.

The lesion is composed of nests of large epithelioid cells and/or spindle-shaped melanocytes with abundant eosinophilic cytoplasm arranged in interlacing bundles or in clusters. Superficial nevus cells may display some mitotic figures but deeper nevus cells display maturation.

Other features are acanthosis, degenerated keratinocytes that may be seen as amorphous pink globules (Kamino bodies) at the dermoepidermal junction.

Ulceration, asymmetry, high number of mitosis, and infiltration into the subcutaneous fat may be seen, which are considered atypical and are termed as "spitzoid melanoma" or "atypical spitzoid tumor of unknown malignant potential".

Histologically, differentiation from malignant melanoma is often very difficult. Immunohistochemistry, fluorescence *in situ* hybridization, and comparative genomic hybridization may aid confirmation and differentiation from melanoma.

Some tumors show recurrence after excision creating diagnostic confusion.

## Treatment

There is no well accepted guideline of management. Some prefer wait and watch policy. Others prefer early excision with 1-2 mm margin. This may result in visible scarring. Presence of atypical feature is often considered indication for early surgery. Some tumors show recurrence after excision.

## SUGGESTED READINGS


1. Clark WH Jr, Reimer RR, Greene M, et al. Origin of familial malignant melanomas from heritable melanocytic lesions. 'The B-K mole syndrome'. Arch Dermatol. 1978;114:732-8.
2. Cribier B, Santinelli F, Grosshans E. Lack of clinical-pathological correlation in the diagnosis of congenital naevi. Br J Dermatol. 1999;141:1004-9.
3. Elder DE, Goldman LI, Goldman SC, et al. Dysplastic nevus syndrome: A phenotypic association of sporadic cutaneous melanoma. Cancer. 1980;46: 1787-94.
4. Groesser L, Herschberger E, Sagrera A, et al. Phacomatosis pigmentokeratotica is caused by a postzygotic HRAS mutation in a multipotent progenitor cell. J Invest Dermatol. 2013;133:1998-2003.
5. Happle R, Hoffmann R, Restano L, et al. Phacomatosis pigmentokeratotica: A melanocytic-epidermal twin nevus syndrome. Am J Med Genet. 1996;65:363-5.
6. Hui P, Perkins A, Glusac E. Assessment of clonality in melanocytic nevi. J Cutan Pathol. 2001;28:140-4.
7. NIH Consensus conference. Diagnosis and treatment of early melanoma. JAMA. 1992;268:1314-9.
8. Quaba AA, Wallace AF. The incidence of malignant melanoma (0 to 15 years of age) arising in "large" congenital nevocellular nevi. Plast Reconstr Surg. 1986;78:174-81.
9. Requena C, Rubio L, Traves V, et al. Fluorescence in situ hybridization for the differential diagnosis between Spitz naevus and spitzoid melanoma. Histopathology. 2012;61(5):899-909.
10. Sarma N, Ankad B. Dermoscopy in Nevoid Disorders. In: Chatterjee M, Neema S, Malakar S eds. Dermoscopy in Darker Skin. Jaypee Brothers Medical Publishers (P) Ltd. New Delhi. 2017, 127-133.
11. Sarma N, Chakraborty S. Birthmarks or clinical significance. In. Sarkar R, Inamadar AC, Palit A. Eds: Advances in Pediatric Dermatology - 2: Neonatal Dermatology. Jaypee Brothers Medical Publishers (P) Ltd. New Delhi. 2014,198-221.
12. Sarma N, Chakraborty S. Nevi and nevoid disorders. In: Inamader AC, Palit A, Rghunatha S. Eds. Textbook of pediatric dermatology, (2nd ed). Jaypee Brothers Medical Publishers (P) Ltd. New Delhi.2014,460-494.
13. Sarma N. Developmental, nevoid, genetically determined and neurocutaneous pigmentary disorders. In: Lahiri K, Chatterjee M, Sarkar R Eds. Pigmentary disorders- A comprehensive compendium. Jaypee Brothers Medical Publishers (P) Ltd. New Delhi.2014,40-52.
14. Sarma N. Pigmentary nevi on face have unique patterns and implications: The concept of Blaschko's lines for pigmentary nevi. Indian J Dermatol. 2012;57: 30-4.
15. Tadini G, Restano L, Gonzales-Perez R, et al. Phacomatosis pigmentokeratotica: Report of new cases and further delineation of the syndrome. Arch Dermatol. 1998;134:333-7.
16. Tannous ZS, Mihm MC, Sober AJ, et al. Congenital melanocytic nevi: Clinical and histopathologic features, risk of melanoma, and clinical management. J Am Acad Dermatol. 2005;52:197-203.
17. Tucker MA, Halpern A, Holly EA, et al. Clinically recognized dysplastic nevi. A central risk factor for cutaneous melanoma. JAMA. 1997;277:1439-44.
18. Vidaurri-de la Cruz H, Happle R. Two distinct types of speckled lentiginous nevi characterized by macular versus papular speckles. Dermatology. 2006; 212:53-8.

# 24 CHAPTER Genetic Pigmentary Disorders

*Gan Yiping Emily, Boon Kee Goh*

## INTRODUCTION

Pigmentary genodermatoses are diverse, ranging from hypo- to hyperpigmented to mixed pigmentary disorders. They can occur as isolated traits or form components of inherited syndromes.

## APPROACH TO THE CLASSIFICATION OF GENETIC PIGMENTARY DISORDERS

Flowchart 1 is a summary table of various genetic pigmentary disorders classified according to clinical morphology. This serves as a practical tool for clinicians when handling patients with suspected inherited pigmentary disorders.

## SPECIFIC MORPHOLOGIES

### Café au lait Macules

Café au lait macules (CALMs) are well circumscribed, round or oval, uniformly pigmented brown patches, which range from light classic coffee-colored to darker brown tones with smooth or jagged border, the latter described as a "coast of Maine" appearance. CALMs are commonly seen at birth or in early infancy and have been described in up to 36% of the general population. Histologically, CALMs demonstrate increased melanin within melanocytes and basal keratinocytes without melanocytic proliferation.

Café au lait macules are characteristically found in several syndromes, the most common of which is neurofibromatosis type 1 (NF1) (Table 1). However, most have no associated abnormalities.

Various lasers such as the Q-switched ruby, frequency doubled Q-switched neodymium:yttrium aluminum garnet (Nd:YAG) and erbium-doped yttrium aluminium garnet (Er:YAG) lasers have been used to treat CALMs but responses can be unpredictable.

### Poliosis

Poliosis is defined as circumscribed hypomelanosis of hair, which can involve any hair-bearing area of the body, including the scalp, eyebrows, and eyelashes. Histologically, there is decreased or absent melanin and/or melanocytes in the hair bulbs of the affected hair follicles.

Poliosis may be seen in Piebaldism and Waardenburg syndrome. It can however also occur in many acquired conditions such as Vitiligo and Vogt–Koyanagi–Harada syndrome, neoplastic lesions and rarely may be drug-induced (Table 2).

## DIFFERENT GENETIC PIGMENTARY CONDITIONS

### Oculocutaneous Albinism

Oculocutaneous albinism (OCA) is a group of rare congenital diseases characterized by poor vision and a variable hypopigmentation phenotype. Syndromic forms of albinism (e.g., Hermansky–Pudlak and Chediak–Higashi syndromes) also exist.

#### Pathogenesis

Mutations in various genes affecting melanin biosynthesis are responsible for OCA. This includes genes that encode key melanogenic enzymes (*TYR* and *TYRP1*), specific receptor/solute carrier/integral proteins found in melanosomes (*OCA2, SLC45A2, GPR143*), and a large family of proteins involved in the biogenesis of lysosome-related organelles such as melanosomes (*HPS1, AP3B1, HPS3* etc). More recently, a locus mapped to 4q24 human chromosomal region, *SLC24A5* and *C10orf11* have been respectively identified as genes causing the following new subtypes of albinism, OCA5, OCA6, and OCA7. OCA is mostly inherited in an autosomal recessive manner except for one autosomal dominant form and an X-linked recessive OA.

#### Clinical Features

Pigmentation of the skin, hair, and eyes is variably reduced in the different types of OCA. All types of OCA and OA have similar ocular findings, including congenital nystagmus, iris hypopigmentation and translucency, reduced pigmentation of the retinal pigment epithelium, foveal hypoplasia, reduced visual acuity, impaired color vision, and photophobia (Fig. 1). Misrouting of the optic nerves can lead to strabismus and reduced stereoscopic vision. Patients with OCA1A (tyrosinase negative), have the highest susceptibility to sunburn, actinic damage, and malignant skin tumors (basal and squamous cell carcinomas, melanomas). These are almost always seen in affected young adults and may present in childhood if the skin and eyes are not protected.

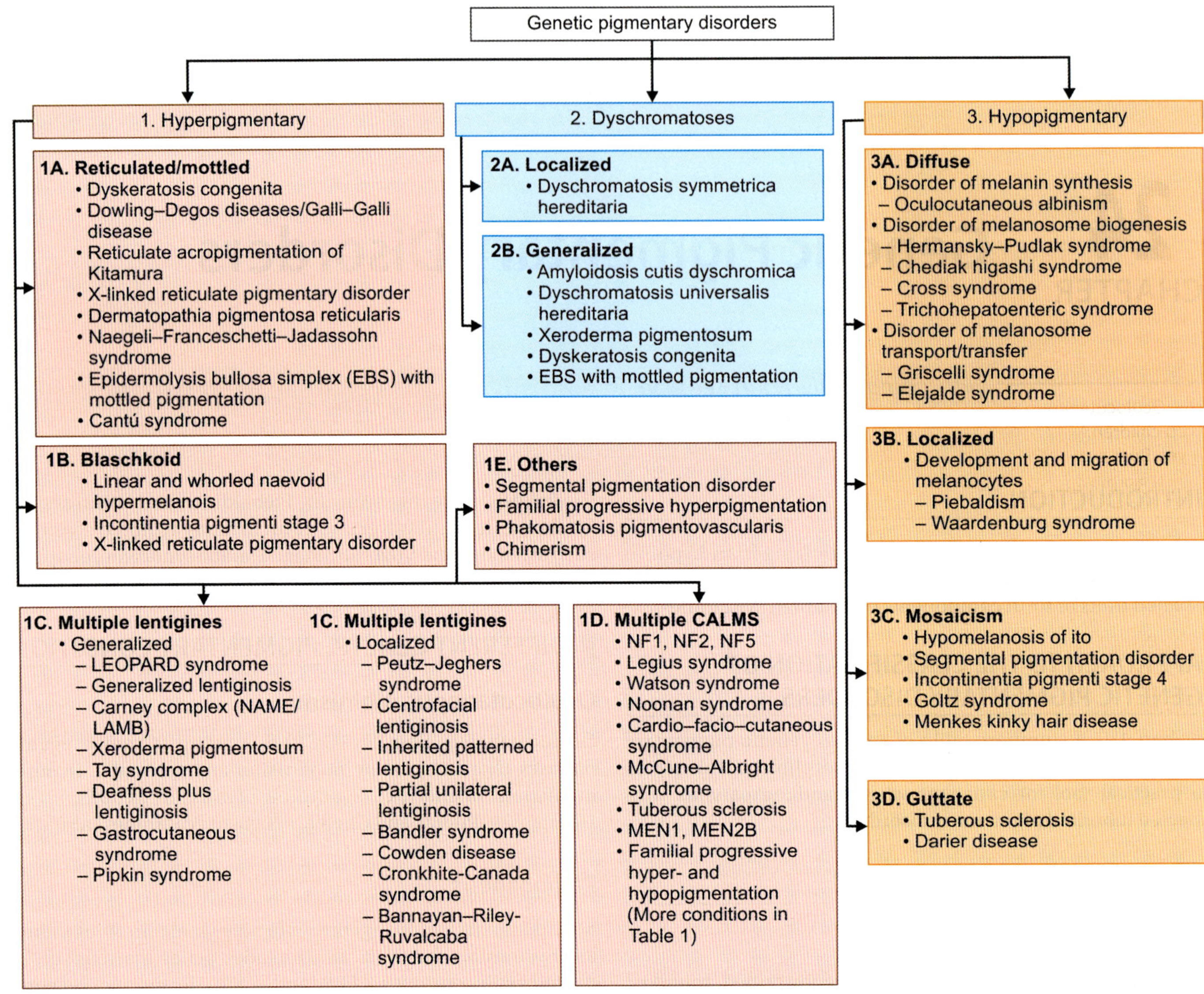


CALM, Café au lait macule.

**FLOWCHART 1:** Classification of genetic pigmentary disorders according to clinical morphology.

**TABLE 1: Disorders with multiple café au lait macules**

| Neurofibromatosis (NF) and related disorders | Other disorders |
|---|---|
| • NF1, NF2, NF5 (segmental NF)<br>• Legius syndrome (NF-1 like syndrome)<br>• Watson syndrome<br>• Noonan syndrome<br>• Cardiofaciocutaneous syndrome<br>• Juvenile xanthogranulomas with multiple CALMs | • McCune–Albright syndrome<br>• Tuberous sclerosis<br>• Familial progressive hyper- and hypopigmentation<br>• LEOPARD syndrome<br>• Partial unilateral lentiginosis<br>• Ataxia telangiectasia<br>• Bannayan–Riley–Ruvalcaba syndrome<br>• Bloom syndrome<br>• Fanconi's anemia<br>• Russell–Silver syndrome<br>• Multiple endocrine neoplasia 1 and 2B |

CALMs, Café au lait macules.

**TABLE 2: Disorders associated with poliosis**

| Congenital | Acquired |
|---|---|
| • Piebaldism<br>• Waardenburg syndrome<br>• Tuberous sclerosis<br>• Neurofibromatosis type 1<br>• Isolated white forelock<br>• Isolated occipital white lock (X-linked recessive)<br>• White forelock with osteopathia striata (autosomal or X-linked dominant)<br>• White forelock with multiple malformations (autosomal or X-linked recessive)<br>• Marfan syndrome<br>• Tietze syndrome<br>• Prolidase deficiency | • Vitiligo<br>• Vogt–Koyanagi–Harada syndrome<br>• Alopecia areata<br>• Alezzandrini syndrome<br>• Post-inflammatory or post-traumatic<br>• Sarcoidosis (associated with uveitis)<br>• Neoplastic–congenital and acquired melanocytic nevi, melanoma, neurofibromas<br>• Drug induced, e.g., topical prostaglandin analogs, topical Imiquimod, topical chloramphenicol and systemic administration of acitretin, chloroquine, cetuximab or tumor-infiltrating lymphocyte immunotherapy |

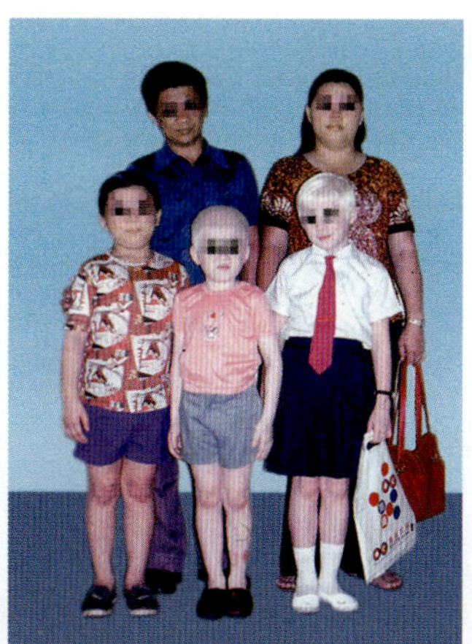

FIG. 1: Oculocutaneous albinism. This figure shows a family with two affected children, who have OCA1 and loss of pigment in their skin, hair, and eyes. Both parents and one brother are unaffected.
*Courtesy*: National Skin Centre, Singapore

### Diagnosis

This is essentially clinical supported by molecular diagnosis.

### Management

Genetic counseling and sun protection are important. Carrier detection and prenatal diagnosis are possible when mutations are known.

## Hermansky–Pudlak Syndrome

Hermansky-Pudlak syndrome (HPS) is a rare autosomal recessive genodermatosis with 9 subtypes (HPS-1 through HPS-9). HPS-1 is the most common HPS subtype, accounting for 50% of non-Puerto Rican cases and occurring at a frequency of 1 in 1,800 in northwest Puerto Rico, attributed to founder effects.

### Pathogenesis

Hermansky-Pudlak syndrome is due to mutations in genes (*HPS1, AP3B1, HPS3* to *HPS8, PLDN*) leading to defects in the formation or function of lysosome-related organelles, such as melanosomes in melanocytes, platelet dense granules, lung lamellar bodies and/or lytic granules of cytotoxic T-cells. HPS gene products have been identified as subunits of at least three multiprotein complexes, named biogenesis of lysosome-related organelles complex (BLOC)-1 to -3. Deficiency of any of these BLOC complexes influences intracellular protein trafficking.

### Clinical Features

It is characterized by oculocutaneous albinism (pigment dilution of the skin, hair, and eyes) and platelet storage disease with additional variable manifestations. Other findings are restrictive lung disease, granulomatous colitis, neutropenia, recurrent infections (HPS-2 and HPS-9), conductive hearing loss, epistaxis, easy bruising and metastatic cutaneous granulomatous involvement.

### Diagnosis

Diagnosis can be made by a wet mount electron microscopic examination of platelets demonstrating absent or greatly decreased numbers of platelet dense granules. Ophthalmologic examination is also useful, whereby iris transillumination, fundus hypopigmentation, presence of nystagmus and reduced visual acuity can be demonstrated. Confirmation of diagnosis and subtyping of HPS is carried out by molecular analysis demonstrating mutation in one of the HPS genes.

### Management

There is currently no cure for HPS. Patients with HPS are managed with symptomatic treatment. Variable response to desmopressin (1-desamino-8-D-arginine vasopressin, DDAVP) treatment has been reported for bleeding time correction.

# SILVERY HAIR SYNDROMES: CHEDIAK–HIGASHI SYNDROME, GRISCELLI SYNDROME

## Chediak–Higashi Syndrome

Chediak-Higashi syndrome (CHS) is a rare autosomal recessive congenital immunodeficiency syndrome caused by mutations in *CHS1*. Less than 500 cases have been reported worldwide in the last 20 years.

### Pathogenesis

The *CHS1* gene encodes the protein CHS1, which is thought to be involved in regulating lysosome-related organelle size, fission, and secretion. The exocytic pathway of secretory lysosomes is defective and plasma membrane repair mechanisms are impaired. CHS patients have profound defects in the function of neutrophils, platelets, cytotoxic and NK cells and giant inclusion bodies occur in virtually all granulated cells.

### Clinical Features

Chediak-Higashi syndrome is a heterogeneous disorder, characterized by variable degrees of oculocutaneous albinism, recurrent pyogenic infections, enhanced tendency for bruising and neurologic dysfunction. A speckled or diffuse hyperpigmentation of sun-exposed skin may rarely be seen in the darker skin phototypes, leading to delay in diagnosis. Hair color may be blond, gray or white, often with a silvery or metallic sheen. The accelerated phase of CHS, termed hemophagocytic lymphohistiocytosis (HLH), develops in 50–85% of patients within the first decade of life and is lethal unless allogeneic transplantation is performed. About 10–15% of patients have a less severe clinical course. They demonstrate subtle hypopigmentation, a lower frequency of infections, mild bleeding manifestations and survive until adulthood without going through an accelerated phase. During adolescence and adulthood, they however develop progressive neurologic dysfunction, including dementia, peripheral neuropathy and parkinsonism.

### Diagnosis

Correlation between clinical features and laboratory findings are important. Giant granules are seen in neutrophils (also in lymphocytes and natural killer cells) on peripheral blood smear, derived from the coalescence of azurophilic and secondary granules. Bone marrow aspirates show large azurophilic or eosinophilic cytoplasmic inclusion bodies in cells of myeloid lineage which react strongly to peroxidase staining. Hair microscopy reveals evenly distributed small granular melanin aggregates along the hair shaft. Molecular genetic testing of *CHS1* provides the definitive diagnosis.

Important differential diagnoses include other hypopigmentation disorders with immunodeficiency, such as Griscelli syndrome type 2, HPS-2, HPS-9 and MAPBP-interacting protein deficiency syndrome.

### Management

Multidisciplinary management is needed. Hematopoietic stem cell transplantation (HSCT) is a definitive therapy. However, there is no evidence that it is efficacious in delaying or preventing progressive neurologic dysfunction. Granulocyte colony-stimulating factor (G-CSF) can be used to improve neutropenia and reduce infections. Aspirin and nonsteroidal inflammatory drugs (NSAIDs) should be avoided.

## Griscelli Syndrome

Griscelli syndrome (GS) is characterized by pigmentary dilution of the skin and hair with variable cellular and humoral immunodeficiency. It is a rare autosomal recessive disorder with three subtypes.

### Pathogenesis

Griscelli syndrome 1 results from mutations in *MYO5A* gene. Griscelli syndrome 2 is caused by mutations in *RAB27A* gene and GS3 is due to *MLPH* gene mutations. Myosin Va is expressed in melanocytes and neurons, and binds the actin cytoskeleton at one end and an organelle, such as a melanosome at the other end. In melanocytes it has a key role in the transfer of melanosomes from melanocytes to keratinocytes. RAB27A is a small Ras-like GTPase, one of the key regulators of intracellular vesicular trafficking and modifies the exocytosis of cytolytic granules in cytotoxic T lymphocytes and natural killer cells. It is expressed in hematopoietic cells and melanocytes. The *MLPH* gene encodes melanophilin which links myosin Va to RAB27A, and this is only expressed in melanocytes.

### Clinical Features

All three subtypes of GS are characterized by pigmentary dilution of the skin and silvery-gray hair due to pigment clumping within melanocytes (Fig. 2). Patients with GS1 exhibit primarily neurological impairment. GS2 patients have recurrent episodes of fever and lymphohistiocytic infiltration of organs, triggered by viral infections. In most GS2 patients, the development of HLH (accelerated phase) occurs from 6 to 12 months of age. GS3 patients only demonstrate diffuse pigmentary dilution and silvery hair. Cetica et al. recently reported the absence of skin pigmentary dilution in six patients with familial HLH, of whom, only 2 had "light" or "blond" hair. They had novel RAB27A mutations, which did not impair the interaction between melanophilin and RAB27A, therefore accounting for the difference in phenotype.

### Diagnosis

A history of parental consanguinity and familial deaths should be sought for. Light microscopic examination of hair shafts

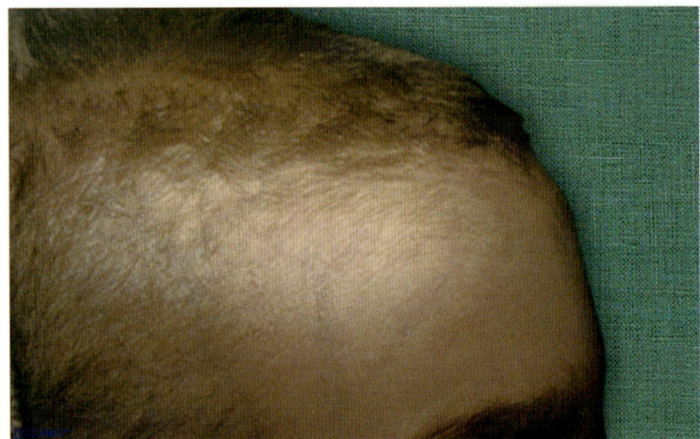

**FIG. 2:** Griscelli syndrome. Close-up view of the light silvery hair in a Caucasian male patient.

*Courtesy*: Professor Jo Lambert, Department of Dermatology, Ghent University Hospital, Belgium.

shows large, unevenly distributed melanin aggregates. Electron microscopic examination of skin specimens shows epidermal melanocytes filled with numerous stage IV melanosomes with few melanosomes in adjacent keratinocytes. Giant granules are absent in peripheral leukocytes.

### Management

In GS2 patients, HLH is treated with immunosuppressive therapy for palliation of symptoms or for induction of remission till definitive treatment with HSCT is performed.

## Piebaldism

Piebaldism is a rare autosomal dominant disorder with leukoderma and poliosis on the frontal scalp, forehead, ventral trunk and extremities.

### Pathogenesis

Most cases of piebaldism are due to mutations in the *KIT* gene which affect melanoblast migration in the embryo, leading to significant or complete loss of melanocytes in the ventral white patches and white hair. Phenotypic severity correlates with the site and type of mutation in the *KIT* gene.

Mutation of the *SLUG* gene on chromosome 8 has also been implicated. The *SLUG* gene encodes Slug, a zinc-finger neural crest transcription factor critical for development of melanoblasts, hematopoietic stem cells and germ cells.

### Clinical Features

The depigmented patches and areas of poliosis are congenital, spare the posterior midline and are typically symmetrical, found on the central anterior trunk and mid extremities, forehead and scalp (white forelock of poliosis), the areas of leukoderma milk-white, irregular in shape but well demarcated. Normally pigmented and hyperpigmented macules and patches are present within the leukodermic patches (Fig. 3). The most distinctive feature of piebaldism is the white forelock, present in up to 90% of affected individuals. However, its absence does not exclude the diagnosis. Multiple CALMs and intertriginous freckling may be present. Loss of function of SPRED1

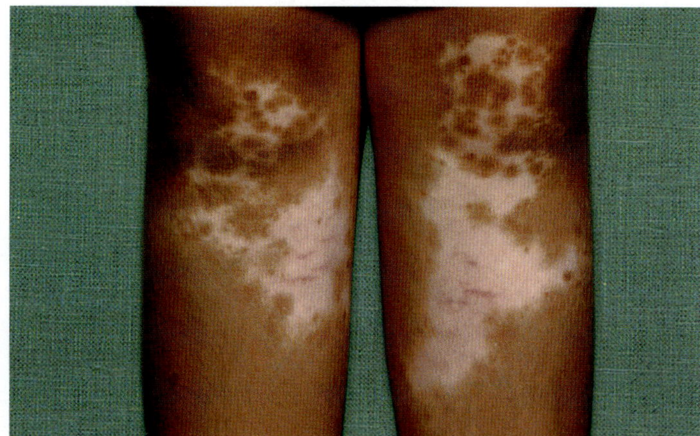

**FIG. 3:** Piebaldism. Depigmented patches on the extensor aspects of both knees and shins with concomitant leukotrichia in affected sites, in an 8-year-old female. The islands of normally pigmented macules within the leukoderma are a hallmark of piebaldism.

*Courtesy*: National Skin Centre, Singapore.

(Sprouty-related, Ena/vasodilator-stimulated phosphoprotein homology-1 domain containing protein 1) due to inadequate phosphorylation of the KIT-binding domain by KIT is believed to be the cause of the hyperpigmented lesions in these individuals.

### Diagnosis

Histological examination shows absence of melanocytes in the interfollicular epidermis and the hair follicles of the amelanotic skin. The hyperpigmented areas in contrast are characterized by an abundance of melanosomes in the melanocytes and keratinocytes.

### Management

Genetic counseling is important. Grafting of the amelanotic areas has been carried out in patients with piebaldism, resulting in successful repigmentation.

## Waardenburg Syndrome

Waardenburg syndrome (WS) is an uncommon genetic disorder or neurocristopathy due to mutations in genes that affect neural crest cells. It accounts for 2–5% of cases of congenital deafness and gives rise to pigmentation abnormalities of the skin, hair, and iris.

### Pathogenesis

Waardenburg syndrome is genetically heterogeneous, with six genes known to be involved (*PAX3, MITF, SOX10, EDN3, EDNRB, SNAI2*) (Table 3). *PAX3* gene encodes the paired box 3 transcription factor, which is a DNA-binding transcription factor expressed in neural crest cells. It is important in the migration and differentiation of melanocytes, which originate from the embryonic neural crest. *MITF* (microphthalmia-associated transcription factor) gene encodes a key transcription factor, MITF, in melanocyte development; *SOX10* (Sry bOX10) encodes an important transcription factor which regulates neural crest development, stem cell maintenance and cell lineage progression. The *EDN3* gene encodes endothelin-3, which controls the migration of neural crest cells, including those that migrate to the Auerbach plexus.

**TABLE 3: Waardenburg syndrome (WS)—four subtypes**

| WS type | Inheritance | Genes involved | Clinical findings |
|---|---|---|---|
| I | AD | *PAX3* | Piebald-like hypopigmented patches, heterochromia irides, broad nasal root, dystopia canthorum, sensorineural deafness, synophrys |
| II | AD | *MITF, SNAI2* | WS I without dystopia canthorum. Most likely to have sensorineural deafness |
| III | AD | *PAX3* | WS I plus musculoskeletal abnormalities |
| IV | AR | *EDN3, EDNRB, SOX10* | WS I plus Hirschsprung's disease |

### Clinical Features

The classical features are that of a white forelock, hypertrophy of the nasal root, sensorineural deafness and partial or total heterochromia of the iris. Additional features, such as lateral displacement of the medial canthi (dystopia canthorum), limb musculoskeletal defects and Hirschsprung disease are found in specific subtypes (Table 3).

### Diagnosis

Early diagnosis and institution of multidisciplinary care is needed with prompt referrals to the otorhinolaryngologist, audiologist and ophthalmologist. A combination of clinical features increases suspicion for the diagnosis of WS. Molecular genetic analysis determines the exact genes involved and therefore the specific subtype of WS.

### Management

No curative treatment is available for WS. Other specialists, such as the orthopedic surgeon and general surgeon can manage their respective limb and gastrointestinal anomalies appropriately.

## Hypomelanosis of Ito

Hypomelanosis of Ito is a condition of genetic mosaicism represented by lines of blaschkoid hypopigmentary changes. The term "blaschkoid dyspigmentation" has been recently suggested as an umbrella name that encompasses the group of blaschkoid hyper- and hypopigmentation disorders.

### Pathogenesis

Genetic mosaicism resulting in pigmentary changes along Blaschko's lines can arise from a multitude of genetic defects, including chromosomal nondysjunction, lyonization, and chimerism. The extent of cutaneous involvement and risk of extracutaneous anomalies increases when mutations occur early in fetal development.

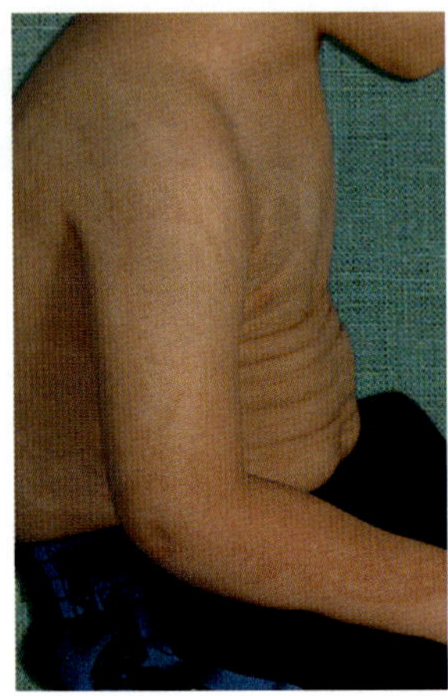

FIG. 4: Hypomelanosis of Ito. Swirls of hypopigmented macules are present along the lines of Blaschko on the left upper limb and trunk of this 5-year-old Chinese male.

*Courtesy*: National Skin Centre, Singapore.

### Clinical Features

Clinically, patients have macular hypopigmentation following lines of Blaschko, giving rise to a whorled shape on the trunk, a V-shape on the back and waves on the vertex scalp (Fig. 4). It has been associated with extracutaneous defects like mental retardation, epilepsy, learning disabilities, vesicoureteric reflux, musculoskeletal deformities and ophthalmological abnormalities.

### Diagnosis

The diagnosis is made clinically, based on the presence of hypopigmented macules along the lines of Blaschko.

### Management

No specific treatment is available for the hypopigmentation.

## Tuberous Sclerosis

Tuberous sclerosis complex (TSC) is a genetic disease with variable manifestations in multiple organs, including cognitive impairment, seizures, and hamartomas of the skin, brain, eyes, kidneys, heart, and lungs. The birth incidence is estimated to be 1:5800.

### Pathogenesis

Mutations in either *TSC1* or *TSC2*, which are genes encoding hamartin (*TSC1*) and tuberin (*TSC2*), are known to cause TSC. The two proteins form a regulatory complex that is responsible for limiting the activity of an important intracellular regulator of cell growth and metabolism known as mammalian target of rapamycin complex 1 (mTORC1) via inhibition of the small GTPase ras homolog enriched in brain (Rheb).

### Clinical Features

Tuberous sclerosis complex can affect multiple organs and these manifestations have typical ages of onset and periods for regression, stabilization and in some cases, spontaneous resolution. Here we will focus on the skin and oral manifestations.

Hypomelanotic macules typically present within the first few years of life, remain stable for decades and become less obvious in late adulthood. This takes the form of the typical ash-leaf macule and/or generalized guttate hypopigmented macules. Angiofibromas start to appear at 3–4 years of age, increasing in adolescence and stabilizing in adulthood. A large shagreen patch is characteristic of TSC but sometimes patients may present with multiple collagenomas, usually appearing in early to mid-childhood. Subungual fibromas usually appear late, typically during adolescence or adulthood. Some patients also develop multiple CALMs. Intraoral fibromas are a less specific finding in TSC and if acquired, are usually multiple and secondary to antiepileptic medications, such as phenytoin.

### Diagnosis

According to the recommendations of the 2012 International Tuberous Sclerosis Complex Consensus Conference, a definite diagnosis of TSC requires at least 2 major features or 1 major and 2 or more minor features (Table 4). A pathological mutation in *TSC1* or *TSC2* in normal tissue is now diagnostic, independent of clinical manifestations. However, genetic testing may not identify a mutation in up to 25% of patients with TSC and a normal gene test does not exclude the disease.

### Management

Genetic testing and counseling must be offered. Dermatologists should collaborate with a geneticist, pediatrician, internist, or relevant specialist to ensure that the various organs systems are managed appropriately.

Intervention may be indicated for TSC skin or oral lesions which are bleeding, symptomatic, disfiguring or disturbing function. Options include surgical excision, pulsed dye laser to

**TABLE 4: Clinical diagnostic criteria for tuberous sclerosis complex**

| | |
|---|---|
| Major features | • Angiofibromas (≥3) or fibrous cephalic plaque<br>• Hypomelanotic macules (≥3, at least 5 mm in diameter)<br>• Ungual fibromas (≥2)<br>• Shagreen patch<br>• Multiple retinal hamartomas<br>• Cortical dysplasias<br>• Subependymal nodules<br>• Subependymal giant cell astrocytoma<br>• Cardiac rhabdomyoma<br>• Lymphangioleiomyomatosis*<br>• Angiomyolipomas (≥2)* |
| Minor features | • Dental enamel pits (≥3)<br>• Intraoral fibromas (≥2)<br>• "Confetti" skin lesions<br>• Nonrenal hamartomas<br>• Multiple renal cysts<br>• Retinal achromic patch |

*A combination of lymphangioleiomyomatosis and angiomyolipomas without other features does not meet criteria for a definite diagnosis.

reduce erythema or use of a mammalian target of rapamycin (mTOR) inhibitor.

Case studies or case series have shown promising results with topical sirolimus for facial angiofibromas with decreased erythema and flattening of the lesions and complete resolution in some individuals, especially children. Oral forms of mTOR inhibitors, such as sirolimus or everolimus may be considered on a case-by-case basis, for individuals whose facial angiofibromas pose serious medical risk, such as recurrent bleeding or obstructed nasal breathing or where surgical risks outweigh the risks of mTOR inhibitors. The hypopigmented macules have also been treated with topical rapamycin in a small study of 6 patients, noting improvement which started at 12 weeks.

## Darier Disease

Darier disease is an autosomal dominant genodermatosis with several characteristic mucocutaneous findings.

The disease usually presents before the age of 30 years with a peak onset at puberty. Guttate leukoderma is a lesser known feature of Darier disease. This observation has however been described in Chinese, Malay, Japanese, and individuals of Negroid-African descent. In a patient with a lighter skin type, this may be easily missed as the hypopigmented macules are inconspicuous (Fig. 5).

## Neurofibromatosis Type 1

Neurofibromatosis type 1 is an autosomal dominant, multisystem disorder which affects 1 in 3,500 persons. Almost half of the cases are due to spontaneous mutations and the rest are inherited. There is 100% penetrance by age 20. Expressivity can be highly variable even among family members with the same mutation.

### Pathogenesis

The *NF1* gene is located on chromosome 17q11.2 and encodes the tumor suppressor protein neurofibromin. Neurofibromin is a regulator of Ras guanosine triphosphatase activity (GTPase-activating protein), controlling signals for cell proliferation and differentiation. Loss of function of neurofibromin leads to uncontrolled cell proliferation involving primary neurons, glial, Schwann cells and melanocytes.

### Clinical Features

The first sign of NF1 is frequently the CALM, which occurs in 99% of NF1 patients within the first year of life (Fig. 6). These CALMs may fade in adulthood. Skin fold freckling (in either the axillae and/or groin) is the most specific of the cardinal criteria for NF1 and is nearly pathognomonic. Generalized hyperpigmentation has also been noted. Cutaneous neurofibromas usually do not become apparent until puberty and are progressive. Blue-red macules and pseudoatrophic macules have been reported to represent unusual variants of cutaneous neurofibromas, appearing before or during puberty, primarily on the trunk. Plexiform neurofibromas are congenital and may be accompanied by overlying hyperpigmentation, hypertrichosis or thickening of the skin.

Other reported associated cutaneous findings are generalized pruritus, juvenile xanthogranuloma, multiple glomus tumors, melanoma, and nevus anemicus.

Other organ systems can be affected. This includes the skeletal (e.g., dysplasia of the long bone or sphenoid), neurologic (learning disabilities are the most common complication in NF1 children), ophthalmologic (Lisch nodules and optic glioma), cardiovascular, endocrine and gastrointestinal systems.

Legius syndrome, formerly known as NF1-like syndrome, has been recently described, where patients have multiple CALMs, with or without freckling and an absence of typical NF1-associated tumors, such as neurofibromas, optic pathway gliomas and Lisch nodules. This is due to a mutation in the *SPRED1* gene.

### Diagnosis

There are seven cardinal diagnostic criteria for NF1, of which two must be met in order to diagnose an individual with NF1.

### Management

Currently, neurofibromas can be managed by surgical removal. Sirolimus (mTOR inhibitor) should not be considered a treatment

**FIG. 5:** Darier disease. Widespread guttate hypopigmented macules on the central chest of this Malay male with the characteristic erythematous keratotic papules of Darier disease.
*Courtesy*: National Skin Centre, Singapore.

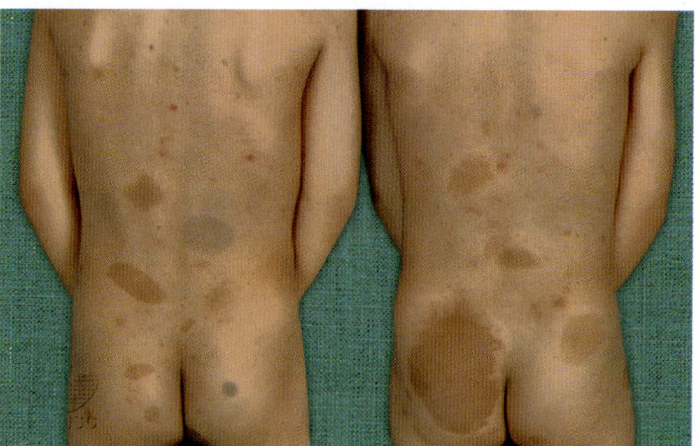

**FIG. 6:** Neurofibromatosis type 1. This is a pair of six-year-old identical twin boys with multiple café au lait macules of varying sizes, soft skin-colored neurofibromas and concomitant Mongolian blue spots.
*Courtesy*: National Skin Centre, Singapore.

option for plexiform neurofibromas. Imatinib mesylate, on the other hand, has shown some improvement in shrinking the volume of plexiform neurofibromas in NF1.

## Peutz–Jeghers Syndrome

Peutz–Jeghers syndrome (PJS) is a hamartomatous polyposis syndrome characterized by mucocutaneous melanosis, polyposis of the gastrointestinal tract, luminal gastrointestinal cancer, and extraintestinal cancer.

### Pathogenesis

Peutz-Jeghers syndrome is inherited in an autosomal dominant manner. Germline mutations can be found in *STK11*, which is a tumor suppressor gene affecting the mTOR pathway.

### Clinical Features

Patients often present in infancy or early childhood with mucocutaneous pigmentations, rectal bleeding, intestinal invagination, and anemia. Dark brown to gray macules occur in 95% of patients on the lips, buccal mucosa, palate, tongue, acral, and perianal areas (Fig. 7). The pigmented macules may fade after puberty but tend to persist on the buccal mucosa. Hamartomatous polyps may occur anywhere along the gastrointestinal tract and also extra-intestinally, e.g., in the gallbladder, bronchi, urinary bladder, and ureter. There is an increased risk of visceral malignancy including small intestinal, colon and pancreatic adenocarcinomas.

### Diagnosis

Diagnosis of PJS requires presence of one of four criteria:

1. Two or more histopathologically confirmed hamartomatous polyps
2. Any number of PJS polyps in an individual who has a family history of PJS in close relative(s)
3. Characteristic mucocutaneous pigmentation in an individual who has a family history of PJS in close relative(s)
4. Any number of PJS polyps in an individual who also has characteristic mucocutaneous pigmentation.

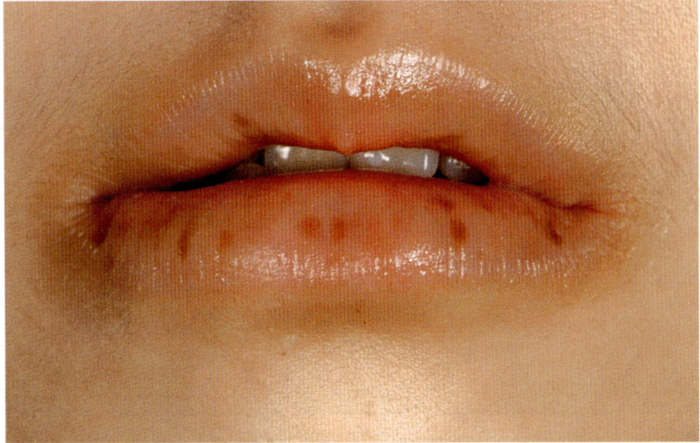

**FIG. 7:** Peutz–Jeghers syndrome. Multiple hyperpigmented macules on the upper and lower lips of an affected female.
*Courtesy*: National Skin Centre, Singapore.



### Management

Periodic surveillance for gastrointestinal polyps and lifelong cancer surveillance is recommended. Genetic counseling should be performed for all patients and their families. Q-switched laser or intense pulsed light can be considered for the pigmented lesions. Rapamycin, an mTOR inhibitor, has shown promising results in mouse models of Peutz-Jeghers, for effective suppression of polyposis, representing a potential new treatment target.

## Dyskeratosis Congenita

Dyskeratosis congenita (DKC) is a rare genodermatosis and inherited bone marrow failure syndrome characterized by a triad of reticular pigmentation, nail dystrophy, and oral leukoplakia. Most cases are males but carrier females with X-linked disease may have limited mucocutaneous findings.

### Pathogenesis

Dyskeratosis congenita is a disease of defective telomere maintenance and can be inherited in X-linked, autosomal dominant or autosomal recessive patterns. Mutations in at least 10 telomere and telomerase associated genes have been described including *DKC1* which encodes dyskerin, *TERC* (telomerase RNA component) and *TERT* (telomerase). There is premature telomere shortening and subsequent replicative senescence leading to premature stem cell exhaustion and tissue failure.

### Clinical Features

The onset of symptoms and signs usually occurs in childhood. Dystrophic nail changes comprise ridging, longitudinal grooving, shortening and pterygium formation. Skin changes present as reticulated grayish-brown hyperpigmentation with surrounding hypopigmented atrophic, telangiectatic patches, predominantly affecting the face, neck, shoulders, upper back, and thighs (Fig. 8). The mucous membranes are affected too, with leukoplakia and rarely blisters and erosions of the oral and anal mucosae, conjunctivae, esophagus, and urethra. Resultant atresia of lacrimal ducts, epiphora, chronic blepharitis, conjunctivitis, and ectropion can occur. Periodontitis may develop and there is increased incidence of cutaneous malignancy, predominantly squamous cell carcinoma in areas of leukoplakia.

Dyskeratosis congenita is a multisystem disease and numerous systemic complications may occur, such as bone marrow failure, pulmonary fibrosis, liver cirrhosis, osteoporotic fractures, avascular necrosis, dysphagia, corneal abrasions and infections.

Patients are predisposed to malignancies, with an increased risk for squamous cell carcinoma and hematolymphoid neoplasms.

### Diagnosis

Diagnosis is based on two of four major features of the disease (mucocutaneous triad and bone marrow failure) and at least two multisystem features of the disease. Screening for DKC is best performed by analyzing telomere lengths via flow cytometry and fluorescence in situ hybridization of leukocyte subsets. Genetic analysis for *DKC* genes should then be carried out in individuals

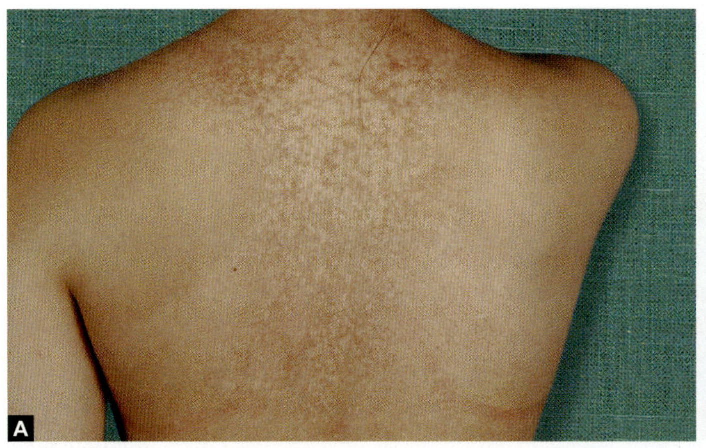


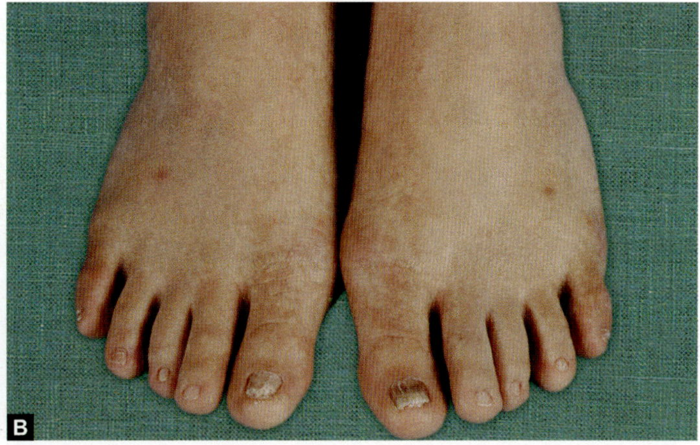


**FIG. 8:** Dyskeratosis congenita. **A,** Reticulated grayish-brown hyperpigmentation with surrounding atrophic, telangiectatic macules on the upper back of an affected 24-year-old female; **B,** Reticulated hyperpigmentation on the dorsum and sides of the feet with concomitant nail abnormalities in the same patient. Nail changes in dyskeratosis congenita comprise ridging, longitudinal grooving, shortening, and pterygium formation.
*Courtesy*: National Skin Centre, Singapore.

with telomere lengths below the first percentile of telomere length in healthy controls.

### Management

Allogeneic hematopoietic stem cell transplantation is the only curative treatment for bone marrow failure. Oral or topical retinoids may be useful for the leukoplakia. Lifelong surveillance for early detection of mucocutaneous malignancies should be enforced.

## Dowling–Degos Disease

Dowling–Degos disease (DDD) is an autosomal dominant genodermatosis, also known as reticulate pigment anomaly of the flexures.

### Pathogenesis

Loss-of-function mutations have been detected in the *KRT5* gene (12q13.13) and more recently, various mutations in the *POGLUT1* and *POFUT1* genes have been described.

### Clinical Features

It can affect both sexes, with onset typically in the third to fourth decades of life. Affected individuals develop a progressive reticulate hyperpigmentation with small keratotic dark-brown papules which affect the flexures mainly, but can also spread to involve the face, trunk and extremities (Fig. 9). Pitted acneiform facial scars, epidermal cysts and genital or perianal reticulated pigmented lesions have also been described. Hidradenitis suppurativa and reticulate acropigmentation of Kitamura have been associated with DDD.

Galli–Galli disease is the rare acantholytic variant of DDD and is characterized by reticulated hyperpigmentation predominantly affecting the flexures along with pruritic, erythematous, scaly papules in the same distribution, as well as on the trunk and proximal extremities.

### Diagnosis

In DDD, the typical histopathological features are presence of elongated and branched (antler-like) epidermal rete ridges with increased melanin at the tips of the rete ridges and preservation of melanocyte number. In Galli–Galli disease, focal suprabasal acantholysis without dyskeratosis is observed.

### Management

Genetic counseling is important. Treatment is generally unsatisfactory. Topical corticosteroids can be used to relieve pruritus. Erbium:YAG laser ablation has been reported to have good clinical results in anecdotal cases.

## Reticulate Acropigmentation of Kitamura

Reticulate acropigmentation of Kitamura (RAPK) is an uncommon genodermatosis with majority of reported cases coming from Japan, although there have been cases reported worldwide. There is an autosomal dominant pattern of inheritance and a high penetration rate.

### Pathogenesis

Truncating, splice site, and missense loss-of-function mutations in the *ADAM10* gene, which encodes a zinc metalloprotease, a disintegrin and metalloprotease domain-containing protein 10 (ADAM10), have been found in patients with RAPK. ADAM10 is involved in the ectodomain shedding of various skin substrates including E-cadherin, N-cadherin, CD30, L1 cell adhesion molecule (L1-CAM), CD44 and IL-6R. Mutations in *POFUT1* have been shown to underlie the genetic defect in patients with DDD-RAPK clinical overlap.

### Clinical Features

The age of onset is during childhood or in the first to second decades of life. Hyperpigmented, sharply demarcated, atrophic

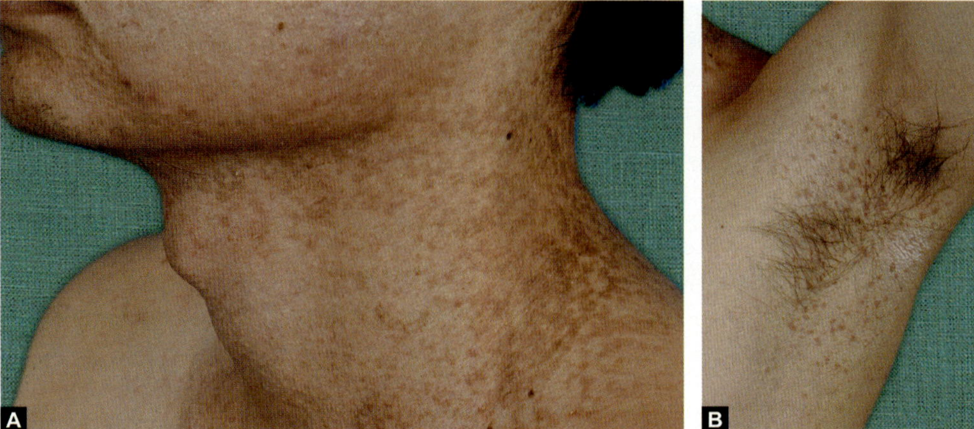

FIG. 9: Dowling–Degos disease. **A,** There are hyperpigmented macules in a reticulate distribution on the neck and lower cheeks, with multiple scattered small keratotic dark-brown papules. In this case, subsequent histological analysis confirmed that this patient had the acantholytic variant of Dowling–Degos disease, Galli–Galli disease; **B,** Reticulate hyperpigmentation and keratotic papules on the axilla of a 28-year-old male.
*Courtesy*: National Skin Centre, Singapore.

macules appear in a reticular pattern on the dorsa of the hands and feet and then spread proximally along the limb to the trunk, darkening over time. There is an absence of hypopigmented macules. Palmoplantar pitting and disrupted dermatoglyphics may also be present. Overlaps cases of RAPK and DDD have been described.

## Diagnosis

Light microscopic examination of the brown macules shows pigmentation at the tip of rete ridges with epidermal thinning, elongation and thinning of rete ridges and slight hyperkeratosis without parakeratosis. There is sparse dermal inflammatory infiltrate and no pigmentary incontinence.

## Management

There is no consistently effective treatment for this condition. Reports have however shown improvement with topical azelaic acid and the 532 nm Q-switched Nd:YAG laser.

# X-linked Reticulate Pigmentary Disorder

X-linked reticulate pigmentary disorder with systemic manifestations, originally called familial cutaneous amyloidosis or X-linked cutaneous amyloidosis, was first described in a Canadian family in 1981. So far, four families, three multiplex with affected relative pairs and one singleton have been reported in the literature.

## Pathogenesis

Genetic linkage studies have mapped the mutated gene to the interval chromosome Xp22.11-21.3. However, the exact gene remains unknown. It is believed that the mutation is most likely within the linked interval, not affecting currently annotated coding exons. In females, penetrance is incomplete and manifestations are limited to the skin.

## Clinical Features



Affected males develop generalized, reticulate hyperpigmentation in early childhood with coarse, unruly hair, upswept eyebrows, and hypohidrosis. Extracutaneous manifestations include corneal dyskeratosis with photophobia, failure to thrive, chronic pulmonary disease, and colitis. In females, there is patchy linear hyperpigmentation in a blaschkoid distribution, morphologically resembling stage III incontinentia pigmenti (Fig. 10). This manifests at birth or a few weeks thereafter and may fade in adulthood.

## Diagnosis

The histopathology of affected skin in females and males is similar although the changes are not specific. Histological findings include increased epidermal melanin, pigmentary incontinence, dermal melanophages and dyskeratosis. The presence of amyloid deposits has been sometimes reported.

## Management

Genetic counseling is important in this condition. Comanagement with the pediatrician is required for the various complications seen in affected males.

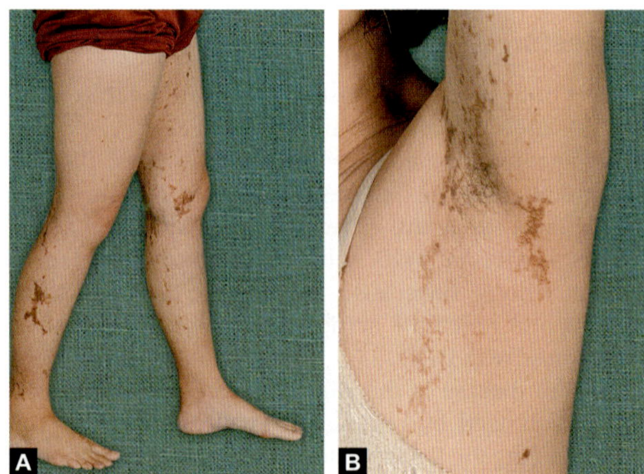

FIG. 10: X-linked reticulate hyperpigmentary disorder. **A,** Hyperpigmented macules and papules in a blaschkoid distribution on the legs of a 47-year-old female; **B,** Blaschkoid streaky hyperpigmentation in the left axilla of the same patient.
*Courtesy*: National Skin Centre, Singapore.

## Dermatopathia Pigmentosa Reticularis

Dermatopathia pigmentosa reticularis (DPR) is an autosomal dominant ectodermal dysplasia syndrome with reticulated hyperpigmentation, hypo- or aplastic dermatoglyphics, palmoplantar keratoderma, hypohidrosis and developmental anomalies of the teeth, hair, and skin. It is allelic to Naegeli–Franceschetti–Jadassohn syndrome (NFJS).

### Pathogenesis

Mutations in keratin 14 (*KRT 14*) are responsible for this condition. Both nonsense and missense mutations have been reported to occur. The hyperpigmentation may be related to melanosome trafficking or due to basal keratinocyte apoptosis leading to pigmentary incontinence.

### Clinical Features

Patients present with dark-brown macular hyperpigmentation at birth or in early childhood (usually by about 2 years of age), which coalesces to form a reticulate pattern and is typically found on the neck, trunk and proximal limbs (Fig. 11). The pigmentation persists throughout life. Other dermatological findings include hypo- or hyperhidrosis, reduced dermatoglyphics, onychodystrophy, diffuse or punctate palmoplantar hyperkeratosis, acral skin fragility, mucosal pigmentation and fine punctate superficial corneal spots.

### Diagnosis

Diagnosis is based on a combination of clinical features and supported by genetic testing with a positive mutation in *KRT14* (Fig. 11).

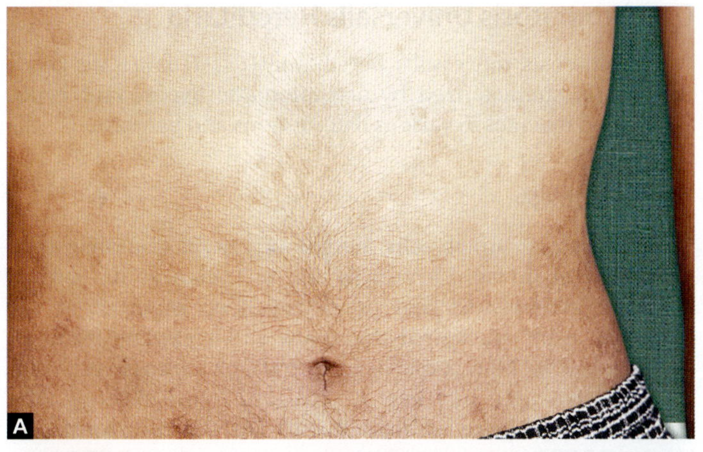


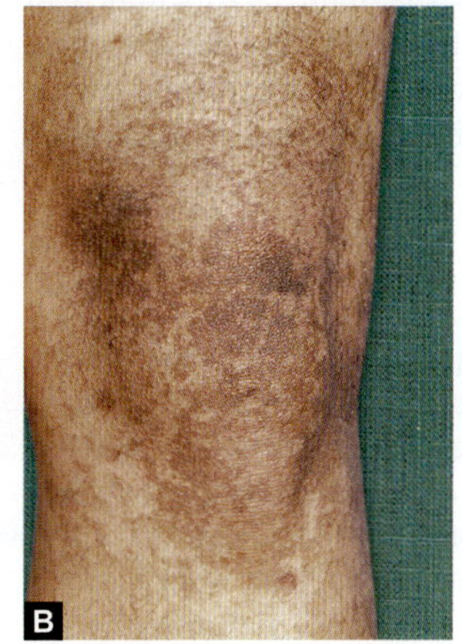


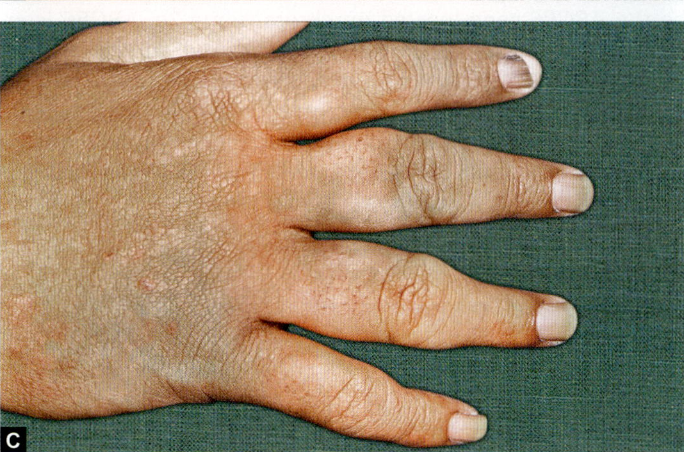


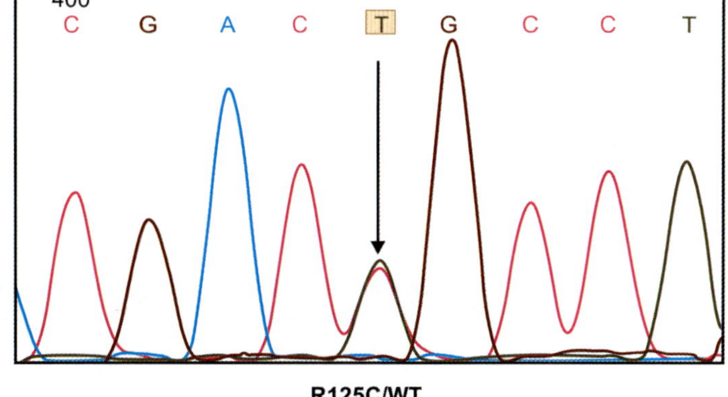


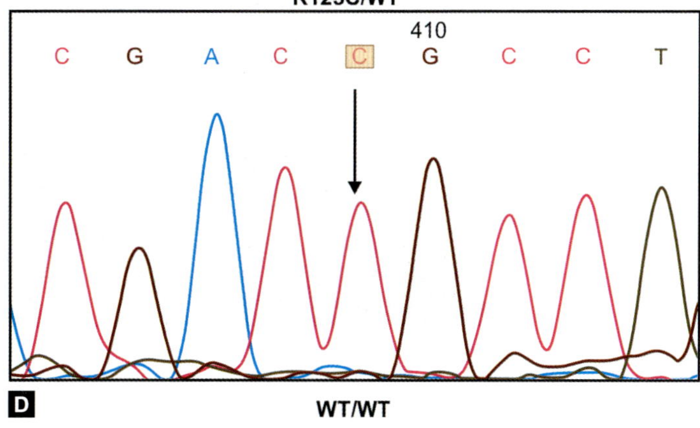


**FIG. 11:** Dermatopathia pigmentosa reticularis (DPR). **A,** Blotchy hyperpigmentation on the lower abdomen of a 20-year-old Malay male. Figures 11B and 11C highlight the various clinical features in this patient; **B,** Coalescent hyperpigmented macules on the knee with a "splashed paint" appearance. **C,** Fusiform fibromatous skin thickening of the digits with healing erosions present on the dorsum of the hand, highlighting the skin fragility in this condition. **D,** In this patient, genetic analysis of *KRT14* showed a heterozygous nucleotide change of c373C -> T (arrows), resulting in the amino acid change p.R125C. This was a sporadic case of DPR.

*Courtesy*: National Skin Centre, Singapore

### Management

No specific treatment is available for DPR. Topical retinoids and keratolytics may be beneficial for the hyperkeratosis. The nonscarring blisters are usually transient and self-healing.

## Amyloidosis Cutis Dyschromica

Amyloidosis cutis dyschromica (ACD) is a rare subtype of primary cutaneous amyloidosis characterized by generalized hyper- and hypopigmented macules (i.e., dyschromatosis) and lichenoid papules. There may be a positive family history.

### Pathogenesis

Amyloidosis cutis dyschromica is a familial disorder with unclear pathogenesis. Environmental factors, such as excessive sun exposure and a genetic predisposition have been suggested to be the underlying trigger and cause. Genetic factors may lead to reduced repair of ultraviolet B induced damage, keratinocyte destruction and triggering of apoptosis. After keratinocyte death, phagocytosis of cytokeratin by histiocytes or fibroblasts leads to amyloid formation.

### Clinical Features

Patients usually present before puberty with non-pruritic generalized hyper- and hypopigmented macules in the absence of systemic features. Lichenoid papules may be present on the trunk and extremities, which also demonstrate amyloid deposits on biopsy (Fig. 12). In some patients, simultaneous manifestation of the various morphological subtypes of primary cutaneous amyloidosis may be seen, including lichen amyloidosis, "dyschromic amyloidosis" and even bullous and poikilodermatous forms.

### Diagnosis

Histological examination of a hyperpigmented macule reveals deposition of an amorphous eosinophilic material in the papillary dermis with increased melanin in the basal layer and pigmentary incontinence in the papillary dermis. The eosinophilic masses stain positively with Congo red stain and demonstrate apple-green birefringence under polarized light.

### Management

Variable success has been reported with different treatment modalities used in ACD. Systemic retinoids have been reported to show some efficacy. Retinoids are potent inducers of apoptosis and therefore decrease the amount of apoptotic basal keratinocytes available for transformation into amyloid and also stimulate macrophages to phagocytose and remove amyloid deposits in the dermis. Avoidance of excessive sun exposure, and use of sunscreen, keratolytics, topical corticosteroids, capsaicin, dimethyl sulfoxide, and carbon dioxide laser have been tried with variable results.

## Dyschromatosis Universalis Hereditaria

Dyschromatosis universalis hereditaria (DUH) is a rare genodermatosis characterized by asymptomatic hyper- and hypopigmented macules in various distributions and patterns.

### Pathogenesis

Dyschromatosis universalis hereditaria is attributable to a deficiency of melanin synthesis and/or melanosome sorting. Different genetic loci had previously been reported in the literature, with autosomal dominant and recessive forms of DUH linked to 6q24.2-q25.2 and 12q21-q23 respectively, but no causative gene had been found until more recently. The first pathologic gene associated with DUH is now known to be the *ABCB6* gene located on chromosome 2q. ABCB6 is an ATP-binding cassette transporter expressed in the human epidermis and also in exosomes. The melanosome transport machinery is related to exosome secretion as many melanogenic proteins are sorted in exosomes. Therefore, a mutant ABCB6 protein is thought to disrupt melanosome transport and cause DUH.

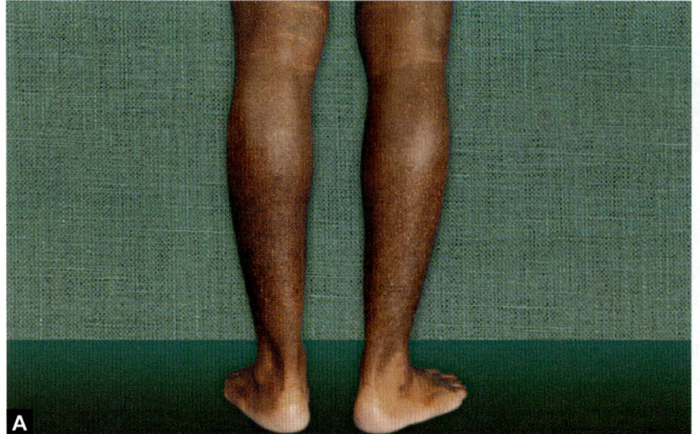


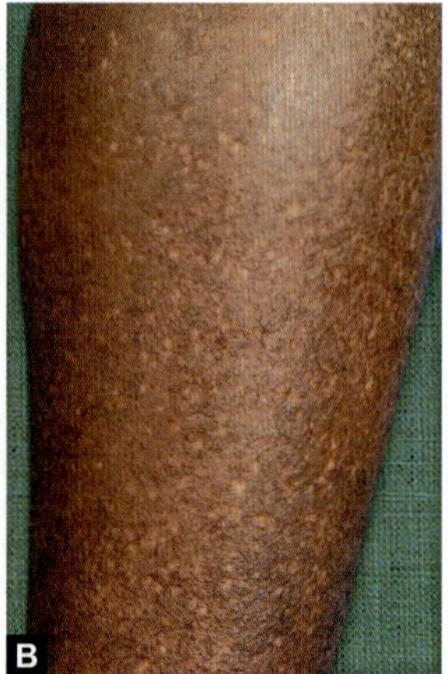


**FIG. 12:** Amyloidosis cutis dyschromica. **A,** Both hyper- and hypopigmented macules are distributed on the lower legs of this Indian male, who has a strong family history of this condition; **B,** Close-up view of the leg shows the hyper- and hypopigmented macules interspersed with lichenoid papules, a known feature of this condition.
*Courtesy*: National Skin Centre, Singapore

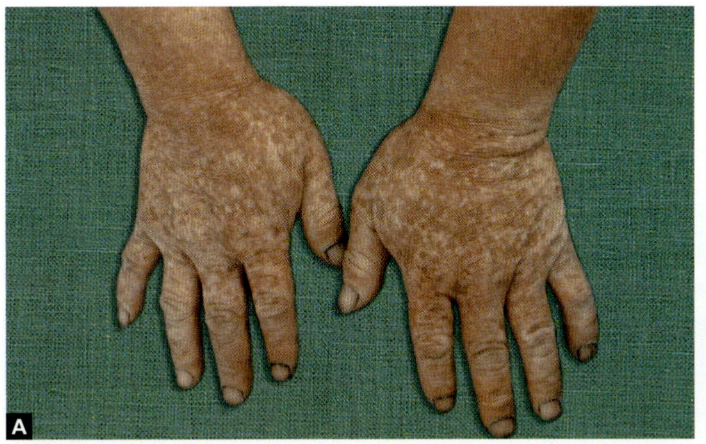

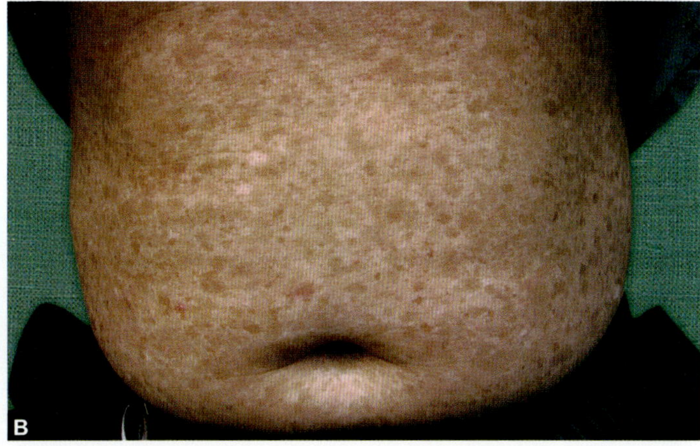

FIG. 13: Dyschromatosis universalis hereditaria. **A,** Numerous hyper- and hypopigmented macules of varying sizes on the dorsum of the hands of this middle-aged patient; **B,** Asymptomatic hyper- and hypopigmented macules predominantly distributed on the abdomen of a Chinese male patient.

*Courtesy*: Dr Zhang Furen, Shandong Provincial Institute of Dermatovenereology, China.

### Clinical Features

Affected individuals develop asymptomatic hyper- and hypopigmented macules of irregular size and shape, in a generalized distribution on the trunk, limbs, and face (Fig. 13). These lesions arise in infancy or early childhood. The trunk and extremities are the dominant sites with the skin changes and facial lesions are seen in about 50% of affected individuals. Abnormalities of the hair and nails have also been reported. Most DUH patients do not have systemic abnormalities although there have been cases in the literature with other features, such as ocular abnormalities, high tone deafness, mental retardation, learning difficulties, epilepsy, and short stature.

### Diagnosis

Diagnosis is established based on clinical features. A skin biopsy can be carried out to exclude other dyschromatoses, such as ACD. A focal increase or decrease in the melanin content of the basal layer is seen in the hyper- and hypopigmented areas, respectively.

### Management

There is no specific treatment for this disorder.

## Xeroderma Pigmentosum

Xeroderma pigmentosum (XP) is a rare autosomal recessive disorder of DNA repair with 100% penetrance. It is characterized by photosensitivity, an increased risk of UV radiation-induced skin and mucous membrane cancers and in some patients, progressive neurological degeneration.

### Pathogenesis

Classical XP patients have a defect in one of eight genes. The products of seven of these genes (*XPA* through to *XPG*) are involved in the repair of UV-induced photoproducts in DNA by the process of nucleotide excision repair (NER). Defects in the eighth XP gene (*XPV* gene) do not affect NER. The *XPV* gene encodes DNA polymerase, one of the specialized enzymes required for replication past damaged sites (translesion synthesis). XP-C is the most common subtype worldwide, comprising 25–40% of cases.

### Clinical Features

The skin is normal at birth. Patients may either present with exaggerated responses to ultraviolet radiation (UVR), with significant burning and blistering on minimal exposure to sunlight or have a normal acute response to sun exposure. All patients develop "freckling" in sun-exposed areas, typically before the age of 2 years. With time, this evolves into poikiloderma. The UVR exposed areas of the skin, tongue, and eyes have an increased cancer risk (e.g., melanoma). Other ocular abnormalities include keratitis with corneal opacification and vascularization and photophobia. They are at increased risk of cancers of the brain and other organs of the central nervous system.

Progressive neurological degeneration is seen in roughly 25% of XP patients. These patients have defects in the *XPA, XPB, XPD* or *XPG* genes. The first clinical signs are usually absent deep tendon reflexes and high-frequency hearing loss. Other abnormalities include delayed developmental milestones, progressive intellectual impairment, loss of ability to walk, and difficulty swallowing.

### Diagnosis

The most commonly used test for defective DNA repair involves taking a skin and the measurement of unscheduled DNA synthesis in cultured skin fibroblasts. XP variants do not show this defect in unscheduled DNA synthesis, however caffeine specifically sensitizes XP-V cells to killing by UV. Therefore, to diagnose XP-V cells, fibroblast cultures are exposed to UV, incubated in caffeine for a few days and their viability is compared to that of normal cells.

### Management

Genetic counseling and psychological support are crucial in the management of XP patients and their families. There are numerous XP support groups worldwide, e.g., Enfants de la Lune in France. Photoprotective measures, such as use of sunscreens, custom-made face shields, UV dosimeters and protective UV-resistant film on windows together with restriction of outdoor activities to the night reduce overall UV exposure. Quarterly surveillance for skin cancer by a dermatologist is recommended.

High-dose oral retinoids such as isotretinoin, have been used to reduce the rate of development of skin cancers in XP patients but the use is limited due to side effects including bone abnormalities, mucocutaneous toxicity, abnormal lipid and liver function tests. Lambert et al. recently proposed using topical 5-fluorouracil and topical imiquimod as prophylactic treatments for XP-induced skin cancers, however further clinical studies are needed to provide more evidence for efficacy.

## Phakomatosis Pigmentovascularis

Phakomatosis pigmentovascularis (PPV) refers to the association of a vascular nevus with an extensive pigmentary nevus.

### Pathogenesis

The genetic model explaining PPV is twin spotting or didymosis (from the Greek didymos = twin). Twin spots are two different cutaneous lesions that are adjacent to each other, formed by mutant tissues that also differ from the rest of the normal tissue surrounding them and believed to appear as a result of loss of the cells' genetic heterozygosity.

### Clinical Features

A new classification for PPV was recently proposed by Happle and divides PPV into four groups:

- Phakomatosis cesioflammea - Mongolian blue spot and nevus flammeus
- Phakomatosis spilorosea - Nevus spilus and pale-pink nevus
- Phakomatosis cesiomarmorata - Mongolian blue spot and cutis marmorata telangiectatica congenita
- Unclassifiable PPV.

The vascular component is generally extensive in PPVs. For the pigmentary component, in phakomatosis cesioflammea, the pigmentary nevus can correspond to nevus of Ota, nevus of Ito or Mongolian blue spot. The most common dermal melanoses in the published literature are aberrant Mongolian blue spots and nevus of Ota (Fig. 14). In the unclassifiable PPV, large café-au-lait spots have been described.

Other reported cutaneous findings are nevus anemicus, generalized vitiligo and congenital triangular alopecia. Systemic involvement occurs in 50% of patients and includes ocular anomalies (ocular melanosis), neurologic anomalies and vascular anomalies such as Sturge-Weber and Klippel-Trenaunay syndromes.

### Diagnosis

The diagnosis of PPV is primarily clinical.

### Management

Phakomatosis pigmentovascularis without systematic complications is benign and requires no treatment. Nevus flammeus can be treated with a pulsed dye laser and the pigmentary nevi can be treated with Q-switched lasers.

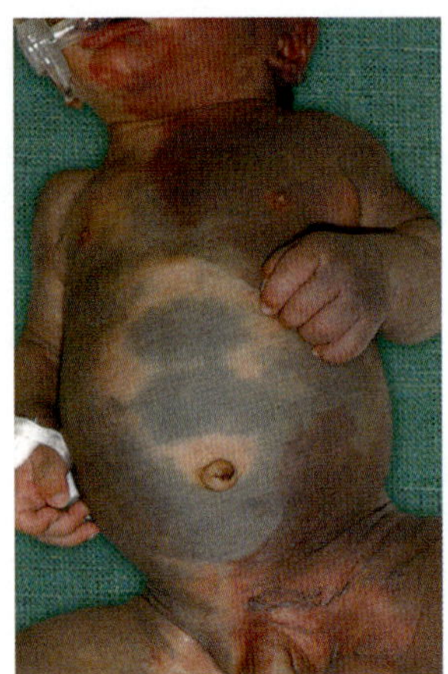

**FIG. 14:** This baby has a large port wine stain or nevus flammeus involving the left side of the face and trunk as well as left upper and lower limb. He also has extensive dermal pigmentation (Mongolian blue spot) involving the trunk and four limbs.

*Courtesy*: Dr Mark Koh, Dermatology Service, KK Women's and Children's Hospital, Singapore.

## CONCLUSION

Our understanding of the diverse range of inherited pigmentary disorders has improved over the years with the advances in genetic research. Unfortunately, there are no specific treatments for many of these disorders. It is important to carry out genetic counseling for families of affected individuals and to carefully exclude syndromes or systemic features in all cases of inherited pigmentary disorders.

## ACKNOWLEDGMENTS

We would like to thank Professor Jo Lambert (Department of Dermatology, Ghent University Hospital, Belgium) for contributing Figure 3, Dr Zhang Furen (Shandong Provincial Institute of Dermatovenereology, China) for figure 13 and Dr Mark Koh (Dermatology Service, KK Women's and Children's Hospital, Singapore) for figure 14.

## SUGGESTED READINGS

1. Bradford PT, Goldstein AM, Tamura D, et al. Cancer and neurologic degeneration in xeroderma pigmentosum: long term follow-up characterises the role of DNA repair. J Med Genet. 2011;48:168-76.
2. Brems H, Legius E. Legius syndrome, an update. Molecular pathology of mutations in SPRED1. Keio J Med. 2013;62:107-12.
3. Cetica V, Hackmann Y, Grieve S, et al. Patients with Griscelli syndrome and normal pigmentation identify RAB27A mutations that selectively disrupt MUNC13-4 binding. J Allergy Clin Immunol. 2015;135:1310-8.
4. Dokai I. Dyskeratosis congenita. Hematology Am Soc Hematol Educ Program. 2011;2011:480-6.
5. Fassihi H. Spotlight on xeroderma pigmentosum. Photochem Photobiol Sci. 2013;12:78-84.
6. Horner ME, Abramson AK, Warren RB, et al. The spectrum of oculocutaneous disease: Part I. Infections, inflammatory, and genetic causes of oculocutaneous disease. J Am Acad Dermatol. 2014;70:795.e1-25.

7. Kiss K, Brozik A, Kucsma N, et al. Shifting the paradigm: the putative mitochondrial protein ABCB6 resides in the lysosomes of cells and in the plasma membrane of erythrocytes. PLoS One. 2012;7:e37378.
8. Kono M, Sugiura K, Suganuma M, et al. Whole-exome sequencing identifies ADAM10 mutations as a cause of reticulate acropigmentation of Kitamura, a clinical entity distinct from Dowling-Degos disease. Hum Mol Genet. 2013;22:3524-33.
9. Krueger DA, Northup H, International Tuberous Sclerosis Complex Consensus Group. Tuberous sclerosis complex surveillance and management: recommendations of the 2012 International Tuberous Sclerosis Complex Consensus Conference. Pediatr Neurol. 2013;49:255-65.
10. Landau M, Krafchik BR. The diagnostic value of café-au-lait macules. J Am Acad Dermatol. 1999;40:877-90.
11. Lozano ML, Rivera J, Sanchez-Guiu I, et al. Towards the targeted management of Chediak-Higashi syndrome. Orphanet J Rare Dis. 2014;9:132.
12. Montoliu L, Gronskov K, Wei AH, et al. Increasing the complexity: new genes and new types of albinism. Pigment Cell Melanoma Res. 2013;27:11-8.
13. Northrup H, Krueger DA, International Tuberous Sclerosis Complex Consensus Group. Tuberous sclerosis complex diagnostic criteria update: recommendations of the 2012 International Tuberous Sclerosis Complex Consensus Conference. Pediatr Neurol. 2013;49:243-54.
14. Oiso N, Fukai K, Kawada A, et al. Piebaldism. J Derm. 2013;40:330-5.
15. Salvaggio HL, Graeber KE, Clarke LE, et al. Mucocutaneous granulomatous disease in a patient with Hermansky-Pudlak syndrome. JAMA Dermatol. 2014;150:1083-7.
16. Sarma N, Chakraborty S, Bhanja DC, et al. Piebaldism with non-intertriginous freckles: what does it mean? Indian J Dermatol Venereol Leprol. 2014;80(2):163-5.
17. Teng JM, Cowen EW, Wataya-Kaneda M, et al. Dermatologic and dental aspects of the 2012 International Tuberous Sclerosis Complex Consensus Statements. JAMA Dermatol. 2014;150:1095-101.
18. van Steensel MA, Lemmink HH. A missense mutation in KRT14 causing a dermatopathia pigmentosa reticularis/Naegeli-Franceschetti-Jadassohn phenotype. J Eur Acad Dermatol Venereol. 2010;24:1116-7.
19. Wataya-Kaneda M, Tanaka M, Yang L, et al. Clinical and histological analysis of the efficacy of topical rapamycin therapy against hypopigmented macules in Tuberous sclerosis complex. JAMA Dermatol. 2015;151:722-30.

# 25 CHAPTER Vitiligo

*Nilendu Sarma*

## INTRODUCTION

Vitiligo is an acquired, hypopigmentation disorder that occurs due to progressive loss of melanocytes caused by multiple factors those are mostly unknown. This is the most common hypopigmentation disorder observed in clinical practice. Worldwide, its prevalence is 0.5–1% among general population, but this may be as high as 8%. It affects both sexes almost equally. Vitiligo has tremendous psychological impact on the sufferers especially in the darker races.

## PATHOGENESIS

Since many years, vitiligo is suggested to be mediated through autoimmune and cytotoxic mechanisms, biochemical destruction through defective metabolism leading to abnormal free radical collection within the cell or some neuroendocrine or cytokine induced exaggerated, and abnormal inflammatory response. Significant advances have been made in our understanding in this field. Presence of various autoantibodies is regularly detected in vitiligo patients. Thyroid abnormality and antithyroid antibodies are commonly detected. These findings have been the basis of autoimmune destruction theory of vitiligo. However, our knowledge has progressed much beyond this simple theory. Pathogenesis of vitiligo is now understood to be more complex process than initially thought. Various proposed mechanisms work in an interconnected and orchestrated fashion that finally culminate into targeted destruction of melanocytes.

Initiating event of melanocyte destruction in vitiligo is yet to be identified. Many believes damage of the melanocytes is the primary event that results in development of a cascade of pathway leading to widespread subsequent melanocytic destruction through autoimmune and cytotoxic mechanism. Mechanisms through which melanocytic antigens are expressed may result from external (trauma, infection) or internal factors (abnormal redox status). Subsequent to this, antibodies are formed against melanocytes, also a nonspecific proinflammatory state develops. The latter seems to aggravate the development of autoimmunity which further lead to more damage.

Presence of dendritic cells, interleukin (IL)-17 cells, and cytotoxic CD8+ cells are present in and around vitiligo patches indicating the lesional proinflammatory status. Interleukin-17 cells that are stimulated by the dendritic cells are also detected further suggesting the active role of dendritic cells in the development of proinflammatory process. There is increased expression of *NLRP1* inflammosome. The finding that regulatory T-cells prevent cytotoxic damage are reduced in number, is considered significant in supporting this theory.

Initial and subsequent destruction of melanocytes leads to development of autoimmune destruction of melanocytes. Damage to the melanocytes through formation of apoptotic blebs exposes the self-antigens making them antigenic. Cell damage due to oxidative stress releases macro and small molecules of melanocytes that form highly active antigens. These are called neoantigens. With time and disease progression, new neoantigens are formed through a mechanism called antigen spreading. Tyrosinase and melan-A are the two most important neoantigens. Damage-associated molecular factors in turn activates innate immunity against various innate pattern recognition receptors like toll-like receptors (TLR). Stimulation of innate immunity is thought to play a major role in damage of the melanocytes.

Despite much progress in the mechanism of melanocytic damage as mentioned above, it is yet unknown what makes some individual prone to such events. Possibly, this is controlled genetically. Susceptibility to easy destruction of the melanocytes by different internal and external events is possibly genetically regulated. Vitiligo is a polygenic disease where most of the genes are still unknown. Thus, confirmation of such hypothesis is not easy. Susceptibility loci may be located on chromosomes 1, 4, 6, 7, 8, 17e, and 22. Genes found to be important in pathogenesis of vitiligo are *NLRP1 (17p13), XBP1 (22q12), PTPN22, CTLA4, MTHFR, FOXP1,* and *FOXP3.*

Both human leukocyte antigen class I and II has been found to be associated in vitiligo. Some alleles and amino acid signature of the DR β-chain seemed to be protective. A study among Indians in North India found significant association of haplotype A*02:01-B*44:03-DRB1*07:01 in both generalized and localized vitiligo.

Another age-old yet interesting theory is neural theory of vitiligo. There has been lot of progress in our understanding of neural pathogenesis that extends much beyond our initial concept where neural mechanism was thought to be the mechanism of segmental vitiligo (SV). Detection of increased amount of neuropeptide Y in and around vitiligo patches and increased norepinephrine levels in the patches, as well as in urine and plasma among patients with generalized nonsegmental vitiligo (NSV) are strong evidence in favor of a neural mechanism in vitiligo pathogenesis.

Neural mechanism has been found to play very important role in another important pathogenic mechanism, i.e., free radical theory. It has been shown that norepinephrine may destroy melanocytes directly through cellular sulfhydryl groups, enzyme inhibition, impairing mitochondrial calcium uptake, and formation of free radicals or through many undefined manner.

Vasoconstriction and subsequent hypoxia and extracellular acidosis can be damaging to the melanocytes. The abnormal biochemical milieu thus formed stimulates nuclear factor-κB and other cytokines (tumor necrosis factor-α, IL-1), various adhesion molecules, and may stimulate expression of almost 400 different genes including inducible nitric oxide synthase enzyme.

There are other proposed mechanisms that can lead to formation of free radicals. Homocysteine that is found to be high in active and bilateral vitiligo is associated with free radical formation via activation of p38 mitogen-activated protein kinase. Methylenetetrahydrofolate reductase (*MTHFR*) gene that regulates homocysteine metabolism is found to be defective in such cases of vitiligo.

Free radicals and other mechanism selectively destroy the melanocytes. It has been recently proposed that damaged (not necessarily dead) melanocytes migrate to dermis (transepidermal migration). This has been defined as melanocytorrhagy. Thus, indicates defect in anchoring of melanocytes with cells of basal layer and basement membrane. Genetic defect involving the PRiMA anchoring proteins called discoidin domain receptor-1 and CCN3 (nephroblastoma overexpressed gene) has been detected.

## CLINICAL FEATURE

Clinically, vitiligo patch appears as depigmented macules of variable sizes. Smaller macules merge to form bigger patches. Some patients may complain of itching, especially during a progressive stage. Active disease may also manifest with development of depigmented linear lesion following scratch (Koebner's phenomena). Despite popular belief, there is no evidence for the relationship of food with vitiligo.

Vitiligo may develop over a wide range of ages. It may start even during few months after birth or even in old ages (Fig. 1).

## CLASSIFICATION

Recent classification system recognizes two primary subtypes—SV and NSV (Fig. 2). Both forms may coexist, and this is called mixed vitiligo. There is another type called focal vitiligo. By definition, this is a single small patch that lacks features to be classified as either SV or NSV and this can progress to develop either form.

Segmental vitiligo refers to vitiligo that develops in one or more segments of the body. Mostly these are unilateral and unisegmental but bilateral and multisegmental vitiligo is also seen. They appear early in childhood but occasional cases may develop later. They have minimal chance of progressive disease.

Nonsegmental vitiligo, on the other hand, generally involves bilaterally and usually symmetrically. Progressive disease is common. It starts as a small patch and progress to involve larger areas. Progression speed, timing, and final extent of the disease is unpredictable.

Nonsegmental vitilgo may involve any area of the body but it can affect some areas preferentially in some patients. Overall, acral areas, lips and areas around lips, nares, and eyes are the common sites (Figs 3 and 4).

Nonsegmental vitilgo is traditionally classified in different subtypes based on the area of involvement. Generalized vitiligo is the term used for most common type with the clinical presentation. Symmetrical involvement is typical of this form (Fig. 5).

Mucosal vitiligo is vitiligo that involves only mucosa. Acrofacial vitiligo involves hand, feet, and head/face (mostly lips).

When vitiligo involves more than 80–90% of body surface areas, it is called universal vitiligo.

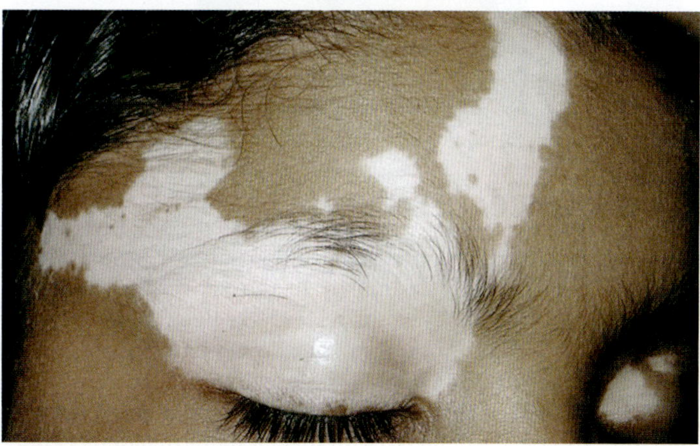

**FIG. 2:** Segmental vitiligo of right side along with nonsegmental vitiligo of eyelids of other side (mixed vitiligo).

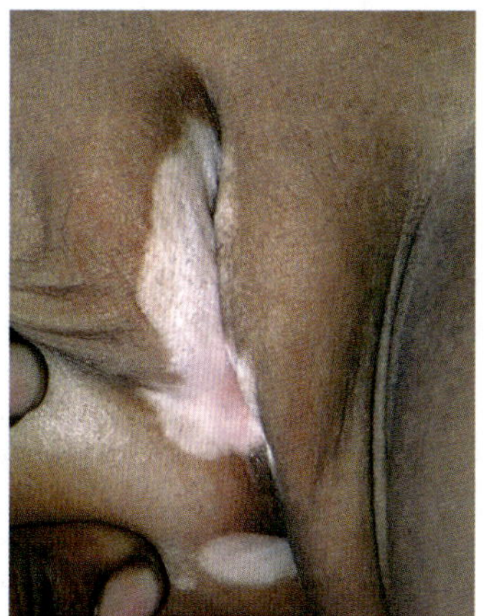

**FIG. 1:** Vitiligo on the vulva and perianal area in an infant.

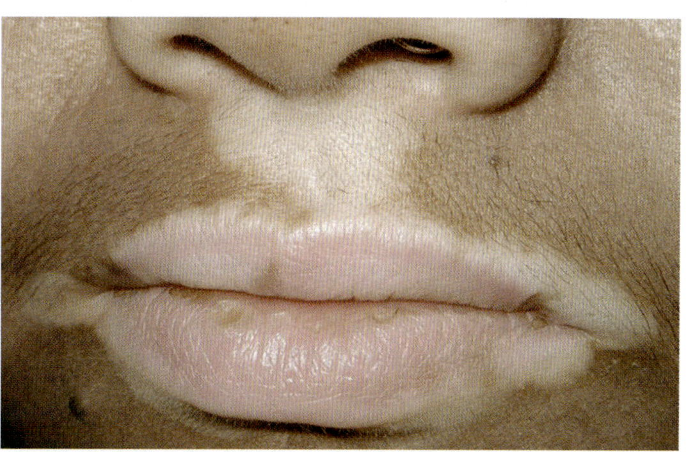

**FIG. 3:** Nonsegmental vitiligo involving lips, philtrum, and around nares.

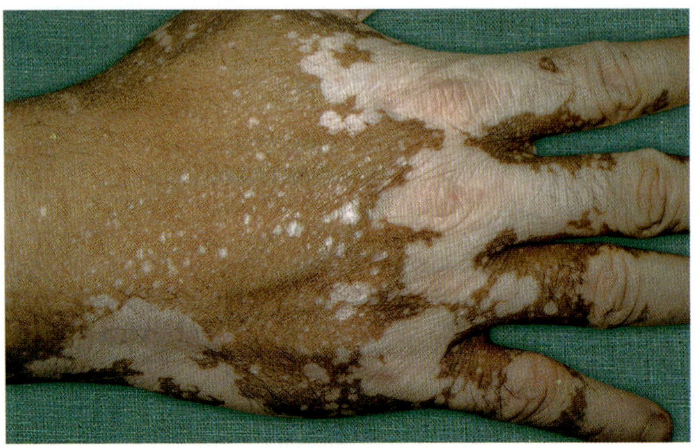

FIG. 4: Acral involvement in nonsegmental vitiligo.

**BOX 1 Differential diagnosis of vitiligo**

- Tinea versicolor
- Leishmaniasis
- Hansen's disease
- Onchocerciasis
- Pinta and syphilis
- Chemical leukoderma
- Pityriasis alba
- Nevus anemicus and nevus depigmentosus
- Piebaldism
- Tuberous sclerosis
- Vogt-Koyanagi-Harada syndrome
- Waardenburg syndrome
- Postinflammatory hypopigmentation
- Halo nevus
- Mycosis fungoides
- Idiopathic guttate hypomelanosis
- Lichen sclerosus et atrophicus
- Lichen striatus

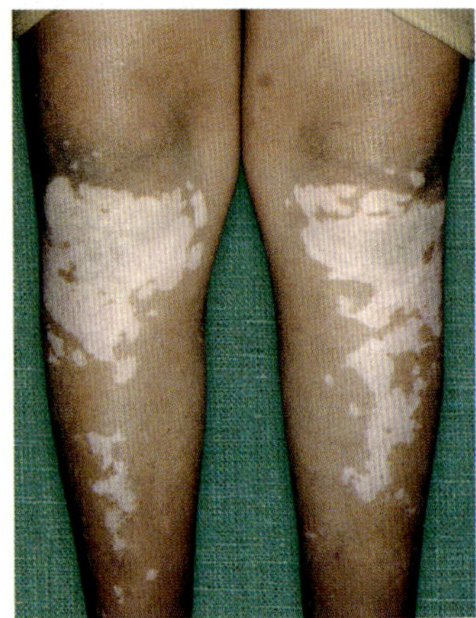

FIG. 5: Symmetrical involvement in nonsegmental vitiligo.

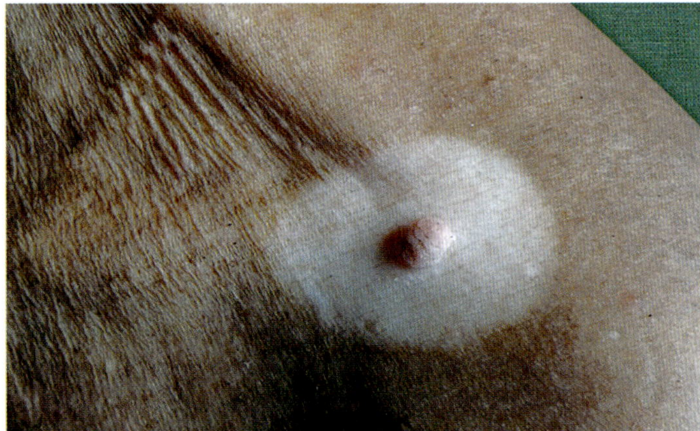

FIG. 6: Halo nevus.

## HISTOLOGICAL FEATURES

Histology is often unremarkable in vitiligo patches. Inflammatory infiltrate may be detected mostly in the active margin of the disease. CD4+ and CD8+ lymphocytes have been demonstrated. Melanocytes are absent in a well-developed patch. However, in the pigmented margin, melanocytes are detected that are larger, vacuolated, and may contain long dendritic processes filled with melanin. This can be detected with special stains that detect either melanin (Fontana-Masson) or functional melanocytes (DOPA stain). Immunohistochemistry studies can detect antibodies against various melanocytic antigenic components.

## DIAGNOSIS

This is diagnosed clinically. Wood's lamp may be useful. Many diseases may appear similar in appearance and may pose difficulty in diagnosis, especially when vitiligo patches are in evolution and not completely depigmented (Box 1). Allergic contact dermatitis may result in development of leucoderma at the contact site. This may clinically mimic vitiligo.

Halo nevi, in which vitiligo-like depigmentation develops around melanocytic nevi, may actually represent a vitiligo lesion (Fig. 6). This is possibly immune mediated destruction of melanocytes of and around the nevi. Sometimes, development of this precedes the onset of progressive vitiligo elsewhere in the body. Some advocates excision of halo nevi to stop vitiligo progression. However, the benefit of this is not proven.

## TREATMENT

Treatment of vitiligo is dependent upon many factors like extent, type, stability, site of involvement, and age of the patient. Also, the response is variable.

Generally, treatment is started with topical drugs. Topical corticosteroids (CS) are considered to be one of the first-line therapies for localized vitiligo. Mid-potent topical CS (class 2, 3, and 4) are generally used for 2–3 months on areas other than face. Topical steroid should be used for shorter period for areas like groin and other fluxures. Side effects like skin atrophy are a major concern.

Topical calcineurin inhibitors (tacrolimus and pimecrolimus) are less potent than topical CS but has better safety profile. These are preferred on areas where topical CS cannot be used and they can also be used for much longer periods (about 6 months). They can be combined with ultraviolet B (UVB) therapy and excimer laser as the benefit may be synergistic.

Topical vitamin D3 analogs (calcipotriol, tacalcitol) have been used but found to be of limited efficacy. Addition of UVB therapy may be superior to monotherapy.

Phototherapy is considered the mainstay in the treatment of vitiligo. Both UVA and UVB can induce significant repigmentation.

Psoralen and ultraviolet A [photochemotherapy (PUVA), oral psoralens and UVA] are approved by the Food and Drug Administration for the treatment of vitiligo. It induces hypertrophy of melanocytes and hyperactive melanosomes. In resource-poor setting, sun-light can be an effective alternative to PUVA. This is often called PUVAsol. Psoralens have adverse effects on eye when used for long time.

Ultraviolet A can also be used along with topical solution of psoralens (topical PUVA/PUVAsol). This can avoid many side effects of oral psoralens.

Recently, high dose UVA (15 J/cm$^2$) without psoralens has been found to be effective.

Ultraviolet B is often preferred over PUVA as it does not require psoralens. Narrow band UVB (310–312 nm) and monochromatic excimer light (MEL, 308 nm) are even much better than broad band UVB which has also been recently shown to be effective.

To avoid unnecessary exposure to the unaffected areas, targeted phototherapies [such as monochromatic excimer light (MEL, 308 nm), excimer laser, helium-neon laser] have been devised.

## Systemic Treatment

Systemic CS are used in fast progressive disease. However, this is associated with significant side effects and long-term benefit may not be satisfactory. The drug, dosage, and ideal duration of therapy is yet to be defined. Smallest possible dose and duration has to be chosen. Pulse dosage style can reduce side effects.

Low-dose oral mini-pulse dexamethasone therapy (2.5 mg/day on 2 consecutive days) in progressive unstable vitiligo was found to be effective and safer than higher dose.

## Newer Drugs

Only limited published reports propose efficacy of azathioprine, cyclosporine, JAK inhibitors (oral/topical tofacitinib, topical ruxolitinib) in vitiligo.

Latanoprost, a prostaglandin F2-α analog mainly used in glaucoma has been reported to be effective in vitiligo. Efficacy is increased when combined with narrow band UVB.

## Surgical Treatment

Surgical treatment is preferred over medical when there is an urgency of improvement, where response to medical treatment is unfavorable as in acrofacial areas or in segmental types or when medical management has failed. However, successful repigmentation following surgical therapy depends on disease activity. There is no well-accepted and full-proof disease activity or stability assessment tool. Clinical stability or nonprogression of disease for at least 1 year is considered a rational prerequisite for surgical treatment.

# SUGGESTED READINGS


1. Alhowaish AK, Dietrich N, Onder M, et al. Effectiveness of a 308-nm excimer laser in treatment of vitiligo: A review. Lasers Med Sci. 2013;28:1035-41.
2. Birlea SA, Jin Y, Bennett DC, et al. Comprehensive association analysis of candidate genes for generalized vitiligo supports XBP1, FOXP3, and TSLP. J Invest Dermatol. 2011;131:371-81.
3. Chen JX, Shi Q, Wang XW, et al. Genetic polymorphisms in the methylenetetrahydrofolate reductase gene (MTHFR) and risk of vitiligo in Han Chinese populations: A genotype–phenotype correlation study. Br J Dermatol. 2014;170:1092-9.
4. Ezzedine K, Lim HW, Suzuki T, et al. Revised classification nomenclature of vitiligo and related issues: The Vitiligo Global Issues Consensus Conference. Pigment Cell Melanoma Res. 2012;25:E1-13.
5. Jin Y, Birlea SA, Fain PR, et al. Genome-wide association analyses identify 13 new susceptibility loci for generalized vitiligo. Nat Genet. 2012;44:676-80.
6. Klarquist J, Denman CJ, Hernandez C, et al. Reduced skin homing by functional Treg in vitiligo. Pigment Cell Melanoma Res. 2010;23:276-86.
7. Lahiri K, Malakar S, Banerjee U, Sarma N. Clinico-cellular stability of vitiligo in surgical repigmentation: an unexplored frontier. Dermatology. 2004;209(2):170-1.
8. Lahiri K, Malakar S, Sarma N, Banerjee U. Inducing repigmentation by regrafting and phototherapy (311 nm) in punch grafting failure cases of lip vitiligo: a pilot study. Indian J Dermatol Venereol Leprol. 2004 May-Jun;70(3):156-8.
9. Lahiri K, Malakar S, Sarma N, Banerjee U. Repigmentation of vitiligo with punch grafting and narrow-band UV-B (311 nm)--a prospective study. Int J Dermatol. 2006 Jun;45(6):649-55.
10. Lan CC, Wu SB, Wu CS, et al. Induction of primitive pigment cell differentiation by visible light (helium-neon laser): A photoacceptor-specific response not replicable by UVB irradiation. J Mol Med (Berl). 2012;90:321-30.
11. Levandowski CB, Mailloux CM, Ferrara TM, et al. NLRP1 haplotypes associated with vitiligo and autoimmunity increase interleukin-1b processing via the NLRP1 inflammasome. Proc Natl Acad Sci USA. 2013;110:2952-6.
12. Ricard AS, Pain C, Daubos A, et al. Study of CCN3 (NOV) and DDR1 in normal melanocytes and vitiligo skin. Exp Dermatol. 2012;21:411-6.
13. Sarma N, Chakraborty S. Vitiligo: Medical treatment. In: Majid I, ed. IADVL Recent advances in dermatology. Jaypee Brothers Medical Publishers (P) Ltd. New Delhi. 2016, 197-205.
14. Sarma N, Poojary S, Chakraborty S. Vitiligo: Recentadvances in pathogenesis. In: Majid I, ed. IADVL Recent advances in dermatology. Jaypee Brothers Medical Publishers (P) Ltd. New Delhi. 2016, 183-190.
15. Sarma N, Singh AK. Topical calcipotriol in childhood vitiligo: An Indian experience. Int J Dermatol. 2004 Nov;43(11):856-9.
16. Spritz RA. Recent progress in the genetics of generalized vitiligo. J Genet Genomics. 2011;38:271-8.
17. Taieb A, Alomar A, Bohm M, et al. Vitiligo European Task Force (VETF), and the European Academy of Dermatology and Venereology (EADV), and the Union Européenne des Médecins Spécialistes (UEMS). Guidelines for the management of vitiligo: The European Dermatology Forum Consensus. Br J Dermatol. 2013; 168:5-19.
18. Taieb A, Picardo M; the VETF Members. The definition and assessment of vitiligo: A consensus report of the Vitiligo European Task Force. Pigment Cell Res. 2007;20:27-35.
19. Wang CQ, Cruz-Inigo AE, Fuentes-Duculan J, et al. Th17 cells and activated dendritic cells are increased in vitiligo lesions. PLoS One. 2011;6 article e18907.

# 26 CHAPTER Disorders of Hyperpigmentation

*Rashmi Sarkar, Samujjala Deb*

## INTRODUCTION

The pigmentation of human skin is genetically determined and is one of the most common criteria for racial identification. Skin pigmentation also depends on the extent of sun exposure, climate, choice of clothing, occupation and anatomic location. One of the most widely used classifications for skin color is the Fitzpatrick classification (I to VI). Another commonly used classification is the Obagi classification. Recently a new classification system—"Genetico-racial classification" has been proposed which takes into consideration the person's genetic constitution and racial ancestry apart from skin color to determine an individuals' susceptibility for having hyperpigmentary disorder.

Hyperpigmentation is a common complaint among patients presenting to a dermatologist. In a study from Western India, 10.8% of all dermatology consultations were for pigmentary disorders alone. Recently the Pigmentary Disorders Academy (PDA) has proposed newer terminology and lexicon for disorders of pigmentation. Terms like "hyperpigmentation", "hyperchromia", "melanosis", and "melanocytosis" are often used interchangeably but each of these terms has a unique pathophysiology and it is important to know the difference.

Hyperchromia signifies macular darkening of the skin from any cause (Flowchart 1). It is thus a broad term and can be further subdivided into melanotic and non-melanotic types. The PDA proposes that the term "hyperpigmentation" can be used for melanotic types of hyperchromias only. Non-melanotic hyperchromia is caused by deposition of endogenous deposits (porphyrin, hemoglobin, ochronosis, etc.) and exogenous deposits (drugs, metals, foreign particles, etc.). Drugs can cause hyperchromia by both melanotic and non-melanotic pathways. Another cause for hyperchromia is the thickening of the epidermis and the stratum corneum. A schematic classification is given later. Till this classification is more widely accepted, and for the sake of avoiding confusion, the term hyperpigmentation will be used in this chapter for ease of understanding.

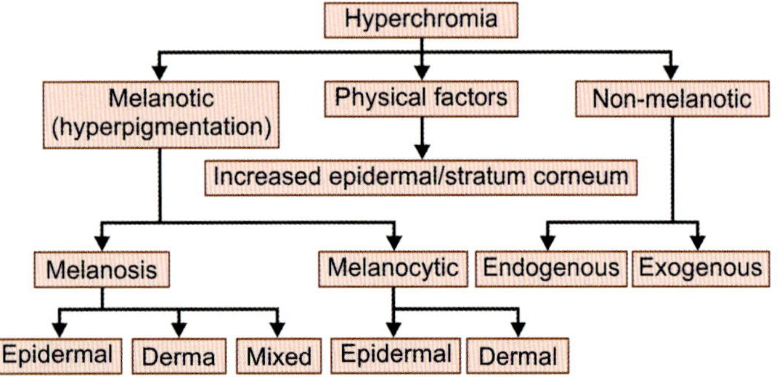


**FLOWCHART 1:** A simplified classification of hyperchromia.

## CLASSIFICATION

Classification of disorders of hyperpigmentation is extensive and exhaustive. A number of classifications have been proposed and the most widely accepted one was proposed by Moscher et al., which is an etio-clinicopathologic classification and distinguishes between epidermal (brown) and dermal (blue) hyperpigmentation. A simplified classification is given in the box 1.

## MELASMA

Melasma ("melas" meaning black in Greek) is a common disorder characterized by appearance of symmetric hyperpigmented macules primarily on the face. They can vary from light to dark, brown to brownish gray in color. When it occurs during pregnancy it is known as chloasma ("Chloazein" meaning green in Greek). The prevalence of melasma varies from 1.5 to 33.3% depending on the population and in pregnancy it is about 33%. Common predisposing factors include genetic makeup (Fitzpatrick skin type IV-VI), female sex although men can also suffer from melasma, sun exposure, pregnancy, and drugs (e.g., phenytoin). A study by Sarkar et al. showed that 20.5% of melasma patients were men and they were similar to females with respect to clinical features and histopathology.

### Pathogenesis

Traditionally, melasma is believed to be associated with pregnancy, oral contraceptive use, family history, menstruation, diphenylhydantoin use, high intensity visible light exposure, thyroid dysfunction, photosensitizing agents, chronic diseases, cosmetics, and sun exposure. It is known that ultraviolet radiation and genetics are most significantly associated with melasma, which supports the theory revolving around melanocortin

**BOX 1 Different causes of epidermal and dermal hyperpigmentation**

*Epidermal Hyperpigmentation*
- Melanocytotic
  - Hereditary/Developmental
    - Lentigines
    - Multiple Lentigines syndrome
    - Centrofacial Lentiginosis
    - Moynihan's syndrome
  - Physical
    - Solar/actinic lentigo
- Melanotic
  - Hereditary/Developmental
    - Ephelides/Freckles
    - Café-au-lait macule
    - Neurofibromatosis
    - Becker melanosis
    - Familial periorbital hyperpigmentation
    - Familial progressive hyperpigmentation
    - Fanconi syndrome
    - Acropigmentation of Dohi
    - Acropigmentation of Kitamura
    - Dowling-Degos disease
    - Dyskeratosis congenita
    - Dermatopathia pigmentosa reticularis
  - Metabolic
    - Hemochromatosis
    - Porphyria cutanea tarda
    - Biliary cirrhosis
    - Gaucher disease
    - Niemann–Pick disease
  - Endocrine
    - Melasma
    - ACTH and MSH-tumors
    - ACTH therapy
    - Addison's disease
    - Pregnancy
    - Contraceptive pill and estrogens
  - Chemicals/Drugs
    - Arsenic
    - Busulfan
    - Bleomycin
    - Berloque dermatitis
    - Phytophotodermatitis
    - Cyclophosphamide
    - Psoralens
    - Tar
  - Physical
    - UV light
    - Ionizing radiation
    - Trauma
  - Nutritional
    - Kwashiorkor
    - Pellagra
    - Vitamin B12 deficiency
  - Inflammation/Infection
    - Eczema
    - Lichen planus
    - Lupus erythematosus
    - Lichen simplex chronicus
    - Psoriasis
    - Pityriasis Versicolor
  - Neoplastic
    - Malignant melanoma
    - Mastocytosis
    - Acanthosis nigricans with adenocarcinoma or lymphoma

*Dermal*
- Melanocytotic
  - Hereditary/Developmental
    - Mongolian spot
    - Nevus of Ota
    - Nevus of Ito
    - Blue melanocytic nevus
  - Neoplastic
    - Melanoma metastasis
- Melanotic
  - Hereditary/Developmental
    - Incontinentia Pigmenti
    - Naegeli-Franceschetti-Jadassohn syndrome
  - Metabolic
    - Hemochromatosis
    - Macular amyloidosis
  - Endocrinal
    - Melasma
  - Nutritional
    - Chronic nutritional deficiency
  - Chemicals/drugs
    - Fixed drug eruptions
  - Physical
    - Erythema ab igne
  - Inflammation/infection
    - Pinta
    - EDP
    - Riehl's melanosis
    - LPP
  - Neoplasms
    - Melanoma and melanguria
- Non-melanotic
  - Metabolic
    - Alkaptonuria
  - Xanthodermas
    - Exogenous (mepacrine, beta-carotene, picric acid)
    - Endogenous (secondary carotenemia, bilirubin)
  - Chemicals/drugs
    - Heavy metals-gold, silver, mercury, bismuth, lead, iron
    - Antimalarials
    - OCP
    - Phenothiazine
    - Minocycline
    - Amiodarone
    - Tattoos
    - Exogenous ochronosis-hydroquinone

ACTH, adrenocorticotropic hormone; MSH, melanocyte-stimulating hormone; EDP, erythema dyschromicum perstans; LPP, Lichen planus pigmentosus; OCP, oral contraceptive pill.

production within keratinocytes and melanocytes upon sun exposure. Estrogen and progesterone may play a greater role in females, if at all in males, in the development of melasma. In fact, one study has identified subclinical ovarian dysfunction in female melasma patients. Increase in vascular endothelial growth factor (VEGF) which leads to increased vascularization in lesions of melasma has been proposed. Many genes are also upregulated in melasma like *TYR, MITF, SILV, TYRP1*. Inducible nitric oxide synthesis (iNOS) is also upregulated along with nuclear factor kβ while genes like *H19* gene, Peroxisome proliferator-activated receptor (PPAR), arachidonate 15-LOX, PPAR-γ coactivator-1α, type B (ALXO15B), diacylglycerol o-acyltransferase 2-like 3 are downregulated.

## Clinical Presentations and Classification

Melasma presents as light brown to dark brown or brown-gray patches with irregular borders primarily over the face. Three classical clinical patterns are seen—centrofacial, malar, and mandibular (Fig. 1). It can also be seen on extensor aspect of arms and mid upper chest less commonly.

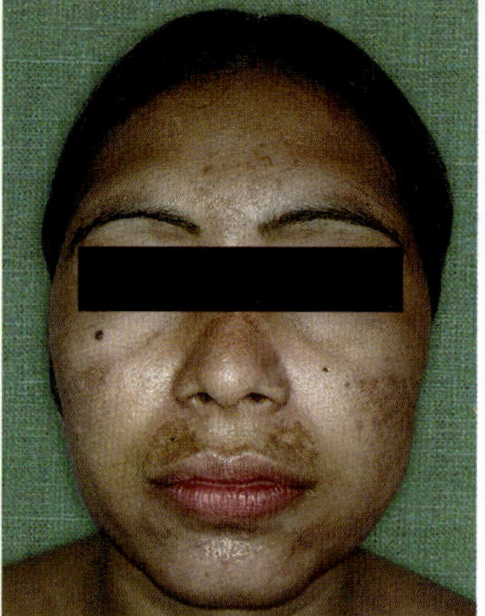

**FIG. 1:** Brown macules and patches of melasma over the forehead, bridge of nose, malar prominence, upper lip, and jaw.

Three histologic subtypes of melasma exist—epidermal, basal, and mixed. Epidermal melasma is characterized by increased melanin deposition in the basal and suprabasal layer.

Evaluation of depth with Wood's lamp examination often shows poor correlational with histopathologic examination. Reflectance confocal microscopy (RCM) can provide real-time en face images that correlate nicely with histopathologic findings. RCM helps classify melasma according to pigment chances. It also helps determine the prognosis and response to treatment.

## Diagnosis

Melasma is usually diagnosed by the typical clinical presentation. Wood's lamp examination can help determine the level of pigment deposition. Dermoscopy is also useful in identifying lesions of melasma which are seen as reticular pigmentation in varying shades of brown with sparing of follicular openings. RCM, of course, is the best tool for diagnosis as well for observing response to treatment.

*Differential diagnosis*: This includes post-inflammatory hyperpigmentation, exogenous ochronosis, pigmented cosmetic dermatitis, Hori's nevus, etc.

## Management

Photoprotection is the cornerstone of management of melasma and a broadspectrum sunscreen should be prescribed to all patients. The various treatment modalities available for melasma are discussed as follows.

Topical agents used in the treatment of melasma are given in table 1.

Newer agents include tranexamic acid, 4-n-butylresorcinol, oligopeptides, silymarin, and orchid extracts. Chemical peels which have been tried are salicylic acid and glycolic acid. Newer peels include tretinoin peels (1%), amino fruit acid peel, and Obagi Blue Peel to name a few.

Botanical extracts that have been tried in the treatment include grape seed extract, pycnogenol, aloe vera extract, marine algae extract, cinnamic acid, green tea extracts, coffee berry, etc.

Lasers that have been tried in the treatment of melasma include—Flashlamp-pumped pulsed dye laser (510 nm), frequency doubled Q-switched neodymium: Yttrium aluminium garnet-532 nm (QS Nd: YAG), Q-switched ruby (694 nm), Q-switched alexandrite (755 nm), QS Nd: YAG (1064 nm), and fractional laser 1550.

**TABLE 1: Various topical agents in the treatment of melasma**

| Molecules | Proposed mechanisms |
|---|---|
| • Azelaic acid, arbutin, deoxyarbutin, aloesin, kojic acid, flavonoids, saponin, orgonon, yohimbine, glabridine, mulberry<br>• Hydroquinone (HQ), derivatives of HQ (mequinol, N-acetyl 4-S cysteaminylphenol, gentisic acid), glutathione | Tyrosine inhibition |
| Niacinamide, soy | Reduce melanosome transfer |
| p-Coumaric acid | Reduce tyrosine oxidation |
| Ascorbic acid, ellagic acid | Copper chelation, antioxidant |
| Retinoids, liquitin | Multiple mechanisms |

# IDIOPATHIC CUTANEOUS HYPERCHROMIA AT THE ORBITAL REGION

Idiopathic cutaneous hyperchromia at the orbital region (ICHOR), also referred as periorbital pigmentation, periorbital melanosis (POM), dark circles, or infraorbital pigmentation, is a fairly common complaint among patients presenting to a dermatologist.

## Etiopathogenesis

A number of etiologic factors can contribute toward the development of POM. They can range from individual factors (e.g., genetic predisposition, skin type, sun exposure, chronic fatigue and lack of sleep, and anatomic aberrances), co-existing dermatologic diseases (e.g., atopic dermatitis, eyelid eczema, allergic dermatitis, and airborne contact dermatitis), medications (bimatoprost, travoprost), cosmetics (Kohl pencils, fragrance, and preservatives) and inherited pigmentary disorders (nevus of Ota, Hori's nevus) and many more (Box 2).

## Clinical Presentations and Classification

Periorbital pigmentation presents as diffuse, bilaterally symmetrical, asymptomatic hyperpigmentation of the periocular region extending up to the eyebrows and malar prominences in severe cases (Fig. 2). The skin may be normal or have features of the associated dermatological condition. If there is associated anatomic abnormality (e.g., tear trough), the pigmentation disappears on stretching the skin (stretch test) while it does not in other cases.

**BOX 2 Pathomechanism of periorbital pigmentation**

- Post inflammatory pigmentation
- Extension of pigmentary demarcation line-F
- Periorbital edema
- Increased melanin deposition
- Increased visibility of blood vessels
- Increased skin laxity (dermatochalasis)
- Prominent tear trough

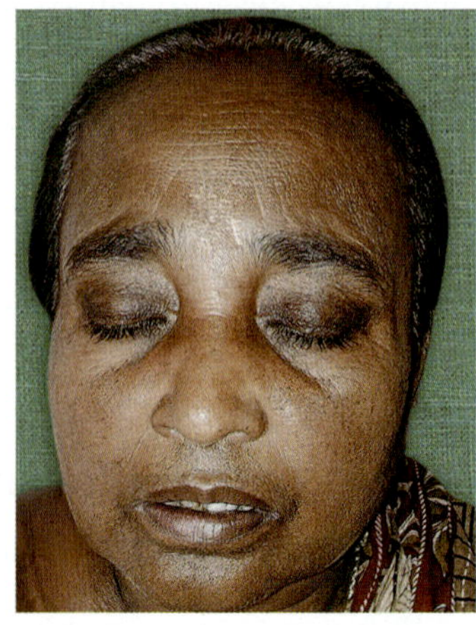

FIG. 2: Hyperpigmentation over the upper eyelids.

**TABLE 2: Various treatment modalities for periorbital pigmentation**

| Medical therapy | Procedural management |
|---|---|
| • Topical depigmenting agents—hydroquinone, Kligman formula, ascorbic acid, azelaic acid, kojic acid, pidobenzone<br>• Newer agents like *Pfaffia paniculata, Ptychopetalum olacoides, Lilium candidum L*-associated compound | • Chemical peeling with arginine peel, lactic acid peel<br>• Transconjunctival blepharoplasty<br>• Autologous fat transplantation<br>• Injectable fillers<br>• Laser therapy with Q-switched Ruby, Q-switched Nd: YAG, fractional $CO_2$, etc. |

Periorbital pigmentation may be classified into primary and secondary types. Primary type is characterized by darkening of the periorbital skin in the absence of any local or systemic abnormality while the secondary type has a multifactorial etiopathogenesis.

## Diagnosis

Diagnosis is mainly clinical. Histopathologic examination reveals dermal melanophages along with dermal melanocytosis. Verschoore et al. have shown using SIAscopy that blood deposits along with melanin plays a role in the pathogenesis of periorbital hyperpigmentation.

## Management

Periorbital melanosis is resistant to treatment. A number of treatment modalities have been tried with varying degrees of success (Table 2).

# POST-INFLAMMATORY HYPERPIGMENTATION

Post-inflammatory hyperpigmentation (PIH) is a clinical condition where there is acquired excess of melanin in the skin following cutaneous injury and inflammation. PIH occurs more frequently in darker skin types.

## Etiopathogenesis

Post-inflammatory hyperpigmentation can be caused by disease, injury, or iatrogenic. Common conditions include acne vulgaris, atopic dermatitis, psoriasis, impetigo and herpes zoster (Fig. 3), fixed drug eruptions (Fig. 4), lichenoid disorders, discoid lupus erythematosus, Stevens-Johnson syndrome, and chemical peel, laser, surgical procedure or other treatment.

Hyperpigmentation results due to increased melanin content. When there is increased production and subsequent transfer to keratinocytes, it results in epidermal hyperpigmentation. If there is destruction of the basal cell layer, leading to dropping off of the melanin into the underlying dermis, it is phagocytosed by the macrophages (melanophages). This leads to dermal hyperpigmentation. There may be increased production of prostaglandin D2 and E2 along with leukotrienes (LTs) and thromboxanes (TXs) which enhance melanin production.

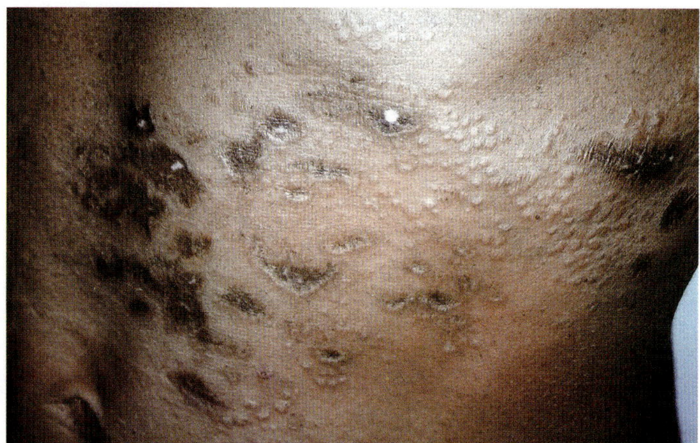

**FIG. 3:** Hyperpigmentation over old healed lesions of herpes zoster.

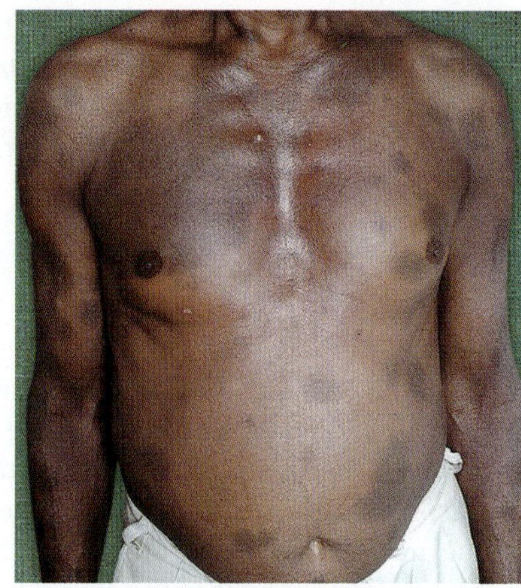

**FIG. 4:** Post-inflammatory hyperpigmentation in areas of recurrent multiple fixed drug eruptions.

## Clinical Presentation and Classification

Asymptomatic hyperpigmented macules and patches with colors varying from light to dark brown (epidermal) or blue-gray to gray-brown can be seen on sites of injury or inflammation. The dermatological condition causing the hyperpigmentation may be present simultaneously. Sometimes the sites and patterns of hyperpigmentation can give an idea about the underlying etiology.

Hyperpigmentation can be subdivided into basically two types—epidermal and dermal, on the basis of the accumulation of melanin and prognosis.

## Differential Diagnosis

Melasma, pityriasis versicolor, ephelids, lentigenes, and erythema dyschromicans perstans.

## Diagnosis

Diagnosis is clinical. Wood's lamp examination and infrared photography may accentuate subtle hyperpigmentation. Sometimes a biopsy may be needed to determine the level of melanin deposition and to rule out other conditions.

## Management

Management of PIH essentially begins with preventing it from occurring in susceptible individuals. Early diagnosis and treatment helps to resolves most cases of epidermal hyperpigmentation. Dermal pigmentation is more difficult to treat.

Use of broadspectrum sunscreen is imperative. Topical treatment includes hydroquinone (2–4%), tretinoin in combination with corticosteroid and hydroquinone, azeleic acid, and peeling with alpha-hydroxy acids. Lasers should be used with caution in darker skin types. Q-switched ruby, alexandrite, and Nd:YAG lasers have been used in dermal hyperpigmentation with varying success.

# DRUG-INDUCED HYPERPIGMENTATION

Drug-induced hyperpigmentation is often an unavoidable consequence of therapy. It accounts for about 10–20% of all causes of hyperpigmentation. All ages and sexes can be affected. Although a number of drugs can cause hyperpigmentation, the most common ones are minocycline, antimalarials, chemotherapeutic agents and zidovudine.

## Pathogenesis

Drug-induced pigmentation or discoloration can occur as a result of a number of pathologic mechanisms. They are mostly not immunologically mediated. The three possible mechanisms are—deposition of the drug or its metabolite in the epidermis and dermis, increased synthesis of melanin with or without an associated increase in the number of melanocytes, and drug-induced post-inflammatory changes in the skin.

## Clinical Presentation and Classification

Drug-induced pigmentation can present in a myriad form of clinical manifestations (Box 3). Onset is usually insidious and progressive. Any part of the body may be involved. Drug-induced hyperpigmentation can be classified in the following manner—generalized or localized pigmentation, linear pigmentation (e.g., supravenous serpentine pigmentation with 5-fluorouracil), patterned pigmentation (e.g., flagellate pigmentation seen with bleomycin), reticulate pigmentation (e.g., diltiazem, 5-fluorouracil), patchy pigmentation, and pigmentation limited to mails and mucous membranes (e.g., zidovudine). Clofazimine is very well-known drug causing pigmentation (Fig. 5).

**BOX 3 Drugs showing characteristic pigmentation**

| *Drug* | *Color* |
|---|---|
| • Minocycline | • Blue-black |
| • Clofazimine | • Red |
| • Amiodarone | • Slate gray |
| • Quinacrine | • Yellow |
| • Arsenic | • Bronze |
| • Iron | • Brown |

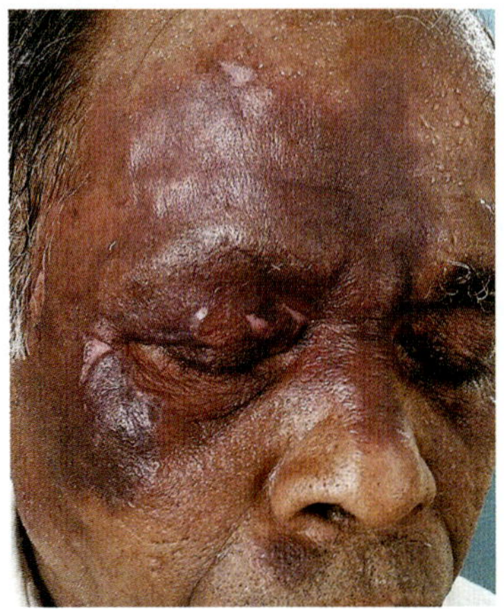

**FIG. 5:** Clofazimine induced dyspigmentation over a plaque of borderline tuberculoid leprosy over the face.

## Differential Diagnosis

Drug-induced hyperpigmentation need to be differentiated from other causes of hyperpigmentation like PIH, ephelids, and melasma.

## Diagnosis

Drug-induced hyperpigmentation often has a characteristic distribution—like in sites of scars and inflammation, pretibial areas, sites of sun exposure, etc. Color of the macule or patch may also provide a clue to the diagnosis.

Histopathologic examination shows basal cell hyperpigmentation, pigment incontinence along with accumulation of melanophages around the blood vessels, and eccrine glands. They stain positive for Fontana-Masson stain and/or Perls Prussian blue stain.

## Management

This includes identification and prompt discontinuation of treatment with the offending drug. Most of the drug-induced hyperpigmentation is reversible and fades away with time. In case a number of drugs are under suspicion or stopping a life-saving drug is not feasible, then the patient must be adequately counseled.

Additionally, sun exposure usually worsens any hyperpigmentary disorder hence strict photoprotection must be advocated. Alongside topical depigmenting agents in conjunction with other modalities of treatments like laser therapy may also be explored and tried.

# INHERITED DISORDERS OF PIGMENTATION

A number of inherited disorders can present with hyperpigmentation. Some of them are discussed in the tables 3 and 4.

**TABLE 3: Inherited disorders of pigmentation**

| | |
|---|---|
| Lentigines | Solitary or multiple, annular or polycyclic, macular or slightly raised lesions over covered/uncovered parts of the body |
| Multiple Lentigines syndrome | LEOPARD syndrome (lentigines, electrocardiographic abnormalities, ocular hypertelorism, pulmonary stenosis, abnormalities of the genitalia, retardation of growth and deafness) |
| Café-au-lait macule (CALM) | Brown-colored macules with distinct margin. Multiple CALMs associated with syndromes like NF-1, TSC, McCune-Albright, Bloom, Watson syndrome, etc. |

*Continued*

*Continued*

| | |
|---|---|
| Neurofibro-matosis | Multiple CALMs, axillary freckling, neurofibromas, Lisch nodules, skeletal deformities |
| Becker's melanosis | Asymptomatic, well demarcated, hyperpigmented and occasionally hypertrichotic patch over the body (Fig. 6) |
| Acropigmen-tation of Dohi | AD, eticulate pigmentation over dorsa of hands and feet |
| Acropig-mentation of Kitamura | AD, eticulate pigmentation over dorsa of hands and feet, palmoplantar pits |
| Dowling-Degos disease | AD, eticulate pigmentation of the flexures, comedone like lesions, pitted facial scars (Fig. 7) |
| Dyskeratosis congenita | XLR, reticulate pigmentation, nail dystrophy and leucoplakia |
| Derma-topathia pigmentosa reticularis | AD, truncal hyperpigmentation with non-scarring alopecia |
| Poikiloderma-tous disorders | Kindler syndrome (Fig. 8), Rothmund–Thomson syndrome, hereditary acrokeratotic poikiloderma, hereditary sclerosing poikiloderma. |

AD, autosomal dominant; XLR, X-linked recessive; TSC, tuberous sclerosis complex.

**TABLE 4: Inherited disorders of pigmentation of the face**

| | |
|---|---|
| Mongolian spot | Common in oriental population. Occur due to failure of migration of melanocytes from neural crest cells to basal layer |
| Nevus of Ota | Blue-gray pigmented macules on the upper half of face. Failure of migration of melanocytes like Mongolian spot (Fig. 9) |
| Nevus of Ito | Blue-gray pigmented macules over the clavicular and scapular region |
| Blue melanocytic nevus | Nevus derived from dermal melanocytes |
| Incontinentia pigmenti | XLD disorder, characterized by vesiculobullous,verrucous, hyperpigmented and hypopigmented lesions along lines Blaschlo. Associated defect of hair, nail, and eyes |
| Naegeli-Franceschetti-Jadassohn syndrome | AD, reticulate pigmentation, dental anomalies, hypohidrosis, dystrophic nails |

AD, autosomal dominant; XLD, X-linked dominant.

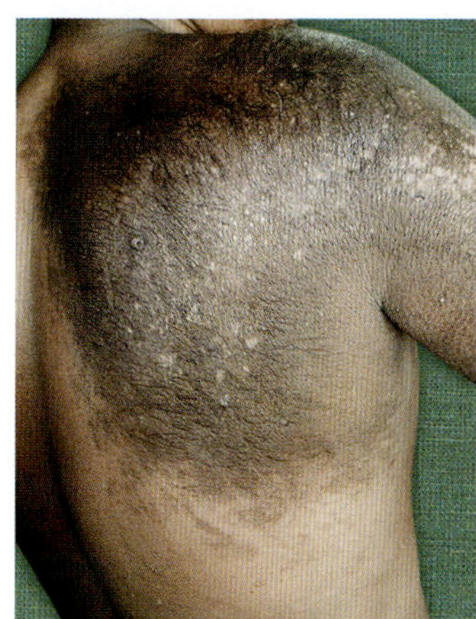

**FIG. 6:** Lesion of giant Becker nevus involving the right arm, shoulder, and part of the trunk with hypertrichosis.

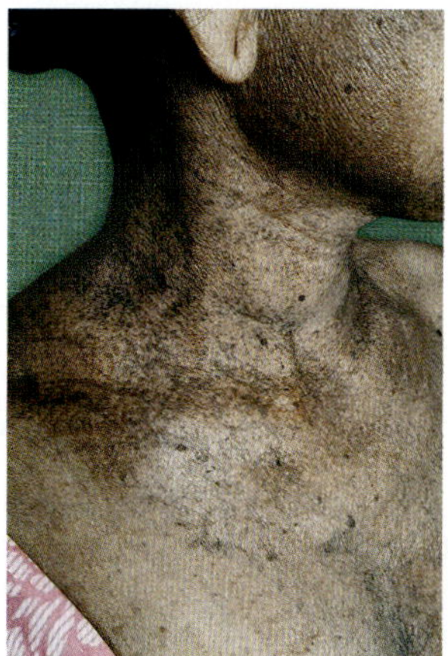

**FIG. 7:** Reticulate pigmentation involving the flexural areas in Dowling-Degos disease.

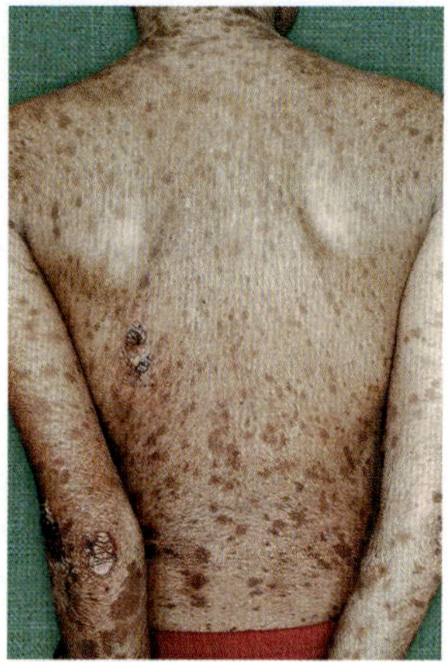

**FIG. 8:** Poikilodermatous changes in a girl with Kindler syndrome.

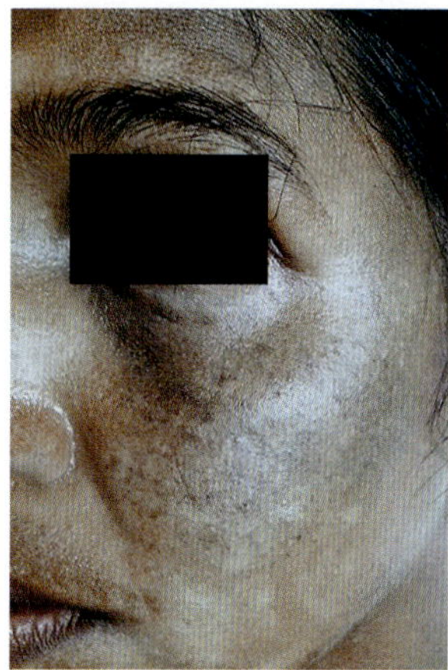

**FIG. 9:** Blue-gray macules of nevus of Ota involving the left upper face and conjunctiva.

## SUGGESTED READINGS

1. Altaei T. The treatment of melasma by silymarin cream. BMC Dermatol. 2012; 12:18.
2. Cestari TF, Dantas LP, Boza JC. Acquired Hyperpigmentations. An Bras Dermatol. 2014;89(1):11-25.
3. Fanous N, Cote V, Fanous A. The new genetico-racial skin classification: how to maximize the safety of any peel or laser treatment on any Asian, Caucasian or Black patient. Can J Plast Surg. 2011;19:9-16.

4. Goldberg DJ. Laser treatment of pigmented lesions. Dermatol Clin. 1997;15:397-407.
5. Grimes PE, Yamada N, Bhawan J. Light microscopic, immunohistochemical, and ultrastructural alterations in patients with melasma. Am J Dermatopathol. 2005;27:96-101.
6. Hantash BM, Jimenez F. Treatment of mild to moderate facial melasma with the Lumixyl topical brightening system. J Drugs Dermatol. 2012;11:660-2.
7. Hong SP, Han SS, Choi SJ, et al. Split-face comparative study of 1550 nm fractional photothermolysis and trichloroacetic acid 15% chemical peeling for facial melasma in Asian skin. J Cosmet Laser Ther. 2012;14:81-6.
8. Hori Y, Yasuo K. Acquired circumscribed hypermelanotic disorders. Dermatol Sinica. 1993;11:1-19.
9. Ilknur T, Biçak MU, Demirtaşoğlu M, et al. Glycolic acid peels versus amino fruit acid peels in the treatment of melasma. Dermatol Surg. 2010;36:490-5.
10. Jang YH, Lee JY, Kang HY, et al. Oestrogen and progesterone receptor expression in melasma: an immunohistochemical analysis. J Eur Acad Dermatol Venereol. 2010;24:1312-6.
11. Jo HY, Kim CK, Suh IB, et al. Co-localization of inducible nitric oxide synthase and phosphorylated Akt in the lesional skins of patients with melasma. J Dermatol. 2009;36:10-6.
12. Kang HY, Bahadoran P, Suzuki I, et al. In vivo reflectance confocal microscopy detects pigmentary changes in melasma at a cellular level resolution. Exp Dermatol. 2010;19:e228-33.
13. Kang HY, Suzuki I, Lee DJ, et al. Transcriptional profiling shows altered expression of wnt pathway- and lipid metabolism-related genes as well as melanogenesis-related genes in melasma. J Invest Dermatol. 2011;131:1692-700.
14. Kim NH, Lee CH, Lee AY. H19 RNA downregulation stimulatedmelanogenesis in melasma. Pigment Cell Melanoma Res 2010;23:84-92.
15. Kubba A, Batrani M. Histopathological evaluation of melasma and other facial hyperchromias. In: Lahiri K, Chatterjee M, Sarkar R (Eds). Pigmentary Disorders, 1st edition. New Delhi: Jaypee Brothers Medical Publishers (P) Ltd.; 2014. pp. 287-98.
16. Levine N. Pigmentary abnormalities. In: Schachner L, Hansen R (Eds). Pediatric Dermatology, 4th edition. New York: Churchill Livingstone; 2011. pp. 539-82.
17. Lowe NJ, Wieder JM, Shorr N, et al. Infraorbital pigmented skin. Preliminary observations of laser therapy. Dermatol Surg. 1995;21:767-70.
18. Malakar S, Lahiri K, Banerjee U, et al. Periorbital melanosis is an extension of pigmentary demarcation line-F on face. Indian J Dermatol Venereol Leprol. 2007;73:323-5.
19. Miot LD, Miot HA, Silva MG, et al. Physiopathology of melasma. An Bras Dermatol. 2009;84:623-35.
20. Nordlund JJ, Ortane JP, Cestari T, et al Confusions about color: formulating a more precise lexicon for pigmentation, pigmentary disorders and abnormalities of "chromatics". J Am Acad Dermatol. 2006;54:S291-7.
21. Pandya AG, Guevara IL. Disorders of hyperpigmentation. Dermatol Clin. 2000; 18(1):91-8.
22. Pichardo R, Vallejos Q, Feldman SR, et al. The prevalence of melasma and its association withquality of life in adult male Latino migrant workers. Int J Dermatol. 2009;48:22-6.
23. Pérez M, Sánchez JL, Aguiló F. Endocrinologic profile of patients with idiopathic melasma. J Invest Dermatol. 1983;81:543-5.
24. Rigopoulos D, Gregoriou S, Katsambas A. Hyperpigmentation and melasma. J Cosmet Dermatol. 2007;6:195-202.
25. Rito C, Pineiro-Maceira J. Reflectance confocal microscopy in the diagnosis of cutaneous melanoma. An Bras Dermatol. 2009;84:636-42.
26. Roh MR, Chung KY. Infraorbital dark circles: Definition, causes, and treatment options. Dermatol Surg. 2009;35:1163-71.
27. Ruiz-Maldonado R, Orozco-Covarrubias ML. Post-inflammatory hypopigmentation and hyperpigmentation. Semin Cutan Med Surg. 1997;16:36-4.
28. Sarkar R. Idiopathic cutaneous hyperchromia at the orbital region or periorbital hyperpigmentation. J Cutan Aesthet Surg. 2012;5:183-4.
29. Sarkar R, Arora P, Garg KV. Cosmeceuticals for hyperpigmentation: what is available? J Cutan Aesthet Surg. 2013;6:4-11.
30. Sarkar R, Arora P, Garg VK, et al. Melasma update. Indian Dermatol Online J. 2014;5:426-35.
31. Sarkar R, Jain RK, Puri P. Melasma in Indian males. Dermatol Surg. 2003;29:204.
32. Sarkar R, Puri P, Jain RK, et al. Melasma in men: a clinical, aetiological and histological study. J Eur Acad Dermatol Venereol. 2010;24;768-72.
33. Sarma N, Chakraborty S, Bhattacharya SR. Acquired, Idiopathic, Patterned Facial Pigmentation (AIPFP) including periorbital pigmentation and pigmentary demarcation lines on face follows the lines of blaschko on face. Indian J Dermatol. 2014;59:41-8.
34. Schmutz JI, Barbaud A, Trechot P. Periocular hyperpigmentation following travoprost application. Ann Dermatol Venereol. 2008;135(6-7):537.
35. Sheth VM, Pandya AG. Melasma: a comprehensive update: part I. J Am Acad Dermatol. 2011;65:689-97.
36. Shin J, Kim JH, Kim EK. Repeated exposure of human fibroblasts to UVR induces secretion of stem cell factor and senescence. J Eur Acad Dermatol Venereol. 2012;26:1577-80.
37. Tomita Y, Maeda K, Tagami H. Leukotrienes and thromboxane B2 stimulate normal human melanocytes in vitro: possible inducers of postinflammatory pigmentation. J Exp Med. 1988;156:303-4.
38. Verschoore M, Gupta S, Ortonne JP, et al. Determination of melanin and haemoglobin in the skin of Idiopathic Cutaneous Hyperchromia of the Orbital Region (ICHOR): a study of Indian patients. J Cutan Aesthet Surg. 2012;5:176-82.
39. Victor FC, Gelber J, Rao B. Melasma: a review. J Cutan Med Surg. 2004;8:97-102.
40. Walia NS, Deb S. Dermatology referrals in the hospital setting. Indian J Dermatol Venereol Leprol. 2004;70:285-7.
41. Werlinger KD, Guevara IL, González CM, et al. Prevalence of self-diagnosed melasma among premenopausal Latino women in Dallas and Fort Worth, Tex. Arch Dermatol. 2007;143:424-5.

# 10 SECTION Papulosquamous Disorders and Arthritis

# 27 CHAPTER Psoriasis

*Smriti K Raychaudhuri, Suravi Raychaudhuri, Sayantani Chakraborty, Siba P Raychaudhuri*

## INTRODUCTION

Psoriasis is a chronic progressive inflammatory cutaneous disease with multiple systemic manifestations which affects about 2–5% of the world population. Psoriasis can appear at any age, from a newborn to an elderly person.

There is no cure for psoriasis and its associated inflammatory psoriatic arthritis. Although mortality from psoriatic disease is low, but it is associated with atherosclerosis, type 2 diabetes, and metabolic syndrome, the leading causes of mortality in the Western world. Psoriasis is associated with a high degree of morbidity; patients with psoriasis have reduced levels of employment and they have decreased quality of life.

Psoriasis is the most prevalent autoimmune disease in human. The overall belief is that immune-mediated inflammation induces hyperproliferation of epidermal keratinocytes, and that generates the erythematous, scaly patches and plaques, the hallmark features of psoriasis.

## PSORIASIFORM DISORDER

As discussed subsequently, diagnosis of psoriasis is clinical and generally straightforward. Neither histopathological examination nor any specific blood tests are recommended for the diagnosis of psoriatic disease. However, some cases may be closely mimicked by other psoriasiform disorders.

### Clinical Mimicker of Psoriasis

Seborrheic dermatitis, pityriasis rubra pilaris, contact dermatitis, nummular dermatitis, lichen simplex chronicus, pityriasis rosea, dermatophytosis, secondary syphilis, mycosis fungoides and parapsoriasis, psoriasiform drug rash, leprosy with type 1 reaction, subacute lupus, and possibly many other conditions (Fig. 1).

### Histopathological Mimickers

Several classifications have been proposed for psoriasiform disorders. Among these, clinicians are more familiar with the classification of Farmer and Hood as this is chiefly based on the presence of a characteristic pattern of epidermal hyperplasia (Box 1).

In a recent clinical and histopathological correlation study of psoriasiform dermatoses, it was observed that psoriasis was the most common of all psoriasiform dermatoses (31%) followed

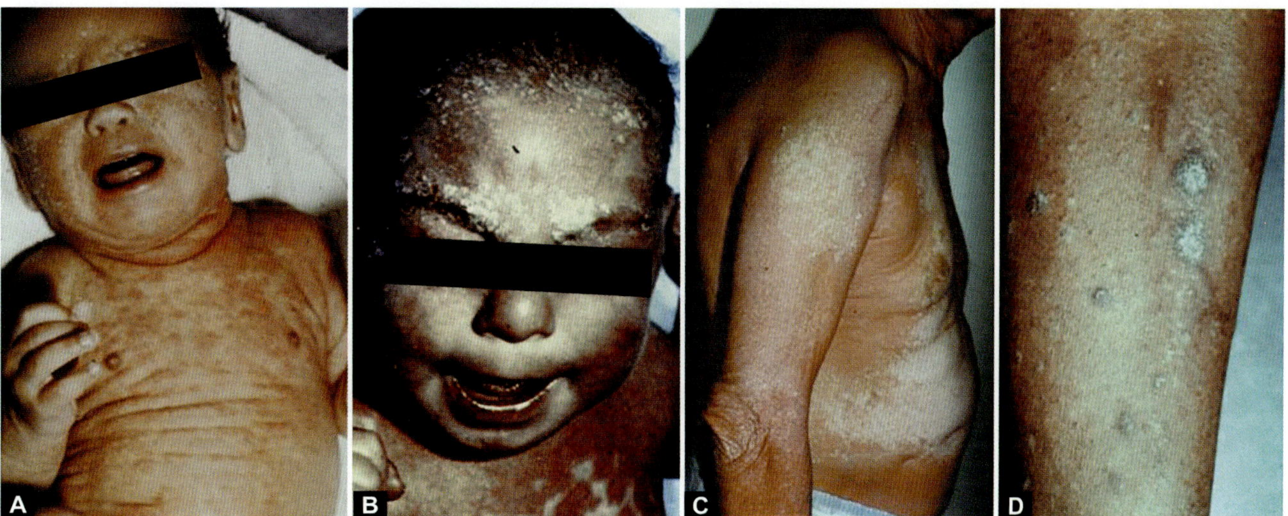


**FIG. 1:** Few clinical variants of psoriasiform dermatitis. **A,** Infantile psoriasis; **B,** Childhood seborrheic dermatitis; **C,** Pityriasis rubra pilaris with the characteristic feature of "islands of sparing"; **D,** Lichen simplex chronicus.

**BOX 1 Farmer and Hood classification of psoriasiform dermatitis**

**Group-1**

Diseases showing psoriasiform epidermal hyperplasia as a characteristic feature

a. Psoriasis
b. Reiter's disease
c. Lichen simplex chronicus
d. Pityriasis rubra pilaris
e. Pellagra
f. Inflammatory linear verrucous epidermal nevus
g. Associated with acquired immuno deficiency syndrome (AIDS)
h. Acrodermatitis enteropathica
i. Necrolytic migratory erythema

**Group-2**

Diseases showing psoriasiform epidermal hyperplasia as a frequent feature

a. Contact dermatitis
b. Nummular dermatitis/eczema
c. Seborrheic dermatitis
d. Psoriasiform syphlids
e. Mycosis fungoides
f. Pityriasis rosea

**Group-3**

Diseases showing psoriasiform epidermal hyperplasia as an occasional feature

a. Dermatophytoses
b. Candidiasis
c. Norwegian scabies

by lichen planus (23%), lichen nitidus (9%), pitryasis rosea (7%), and seborrheic dermatitis (6%). The remaining dermatoses like lichenoid drug eruptions, parapsoriasis, Reiter's disease, mycosis fungoides, pitryriasis rubra pilaris, lichen striatus, and lichen simplex chronic were uncommon.

## Pathogenesis

The etiology of psoriasis remains poorly understood, psoriasis is thought to result from a complex interplay between genetics, environment, skin barrier disruption, and immune dysfunction. Elder and his colleagues have reviewed the single nucleotide polymorphism analyses of several major studies in this field to provide collective information about an association between psoriasis and various loci of the immune system, such as the TH17 pathway (*IL12B, IL23A, IL23R, TRAF3IP2, TYK2)*, innate immunity (NFκB and IFN), signaling pathways (*TNFAIP3, TNIP1, NFKBIA, REL, TYK2, IFIH1, IL23RA*) and β-defensin, the TH2 pathway (*IL4, IL13*), and adaptive immunity involving CD8 T-cells (*ERAP1, ZAP70*).

## Histopathology

A psoriatic plaque is characterized by marked thickening of the epidermis, elongated epidermal rete pegs, parakeratosis, loss of the granular layer, suprapapillary thinning, microabscess of Munro (collection of neutrophils in the stratum corneum), spongiform pustule of Kogoj (epidermal spongiotic pustule with neutrophilic infiltration), dermal or epidermal CD3+ T-cell infiltrates (Fig. 2) with epidermotropism of CD8+ T-cells. The histology of psoriatic subtypes may share classic dermal and epidermal features of plaque psoriasis however they may also display distinct histopathologic characteristics.

Although CD4+ T-cells are predominant in these tissues, this ratio is reversed in the epidermis, synovial fluid compartment, and at the enthesis, where CD8+ T-cells are more common. This differential tropism of CD8+ T-cells suggests that CD8+ T-cells may be driving the immune response in the joint and skin. This is supported by an association of psoriasis with human leukocyte antigen (HLA) class 1.

Cytokines (Th1, Th17, and Th22), chemokines, adhesion molecules, growth factors like NGF, neuropeptides, and specific T-cell subpopulations along with their receptors all act in an integrated way to evolve into unique inflammatory and proliferative processes typical for psoriasis.

## The Clinical Spectrum, Classification, and Diagnosis of Psoriasis

Psoriasis is a systemic disease and thus, the disease is not restricted to skin and nails. The primary skin lesions may vary from macules, papules, plaques to pustules.

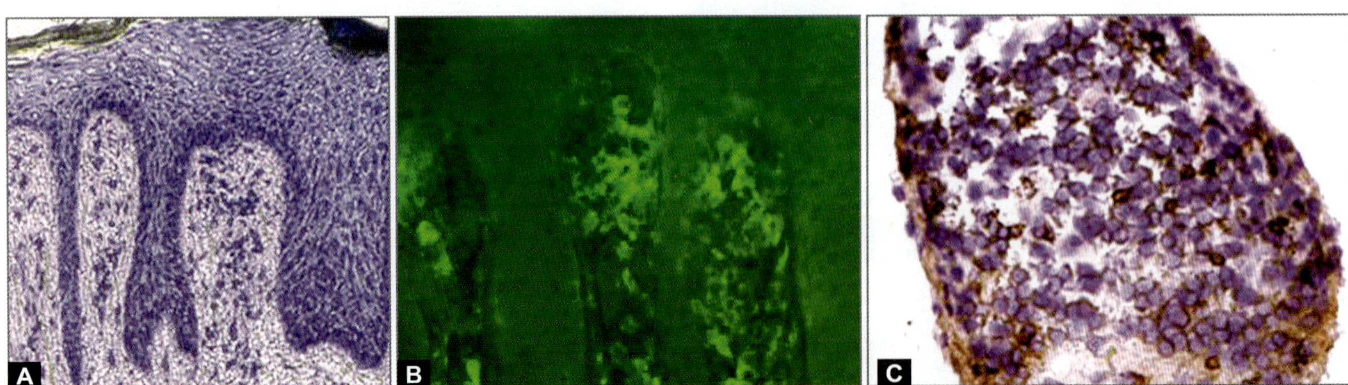


**FIG. 2:** Histopathological features of psoriatic disease. **A,** A psoriasis plaque demonstrating some of the unique histological features of psoriasis—parakeratosis, loss of stratum granulosum, suprapapillary thinning, elongated rete pegs, diffuse superficial, and deep dermal infiltrates; **B,** A psoriasis plaque stained with an anti-CD3 antibody demonstrates diffuse infiltration of CD3+ T-cells in the deep and superficial dermis; **C,** Synovial tissue collected from knee joint of a psoriatic arthritis patient; stained with an anti-CD3 antibody and counter stained with hematoxylin demonstrates marked infiltrations of CD3+ T lymphocytes.

About 30% of patients may develop an inflammatory arthritis; and on occasions patients with psoriatic disease may also develop uveitis and inflammatory bowel disease.

## Disease Classification

Based on the morphology of a specific lesion, anatomic location of psoriasis, age of onset, and the degree of the skin involvement psoriasis has been classified into various clinical phenotypes. Clinical features of the different psoriasis subtypes are described in details by Farber and Nall. Table 1 outlines the various clinical phenotypes that can be seen.

**TABLE 1: Clinical classification of psoriasis**

| Classification criteria | Clinical phenotypes |
|---|---|
| Age of onset | • Infantile psoriasis<br>• Childhood psoriasis<br>• Type I psoriasis—age of onset before 40 years<br>• Type II psoriasis—age of onset before 40 years |
| Degree of severity according to body surface area (BSA) involvement or number of sites | • Mild psoriasis: <5% BSA<br>• Moderate psoriasis: 5–10% BSA<br>• Severe psoriasis: >10% BSA<br>• Localized psoriasis or widespread psoriasis |
| Pattern of distribution | • Inverse, flexor, and seborrheic |
| Morphology | • Plaque, guttate, erythrodermic, pustular (generalized/localized), rupioid, elephantine |
| Anatomical site | • Scalp psoriasis, palmoplantar psoriasis, genital psoriasis, nail psoriasis, and anal psoriasis |
| Stage of development | • Stable plaque psoriasis<br>• Unstable eruptive psoriasis |

## Clinical Phenotypes of Psoriasis

### *Plaque Psoriasis*

Plaque psoriasis also known as psoriasis vulgaris represents almost 90% of psoriatic patients. Morphologic characteristics of psoriasis vulgaris are—symmetrical, circumscribed erythematous scaly indurated plaques, and dry and loosely adherent silvery white scales (Fig. 3). The lesions usually begin as erythematous macules or papules, extend peripherally, and coalesce to form plaques. Elbows, knees, and scalp are the most common site of involvement (Fig. 4a to c).

New lesions may appear following direct cutaneous trauma, which is known as the Koebner phenomenon (Fig. 4e). Removal of the surface scales shows presence of in pinpoint bleeding (Auspitz phenomenon).

## Guttate Psoriasis

Onset of guttate psoriasis many a times is associated with streptococcal infection or an upper respiratory tract infection. Guttate psoriasis frequently affects children and adolescents. The characteristic features of guttate psoriasis are—sudden onset, the lesions appear as droplets ('gutta'), round erythematous exanthem (<1 cm) over the trunk and extremities in a centripetal fashion, and monomorphic lesions at the same stage of evolution. Generally the disease is self-limiting, but a certain percentage of individuals with guttate psoriasis may progress to chronic plaque psoriasis and patients who have complete recovery still have a significantly higher risk for developing plaque psoriasis in the future. Chronic plaque psoriasis and guttate psoriasis are genetically similar, both with a strong association with the PSORS1 genetic locus.

### *Pustular Psoriasis*

Pustular psoriasis is characterized by sterile pustules with an underlying, blotchy, and erythematous base (Fig. 4f). Pustular

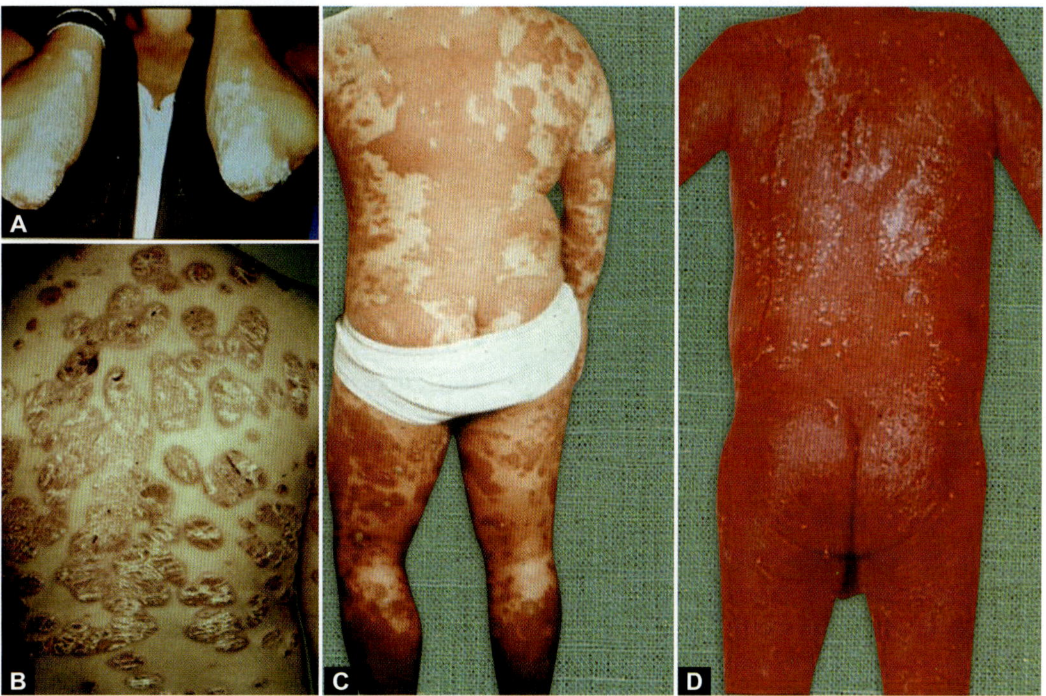

FIG. 3: Plaque psoriasis and erythrodermic psoriasis. **A,** Localized plaques psoriasis on elbows; **B,** Stable widespread plaques with characteristic features of psoriasis—circumscribed erythematous indurated lesions with loosely adherent silvery white scales; **C,** Unstable widespread psoriasis progressing to erythrodema; **D,** Erythrodermic psoriasis.

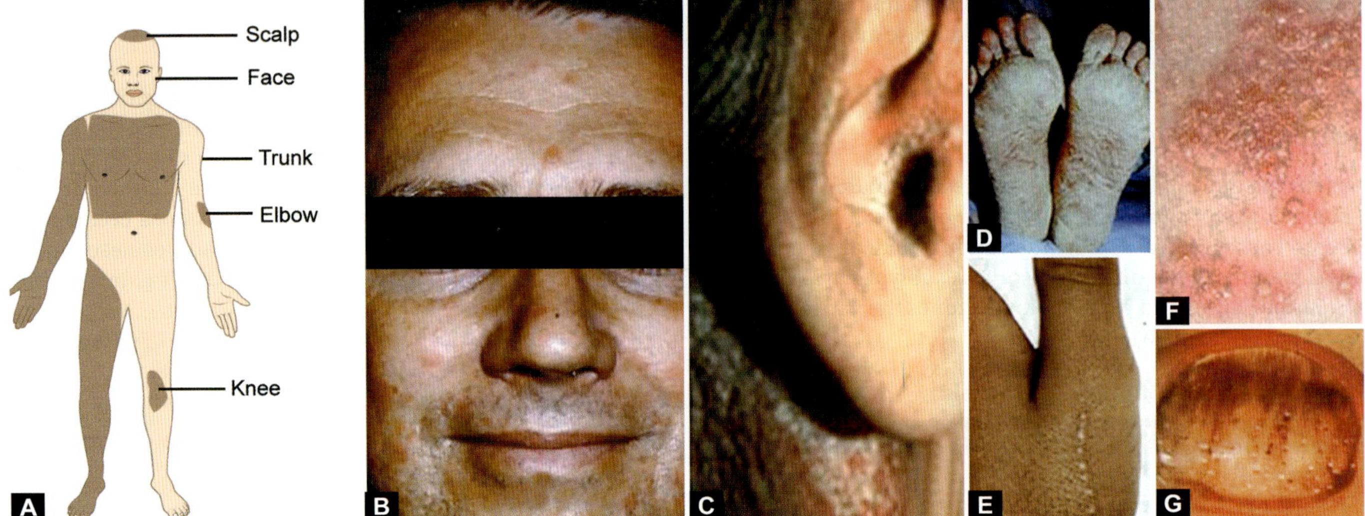


**FIG. 4:** Clinical phenotypes of psoriasis. **A,** Common sites of psoriasis; **B,** Facial psoriasis—a clinical challenge, many a times difficult to treat; **C,** Scalp and ear psoriasis; **D,** Plantar psoriasis; **E,** Koebner phenomenon—in a known patient of psoriasis after a cat scratch; **F,** Pustular psoriasis—initial discrete pustular lesions on an erythematous base, lesions are often tender; **G,** Classical nail pitting on a finger nail, nail changes are a frequent feature of psoriasis.

psoriasis can be generalized (von Zumbusch) or localized. Histologically, the lesions show diffuse dermal neutrophilic infiltration and intraepidermal micropustules.

Palmoplantar pustulosis and acrodermatitis continua of Hallopeau are two distinct forms of localized pustular psoriasis. It has been reported that 20% of chronic plaque psoriasis patients may have pustular lesions during the course of the disease.

Palmoplantar pustular psoriasis manifests *as* pustules on the palms and soles on an erythematous base and scaling. Plaque formation is not typically seen in palmoplantar pustulosis, but it may be associated with psoriasis vulgaris.

Generalized pustular psoriasis (von Zumbusch) is another rare serious life-threatening dermatological condition. This condition may appear *de-novo*; however, well-known precipitating factors for this severe condition are—infection, pregnancy, drugs, hypocalcemia, irritant topical treatment of plaque psoriasis such as with anthralin, and abrupt corticosteroid withdrawal. Generalized pustular psoriasis is a systemic disease, often associated with fever, myalgia, nausea, leukocytosis, and characterized by erythematous tender skin. There may be geographic tongue, polyarthritis, and cholestasis associated with generalized pustular psoriasis. Infrequently pustular psoriasis can appear during the first 6 months of pregnancy, which is then referred to as impetigo herpetiformis.

Generalized pustular psoriasis is an aggressive disease. Within hours of onset, innumerable pustules appear on an erythematous base (Fig. 4f) and later pustules may confluent to create sheets of superficial pus. The pustules eventually desiccate and the lesions sloughs off leaving a shiny erythematous surface where new crops of pustules might appear. Patients with generalized pustular psoriasis are often severely sick, require hospitalization, and require close monitoring of their liver function, hypocalcemia, and hydration. With supportive care and aggressive treatment pustular psoriasis may go into remission.

### Erythrodermic Psoriasis

Erythrodermic psoriasis is characterized by generalized erythema, (Fig. 3d). Precipitating factors for erythrodermic psoriasis are—poor control of existing psoriasis, abrupt withdrawal of systemic medication, such as corticosteroids, drug reaction, such as with lithium or antimalarial drugs, and underlying systemic infection.

Erythroderma can be a life-threatening condition and the differential diagnosis of erythroderma is broad—psoriasis, drug rash, and atopic dermatitis especially in children, airborne contact dermatitis, Sézary syndrome, and pityriasis rubra pilaris.

Pre-existing psoriasis lesion and nail changes may offer vital clinical clues to the diagnosis. Also skin biopsy may be helpful for diagnosing.

### Localized Psoriasis

Specific phenotypes according to anatomical locations—

- *Scalp psoriasis*: The scalp is a common site for psoriasis (Figs 4a and c). Because of its visibility scalp psoriasis impairs quality of life and needs special attention. Particular challenges in managing scalp psoriasis include choosing an appropriate treatment option, difficulties of applying topical treatments, and deciding how to treat severe disease which includes use of biologics in appropriate condition
- *Inverse or flexural psoriasis*: Inverse psoriasis or flexural psoriasis is the psoriasis of flexor surfaces and the skin folds such as on perineal, inframammary, axillary, inguinal, and intergluteal areas. As these areas are moist, psoriasis is less scaly than the plaque form of psoriasis
- *Palmoplantar psoriasis*: Palmoplantar psoriasis is characterized by thickening of the palmoplantar skin (Fig. 4d). This can be a disabling condition with thick scales and painful fissures. Palmoplantar psoriasis may be associated with severe impairment of health-related quality of life. Treatment of recalcitrant palmoplantar psoriasis can be difficult
- *Genital psoriasis*: Genital involvement is common (>30%) in patients with psoriasis. Sexual distress and dysfunction are particularly prominent in women. A special attention is required to this form of psoriasis as it significantly affects quality of life in both men and women

- *Nail psoriasis*: Nails are commonly involved in psoriasis and on occasions their characteristic changes can fetch the diagnosis of psoriasis. Pitting (Fig. 4g) and onycholysis of nails are the most common and characteristic feature of psoriasis. Whereas, "oil spots" or orange-yellow areas beneath the nail plates indicate involvement of the nail beds. In addition, the nail plate may become thickened, dystrophic, discolored, and yellow. Current treatment options for nail psoriasis are limited and often poorly efficacious.

## TREATMENT

### Topical Therapy

Topical therapies are the mainstay for mild disease either as monotherapy or in combination, and are also commonly used in conjunction with phototherapy, traditional systemic agents, or biologic agents for moderate-to-severe disease. The main molecules used for topical therapy of psoriasis are emollients, coal tar, topical corticosteroids, dithranol, vitamin D and its analog, and retinoids.

### Topical Corticosteroids

Mild-to-moderate potency topical corticosteroids are the mainly used. They should be avoided in genital and flexural psoriasis and psoriasis involving face.

Intralesional therapy is used for nail psoriasis, though the treatment is very painful and less endurable.

Topical corticosteroid treatment of limited plaque psoriasis has been found to achieve good results. However, continuous use of it for more than 2–3 weeks may induce tachyphylaxis. Topical corticosteroids are often combined with other topical drugs like vitamin D3 analog, keratolytics like salicylic acids and anthralin to achieve faster and prolonged benefits.

### Tar

Coal tar by virtue of its anti-inflammatory action is found to have effective role in limited plaque psoriasis. Tar shampoos alone or in combination are used in scalp psoriasis. It also has antipruritic role.

### Anthralin

Anthralin has anti-proliferative effect on the keratinocytes. It also has inhibitory effect on the proliferating T-cells and also inhibits neutrophil chemotaxis thereby justifying its anti-inflammatory role in treatment of psoriasis. The use of dithranol for the treatment of psoriasis was first described by Unna in 1916. In the past it used to be recommended as Ingram regimen. Dithranol is recommended as a second-line monotherapeutic topical agent in the treatment of mild-to-moderate psoriasis. It is contraindicated in pustular lesions, unstable lesions, and in erythrodermic phase. Out-patient short-contact dithranol is less effective than Ingram regimen but considering its cost-effectiveness and compliance, short contact therapy with dithranol has replaced Ingram regimen. Irritation and brown staining of the skin are the common side effects and is better to avoid in facial and flexural lesions.

### Vitamin D Analog

The naturally occurring active metabolite of vitamin $D_3$, 1, 25-dihydroxyvitamin $D_3$ (calcitriol), and synthetic analogs—calcipotriol and 1, 24-dihydroxyvitamin $D_3$ (tacalcitol) have all been shown to be effective as topical therapy. Vitamin D induces normal differentiation of hyperproliferating epidermal cells and also inhibits neutrophil function. Vitamin D monotherapy has been found to be quite effective. Efficacy increases when combined with topical corticosteroids. Cream formulation is less effective than ointment. It is recommended as a first-line monotherapy in mild-to-moderate disease. Major contraindications are renal insufficiency, pregnancy, lactation, and patients with bone or calcium metabolism defect. Irritation may occur as common local side effect and there may occur systemic hypercalcemia and hypercalciuria in predisposed individual or in case of overdosing.

It is recommended to restrict the amount of calcipotriol (50 μg/g) ointment to less than 100 g or 50 g/$m^2$ per week, and to monitor serum and urinary calcium levels when doses are exceeded.

### Topical Retinoids

Tazarotene, a synthetic retinoid, whose main metabolite, tazarotenic acid, binds to retinoic acid receptors (RARs) β and γ, is probably best reserved for thick recalcitrant plaques of psoriasis. All-trans retinoic acid is not effective in psoriasis. Tazarotene decreases epidermal proliferation and inhibits keratin 16 and transglutaminase expression. Manufactured as cream as well as gel formulation and recommended to be applied as once or twice daily.

The main drawback of tazarotene is local irritation at the site of application, and so it is frequently alternated with a potent topical corticosteroid.

### Topical Calcineurin Inhibitor

The topical calcineurin inhibitors tacrolimus and pimecrolimus have been shown to be effective for psoriasis affecting the face, neck, flexures, and genitalia. They have steroid sparing anti-inflammatory effect and can be given for long-term use.

### Salicylic Acid

Salicylic acid is a topical keratolytic agent. These effects lead to reduced scaling and softening of psoriatic plaques. Salicylic acid is mostly used in combination with topical corticosteroids. Topical salicylic acid decreases the efficacy of UVB phototherapy because of a filtering effect. It therefore should not be applied before UVB phototherapy.

### Combination Therapy

The combination of topical corticosteroids and salicylic acid may be valuable because of the ability of salicylic acid to enhance the efficacy of corticosteroids by increasing penetration. Due to the potential irritancy of topical tazarotene, adding topical corticosteroids to a regimen of tazarotene is an appropriate option. This combination therapy may increase the duration of treatment benefit as well as length of remission.

## Phototherapy and Photochemotherapy

### Psoralen and UVA

Psoralens bind to DNA and when activated by UVA cause permanent DNA damage with resulting cell death. Photochemotherapy is one of the mainstay in the treatment of moderate-to-severe psoriasis. Psoralens are used either topically or orally in combination with UVA. 8-Methoxypsoralen (8-MOP) is most commonly used for psoriasis and is given in the dose of 0.6 mg/kg 2 hours before UVA therapy. Psoralen-ultraviolet A (PUVA) is usually given as a twice or thrice weekly treatment. The initial dose of UVA is calculated as 70% of the minimal phototoxic dose and 20% increments are given until erythema occurs.

The contraindications to PUVA are genetic and acquired photosensitive disorders, treatment with other immunosuppressants like cyclosporine, pregnancy, lactation, and impaired liver function.

Presently its use is largely declining as there is much safer option yet efficacious is available with narrow-band UVB.

### Narrow-band UVB

Narrow-band UVB therapy (311 nm) is found to be more efficacious than broadband UVB and almost of equal efficacy to PUVA. It can be combined with other systemic therapies like methotrexate and acitretin to achieve faster clearance rate with lesser incidence of side effects due to long-term systemic therapy. NB UVB has less carcinogenic potential than PUVA. It can be safely used in children and in pregnant women.

## Systemic Therapy

### Methotrexate

This is the most commonly prescribed the first-line systemic therapy for psoriasis.

Methotrexate competitively inhibits the enzyme dihydrofolate reductase, thus decreasing the synthesis of folate cofactors needed to produce nucleic acids. Methotrexate was approved by the Food and Drug Administration (FDA) in 1972 for the treatment of severe, recalcitrant, and disabling psoriasis.

The indications of methotrexate are:

- Chronic plaque psoriasis with more than 10% body surface area (BSA) involvement
- Pustular psoriasis
- Erythrodermic psoriasis
- Psoriatic arthritis
- Psoriasis recalcitrant to topical treatments, photo (chemo) therapy or systemic retinoids.

Methotrexate is administered weekly. Single weekly dosage is more convenient than 2–3 doses given at 12 hours interval. Intramuscular injection reduces the gastric side effects. The maximum weekly dose should not exceed 25 mg. Usually a much lower dose is needed in most of the plaque psoriasis cases.

Common and generally minor toxicities of methotrexate include nausea, anorexia, stomatitis, and fatigue that most often occur at the time of methotrexate administration. The major toxicities that are of greatest concern in patients treated with methotrexate are myelosuppression, hepatotoxicity, and pulmonary fibrosis.

The practice of using a single test dose of methotrexate helps to ensure that severe myelosuppression does not occur. However, pancytopenia can rarely happen after an uneventful result following test dose.

Methotrexate-induced liver toxicity resembles nonalcoholic steatohepatitis. Hepatic fibrosis and cirrhosis occur less frequently. Methotrexate is FDA pregnancy category X and is contraindicated in women attempting to conceive.

### Cyclosporine

Cyclosporine (CyA) is a highly effective and rapidly acting systemic agent for the treatment of psoriasis. CyA induces immunosuppression by inhibiting the first phase of T-cell activation. Binding to cyclophillin with the resulting CyA/cyclophilin complex, inhibiting the enzyme calcineurin leading to blockade of signal transduction pathways that are dependent on the transcription factor and nuclear factor of activated T-cells.

Usual dose is 2.5–5 mg/kg/day. It should be tapered after 4–6 weeks. CyA should be administered at a consistent time of the day and in relation to meals to decrease the intraindividual blood level variations.

The CyA solution can be mixed with milk or orange juice but not with grapefruit juice.

The most serious side effects are nephrotoxicity and hypertension. Patients with psoriasis taking CyA may be at increased risk of developing cutaneous squamous cell carcinomas (SCCs).

Hypertriglyceridemia, hypertrichosis, headache, gingival hypertrophy, reduction of seizure threshold, and gastrointestinal symptoms are the other commonly encountered side effects.

This is possibly safe in pregnancy when treatment becomes necessary.

### Acitretin

Etretinate was the first retinoid introduced for the treatment of severe psoriasis and replaced in 1988 by acitretin, the active metabolite of etretinate. Retinoids are known to modulate epidermal proliferation and differentiation and to have immunomodulatory and anti-inflammatory activity. Acitretin may be used as an effective maintenance therapy in chronic plaque psoriasis. Acitretin monotherapy is indicated in erythrodermic and pustular psoriasis.

The efficacy of acitretin is dose-dependent. Acitretin response is relatively slow with a 3–6-month period required to achieve a maximal response. Acitretin is FDA pregnancy category X (highly unsafe during pregnancy). Half-life of acitretin is 49 hours. However, acitretin may transform either spontaneously, or as a result of alcohol ingestion, into etretinate, which has a half-life of 168 days. Based on this long half-life, it can take up to 3 years for etretinate to be eliminated from the body. For these reasons, acitretin is contraindicated in women who plan to become pregnant or who fail to use adequate contraception for 3 years after discontinuing acitretin.

Mucocutaneous side effects of acitretin occur in almost all patients to varying degrees and may include cheilitis, dryness of the eyes, nasal and oral mucosa, epistaxis, xerosis, brittle nails, hair loss, and burning or sticky skin. The most common laboratory abnormality seen in patients treated with acitretin is hyperlipidemia. Elevations of transaminases occur in 13–16% of patients treated with acitretin.

## Targeted Immune Therapy

Biologic therapy was introduced for the treatment of psoriatic arthritis and moderate-to-severe psoriasis. The two major targets are T-cells and the cytokines. The biologics are chosen according to the target of action. The biologics used in psoriasis and psoriatic arthritis are etanercept, alefacept, infliximab, adalimumab, and ustekinumab. Biologics should be reserved for those patients who have failed to respond to one of the classic systemic therapies. There is considerable overlap in the efficacies of the biologic agents and other modes of systemic therapies. However, it is in consensus that the TNF-α inhibitors and the IL-12/23 antibodies show good efficacy in clearing disease and also in maintaining long-term control.

## Second-line Systemic Therapy

### Azathioprine

Azathioprine, a purine analog that blocks purine synthesis, is a commonly used immunosuppressive agent. Few reports suggest beneficial results in psoriasis.

### Hydroxyurea

Hydroxyurea is an antimetabolite used in the treatment of certain cancers and hematologic conditions. It is used for long in the treatment of psoriasis. It is thought to work by inhibiting DNA replication.

The major adverse effect of hydroxyurea is bone marrow toxicity causing leukopenia, anemia, thrombocytopenia, or, less commonly, pancytopenia.

### Fumaric acid esters

Fumaric acid esters (also known as fumarates) are a mixture of dimethylfumarate along with monoethylfumarate salts. Fumarates appear to function by inhibiting T lymphocytes and shifting the cytokine profile from a T-helper 1 to a T-helper 2 phenotype.

The most common adverse effect of the fumarates are gastrointestinal symptoms, including gastric and esophageal pain as well as nausea and vomiting, which may occur in over two-thirds of patients.

Drugs like sulfasalazine, mycophenolate mofetil, leflunomide, 6-thioguanine, etc. have also been tried.

### Newer Agents

Apremilast is an inhibitor of phosphodiesterase-4 that has modulating role on pro-inflammatory production. It has recently been approved in the treatment of psoriasis and psoriatic arthritis.

## Tofacitinib

It is an oral drug which acts by inhibiting Janus kinase JAK1 and JAK 3. It has also shown efficacy in the treatment of psoriasis and psoriatic arthritis.

## SUGGESTED READINGS


1. Cassell SE, Bieber JD, Rich P, et al. The modified Nail Psoriasis Severity Index: Validation of an instrument to assess psoriatic nail involvement in patients with psoriatic arthritis. J Rheumatol. 2007;34:123-9.
2. Chan CS, Van Voorhees AS, Lebwohl MG, et al. Treatment of severe scalp psoriasis: from the Medical Board of the National Psoriasis Foundation. J Am Acad Dermatol. 2009;60:962-71.
3. Chung J, Callis Duffin K, Takeshita J, et al. Palmoplantar psoriasis is associated with greater impairment of health-related quality of life compared with moderate to severe plaque psoriasis. J Am Acad Dermatol. 2014;71:623-32.
4. Datta Mitra A, Raychaudhuri SP, Abria CJ, et al. 1α, 25-Dihydroxyvitamin-D3-3-bromoacetate regulates AKT/mTOR signaling cascades: a therapeutic agent for psoriasis. J Invest Dermatol. 2013;133:1556-64.
5. de Jong EM, Seegers BA, Gulinck MK, et al. Psoriasis of the nails associated with disability in a large number of patients: results of a recent interview with 1,728 patients. Dermatology. 1996;193:300-3.
6. Elder JT, Bruce AT, Gudjonsson JE, et al. Molecular dissection of psoriasis: integrating genetics and biology. J Invest Dermatol. 2010;130(5):1213-26.
7. Farley E, Masrour S, McKey J, et al. Palmoplantar psoriasis: a phenotypical and clinical review with introduction of a new quality-of-life assessment tool. J Am Acad Dermatol. 2009;60:1024-31.
8. Gelfand JM, Neimann AL, Shin DB, et al. Risk of myocardial infarction in patients with psoriasis. JAMA. 2006;296:1735-41.
9. Janagond AB, Kanwar AJ, Handa S. Efficacy and safety of systemic methotrexate vs. acitretin in psoriasis patients with significant palmoplantar involvement: a prospective, randomized study. J Eur Acad Dermatol Venereol. 2013;27(3):e384-9.
10. Jordan CT, Cao L, Roberson ED, et al. PSORS2 is due to mutations in CARD14. Am J Hum Genet. 2012;90(5):784-95.
11. Krishnamurthy K, Walker A, Gropper CA, Hoffman C. To treat or not to treat? Management of guttate psoriasis and pityriasis rosea in patients with evidence of group A Streptococcal infection. J Drugs Dermatol. 2010;9(3):241-50.
12. Leonardi C, Matheson R, Zachariae C, et al. Anti-interleukin-17 monoclonal antibody ixekizumab in chronic plaque psoriasis. N Engl J Med. 2012;366(13):1190-9.
13. Levine D, Gottlieb A. Evaluation and management of psoriasis: an internist's guide. Med Clin North Am. 2009;93(6):1291-303.
14. McInnes IB, Sieper J, Braun J, et al. Efficacy and safety of secukinumab, a fully human anti-interleukin-17A monoclonal antibody, in patients with moderate-to-severe psoriatic arthritis: a 24-week, randomised, double-blind, placebo-controlled, phase II proof-of-concept trial. Ann Rheum Dis. 2014;73(2):349-56.
15. Meeuwis KA, de Hullu JA, de Jager ME, et al. Genital psoriasis: a questionnaire-based survey on a concealed skin disease in the Netherlands. J Eur Acad Dermatol Venereol. 2010;24(12):1425-30.
16. O'Brien M, Koo J. The mechanism of lithium and beta-blocking agents in inducing and exacerbating psoriasis. J Drugs Dermatol. 2006;5:426-32.
17. Papp KA, Leonardi C, Menter A, et al. Brodalumab, an anti-interleukin-17-receptor antibody for psoriasis. N Engl J Med. 2012;366(13):1181-9.
18. Patel M, Liu SW, Qureshi A, et al. The Brigham Scalp Nail Inverse Palmoplantar Psoriasis Composite Index (B-SNIPI): a novel index to measure all non-plaque psoriasis subsets. J Rheumatol. 2014;41:1230-2.
19. Rathod NN, Panicker NK, Gore CR, et al. The clinical and histopathological co-relation of psoriasiform dermatoses. NJIRM. 2012;3(3):52-6.
20. Raychaudhuri SK, Maverakis E, Raychaudhuri SP. Diagnosis and classification of psoriasis. Autoimmun Rev. 2014;13(4-5):490-5.
21. Raychaudhuri SP, Farber EM. The prevalence of psoriasis in the world. J Eur Acad Dermatol Venereol. 2001;15(1):16-7.
22. Raychaudhuri SP, Gross J. Psoriasis risk factors: role of lifestyle practices. Cutis. 2000;66(5):348-52.
23. Raychaudhuri SP, Gross J. A comparative study of pediatric onset psoriasis with adult onset psoriasis. Pediatr Dermatol. 2000;17(3):174-8.
24. Raychaudhuri SP, Jiang WY, Raychaudhuri SK. Revisiting the Koebner Phenomenon: Role of NGF and its receptor system in the pathogenesis of psoriasis. Am J Pathol. 2008;172(4):961-71.
25. Raychaudhuri SP, Smoller BR. Nonspecific inflammatory dermatoses of patients with HIV disease. European J Dermatol. 1993;3:102-4.
26. Raychaudhuri SP, Raychaudhuri SK, Tamura K, et al. FR255734, a humanized, Fc-silent, anti-CD28 antibody improves psoriasis in the SCID mouse-psoriasis xenograft model. J Invest Dermatol. 2008;128(8):1969-76.
27. Raychaudhuri SP. Role of IL-17 in psoriasis and psoriatic arthritis. Clin Rev Allergy Immunol. 2013;44:183-93.
28. Raychaudhuri SP. A Cutting Edge Overview: Psoriatic Disease. Clin Rev Allergy Immunol. 2013;44:109-13.
29. Rongioletti F, Fiorucci C, Parodi A. Psoriasis induced or aggravated by drugs. J Rheumatol Suppl. 2009;83:59-61.
30. Sugiura K, Oiso N, Iinuma S, et al. IL36RN mutations underlie impetigo herpetiformis. J Invest Dermatol. 2014;134:2472-4.
31. Wozel G. Psoriasis treatment in difficult locations: scalp, nails, and intertriginous areas. Clin Dermatol. 2008;26(5):448-59.

# 28 CHAPTER Psoriatic Arthritis

*Nilendu Sarma, Sushila Hansda*

## INTRODUCTION

Psoriatic arthritis (PsA) is a heterogeneous disease in terms of wide range of articular manifestation, severity, response to treatment and also in its involvement of extra-articular manifestations (skin and other organs).

Prevalence of PsA among psoriasis cases varies widely from 6.25 to 48% as reported from some Western countries. This is reported to be much less (1–8%) in many Asian countries, including India. However, prevalence is possibly under-reported from many areas, because of under recognition of this condition.

## PATHOGENESIS

### Genetics

First degree relatives of psoriasis are at higher risk (49 times higher risk). Newer studies suggest that PsA and psoriasis may be regulated by different sets of genes. Although many of human leukocyte antigen (HLA) and many outside the major histocompatibility complex (MHC) region are found to have strong association with psoriasis as well as PsA, some of these show stronger association for either of these two. HLA-B*27 and other HLA-B alleles like B*38, B*08, and polymorphisms in the *IL-13* gene have stronger association with PsA. In contrast HLA-Cw*0602 is associated with more severe skin disease without joint involvement. *TRAF3IP2* gene has stronger association with PsA. Apart from these, many other candidate genes have been found to be associated with psoriasis and PsA like *LCE3, DEFB4, GJB2, TNFAIP3, NFKBIA, REL, TYK2, NOS2, DDX58, ZC3H12C, CARD14, HLA-C, IL12B, IL23R, IL23A, TRAF3IP2, ERAP1, TAGAP* and *STAT3.*

### Immune Dysregulation

Immune dysregulation is one of the major regulating mechanisms in psoriasis and PsA. Many facts are yet to be defined and understood. Activated CD4+ and CD8+ cells and neutrophils infiltrate the affected tissue and causes damage to it. CD4+ cells predominate in dermal papilla and CD8+ predominate in epidermis, and joints especially entheses. Neutrophils are detected in high number in synovial fluid.

The IL-17A secreted by Th17 cells, including neutrophils and mast cells is detected in synovial tissue in PsA as well as in skin lesions in psoriasis. IL23, another important cytokine promotes Th17 phenotype. Similar to IL17A, IL23 is significantly elevated in psoriatic skin and in synovium in PsA.

## RISK FACTORS

- Trauma to the joints, infection (HIV), rubella vaccination (Koebner's phenomena)
- Cardiovascular diseases, dyslipidemia, obesity, type 2 diabetes mellitus, and other components of metabolic syndromes are known to be risk factors of PsA as described later
- Body surface area (BSA) of psoriasis is correlated with chance of PsA. Psoriasis Area Severity Index (PASI) does not correlate with PsA severity.
- Type of psoriasis—scalp psoriasis, nail psoriasis (risk factor for severity of PsA)
- Body mass index (correlates with incidence of PsA among psoriasis patients).

## CLINICAL FEATURES

Psoriatic arthritis involves peripheral joints, digital joints, and axial joints. Generally, PsA starts many months to years after psoriasis (average 12 years) but PsA may precede or start simultaneously with psoriasis in about one-fifth of the cases.

Typically, PsA starts insidiously. In a large number of cases, it may progress to erosive joint deformities (40–57% of all PsA). In as much as 19% of cases, it may lead to functional disability. Even the overall mortality is higher than general population.

In 1973, Moll and Wright proposed criteria for classification of PsA. They classified PsA into five subtypes (Box 1).

This has been placed into a group of disorders characterized by axial arthropathy called spondyloarthropathy [rheumatoid arthritis (RA) factor negative]. Other diseases in this group are ankylosing spondylitis (AS), reactive arthritis (ReA) and inflammatory bowel disease associated arthropathy. Distal interphalangeal joint involvement although not seen in many cases of PsA is a typical feature of this condition. Enthesitis is another diagnostic presentation.

| **BOX 1** | **Moll and Wright classification criteria of psoriatic arthritis (PsA)** |
|---|---|
| • Polyarticular, symmetric arthritis (rheumatoid arthritis like)<br>• Oligoarticular, asymmetric arthritis | • Spondylitis predominant<br>• Arthritis mutilans<br>• Distal interphalangeal joint predominant |

Unless there is presence of psoriasis, diagnosis of PsA may be difficult even by the experts. It is frequently confused with other rheumatological conditions like RA, ReA, AS, osteoarthritis (OA) and gout. These conditions may coexist with PsA further complicating the situation. No laboratory test is available to confirm the diagnosis. Clinical diagnosis is the only way to diagnose PsA. Meticulous clinical examination is the most helpful tool for diagnosis of PsA.

Enthesitis, a condition defined as inflammation at the site of tendon or ligament insertion at the bone is another very classical and common feature of PsA. This is different from synovitis, which is typically found in RA. This is seen in about 42% of all PsA.

Pattern of joint involvement has been traditionally considered as helpful signs for diagnosis of PsA as proposed in Moll and Wright criteria. Predominant distal interphalangeal joint (DIP) involvement is considered a unique feature of PsA (Figs 1 and 2). However, this is seen in just 5–10% of all cases, mostly men.

Involvement of all three joints of a single finger along with tenosynovitis may result in "dactylitis" that manifests as swollen finger (sausage digit) or toe (Fig. 3). This is rarely seen in other conditions. ReA may occasionally develop dactylitis and gouty tophi may sometimes mimic it.

Clinical presentation may simulate RA (Fig. 4). Presence of classical psoriasis elsewhere is considered a helpful sign.

Psoriatic arthritis involves spinal joints (spondylitis, i.e., inflammation of spinal apophyseal joints and/or sacroiliitis. Spondylitis alone or in association with peripheral joints may be seen in about 40% of all cases. Cervical and lower spinal with relative sparing of thoracolumbar spinal joint involvement is seen in PsA. PsA is characterized by oligoarthritis (4 or less) that subsequently becomes polyarticular. Asymmetrical involvement even at late stage, for both peripheral and spinal joints is very typical finding in PsA. Pattern of joint involvement in PsA was first described by Moll and Wright. Although this is very important to understand the disease manifestation and diagnosis, too much dependence only on patterns in joint involvement may lead to misdiagnosis.

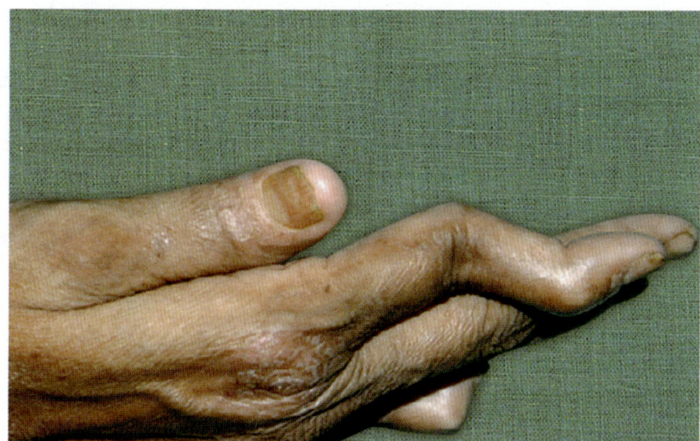

**FIG. 1:** Classical distal interphalangeal joint involvement in psoriatic arthritis.

*Courtesy*: Dr Shekhar Neema, Assistant Professor, Department of Dermatology, Command Hospital, Kolkata, West Bengal.

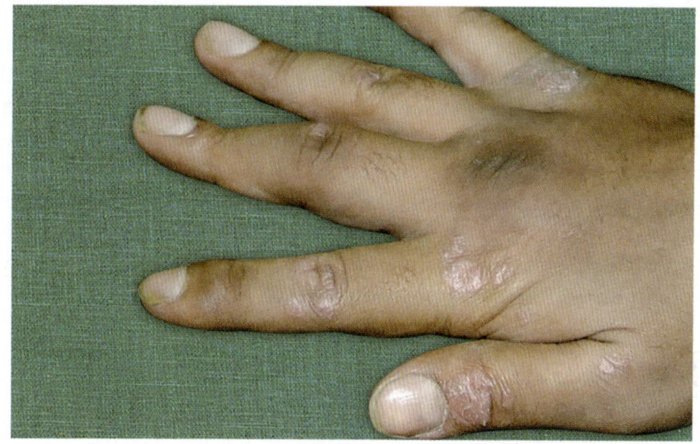

**FIG. 3:** Sausage-shaped middle finger due to psoriatic dactylitis.

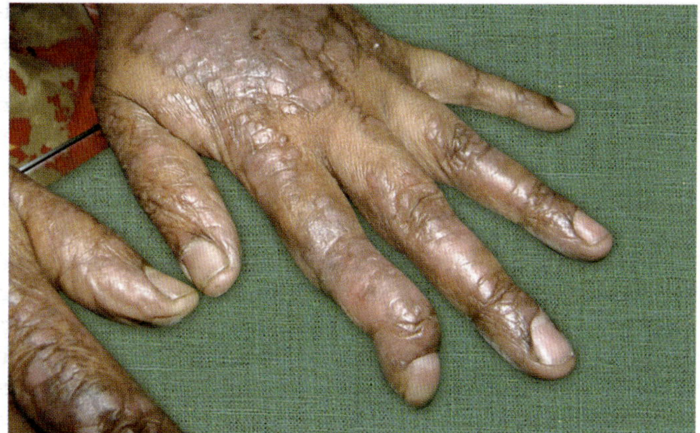

**FIG. 2:** Distal interphalangeal joint involvement psoriatic arthritis and typical psoriasis lesion on hands.

*Courtesy*: Dr Brijesh Nair, Consultant Dermatologist, Military Hospital, Jaipur, Rajasthan.

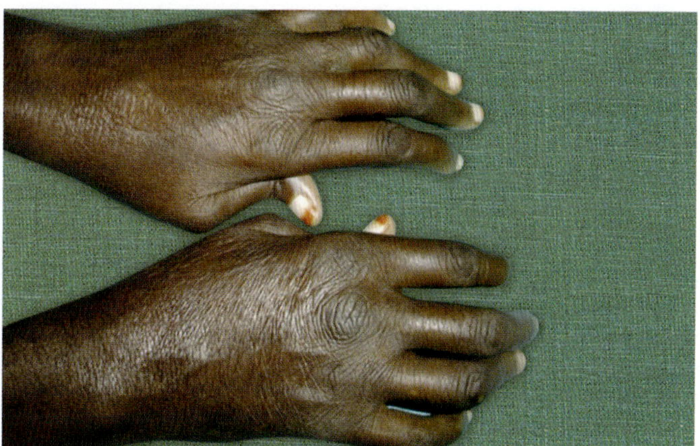

**FIG. 4:** "Rheumatoid arthritis"-like psoriatic arthritis; bilateral symmetrical proximal interphalangeal joint involvement.

*Courtesy*: Dr Aprana Palit, Dr Arun C Inamadar, Department of Dermatology, Venereology and Leprosy, Shri B.M. Patil Medical College, Hospital & Research Center, BLDE University, Vijayapur, Karnataka.

Psoriatic arthritis is also characterized by simultaneous bone erosion and new bone formation (periostitis). Erosion is initially marginal (marginal areas or articular cartilage) and then it spread centrally. Central erosion leads to formation of pencil in cup/telescoping/opera glass deformity of digit. Extreme erosion leads to bone shortening at the end stage of so called arthritis mutilans. New bone formation/periostitis is seen close to erosion and is most prominent at the insertion site of tendons/ligaments. There is simultaneous bone formation in the form of "syndesmophyte" which is thicker and larger than seen in AS and is also different from osteophytes seen in OA. Moreover, in contrast to AS that involves the spines continuously, PsA leads to skipped involvement of the spinal joints. Erosion is not a feature of OA. Nodes around the joints (Heberden and Bouchard node), classical features of OA is not seen in PsA.

There are some helpful clues for the diagnosis of PsA. As mentioned earlier, presence of psoriasis elsewhere is very helpful in suspecting PsA as the etiology of inflammatory joint. Psoriatic nail involvement is very common (>80%) when PsA is present. In psoriasis without PsA it is present in less than 50% cases.

### Systemic Illness

Similar to psoriasis, PsA is also associated with higher prevalence of various systemic illness related to metabolic syndrome like cardiovascular morbidity, obesity, glucose intolerance, type-2 diabetes mellitus, hyperlipidemia, hypertension, coronary heart disease, congestive heart failure, cerebrovascular disease, peripheral vascular disease, and subclinical atherosclerosis. The relationship is bidirectional, i.e., both PsA and these conditions increase risk of each other. The association is stronger than with psoriasis. Presence of many of these conditions like obesity may impart unfavorable response to therapy.

## DIAGNOSIS

Joint stiffness in the morning or after periods of inactivity and that last more than 30–45 min is a helpful symptom. Presence of dactylitis, enthesitis, nail changes also help in diagnosis. Clinical examination should be supplemented with radiological examination whenever required. RA factor is generally negative except in a small subset (<10% of cases). HLA*B27 is positive in good number of cases (15–70%). Opinion of rheumatologists is invaluable in many occasions especially in many mild cases. This is important because missing cases at early stages correlates with poor prognosis. Laboratory parameter like erythrocyte sedimentation rate (ESR) is generally elevated and is known for its positive relation with disease score. C-reactive protein (CRP) is also often elevated.

Plain radiograph of the joints shows bone erosion and periostitis (new bone formation). New bone formation is detected at the site of insertion of ligaments. Tendo Achilles insertion at calcaneus is often the site of choice for detection of periostitis. Plain radiograph cannot detect enthesitis. MRI and ultrasound are required for this. In advanced stages, gross erosion results in pencil in cup deformity.

To ensure uniformity in diagnosis, CASPAR criteria that have specificity of 98.7% and sensitivity of 91.4% is used. Individual with presence of inflammatory arthritis having three or more of the features is considered having PsA:

1. Psoriasis: Active disease, or personal/family history in first or second degree relative
2. Psoriatic nail dystrophy
3. Negative RA factor
4. Dactylitis: Active disease or history
5. Radiographic evidence of juxta-articular new bone formation.

## MANAGEMENT

Management of PsA is dependent on severity of the condition, distribution and number of the joints involved (dactylitis or spinal disease), presence of enthesitis, associated skin lesions, and systemic illness.

## TREATMENT EFFICACY ASSESSMENT

Measurement of disease response to treatment can be done with many of the proposed scoring tools like the American College of Rheumatology (ACR) score, the modified disease activity score (DAS), PsA response criteria (PsARC). However, these are used only in clinical trials.

The ACR20 improvement criteria were proposed to measure the improvement after treatment in RA and now also used in PsA. "ACR response criteria" were proposed to measure the persistence in the improvement of various determinants for at least 2 months.

The ACR20 response criteria was defined as at least 20% improvement in the following parameters:

1. Swollen joint count
2. Tender joint count
3. Pain (visual analog scale)
4. Patient global disease activity
5. Physician global disease activity
6. Physical function
7. Acute-phase reactants (ESR or CRP).

[Points 1 and 2 are mandatory and there should be 3 out of the rest 5 points (3–7)].

Similarly ACR50 and ACR70 were proposed later to measure more satisfactory response.

### Drugs

There are many international guidelines on the management of PsA. Some of the most widely used are guidelines from European League against Rheumatism (EULAR), Scottish Intercollegiate Guidelines Network (SIGN), Group for Research and Assessment of Psoriasis and Psoriatic Arthritis (GRAPPA), and American Academy of Dermatology (AAD).

Treatment scheme of PsA is governed by the distribution of the disease. Most guidelines classify disease in categories like peripheral joint disease, dactylitis, spinal disease, and enthesitis. In each category, drugs are recommended as first line, second line, third line, and fourth line based on the severity in terms of symptoms, number of joints, progression, and objective signs of disease severity. Thus disease is sub-categorized as mild, moderate, and severe disease. Number of affected joints less than five is sometimes used as a guide to define mild disease.

Nonsteroidal anti-inflammatory drugs (NSAIDs) are the first-line drugs for mild disease in all the categories. Intra-articular corticosteroid injections are also recommended as first or second-line treatment. Disease-modifying antirheumatic drugs (DMARDs) are used in moderate to severe PsA generally in nonaxial diseases. Biologicals are recommended to be used in severe diseases.

Few important facts that should be kept in mind while managing a case of PsA. NSAIDs and acetaminophen are reported to aggravate PsA and also psoriasis (acetaminophen) when used for long term. Moreover, long-term use of NSAIDs may increase the chance of development of cardiovascular disease and inflammatory bowel diseases. Both have strong association with PsA.

The NSAIDs and all of the DMARDs do not halt the disease progression in a major subset of patients. Beyond guidelines, methotrexate (MTX) is the most commonly used DMARDs in PsA in clinical practice. This improves joint tenderness, swelling, and global symptoms of PsA. However, blinded control trials on the efficacy of MTX and other DMARDs in modifying disease activity after long-term use in PsA are lacking. Despite these facts, NSAIDs and DMARDs still find place in most of the available guidelines. Only TNF-α inhibitors are reported in few studies to halt the disease progression or even reverse. High cost is however prohibitive in most cases. Long-term studies are also lacking.

There are some other indirect advantages of the use of MTX is PsA. Methotrexate reduces the chance of development of antibody against TNF-α inhibitors, increases serum level of TNF-α inhibitors like infliximab and adalimumab. These facts support the advantages of MTX cotherapy along with TNF-α inhibitors. Another advantage of MTX use in PsA is its capacity to significantly reduce mortality rate from cardiovascular diseases, one frequently associated important systemic condition in PsA.

Sulfasalazine is another DMARD that has shown to be effectively improve PsA clinically. It has no beneficial role in psoriasis. Main difficulty in its use is its associated gastrointestinal intolerance. This is also not used in case of urinary obstruction, porphyria, breastfeeding mothers, liver or renal diseases, and hypersensitivity to sulfonamides or salicylates.

Leflunomide can improve PsA as well as psoriasis. Similar to MTX, it is hepatotoxic, teratogenic, and immunosuppressant.

Cyclosporine is less effective in PsA than in psoriasis. Similar to DMARDs, there is no evidence of its efficacy in modifying disease activity in PsA. This should be avoided in breastfeeding mothers, in presence of renal diseases, uncontrolled hypertension, lymphoproliferative, and skin malignancy and cotherapy is not recommended along with MTX, phototherapy, tar, and other immnosuppressants. It can cause low birth weight if used in pregnancy.

At present, five TNF inhibitors adalimumab, etanercept, golimumab, infliximab and certolizumab pegol and one IL-12/IL-23 inhibitor, ustekinumab are approved for treatment of PsA. All these TNF inhibitors increase the risk of opportunistic infections. They should be avoided in presence of active infection, immunosuppression (by drugs or diseases). Live vaccine should be avoided. Breastfeeding is better avoided. They can exacerbate demyelinating disease, congestive heart failure, and psoriasis.

All the five TNF inhibitors and ustekinumab are pregnancy category B drugs.

Newer biological and smaller molecules that have shown some promise in the management of PsA are abatacept, tocilizumab (IL-6 inhibitors), secukinumab and ixekizumab, and brodalumab (all IL-17 inhibitors), apremilast (phosphodiesterase-4 inhibitor) and tofacitinib (selective Janus kinase inhibitor).

## SUGGESTED READINGS


1. Boehncke WH, Kirby B, Fitzgerald O, et al. New developments in our understanding of psoriatic arthritis and their impact on the diagnosis and clinical management of the disease. J Eur Acad Dermatol Venereol. 2014;28:264-70.
2. Boehncke WH, Qureshi A, Merola F, et al. Diagnosing and treating psoriatic arthritis: an update. Br J Dermatol. 2014;170:772-86.
3. Chou R, Helfand M, Peterson K, et al. Drug Class Review: Cyclo-oxygenase (COX)-2 Inhibitors and Non-steroidal Anti-inflammatory Drugs (NSAIDs): Final Report Update 3. Portland (OR): Oregon Health & Science University; 2006.
4. de Vlam K, Gottlieb AB, Mease PJ. Current concepts in psoriatic arthritis: pathogenesis and management. Acta Derm Venereol. 2014;94:627-34
5. Eder L, Chandran V, Pellett F, et al. IL13 gene polymorphism is a marker for psoriatic arthritis among psoriasis patients. Ann Rheum Dis. 2011;70:1594-8.
6. Felson DT, Anderson JJ, Boers M, et al. American College of Rheumatology. Preliminary definition of improvement in rheumatoid arthritis. Arthritis Rheum. 1995;38:727-35.
7. Garg A, Gladman D. Recognizing psoriatic arthritis in the dermatology clinic. J Am Acad Dermatol. 2010;63:733-48.
8. Gossec L, Smolen JS, Gaujoux-Viala C et al. European League against Rheumatism recommendations for the management of psoriatic arthritis with the pharmacological therapies. Ann Rheum Dis. 2012;71:4-12.
9. Gottlieb A, Korman NJ, Gordon KB, et al. Guidelines of care for the management of psoriasis and psoriatic arthritis. Section 2. Psoriatic arthritis: Overview and guidelines of care for treatment with an emphasis on the biologics. J Am Acad Dermatol. 2008;58:851-64.
10. Kingsley GH, Kowalczyk A, Taylor H, et al. A randomized placebo-controlled trial of methotrexate in psoriatic arthritis. Rheumatology (Oxford). 2012;51:1368-77.
11. Maini RN, Breedveld FC, Kalden JR, et al. Therapeutic efficacy of multiple intravenous infusions of anti-tumor necrosis factor alpha monoclonal antibody combined with low-dose weekly methotrexate in rheumatoid arthritis. Arthritis Rheum. 1998;41:1552-63.
12. Maneiro JR, Salgado E, Gomez-Reino JJ. Immunogenicity of monoclonal antibodies against tumor necrosis factor used in chronic immune-mediated inflammatory conditions: systematic review and meta-analysis. JAMA Intern Med. 2013;173:1416-28.
13. Micha R, Imamura F, Wyler von Ballmoos M, et al. Systematic review and meta-analysis of methotrexate use and risk of cardiovascular disease. Am J Cardiol, 2011;108:1362-70.
14. Moll JM, Wright V. Psoriatic arthritis. Semin Arthritis Rheum. 1973;3:55-78.
15. Rahman P, Elder JT. Genetics of psoriasis and psoriatic arthritis: a report from the GRAPPA 2010 annual meeting. J Rheumatol. 2012;39:431-3.
16. Ritchlin CT, Kavanaugh A, Gladman DD, et al. Treatment recommendations for psoriatic arthritis. Ann Rheum Dis, 2009;68:1387-94.
17. Scottish Intercollegiate Guidelines Network (SIGN). Diagnosis and management of psoriasis and psoriatic arthritis in adults. Edinburgh: SIGN; 2010.
18. Shaowei WU, Jiali HA, Qureshi AA. Use of Aspirin, Non-steroidal Anti-inflammatory Drugs, and Acetaminophen (Paracetamol), and Risk of Psoriasis and Psoriatic Arthritis: A Cohort Study. Acta Derm Venereol. 2015;95:217-22.
19. Torre Alonso JC, Rodriguez Perez A, Arribas Castrillo JM, et al. Psoriatic arthritis (PA): a clinical, immunological and radiological study of 180 patients. Br J Rheumatol. 1991;30:245-50.
20. Tsoi LC, Spain SL, Knight J, et al. Identification of 15 new psoriasis susceptibility loci highlights the role of innate immunity. Nat Genet, 2012;44:1341-8.
21. Van Gestel AM, Prevoo ML, van Rijswijk MH, et al. Development and validation of the European League against Rheumatism response criteria for rheumatoid arthritis: comparison with the preliminary American College of Rheumatology and the World Health Organization/International League against Rheumatism Criteria. Arthritis Rheum. 1996;39:34-40.
22. Winchester R, Minevich G, Steshenko V, et al. HLA associations reveal genetic heterogeneity in psoriatic arthritis and in the psoriasis phenotype. Arthritis Rheum. 2012;64:1134-44.

# 29 CHAPTER Reactive Arthropathy

*Nilendu Sarma*

## INTRODUCTION

Reactive arthritis (ReA), (earlier name Reiter's syndrome/ Reiter's disease) is a condition characterized by a triad of conditions arthritis, urethritis, and eye inflammation (uveitis, conjuctivitis). However, other signs and symptoms in addition to this triad are also seen. Reactive arthritis is considered to be caused by an immunological reaction following a gastrointestinal or urogenital tract infection. Arthritis is negative for rheumatoid factor (seronegative arthritis). As spinal joints are also affected in addition to peripheral joints, this is often grouped along with other seronegative spondyloarthropathies (Box 1). ReA is characterized by predominantly peripheral joint involvement (see diagnostic criteria by American Colleague for Rheumatology later).

**BOX 1 Seronegative spondyloarthropathies**

- Ankylosing spondylitis
- Psoriatic arthritis
- Reactive arthritis
- Arthritis associated with inflammatory bowel diseases

## EPIDEMIOLOGY

Reactive arthritis is seen worldwide. Males have higher prevalence. Although, children are also affected, adults are commonly affected. Mean age of onset is third decade.

**BOX 2 Etiologies for reactive arthritis**

- *Chlamydia trachomatis*
- *Chlamydophila pneumonia*
- *Campylobacter jejuni*
- *Ureaplasma urealyticum*
- *Shigella flexneri*
- *Salmonella enteritidis*
- *Salmonella typhimurium*
- *Salmonella muenchen*
- *Yersinia enterocolitica*
- *Yersinia pseudotuberculosis*
- *Clostridium difficile*
- Immunization with Bacillus Calmette-Guérin vaccine
- *Helicobacter pylori*
- *Streptococcus beta-haemolyticus*
- *Propionibacterium acnes*
- *Neisseria gonorrhoeae*
- *Escherichia coli*
- *Borrelia burgdorferi*
- Interferon alpha

## PATHOGENESIS

Infectious gastroenteritis or urogenital infections are the primary inciting event. The disease manifests after a gap that may range from few weeks to many months. Children generally develop ReA following gastroenteritis infection or dysentery and adults after urogenital infections following sexual exposure. Chlamydia trachomatis is the most common etiology for the adult onset post venereal ReA and *Salmonella*, *Shigella*, *Campylobacter*, and *Yersinia* are the most common organisms implicated in postdysentery cases those are common in children (Box 2). The mechanism how infection activates immune system is unknown. Role of toll-like receptors have been proposed in this pathway.

There is known association with human leukocyte antigen (HLA) B27 as found in many cases (70–90%). Presence of HLA B27 increases the risk of severity and possibly also susceptibility. Human immunodeficiency virus increases the risk and severity of ReA.

Although, the arthritis in ReA is considered noninfectious and joint synovial fluid is sterile as detected in standard methods, recent development of more sophisticated methods have questioned this. Synovial fluid and tissue polymerase chain reaction studies have detected presence of chlamydial deoxyribonucleic acid (DNA). However, chlamydial DNA is also detected occasionally in some normal individuals. Persistent chlamydial infection is suggested by detection of persistent upregulation of chlamydial heat shock proteins with absence of other markers of acute chlamydial infection (Gerard et al., 2002).

## CLINICAL FEATURES

Reactive arthritis is characterized by classical triad of arthritis, urethritis, and uveitis/ conjuctivitis.

Arthritis is typically asymmetrical polyarthritis similar to psoriatic arthropathy. This involves larger joints like knee, ankle joints, and spine including sacroiliac joints. Lower limbs are more commonly affected than upper. Smaller hand joints like distal interphalangeal joints are also affected in lesser number of cases. Dactylitis that manifest as fusiform swelling of entire finger may be seen. Enthesitis that is defined as inflammation of the insertion of ligaments and tendon on bones is also a common feature of ReA. Arthritis generally persists for few months. It may be relapsing and cause progressive disability.

Eye: Bilateral conjunctivitis is a classical and common feature of ReA. Keratitis and uveitis can also develop. Uveitis, that generally involves one eye at a time, may lead to blindness.

Typical skin manifestations are well-defined scaly plaques. There may be vesiculopustular lesions on the keratotic lesions mimicking pustular psoriasis. Scaly plaques, also known as keratoderma blenorhagicum, are classically present over palms and soles but may be seen on the dorsal surfaces, over finger joints, scrotum, scalp and different other body areas (Figs 1 and 2).

Nail changes are similar to psoriasis. It shows onycholysis and subungual hyperkeratosis.

Geographic tongue and asymptomatic oral erosions are seen in some patients.

Circinate balanitis is a common manifestation in males (about 50%). In uncircumcised males, it appears as superficial erosions that transforms to well-defined serpiginous erosion (Fig. 3). In circumcised persons, these become hyperkeratotic plaques. In females, there may be ulcerative vulvitis.

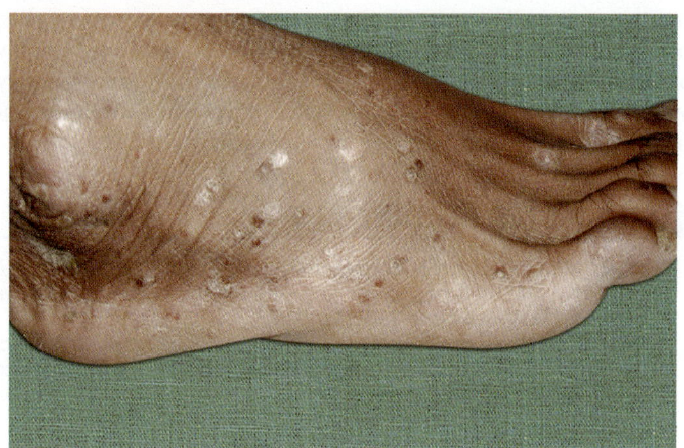

**FIG. 1:** Small scaly plaques on the dorsum of foot in a patient with Reiter's syndrome.

*Courtesy*: Dr Raghunatha Shivanna, Professor and Head, Department of Dermatology, Venereology and Leprosy, ESIC Medical College and PGIPSR, Rajajinagar, Bengaluru.

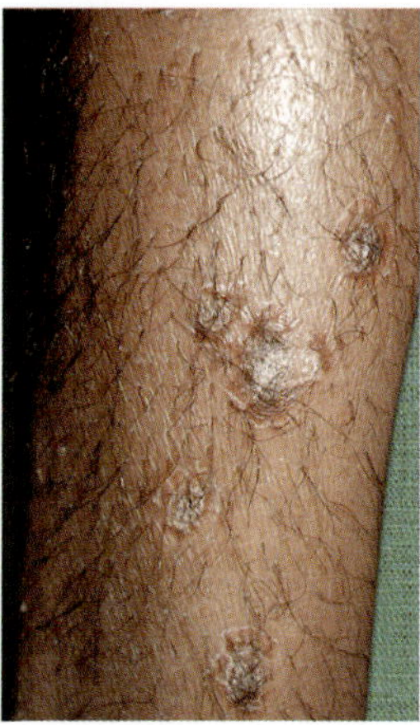

**FIG. 2:** Well-defined scaly plaques on leg in a patient with Reiter's syndrome.

*Courtesy*: Dr Raghunatha Shivanna, Professor and Head, Department of Dermatology, Venereology and Leprosy, ESIC Medical College and PGIPSR, Rajajinagar, Bengaluru.

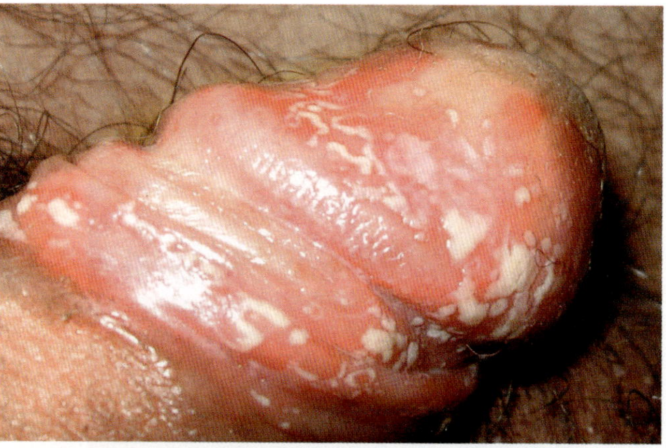

**FIG. 3:** Typical circinate balanitis in a patient with Reiter's syndrome.

*Courtesy*: Dr Raghunatha Shivanna, Professor and Head, Department of Dermatology, Venereology and Leprosy, ESIC Medical College and PGIPSR, Rajajinagar, Bengaluru.

There may be persistent or recurrent fever, lymphadenopathy, weight loss, and fatigue. These are features of systemic inflammation. Less commonly, ReA may cause cardiac conduction abnormalities, myocarditis, pericarditis, aortitis, aortic regurgitation, aortic insufficiency (late complication), proteinuria, microhematuria, amyloid deposits immunoglobulin A nephropathy, myelopathy, and neurologic complication.

## DIAGNOSIS

Reactive arthritis lacks specific diagnostic criteria, both clinical as well as laboratory. There are many hurdles in the diagnosis of ReA. Disease may manifest after a variable period after primary infection. Thus, history of such events is frequently not properly recalled by the patients. Classic triad is seen only in about one-third of the patients. Individual features may develop at different times. And finally lack of a definitive diagnostic test is a big challenge.

Clinically, cutaneous and joint involvement in ReA appears very similar to psoriasis. In the presence of persistent arthritis (>1 month) of peripheral joints when associated with (or along with a definite history of) urethritis, cervicitis, or diarrhea diagnosis is highly likely. This diagnostic criterion was adopted by the American Rheumatism Association in 1981.

Children affected with ReA who have persistent fever, lymphadenopathy, involvement of conjunctiva, and oropharyngeal mucosa may mimic Kawasaki disease.

Laboratory abnormalities (serology, cultures of suitable medium like blood, urine, stool, cervix, and urethral swab) include elevated erythrocyte sedimentation rate and C-reactive protein. Infectious agents may be detected during initial infectious stage. Human immunodeficiency virus should be ruled out.

Radiography can be helpful for the diagnosis of ReA. Plain X-ray, computed tomography (CT) and MRI may have suggestive changes.

X-ray is generally normal in early stage. Overall, the changes may be similar to are similar to those of psoriatic arthritis. However, characteristic changes in ReA are found in small joints of the foot, the ankle, the calcaneus, the knee, and the sacroiliac joint.

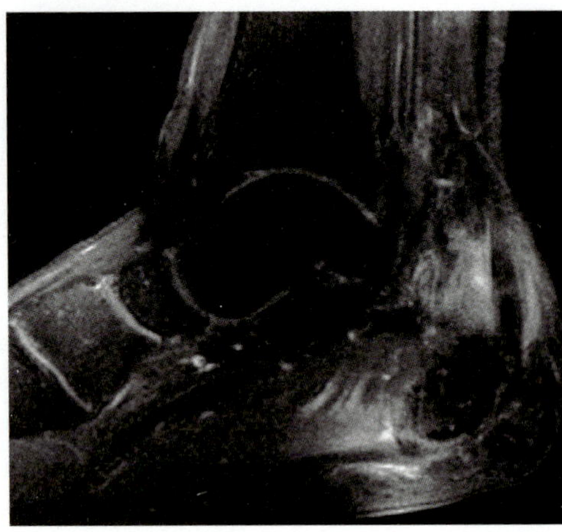

**FIG. 4:** Magnetic resonance imaging shows left ankle achilles tendinitis and plantar fasciitis.

*Courtesy*: Dr Siba P Raychaudhuri, VA Sacramento Medical Center, Northern California Health Care System, Mather, CA.

Periarticular osteoporosis (acute stage), loss of the articular space and bone erosions (starts at the margin to reach centre) are found.

Bone proliferation is common similar to all seronegative spondyloarthropathies (absent in rheumatoid arthritis). These manifest with linear and fluffy periosteal bone proliferations and calcification at the insertion site of tendon/ ligaments.

The CT scan can yield the changes better than plain X-ray especially the sacroilitis, enthesopathy

The MRI may be able to detect presence of bursitis and tenosynovitis, presence of complications like synovial cysts. (Fig. 4)

## TREATMENT

Most of the treatment used in ReA are not based on any evidence-based recommendation.

Antibiotics like lymecycline, ciprofloxacin, azithromycin, and doxycycline are used. However, there is no consensus regarding the duration and efficacy of the antibiotics in reducing disease severity or short- or long-term complications. Rifampicin has been shown to reduce chlamydial heat shock protein. A prospective, randomized study has shown that a combination therapy using rifampicin along with doxycycline for 9 months in suspected postchlamydial ReA. This has shown significantly better improvement in comparison to doxycycline alone.

Anti-inflammatory agents paracetamol, nonsteroidal anti-inflammatory drugs, and systemic corticosteroids are also known to be useful but lacks data to support their definite role. Systemic corticosteroids are possibly effective in many nonarthritic manifestations of ReA like eye, keratoderma, and balanitis. Even intra-articular injection is used with some benefits. Peripheral joints respond better than spinal joints.

Some studies have supported role of sulfasalazine, which is more effective in chronic disease than acute stage. Other disease-modifying antirheumatic drugs like methotrexate, azathioprine, and cyclosporine are also used but significantly lacks evaluation of their efficacy.

Acitretin are also known to be effective to some extent for the joints as well as skin involvement. Systemic corticosteroids, methotrexate, and other immunosuppressants are usually avoided in ReA associated with acquired immunodeficiency syndrome. Tumor necrosis factor-α like infliximab and etanercept blockers have been used in severe joint diseases in ReA.

## SUGGESTED READINGS


1. Ajene AN, Fischer Walker CL, Black RE. Enteric pathogens and reactive arthritis: A systematic review of Campylobacter, Salmonella and Shigella-associated reactive arthritis. J Health Popul Nutr. 2013;31:299-307.
2. Carter JD, Valeriano J, Vasey FB. A prospective, randomized 9-month comparison of doxycycline vs. doxycycline and rifampin in undifferentiated spondyloarthritis with special reference to Chlamydia-induced arthritis. J Rheumatol. 2004;31:1973-80.
3. Engel JN, Pollack J, Perara E, et al. Heat shock response of murine Chlamydia trachomatis. J Bacteriol. 1990;172:6959-72.
4. Pope JE, Krizova A, Garg AX, et al. Campylobacter reactive arthritis: A systematic review. Semin Arthritis Rheum. 2007;37(1):48-55.
5. Wu IB, Schwartz RA. Reiter's syndrome: The classic triad and more. J Am Acad Dermatol. 2008;59:113-21.

# 30 CHAPTER Lichen Planus and Lichenoid Disorders

Nirmal B

## INTRODUCTION

Lichen planus (LP) is a common inflammatory disorder with characteristic clinical and histopathologic features. Apart from skin and mucosa, the disease can also involve hair and nails. The word "lichen planus" is derived from the Greek word *leichen* meaning tree moss and Latin word *planus* meaning flat. Clinical features of LP can be recalled with the mnemonic of 4Ps—purple, polygonal, pruritic, and papule. Lichenoid disorders are the clinical entities that share similar morphological and histopathological features with LP.

## EPIDEMIOLOGY

Lichen planus has a prevalence of less than 1% worldwide without any racial or sex predilection. More than two-thirds are affected between 3$^{rd}$ and 6$^{th}$ decades with males manifesting the disease relatively earlier when compared to females. LP is uncommon in children constituting only 1–3%. Human leukocyte antigen (HLA)-Bw35 is strongly associated with cutaneous LP and HLA-B8 with isolated oral LP (OLP). More than two-thirds of patients with vulvovaginal-gingival syndrome have HLA-DQB1*0201 gene association.

## ETIOPATHOGENESIS

Lichen planus is an immunological mediated disorder where cell-mediated immunity plays the major role and humoral immunity is a secondary response. Pathogenesis includes the following three stages:

- Lichen planus-specific antigen recognition
- Cytotoxic lymphocyte activation
- Keratinocyte apoptosis.

Both CD4+ and CD8+ T-cells accumulate in the dermis, while CD8+ T-cells infiltrating the epidermis recognize LP-specific antigen associated with major histocompatibility complex (MHC) class I on lesional keratinocytes. The antigen is currently unknown and postulated to be an autoreactive peptide or of exogenous origin which includes drug, contact allergen, infection, or altered protein. Hepatitis C virus (HCV), human herpesvirus-7 (HHV-7), human immunodeficiency virus (HIV), human papillomavirus (HPV), herpes simplex virus-2 (HSV-2), *Helicobacter pylori*, syphilis, amebiasis, and bladder infections are the infections proposed to be provocative factors for LP.

Following antigen recognition, CD8+ T-cells are activated to upregulate cytokines associated with a T helper 1 (Th1) immune response, such as interferon-gamma (IFN-$\gamma$), tumor necrosis factor-alpha (TNF-$\alpha$), interleukin (IL)-1-alpha, IL-6, and IL-8. Increased expression of vascular endothelial adhesion molecules [intercellular adhesion molecule-1 (ICAM-1) and vascular cell adhesion molecule-1 (VCAM-1)] and mast cell degranulation has also been observed. Overexpression of matrix metalloproteinase-9 (MMP-9) results in disruption of basement membrane thus enabling the transit of T lymphocytes into the epidermis.

Keratinocyte apoptosis takes place due to TNF-$\alpha$, T-cell surface Fas ligand, and granzyme B secreted by T-cells. Perforin forms pores in the target cell membrane and thus enables entry of granzymes, responsible for DNA degradation and apoptosis of target cells.

## CLINICAL FEATURES

Classical LP lesions are characterized by purplish, plane-topped, polygonal, papules and plaques, (Fig. 1). Fine whitish network traversing the surface of papules are known as Wickham striae (WS) are characteristic and are more easily observed after

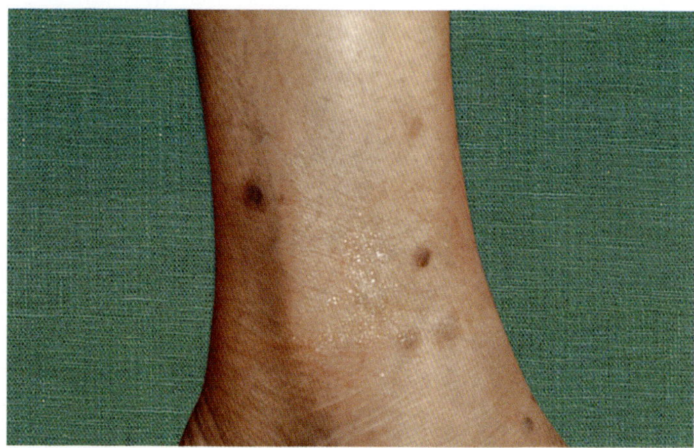

**FIG. 1:** Classical lichen planus.

application of oil or water with the help of magnifying glass or dermatoscope. Wickham striae have been postulated to occur due to:

- Increase in granular cell layer
- Focal increase in epidermal activity due to abnormal keratinocyte function
- Reduction of dermal vessels.

The onset is usually insidious with lesions being distributed symmetrically with flexural predominance mostly seen over volar aspect of wrist, ankles, and lumbar region. A few cases can evolve rapidly with widespread dissemination. The papules eventually flatten with hyperpigmentation, especially in dark skin. Inverse LP involves axilla, groin, and inframammary region. Itching is fairly a consistent feature in LP but the patient rubs rather than scratches for relief from itch. Koebner phenomenon of isomorphic lesions along lines of trauma is usually observed in evolving stage.

## VARIANTS (BOX 1)

### Mucosal Lichen Planus

Mucous membrane lesions in LP are very common occurring in up to 70% of cases (Fig. 2). Isolated oral lesions without skin involvement are seen in 20–30% patients. OLP has a slight elderly female predilection. The buccal mucosa, gingiva, and tongue are most often involved. Very rarely, larynx, and esophagus can be involved resulting in strictures. Clinical subtypes include:

- Reticular
- Plaque-like
- Atrophic
- Papular
- Erosive
- Ulcerative
- Bullous.

Malignant transformation to squamous cell carcinoma in oral lesions is rare but a potential complication seen especially with ulcerative OLP due to increased expression of cyclooxygenase (COX)-2. Desmocollin-1 and E-cadherin have been found to be predictors of malignant transformation.

In young men, genital lesions may be present on shaft of penis, glans, prepuce, or scrotum. The association of erosive LP of vulva and vagina with desquamative gingivitis has been termed as "vulvovaginal-gingival syndrome", the spectrum varying from fine reticulate lesions to severe erosions resulting in scarring.

**BOX 1 Classification of lichen planus (LP)**

- Based on morphology
  - Classical
  - Lichen planus pigmentosus
  - Hypertrophic LP
  - Atrophic LP
  - Linear LP
  - Annular LP
  - Guttate LP
  - Bullous LP
- Based on site of involvement
  - Cutaneous LP
  - Mucosal LP
  - Lichen planus of palms and soles
  - Lichen planopilaris
  - Nail LP
- Special forms
  - Lichenoid contact dermatitis
  - Lichenoid drug eruption
  - Lichenoid graft versus host disease (GVHD)
  - Lichen planus pemphigoides
  - Lichen planus-lupus erythematosus (LP-LE) overlap

### Lichen Planus of Palms and Soles

Palmoplantar LP lacks the characteristic color and morphology of lesions elsewhere, rarely itch, and are yellowish in color. Clinical morphological types include:

- Hypertrophic
- Diffuse broad sheeted
- Punctate keratoses with pits/umbilicated papules
- Vesicle-like papules
- Erosive/ulcerative
- Pigmented macular variant.

### Lichen Planus Pigmentosus

Lichen planus pigmentosus is a pigmentary disorder with clinical lesions different from classical LP papules, characterized by slate-gray macules involving face, neck, and upper limbs predominantly (Fig. 3). Similar lesions seen in flexural folds are termed "lichen planus pigmentosus-inversus". This pigmentary disorder is seen in individuals with darker skin in India, Latin America, and Middle East. The forms include:

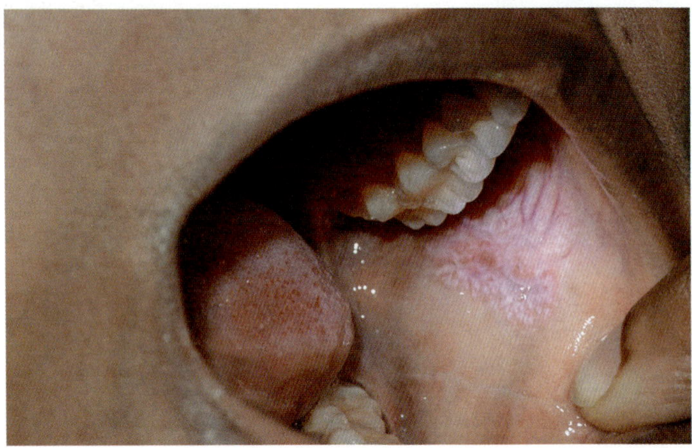

**FIG. 2:** Oral lichen planus.

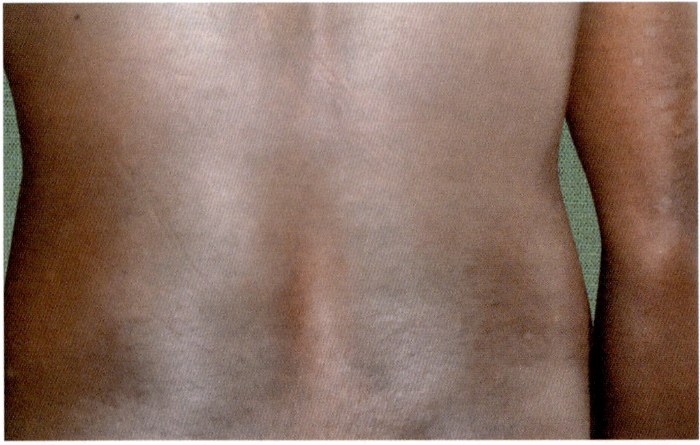

**FIG. 3:** Lichen planus pigmentosus.

- Diffuse
- Reticular
- Blotchy
- Perifollicular
- Linear.

## Lichen Planopilaris

Lichen planus of scalp is one of the most common causes of scarring alopecia with three clinical variants:
- Lichen planopilaris
- Graham-Little syndrome
- Frontal fibrosing alopecia.

Lichen planopilaris clinically presents as itchy areas of hair loss clinically showing perifollicular erythema and scaling to start with and scarring eventually ensues with loss of follicular orifices (Fig. 4). Features of Graham-Little-Piccardi-Lassueur syndrome include cicatricial alopecia of scalp, nonscarring alopecia of axillary and pubic hair, and keratosis pilaris. Frontal fibrosing alopecia of Kossard typically affects postmenopausal women, with recession of frontal hairline in a straight line involving eyebrows also frequently.

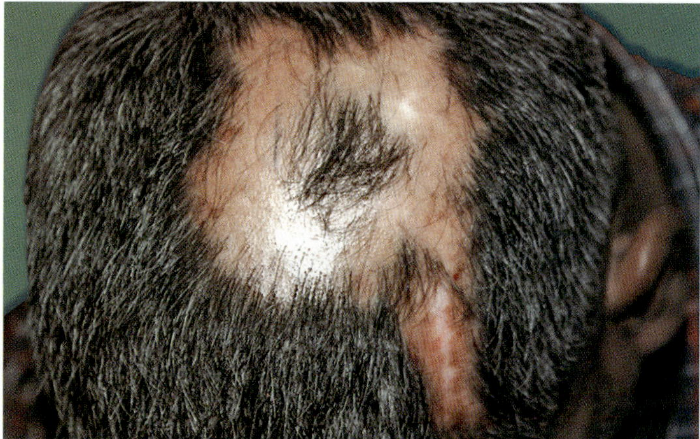

**FIG. 4:** Lichen planopilaris.

## Nail Lichen Planus

Nail LP occurs commonly later in life at $5^{th}$–$6^{th}$ decades (Fig. 5). Nail involvement in childhood is rare but LP can overlap with idiopathic trachyonychia. Nail finding is a minor feature of LP occurring in 10% of the patients. Isolated nail LP is seen only in 1–2%.
- Nail fold—paronychia
- Nail matrix—onychorrhexis, pitting, chromonychia, pterygium, and atrophy
- Nail bed—subungual hyperkeratosis, and onycholysis.

The most common nail finding in LP is exaggeration of linear longitudinal lines. Angel wing deformity is due to thinning of the nail plate. Pup tent sign is due to elevation of nail plate in the center and peripheries remain depressed. Pterygium unguis is observed as a result of adhesion between dorsal nail fold and nail bed.

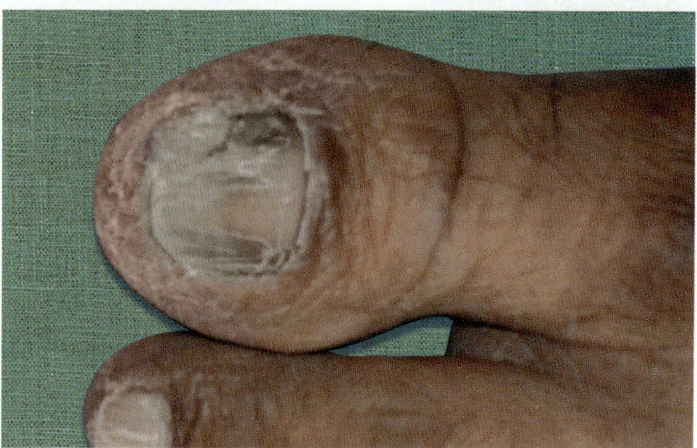

**FIG. 5:** Nail lichen planus.

## Actinic Lichen Planus

*Synonyms*: Summertime actinic lichenoid eruption (SALE), lichenoid melanodermatitis, LP tropicus, and LP subtropicus.

The disease is usually seen in children and young adults. Most common site of involvement is the sun-exposed region of the face. Lesions are usually annular with hyperpigmentation in the center and characteristic hypopigmentation around it.

## Hypertrophic Lichen Planus

*Synonym*: Lichen planus verrucosus.

They most often occur on the lower limbs, especially around the ankles (Fig. 6). Venous stasis has been put forward as an explanation. The development of hypertrophic lesions may persist for many years. When lesions eventually clear, pigmentation, atrophy, and scarring may remain. Multiple cutaneous horns, keratoacanthoma, verrucous carcinoma, and squamous cell carcinoma can arise in hypertrophic LP.

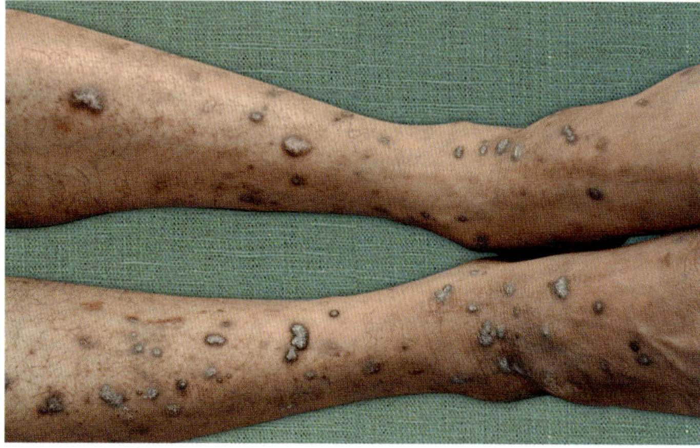

**FIG. 6:** Hypertrophic lichen planus.

## Atrophic Lichen Planus

Atrophic LP manifests as annular lesions with atrophy in the center or resolved hypertrophic lesions. Most common sites of involvement are trunk and lower legs. Lesions clinically resemble porokeratosis or lichen sclerosus et atrophicans.

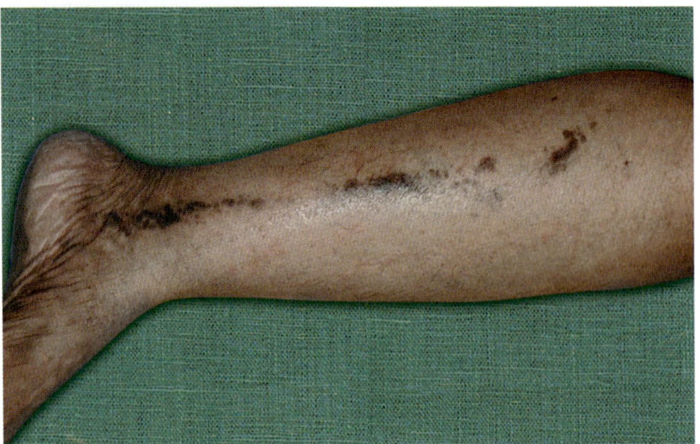

FIG. 7: Linear lichen planus.

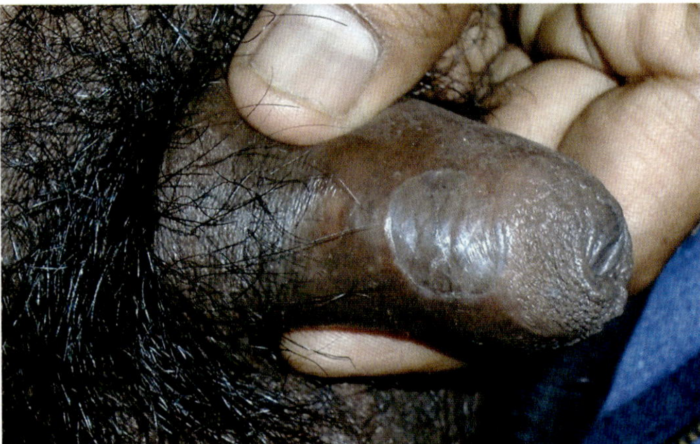

FIG. 8: Annular lichen planus.

### Linear Lichen Planus

Linear lesions in LP can arise as a result of Koebner effect or rarely as isolated lesions along the lines of Blaschko (Fig. 7). Blaschkoid LP is common in children. Linear LP can also arise as isotopic phenomenon in sites of healed herpes zoster.

### Annular Lichen Planus

Annular LP is commonly seen in penis and scrotum (Fig. 8). Mostly lesions of actinic LP are annular in shape. They are usually small measuring less than 2 cm and have a depressed center with raised edge.

### Guttate Lichen Planus

Lesions are usually discrete and widespread resembling guttate psoriasis. Individual lesions are commonly smaller measuring 1–2 mm and rarely large up to 1 cm across.

### Bullous Lichen Planus

Blisters in bullous LP occur as a result of severe basal cell liquefactive degeneration arising from the papules and plaques of LP or near those lesions. They rarely appear from normal looking skin. Lesions commonly appear over the extremities.

## SPECIAL FORMS

### Lichenoid Contact Dermatitis

It is a type of noneczematous contact dermatitis clinically resembling LP affecting both skin and mucous membrane. The agents responsible include color developers containing substituted paraphenylenediamines (PPDs), PPD in hair color, methacrylic acid esters used in dental devices and car industries, mercury in dental amalgam fillings, epoxy resin, musk ambrette, nickel, aminoglycoside antibiotics, and gold. Onset is acute, while the course is prolonged leaving behind intense pigmentary changes.

### Lichenoid Drug Eruption

The latency between drug intake and appearance of lichenoid eruption varies from several weeks to months. Resolution is also slow after cessation of the drug. Eruption tends to be symmetric and extensive appearing more psoriasiform unlike classical LP. Lesions lack WS, are often photodistributed and spare the oral cavity. On resolution, hyperpigmentation, alopecia, anhidrosis, and skin atrophy may develop.

*Common inducers*:
- Beta-blockers
- Diuretics—thiazide, furosemide, spironolactone
- Antimalarials
- Penicillamine
- Gold.

*Less common*:
- Angiotensin-converting enzyme (ACE) inhibitors
- Calcium channel blockers
- Sulfonylurea
- Nonsteroidal anti-inflammatory drugs (NSAIDs)
- Ketoconazole.

*Oral*:
- Dental restorative materials
- Gold
- ACE inhibitors
- Sulfonylurea
- NSAIDs
- Ketoconazole
- Penicillamine.

### Lichenoid Graft versus Host Disease

Lichenoid graft versus host disease (GVHD) is a chronic GVHD occurring after 100 days following transplant involves predominantly trunk, oral cavity, palms, and soles (Fig. 9). Lesions may be localized or generalized, starts as hyperpigmented nodular papules and plaques which eventually becomes atrophic.

### Lichen Planus Pemphigoides

This entity was first described by Kaposi in 1892 where LP coexists with subepidermal bullous lesions. The damage to the basal layer as a result of marked basal cell vacuolation and intense inflammation in LP exposes a basement membrane antigen. The target antigen is MCW-4 epitope within the C-terminal of NC16A domain of BP180 type XVII collagen and also a 200 kDa antigen. Antibodies are formed against the antigen leading to the blister formation. LP lesions are usually acute in onset and are also generalized. They are followed by appearance of tense bullae mostly on the extremities developing on both normal skin and involved skin. Oral cavity involvement is rare. The age of involvement is lesser than bullous pemphigoid and the course is also less severe.

### Lichen Planus—Lupus Erythematosus Overlap

This syndrome is characterized by overlapping features of both LP and lupus erythematosus. Lupus erythematosus is usually chronic cutaneous or systemic rarely subacute cutaneous. Chronic atrophic discoid lupus erythematosus-like plaques with telangiectasia and minimal scaling may develop on the head, neck, and upper trunk. Lichenoid lesions commonly over extremities with lacy reticular oral lesions coexist. Lesions tend to have a prolonged course and are treatment refractory.

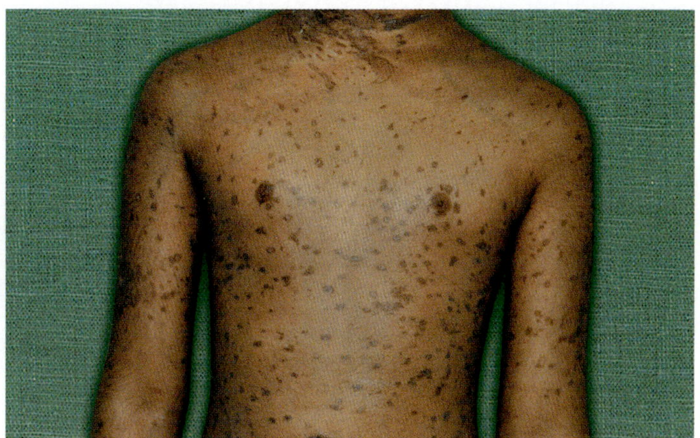

FIG. 9: Lichenoid graft versus host disease.

## DERMATOSCOPY

The light of a dermatoscope can reach the depth of histopathologic changes in LP. Dermatoscopic patterns in LP should account for WS, vascular, and pigment patterns.

The various forms of WS include (Fig. 10):

- Reticular
- Annular
- Linear
- Radial streaming
- Leaf venation pattern
- Starry-sky pattern.

In leaf venation pattern, fine secondary striae branched from the main center WS. Starry-sky pattern signifies follicular white dots of WS clustered together.

Vascular pattern includes red dots and lines, have a peripheral arrangement. Red fine lines run parallel to thin white radiating lines at the periphery of WS. Pigmented streaming lines can also be seen near the disappearing WS.

Grayish blue pigmented dots or granules in a reticular pattern corresponding to the dermal melanophages are seen

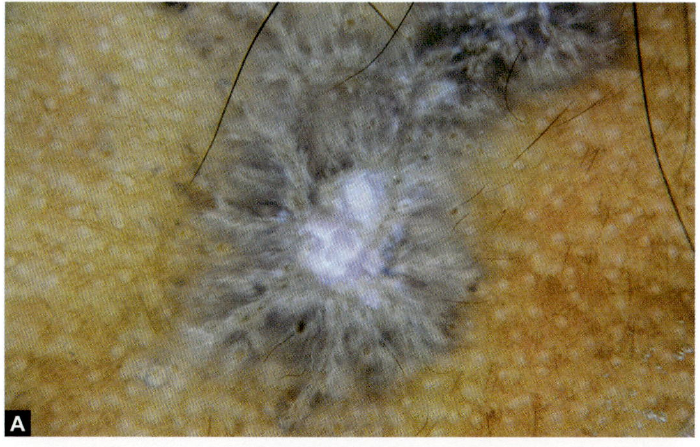


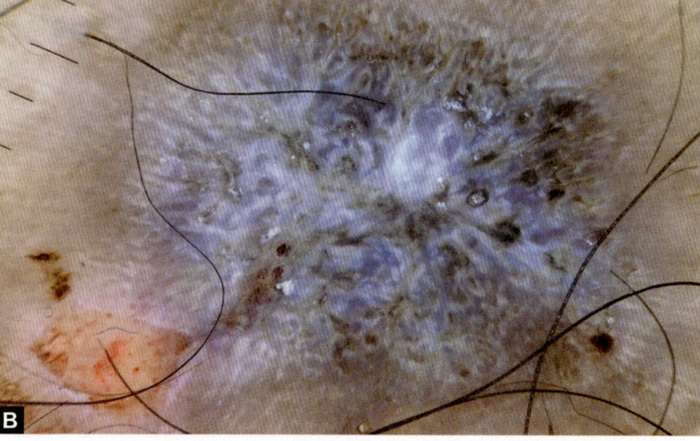


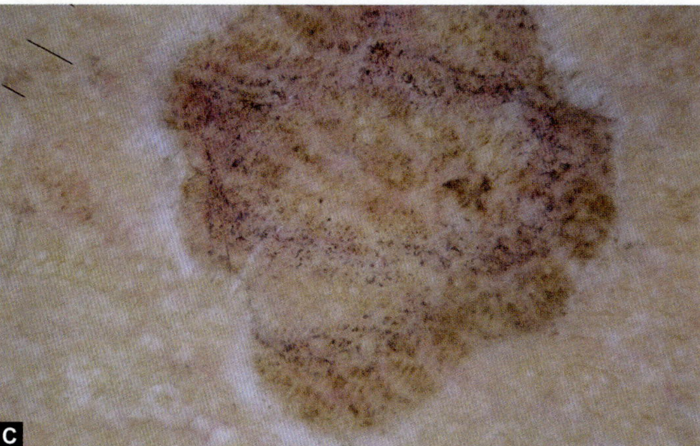


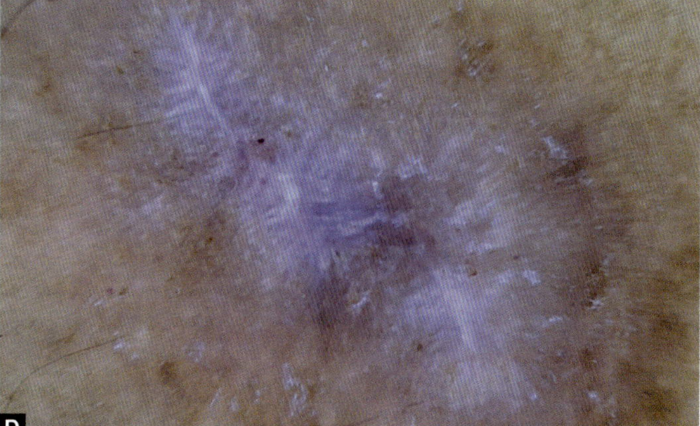


FIG. 10: Dermatoscopy of lichen planus with various types of Wickham striae (WS). **A,** Radial WS; **B,** Reticular WS; **C,** Annular WS; **D,** Leaf venation WS.

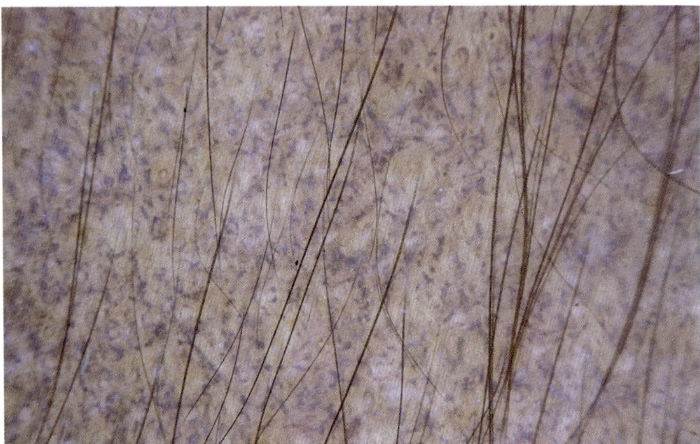

FIG. 11: Dermatoscopy of lichen planus pigmentosus.

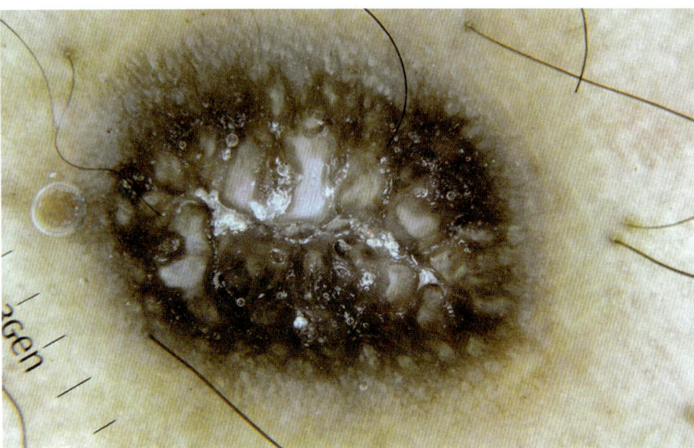

FIG. 12: Dermatoscopy of hypertrophic lichen planus.

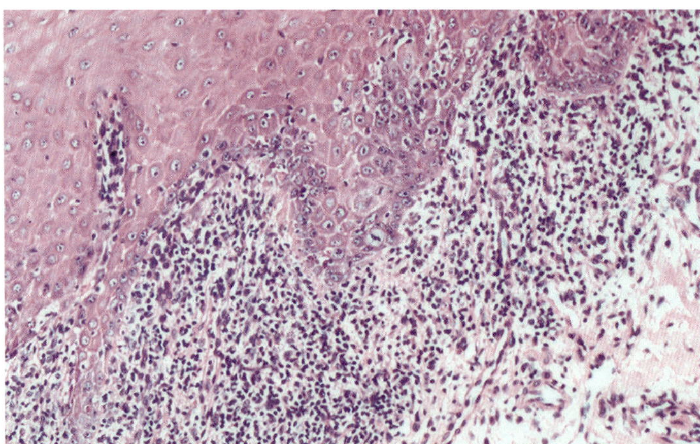

FIG. 13: Histopathology of classical lichen planus.

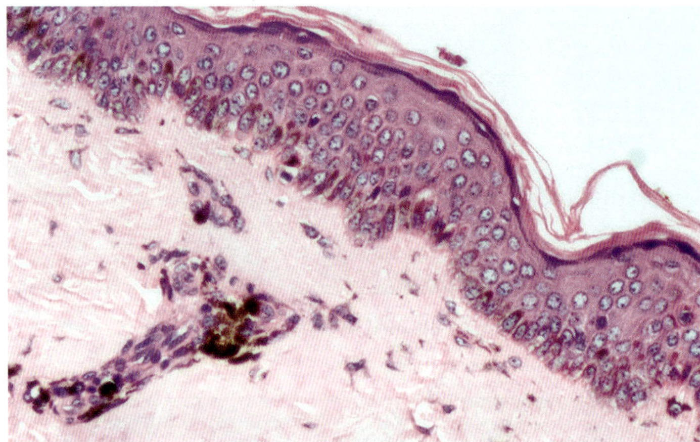

FIG. 14: Histopathology of lichen planus pigmentosus.

in LP pigmentosus (Fig. 11). A hem-like pattern has also been described over the extremities.

Hypertrophic LP shows comedo-like structures with corn pearls which correspond to keratin filled craters, and may show WS and vascular patterns in early lesions (Fig. 12).

## HISTOPATHOLOGY

- *Classic LP*: The characteristic histological changes seen in LP are (Fig. 13):
  - Compact hyperkeratosis
  - Irregular acanthosis of epidermis
  - Irregular thickening of granular layer
  - Rete ridges appear flattened or effaced ("saw-tooth" appearance)
  - Vacuolar alteration of basal layer epidermal cells is transformed into colloid bodies (15–20 μm diameter)
  - Clefting along the dermal-epidermal junction (DEJ) focal separation from the dermis may lead to Max-Joseph spaces
  - Perivascular infiltrate of lymphocytes and histiocytes impinging on the DEJ.
  - Pigmentary incontinence with dermal melanophages.
- *Hypertrophic LP*: Pseudoepitheliomatous hyperplasia of the epidermis with irregular acanthosis is seen. Infiltrates are less dense and are not band like. In older lesions, dermal fibrosis is usually present along with inflammation
- *Atrophic LP*: Compact hyperkeratosis is relatively preserved. Epidermis is thinned out markedly in atrophic
- *Actinic LP*: Three forms in a spectrum all sharing marked pigment incontinence include:
  - Form with classical LP
  - Intermediate form with spongiosis and parakeratosis called lichenoid melanodermatitis
  - Predominantly eczematous form.
- *Lichen planus pigmentosus*: Histopathologically LP pigmentosus has two patterns representing ends of spectrum of the disease:
  - *Early pattern*: Frequent keratinocyte apoptosis, marked basal cell vacuolar degeneration, and band-like lymphohistiocytic inflammatory infiltrate with mild-to-moderate melanin incontinence
  - *Late pattern*: Few apoptotic keratinocytes, focal or absent vacuolar degeneration, and superficial mild perivascular lymphohistiocytic inflammatory infiltrate with dense melanin incontinence (Fig. 14).
- *Lichen planus pilaris*: In lichen planopilaris, there is a lichenoid reaction pattern involves basal layer of infundibulum and isthmus of hair follicle epithelium, with an associated dense perifollicular infiltrate of lymphocytes and a few macrophages. Scarring alopecia develops when there is perifollicular fibrosis and loss of arrector pili and sebaceous glands. Fibrosis may also be present in the papillary dermis. Some mucins may be present in the perifollicular fibroplasia.

Unlike lupus erythematosus, the infiltrate does not extend around blood vessels of the mid and deep plexus and mucin is not present in the interfollicular dermis

- *Mucosal LP*: Parakeratosis is present with thinned out epidermis. Plasma cells are present in the band-like dense infiltrate. Colloid bodies are fewer. Neutrophils are present in erosive OLP. Epithelial dysplasia is a risk for transformation into malignancy
- *Bullous LP*: Subepidermal bulla formation is present with typical changes of classical LP. Direct immunofluorescence (DIF) and indirect immunofluorescence (IIF) are negative
- *Lichen planus pemphigoides*: The histology of LP pemphigoides shows a cell poor subepidermal bulla with mild perivascular infiltrate of lymphocytes, neutrophils, and eosinophils. DIF shows immunoglobulin G (IgG) and C3 in the basement membrane zone. IIF shows binding to the roof of the split
- *Lichenoid drug eruption*: The following features differentiate it from classical LP:
    - Focal parakeratosis
    - Focal interruption of the granular layer
    - Cytoid bodies situated higher in granular and cornified layers
    - Exocytosis of lymphoid cells into upper epidermis
    - Cellular infiltrate tends to be more pleomorphic and less dense
    - Presence of few eosinophils
    - Deeper perivascular infiltrate
    - More melanin incontinence.

## TREATMENT

### Oral Lichen Planus

Dental care and good oral hygiene practices must be encouraged. Replacing metal dental restorative materials with composite materials should be considered. Topical anesthetics provide symptomatic relief from pain and burning.

The first-line drugs in treating OLP include topical corticosteroids and topical calcineurin inhibitors. However, there is no evidence to suggest that pimecrolimus is better than placebo in reducing symptoms of OLP. Evidence is also insufficient to suggest the superiority of any specific steroid. Other topical agents used include: tretinoin gel, topical tetracycline, and topical cyclosporine but not of these have been proven to be better than topical corticosteroids. Intralesional steroid injections are also effective.

Extensive oral and vulvovaginal lesions should be treated with systemic steroid preparations at doses higher than that used for cutaneous LP. Oral retinoids are the next group of first-line drugs used for OLP with almost two-thirds of the patients showing marked improvement in 8 weeks. Second-line drugs for OLP include cyclosporine, dapsone, hydroxychloroquine, thalidomide, griseofulvin, azathioprine, mycophenolate mofetil, and cyclophosphamide. Treating secondary colonization of OLP with antifungals may be useful especially when treating with systemic steroids.

Other treatment modalities for OLP include extracorporeal photochemotherapy, photodynamic therapy, $CO_2$ laser, neodymium-doped yttrium aluminum garnet (Nd:YAG) laser and excimer laser. Malignant transformation warrants surgical excision combined with radiotherapy.

**TABLE 1: Treatment of lichen planus**

| Drugs | Level of evidence |
|---|---|
| **Topical** | |
| Steroids | B |
| Calcineurin inhibitors | C |
| Calcipotriol | C |
| **Systemic** | |
| Retinoids | A |
| Phototherapy—NBUVB, PUVA | B |
| Corticosteroids | B |
| Dapsone | B |
| Methotrexate | C |
| Cyclosporine | C |
| Azathioprine | C |
| Mycophenolate mofetil | C |
| Hydroxychloroquine sulfate | D |

NBUVB, narrowband ultraviolet B; PUVA, psoralen plus ultraviolet A.

### Cutaneous Lichen Planus (Table 1)

Topicals used in LP include potent topical steroids and topical calcineurin inhibitors. Hypertrophic LP can be treated with topical steroids under occlusion and intralesional steroids. While injecting steroids in a hypertrophic LP, the solution jets out and this is called "fountain sign".

Systemic steroids are used in extensive cutaneous lesions, symptomatic lesions not responding to topicals, progressive nail involvement and cicatricial alopecia. They are effective at doses greater than 20 mg/day of oral prednisolone. Retinoids both acitretin (25 mg/day) and isotretinoin (20–40 mg/day) can be used for their anti-inflammatory effect. Psoralen with ultraviolet A (UVA) can be used along with steroids or retinoids for quicker resolution.

Second-line systemic drugs include cyclosporine, dapsone, hydroxychloroquine, low-molecular-weight heparin, metronidazole, IFN-α, methotrexate, cyclophosphamide, thalidomide, sulfasalazine, azathioprine, mycophenolate mofetil, alefacept and basiliximab. Low-molecular-weight heparin is effective in low doses that have no anticoagulant effect. Enoxaparin 20 mg subcutaneously weekly appears to play an immunomodulatory role by blocking T-cell heparinase and inhibiting T-cell migration. Tetracycline and nicotinamide have been used in LP pemphigoides.

## SUGGESTED READINGS


1. Al-Mutairi N, El-Khalawany M. Clinicopathological characteristics of lichen planus pigmentosus and its response to tacrolimus ointment: an open label, non-randomized, prospective study. J Eur Acad Dermatol Venereol. 2010;24:535-40.
2. Birkenfeld S, Dreiher J, Weitzman D, et al. A study on the association with hepatitis B and hepatitis C in 1557 patients with lichen planus. J Eur Acad Dermatol Venereol. 2011;25:436-40.
3. Breathnach SM. Lichen planus and lichenoid disorders. In: Burns T, Breathnach S, Cox N, Griffiths C (Eds). Rook's Textbook of Dermatology, 8th edition. West Sussex: Wiley-Blackwell Publishers; 2010. pp. 41.1-4.
4. De Jong EM, Van De Kerkhof PC. Coexistence of palmoplantar lichen planus and lupus erythematosus with response to treatment using acitretin. Br J Dermatol. 1996;134:538-41.

5. Dhar S. Fountain sign in lichen planus hypertrophicus. Indian J Dermatol Venereol Leprol. 1997;63:210.
6. Gaertner E, Elstein W. Lichen planus pigmentosus-inversus: case report and review of an unusual entity. Dermatol Online J. 2012;18:11.
7. Gutte R, Khopkar U. Predominant palmoplantar lichen planus: a diagnostic challenge. Indian J Dermatol. 2014;59:343-7.
8. Holzberg M, Baran R. The nail in dermatological disease. In: Baran R, de Berker DA, Holzberg M, Thomas L (Eds). Diseases of the Nails and their Management, 4th edition. West Sussex: Wiley-Blackwell Publishers; 2012. pp. 282-9.
9. Kirtschig G, Wakelin SH, Wojnarowska F. Mucosal vulval lichen planus: outcome, clinical and laboratory features. J Eur Acad Dermatol Venereol. 2005;19: 301-7.
10. Lodi G, Carrozzo M, Furness S, et al. Interventions for treating oral lichen planus: a systematic review. Br J Dermatol. 2012;166:938-47.
11. Lyakhovitsky A, Amichai B, Sizopoulou C, et al. A case series of 46 patients with lichen planopilaris: demographics, clinical evaluation, and treatment experience. J Dermatolog Treat. 2015;26:275-9.
12. Mattila R, Alanen K, Syrjänen S. Desmocollin expression in oral atrophic lichen planus correlates with clinical behavior and DNA content. J Cutan Pathol. 2008;35:832-8.
13. Pittelkow MR, Daoud MS. Lichen planus. In: Wolff K, Goldsmith LA, Katz SI, Gilchrest BA, Paller AS, Leffell DJ (Eds). Fitzpatrick's Dermatology in General Medicine, 7th edition. New York: McGraw-Hill Companies Inc.; 2008. pp. 244-6.
14. Prpić Massari L, Kastelan M, Gruber F, et al. Perforin expression in peripheral blood lymphocytes and skin-infiltrating cells in patients with lichen planus. Br J Dermatol. 2004;151:433-9.
15. Sachdeva S, Sachdeva S, Kapoor P. Wickham striae: etiopathogenensis and clinical significance. Indian J Dermatol. 2011;56:442-3.
16. Setterfield JF, Neill S, Shirlaw PJ, et al. The vulvovaginal gingival syndrome: a severe subgroup of lichen planus with characteristic clinical features and a novel association with the class II HLA DQB1*0201 allele. J Am Acad Dermatol. 2006;55:98-113.
17. Tan C, Min ZS, Xue Y, et al. Spectrum of dermoscopic patterns in lichen planus: a case series from China. J Cutan Med Surg. 2014;18:28-32.
18. Wagner G, Rose C, Sachse MM. Clinical variants of lichen planus. J Dtsch Dermatol Ges. 2013;11:309-19.
19. Weedon D. The lichenoid reaction pattern ('interface dermatitis'). In: Weedon D (Ed). Skin Pathology, 3rd edition. China: Elsevier; 2010. pp. 38-45.
20. Zillikens D, Caux F, Mascaro JM, et al. Autoantibodies in lichen planus pemphigoides react with a novel epitope within the C-terminal NC16A domain of BP180. J Invest Dermatol. 1999;113:117-21.

# 11 SECTION Disorders of Cornification

# 31 CHAPTER Basics of Disorders of Keratinization and Introduction to MEDOC

*Nilendu Sarma*

## INTRODUCTION

Keratinization is a continuous process by which keratinocytes proliferate and then differentiate. Basal keratinocytes are the only proliferating cell in epidermis. In a stepwise manner, newly formed daughter cells from basal layer successively form spinous cell layer, granular cell layer and then terminally differentiates to form an acellular keratin structure. This final step is called cornification. Adhesion molecules that bind corneocytes are lysed by the proteases.

Among the various functions of skin, protection of the internal organs and a barrier function is very important. The tensile strength of the skin is imparted by the adhesion of keratinocytes in various layers. Keratinocytes have many junctional molecules like desmosomes, gap junctions (connexins), tight junctions and calcium pump that assist exchange of smaller molecules and ions. These also have important role in epidermal integrity and keratinocyte differentiation (Table 1 and Box 1).

The barrier function of the skin is mostly exerted by the outermost acelluar cornified layer and also granular cell layer. Granular cells have "cornified cell envelope" in the cytoplasm that has powerful barrier property. This cornified cell envelope (10 nm thick) is composed of highly cross-linked insoluble proteins like keratin, loricrin, filaggrin, involucrin and transglutaminase 1 and lipid called ceramides. At the outermost cornified layer important changes take place. In this layer, granular cells are transformed in dead corneocytes. Intracellular lipids come out to extracellular space by a structure called "lamellar body". This lipids

**TABLE 1: Keratinization disorders**

| | Defective protein/ function | Disease |
|---|---|---|
| Adhesion molecules | Desmosomes | Mostly manifest with striate keratoderma and sometimes blisters. Examples include—ectodermal dysplasia/skin fragility syndrome, dilated cardiomyopathy with wooly hair and keratoderma and Naxos disease |
| | Hemidesmosomes | Mostly manifest with epidermolysis bullosa. Some of these also feature PPK. Examples: EBS (Dowling-Meara), EBS with muscular dystrophy, non-Herlitz JEB, generalized, Kindler syndrome |
| | Connexins (gap junction) | • KID syndrome<br>• EKV<br>• Vohwinkel keratoderma<br>• Hidrotic ectodermal dysplasia |
| | Corneodesmosome | • Peeling skin syndrome<br>• Ichthyosis hypotrichosis syndrome |
| | Tight junction | • Ichthyosis-hypotrichosis-sclerosing<br>• Cholangitis |
| | Calcium pump | • Darier disease<br>• Hailey–Hailey disease |
| Keratinocyte structural and barrier molecules | Keratins | • Epidermolytic ichthyosis<br>• Epidermolytic palmoplantar keratoderma<br>• Pachyonychia congenita<br>• Ichthyosis bullosa of siemens |
| | Cell envelope precursor | • Camisa keratoderma<br>• PSEK (loricrin keratoderma) |
| | Cell envelope | • Lamellar Ichthyosis<br>• Ichthyosis vulgaris (filaggrin) |

*Continued*

*Continued*

| | Defective protein/ function | Disease |
|---|---|---|
| Molecules involved in metabolic pathway | Lipid metabolism | • Autosomal recessive congenital ichthyosis<br>• CEDNIK syndrome, MEDNIK syndrome<br>• X-linked ichthyosis<br>• Conradi–Hünermann–Happle syndrome<br>• Ichthyosis follicularis, alopecia, and photophobia syndrome<br>• Neutral lipid storage disease<br>• Sjögren–Larsson syndrome<br>• CHILD syndrome |
| | Peroxisome (lipid metabolism) | • Rhizomelic chondrodysplasia punctata type-I<br>• Refsum disease |
| | Sulfatase | • X-linked ichthyosis<br>• X-linked recessive chondrodysplasia punctata<br>• Kallmann syndrome or other contiguous gene deletion syndromes on Xp<br>• Multiple sulfatase deficiency |
| | Proteinase | • Netherton syndrome<br>• Papillon–Lefèvre syndrome |
| | Amino acid metabolism | Richner–Hanhart syndrome |
| Repair mechanism | Nucleotide excision repair | Trichothiodystrophy |

PPK, palmoplantar keratosis; EBS, epidermolysis bullosa simplex; JEB, junctional epidermolysis bullosa; KID, keratitis-ichthyosis-deafness; EKV, erythrokeratodermia variabilis; PSEK, progressive symmetric erythrokeratoderma; CEDNIK, cerebral dysgenesis, neuropathy, ichthyosis and keratoderma; MEDNIK, mental retardation, enteropathy, deafness, peripheral neuropathy, ichthyosis and keratoderma; CHILD, congenital hemidysplasia with ichthyosiform erythroderma and limb defects.

**BOX 1 Important structural components of keratinocytes**

*Desmosome*: This is the cell-to-cell adhesion molecule present in keratinocytes and myocardial cells

*Components*:

- Desmogleins 1–4 (DSG1-4)
- Desmocollins 1–3 (DSC1-3)
- Plakoglobin (PG)
- Plakophillins (PKP1-4)
- Desmoplakin (DSP)
- Envoplakin
- Periplakin
- Corneodesmosin (*CDSN* gene; CDSN)

Defect leads to mostly palmoplantar keratoderma and sometimes blistering disease

*Hemidesmosomes*: This connect epithelial cells with extracellular matrix proteins (collagen IV, VII and laminin-332)

*Components*:

- Intracellular: keratin 5/keratin 14 complex, plectin, and BP230
- Transmembrane: BP180 (collagen XVII) and α6β4 integrin

Defect leads to mostly epidermolysis bullosa and sometimes palmoplantar keratoderma

*Keratins*: These cytoskeletal proteins act as major structural protein. More than 50 types are keratins are present. Important keratins with their locations are:

- Keratin 5, 14: Basal keratinocyte
- Keratin 1, 10: Suprabasal layer
- Keratin 9: Suprabasal layer in palmoplantar skin
- Keratin 2: Uppermost layers of epidermis
- Keratin 6, 16, 17: Hair, nail, appendages, palmoplantar epidermis, healing wounds

are transformed into a powerful lipid envelope through various enzymatic and nonenzymatic steps. There is another structure in the cornified layer called corneodesmosomes that also play important role in barrier function.

## KERATINIZATION DISORDERS

This process of keratinization is regulated by various key genes and proteins. Abnormality of the key proteins results in various disease that manifest as keratinization disorders. Known defects involve cornified envelope proteins, adhesion molecules like desmosomes, hemidesmosomes and corneodesmosomes, keratins, junctional molecules, proteolytic enzymes, proteins involved in lipid metabolism, and for DNA repair.

Many of these proteins have different functions in addition to keratinization like adhesion, signaling and intercellular exchange of smaller molecules. Thus mutations affecting these proteins may frequently result in diverse and overlapping phenotypic expression of keratoderma, ichthyosis, (Figs 1 and 2) skin fragility, and blistering disease. It is easy to understand that most if not all these disorders have defective barrier function. Colonization of the infective organisms on the epidermis is also seen. Major cause of death in keratitis-ichthyosis-deafness (KID) syndrome is severe septicemia that occurs due to colonization with opportunistic organisms.

Desquamation of cells at the final step requires lysis of corneodesmosome which is the adhesion molecules in corneocytes. Extracellular part of corneodesmosome is composed of desmoglein 1 (DSG1), desmocollin 1 (DSC1) and corneodesmosin (CDSN). The lysis of these adhesion molecules is mediated through various proteases. The stratum corneum chymotryptic enzyme (SCCE) and the stratum corneum tryptic enzyme (SCTE) are two important epidermal proteases that facilitate this action. Netherton's syndrome that occurs due to mutation in *SPINK5* gene that encodes a protein called LEKTI (lymphoepithelial Kazal-type related inhibitor), a protease inhibitor that regulates these protease function share many clinical phenotype with peeling skin syndrome that occurs due to mutation in CDSN.

Despite tremendous advancement in the understanding of the ultrastructural alterations in keratinization disorders, many aspects remained unexplained. There is significant phenotypic heterogeneity hindering understanding the disease and its

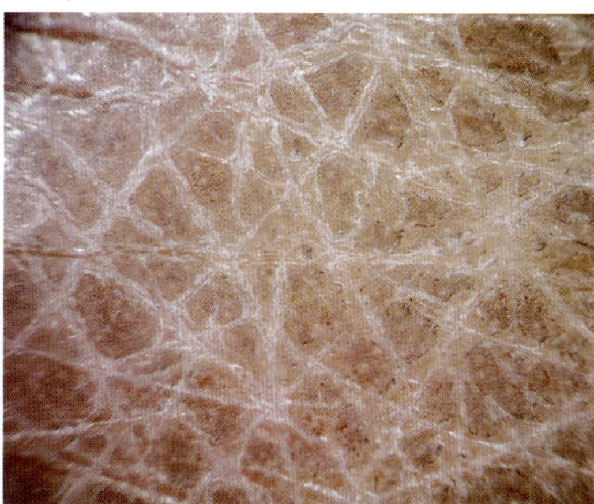

FIG. 1: Mild ichthyosis vulgaris seen under dermoscope (non-polarized, 10x).

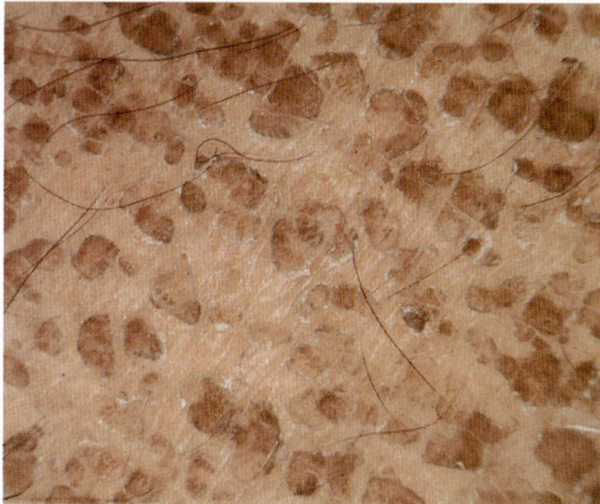

FIG. 2: X-linked recessive ichthyosis seen under dermoscope (polarized, 10x).

classification. Genotype-phenotype correlation is also not straightforward in many occasions.

Many of the genetic disorders of keratinization are due to single gene mutation and follow simple Mendelian rules of inheritance. This has greatly helped us to understand and characterize the conditions. Table 1 shows various proteins and mutations and resulting keratinization disorders.

## MENDELIAN DISORDERS OF CORNIFICATION

Mendelian disorders of cornification (MEDOC) is an umbrella term that includes all disorders that result from genetic disorders (following Mendelian rule) of cornification. This is a new and evolving concept and has been initiated with the purpose to include a large number of diseases under single heading based on the pathophysiological alteration, i.e., the cornification disorders. This is not easy as all diseases having a defect in cornification have a well-defined and distinct phenotypic character.

Basic defect in all disorders in MEDOC is impairment in skin barrier function. Thus, a diverse array of mutations that have been identified so far (and many unidentified) results in a similar type of barrier abnormality. Ultrastructurally however, different molecular defects are found for this apparently uniform phenotype of altered epidermal barrier function.

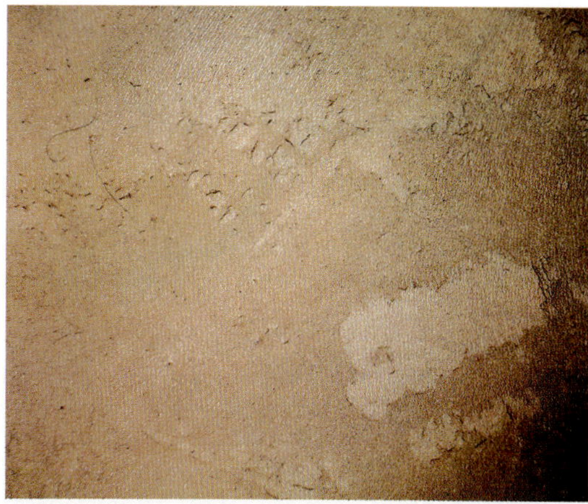

FIG. 3: Superficial skin peeling in peeling skin syndrome.

Keratinocytes are surrounded by a water-impermeable lipid enriched extracellular layer formed by cholesterol, free fatty acids, and ceramides. Keratinocytes have a well formed envelope protein and are themselves tightly adhered by the way of junctional molecules. The barrier formed by the keratinocytes and the surrounding lipid layer maintain fluid homeostasis of body. Additionally, it prevents all forms of external noxious substances and infective agents from entering the body. Eventually, enzymatic dissolution of the keratinocyte junctional molecules results in desquamation. Mutation may affect each step in the physiological maintenance of barrier function starting from formation of structural protein (cornified envelope proteins), junctional molecules, proteolytic enzymes, defect in lipid layer formation, defect in repair mechanism, and many more.

Disease with ichthyosis phenotype is the major condition under MEDOC (Figs 1 and 2). Other diseases that have been included are erythrokeratodermia, palmoplantar keratosis (PPK), peeling skin syndrome (Fig. 3) and many ichthyosis-related disorders (Box 2). Newer diseases are still being included in the list.

## INTRODUCTION TO REVISED CLASSIFICATION OF NOMENCLATURE OF ICHTHYOSIS

Ichthyosis is an age old term and considered vague and even inaccurate. Thus this is not universally accepted. Often the stages and clinical expression of the disease controlled the nomenclature of the diagnosis. Epidermolytic hyperkeratosis, bullous congenital ichthyosiform erythroderma (CIE), or bullous ichthyosis is used interchangeably for a single entity based on the choice of the physician or the stage and clinical manifestation of the disease. However, in the recently proposed revised nomenclature and classification of inherited ichthyosis, the term "ichthyosis" is kept unmodified for practical reasons. Specific definitions and more descriptive terminology have been proposed.

In this proposed classification, ichthyosis has been classified into inherited (under MEDOC) and acquired. Ichthyosis is defined as a disease that affects all or most of the integument and is clinically characterized by hyperkeratosis, scaling, or both.

Age of onset of ichthyosis (congenital vs late onset) has not been given much importance in classification as many form of ichthyosis may be subtle at birth that may be missed or some forms may have variable onset age. Classification is primarily

**BOX 2 Diseases included under Mendelian disorders of cornification**

*Ichthyosis*

- Non-syndromic ichthyosis
  - *Common ichthyosis*: Ichthyosis vulgaris(IV), X-linked recessive ichthyosis (XLRI)
  - *Autosomal recessive congenital ichthyosis (ARCI)*: Harlequin ichthyosis (HI), lamellar ichthyosis (LI), congenital ichthyosiform erythroderma (CIE)
  - *Keratinopathic ichthyosis (KPI)*: Epidermolytic ichthyosis (IE), superficial epidermolytic ichthyosis (SEI), ichthyosis Curth-Macklin (ICM), congenital reticular ichthyosiform erythroderma (CRIE)
  - *Other non-syndromic ichthyosis*: Erythrokeratodermia variabilis (EKV), keratosis linearis ichthyosis congenital keratoderma (KLICK), loricrin keratoderma (LK), peeling skin disease (PSD)
- Syndromic ichthyosis
  - *X-linked ichthyosis syndromes*: Ichthyosis follicularis, atrichia, and photophobia syndrome (IFAP) syndrome, Conradi-Hünermann-Happle syndrome (CDPX2)
  - *Autosomal ichthyosis syndromes with prominent hair abnormalities*: Ichthyosis hypotrichosis syndrome HIS, ichthyosis hypotrichosis sclerosing cholangitis (IHSC), Netherton syndrome (NS)
  - *Autosomal ichthyosis syndromes with prominent hair abnormalities and/or prominent neurologic signs*: Trichothiodystrophy TTD Sjögren-Larsson syndrome (SLS) Refsum syndrome (HMSN4), mental retardation, enteropathy, deafness, neuropathy, ichthyosis, keratodermia (MEDNIK) syndrome
  - *Autosomal recessive ichthyosis syndromes with fatal disease*: Gaucher syndrome type 2, multiple sulfatase deficiency, cerebral dysgenesis neuropathy ichthyosis palmoplantar keratoderma (CEDNIK) syndrome and arthrogryposis renal-dysfunction cholestasis (ARC) syndrome
- *Other conditions*: KID syndrome, neutral lipid storage disease with ichthyosis/Chanarin-Dorfman syndrome, ichthyosis prematurity syndrome (IPS) erythrokeratoderma, palmoplantar keratoderma (PPK)

dependent on presence (syndromic ichthyosis) or absence (nonsyndromic ichthyosis) of systemic involvement. A more detailed discussion on ichthyosis is available in chapter on Ichthyotic Disorders.

While including new diseases in MEDOC, both phenotypic features and genotypic parameters (genes involved) are considered. While diagnosing and classifying the conditions under MEDOC, clinical parameters are crucial. Scales and hyperkeratosis has been defined. Quality of the scales, distribution of scaling and hyperkeratosis, syndromic (with extracutaneous involvement) and nonsyndromic (only skin involvement), congenital onset versus delayed onset, inheritance pattern are all important parameters that need to be evaluated. However, it should be remembered that classification of diseases under MEDOC should ideally be based on pathogenic mechanism.

## SUGGESTED READINGS


1. Caubet C, Jonca N, Brattsand M, et al. Degradation of Corneodesmosome Proteins by Two Serine Proteases of the Kallikrein Family, SCTE/KLK5/hK5 and SCCE/KLK7/hK7. J Invest Dermatol. 2004;122:1235-44.
2. Hamada T, Tsuruta D, Fukuda S, et al. How do keratinizing disorders and blistering disorders overlap? Experiment Dermatol. 2013;22:83-7.
3. Hohl D. Towards a better classification of erythrokeratodermias. Br J Dermatol. 2000:143:1133.
4. Martin PE, Easton JA, Hodgins MB, et al. Connexins: Sensors of epidermal integrity that are therapeutic targets. FEBS Lett. 2014;588:1304-14.
5. Oji V, Tadini G, Akiyama M, et al. Revised nomenclature and classification of inherited ichthyoses: results of the First Ichthyosis Consensus Conference in Sore`ze 2009. J Am Acad Dermatol. 2010;63:607-41.
6. Sarma N, Boler AK, Bhanja DC. Peeling skin syndrome in eight cases of four different families from India and Bangladesh. Indian J Dermatol Venereol Leprol. 2012;78:625-31.
7. Sbidian E, Feldmann D, Bengoa J, et al. Germline mosaicism in keratitis–ichthyosis–deafness syndrome: pre-natal diagnosis in a familial lethal form. Clin Genet. 2010;77:587-92.
8. Schmuth M, Martinz V, Janecke AR, et al. Inherited ichthyoses/generalized Mendelian disorders of cornification. Eur J Hum Genet. 2013;21:123-33.
9. Serre G, Mils V, Haftek M, et al. Identification of late differentiation antigens of human cornified epithelia, expressed in reorganized desmosomes and bound to cross-linked envelope. J Invest Dermatol. 1991;97:1061-72.
10. Hamada T, Tsuruta D, Fukuda S, et al. How do keratinizing disorders and blistering disorders overlap? Exp Dermatol. 2013;22(2):83-7.
11. Oji V, Tadini G, Akiyama M, et al. Revised nomenclature and classification of inherited ichthyoses: Results of the First Ichthyosis Consensus Conference in Sore`ze 2009. J Am Acad Dermatol 2010;63:607-41.

# 32 CHAPTER Ichthyotic Disorders of Skin

Arun C Inamadar, Aparna Palit

## INTRODUCTION

Ichthyotic disorders are mostly congenital and manifest at or around birth. However, some systemic diseases and exogenous factors like drugs, may give rise to ichthyotic changes in skin.

These are designated as secondary ichthyotic disorders. The discussion in this chapter will primarily highlight the congenital ichthyotic disorders.

The term "ichthyosis" is descriptive of "fish-scale", derived from the Greek word "ichthys". Congenital ichthyoses are characterized by variable degree of generalized, persistent scaling, with a chronic course throughout the life.

Ichthyotic disorders are characterized by either increased stratum corneum production or abnormal corneocyte shedding along with altered skin barrier function. Clinical expression is highly variable ranging from mild ichthyosis vulgaris (IV) to severe, lethal harlequin ichthyosis (HI). Categorizing the ichthyosis subtypes is often difficult without genetic studies.

## CONGENITAL ICHTHYOSIS

### Classification

The current system being followed for classification of congenital ichthyoses has been derived from the "2009 Ichthyosis Consensus Conference on Terminology and Classification of Inherited Ichthyosis." The classification of ichthyosis has been presented in table 1.

**TABLE 1: Classification of ichthyosis**

| Nonsyndromic forms | | Syndromic forms | |
|---|---|---|---|
| Common ichthyosis | • Ichthyosis vulgaris (IV)<br>• Recessive X-linked ichthyosis (RXLI), nonsyndromic | X-linked ichthyosis syndromes | • RXLI (Syndromic form)<br>• IFAP syndrome<br>• Conradi–Hünermann–Happle syndrome |
| Autosomal recessive congenital ichthyosis (ARCI) | Major types<br>• Harlequin ichthyosis (HI)<br>• Lamellar ichthyosis (LI)<br>• Congenital ichthyosiform erythroderma (CIE)<br>Minor variants<br>• Self healing collodion baby (SHCB)<br>• Acral SHCB<br>• Bathing suit ichthyosis (BSI) | Autosomal ichthyosis syndromes | • *Prominent hair abnormalities*:<br>○ Netherton syndrome (NS)<br>○ Ichthyosis-hypotrichosis syndrome (IHS)<br>○ Ichthyosis-hypotrichosis-sclerosing cholangitis (IHSC) syndrome<br>○ Trichothiodystrophy (TTD) syndrome<br>• *Prominent neurologic signs*:<br>○ Sjögren–Larsson syndrome (SLS)<br>○ Refsum syndrome<br>○ Mental retardation-Enteropathy-deafness-neuropathy-ichthyosis-keratoderma (MEDNIK) syndrome<br>• *Fatal disease course*:<br>○ Gaucher syndrome type 2<br>○ Multiple sulfatase deficiency (MSD)<br>○ Cerebral dysgenesis, neuropathy, ichthyosis, and palmoplantar keratoderma (CEDNIK) syndrome<br>○ Arthrogryposis-renal dysfunction-cholestasis (ARC) syndrome |

*Continued*

*Continued*

| Nonsyndromic forms | | Syndromic forms | |
|---|---|---|---|
| Keratinopathic ichthyosis (KPI) | • Major types<br>○ Epidermolytic ichthyosis (EI)<br>○ Superficial EI (SEI)<br>• Minor Variants<br>○ Annular EI (AEI)<br>○ Ichthyosis Curth-Macklin (ICM)<br>○ Autosomal recessive EI (AREI)<br>○ Epidermolytic nevi | Other associated syndromes | • Keratitis-ichthyosis-deafness (KID) syndrome<br>• Neutral lipid storage disease with ichthyosis<br>• Ichthyosis prematurity syndrome (IPS) |
| Other forms | • Loricrin keratoderma (LK)<br>• Erythrokeratodermia variabilis (EKV)<br>• Peeling skin disease (PSD)<br>• Congenital reticular ichthyosiform erythroderma (CRIE)<br>• Keratosis linearis–ichthyosis congenita-sclerosing keratoderma (KLICK) | – | – |

IFAP, ichthyosis follicularis, atrichia, and photophobia.

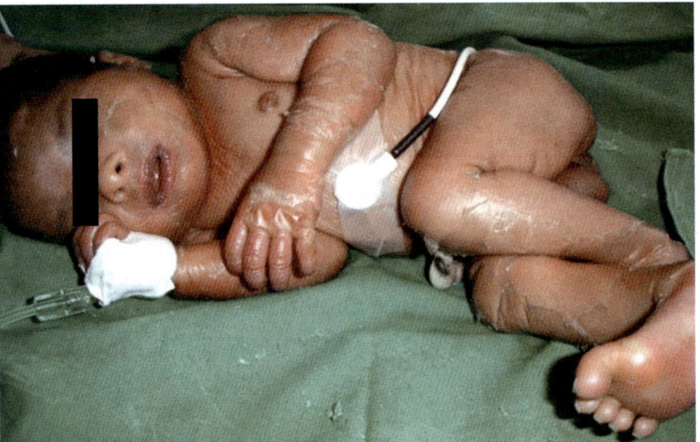

**FIG. 1:** Collodion baby with partial shedding of the membrane at places.

*Collodion baby (Fig. 1)*: Neonates born with some congenital ichthyosis are found encased in a shiny, parchment-thin, yellowish, and plastic-like taut membrane, with tethering at the body orifices. This sheds thereafter and gradually clinical features of a definitive ichthyosis become apparent. There is associated ectropion, eclabium, flat pinna, absence of skin creases, and sausage-shaped digits. Limb movements and respiratory movements are restricted and feeding is impaired. Congenital ichthyosiform erythroderma (CIE) is the most common ichthyosis (60–80%) presenting as collodion baby, followed by lamellar ichthyosis (LI). Some ichthyosiform syndromes like, Sjögren–Larsson syndrome (SLS), Conradi–Hünermann syndrome, and trichothiodystrophy (TTD) may also present with collodion membrane at birth.

## NONSYNDROMIC FORMS OF ICHTHYOSIS

Salient features of the nonsyndromic congenital ichthyoses have been presented in table 2.

### Ichthyosis Vulgaris

Ichthyosis vulgaris is a common disease, often associated with atopy. It is an autosomal semidominant condition with variable penetrance.

#### Pathogenesis

There is mutation in *FLG* gene located on chromosome 1q21.3. The defect involves keratohyalin, a keratinocyte protein. The skin is deficient in histidine, a basic molecule necessary for synthesis of profilaggrin and filaggrin. In addition, stratum corneum ceramide is low. *FLG* gene is also seen in atopic individuals that may coexist.

#### Clinical Features

Clinical presentation of IV occurs during 2–6 months after birth. The scales are fine, light gray colored, involving extensor extremities, and trunk (Fig. 2). Flexural areas like—axillae, groins and antecubital, and popliteal fossae are spared (Fig. 3). This is usually asymptomatic with multiple affected family members, improves with age and in summer. Atopic dermatitis, keratosis pilaris, hyperlinearity of palms and soles, and pruritus are frequently associated.

#### Investigations

##### *Histopathology*

There is orthohyperkeratosis and absence of granular layer. Eccrine sweat and sebaceous glands are small and decreased in number. There may be mononuclear infiltrate in the upper dermis. Electron microscopy (EM) shows fragmented, small, or only rudimentary keratohyaline granules.

Antigen mapping demonstrates reduced or negative filaggrin staining.

### Recessive X-linked Ichthyosis

Recessive X-linked ichthyosis (RXLI) is the second common variant of ichthyotic disorders. This may be associated with extracutaneous manifestations (syndromic ichthyosis).

#### Pathogenesis

Recessive X-linked ichthyosis results from deletion (>90%) or point mutation of the steroid sulfatase (*STS*) gene, located

**TABLE 2: Salient features of nonsyndromic congenital ichthyoses**

| Type of ichthyosis | Inheritance pattern | Genetic defect | Clinical feature | Distinguishing feature |
|---|---|---|---|---|
| Ichthyosis vulgaris | Autosomal semidominant | Mutation at Filaggrin gene, *FLG* (1q21.3) | • Onset around 6 months of age<br>• *Scales*: Fine, light-gray, over extensor extremities, and trunk | • Sparing of flexures<br>• Atopy may be associated |
| Recessive X-linked ichthyosis | X-linked recessive | • Deletion at steroid sulfatase gene, (Xp22.3)<br>• Sometimes point mutation | • Present soon after birth, often born with collodion membrane.<br>• *Scales*: Large, polygonal, dark and adherent, over the extremities, neck, and pre-auricular area | • Rhomboid scales<br>• Extracutaneous manifestations |
| Harlequin ichthyosis | • Autosomal recessive<br>• Sporadic cases may occur | Mutation at *ABCA12* gene (2q35) | • Present at birth<br>• *Scales*: Thick, yellow, plate-like, with deep red fissuring; generalized distribution | Grotesque appearance |
| Lamellar ichthyosis | • Autosomal recessive<br>• Rarely, autosomal dominant | Mutation at *TGM1* gene (14q11) | • Collodion membrane at birth.<br>• *Scales*: Dark-brown, large plate like, with deep fissures in between. Free and raised at margin and adherent at center; generalized distribution | Tree-bark appearance of the skin |
| Congenital ichthyosiform erythroderma | • Autosomal recessive<br>• Sometimes, autosomal dominant | Mutation at *TGM-1* gene | Collodion membrane at birth. Since childhood, persistent erythroderma with thin, white, small, semiadherent scales; generalized distribution | • Persistent erythroderma, with fine, white scales<br>• Palmoplantar hyperkeratosis and digital contractures |
| Epidermolytic ichthyosis | • Autosomal dominant;<br>• Sometimes, autosomal recessive/ sporadic | Mutations at epidermal *KRT 1/KRT 10* genes | • Generalized flaccid bullae and widespread denudation present at birth<br>• Blistering improves with age and hyperkeratotic lesions appear; distribution over joints, flexures, back, scalp, periumbilical and peri-areolar regions | Dirty brown ridges and minute spiny projections. Occasional focal vesiculation over these areas, induced by friction |

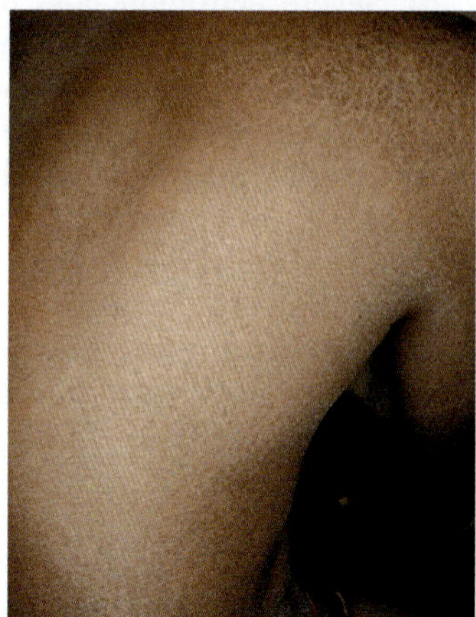

**FIG. 2:** Fine, branny scale of ichthyosis vulgaris.

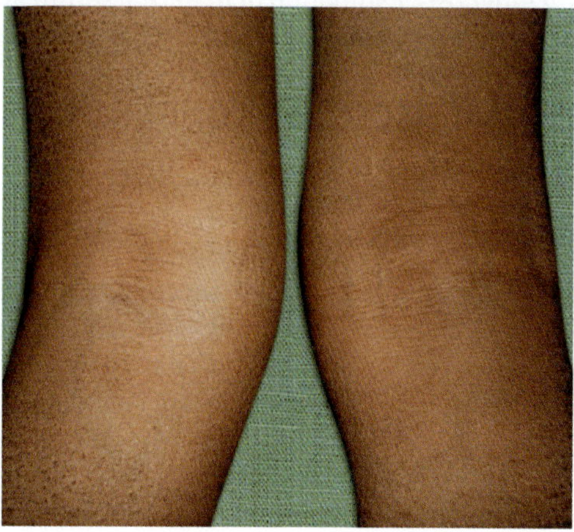

**FIG. 3:** Sparing of the popliteal fossae in a child with ichthyosis vulgaris.

at Xp22.3.The pathomechanism of RXLI is two-fold. There is lack of STS (isomer of aryl sulfatase C, a membrane-bound microsomal enzyme), an enzyme present normally in various cells. STS converts cholesterol sulfate to cholesterol by hydrolytic pathway. Deficiency of STS leads to cholesterol sulfate accumulation in the epidermis. The excess cholesterol sulfate delays corneodesmosome degradation; the ultimate results are epidermal barrier instability and corneocyte retention.

Recessive X-linked ichthyosis is also found to result into contiguous gene syndromes associated with Kallmann syndrome, ocular albinism type 1, X-linked recessive chondrodysplasia punctata, short stature, and mental retardation.

## Clinical Features

Manifestations start within few weeks of birth and are persistent. Often the affected child is born with collodion membrane. The scales in RXLI are large, polygonal (rhomboid), dark, and adherent especially over the extremities (Fig. 4A), forehead (Fig. 4B), neck, and preauricular area (Fig. 4C). Flexural involvement may be seen in some cases. Palms and soles are spared.

Extracutaneous manifestations of RXLI are corneal opacities (25–50%) and cryptorchidism (10–20%). Numerous corneal opacities (dots or commas), without hampering the vision are present in adult patients and carrier females.

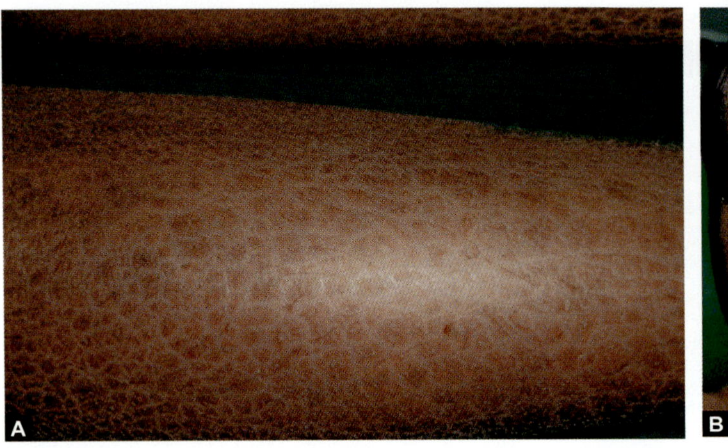


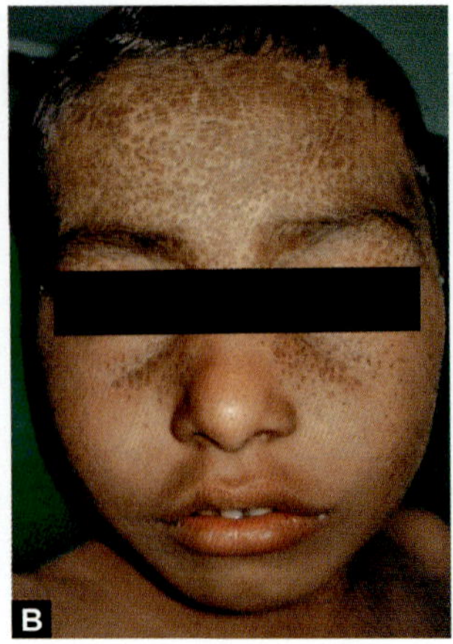


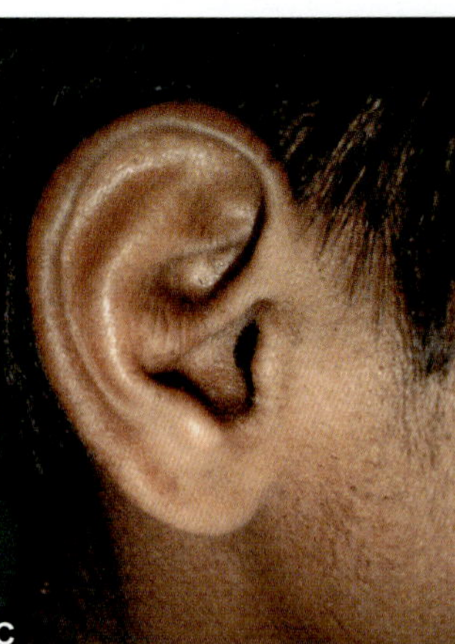


**FIG. 4: A,** Dark, polygonal scales of recessive X-linked ichthyosis (RXLI); **B,** Distribution of scales on forehead in RXLI; **C,** Distribution of scales on preauricular area and external ear in RXLI.

Improvement may occur in summer season. Deficient placental STS causes prolonged labor even in carrier females. Risk of testicular cancer is higher.

### Investigations

Histopathology is nonspecific with normal or prominent granular layer. Electron microscopy shows numerous keratohyalin granules that are normal or may be smaller.
Slit lamp examination shows corneal opacities.

Absence of STS activity in leukocytes and fibroblasts may be detected. Blood cholesterol sulfate level is usually high. Fluorescence *in situ* hybridization test identifies STS deletion.

*Prenatal diagnosis*: Estimation of maternal serum and urinary estriol levels; fetal STS deficiency leads to low levels.

# AUTOSOMAL RECESSIVE CONGENITAL ICHTHYOSIS

## Harlequin Ichthyosis

Harlequin ichthyosis is a rare and severe form of congenital ichthyosis with high perinatal mortality. The inheritance pattern is autosomal recessive, but may be sporadic.

### Pathogenesis

There is abnormal localization of epidermal lipids and defective lipid barrier in stratum corneum. The mutation lies in *ABCA12* gene on 2q35. ABCA12 encodes an adenosine triphosphate-binding cassette (ABC) transporter, which regulates lipid transport in lamellar granules.

Harlequin ichthyosis is a disorder with genetic heterogeneity. Three types are described:

- Type I (normal keratin, profilaggrin staining present)
- Type II (hyperproliferation of suprabasal keratin, K6/K16)
- Type III (hyperproliferation of suprabasal keratin, K6/K16 and negative profilaggrin staining).

### Clinical Features

The baby is born encased in "armor"-like thick, yellow plate-like scales, deep red fissuring, and tight skin over face (grotesque appearance) (Fig. 5). Severe ectropion, loss of eyelashes and eyebrows, severe eclabium, flat nose, and flattening or synechiae of the ears are the other features. There are constriction bands around the limbs and flexion deformity of the digits; constant pressure from these bands may lead to hypoplastic and rudimentary digits.

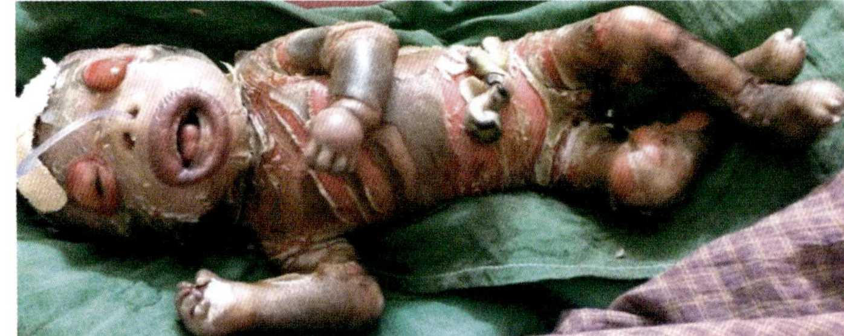

**FIG. 5:** Neonate born with "armor"-like thick encasement, deep fissuring, extensive ectropion, and eclabium; a Harlequin baby.

Preterm delivery and stillbirth are usual in these cases. Postnatal period is complicated by hypoglycemia, dehydration, respiratory distress due to chest wall constriction, electrolyte imbalance, thermoregulatory imbalance, infections, and death. Morbidity in survivors is very high.

### Investigations

Histopathology shows nonspecific features. There are vesicular lamellar body ghosts and sparsely secreted lamellar structures in the stratum corneum in EM.

## Lamellar Ichthyosis

Lamellar ichthyosis is recessively inherited (rarely dominant) and severe form of congenital ichthyosis. These forms are indistinguishable clinically.

### Pathogenesis

Mutation occurs in *TGM1* gene located on chromosome 14q11. There is abnormal keratinocyte transglutaminase 1 (TGase1) enzyme which is responsible for formation of impermeable layers of epidermal cell envelope.

### Clinical Features

The affected children are born as collodion babies. Subsequently, there is generalized ichthyosis involving face, flexures, palms, and soles. The scales are dark-brown in color, quadrilateral, large plate-like, which are free and raised at the edges and adherent at the center (Fig. 6). There are deep fissures in between the scales with an appearance of tree bark (Fig. 7). There is associated ectropion, eclabium, hypoplasia of nose (Fig. 8) and pinna, and flexion contracture of limb joints and digits. There is lack of sweating and heat intolerance due to blockage of sweat ducts, scarring alopecia along the scalp margins, and nail changes like ridging, thickening, and gross dystrophy. The disease is stable and persistent.

### Investigations

Histopathological study reveals marked orthohyperkeratosis, mild acanthosis, and regular papillomatosis. Electron microscopic study shows elongated cholesterol clefts and lipid droplets in the stratum corneum. There may be attenuated or absent cornified cell envelope.

## Congenital Ichthyosiform Erythroderma

Congenital ichthyosiform erythroderma (nonbullous ichthyosiform erythroderma) is an autosomal recessive disorder. (autosomal dominant has been form reported).

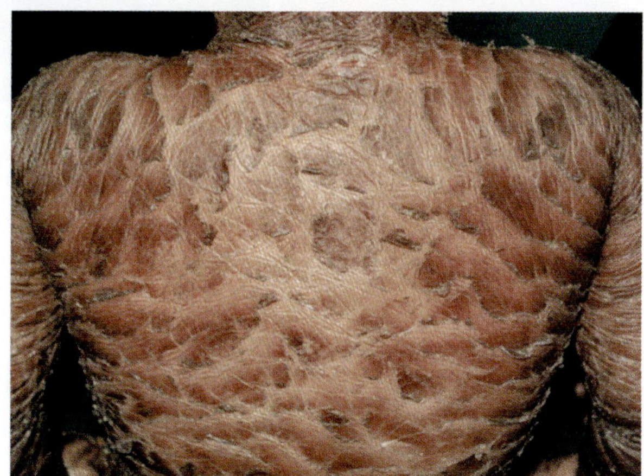

**FIG. 6:** Large, dark, plate-like scales of lamellar ichthyosis.

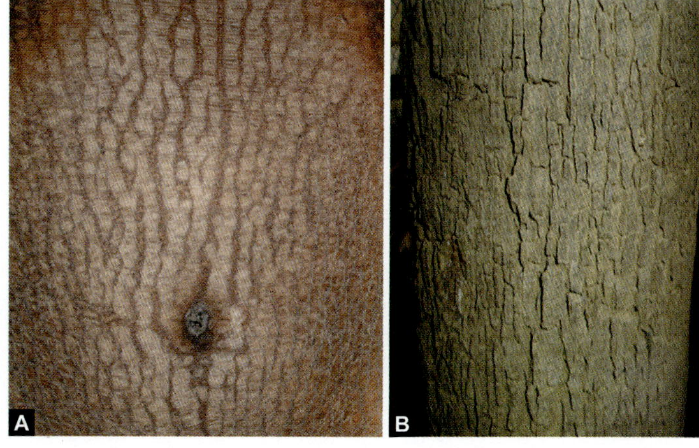


**FIG. 7: A,** Lamellar ichthyosis; **B,** Appearance like the bark of a tree.

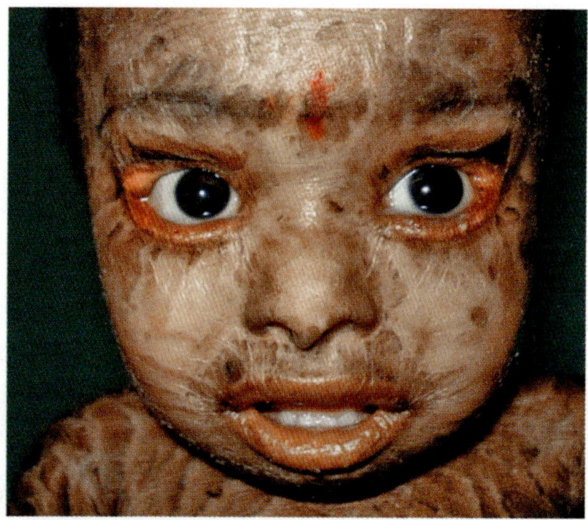

**FIG. 8:** Ectropion, eclabium, and hypoplastic nose in a child with lamellar ichthyosis.

### Pathogenesis

Congenital ichthyosiform erythroderma is a disorder with extensive genetic heterogeneity. Some patients show mutation in *TGM-1.*

### Clinical Features

Congenital ichthyosiform erythroderma mostly starts with collodion membrane at birth (90%). Thereafter, there is a persistent variable erythroderma with thin, white, small, and semiadherent scales till adulthood (Fig. 9). Associated appendageal involvement may lead to scarring alopecia, nail dystrophy, hypohidrosis, and heat intolerance.

### Investigations

Light microscopic findings are nonspecific. Electron microscopy shows lipid droplets in the stratum corneum due to retained, abnormal lamellar bodies in the corneocytes along with disorganization of the intercellular lipid lamellae.

## Self-healing Collodion Baby or Lamellar Ichthyosis of the Newborn

This occurs in 10–20% of the neonates born with collodion membrane. The condition is short-lasting and as the membrane is shed, the child gradually develops normal skin by 3 months of life.

## Bathing Suit Ichthyosis

Bathing suit ichthyosis (BSI) is a recently described recessive disorder, reported mostly from South Africa. There is mutation in *TGM1*. The child may be born with collodion membrane. The distribution of scaling is unique as there is diffuse scaling of scalp, trunk, and proximal parts of the upper limbs sparing warmer skin areas like face and distal extremities (Fig. 10).

# KERATINOPATHIC ICHTHYOSIS

## Epidermolytic Ichthyosis

Epidermolytic ichthyosis (EI), earlier designated as "epidermolytic hyperkeratosis" or "bullous CIE", is transmitted as autosomal

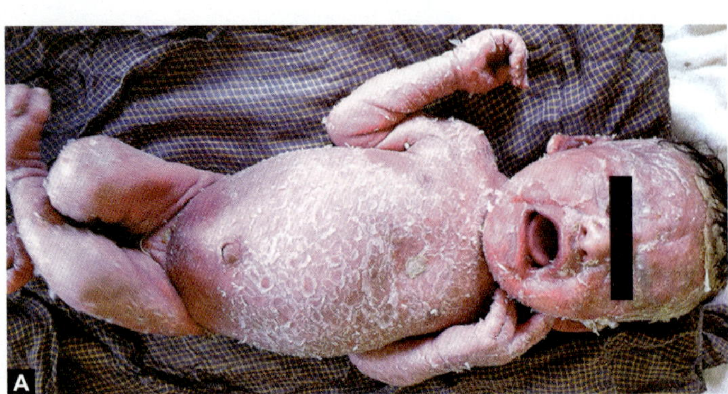

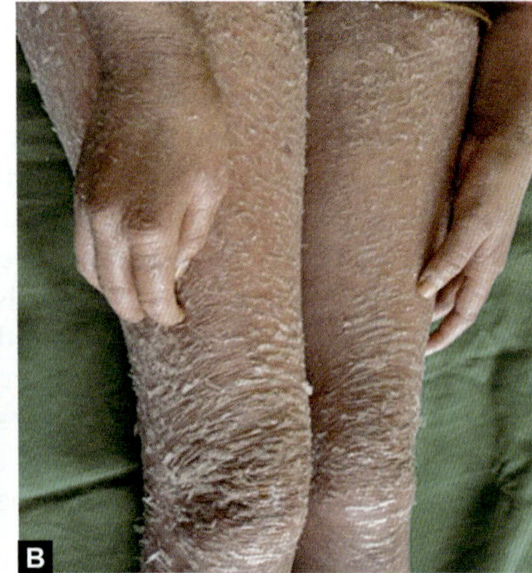

FIG. 9: **A,** A neonate with congenital ichthyosiform erythroderma; **B,** Thin, small, white, semi-adherent scales of congenital ichthyosiform erythroderma in an older child.

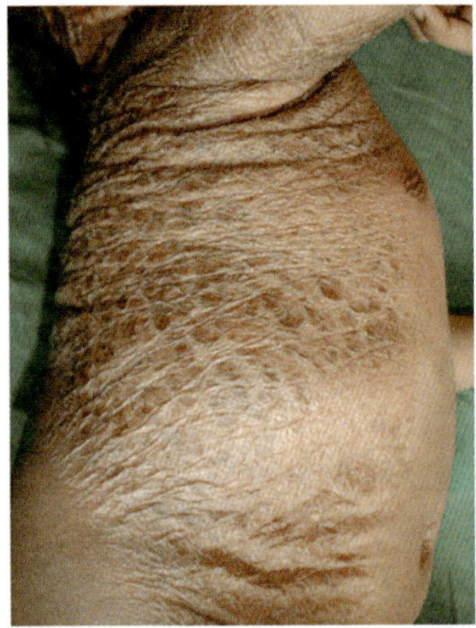

FIG. 10: Bathing suit ichthyosis; note the surrounding normal skin.

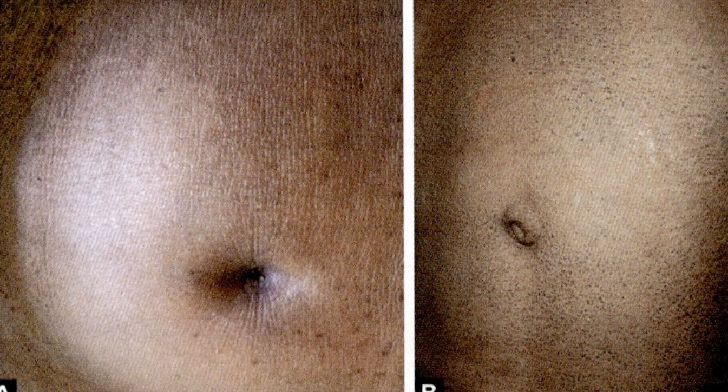

FIG. 11: **A,** Dirty brown ridges in peri-umbilical area in a child with epidermolytic ichthyosis; **B,** Brownish, spiny projections on peri-umbilical area in a child with epidermolytic ichthyosis.

dominant disorder. Sometimes also as autosomal recessive, and sporadic forms may occur. Epidermolytic ichthyosis is unique among the congenital ichthyoses because of blister formation.

## Pathogenesis

Epidermolytic ichthyosis results from mutations in the epidermal keratin 1 or keratin 10 (*KRT1* or *KRT10*) genes. These keratins are the components of the intermediate filaments of suprabasal keratinocytes. The autosomal recessive variant of the disease results from *KRT* 10 mutation.

## Clinical Features

Generalized flaccid bullae and widespread denudation are present at birth. The friction during passage through the birth canal precipitates the denudation. Over the time, tendency to blistering is improved and replaced by hyperkeratotic skin lesions. The classical lesions in older children, adolescents, and adults are dirty brown ridges and minute spiny projections, predominantly distributed over the joints, flexures, back, scalp, periumbilical (Fig. 11), and periareolar regions. Occasional focal vesiculation is common, induced by friction, trauma, or infection (Fig. 12). Diffuse palmoplantar keratoderma with sharply demarcated, erythematous border, with or without fissuring

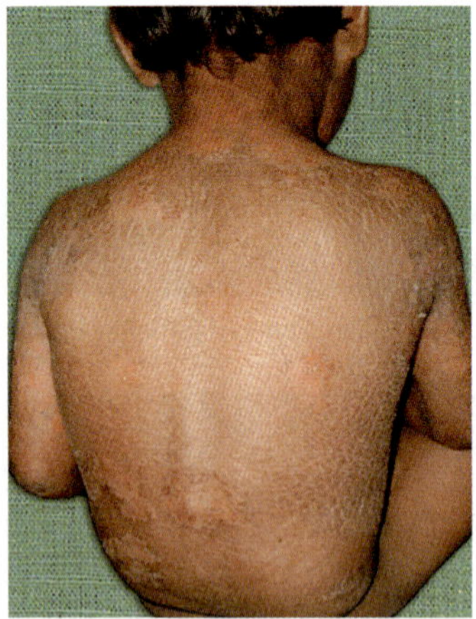

FIG. 12: Areas of superficial erosions in between ichthyotic skin in a child with epidermolytic ichthyosis.

(rarely a cerebriform pattern) may be associated. Severe scalp involvement occurs commonly with encasement of hair shafts with scales. Nails may be dystrophic but mucosae and teeth are normal.

Epidermolytic ichthyosis runs a chronic recalcitrant course, with frequent episodes of infection involving eroded areas, giving rise to foul body odor. During neonatal period, sepsis, and fluid-electrolyte imbalance are the important causes of mortality.

## Investigations

Epidermis shows marked hyperkeratosis, acanthosis, perinuclear vacuoles, large clumps of keratohyaline granules in granular and upper spinous layer and suprabasal splits. These features are known as "epidermolytic hyperkeratosis". Scanty perivascular lymphocytic infiltrate may be present in the upper dermis.

Epidermolytic ichthyosis reveals perinuclear clumping of tonofilaments in suprabasal cells and variable desmosomal dissolution with cleft formation.

## Superficial Epidermolytic Ichthyosis or Ichthyosis Bullosa of Siemens

This is a superficial variant of EI.

### *Pathogenesis*

There are autosomal dominant mutations involving *K2e* gene and the sites of clinical lesions correspond to the sites of expression of this gene.

### *Clinical Features*

Symptoms start during neonatal period with superficial bullae which rupture shortly with collarette-like scaling (mauserung or moulting). Subsequently, circumscribed areas with grayish, rippled scales develop. Flexures, shin, and lower abdomen are commonly involved areas (Fig. 13). Erythema and palmoplantar keratoderma are absent in these cases. Rarely, hypertrichosis and palmoplantar blistering with hyperhidrosis may be associated.

## Investigations

Histopathological features are similar to classic epidermolytic hyperkeratosis, but are more superficial, located to granular and upper spinous layers with normal suprabasal and basal cells. Bullous areas show intracorneal split surrounded by orthohyperkeratosis.

Electron microscopy reveals cytolysis in granular cells without any keratin clumping.

## Annular Epidermolytic Ichthyosis

This is a variant of EI. Numerous annular, polycyclic, erythematous, and scaly plaques develop on the trunk and extremities . The lesions progress slowly, and then resolve.

## Ichthyosis Curth–Macklin

Ichthyosis Curth–Macklin (ICM) is considered as a variant of a broad heterogenous group designated as ichthyosis hystrix (IH).

## Clinical Features

Skin lesions are present at birth or may appear by childhood. There is localized, muddy, and spiny hyperkeratosis (scales) distributed on extensor extremities and trunk with or without mild erythema (Fig. 14). The lesions simulate EI, but skin fragility or bullae formation are absent. Lesions may follow Blaschko's lines. Diffuse, mutilating palmoplantar keratoderma may be a part of the disease (Fig. 15).

## Investigations

Histopathology shows vacuolated and binucleate cells in the upper epidermis. This is a characteristic feature of this disorder (Fig. 16). There is no evidence of epidermolysis.

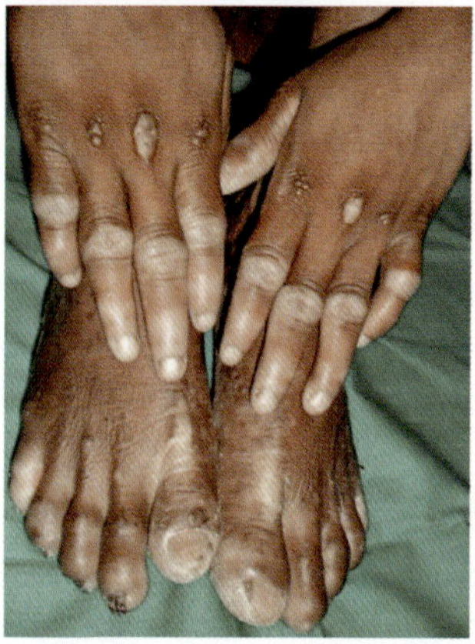

**FIG. 14:** Spiny hyperkeratosis on the dorsal surface of hands in a case of "Ichthyosis Curth–Macklin".

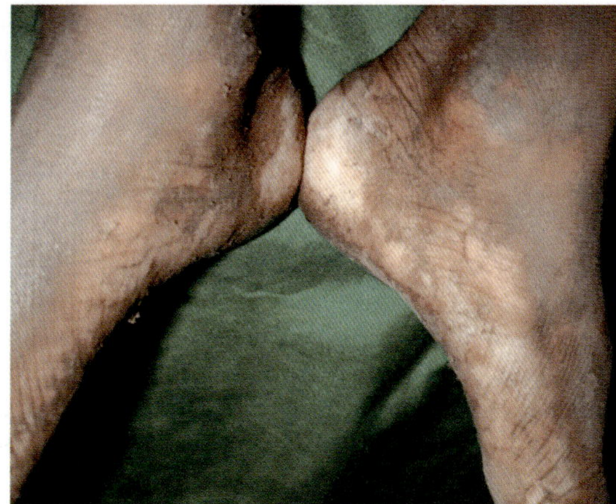

**FIG. 13:** "Mauserung" in a patient with ichthyosis bullosa of Siemens.

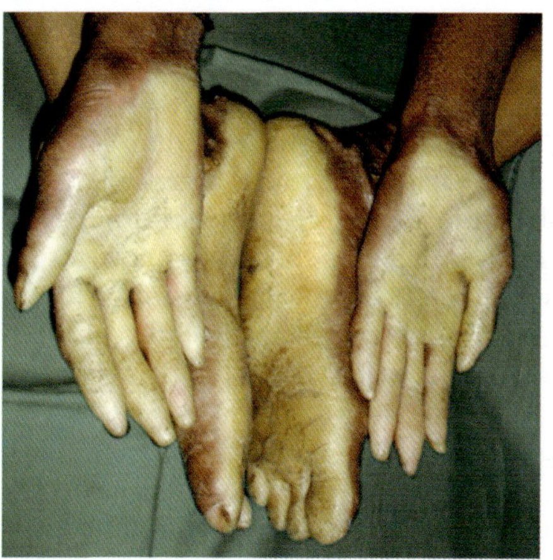

**FIG. 15:** Diffuse palmoplantar keratoderma in a case of "Ichthyosis Curth–Macklin."

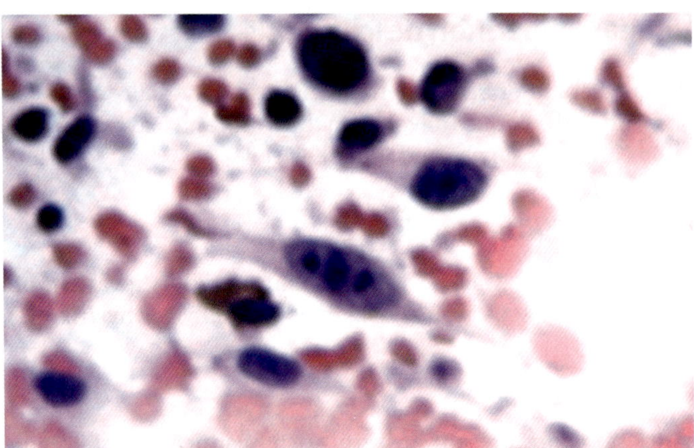

**FIG. 16:** Histopathology (H&E, 40x) showing typical binucleate cells in epidermis in a case of "Ichthyosis Curth–Macklin."

Electron microscopic findings are evident in granular and upper spinous cell layers. There are perinuclear tonofilament shells forming cytoplasmic compartments, surrounded by a ribosome-rich region.

### Epidermolytic nevi

Nevoid form of EI resembling ichthyosis hystrix may be present over flexures, extremities, and genitalia.

# ICHTHYOSIFORM SYNDROMES

## X-linked Ichthyosis Syndromes

### Syndromic form of RXLI

The RXLI is regarded as syndromic when accompanied by associated manifestation such as testicular maldescent. Rarely, mental deficiency or hypogonadism may be present.

## IFAP Syndrome

The IFAP is the acronym for *i*chthyosis *f*ollicularis, *a*lopecia, and *p*hotophobia. It is an X-linked recessive disease.

### Clinical Features

The child presents at birth with collodion membrane. There is generalized, mild to moderate, whitish scales with scalp involvement, like follicular keratosis and congenital atrichia. Various extracutaneous manifestations include severe photophobia, psychomotor retardation, cerebral anomalies (brain atrophy, temporal lobe malformation, hypoplasia of corpus callosum), failure to thrive, atopic manifestations, inguinal hernia, aganglionic megacolon, and testicular or renal abnormalities. Female carriers may present with milder clinical features such as linear follicular ichthyosis, atrophoderma, hypotrichosis, and hypohidrosis.

### Investigations

Histopathology shows numerous atrophic hair follicles and absence of sebaceous glands.

## Conradi–Hünermann–Happle Syndrome or X-linked Dominant Chondrodysplasia Punctata

Conradi-Hünermann-Happle syndrome (CHH) is a rare, X-linked-dominant, multisystem disorder, affecting skin, bone, and eye. An autosomal dominant form may exist.

### Pathogenesis

There is mutation at the *ARSE* gene, located at Xp11.23. Exact pathogenesis is unknown.

### Clinical Features

Usually erythroderma is present at birth. Frequently the scales are arranged along the lines of Blaschko, in swirls and whorls. The scaling improves by first few months of life and persists as mild ichthyosis on the limbs. Unilateral and sectorial cataracts, follicular atrophoderma, hyper- and hypopigmentation and localized scarring alopecia of the scalp, asymmetrical skeletal, and ocular involvements are the characteristic other cutaneous features. Skeletal manifestations appear later and present with limb length discrepancies, severe kyphoscoliosis, and congenital dislocation of hip and facial dysplasia.

### Investigations

Serum gas chromatography-mass spectrometry reveals high 8-dehydrocholesterol and cholesterol levels.

Radiologically, there is punctate calcification of the epiphysis of the long bones.

# AUTOSOMAL ICHTHYOSIS SYNDROMES

## Netherton Syndrome

Netherton syndrome (NS) is a rare autosomal recessive disorder characterized by ichthyosis, hair shaft disorder, and atopy.

### Pathogenesis

There is mutation in *SPINK5*, located at 5q. 32, which encodes LEKTI (*l*ympho *e*pithelial *K*azal-*t*ype-related *i*nhibitor). Deficiency of LEKTI results in altered lamellar body membrane and cutaneous barrier function. Altered barrier function enhances penetration of exogenous allergen and exacerbation of atopy.

### Clinical Features

Disease presents at birth with congenital or neonatal erythroderma (Fig. 17). Subsequently, erythematous, polycyclic lesions develop with double-edged scaling, classically known as ichthyosis linearis circumflexa (Fig. 18). Atopic features and intense pruritus are common in these patients. Trichorrhexis invaginata (bamboo hair) is classical and develops during childhood (Fig. 19). Other hair anomalies include helical hairs or tulip-like invaginations of the hair shaft. Other features are recurrent sinopulmonary infections, bacterial and viral skin infections, malnutrition, and growth retardation.

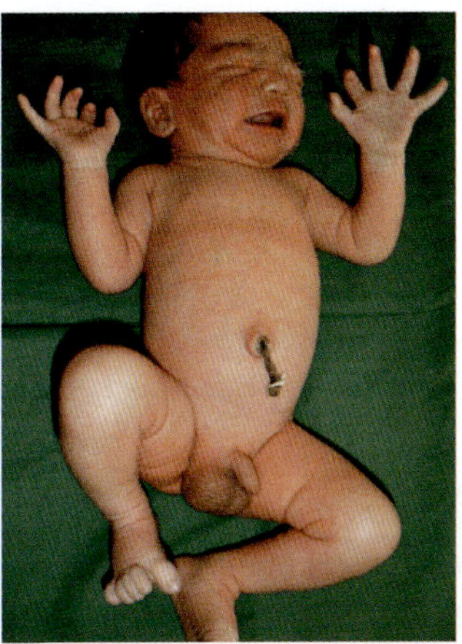

FIG. 17: Neonatal erythroderma in a case of Netherton syndrome.

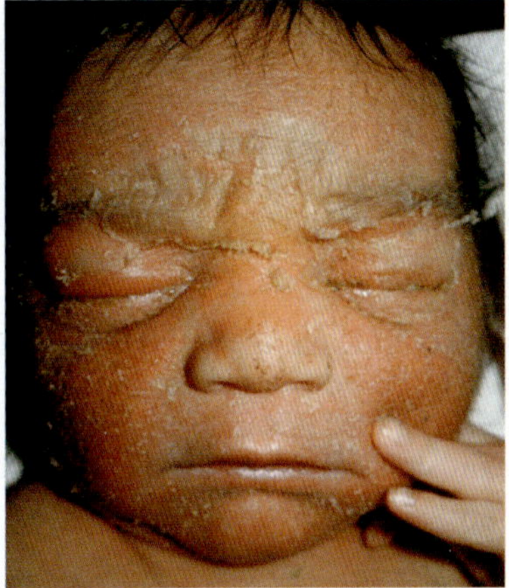

FIG. 18: Typical double-edged scales (ichthyosis linearis circumflexa) over forehead and peri-ocular area in a neonate with Netherton syndrome.

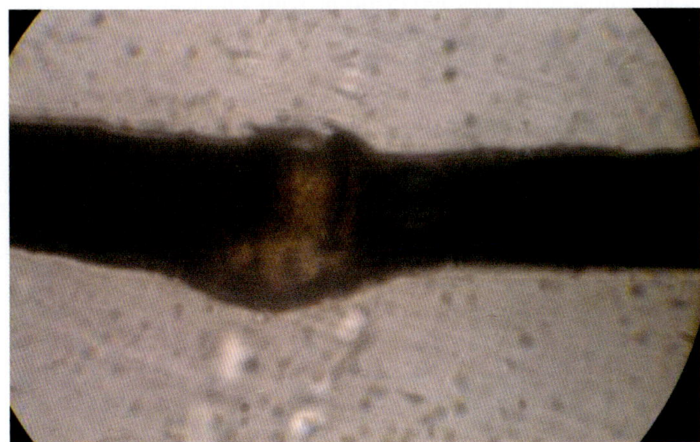

FIG. 19: Trichorrhexis nodosa with a linear split seen in case of Netherton syndrome (Light microscopy, 20x).

## Investigations

Light microscopy of plucked scalp or eyebrow hairs help in early and easy diagnosis of trichorrhexis nodosa and other hair shaft anomalies. Scanning EM gives a clearer picture of hair anomalies. Elevated serum IgE level may be present.

# Trichothiodystrophy or IBIDS Syndrome

Trichothiodystrophy is a heterogenous disorder and several genotypes and phenotypes exist.

## Pathogenesis

Most affected individuals have mutations in *ERCC2* or *XPD* gene, located on 19q13.32. However, genetic heterogeneity is common. Defect may lie in the UV-induced DNA repair pathway. There is reduced sulfur content, resulting in frequent breakage of hair shaft.

## Clinical Features

The typical clinical features comprised of photosensitivity, ichthyosis, brittle hair (Fig. 20), developmental delay, and/or short stature, infertility, and a varying combination of these. The ichthyosis may be mild or similar to LI. Depending upon the clinical features present, it can be categorized as PIBIDS, IBIDS, and BIDS.

## Investigation

Undulating contour of hair shaft with wavy melanin may be seen under light microscopy of hair. Fractured hair shaft is a frequent finding (Fig. 21).

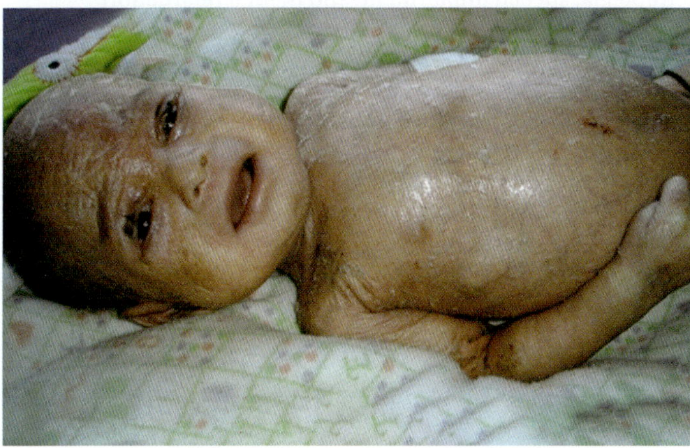

FIG. 20: A neonate with ichthyosiform erythroderma and sparse scalp hair, eyebrows and eyelashes; a case of trichothiodystrophy.

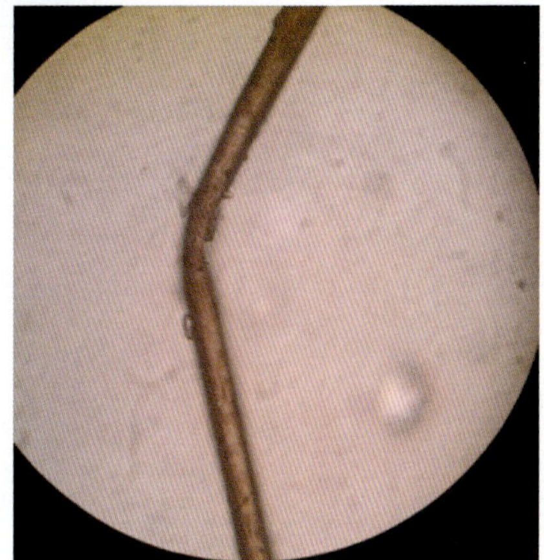

FIG. 21: Fractured hair shaft in a case of trichothiodystrophy (Light microscopy, 10x).

Banded appearance (tiger-tail) of the hair shaft seen in polarized microscopy is characteristic of TTD.

Trichothiodystrophy can be identified by demonstrating UV sensitivity in cultured fibroblasts.

## Sjögren–Larsson Syndrome

Sjögren–Larsson syndrome is a rare autosomal recessive ichthyosiform syndrome in association with neurological manifestation.

### Pathogenesis

There is mutation of the *ALDH3A2* gene (17p11.2), which encodes fatty aldehyde dehydrogenase (FALDH) that catalyzes oxidation of medium and long chain fatty aldehydes to fatty acids. There is abnormal lipid accumulation in skin and brain.

### Clinical Features

Sjögren–Larsson syndrome is a triad of congenital ichthyosis, neurological impairment, and mental retardation. Ichthyosis is present at birth, rarely there is collodion baby. Nature of scales varies from fine, white to large, plate-like (Fig. 22). A characteristic feature of SLS is associated pruritus. Neurological manifestations appear by 2–3 years of age as progressive, spastic, diplegia or tetraplegia, speech impairment, and mental retardation.

### Investigations

Perifoveal glistening white dots in the retina are a pathognomonic feature of SLS. Measurement of FALDH in cultured fibroblasts from skin biopsies helps in diagnosis.

Mutation analysis is confirmatory.

Sjögren–Larsson syndrome can be diagnosed *in utero* by using above techniques.

## Refsum Syndrome

Refsum syndrome (RS) is the other name for "hereditary motor and sensory neuropathy type IV". It is an autosomal recessive neurocutaneous disorder.

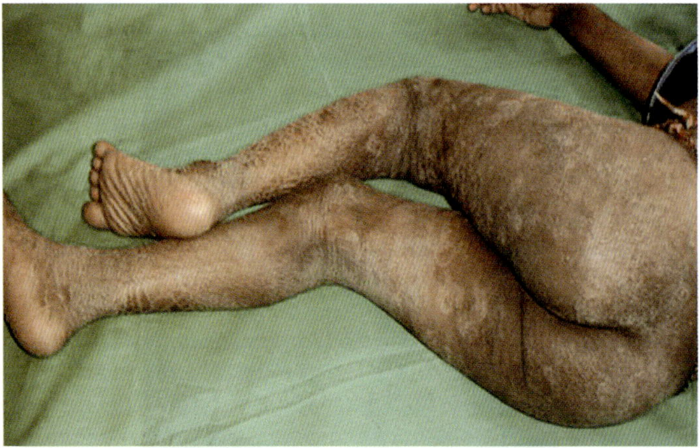

**FIG. 22:** A child with spastic diplegia and ichthyosis; a case of Sjögren–Larsson syndrome. Note large plate-like scales in legs and fine, white scales higher up.

### Pathogenesis

Two genes, *PHYH (PAHX)* located on chromosome 10p13, and *PEX7* have been identified to cause RS. There is deficiency of peroxisomal enzyme phytanoyl-CoA hydroxylase leading to inability to degrade phytanic acid, derived from dietary chlorophyll (plant products). This metabolic defect leads to accumulation of excessive phytanic acid in blood (5–30% of total serum lipid), fatty tissues and body fluids, mostly affecting nervous system and skin.

### Clinical Features

Characteristic neurological manifestations are cerebellar ataxia, peripheral polyneuropathy, and atypical retinitis pigmentosa. Patients present with night blindness, anosmia, and progressive deafness during childhood. Ichthyosis simulates IV and appears in adult life. RS runs a progressive course with periods of exacerbation and remission.

### Investigation

Histopathology shows lipid containing vacuoles in basal keratinocytes.

Liquid gas chromatography of plasma shows very high levels of phytanic acid.

Phytanic acid oxidase activity is greatly reduced in cultured fibroblasts of patients and heterozygous carriers. However, serum phytanic acid level is normal in carriers in contrast to the patients. Elevated protein is detected in cerebrospinal fluid.

Prenatal diagnosis is done by phytanic acid oxidation assay in cell culture (chorionic villus biopsy or amniocentesis).

## MEDNIK syndrome

The MEDNIK syndrome stands for *m*ental retardation-*e*nteropathy-*d*eafness-*n*europathy-*i*chthyosis-*k*eratoderma. It is an autosomal recessive disorder with onset at or soon after birth and progressive thereafter. The skin lesions are transient and erythematous simulating erythrokeratoderma variabilis. Diarrhea present since birth may prove life-threatening, causing death. Increased blood level of very long chain fatty acids is helpful in diagnosis.

## Multiple Sulfatase Deficiency

The inheritance pattern is autosomal recessive.

Neurological manifestations predominate clinical picture; these start by second year of life as progressive psychomotor retardation, limb hypotonia, and unsteady gait. Subsequently, the child is blind, bed-bound, and death may supervene in first year of life. The condition simulates late infantile metachromatic leukodystrophy. Ichthyosis mimicks mild RXLI.

There is deficiency of all the seven types of sulfatases; partial deficiency of STS explains milder ichthyosis. Estimation of urinary metabolites may be diagnostic.

## KID Syndrome

This very rare syndrome manifests with *k*eratitis, *i*chthyosis, and *d*eafness. Most cases are sporadic, but autosomal dominant and recessive modes of inheritance have been reported.

### Pathogenesis

There is mutation in the connexin gene (*GJB2*, located on 13q11.12, or, rarely *GJB6*), which may be involved in the pathogenesis of this condition.

### Clinical Features

Cutaneous involvement is varied; there is a transient erythroderma at or soon after birth. Thereafter, well-defined, fixed, hyperkeratotic plaques on erythematous base develop on elbows, knees, palms and soles, and sometimes on face. Generalized, rippled hyperkeratosis, and palmoplantar keratoderma or cobblestone type of scaling may be present. Scarring alopecia involving the entire scalp is a constant feature. Leukonychia and nail dystrophy may be present. Squamous cell carcinoma arising over the hyperkeratotic plaques is frequent in these patients.

Extracutaneous manifestations include congenital, bilateral, sensorineural deafness, and keratitis resulting in progressive photophobia. Corneal vascularization and blindness are the sequelae.

## Neutral Lipid Storage Disease with Ichthyosis or Chanarin–Dorfman Syndrome

It is a rare, autosomal recessive disease with ichthyosis (Fig. 23).

### Pathogenesis

There is mutation of *CGI-58* gene (3p21), leading to collection of triglycerides in all tissues.

### Clinical Features

This is characterized by congenital generalized ichthyosis, "rhomboid lichenification" of neck and extracutaneous features like sensorineural deafness, cataract, myopathy, hepatosplenomegaly, and growth retardation.

### Disease Course

Extent of hepatic involvement determines the prognosis of the disorder.

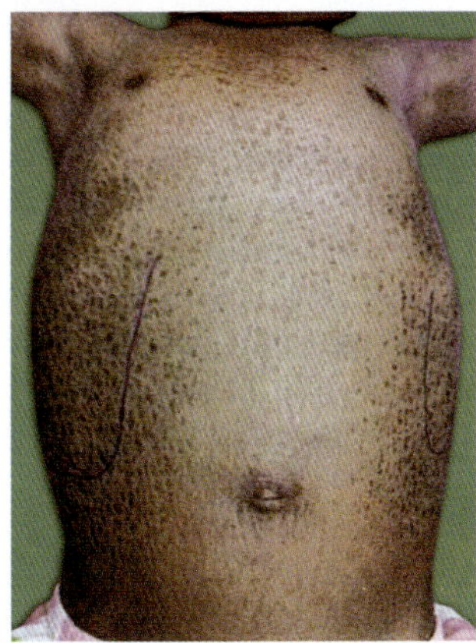

FIG. 23: Generalized ichthyosis with hepato- splenomegaly in a child with neutral lipid storage disease.

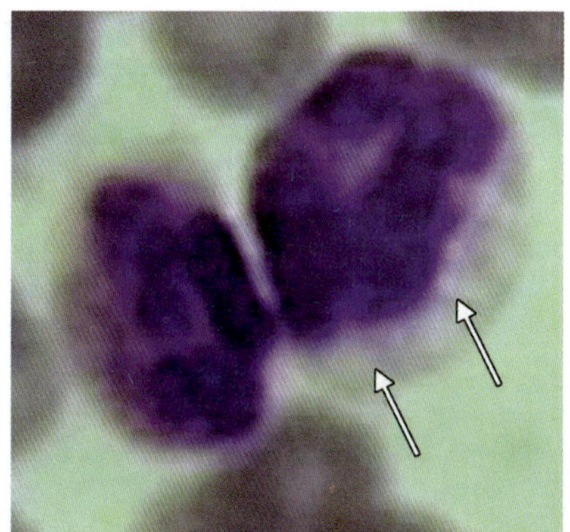

FIG. 24: Lipid-vacuoles in neutrophils (Jordan anomaly in peripheral blood smear) in a case of neutral lipid storage disease (Light microscopy, 100x).

### Investigations

Freshly prepared peripheral blood smear shows numerous lipid-vacuoles (Jordan anomaly) (Fig. 24) in the circulating granulocytes and monocytes. This is the diagnostic feature of this disorder.

*Skin biopsy*: Special staining of fresh, frozen specimen of skin shows cytoplasmic lipid droplets in epidermal and dermal cells.

Molecular defects and characteristic features of some of the syndromic congenital ichthyoses have been presented in table 3.

## ACQUIRED ICHTHYOSIS

All late-onset ichthyosis should be enquired or investigated for an underlying cause as these are usually acquired cases. Various causes of acquired ichthyoses have been presented in table 4. Management of acquired ichthyosis is elimination of the underlying cause and most of the cases are reversible.

## COMPLICATIONS

Known common complications are ectropion leading to epiphora, exposure keratitis, corneal opacity, and eclabium; difficulty in feeding of neonates and infants; shedding of hair, nail and scarring alopecia, bacterial colonization and systemic infections, autoamputation of digits; vitamin D deficiency and rickets, anemia, malnutrition. In erythrodermic stage; fluid and electrolyte imbalance, hypovolemic shock, acute renal shut down, hypothermia, protein loss through scales leading to dependent edema and negative nitrogen balance.

## MANAGEMENT

Initial categorization of congenital ichthyoses to "syndromic" or "nonsyndromic" form is essential. Simple histopathological examination of skin is often inconclusive. EM and genetic mapping are required for confirmation of diagnosis. Various investigations helpful in the diagnosis of nonsyndromic and syndromic ichthyoses have been presented in tables 5 and 6.

### General Measures

A humid and cool environment, daily bath and extended soaking (up to 1 h) ensures softening and easy removal of the scales. Mineral oil may be added in the bath water (liquid paraffin, half

**TABLE 3: Salient features of syndromic forms of congenital ichthyoses**

| Syndrome | Inheritance pattern | Genetic defect | Cutaneous feature | Systemic feature | Distinguishing feature |
|---|---|---|---|---|---|
| Ichthyosis follicularis with alopecia and photophobia syndrome | X-linked recessive | Mutation at *MBTPS2* gene (Xp22.12-p22.11) | • Mild-collodion membrane and atrichia at birth<br>• Later generalized mild to moderate ichthyosis and follicular keratosis | Photophobia, psychomotor retardation, cerebral anomalies, aganglionic megacolon, testicular or renal abnormalities | Follicular ichthyosis, congenital atrichia |
| Conradi–Hünermann–Happle syndrome | • X-linked-dominant<br>• Autosomal dominant form may occur | Mutation at *ARSE* gene (Xp11.23) | Erythroderma at birth. Mild ichthyosis in later life. Follicular atrophoderma, hyper- and hypopigmentation, localized scarring alopecia of scalp | Limb length discrepancies, kyphoscoliosis, congenital dislocation of hip, facial dysplasia, and cataracts | Frequently scales are in swirls and whorls, along lines of Blaschko, unilateral and sectorial cataracts |
| Netherton syndrome | Autosomal recessive | Mutation at *SPINK5* (5q. 32) | Congenital/neonatal erythroderma. Later, polycyclic lesions with double-edged scaling. Atopic features, trichorrhexis invaginata | Asthma, recurrent sinopulmonary infections, bacterial and viral skin infections | • Ichthyosis linearis circumflexa, associated with pruritus<br>• Trichorrhexis invaginata |
| Trichothiodystrophy (IBIDS syndrome) | Autosomal recessive | Mutations at *ERCC2/XPD* gene (19q13.32) | Mild to moderate ichthyosis, may simulate lamellar ichthyosis. Brittle hair | Photosensitivity, growth retardation | Brittle hair, tiger-tail appearance under polarized microscope |
| Sjögren–Larsson syndrome | Autosomal recessive | Mutation at *ALDH3A2* gene (17p11.2) | Congenital ichthyosis, rarely collodion membrane at birth. Variable ichthyosis in later life; scales fine white to large, plate-like (on legs)<br>Verrucous hyperkeratosis on flexures by 1 year of age | Progressive, spastic, diplegia/tetraplegia, speech impairment, and mental retardation | • Ichthyosis associated with pruritus<br>• Spastic diplegia/ tetraplegia |
| Refsum syndrome | Autosomal recessive | Mutation at *PHYH* (10p13) and *PEX7* | Mild ichthyosis in adult life, simulate ichthyosis vulgaris | Cerebellar ataxia, peripheral polyneuropathy, atypical retinitis pigmentosa | Predominant neurological features, adult-onset ichthyosis |
| Mental retardation, enteropathy, deafness, neuropathy, ichthyosis, keratoderma (MEDNIK) syndrome | Autosomal recessive | Homozygous mutation at *AP1S1* gene (7q22.1) | Skin lesions simulating erythrokeratoderma variabilis (EKV) | Diarrhea, deafness, and neuropathy | Life-threatening diarrhea since birth. Transient skin lesions simulating EKV |
| Keratitis-ichthyosis-deafness (KID) syndrome | Sporadic, autosomal dominant/ recessive | Mutation at connexin gene *GJB2*, (13q11.12), or, rarely *GJB6* | • Transient erythroderma at birth. Later, fixed hyperkeratotic plaques, rippled hyperkeratosis, and palmoplantar keratoderma<br>• Scarring alopecia | • Bilateral sensorineural deafness<br>• Keratitis leading to blindness | • Fixed hyperkeratotic plaques<br>• Scarring alopecia involving entire scalp |
| Chanarin–Dorfman syndrome | Autosomal recessive | Mutation at *CGI-58* gene (3p21) | Generalized ichthyosis since birth | Sensorineural deafness, cataract, myopathy, hepato-splenomegaly, growth retardation | • Ichthyosis in combination with hepatosplenomegaly<br>• Lipid vacuoles in peripheral blood smear (Jordan anomaly) |

to one cup during each bath). Emollients and keratolytics should be applied soon after bath.

All patients with ichthyosis require protein supplementation, especially during erythrodermic phase.

## Topical Therapy

The aims of topical therapy in patients with ichthyosis are hydration and softening of skin as well as removal of the scales. Main modalities of topical treatment are emollients (white soft

**TABLE 4: Various causes of acquired ichthyosis**

| | |
|---|---|
| Drugs | • 3-hydroxy-3-methylglutaryl (HMG)-CoA reductase inhibitors<br>• Clofazimine<br>• Allopurinol<br>• Nicotinic acid<br>• Cimetidine<br>• Maprotiline |
| Infections | • Leprosy (Fig. 25)<br>• HIV infection |
| Systemic illness | • Sarcoidosis<br>• Collagen vascular disorder (Systemic lupus erythematosus, dermatomyositis)<br>• Shwachman–Diamond syndrome (pancreatic insufficiency)<br>• Renal failure ± secondary hyperparathyroidism |
| Malignancy | • Hodgkin's lymphoma<br>• Non-Hodgkin's lymphoma<br>• Multiple myeloma<br>• Solid-organ malignancy (breast, lungs, liver, cervix)<br>• Mycosis fungoides<br>• Sarcoma |
| Dietary deficiency | • Protein energy malnutrition<br>• Malabsorption syndromes<br>• Essential fatty acid deficiency |
| Endocrine disorders | Hypo- and hyperthyroidism |
| Miscellaneous causes | • Post-bone marrow transplant<br>• Haber's syndrome<br>• Eosinophilic fasciitis |

HIV, human immunodeficiency virus.

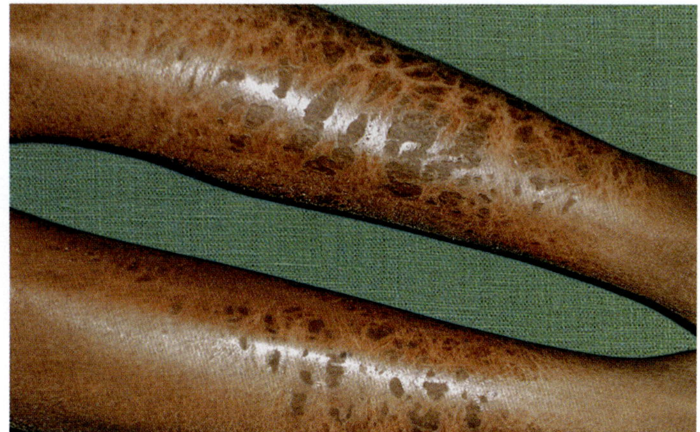

**FIG. 25:** Acquired ichthyosis in a patient with lepromatous leprosy. The dark brown color of the scales is due to clofazimine intake.

paraffin, liquid paraffin), humectants [propylene glycol (50%), urea cream (20–40%), glycerin], keratolytics [glycolic acid (5–10%), lactic acid (12%), beta-OH acid, salicylic acid (2–6%)], and topical retinoids (tretinoin 0.025–0.1%, adapalene 0.1%, tazarotene 0.5–0.1%).

Topical retinoids can be used for milder ichthyosis. Ectropion associated with severe ichthyosis respond rapidly to daily application of tazarotene and the effect is persistent.

### Systemic Therapy

Oral retinoids are the mainstay of maintenance therapy. These drugs improve ichthyotic skin significantly, but their use in these patients is associated with some difficulties. These patients require life-long therapy, with risk of the usual drug-related side effects and cannot be advised in female patients of child-bearing age. Retinoids cause cutaneous and mucosal dryness, which may be additive to the symptoms of ichthyosis. Moreover, the drug affects growth of long bones causing stunted growth in children, making long-term therapy difficult.

Scaling, ability to sweat, ectropion, and constriction bands improve within 2 weeks to 1 month of starting treatment and complete clearance may be achieved, but recurrence is common as soon as the therapy is stopped. Both monoaromatic and polyaromatic retinoids can be used in patients with ichthyosis; isotretinoin (0.5–1 mg/kg) or acitretin (0.5 mg/kg) may be used to treat ichthyosis, with comparable risk: benefit ratio. High dose of systemic retinoid increases the blistering in EI, and gradual dose-escalation is recommended. Oral alitretinoin (30 mg/day) may also be used.

## MANAGEMENT OF ICHTHYOSIFORM SYNDROMES

This group of patients require multispecialty approach, as they have variable systemic involvement. Milder cases are amenable to topical therapy.

### Dietary Modification

Some patients with SLS may improve with reduced dietary fat (<30% of total calorie) and increased essential fatty acids.

Patients with Refsum disease should take a diet totally free of green vegetables (contains phytanic acid) and animal fat (phytol). Strict, life-long, dietary restriction with total dietary intake of phytanic acid less than 5 mg/day (normal 50 mg /day) is essential. Ichthyosis and neurological symptoms generally improve with variable effect on visual and hearing impairment. Rapid wasting may mobilize tissue phytanic acid to blood and must be avoided in these patients. Reappearance of ichthyosis in these patients is a marker of rise in serum phytanic acid.

In patients with neutral lipid storage disease, long-chain fatty acids should be restricted and medium-chain fatty acids may be given.

### Topical Therapy

The basic principle for topical therapy for ichthyoses remains same for these patients except in few circumstances.

### Systemic Therapy

Patients with NS may show aggravation of atopic features after oral retinoids and should better be avoided. Patients with KID syndrome responds variably to retinoids and there is risk of exacerbation of corneal neovascularization. Oral alitretinoin has also been used successfully in these patients.

In SLS, the intractable and persistent pruritus may be due to the elevated level of leukotriene B4. Severe pruritus in SLS can be managed with antihistamines, 5-lipoxygenase inhibitor zileuton, or leukotriene antagonist montelukast.

## MANAGEMENT OF EMERGENCY SITUATION

Collodion baby and HI are important causes of neonatal dermatological emergency. These patients present at birth with ectropion, eclabium, rigid, fixed position of the limbs, feeding difficulty, and respiratory distress due to restricted chest movement. These babies must be nursed in intensive care unit in a high humidity incubator.

**TABLE 5: Investigations helpful in diagnosis of non-syndromic ichthyoses**

| Disorder | Light microscopy | Electron microscopy | Biochemical estimation | Others |
|---|---|---|---|---|
| Ichthyosis vulgaris | Compact orthohyperkeratosis and absence of granular layer | Fragmented, small or rudimentary keratohyaline granules | – | Antigen mapping demonstrates reduced or negative filaggrin staining |
| Recessive X-linked ichthyosis | Nonspecific with normal or prominent granular layer | Numerous normal or smaller keratohyaline granules. Prominent corneal melanosomes and desmosomes are more persistent than normal | *Serum lipoprotein electrophoresis*:<br>• Raised serum cholesterol sulfate, demonstrable as fast band<br>• Absent steroid sulfatase activity in leukocytes or skin fibroblasts<br>• Low level of maternal serum and urinary estriol levels (prenatal diagnosis) | *Slit-lamp examination*: Corneal opacities. |
| Harlequin ichthyosis | Marked, compact orthohyperkeratosis, extending to dilated hair follicles, and pilosebaceous unit | Vesicular lamellar body ghosts and sparsely secreted lamellar structures in stratum corneum | – | • Prenatal diagnosis by electron microscopy of corneocytes collected through amniocentesis<br>• *Maternal ultrasonography*: Amniotic fluid debris is suggestive |
| Lamellar ichthyosis | Marked orthohyperkeratosis, mild acanthosis and regular papillomatosis | Elongated cholesterol clefts, crystals and lipid droplets in stratum corneum. Attenuated or absent cornified cell envelope | – | – |
| Congenital ichthyosiform erythroderma | Compact hyperkeratosis, mild parakeratosis and acanthosis, normal or prominent granular layer, broad rete ridges | Retained, abnormal lamellar bodies in the corneocytes resulting in lipid droplets in the stratum corneum. Disorganization of intercellular lipid lamellae | – | – |
| Epidermolytic ichthyosis (EI) | Marked hyperkeratosis and acanthosis. Perinuclear vacuoles and large clumps of keratohyaline granules in granular and upper spinous layer cells. Suprabasal splits present | Perinuclear clumping of tonofilaments in suprabasal cells and desmosomal dissolution with cleft formation | – | – |
| Superficial epidermolytic ichthyosis | Features are similar to classic EI, but more superficial | Cytolysis of granular cells without keratin clumping | – | – |
| Ichyhyosis Curth-Macklin | Vacuolated and binucleate cells in the upper epidermis | Granular and upper spinous cell layers show perinuclear tonofilament shells forming cytoplasmic compartments, surrounded by a ribosome-rich region | – | – |

**TABLE 6: Investigations helpful in diagnosis of syndromic ichthyoses**

| Disorder | Light microscopy | Electron microscopy | Biochemical estimation | Others |
|---|---|---|---|---|
| Ichthyosis follicularis with alopecia and photophobia syndrome | • Orthohyperkeratosis with follicular plugging, normal granular layer. Rete ridges are effaced<br>• Numerous atrophic hair follicles and absent sebaceous glands. Thinned dermis | No specific finding | – | – |
| Conradi–Hünermann–Happle Syndrome | Similar to IV. Older lesions, prominent perifollicular atrophy, epidermal calcification and needle-like inclusions in granular cells | Persistent desmosomes in stratum corneum, abnormal mitochondria, vacuolated lamellar bodies. | Serum gas chromatography-mass spectrometry: High 8-dehydrocholesterol and cholesterol levels | Radiology: Punctate calcification of the epiphysis of the long bones |
| Netherton syndrome | • *Skin*: Mild hyperkeratosis, parakeratosis and reduced or absent granular layer at borders of lesions<br>• Plucked scalp or eyebrow hairs: Trichorrhexis nodosa or invaginata | • Suprabasal keratinocytes with inclusion bodies containing fine granular material. Decreased tonofilament-keratohyaline structures, desmosomes and abnormal lamellar bodies<br>• Clearly demonstrates the hair anomalies | – | High serum IgE level |
| Trichothiodystrophy or IBIDS syndrome | • *Skin*: Similar to congenital ichthyosiform erythroderma; Hyperkeratosis, mild parakeratosis and acanthosis, normal or prominent granular layer<br>• *Plucked hair*: Undulating contour of hair shaft with wavy melanin | Perinuclear vacuoles and tonofilament abnormalities | – | • *Polarized microscopy*: Banded appearance (tiger-tail) of hair shaft<br>• Ultraviolet sensitivity in cultured fibroblasts |
| Sjögren–Larsson syndrome | Orthohyperkeratosis, acanthosis and papillomatosis. Normal or increased granular layer | Atypical membranous structures in granular and upper spinous layers. Numerous, large lamellar bodies | – | • *Immunohistochemistry on skin and jejunal mucosa*: negative staining for alcohol dehydrogenase; diagnostic<br>• Ophthalmoscopy<br>• Perifoveal glistening white dots in retina are a pathognomonic feature<br>• Estimation of FALDH activity in cultured fibroblasts from skin biopsy specimen |
| Refsum syndrome | Similar to IV; in addition, there are lipid-containing vacuoles in basal and suprabasal keratinocytes | Enlarged and disorganized mitochondria | Cerebrospinal fluid; analysis: elevated protein level | • Liquid gas chromatography of plasma: very high level of phytanic acid<br>• Cultured fibroblasts from skin biopsy<br>• Phytanic acid oxidase activity is greatly reduced<br>• *Prenatal diagnosis*: Phytanic acid oxidation assay in cell-culture (chorionic villus biopsy or amniocentesis) |

*Continued*

*Continued*

| Disorder | Light microscopy | Electron microscopy | Biochemical estimation | Others |
|---|---|---|---|---|
| Keratitis-ichthyosis-deafness syndrome | Marked orthohyperkeratosis, acanthosis, focal parakeratosis and papillomatosis | Irregular clumps of tonofilaments in lower epidermis, located in perinuclear area in granular cells. Indented keratinocyte nuclei | – | – |
| Chanarin–Dorfman syndrome | • Oil red O or Sudan black staining of fresh, frozen specimen of skin: Cytoplasmic lipid droplets in epidermal and dermal cells, around appendages<br>• Lipid vacuoles are also seen in muscle fibers, bone marrow and other viscera | Globular electron-lucent inclusion bodies present in lamellar bodies and intercellular lipid lamellae are disrupted | – | *Freshly prepared peripheral blood smear*:Numerous lipid-vacuoles (Jordan anomaly) |

IV, ichthyosis vulgaris; FALDH, fatty aldehyde dehydrogenase.

**TABLE 7: Pathogenesis-based targeted therapy in various congenital ichthyosis and syndromic ichthyosis**

| Disorder | Defect | Accumulated substance | Deficient substance | Proposed therapy (theoretical) |
|---|---|---|---|---|
| Sjogren-Larsson syndrome | Disorder of fatty acid (FA) metabolism, deficient enzyme FALDH | Fatty aldehyde | Free fatty acids (FFA) | Topical FFAs and/or farnesoic acid + acetyl-CoA carboxylase (ACC) or fatty acid synthase (FAS) inhibitor |
| Neutral lipid storage disease with ichthyosis | Triacylglycerol and sphingolipid metabolism | Triacylglycerol | Acyl ceramide | Topical acyl ceramide |
| Refsum disease | Disorder of FA metabolism (defect in plant-derived, branched fatty acids utilization) | Phytanic acid from dietary source | Acyl ceramide | FFA or acyl ceramide with or without a topical inhibitor of diacylglycerol or triacylglycerol synthesis |
| Type II Gaucher disease | Loss-of-function mutations in β-glucocerebrosidase | Glucosylceramide | Decreased production of ceramide | Glutamylcysteine synthase inhibitor and topical ceramide |
| Some variants of autosomal recessive congenital ichthyosis | Epidermal lipoxygenase-3 (*eLOX3*) or 12R-lipoxygenase (*12R-LOX*) mutation | – | – | Topical ω-OH-ceramide |
| Harlequin ichthyosis | ATP-binding cassette subfamily A member 12 (*ABCA12*) missense mutations | – | – | Topical glucosylceramide |

FALDH, fatty aldehyde dehydrogenase; ATP, adenosine triphosphate.

*Source*: Reproduced with permission from Inamadar AC, Palit A. Congenital ichthyosis: insight into management. What's new in Dermatology? 2013;75:2-12.

## RECENT ADVANCES AND FUTURE DIRECTIONS IN THE THERAPY OF ICHTHYOSIS

### Retinoic Acid Metabolism Blocking Agents

Liarozole and rambazole (imidazole derivative) are the members of this group of drugs and they inhibit the metabolism of endogenous retinoids.

### Pathogenesis-based Targeted Therapy

Some of the proposed pathogenesis-based therapeutic modalities in various ichthyosis have been presented in table 7.

## GENE-BASED THERAPY

The "replacement technique" is usually adopted in ichthyoses with specific mutations. Gene therapy has been attempted in RXLI, LI, and NS.

## SUGGESTED READINGS

1. Akiyama M, Sawamura D, Shimizu H. The clinical spectrum of nonbullous congenital ichthyosiform erythroderma and lamellar ichthyosis. Clin Exp Dermatol. 2003;28:235-40.
2. Akiyama M. FLG mutations in ichthyosis vulgaris and atopic eczema: spectrum of mutations and population genetics. Br J Dermatol. 2010;162:472-7.
3. Boeshans KM, Mueser TC, Ahvazi B. A three-dimensional model of the human transglutaminase 1: insights into the understanding of lamellar ichthyosis. J Mol Model. 2007;13:233-66.

4. Braverman N. Conradi-Hunnermann syndrome. NORD Guide To Rare Disorders. Philadelphia: Lippincott, Williams & Wilkins; 2003. pp. 173-4.
5. Craiglow BG, Choate KA, Milstone LM. Topical tazarotene in the treatment of ectropion in ichthyosis. JAMA Dermatol. 2013;149:598-600.
6. Digiovanna JJ, Mauro T, Milstone LM, et al. Systemic retinoids in the management of ichthyoses and related skin types. Dermatol Ther. 2013;26:26-38.
7. Elias PM, Crumrine D, Paller A, et al. Pathogenesis of the cutaneous phenotype in inherited disorders of cholesterol metabolism. Dermatoendocrinol. 2011;3:100-6.
8. Elias PM, Williams ML, Feingold KR. Abnormal barrier function in the pathogenesis of ichthyosis: therapeutic implications for lipid metabolic disorders. Clin Dermatol. 2012;30:311-22.
9. Elias PM, Williams ML, Holleran WM, et al. Pathogenesis of permeability barrier abnormalities in the ichthyoses: inherited disorders of lipid metabolism. J Lipid Res. 2008;49:697-714.
10. Fleckman P, Newell BD, van Steensel MA, et al. Topical treatment of ichthyosis. Dermatol Ther. 2013;26:18-25.
11. Fontao L, Laffitte E, Briot A, et al. Infliximab infusions for Netherton syndrome: sustained clinical improvement correlates with a reduction of thymic stromal lymphopoietin levels in the skin. J Invest Dermatol. 2011;131:1947-50.
12. Gordon N. Sjögren-Larsson syndrome. Dev Med Child Neurol. 2007;49:152-4.
13. Gånemo A, Sommerlund M, Vahlquist A. Oral alitretinoin in congenital ichthyosis: a pilot study shows variable effects and a risk of central hypothyroidism. Acta Derm Venereol. 2012;92:256-7.
14. High WA, Miller MD. Localized epidermolytic hyperkeratosis of the female genitalia: a case report and review of an under appreciated disorder of women. Med Gen Med. 2005;7:33.
15. Inamadar AC, Palit A. Congenital ichthyosis: insight into management. What's new in Dermatology? 2013;75:2-12.
16. Inamadar AC, Ragunatha S. Inherited ichthyosis and other hereditary disorders of keratinization. In: Inamadar AC, Palit A, Ragunatha S (Eds). Textbook of Pediatric Dermatology, 2nd edition. New Delhi: Jaypee Brothers Medical Publishers Pvt Ltd; 2014. pp. 89-111.
17. Kathuria S, Arora S, Ramesh V. Sjogren-Larsson syndrome: Importance of early diagnosis and aggressive physiotherapy. Dermatology Online J. 2012;18(9):11.
18. Merino De Paaz N, Rodgriguez-Martin M, Contreras-Ferrer P, et al. Topical treatment of CHILD nevus and Sjögren-Larsson Syndrome with combined lovastatin and cholesterol. Eur J Dermatol. 2011;21:1026-7.
19. Oji V, Tadini G, Akiyama M, et al. Revised nomenclature and classification of inherited ichthyoses: results of the First Ichthyosis Consensus Conference in Sorèze 2009. J Am Acad Dermatol. 2010;63:607-41.
20. Oji V, Traupe H. Ichthyosis: clinical manifestations and practical treatment options. Am J Clin Dermatol. 2009;10:351-64.
21. Palit A, Inamadar AC. Genodermatoses. In: Inamadar AC, Palit A, Ragunatha S (Eds). Textbook of Pediatric Dermatology, 2nd edition. New Delhi: Jaypee Brothers Medical Publishers Pvt Ltd; 2014. pp. 28-88.
22. Paller AS, Rodgriguez-Martin M, Van Steensel M, et al. SID 2011 Annual Meeting. Phoenix AZ: 2011. Pathogenesis (Pathway)-based therapy and genetic basis for lateralization in CHILD syndrome.
23. Pirgon O, Aidyn K, Atabek ME. Proton magnetic resonance spectroscopy findings and clinical effects of montelukast in a case with Sjogren-Larsson syndrome. J Chil Neurol. 2006;21:1092-5.
24. Prado R, Ellis LZ, Gamble R, et al. Collodion baby: an update with a focus on practical management. J Am Acad Dermatol. 2012;67:1362-74.
25. Rajpopat S, Moss C, Mellerio J, et al. Harlequin ichthyosis: a review of clinical and molecular findings in 45 cases. Arch Dermatol. 2011;147:681-6.
26. Richard G, Choate K, Milstone L, et al. Management of ichthyosis and related conditions gene-based diagnosis and emerging gene-based therapy. Dermatol Ther. 2013;26:55-68.
27. Rizzo WB. Sjögren-Larsson syndrome: molecular genetics and biochemical pathogenesis of fatty aldehyde dehydrogenase deficiency. Mol Genet Metab. 2007;90:1-9.
28. Rossi G, Mesia D. Management of Harlequin ichthyosis in low-income countries. Ann Trop Paediatr. 2011;31:247-9.
29. Sahoo B, Handa S, Kaur I, et al. KID syndrome: response to acitretin. J Dermatol. 2002;29:499-502.
30. Sakai K, Akiyama M, Yanagi T, et al. An Indian family with Sjögren-Larsson syndrome caused by a novel ALDH3A2 mutation. Int J Dermatol. 2010;49:1031-3.
31. Smith FJ, Irvine AD, Terron-Kwiatkowski A, et al. Loss-of-function mutations in the gene encoding filaggrin cause ichthyosis vulgaris. Nat Genet. 2006;38:337-42.
32. Werchau S, Toberer F, Enk A, et al. Keratitis-Ichthyosis-Deafness syndrome: response to alitretinoin and review of literature. Arch Dermatol. 2011;147:993-5.
33. Willemsen MA, Lutt MA, Steijlen PM, et al. Clinical and biochemical effects of zileuton in patients with Sjogren-Larsson syndrome. Eur J Pediatr. 2001;160:711-7.
34. Zhang X, He Y, Zhou H, et al. Severe ichthyosis-related disorders in children: response to acitretin. J Dermatolog Treat. 2007;18:118-22.

# 33 CHAPTER Palmoplantar Keratoderma

*Nilendu Sarma, Dipti Das*

## INTRODUCTION

Palmoplantar keratodermas (PPK) are a group of keratinization disorders characterized by hyperkeratotic thickening of palms and soles. It can be classified as genetic or hereditary and acquired.

There is no universally acceptable classification of hereditary PPK. Most acceptable classification is according to the pattern of hyperkeratotic lesions observed clinically and classified as diffuse, focal, striate, spiny, marginal, and punctuate with some expected overlap (Table 1). Pattern of involvement is the primary clinical criteria for classification of PPK. Generally, diseases can be grouped into different category based on the pattern. However, practical aspects should not be overlooked. Multiple focal keratoderma may sometimes merge in severe cases to appear as diffuse keratoderma. This is seen mostly in sole. Palmar lesions may still show focal keratoderma.

There are many other clinical features that need attention while evaluating a case of PPK. Keratoderma may develop into a constricting band (ainhum) that may lead to autoamputation of digits. This is a striking feature and is considered the sign of "mutilating keratoderma." Presence of this helps to narrow down the differential diagnosis of PPK (Box 1).

**TABLE 1: Important diseases, genetic defect, and inheritance pattern in major clinical subtypes of hereditary palmoplantar keratodermas**

| Disease | Inheritance | Mutation |
|---|---|---|
| **Diffuse palmoplantar keratodermas** | | |
| EPPK (Voerner keratoderma) | AD | KRT9 (keratin 9), rarely KRT1 (keratin 1) |
| Mal de Meleda | AR | SLURP1 (secreted Ly-6/uPAR-related protein 1) |
| NEPPK (Nagashima type) | AR | SERPINB7 (serine protease) |
| NEPPK (Greither disease) | AD | K1 (keratin 1) |
| NEPPK (Bothnia type) | AD | AQP5 (aquaporin) |
| Vohwinkel syndrome | AD | GJB2 (connexin 26) |
| Camisa syndrome/Loricrin keratoderma (ichthyosiform variant of Vohwinkel syndrome) | AD | LOR (loricrin) |
| Papillon–Lefèvre syndrome | AR | CTSC (cathepsin C) |
| Clouston syndrome | AD | GJB6 (connexin 30) |
| Howel–Evans syndrome | AD | RHBDF2 (rhomboid protease family) |
| Huriez syndrome | AD | Unknown |
| Olmsted syndrome | AD/AR/XLR | TRPV3 (transient receptor potential vanilloid 3)<br>MBTPS2 (membrane-bound transcription factor protease, site 2) |
| Keratitis–ichthyosis–deafness syndrome | AD | GJB2 (connexin 26 and Connexin 30) |
| Focal palmoplantar keratodermas | | |
| Richner–Hanhart syndrome | AR | Tyrosine aminotransferase |
| Howel–Evans' syndrome | AD | RHBDF2 (rhomboid protease family) |
| Focal keratoderma with oral leukokeratosis | AD | K16 (keratin 16) |

*Continued*

*Continued*

| Disease | Inheritance | Mutation |
|---|---|---|
| Pachyonychia congenita | AD | K6A/6B/6C/16/17 |
| Punctate palmoplantar keratodermas | | |
| Punctate keratoderma of Brauer-Buschke-Fischer | AD | AAGAB (alpha-and gamma-adaptin binding protein) |
| Punctate keratoderma of palmar creases | AD | – |
| Marginal papular keratoderma/acrokeratoelastoidosis of Costa | AD | – |
| **Striate keratoderma** | | |
| SPPK 1–3 types | AD | Desmoglein 1, desmoplakin, KRT1 |
| Naxos syndrome | AR (or AD) | Plakoglobin |
| Carvajal–Huerta syndrome | AR (or AD) | Desmoplakin |

EPPK, epidermolytic palmoplantar keratoderma conditions; NEPPK, nonepidermolytic palmoplantar keratoderma; SPPK, striate palmoplantar keratoderma.

**BOX 1 Mutilating palmoplantar keratodermas**

- Vohwinkel syndrome
- Loricrin keratoderma
- Mal de Meleda (often pseudoainhum)
- NEPPK of Sybert type

NEPPK, nonepidermolytic palmoplantar keratoderma.

**BOX 2 Transgradient keratoderma**

- Nonepidermolytic keratoderma
- Most of the syndromic keratoderma
- Papillon–Lefèvre syndrome
- Huriez syndrome

Ainhum is found in Vohwinkel syndrome and loricrin keratoderma. The later has a highly characteristic presentation of honeycomb pattern of keratoderma leading to diffuse keratoderma with transgrediens. Transgrediens is another conspicuous presentation defined as involvement of adjoining skin beyond palms and soles like dorsum, ankle, and wrist. There are few conditions that show presence of transgrediens (Box 2). Character of the lesion at the margin also helps differentiate diseases. Loricrin keratoderma has a diffuse edge, whereas Vohwinkel keratoderma has sharper margin often having a highly characteristic “star-fish” appearance.

Histological presence of epidermolysis is now used to classify diffuse hereditary PPK into two major subtypes—epidermolytic and nonepidermolytic PPK. Recent progress in the genetic analysis has helped identify multiple conditions under each of these types.

Palmoplantar keratodermas in hereditary conditions may be the sole manifestation (primary) or it may be an associated finding in other conditions like ichthyosis (ichthyosis vulgaris, epidermolytic ichthyosis), ectodermal dysplasia, erythrokeratoderma, and pachyonychia congenita. It may also be a part of a syndrome or even represent a paraneoplastic manifestation (Table 2).

## PATHOGENESIS

Although many things are still unknown, our knowledge on the genetic aspect of hereditary PPK has advanced greatly in recent years. Many of these conditions are caused by single gene mutation (Table 1).

**TABLE 2: List of conditions in syndromic palmoplantar keratodermas**

| | |
|---|---|
| Diffuse PPK: Syndromic | Vohwinkel syndrome |
| | Olmsted syndrome |
| | Huriez syndrome |
| | Papillon–Lefevre syndrome |
| | Haim–Munk syndrome |
| | Clouston syndrome |
| Focal PPK: Syndromic | Howel–Evans syndrome |
| | Striate keratoderma of Brunauer–Fuhs–Siemens |
| | Focal keratoderma with oral leukokeratosis |
| | Carvajal syndrome |

PPK, palmoplantar keratodermas.

## EPIDERMOLYTIC PALMOPLANTAR KERATODERMA

*Synonym:* Vörner's keratoderma, Voerner–Unna–Thost disease.

### Pathogenesis

The disease is autosomal dominantly inherited. It is caused by mutations in the keratin 9 (*KRT9*) gene, which is expressed exclusively in the suprabasal keratinocytes of the palmoplantar epidermis or rarely in *KRT1* gene which is present even beyond palm and soles, and is primarily involved epidermolytic ichthyosis.

### Clinical Features

Palmoplantar keratoderma of Vörner represents the most frequent type of hereditary PPK. The disease manifests in the early months of life. Clinically, it is characterized by diffuse yellowish thickening of the palm and sole. There is no transgradiens and the margin is sharp, sometimes with an erythematous border. Knuckle pads and digital mutilation may be seen rarely. Blistering is not common but may be occasionally present in early life. Epidermolytic ichthyosis may present clinically with similar type

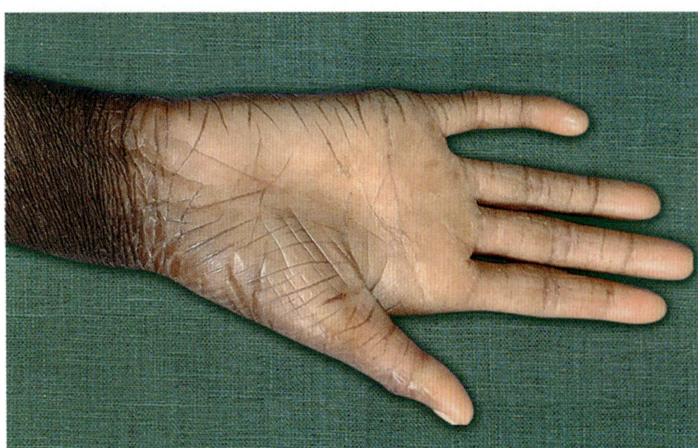

FIG. 1: Palmoplantar hyperkeratosis in epidermolytic ichthyosis.

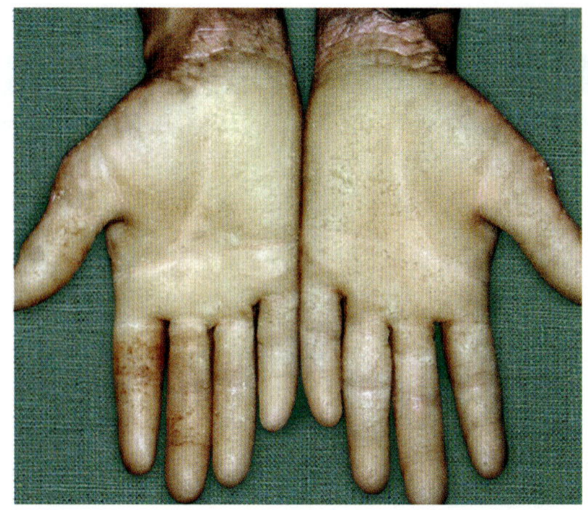

FIG. 2: Waxy yellowish diffuse hyperkeratosis with transgradiens in Mal de Meleda.

**BOX 3 Different nonepidermolytic palmoplantar keratoderma conditions**

- NEPPK—Nagashima type
- NEPPK—Bothnia type
- NEPPK—Kimonis type
- Mal de Meleda
- NEPPK—Sybert type

NEPPK, nonepidermolytic palmoplantar keratoderma.

of palmoplantar hyperkeratosis but is distinguished with more extensive disease, typically the flexures (Fig. 1).

### Diagnosis

Histopathology is very specific which shows epidermolytic hyperkeratosis. Genetic mutation analysis shows *KRT9*, rarely *KRT1* mutation.

## NONEPIDERMOLYTIC PALMOPLANTAR KERATODERMA

Absence of epidermolysis in the superficial epidermis is the key diagnostic and differentiating features of NEPPK. Advancement in genetics has helped identify many conditions fulfil the definition of NEPPK (Box 3).

### Mal de Meleda

#### Pathogenesis

Mutation occurs in the *ARS* gene, encoding *SLURP-1* (secreted lymphocyte antigen-6/urokinase-type plasminogen activator receptor-related protein-1) and inheritance is autosomal recessive.

#### Clinical Features

There is diffuse waxy transgradient keratoderma, psoriasiform plaques on knees, elbows, and hyperhidrosis (Fig. 2). Hyperhidrosis leads to maceration, malodor, and fungal superinfection. Angular cheilitis is also common (Fig. 3).

Palmoplantar keratoderma of the Gamborg-Nielsen type is caused by mutations in the *SLURP1* gene and represents a variant of Mal de Meleda.

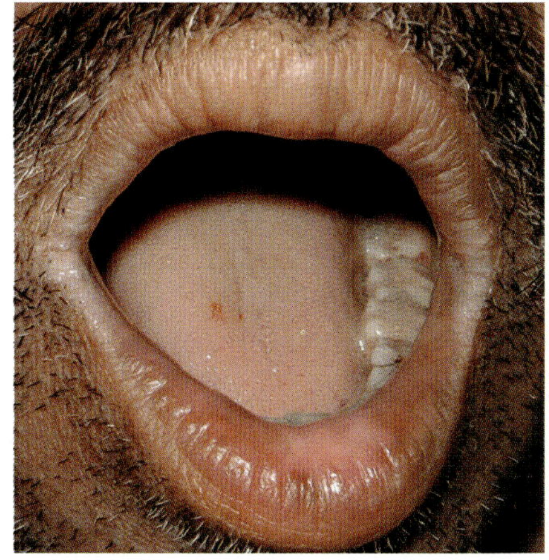

FIG. 3: Angular stomatitis in Mal de Meleda.

### Nonepidermolytic Palmoplantar Keratoderma—Nagashima Type

This was initially considered a milder form of Mal de Meleda keratoderma, which presents with the diffuse autosomal-recessive PPK. However, now it is known that genetics of these two conditions differ. This is reported from Japanese and Chinese families.

#### Pathogenesis

The disease is autosomal recessively inherited and caused by mutations in *SERPINB7*, a member of the serine protease inhibitor superfamily.

#### Clinical Features

This newly described type is characterized by diffuse nonepidermolytic transgradient palmoplantar keratoderma that is well-demarcated reddish, diffuse, and mild.

### Nonepidermolytic Palmoplantar Keratoderma—Bothnia Type

Bothnian-type PPK is similar to Nagashima type showing whitish changes in the palms and soles after water but caused by aquaporin (*AQP5*) mutations and autosomal dominant inheritance.

## Nonepidermolytic Palmoplantar Keratoderma—Greither Disease

*Synonym:* Transgrediens et progrediens palmoplantar keratoderma.

### Pathogenesis

Mutation is in *KRT1* gene and the disease is autosomal dominantly inherited.

### Clinical Features

It shows diffuse transgradient palmoplantar keratoderma and hyperhidrosis. Hyperkeratotic plaques may occur on the elbows and knees.

## Vohwinkel Syndrome

*Synonym*: Keratoderma hereditarium mutilans.

### Pathogenesis

This autosomal dominantly inherited. Vohwinkel syndrome occurs due to mutations in *GJB2*.

### Clinical Features

This type is characterized by triad of mutilating PPK, pseudoainhum, and starfish keratosis on knuckles, elbows, wrists, and knees. Palmoplantar keratoderma is diffuse, transgradient, and honeycomb patterned. Focal variant of Vohwinkel syndrome is also reported. Pseudoainhum or constricting band on digits particularly involves fifth finger and may lead to autoamputation. Other associations described are alopecia, spastic paraplegia, myopathy, nail changes, mental retardation, and seizures. There is associated with sensorineural hearing loss.

### Diagnosis

Histopathology shows hyperkeratosis, parakeratosis, acanthosis, and hypergranulosis. Genetic mutation analysis shows *GJB2* gene mutation.

## Loricrin Keratoderma

*Synonym:* Camisa syndrome.

### Pathogenesis

This is caused by mutation in loricrin gene (*LOR*) but the mutations are heterogeneous. Loricirin is an important component protein of the cornified cell envelope. This is synthesized in the upper granular layer develops late in the differentiation of keratinocytes. Thus, defect in loricrin may result in different keratinization disorders like progressive symmetric erythrokeratoderma, loricrin keratoderma, and congenital ichthyosiform erythroderma. Ultrastructural investigation of the affected skin reveals intranuclear inclusions within the granular layer and these contain loricrin.

### Clinical Features

Dominantly inherited. Usually presents with collodion baby at birth and later manifests as generalized ichthyosis and mild diffuse PPK. Characteristically, PPK has a honeycomb pattern. Similar to Vohwinkel keratoderma, often, ainhum (pseudoainhum) develops. Loricrin keratoderma is frequently considered a milder variant of Vohwinkel keratoderma. Other features are hyperkeratosis on the knuckles (knuckle pad) and dorsum. This is important to know that PPK may be mild and ichthyosis is present in almost all. Thus, some suggest it to be called as loricrin ichthyosis rather the loricrin keratoderma.

Pseudoainhum may be managed surgically. Treatment is supportive. Retinoids may be tried.

## Olmsted Syndrome

*Synonym:* Mutilating palmoplantar keratoderma with periorificial keratotic plaques.

### Pathogenesis

Autosomal dominant, autosomal recessive, and X-linked recessive inheritance are described. Transient receptor potential vanilloid 3 (*TRPV3*) mutation is responsible for autosomal dominant but also recessive OS, and membrane-bound transcription factor protease, site 2 (*MBTPS2*) mutation is responsible for recessive X-linked OS.

### Clinical Features

The disease starts at birth or early infancy and slowly progressive. It is characterized by bilateral mutilating palmoplantar keratoderma and periorificial keratotic plaques. Keratoderma is transgradient, painful, and disabling. Periorificial keratotic plaques involve mouth, nose, eyes, ears, navel, and anus. Association of erythromelalgia, hair abnormality, nail abnormality, oral leukokeratosis, and abnormal dentition are reported.

### Diagnosis

Histopathological findings are nonspecific which shows orthohyperkeratosis, focal parakeratosis, hypergranulosis, acanthosis, and inflammatory infiltration in upper dermis. Molecular genetics analysis reveals *TRPV3/MBTPS2* mutation.

## Papillon–Lefèvre Syndrome

### Pathogenesis

The disease is inherited as an autosomal recessive disorder with mutation in cathepsin C (*CTSC*) gene.

### Clinical Features

It is characterized by PPK with periodontitis and psoriasiform plaques on knees and elbows. (Fig. 4). Periodontitis leads

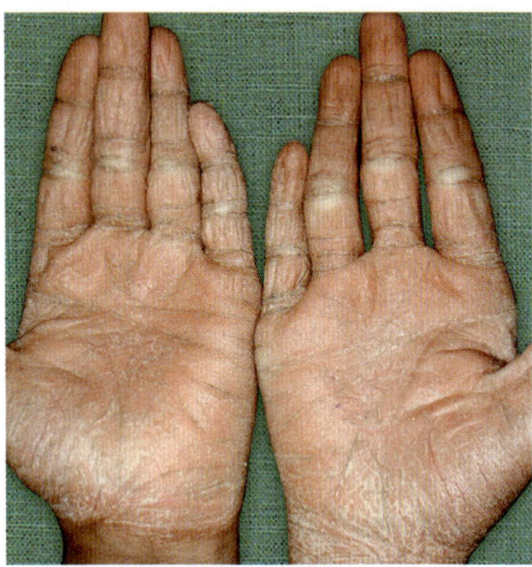

FIG. 4: Psoriasiform hyperkeratosis of palms in Papillon–Lefèvre syndrome.

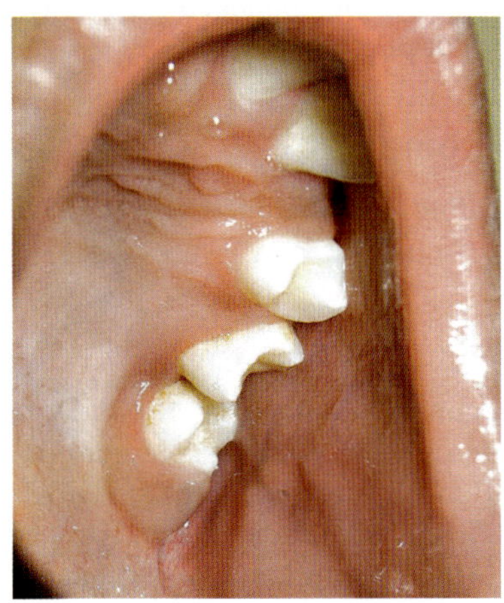

FIG. 5: Loss of teeth due to significant loss of alveolar bone.

to premature loss of primary and permanent teeth due to generalized atrophy of the alveolar ridges along with destruction of the alveolar bone (Fig. 5). There is increased susceptibility to pyogenic skin infection. Consanguinity is a risk factor in the development of Papillon-Lefèvre syndrome.

### Diagnosis

Histopathology shows hyperkeratosis with occasional parakeratotic patches, acanthosis, and slight perivascular infiltrates. Genetic mutation analysis shows *CTSC* gene mutation.

## Huriez Syndrome

*Synonym:* Sclerotylosis.

### Pathogenesis

The disease is autosomal dominantly inherited. The causative gene maps to chromosome 4q23, but has not been identified.

### Clinical Features

It is characterized by the triad of palmoplantar keratoderma, congenital scleroatrophy of the distal extremities, and hypoplastic nails. There is pseudosclerodermatous appearance of the hands and digits. There is high risk for the development of aggressive squamous cell carcinoma in the affected skin.

## Richner–Hanhart Syndrome

*Synonym:* Tyrosinaemia type II or oculocutaneous tyrosinemia.

### Pathogenesis

This is a rare autosomal recessively inherited disorder of amino acid metabolism caused by deficiency of hepatic tyrosine aminotransferase, resulting in elevated plasma and urinary tyrosine concentrations.

### Clinical Features

It is characterized by classical triad of focal palmoplantar keratoderma, ocular changes, and mental retardation. Painful, circumscribed callosities develop on the pressure points of the palm and sole. Ocular changes include photophobia, and corneal erosions. The corneal erosions may progress to corneal ulceration and glaucoma.

### Diagnosis

Histology of the palmoplantar lesions may be helpful diagnostically in demonstrating eosinophilic cytoplasmic inclusions.

## Howel–Evans Syndrome

*Synonym:* Tylosis palmoplantaris with esophageal cancer.

### Pathogenesis

It is an autosomal dominant disorder having mutation in rhomboid protease family (*RHBDF2*) gene.

### Clinical Features

Lesions start during childhood and are more evident in areas of pressure. This rare hereditary disease is characterized by palmoplantar keratoses, squamous cell carcinoma of the esophagus, oral leukoplakia, and keratosis pilaris.

## Striate Keratoderma or Brunauer–Fuhs–Siemens Syndrome

### Pathogenesis

This autosomal dominant genetic disorder has been linked to mutations in desmoglein 1, desmoplakin, and keratin 1.

### Clinical Features

It presents with linear hyperkeratosis on the palms and fingers and focal plaques on the plantar aspects of the feet. Disease usually manifests in early childhood but may be delayed.

### Diagnosis

Histopathologic features include hyperkeratosis, hypergranulosis, and acanthosis with no epidermolysis.

## Pachyonychia Congenita

It is an autosomal-dominant keratin disorder caused by mutations in the keratin genes. Two main subtypes of pachyonychia congenita (PC) have been distinguished—the Jadassohn-Lewandowsky (PC type 1) and Jackson-Lawler syndromes (PC type 2). Recently, such classification is being questioned as there as significant clinical overlap and there is new information available on genetic pathomechanism of the disease.

### Pathogenesis

Four genes are now known to cause the disease. The most common mutated gene is *KRT6A* (41%), followed by *KRT16* (30%), *KRT17* (17%), *KRT6B* (9%) and KRT6C (3%). Pachyonychia congenita has been reclassified into subtypes based on the genes affected like PC-6b, PC-16, PC-17, and PC-U (unknown genes). There is poor genotype-phenotype correlation.

### Clinical Features

Both the types show presence of keratoderma. Pachyonychia congenita type 1 is associated with focal palmoplantar hyperkeratosis, follicular keratosis, and oral leukokeratosis. Pachyonychia congenita type 2 is associated with natal teeth, multiple pilosebaceous cysts, focal palmoplantar keratoderma, follicular keratosis, and hair abnormalities. Plantar keratoderma is much commoner than palmar one. Keratoderma is typically painful that is out of proportion to the keratoderma and disabling. Keratoderma and nail changes are more severe in type 1. Typical nail changes start very early during infancy and are characterized by discoloration, thickening, and dystrophy. Subungual hyperkeratosis is prominently present. Nail changes are important in distinguishing other causes of palmoplantar keratoderma (Fig. 6).

### Treatment

Topical rapamycin has shown encouraging results.

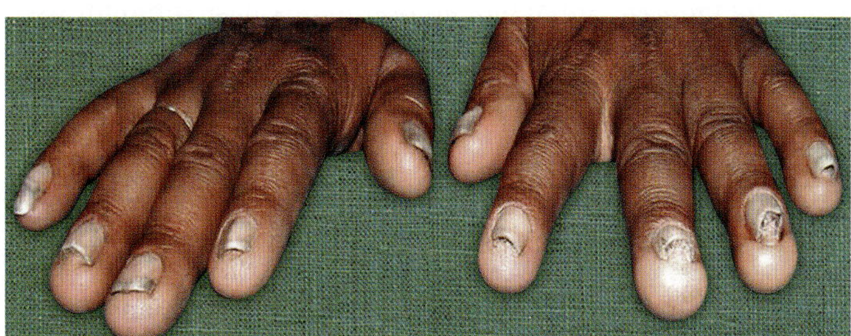

**FIG. 6:** Increased curvature, thickening of the nails, and subungual hyperkeratosis in pachyonychia congenita

*Courtesy*: Dr Archana Singhal, Director, Professor, and Head, Department of Dermatology and STD, University College of Medical Sciences and GTB Hospital, Delhi.

## Focal Keratoderma with Oral Leukokeratosis

This syndrome is characterized by autosomal-dominant inheritance, *KRT16* gene mutation, focal palmoplantar hyperkeratosis, and oral leukokeratosis.

## Punctate Keratoderma of Brauer–Buschke–Fischer

*Synonym:* Brauer-Buschke-Fischer keratoderma palmoplantare punctata or punctate palmoplantar keratoderma type I.

### Pathogenesis

This autosomal dominant disorder is caused by mutations in *AAGAB,* encoding α- and γ-adaptin-binding protein.

### Clinical Features

The disease is manifested bilaterally as asymptomatic, tiny, and hyperkeratotic punctate papules/plaque scattered diffusely on the palmoplantar surface. The disease is circumscribed on the palms and soles; associated abnormalities are unusual.

## Punctate Keratoderma of Palmar Creases

This autosomal dominantly inherited palmoplantar keratoderma is presented as small keratotic papules confined exclusively to the flexion creases of the palms, digits, and uncommonly soles creases (Fig. 7). The etiology is unknown.

## Acrokeratoelastoidosis of Costa

It was first described by the Brazilian dermatologist, Oswaldo Costa.

### Pathogenesis

This rare genodermatosis is either sporadic or familial where the familial cases are mostly autosomal dominant.

### Clinical Features

Clinically, the condition is characterized by multiple yellowish papules, sometimes glossy and keratotic, sometimes umbilicated, and located symmetrically on the sides of the hands and feet.

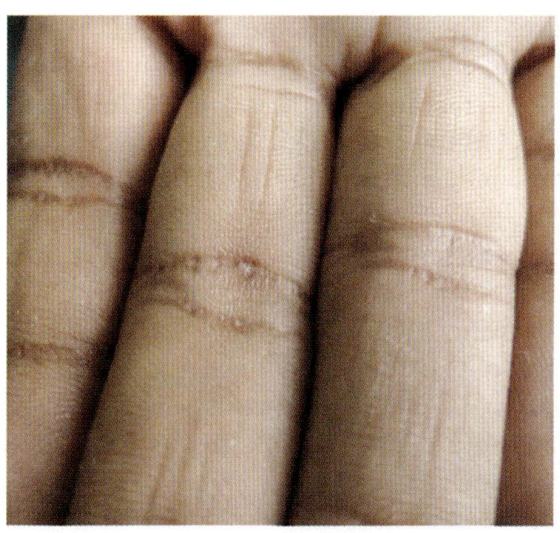

**FIG. 7:** Punctate keratoderma of the palmar creases.

## Diagnosis

Histopathology shows hyperkeratosis, mild acanthosis, and fragmented elastic fibers in the dermis (elastorrhexis).

## Treatment

### *General Treatment*

Response to treatment in most of the genetic PPK is unsatisfactory. Treatment tends to be symptomatic. Salt-water soaks, paring, topical keratolytic (6–10% salicylic acid in white soft paraffin, 35–70% propylene glycol, 20% urea, and 12% ammonium lactate), topical vitamin D analogs, and systemic retinoid have been used to treat hyperkeratosis. Secondary dermatophyte infections should be treated with antifungals.

### *Specific Treatment*

- Reconstructive surgery is needed for the treatment of pseudoainhum
- Dental pathology in Olmsted syndrome is treated by oral hygiene instructions, removable prosthesis and dentures
- One study suggested the possibility of using serum immunoglobulin E as a monitoring index for Papillon-Lefèvre syndrome inflammation level, thus possibility of new target for therapy
- Treatment with a diet low in tyrosine and phenylalanine is needed in Richner-Hanhart syndrome
- Apart from isotretinoin and acitretin, alitretinoin (9-cis-retinoic acid), a new retinoid with immunomodulatory and anti-inflammatory effects, which binds to retinoic acid receptors has been used in punctate keratoderma of Brauer-Buschke-Fischer.

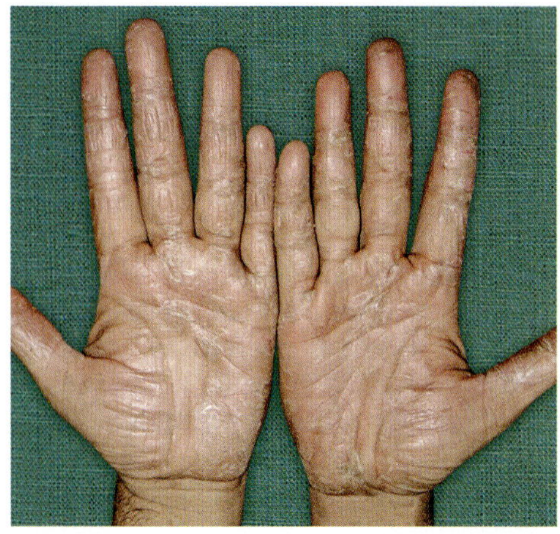

FIG. 8: Psoriasis involving the palms leading hyperkeratosis.

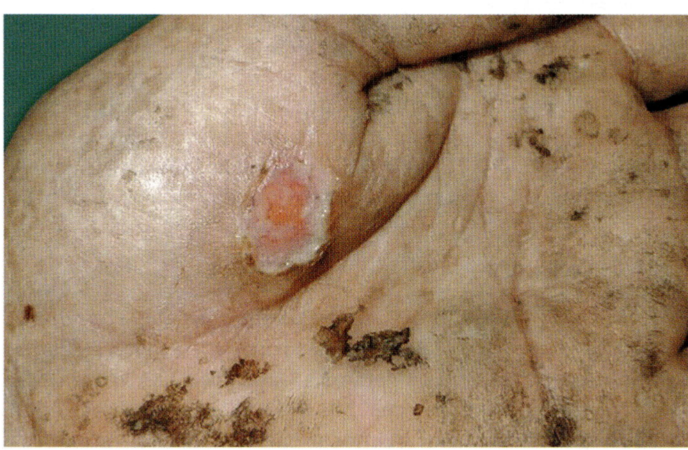

FIG. 9: Arsenical keratosis of palm showing pigmented keratotic papules and an ulcer.

## ACQUIRED PALMOPLANTAR KERATODERMAS

Common causes of acquired PPK are allergic and irritant dermatitis, frictional keratoses, exposure to metals and chemicals like arsenic, chlorinated hydrocarbon fluids, and side effects of some drugs (e.g., beta-glucan, lithium, and chemotherapy agents). Atopic dermatitis can cause palmoplantar hyperlinearity and even PPK. Dyshydrotic eczema is a common cause of PPK. One important etiology of acquired PPK is paraneoplastic PPK. Sézary syndrome, Bazex syndrome, and hereditary Howel-Evans syndrome commonly manifest with acquired PPK. Esophageal carcinoma is a common etiology. Management of the cancer generally helps to improve the PPK.

Various causes of acquired PPK are:

- Keratoderma climactericum is a common condition seen in women at menopause. Hyperkeratosis affects predominantly the palms, but the soles might also be involved. Skin changes may be related to the decline of ovarian hormones
- *Infections*:
  - Bacterial—syphilis
  - Fungal—dermatophyte infection
  - Viral—wart, AIDS
  - Parasitic—Norwegian scabies.
- *Inflammatory diseases*: Psoriasis (Fig. 8), lichen planus, pityriasis rubra pilaris, Reiter's disease, atopic eczema, and hyperkeratotic eczema
- *Endocrine diseases*: Hypothyroidism
- *Toxins*: Arsenical keratosis (Fig. 9)
- *Malignancy*: Mycosis fungoides, Sézary syndrome, Bazex syndrome, tripe palms in gastrointestinal, and other internal organ malignancies
- Aquagenic palmoplantar keratoderma or aquagenic syringeal acrokeratoderma is a rare acquired disorder that predominantly affects young women. It may be associated with a mutation in the cystic fibrosis gene. Abnormal aquaporin 5 has been described in sweat glands. It is characterized by whitish edematous papules, plaques, keratoderma, pruritus, burning, and pain developing after brief exposure to water and resolving shortly after drying
- *Drug induced*: Sorafenib, an oral multikinase inhibitor used in the treatment of renal cell carcinoma has been reported to cause palmoplantar hyperkeratosis.



## SUGGESTED READINGS


1. Bethke G, Kolde G, Bethke G, et al. Focal palmoplantar and oral mucosa hyperkeratosis syndrome. Mund Kiefer Gesichtschir. 2001;5:202-5.
2. Blaydon DC, Lind LK, Plagnol V, et al. Mutations in AQP5, encoding a water-channel protein, cause autosomal-dominant diffuse nonepidermolytic palmoplantar keratoderma. Am J Hum Genet. 2013;93:330-5.
3. Bragg J, Rizzo C, Mengden S. Striate palmoplantar keratoderma (Brunauer-Fohs-Siemens syndrome). Dermatol Online J. 2008;14:26.
4. Corte LD, Silva MV, Oliveira CF, et al. Vohwinkel syndrome, ichthyosiform variant--by Camisa--case report. An Bras Dermatol. 2013;88(6 Suppl 1):206-8.

5. Costa MC, Bornhausen Demarch E, Hertz A, Pereira FB, Azulay DR. Case for diagnosis. Acrokeratoelastoidosis. An Bras Dermatol. 2011;86:1222-3.
6. de Souza CA, Santos Ada C, Santos Lda C, et al. Hereditary tylosis syndrome and esophagus cancer. An Bras Dermatol. 2009;84:527-9.
7. Duchatelet S, Hovnanian A. Olmsted syndrome: Clinical, molecular and therapeutic aspects. Orphanet J Rare Dis. 2015;10:33.
8. Eytan O, Fuchs-Telem D, Mevorach B, et al. Olmsted syndrome caused by a homozygous recessive mutation in TRPV3. J Invest Dermatol. 2014;134:1752-4.
9. Flückiger R, Itin PH. Keratosis extremitatum (Greither's disease): Clinical features, histology, ultrastructure. Dermatology. 1993;187:309-11.
10. Fond L, Perrot JL, Gentil-Perret A, et al. Focal familial palmoplantar keratoderma with punctate hyperkeratosis of the palmar creases. Ann Dermatol Venereol. 1998;125:898-901.
11. Gönül M, Cevirgen Cemil B, Keseroglu HO, et al. New described dermatological disorders. Biomed Res Int. 2014;2014:616973.
12. Guo Y, Shi M, Tan ZP, et al. Possible anticipation in familial epidermolytic palmoplantar keratoderma with the p.R163W mutation of Keratin 9. Genet Mol Res. 2014;13:8089-93.
13. Hinterberger L, Pföhler C, Vogt T, et al. Diffuse epidermolytic palmoplantar keratoderma (Unna-Thost-). BMJ Case Rep. 2012;2012. pii: bcr2012006443.
14. Jijin MJ, Jaishankar HP, Narayaran VS, et al. Papillon-Lefevre syndrome in an adolescent female: A case study. J Clin Diagn Res. 2015;9:ZD23-5.
15. Kabashima K, Shimauchi T, Kobayashi M, et al. Aberrant aquaporin 5 expression in the sweat gland in aquagenic wrinkling of the palms. J Am Acad Dermatol. 2008;59(2 Suppl 1):S28-32.
16. Kim J, Foster R, Lam M, et al. Mycosis fungoides: An important differential diagnosis for acquired palmoplantar keratoderma. Australas J Dermatol. 2015;56:49-51.
17. Kubo A. Nagashima-type palmoplantar keratosis: A common Asian type caused by SERPINB7 protease inhibitor deficiency. J Invest Dermatol. 2014;134: 2076-9.
18. Lee YA, Stevens HP, Delaporte E, et al. A gene for an autosomal dominant scleroatrophic syndrome predisposing to skin cancer (Huriez syndrome) maps to chromosome 4q23. Am J Hum Genet. 2000;66:326-30.
19. Liu WT, Ke HP, Zhao Y, et al. The most common mutation of KRT9, c.C487T (p.R163W), in epidermolytic palmoplantar keratoderma in twolarge Chinese pedigrees. Anat Rec (Hoboken). 2012;295:604-9.
20. Loh TH, Yosipovitch G, Tay YK. Palmar-plantar keratoderma of Unna Thost associated with atopic dermatitis: an underrecognized entity? Pediatr Dermatol. 2003;20:195-8.
21. Lountzis NI, Maroon MS. Sorafenib-induced palmoplantar hyperkeratosis. J Drugs Dermatol. 2008;7:588-9.
22. Madan V, Gupta U. Tyrosinaemia type II with diffuse plantar keratoderma and self-mutilation. Clin Exp Dermatol. 2006;31:54-6.
23. Nellen RG, Steijlen PM, van Geel M, et al. Comment on Zhao et al. "Palmoplantar keratoderma of the Gamborg-Nielsen type is caused by mutations in the SLURP1 gene and represents a variant of Mal de Meleda". Acta Derm Venereol. 2015;95(8):1034-5.
24. O'Toole EA, Kaspar RL, Sprecher E, et al. Pachyonychia congenita cornered: report on the 11th Annual International Pachyonychia Congenita Consortium Meeting. Br J Dermatol. 2014;171:974-7.
25. Pohler E, Cunningham F, Sandilands A, et al. Novel autosomal dominant mutation in loricrin presenting as prominent ichthyosis. Br J Dermatol. 2015;173(5):1291-4.
26. Pohler E, Huber M, Boonen SE, et al. New and recurrent AAGAB mutations in punctate palmoplantar keratoderma. Br J Dermatol. 2014;171:433-6.
27. Rabinowitz LG, Williams LR, Anderson CE, et al. Painful keratoderma and photophobia: Hallmarks of tyrosinemia type II. J Pediatr. 1995;126:266-9.
28. Raone B, Raboni R, Patrizi A. Alitretinoin: A new treatment option for hereditary punctate palmoplantar keratoderma (Brauer-Buschke-Fischer syndrome). J Am Acad Dermatol. 2014;71:e48-9.
29. Rongioletti F, Tomasini C, Crovato F, et al. Aquagenic (pseudo) keratoderma: A clinical series with new pathological insights. Br J Dermatol. 2012;167:575-82.
30. Sarma N, Ghosh C, Kar S, Bazmi BA. Low-dose acitretin in Papillon-Lefèvre syndrome: Treatment and 1-year follow-up. Dermatol Ther. 2015; 28(1):28-31.
31. Sarma N. Arsenicosis- Indian Perspective. In: Ghosh S, Sarma N, De D Eds: Recent advances in Dermatology (Vol 3). Jaypee Brothers Medical Publishers (P) Ltd. New Delhi.2014,134-153
32. Sarma N. Skin manifestations of chronic arsenicosis. In: States JC Ed. Arsenic: Exposure Sources, Health Risks, and Mechanisms of Toxicity. John Wiley and Sons, Inc. New Jersey. 2016,127-136.
33. Schiller S, Seebode C, Hennies HC, Giehl K, Emmert S. Palmoplantar keratoderma (PPK): acquired and genetic causes of a not so rare disease. J Dtsch Dermatol Ges. 2014;12:781-8.
34. Seirafi H, Khezri S, Morowati S, et al. A new variant of Vohwinkel syndrome: A case report. Dermatol Online J. 2011;17:3.
35. Shah AF, Tangade P, Agarwal S. Papillon-Lefevre syndrome: Reporting consanguinity as a risk factor. Saudi Dent J. 2014;26:126-31.
36. Simon M, Hagedorn M. The Clark-Howel-Evans-McConnell syndrome. Observations in one family over 5 generations. Hautarzt. 1997;48:800-5.
37. Sreeramulu B, Shyam ND, Ajay P, et al. Papillon-Lefèvre syndrome: Clinical presentation and management options. Clin Cosmet Investig Dent. 2015;7:75-81.
38. Wang X, Liu Y, Liu Y, et al. Long-term change of disease behavior in Papillon-Lefèvre syndrome: Seven years follow-up. Eur J Med Genet. 2015;58:184-7.
39. Wilson NJ, Messenger AG, Leachman SA, et al. Keratin K6c mutations cause focal palmoplantar keratoderma. J Invest Dermatol. 2010;130:425-9.
40. Xu Cao, Jinghua Yin, Huijun Wang, et al. Mutation in AQP5, encoding aquaporin 5, causes palmoplantar keratoderma Bothnia type. J Invest Dermatol. 2014;134:284-7.
41. Zhao L, Vahlquist A, Virtanen M, et al. Palmoplantar keratoderma of the Gamborg-Nielsen type is caused by mutations in the SLURP1 gene and represents a variant of Mal de Meleda. Acta Derm Venereol. 2014;94:707-10.

# 34 CHAPTER Follicular Keratosis and Erythrokeratodermia

*Dipti Das, Nilendu Sarma*

## FOLLICULAR KERATOSES

Follicular keratoses are a group of disorders of hair follicle keratinization causing follicular inflammation and keratotic follicular papules. This group of disorder includes:

- Keratosis pilaris (KP)
- Lichen spinulosus
- Phrynoderma
- Pityriasis rubra pilaris (PRP)
- Darier disease.

### Keratosis Pilaris

It is an inherited disorder of keratinization characterized by folliculocentric keratotic papules.

### Pathogenesis

The disease is autosomal dominantly inherited. Abnormal follicular keratinization involving the follicular infundibulum is the main cause of KP. Keratosis pilaris is associated with chromosome 18p deletion, which may be related to an alteration in the functioning of the laminin alpha 1 (*LAMA1*) gene. This chromosomal region perhaps regulates follicular keratinization and formation of sebaceous gland structures and thus may play a role in the pathophysiology and in the genetic susceptibility. Filaggrin mutations may also partially account for the KP phenotype.

### Clinical Features

It develops most often in early childhood and may increase during puberty. Lesions are symmetrically distributed, 1–2 mm folliculocentric keratotic papules distributed mainly on extensor surfaces of the upper arms, thighs, buttocks, and cheeks. Papules may have surrounding erythema. Eruptions are usually asymptomatic, or there may be occasional pruritus. Association with atopic dermatitis, ichthyosis vulgaris, and vitamin A deficiency are also described.

### Diagnosis

Diagnosis is mainly clinical. Biopsy reveals hyperkeratosis, hypergranulosis, follicular plugging, and superficial perivascular lymphocytic infiltrates. Dermoscopy shows circular hair shafts mostly within normal-appearing follicular openings, suggesting that the defect in KP may not be of keratinization, but of the circular hair shaft which ruptures the follicular epithelium, leading to inflammation and abnormal follicular keratinization.

### Variants

#### *Keratosis Pilaris Rubra*

It shows more prominent erythema and more widespread areas of skin involvement but without atrophy or hyperpigmentation.

#### *Erythromelanosis Follicularis Faciei Et Colli*

It is characterized by triad of brownish hyperpigmentation, follicular plugging and erythema of face and neck mainly on preauricular and cheek areas.

#### *Keratosis Pilaris Atrophicans*

It is a group of disorders characterized by inflammatory keratotic papules that may result in alopecia and scarring. They include KP atrophicans faciei (also called ulerythema ophryogenes), keratosis follicularis spinulosa decalvans, and atrophoderma vermiculatum.

#### *Keratosis Pilaris Atrophicans Faciei/Ulerythema Ophryogenes*

It shows erythematous follicular papules of the eyebrows, forehead, and cheeks followed by alopecia, scarring, and atrophy. Ulerythema ophryogenes predominantly involves the lateral third of eyebrows. Associations with Noonan syndrome have been described. It is differentiated from erythromelanosis follicularis faciei et colli by the presence of atrophy and scarring.

#### *Keratosis Follicularis Spinulosa Decalvans*

This X-linked genodermatosis is characterized by follicular hyperkeratosis and scarring alopecia. Keratosis follicularis spinulosa decalvans is caused by missense mutations in *MBTPS2*.

#### *Atrophoderma Vermiculata/Folliculitis Ulerythematosa Reticulata*

Atrophoderma vermiculatum is characterized by honeycombed or reticular atrophy of the cheeks and forehead. It predominantly affects children.

### Treatment

Various treatment options for KP are keratolytics (salicylic acid, lactic acid, and urea), vitamin D3 analogs, topical and systemic retinoids, and various laser therapies (pulsed dye laser, intense pulsed light, and diode laser).

## Lichen Spinulosus

*Synonym*: Keratosis spinulosa.

### Clinical Features

It is an idiopathic keratotic disorder characterized by asymptomatic, follicular keratotic papules, and topped by horny spine. Lesions are grouped and symmetrically distributed on neck, buttocks, abdominal wall, and the extensor surfaces of the arms. It mainly occurs in children and adolescents. Generalized form has been described with human immunodeficiency virus (HIV).

### Diagnosis

Diagnosis is made by clinical assessment alone. Dermatoscopy greatly assist in finding the spines (Fig. 1). Biopsy shows hyperkeratosis, follicular plugging, and superficial perivascular lymphocytic infiltrates.

### Treatment

Lesions may resolve spontaneously. Emollients, keratolytics (salicylic acid, lactic acid, and urea) tretinoin, adapalene, or tacalcitol creams may be effective.

## Phrynoderma

This is a nutritional deficiency disorder, also known as "toad skin".

### Pathogenesis

Multiple nutrients deficiency plays role in the pathogenesis of phrynoderma (vitamin A, vitamin B complex, vitamin C, vitamin E, essential fatty acids deficiency).

### Clinical Features

It occurs mainly in children and adolescents. Lesions are multiple, asymptomatic, brown or skin colored, keratotic follicular papules with central keratinous plug, distributed symmetrically on elbows, knees, buttocks, extensor extremities, and rarely on trunk and face (Fig. 2). Ocular manifestations of vitamin A deficiency may be associated. Normal serum levels of nutrients (vitamin A, vitamin B complex, and essential fatty acids) have also been reported in phrynoderma patients.

### Treatment

High dose vitamin A replacement therapy along with replacement of other vitamins like vitamin B complex, vitamin C, and essential fatty acids. Topical keratolytics can also be used for hyperkeratotic lesions.

## Pityriasis Rubra Pilaris

This is a papulosquamous disease of unknown etiology.

### Pathogenesis

Exact etiology is not known. Autosomal dominant inheritance with incomplete penetrance has been described (in most cases of type V). The inherited form of PRP is linked to mutations in *CARD14* gene.

### Clinical Features

Lesions are erythematous follicular keratotic papules; coalesce to form orange-red plaques with island of sparing. Waxy, diffuse palmoplantar keratoderma is commonly associated. According to Griffith's classification, five types of PRP are described (type I–V). An HIV-associated variant (type VI) has been added to this classification system.

Type I or classic adult type is most common, accounting for around 50% of all cases. It starts on the head and neck, and then spreads caudally (Fig. 3).

Type II or atypical adult is characterized by follicular keratosis, ichthyosis of legs, eczematous dermatitis, and alopecia. Type III or classic juvenile is similar to type I. Type IV or circumscribed juvenile

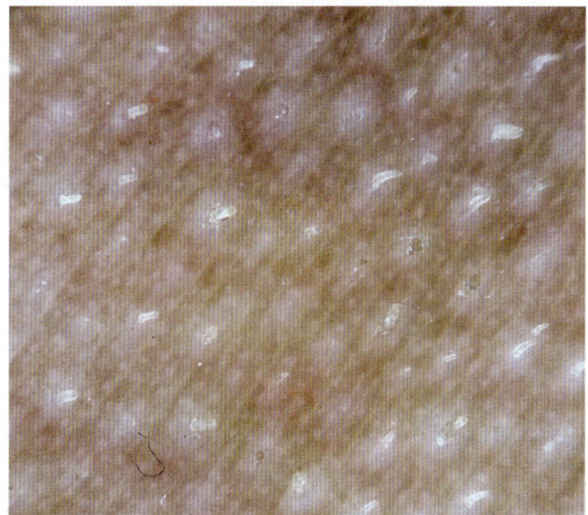

FIG. 1: Dermatoscopy shows spiny follicular projections in lichen spinulosus.

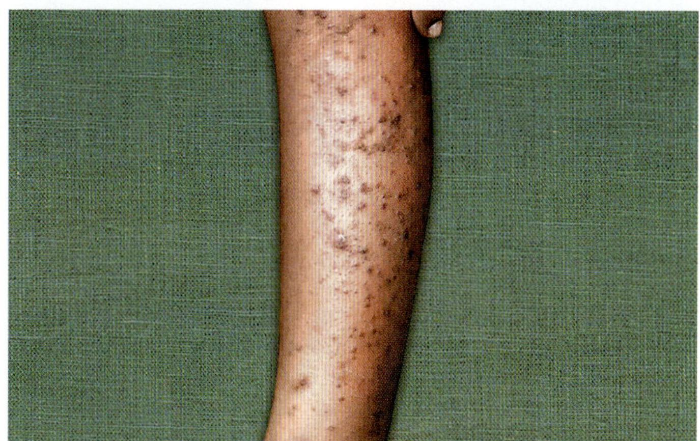

FIG. 2: Horny papules in phrynoderma.

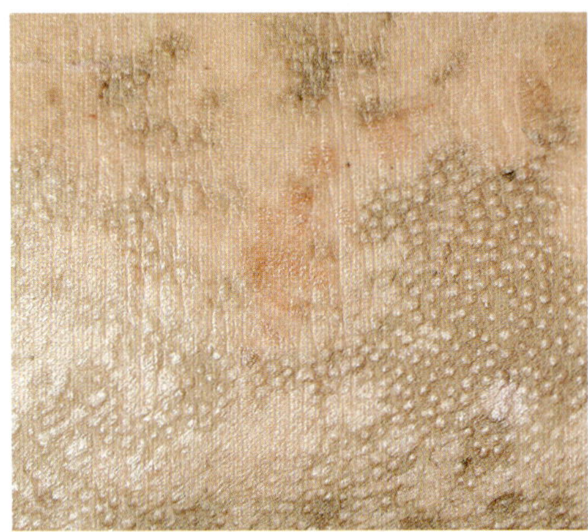

FIG. 3: Grouped perifollicular papules developing into patches of erythema in type I pityriasis rubra pilaris.

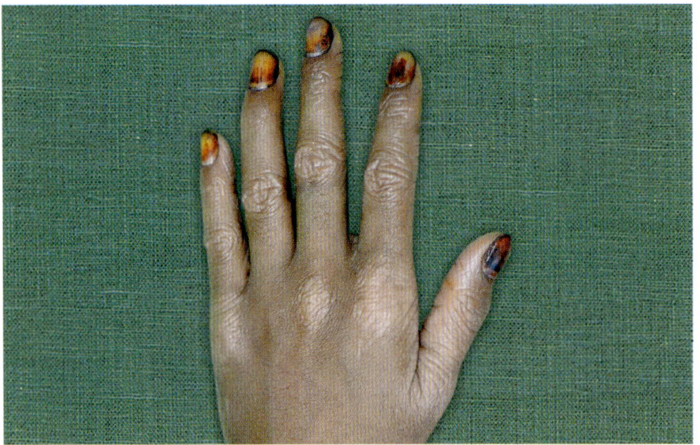

FIG. 4: Localized hyperkeratosis on the knuckles in circumscribed juvenile pityriasis rubra pilaris.

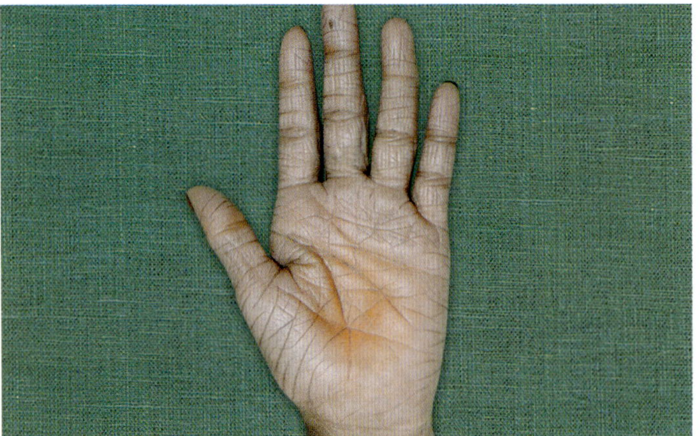

FIG. 5: Localized hyperkeratosis on the palms in circumscribed juvenile pityriasis rubra pilaris.

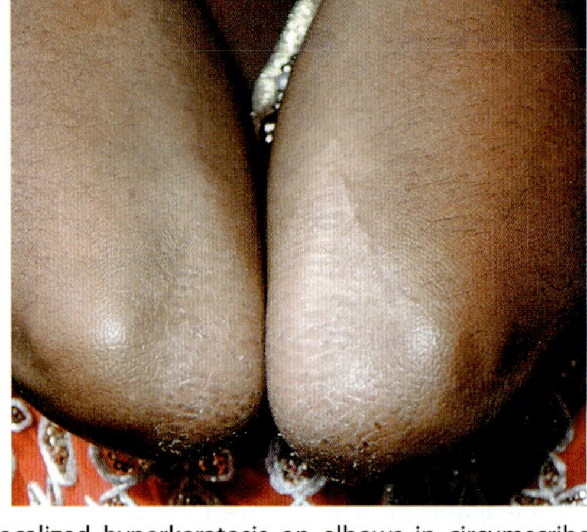

FIG. 6: Localized hyperkeratosis on elbows in circumscribed juvenile pityriasis rubra pilaris.

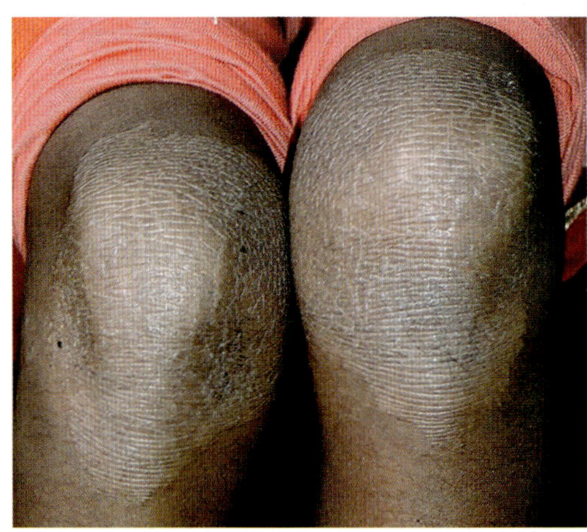

FIG. 7: Localized hyperkeratosis on knees in circumscribed juvenile pityriasis rubra pilaris.

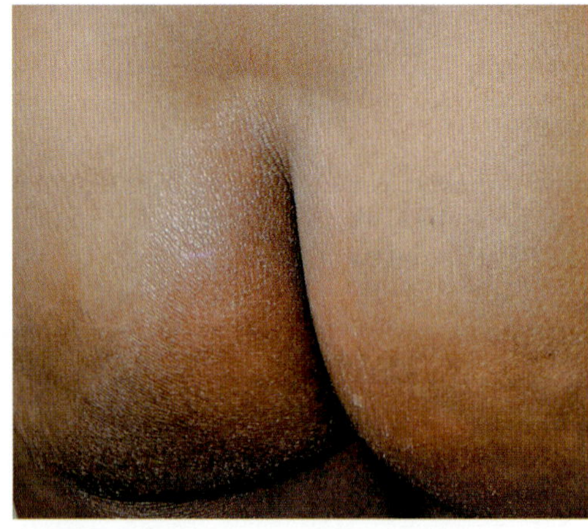

FIG. 8: Localized hyperkeratosis on buttocks in circumscribed juvenile pityriasis rubra pilaris.

is the second most common type and is characterized by follicular keratotic papules and plaques localized to elbows and knees (Figs 4 to 8). Type V or atypical juvenile is characterized by follicular keratosis and sclerodermoid changes of the hands and feet. Type VI or HIV associated is similar to type I. It may be associated with acne conglobata, hidradenitis suppurativa, and lichen spinulosus.

## Diagnosis

Diagnosis is mainly clinical. Biopsy reveals alternating vertical and horizontal orthokeratosis and parakeratosis (checkerboard pattern), follicular plugging, and a mild superficial perivascular lymphocytic infiltrate.

### Treatment

Topical therapy includes emollients, keratolytics, tazarotene, calcipotriol, and corticosteroid. Various systemic therapies are oral retinoids (acitretin, isotretinoin, or alitretinoin), methotrexate, cyclosporine, azathioprine, psoralen ultraviolet A, biologics (infliximab, adalimumab, ustekinumab), and highly active antiretroviral therapy.

## ERYTHROKERATODERMIA

Erythrokeratodermia or erythrokeratoderma is a heterogeneous group of inherited keratinization disorder. This is just a descriptive term to encompass disorders characterized by erythematous lesions and hyperkeratotic plaques. Generally, these manifest at or shortly after birth. Erythema may be present on or at the periphery of the keratoses or separately. These conditions have to be differentiated from other conditions that also manifest with similar features like PRP and congenital ichthyosiform erythroderma.

Erythrokeratodermias have been divided into nonsyndromic type and syndromic type. Progressive symmetric erythrokeratodermia (PSEK) and erythrokeratodermia variabilis (EKV) have characteristic clinical manifestations. The *GJB3* and *GJB4* genes on chromosome 1p35 are associated with EKV. *Loricrin* gene is associated with many cases (mostly Japanese) of PSEK although a specific mutation is yet elusive.

However, it has to be understood that clinical distinction between EKV and PSEK is not always possible. Even electron microscopic ultrastructural studies failed to differentiate them in many occasions. Thus, many consider these two conditions as different phenotypic manifestation of single condition. Further molecular research is required to understand these conditions.

Two main nonsyndromic types are:

1. Erythrokeratodermia variabilis
2. Progressive symmetric erythrokeratodermia.

Erythrokeratodermia may be part of various syndromes such as keratitis, ichthyosis, and deafness (syndrome) and hystrix like ichthyosis-deafness (HID) syndrome.

### Erythrokeratodermia Variabilis

*Synonym*: Mendes da Costa disease.

Erythrokeratodermia variabilis, first described by Mendes da Costa in 1925, is a rare genetic ichthyosiform disorder.

#### Pathogenesis

There are mutations in connexin, which is a gap junction protein. There is mutation of the gene *GJB3* or *GJB4*, coding for a gap junction protein connexin 31 and connexin 30.3 respectively. Erythrokeratodermia variabilis is pathologically heterogeneous. Connexin mutations have been reported to be absent in some cases. The disease is usually inherited in an autosomal dominant fashion, but autosomal recessive transmission has also been reported.

#### Clinical Features

The disease presents at birth or in infancy except some occasional cases that appear during early childhood. Hyperkeratosis may be generalized or more classically limited, involving fixed, localized areas with well-defined hyperkeratotic plaques.

These fixed hyperkeratotic plaques have predilection for the extremities, buttocks, and trunk.

Second characteristic feature of the disease is development of migratory erythema. This migratory erythema that have polycyclic configuration that change size and shape appears for transient period, for minutes to hours, usually following some precipitating factors like trauma, temperature change, or some form of irritation. These lesions are more common on face, buttocks, and extensor surfaces of limbs.

Approximately 50% of patients display a palmoplantar keratoderma. This displays a fine erythematous scaling associated with peeling without hyperkeratosis.

Rare EKV variants include erythroderma en cocardes, known as Degos' disease, reticulate erythrokeratoderma, and EKV with erythema gyratum repens like lesions. The course of the disease is chronic, with remissions and exacerbations throughout life.

#### Diagnosis

Diagnosis is mainly clinical. Histopathology is nonspecific showing orthokeratotic hyperkeratosis or parakeratosis, acanthosis, and papillomatosis. Genetic mutation analysis can be done.

#### Differential Diagnosis

Progressive symmetric erythrokeratoderma, ichthyosis linearis circumflexa (Netherton syndrome), psoriasis.

#### Treatment

Topical emollients, keratolytics ointments (urea, salicylic acid, propylene glycol, and lactic acid), coal tar, tacrolimus, tazarotene, vitamin D analogs, and systemic retinoids can be used.

### Progressive Symmetric Erythrokeratodermia

*Synonym*: Gottron's syndrome.

It is first described by Darier in 1911 and is named after Gottron's article in 1922.

#### Pathogenesis

Predominantly autosomal-dominant inheritance with incomplete penetrance and variable expressivity. Autosomal-recessive transmission and sporadic cases have been observed. Mutations in gene coding for loricrin have been implicated in majority of cases. Loricrin is the major structural component of the cornified cell envelop. Mutation in the *GJB4* gene coding connexin 30.3 has been observed in both EKV and PSEK.

#### Clinical Features

The disease starts in early childhood, progresses for few years, and then becomes stable. Lesions are stable but slow progression is sometimes seen. Even intermittent generalization is reported. Lesions may regress rarely at puberty. Characteristic lesions are well-defined, erythematous, scaly (squamous), or hyperkeratotic plaques distributed symmetrically on extremities and buttocks.

Face may show scaling. The trunk is usually spared. Palmoplantar keratoderma may be present. It differs from EKV in the absence of migratory erythematous lesions, presence of symmetry, and greater incidence of palmoplantar keratoderma. Pseudoainhum is not seen. As discussed, there may be considerable clinical overlap between the two.

## Diagnosis

Biopsy shows hyperkeratosis, often parakeratosis and acanthosis. Lipid-like vacuoles are frequently noted in granular cell layer.

## Differential Diagnosis

Erythrokeratodermia variabilis, psoriasis, pityriasis rubra pilaris.

## Treatment

Topical keratolytics, retinoids, steroids, calcipotriol, and oral retinoids have been used with variable results.

# SUGGESTED READINGS


1. Adnot-Desanlis L, Antonicelli F, Tabary T, et al. Effectiveness of infliximab in pityriasis rubra pilaris is associated with pro-inflammatory cytokine inhibition. Dermatology. 2013;226:41-6.
2. Amann PM, Susic M, Glüder F, et al. Alitretinoin (9-cis retinoic acid) is effective against pityriasis rubra pilaris: A retrospective clinical study. Acta Derm Venereol. 2015;95:329-31.
3. Aten E, Brasz LC, Bornholdt D, et al. Keratosis Follicularis Spinulosa Decalvans is caused by mutations in MBTPS2. Hum Mutat. 2010;31:1125-33.
4. Bilgin I, Bozdað KE, Uysal S, et al. Progressive symmetrical erythrokeratoderma—response to topical calcipotriol. J Dermatol Case Rep. 2011;5:50-2.
5. Carvalho CA, Carvalho AV, Kiss A, et al. Keratosis pilaris and ulerythema ophryogenes in a woman with monosomy of the short arm of chromosome 18. An Bras Dermatol. 2011;86:S42-5.
6. Fuchs-Telem D, Pessach Y, Mevorah B, et al. Erythrokeratoderma variabilis caused by a recessive mutation in GJB3. Clin Exp Dermatol. 2011;36:406-11.
7. Gruber R, Sugarman JL, Crumrine D, et al. Sebaceous gland, hair shaft, and epidermal barrier abnormalities in keratosis pilaris with and without filaggrin deficiency. Am J Pathol. 2015;185:1012-21.
8. Guidry JA, Rees A, Chan AJ, et al. Ulerythema ophryogenes and Noonan syndrome. Dermatol Online J. 2013;19:14.
9. Hong JB, Chen PL, Chen YT, et al. Genetic analysis of CARD14 in non-familial pityriasis rubra pilaris: A case series. Acta Derm Venereol. 2014;94:587-8.
10. Ibrahim O, Khan M, Bolotin D, et al. Treatment of keratosis pilaris with 810-nm diode laser: A randomized clinical trial. JAMA Dermatol. 2015;151:187-91.
11. Inoue N, Dainichi T, Fujisawa A, et al. CARD14 Glu138 mutation in familial pityriasis rubra pilaris does not warrant differentiation from familial psoriasis. J Dermatol. 2016;43(2):187-9
12. Itin PH, Moschopulos M, Richard G. Reticular erythrokeratoderma: A new disorder of cornification. Am J Med Genet A. 2003;120A:237-40.
13. Kim BR, Chae JB, Park JT, et al. Clinical remission of pityriasis rubra pilaris with adalimumab in an adolescent patient. J Dermatol. 2015;42(11):1122-3.
14. Kokotas H, Papagiannaki K, Grigoriadou M, et al. Erythrokeratodermia variabilis: Report of two cases and a novel missense variant in GJB4 encoding connexin 30.3. Eur J Dermatol. 2012;22:182-6.
15. Li K, Ann Thomas M, Haber RM. Ulerythema ophryogenes, a rarely reported cutaneous manifestation of noonan syndrome: case report and review of the literature. J Cutan Med Surg. 2013;17:212-8.
16. Liakou AI, Esteves de Carvalho AV, Nazarenko LP. Trias of keratosis pilaris, ulerythema ophryogenes and 18p monosomy: Zouboulis syndrome. J Dermatol. 2014;41:371-6.
17. Maheswari UG, Chaitra V, Mohan SS. Keratosis follicularis spinulosa decalvans: A rare cause of scarring alopecia in two young Indian girls. Int J Trichology. 2013;5:29-31.
18. Morton CM, Bhate C, Janniger CK, et al. Ulerythema ophryogenes: Updates and insights. Cutis. 2014;93:83-7.
19. Thomas M, Khopkar US. Keratosis pilaris revisited: Is it more than just a follicular keratosis? Int J Trichology. 2012;4:255-8.

# 12 SECTION Dermatoses with Specific Histological Reaction Patterns

# 35 CHAPTER Neutrophilic Dermatoses

Rajiv S Joshi

## INTRODUCTION

The classic neutrophilic dermatoses present with common histopathological findings of dense interstitial nonseptic neutrophilic infiltrates in the dermis without evidence for an infective cause. Many of these show the phenomenon of "pathergy" which is hyperreactivity of the skin to minor trauma with development of papulo-pustules or ulcers at site of minor trauma.

Cutaneous lesions are commonly seen and include vesiculopustules, erythematous edematous plaques, nodules, and ulcers. Many of these conditions are associated with underlying systemic diseases both inflammatory and malignant and may be considered as skin markers of systemic disease.

These all represent an abnormal tissue reaction with dysregulated immune responses that leads to elaboration of factors that are strongly chemotactic to neutrophils. Therapy with corticosteroids is uniformly successful in these diseases but relapses, and chronicity is often the rule in many patients.

## SWEET'S SYNDROME (SYN. ACUTE FEBRILE NEUTROPHILIC DERMATOSIS)

Sweet's syndrome is the classic neutrophilic dermatoses eponymically named after Robert Sweet who in 1964 described "acute febrile neutrophilic dermatosis" in eight middle-aged women who developed erythematous plaques associated with fever and history of respiratory tract or gastrointestinal tract infection. Histopathology showed a dense neutrophilic infiltrate without vasculitis. Whittle et al. in 1968 described two additional cases one of which was a male with lesions on the face and first used the term Sweet's syndrome.

Sweet's syndrome may be divided into:

- *Classical (idiopathic)*: This is more common in middle-aged women. Recurrence is common.
- *Systemic conditions and disorders*: Inflammatory bowel disease, pregnancy, Sjogren's syndrome, Behcet's disease (BD), and connective tissue diseases like systemic lupus erythematosus and rheumatoid arthritis.
- *Infection related*: This is often preceded by upper and lower respiratory tract infection. Bacterial infections like Streptococci, *Staphylococcus, Salmonella, Yersinia enterocolitica, Escherichia coli, Helicobacter pylori, Borrelia burgdorferi,* mycobacteria (*Mycobacterium tuberculosis* and atypical mycobacteria), fungal infections like coccidioidomycosis, sporotrichosis, and infections with human immunodeficiency virus, cytomegalovirus, hepatitis A and B, and parvovirus B19, can induce Sweet's syndrome.
- *Malignancy associated Sweet's syndrome (MASS)*: Most commonly related to acute myelogenous leukemia but has been described in other hematologic and solid cancers. It may be considered as a paraneoplastic syndrome in this setting and may precede or appear along with the malignancy.
- *Drug induced*: Co-trimoxazole, doxycycline, minocycline, all trans-retinoic acid, carbamazepine, oral contraceptives, azathioprine, abacavir, imatinib, granulocyte colony-stimulating factor (G-CSF), and vaccines like bacille Calmette-Guerin, pneumococcal and influenza vaccines.

### Epidemiology

Sweet's syndrome has been described from all parts of the world and while seen most commonly in middle-aged persons (30–60 years) has also been described in infants, children, and elderly individuals. Female are more commonly affected (F:M::4:1) in the classical form of Sweet's syndrome whereas the gender difference in not pronounced in the other forms.

### Pathogenesis

It is now accepted that Sweet's syndrome is a reactive process. A dysregulation of the cytokine milieu involving interleukin (IL)-1, G-CSF, granulocyte, and macrophage colony-stimulating factor (GM-CSF) and interferon gamma has been postulated in the development of Sweet's syndrome. A possible genetic link with human leukocyte antigen (HLA)-B54 has been observed in Japanese. Involvement of genes that affect regulation of granulopoiesis and neutrophil migration may play a role.

### Clinical Features

Skin lesions are well circumscribed, rapidly spreading, tender erythematous papules and plaques, of variable sizes that often show a pseudo-vesicular appearance due to massive subepidermal edema. Plaques may assume a targetoid appearance due to partial resolution of the center of the lesions with a yellowish or pigmented hue. True vesicles or pustules are uncommon although a vesiculobullous variant has been described, commonly associated with myelogenous leukemia and which may progress to ulceration that can resemble pyoderma gangrenosum (PG). An erysipelas-like or abscess-like presentation may be seen and can be difficult to diagnose clinically. Lesions on the dorsum of the hand are not uncommon and are often bullous and ulcerative and the entity neutrophilic dermatosis of the dorsum of hand has been considered to be a localized variant of Sweet's syndrome and atypical PG when it occurs on that site.

Oral aphthae are seen in only about 2% of cases but are more common in patients with associated hematological malignancies.

Usually multiple lesions are seen and appear to favor the head and neck region and the extremities. Pathergy, i.e., appearance of lesions at sites of minor skin trauma as in venepuncture sites may be seen.

It tends to resolve spontaneously within 5–12 weeks but recurrence may be seen in up to 30% of cases, especially the classical type.

Systemic findings are seen in 50–80% of cases and commonly seen are arthralgias, myalgias and arthritis, periorbital edema, conjunctivitis, episcleritis, iritis, keratitis, and choroiditis. Less commonly, cough and chest pain with dyspnea may be seen and pulmonary infiltrates and effusions may be seen on X-ray of the chest. Cardiac, renal, hepatic, and neurological involvement is rare.

A high erythrocyte sedimentation rate (ESR) with leukocytosis and neutrophilia is the most common laboratory finding. Antineutrophil cytoplasmic antibodies (ANCA) have been sometimes found.

## Pathology

The characteristic histological finding is the presence of numerous neutrophils scattered diffusely in the upper and mid-reticular dermis with some leukocytoclasia but no vasculitis. At times, a deeper infiltrate of neutrophils may be seen in the subcutaneous fat giving rise to either an erythema nodosum like septal panniculitis or even a neutrophilic lobular panniculitis. Also seen is prominent subepidermal edema. The epidermis generally is normal but may show mild spongiosis or exocytosis of neutrophils, and intraepidermal pustulation may be seen (Figs 1 and 2).

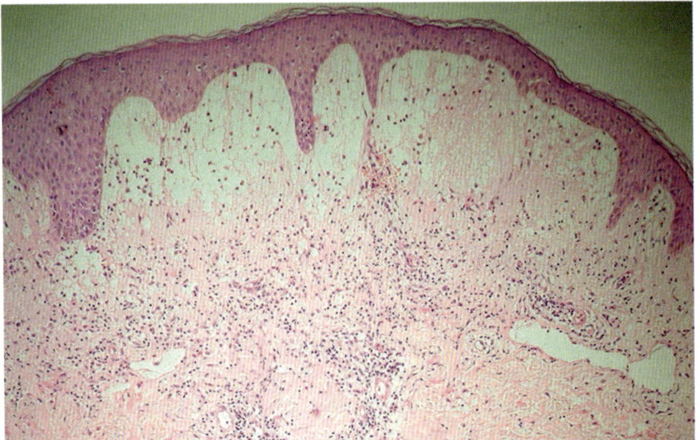

**FIG. 1:** Sweet's syndrome showing marked sub-epidermal edema. (H&E 40x).

A histiocytoid variant of Sweet's syndrome has been described in which the infiltrate is composed of histiocytoid cells that are actually immature myeloid cells expressing myeloperoxidase activity and which must be differentiated from leukemia cutis.

## Diagnostic Criteria for Sweet's Syndrome

Both major and at least two minor criteria are necessary for the diagnosis.

### Major Criteria

- Abrupt onset of typical cutaneous lesions
- Histopathology consistent with Sweet's syndrome.

### Minor Criteria

- Cutaneous eruption preceded by one of the associated infections or vaccinations, accompanied by one of the associated malignancies or inflammatory disorders, associated with drug exposure or pregnancy
- Presence of fever (>38°C) and constitutional signs and symptoms
- Erythrocyte sedimentation rate more than 20 mm, positive C-reactive protein, leukocytosis with left shift
- Excellent rapid response to systemic corticosteroids.

## Treatment

Sweet's syndrome may subside spontaneously in few weeks to months without any scarring. However, recurrences are common and may occur in up to 50% of patients especially in those with associated hematological malignancies.

The most effective and reliable treatment is with oral steroids (Prednisolone in doses of 0.5–1 mg/kg body weight or other steroids in equivalent doses). Steroids may need to be given for few weeks and even months in a low dose to prevent recurrences.

The other drugs used include dapsone (100 mg/day), colchicine (1–1.5 mg/day) and potassium iodide. These may be used as steroid sparing agents especially if therapy needs to be prolonged beyond several weeks. Nonsteroidal anti-inflammatory drugs (NSAIDs) like indomethacin, naproxen, clofazimine, cyclosporine, and thalidomide have also been used in the treatment of Sweet's syndrome.

# PYODERMA GANGRENOSUM

This is an ulcerative skin disease wherein single or multiple ulcers develop rapidly, either spontaneously or in response to cutaneous trauma. This is considered as a cutaneous marker of systemic disease.

First described by Brunsting et al. in 1930, in a series of patients with ulcerative colitis, the term "pyoderma gangrenosum" is a misnomer as it is not a pyoderma due to bacteria nor does it lead to gangrene, but the term has remained historically well entrenched in medical literature.

Greenbaum, in 1941, suggested that phagedena geometrica first used by Brocq, in 1916, may be a more appropriate term to describe this condition as phagedena refers to a burrowing and spreading purulent dissolution of superficial dermal layers, a situation of veracity in PG and not gangrene which refers to necrosis en masse.

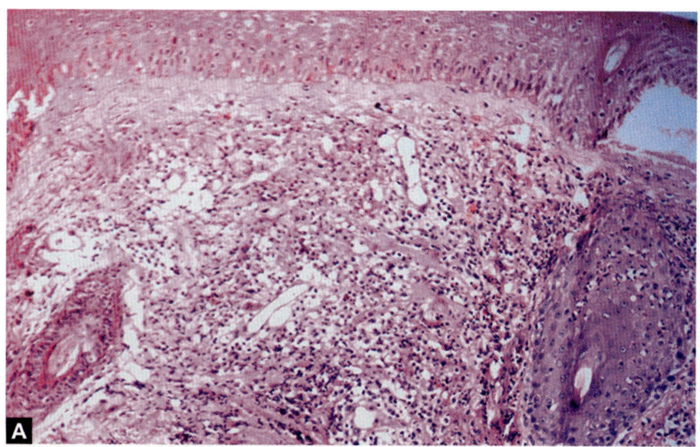
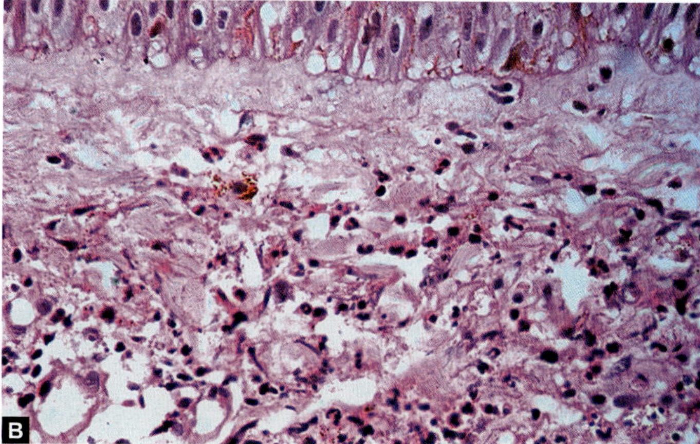

**FIG. 2: A,** Sweet's syndrome showing dense diffuse infiltrate of neutrophils in the upper and mid-dermis. (H&E, 100x); **B,** Sweets syndrome, diffuse infiltrate of neutrophils in upper dermis. (H&E, 400x).

## Epidemiology

Pyoderma gangrenosum occurs most commonly during the third to fifth decades of life although cases have been described in young children as well as patients in their ninth decade. Females are slightly more affected than males and the disease has been described from all over the world.

## Pathogenesis

Although the precise pathogenesis is not known immunological factors, impaired phagocytosis, and abnormal neutrophil trafficking are important factors in the etiopathogenesis. IL-8, which is a potent leukocyte chemotactic agent, is overexpressed. *IL-16* gene and the IL-16 protein are strongly chemotactic to neutrophils and are increased in the "PAPA syndrome" (pyogenic arthritis, pyoderma gangrenosum, and acne). These patients have mutations in the gene encoding CD2 binding protein that leads to abnormal inflammatory responses.

Genetic predisposition is suggested. Several drugs such as propylthiouracil, pegfilgrastim (granulocyte-stimulating factor), gefitinib (epidermal growth factor receptor inhibitor), and isotretinoin are known to be associated with induction of PG.

## Clinical Presentation

Ulcers occur mostly on the extremities and mimic those caused by infection, malignancy, vasculitis, diabetes, trauma, and collagen vascular diseases, and which is why PG is often a diagnosis of exclusion.

The primary lesion in usually a pustule that often is related to a hair follicle and may be single or in small clusters. These pustules rapidly undergo erosion and central necrosis and start extending rapidly at the periphery, giving rise to multiple serpiginous ulcers of varying sizes (1–2 cm to large ulcers that may involve the entire extremity or large part of the abdomen) with well-defined blue-red, shaggy, and extensively undermined edge. Pustules and sometimes bullae are seen at the margins. The advancing undermined edge shows a peripheral rim of erythema. The base of the ulcer is covered by purulent debris. Pathergy, i.e., ulcers developing at sites of minor skin trauma such as sites of venipuncture, infections, and surgical incision, is seen in almost 40% of patients.

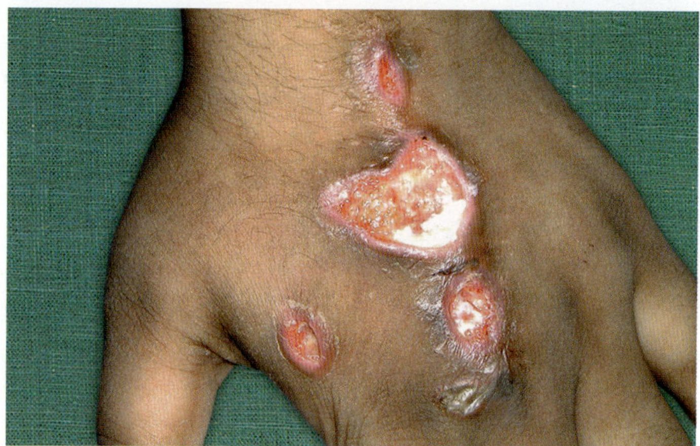

**FIG. 3:** Pyoderma gangrenosum affecting the dorsum of hand.

Pyoderma gangrenosum is most commonly seen on the legs with the pretibial area—the most commonly affected site, but has also been reported on other body sites like the breast, hands (Fig. 3), trunk, head, and neck, with special predilection for peristomal skin. Rarer sites include scrotum (Fig. 4), vulva, tongue, buccal mucosa, and external auditory canal. Extracutaneous manifestations include involvement of eyes, upper airway mucosa, sterile pulmonary infiltrates, involvement of the spleen and neutrophilic myositis. Sterile cortical osteolysis of bone has also been reported.

Pain and tenderness are common and relief from pain is an early sign of healing. Malaise and low-grade fever may occur.

The natural history follows two typical courses—acute rapidly progressive or a chronic long-term course of weeks to months. The ulcers heal with paper-thin atrophic or cribriform scars with hypo- or hyperpigmentation. Repeated cycles of ulceration and healing can occur over months or decades (Fig. 5).

Four major clinical forms of the disease are recognized:

- *Classic (ulcerative) type*: As described above
- *Vesiculobullous or atypical form of PG*: The clinical picture overlaps with the bullous variant of Sweet's syndrome and occurs commonly in association with acute myelogenous leukemia and myeloproliferative diseases. The lesions are vesiculobullous and occur mostly on the dorsae of hands and the face (Fig. 6)

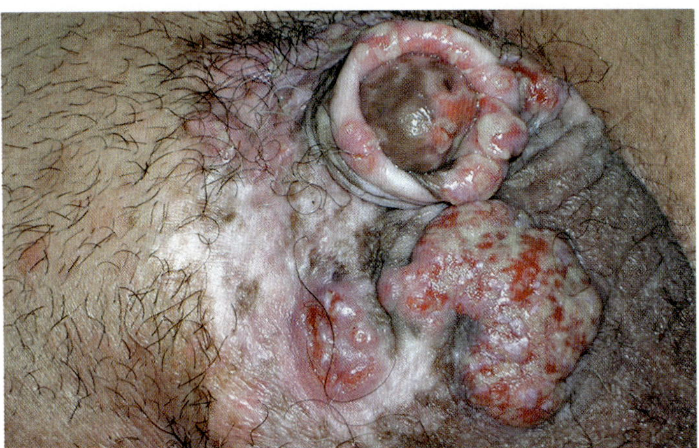

FIG. 4: Pyoderma gangrenosum affecting scrotum and penis.

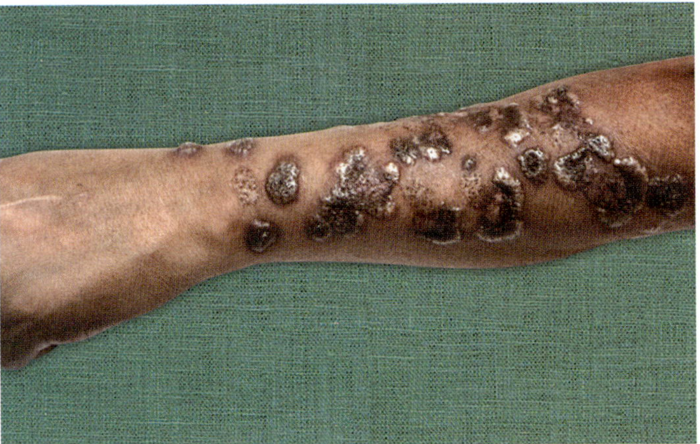

FIG. 5: Superficial scarring pyoderma gangrenosum-ulcers and cribriform scars on forearm.

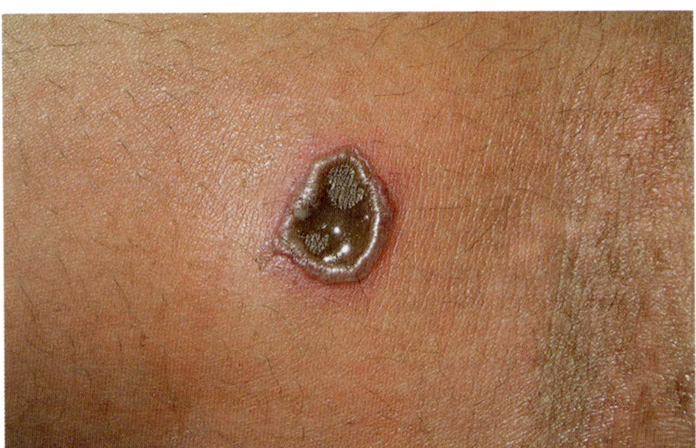

FIG. 6: Early bullous pyoderma gangrenosum.

- Pustular PG presents with multiple small sterile pustules which clear without scarring but may in some cases evolve into classic PG. This type is most often associated with inflammatory bowel disease, BD or bowel-associated dermatitis-arthritis syndrome
- Superficial granulomatous PG has localized, superficial vegetative lesions with a less intense neutrophilic infiltrate but may show localized granulomas.

Pyostomatitis vegetans is considered by some to be a variant of PG with chronic vegetative lesions of the labial and buccal mucosae and associated with inflammatory bowel disease.

## Prognosis and Follow-up

More than 50% of patients with PG tend to have recurrent or chronic disease and need long-term treatment and follow-up.

## Pyoderma Gangrenosum and Systemic Diseases

Almost 50–70% of patients have an associated systemic disease, with PG developing either before, coincidently or subsequent to the disease. Inflammatory bowel disease (ulcerative colitis, Crohn's disease), arthritis (seronegative arthritis, spondylitis, rheumatoid arthritis), hematologic diseases (acute or chronic myelogenous leukemia, hairy cell leukemia, myelodysplasia, and monoclonal gammopathy). In some patients, a good correlation exists between severity and activity of inflammatory bowel disease and skin ulcerations.

## Diagnosis

Diagnosis of PG is often one of exclusion and depends principally on the medical history and the clinical examination of the patient. No specific histologic or laboratory features of this disease have been demonstrated (Figs 7 to 9).

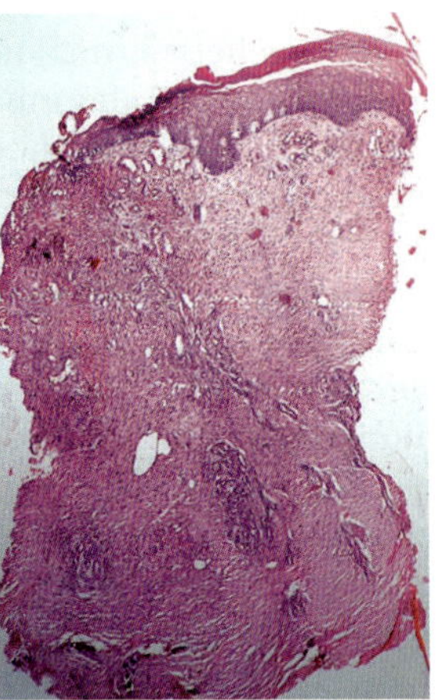

FIG. 7: Pyoderma gangrenosum. Low power (H&E, 20x).

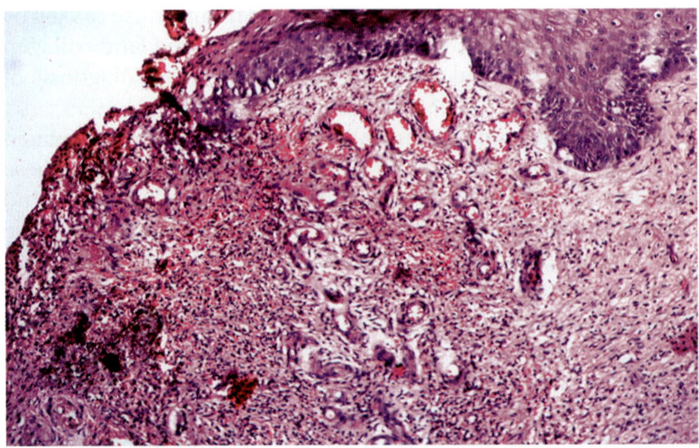

FIG. 8: Pyoderma gangrenosum. Ulcer with neutrophils in upper dermis with angiomatous blood vessels.

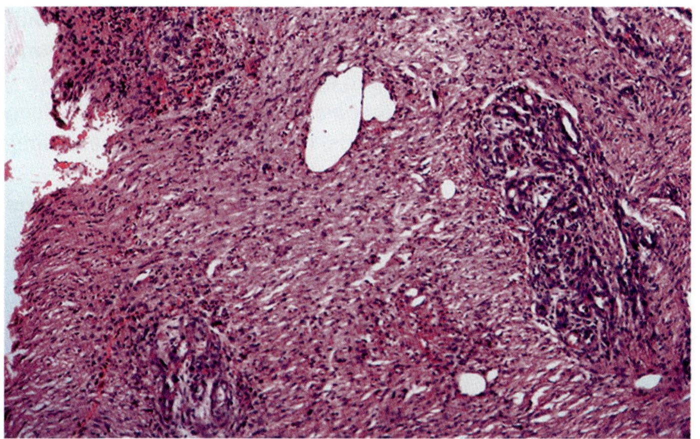

FIG. 9: Pyoderma gangrenosum. Neutrophils and lower and mid dermal fibrosis. (H&E, 400x).

### Criteria for Diagnosis of Pyoderma Gangrenosum

#### *Major Criteria*

- Rapidly progressive painful, necrolytic ulcer with irregular, violaceous undermined borders
- Exclusion of other causes of cutaneous ulceration.

#### *Minor Criteria*

- History of pathergy, clinical finding of cribriform scarring
- Presence of systemic diseases known to be associated with PG
- Histological findings of sterile dermal neutrophilia
- Rapid response to systemic corticosteroids.

## Treatment

Search for underlying systemic disease is important as effective control of that is often linked to healing of the cutaneous ulcerations.

Topical therapy may be attempted in small nonprogressive ulcers with local wound care and dressing, use of superpotent corticosteroids like clobetasol proprionate or calcineurin inhibitors like tacrolimus or pimecrolimus.

Large progressive ulcers with severe pain and morbidity need systemic treatment and oral steroids in the dose of 0.5–1 mg/kg of prednisolone are often the first choice. High-dose pulse steroids with 1 g daily of methylprednisolone are also used. Other systemic drugs include cyclosporine A, mycophenolate mofetil, azathioprine, and dapsone. Thalidomide may be tried if the previously mentioned agents do not control the disease. Tumor necrosis factor-alpha inhibitors like infliximab and others have been tried with good results.

Surgery should as far as possible be avoided in cases of PG as it only tends to worsen the ulceration. Development of new lesions of PG may occur at donor sites of skin grafts taken for skin grafting.

Skin injury should be minimized in patients who tend to have strong pathergy responses. Management of underlying systemic diseases is important to reduce morbidity associated with chronic and persistent ulcerations of PG.

# BEHCET'S DISEASE (ADAMANTIADES-BEHCET'S DISEASE)

Behcet's disease is a complex multisystem disease that shows a genetic predisposition and geographically restricted presentation. Probably mentioned by Hippocrates, it was first described in detail from Turkey in 1937 by Hulusi Behcet who described three cases of recurrent orogenital ulcers with uveitis. Similar cases had earlier been described by Adamantiades so it is also known as Adamantiades-Behcet's disease.

## Epidemiology

Behcet's disease is seen most commonly in the Middle East and is endemic in populations along the historic silk route which extended from East Asia to the Mediterranean basin. It has a strong association with HLA-B51 antigen with a relative risk ranging from 1.38 to 20.70. In the Middle East, young men are most often affected while a slight female predominance has been noted in Japan and Korea. The typical age of onset is in the third and fourth decade of life. Prevalence is estimated to range from a low of 0.3 per 100,000 in Northern Europe to a high of 110–420 per 100,000 in Turkey (highest). Environment too seems to have some effect on the incidence of the disease and migrants from high endemic areas like the Middle East to Europe or North America show lower incidence rates than in their home countries.

## Pathogenesis

An autoimmune process is possibly triggered by an infectious or environmental agent in a genetically predisposed individual. HLA-B51 is strongly associated. There is enhanced neutrophil activation, superoxide release, abnormal neutrophil function. Tissue neutrophilia is seen in the pathergy reactions, pustular folliculitis and orogenital ulcerations. Levels of IL-12 are elevated which leads to Th1 type of T-cell differentiation leading to increased levels of IL-2 and interferons.

Infectious agents both viruses (herpes simplex type 1, parvovirus B19, hepatitis, *Cytomegalovirus, Epstein-Barr virus*) and bacteria (*Streptococcus sanguis, Saccharomyces cerevisiae*, mycobacteria, *B. burgdorferi, H. pylori, E. coli*, and *Mycoplasma fermentans*) may be involved in the pathogenesis of BD. It has been proposed that bacterial antigens such as heat shock proteins are fairly homologous to human counterparts leading to autoimmune pathology due to molecular mimicry.

## Pathology

Two main patterns of inflammation are seen in BD, perivascular and interstitial, and folliculo-centric.

Immune-mediated vasculitis is now considered to be the most common pathology in BD and leukocytoclastic vasculitis with fibrinoid necrosis of postcapillary venules or perivascular neutrophilic accumulations are common in cutaneous lesions of BD.

Papulopustular lesions seen in Behcet's too may show features of vasculitis which helps in differentiating them from folliculocentric papulopustules seen in acne. Intraepidermal and intrafollicular pustules, spongiosis, neutrophil or lymphocyte exocytosis, basal cell vacuolization, dermal edema, and lymphohistiocytic and neutrophilic infiltrates both perivascular and interstitial between collagen fibers are reported as findings in cutaneous lesions of BD.

## Clinical Features

Several mucocutaneous lesions occur in BD and are pointers to the diagnosis.

- Oral apthae are usually the initial clinical manifestation but may be present for several years till the diagnosis of BD is finally made (Pre-diagnostic phase). Recurrent apthous ulcers (RAU) are not specific for BD and for diagnosis of BD; patient should have at least three recurrences in 1 year
- Genital ulcers occur in the majority of patients and are usually larger than oral apthae. Common sites of ulceration are scrotum and shaft of penis in men and labia majora and minora in women. They have irregular borders, are usually deep and heal with scarring. Fistulae extending to the urethra or bladder may form
- *Extragenital ulcers*: Rare and seen in about 3% of BD patients, mostly in children. They occur on the legs, neck and interdigital areas, and are painful and persist for several weeks
- *Erythema nodosum-like lesions*: Painful erythematous nodules occur mainly on legs but also on face and neck and are more common in women. Histologically may show vasculitis and necrobiosis and there is a spectrum of histopathologic changes similar to that seen in typical erythema nodosum which includes lymphocytic vasculitis, septal panniculitis, and even lobular panniculitis with fat necrosis
- *Papulopustular lesions*: These are the most common cutaneous lesions in BD and occur on the trunk, face, and extremities and also develop due to vasculitis. They present as papular lesions on erythematous base progressing to sterile pustules and on the face are similar to inflammatory lesions of acne
- *Thrombophlebitis*: Multiple vessels may be affected and several discrete nodules may develop at different locations over a period of time or sequentially. Superficial thrombophlebitis may coexist with major vessel vasculitis and thrombosis. Large vessel vasculitis occurs in a subgroup of patients with BD. These *vasculo-Behcet's* patients are at risk for multiple vessel-related complications including thromboses, stenoses, occlusions, and aneurysms. The primary reason for clot formation is an inflammatory process in affected vessel walls
- *Other cutaneous lesions*: Other lesions described in BD include erythema multiforme like, polyarteritis nodosa like, pernio like, Sweet's syndrome, necrotizing folliculitis, and necrotizing small vessel vasculitis
- *Pathergy reaction*: Pathergy is one of the diagnostic criteria for BD and may indicate active disease
- *Nailfold abnormalities* are seen in a large percentage of BD patients and include enlarged capillaries and nailfold hemorrhages which may be seen on nailfold capillaroscopy.

## Systemic Manifestations of Behcet's Disease

- *Ophthalmic manifestations*: Occur in 70–85% of patients. Most common is uveitis but vitreous deposits, choroiditis, and retinitis with reduction of visual acuity are also seen
- *Joint involvement*: Seronegative arthritis is common with monoarticular synovitis of knee. Ankylosing spondylitis and sacroiliitis also occur in up to a third of patients
- *Vascular and cardiac involvement*: Superficial and deep thrombophlebitis. Pericarditis, cardiomyopathy, aneurysms, endocardiac fibrosis, and vasculitis of coronary arteries
- *Pulmonary*: Pleural effusions, pulmonary embolism, and fibrosis
- *Renal*: Rare but may show glomerulonephritis and systemic amyloidosis
- *Gastrointestinal*: Ulcerative lesions in terminal ileum and cecum
- *Neurologic and psychiatric*: Meningoencephalitis, mononeuritis multiplex, cranial nerve palsies, and hemiplegia. Fibromyalgia, migraine, anxiety, and depression may occur in more than 50% of patients and stressful events may trigger the psychological complications.

## Diagnosis

No specific tests are useful. Diagnostic criteria have been defined by an International Study Group.

*Major criterion*: Recurrent oral ulceration observed by physician or patient that recurred at least 3 times in one 12-month period.

Plus, at least two of the following criteria:

- Recurrent genital ulcerations
- *Eye lesions*: Anterior uveitis, posterior uveitis, cells in vitreous, and retinal vasculitis.
- *Cutaneous lesions*: Erythema nodosum, pseudofolliculitis, papulopustular lesions, and acneiform nodules in post-adolescent patients not on corticosteroid treatment.
- Positive pathergy test
  Zouboulis et al. in 2007 presented revised criteria wherein a score of 3 points was necessary for the diagnosis of BD
- *Oral aphthae*: 1 point
- *Cutaneous manifestations*: (pseudofolliculitis, cutaneous apthae) 1 point
- *Vascular lesions*: (phlebitis, venous thrombosis, aneurysm, arterial thrombosis) 1 point
- *Positive pathergy test*: 1 point
- *Genital apthae*: 2 points
- *Typical eye involvement*: 2 points.

## Treatment

Treatment of oral ulcers is usually symptomatic with maintenance of oral hygiene. Topical anesthetics may be used. Tacrolimus ointment, cyclosporine solution, and sucralfate suspension may be used instead of steroids.

For patients with systemic involvement or with severe orogenital ulcers oral prednisolone (1 mg/kg), colchicine 1–2 mg/day, dapsone 100–200 mg/day, thalidomide 100–300 mg/day, cyclosporine 5 mg/kg, azathioprine 2 mg/kg may be tried.

## Prognosis

Chronic recurrent painful oral and genital ulceration or blindness due to eye complications leads to severe morbidity. The disease is more severe in HLA-B51-positive men and death may occur in up to 6% of patients. The prognosis is poor if there is severe involvement of central nervous system, lungs, or great arteries.

## NEUTROPHILIC DERMATOSIS OF THE DORSAL HANDS

Strutton et al. in 1995 described under the term pustular vasculitis of the hands, 6 patients with lesions resembling Sweet's syndrome restricted to the dorsum of hands.

There is definite histological features of leukocytoclastic vasculitis in many but not all. Thus, the term neutrophilic dermatosis of the dorsal hands (NDDH) was proposed and it has been suggested that this is localized subset of Sweet's syndrome.

Features in common with Sweet's syndrome include predominance in females, fever, positive pathergy, neutrophilia at time of eruption, and association with inflammatory bowel disease. Clinically, patients present with severely painful plaques and nodules with frequent ulceration and postulation involving predominantly the dorsum of hands. Few lesions have been reported to occur at other sites but the predominant involvement is of the dorsum of hands. Response to systemic antibiotics is usually poor, but a rapid response to systemic corticosteroids is the rule. Recurrences are common.

Biopsy shows dense dermal infiltrates of neutrophils with subepidermal edema similar to Sweet's syndrome (Fig. 10); however, many cases also show in addition abundant neutrophilic nuclear dust and fibrinoid necrosis of vessel walls resembling a true leukocytoclastic vasculitis. Epidermal changes of spongiosis with exocytosis of neutrophils and even intraepidermal pustules may be seen.

## NEUTROPHILIC ECCRINE HIDRADENITIS

Neutrophilic eccrine hidradenitis (NEH) was first described as a distinctive neutrophilic dermatosis associated with chemotherapy for myelogenous leukemia with selective infiltration of eccrine glands with neutrophils leading to eccrine gland necrosis. Subsequently, the term "toxic erythema of chemotherapy" was proposed as it was seen in patients with other malignancies undergoing chemotherapy. It has also been described to occur in patients without malignancies or on chemotherapy and also in children and as a recurrent eruption.

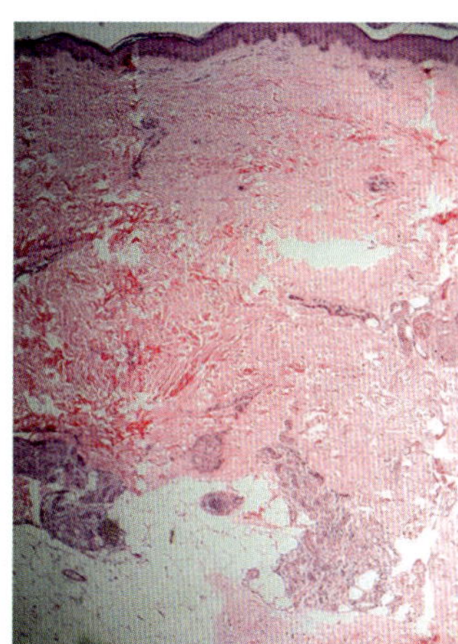

**FIG. 10:** Neutrophilic eccrine hidradenitis, Eccrine glands in deep dermis (H&E, 40x).

### Pathogenesis

The possible pathogenetic mechanisms for NEH include:

- Direct toxic effects of chemotherapeutic agents that may be secreted by or concentrated in the eccrine glands or a generalized reaction to the chemotherapeutic agent
- Abnormal neutrophil functions leading to eccrine gland damage by neutrophils.

Neutrophilic eccrine hidradenitis may be considered to be a disease localized to eccrine glands in the broader spectrum of neutrophilic dermatoses.

### Clinical Features

Most patients have fever followed by appearance of erythematous edematous papules and plaques on the extremities and flexures with a spontaneous resolution after few weeks. Lesions may be purpuric or resemble cellulitis, especially on the face. NEH needs to be differentiated from Sweet's syndrome, other drug reactions urticarial vasculitis and erythema nodosum, if restricted to the legs.

### Histological Findings

There are presence around and infiltration of eccrine glands by neutrophils with eccrine gland necrosis. The density of neutrophils is variable and in neutropenic patients may be sparse but will be accompanied by necrosis of eccrine glands (Figs 11 and 12).

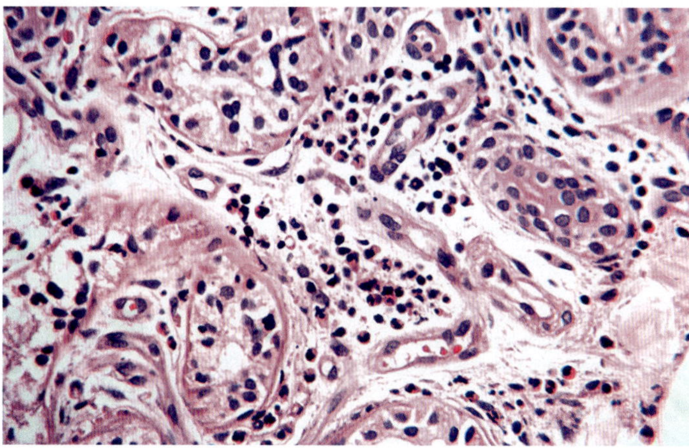

**FIG. 11:** Neutrophilic eccrine hidradenitis, neutrophils surrounding eccrine glands. (H&E, 200x).

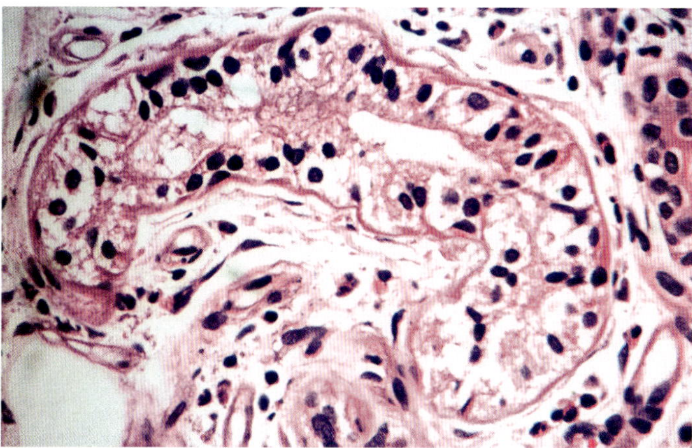

**FIG. 12:** Neutrophilic eccrine hidradenitis, eccrine gland necrosis. (H&E, 400x).

## Treatment and Prognosis

In general, NEH is a self-limiting condition and resolves after the underlying condition has been successfully treated. Oral corticosteroids give rapid resolution of the condition. Dapsone has been tried in a case with recurrent episodes of NEH.

## SUGGESTED READINGS


1. Azizlerli G, Ozarmagan G, Ovul C, et al. A new kind of skin lesion in Behcet's disease: extragenital ulcerations. Acta Dermato-Venereologica. 1992;72:286-8.
2. Behcet H. Uber rezidiveirende aphthose durch ein virus verursachte Geschwure am Mund am Auge und an den Genitalien. Dermatologische Wochenschrift. 1937;105:1152-7.
3. Bolognia JL, Cooper DL, Glusac EJ. Toxic erythema of chemotherapy: A useful clinical term. J Am Acad Dermatol. 2008;59:524-9.
4. Brunsting LA, Goeckermann WH, O'Leary PA. Pyoderma (echthyma) gangrenosum-clinical and experimental observation in five cases occurring in adults. Arch Dermatol. 1930;22:655-80.
5. Calamia KT, Schirmer M, Melikoglu M. Major vessel involvement in Behcet's disease: An update. Curr Opin Rheumatol. 2011;23:24-31.
6. Chun SI, Su WPD, Lee S, et al. Erythema nodosum-like lesions in Behcet's syndrome: A histopathologic study of 30 cases. J Cut Pathol. 1989;16:259-65.
7. Clarke DM. Pyoderma gangrenosum: Discussion of the literature and report of a case and another probable case. Australas J Dermatol. 1955;3:19-26.
8. Cohen PR, Talpaz M, Kurzrock R. Malignancy-associated Sweet' syndrome: review of the world literature. J Clin Oncol. 1988;6:1887-97.
9. Cohen PR. Pregnancy-associated Sweet's syndrome: world literature review. Obstet Gynecol Surv. 1993;48:584-7.
10. Criteria for diagnosis of Behcet's disease. International Study Group for Behcet's disease. Lancet. 1990;335:1078-80.
11. Galaria NA, Junkins-Hopkins JM, Kligman D, et al. Neutrophilic dermatosis of the dorsal hands: Pustular vasculitis revisited. J Am Acad Dermatol. 2000;43:870-4.
12. Giasuddin AS, El-Orfi AH, Ziu MM, et al. Sweet's syndrome: is the pathogenesis mediated by helper T cell type 1 cytokines? J Am Acad Dermatol. 1998;39:940-3.
13. Harrist TJ, Fine JD, Berman RS, et al. Neutrophilic eccrine hidradenitis: a distinctive type of neutrophilic dermatosis associated with myelogenous leukemia and chemotherapy. Arch Dermatol. 1982;118:263-6.
14. Jorizzo JL, Abernathy JL, White WL, et al. Mucocutaneous criteria for the diagnosis of Behcet's disease: An analysis of clinic-pathologic data from multiple international centres. J Am Acad Dermatol. 1995;32:968-76.
15. Kalkan G, Karadag AS, Astarci HM, et al. A histopathological approach: when papulopustular lesions should be in the diagnostic criteria of Behcet's disease? J European Acad Dermatol Venereol. 2009;23:1056-60.
16. Kawakami T, Ohashi S, Kawa Y, et al. Elevated serum granulocyte colony stimulating factor levels in patients with active phase of Sweet's syndrome and patients with active Behcet's disease: implication in neutrophil apoptosis dysfunction. Arch Dermatol. 2004;140:570-4.
17. Kemmet D, Harrison DJ, Hunter JM. Antibodies to neutrophil cytoplasmic antigens: a serological marker for Sweet's syndrome. J Am Acad Dermatol. 1991;24:967-9.
18. Kemmett D, Hunter JA. Sweet's syndrome: a clinic-pathological review of twenty-nine cases. J Am Acad Dermatol. 1990;23:503-7.
19. Lee WJ, Kim CH, Chang SE, et al. Generalized idiopathic neutrophilic eccrine hidradenitis in childhood. Int J Dermatol. 2010;49:75-8.
20. MacCormack M, Phillips T. Behcet's disease: A Clinical Review. Wounds. 2002;14:8.
21. Movasat A, Shahram F, Carreira PE, et al. Nailfold capillaroscopy in Behcet's disease: Analysis of 128 patients. Clin Rheumatol. 2009;28:603-5.
22. Mutlu S, Scully C. The person behind the eponym: Hulusi Behcet (1889-1948). J Oral Pathol Med. 1994;23:289-90.
23. Newell LM, Malkinson FD. Commentary: Pyoderma gangrenosum. Arch Dermatol. 1982;118:769-73.
24. Requena L, Kutzner H, Palmedo G, et al. Histiocytoid Sweet syndrome: a dermal infiltration of immature neutrophilic granulocytes. Arch Dermatol. 2005;141:834-42.
25. Ruocco E, Sangiuliano S, Gravina AG, et al. Pyoderma gangrenosum: An updated review. J Eur Acad Dermatol Venereol. 2009;23:1008-17.
26. Saigal R, Singh Y, Mittal M, et al. Pyoderma Gangrenosum. J Assoc Physicians India. 2010;58:378-83.
27. Shear NH, Knowles SR, Shapiro L, et al. Dapsone in prevention of recurrent neutrophilic eccrine hidradenitis. J Am Acad Dermatol. 1996;35:819-22.
28. Strutton G, Weedon D, Robertson I. Pustular vasculitis of the hands. J Am Acad Dermatol. 1995;32:192-8.
29. Su WP, Davis MD, Weenig RH, et al. Pyoderma gangrenosum: Clinico-pathologic correlation and proposed diagnostic criteria. Int J Dermatol. 2004;43:790-800.
30. Su WPD, Liu HNH. Diagnostic criteria for Sweet's syndrome. Cutis. 1986;37:167-74.
31. Sweet RD. An acute febrile neutrophilic dermatosis. Br J Dermatol. 1964;76:349-56.
32. Tinoci MP, Tamler C, Maciel G, et al. Pyoderma gangrenosum following isotretinoin therapy for nodulocystic acne. Int J Dermatol. 2008;47:953-6.
33. Verity DH, Marr JE, Ohno S, et al. Behcet's disease, the Silk Road and HLA-B51: Historial and geographical perspectives. Tissue Antigens. 1999;54:213-20.
34. Voelter-Mahlknecht S, Bauer J, Metzler G, et al. Bullous variant of Sweet's syndrome. Int J Dermatol. 2005;44:946-7.
35. Von den Driesch P, Manfred FA, Weber MU. Are antibodies to neutrophilic cytoplasmic antigens (ANCA) a serologic marker for Sweet' syndrome? J Am Acad Dermatol. 1993;29:666.
36. Von Den Driesch P. Pyoderma gangrenosum: a report of 44 cases with follow up. Br J Dermatol. 1997;137:1000-5.
37. Walker DC, Cohen PR. Trimethoprim-sulfamethoxazole-associated acute febrile neutrophilic dermatosis: Case report and review of drug-induced Sweet's syndrome. J Am Acad Dermatol. 1996;34:918-23.
38. Walling HW, Snipes CJ, Gerami P, et al. The relationship between neutrophilic dermatosis of the dorsal hands and sweet syndrome: report of 9 cases and comparison to atypical pyoderma gangrenosum. Arch Dermatol. 2006;142:57-63.
39. Whittle CH, Beck GA, Champion RH. Recurrent neutrophilic dermatosis of the face-a variant of Sweet's syndrome. Br J Dermatol. 1968;80:806-10.
40. Yoon TY, Ahn GB, Yang TH, et al. Sweet's syndrome with abscess-like lesions in a patient with acute myelogenous leukemia. J Dermatol. 2000;27:794-7.
41. Zouboulis CC, Schirmer M, Baltac M, et al. Evaluation and revision of the International Criteria for Behcet's disease. Abstract at the 21st World Congress of Dermatology. Buenos Aires, Argentina: World Congress of Dermatology; 2007.

# 36 CHAPTER Histiocytic Disorders of Skin

*Uday Khopkar, Atul Dongre*

## INTRODUCTION

Histiocytoses are rare and constitute a diverse group of disorders that include benign, self-healing as well as malignant conditions. The current concept of histiocytoses includes disorders arising from cells of monocyte/macrophage series or Langerhan cell ( dendritic cell) series or lymphocytes (malignant histiocytosis). Both macrophages and Langerhans or dendritic cells arise from bone marrow (CD34 stem cells).

Exact incidence of histiocytosis in India is not known. According to the Histiocytosis Association of America, 1 in 200,000 children in the United States are born with histiocytosis each year. Large number of patients affected with histiocytosis are children under the age of 10 years and it is rarely seen in adults.

## CLASSIFICATION

Various classifications have been proposed for this diverse group of disorders.

Broadly, histiocytoses may be divided into the following groups:

- X-type histiocytoses (characterized by infiltrates of Langerhans cells)
- Non-X histiocytoses (characterized by infiltrates of monocytes or macrophages).

### X-type Histiocytosis

X-type histiocytoses are group of cutaneous syndromes characterized by infiltrates of Langerhans cells.

Following conditions have been described:

- Letterer–Siwe disease
- Hand–Schüller–Christian disease
- Eosinophilic granuloma
- Congenital self-healing reticulohistiocytosis.

Of these, the first three conditions can overlap clinically.

### Non-X Histiocytosis

Non-X histiocytoses are group of cutaneous syndromes characterized by infiltrates of monocytes or macrophages, as opposed to X-type histiocytoses in which the infiltrates contain Langerhans cells as predominant cells.

Various conditions included under non-X histiocytosis:

- Juvenile xanthogranuloma (JXG)
- Benign cephalic histiocytosis
- Generalized eruptive histiocytoma
- Xanthoma disseminatum (XD)
- Progressive nodular histiocytosis
- Papular xanthoma
- Hereditary progressive mucinous histiocytosis
- Reticulohistiocytosis
- Indeterminate cell histiocytosis
- Sea-blue histiocytosis
- Erdheim–Chester disease.

### World Health Organization: Histiocytosis Classification

#### Class I

- Langerhans cell histiocytosis (LCH)
- Histiocytosis of mononuclear phagocytes other than Langerhans cells.

#### Class II

- Familial and reactive hemophagocytic lymphohistiocytosis (HLH)
- Sinus histiocytosis with massive lymphadenopathy (SHML or Rosai–Dorfman disease)
- Juvenile xanthogranuloma
- Reticulohistiocytoma.

#### Class III

- Malignant histiocytic disorders
- Acute monocytic leukemia (FAB M5)
- Malignant histiocytosis
- True histiocytic lymphoma.

### Histiocyte Society: Histiocytosis Classification

The working group of the Histiocyte Society has divided histiocytic disorders into three groups: (1) dendritic cell histiocytosis; (2) macrophage-related disorders; and (3) malignant histiocytosis.

# X-TYPE HISTIOCYTOSIS

## Langerhans Cell Histiocytosis

Langerhans cell histiocytosis is a rare but most common amongst histiocytic disorders. Langerhans cells are derived from bone marrow and are capable of migrating from skin to lymph nodes. Clonal proliferation and accumulation of Langerhans cells occur manifesting as an isolated bone lesion to a multisystem disease.

In older days, the term histiocytosis X was used for this condition where the word "X" was used to indicate unknown origin of Langerhans cells. But, as origin of Langerhans cell has been proved, the term "Langerhans cell histiocytosis" is generally preferred to the older term, histiocytosis X.

### Prevalence

Langerhans cell histiocytosis usually affects children between 0 years and 15 years of age, with a peak incidence between 5 years and 10 years of age. Among children under the age of 10, yearly incidence is thought to be 1 in 200,000. It is very rare in adults. It is most prevalent in Caucasians, and occurrence is two times more in males as compared to females.

### Pathogenesis

The exact pathogenesis of LCH is a matter of debate. It is still under investigation to determine whether LCH is a reactive or neoplastic process. Activating mutation of a proto oncogene in the RAF family, the *BRAF* gene was detected in some patients. LCH is usually a sporadic and nonhereditary condition but familial clustering has been noted in a few cases.

### Clinical Subtypes of Langerhans Cell Histiocytosis

Langerhans cell histiocytosis encompasses a number of diseases. On one end, the clinical spectrum includes an acute, fulminant, and disseminated disease called Letterer-Siwe disease and, on the other end, solitary or few, indolent, and chronic lesions of bone or other organs called eosinophilic granulomas. The intermediate clinical form called Hand-Schüller-Christian disease is characterized by multifocal, chronic involvement. A congenital, self-healing form called Hashimoto-Pritzker disease has also been described.

Though clinical spectrum of LCH includes several clinical types, overlap of these types are known to occur.

- *Letterer-Siwe disease*: Occurs predominantly in children younger than 2 years. Cutaneous lesions are present in 80% of cases. Multiple scaly or crusted papular eruptions occur which may be accompanied with petechiae leading to hemorrhagic appearance to the papules. Lesions are seen on the scalp, retroauricular areas, face, and trunk. As lesions favor intertriginous areas, it may resemble seborrheic dermatitis or Darier's disease. Rarely, vesicles may be seen. Hemorrhagic papules or vesicles may also be seen over palms or soles and are a poor prognostic indicator. Nail involvement though uncommon is known to occur. Nails may show subungual purpuric streaks, hyperkeratosis, nail deformities, and loss of nail plate. Systemic involvement in the form of fever, anemia, thrombocytopenia due to bone marrow infiltration, hepatic and splenic enlargement, lymphadenopathy and pulmonary infiltrates may occur and carries bad prognosis. Osteolytic lesions in mastoid areas of temporal bone presents as otitis media
- *Hand-Schüller-Christian syndrome*: It is a chronic multifocal form of LCH. It has a peak of onset of disease in children aged 2–10 years. Exophthalmos, diabetes insipidus and osteolytic lesions in the skull bones form classic triad of Hand-Schüller-Christian syndrome. This classic triad is seen in only one-third of patients. Cutaneous lesions occur in one-third patients, and infiltrated nodules or plaques with ulceration in axillae, anogenital region, and mouth is a common cutaneous presentation. Osteolytic lesions occur commonly in cranial bone. Involvement of long bones leads to spontaneous fractures. Extensive eruptions similar to that in infants or xanthomatous lesions are uncommon cutaneous presentations
- *Eosinophilic granuloma*: This localized or chronic focal form of LCH occurs most frequently in children aged 5–15 years. As such, it commonly involves the bones, and cutaneous or mucosal involvement is occasionally seen. Involvement of jaw leading to loose or floating tooth is typical presentation. Bone lesions are sometimes seen eroding through the skin forming a nodule or nodulo-ulcerative lesion in the skin. Cutaneous lesions may heal spontaneously. Rarely cases initially presenting as localized lesion may progress to multifocal or disseminated disease. Hence, such patients with chronic focal LCH should be monitored for systemic involvement
- *Congenital self-healing reticulohistiocytosis (Hashimoto-Pritzker disease)*: It presents at birth or within few weeks after birth as scattered papules and nodules. Nodules break down in the center and form crater-shaped ulcers and heal leaving behind atrophy. In one-fourth of patients, single nodule may be seen. The involution of the lesions begins within 2–3 months and by the end of 12 months, complete regression may be noted. Though lesions are known to regress, in few cases relapses may occur and occasionally case may advance to acute disseminated disease.

## Diagnosis

Skin biopsy along with immunohistochemistry helps to confirm diagnosis.

Histopathological features of LCH can be divided into proliferative, granulomatous, and xanthomatous form. Depending upon the type of clinical lesion, histopathological features may vary. Acute disseminated LCH shows extensive infiltrate of Langerhans cells in the upper dermis (Figs 1 and 3). On light microscopy, Langerhans cells have folded or kidney-shaped nuclei and abundant amphophilic cytoplasm (Figs 2 and 4). Frequently, cells may be impinging upon the epidermis or even infiltrating it (Figs 5 and 6). Ulceration of the epidermis and crusting may be seen. Other cells like eosinophils and lymphocytes are common within the infiltrate.

Granulomatous reaction is seen in the infiltrated nodules and plaques as well as nodules in the internal organs and bones. Extensive infiltration of Langerhans cells with admixture of eosinophils, lymphocytes, plasma cells, neutrophils, and multinucleated giant cell formation is seen (Figs 7 and 8).

Congenital self-healing reticulohistiocytosis shows densely aggregated Langerhans cells with abundant eosinophilic cytoplasm. Giant cell formation is seen with some cells having ground glass appearance.

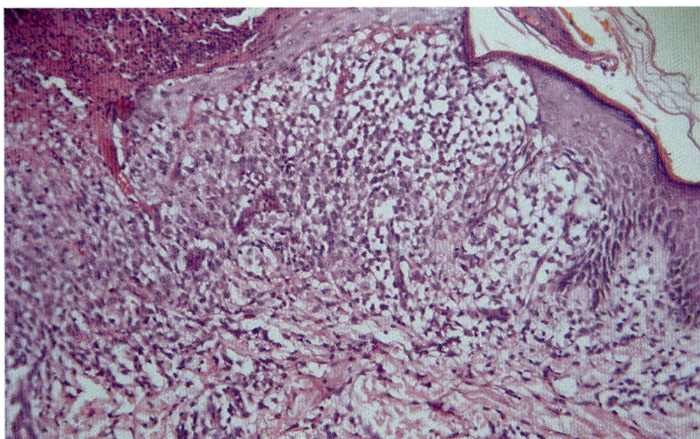

FIG. 1: Wedge-shaped infiltrate in the upper dermis. Epidermis shows ulceration with scale crust.

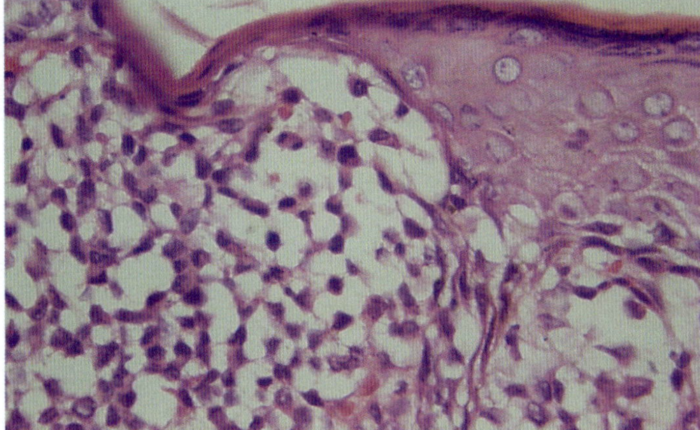

FIG. 2: Langerhans cells with ample amount of eosinophilic cytoplasm and reniform nuclei. (Higher power view of Fig. 1).

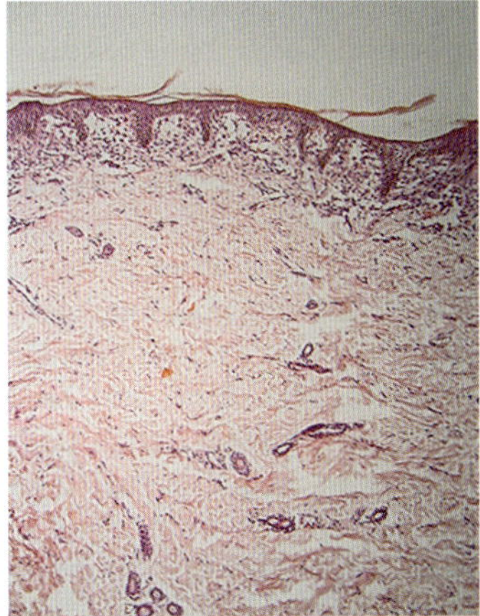

FIG. 3: Lichenoid infiltrate in the papillary dermis.

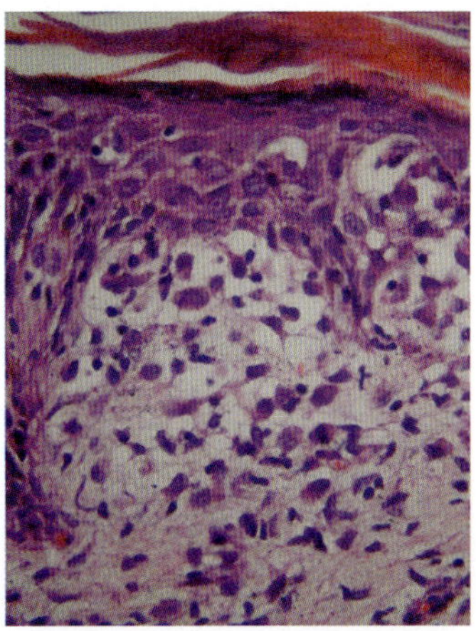

FIG. 4: Langerhans cells with ample amount of eosinophilic cytoplasm and reniform nuclei.

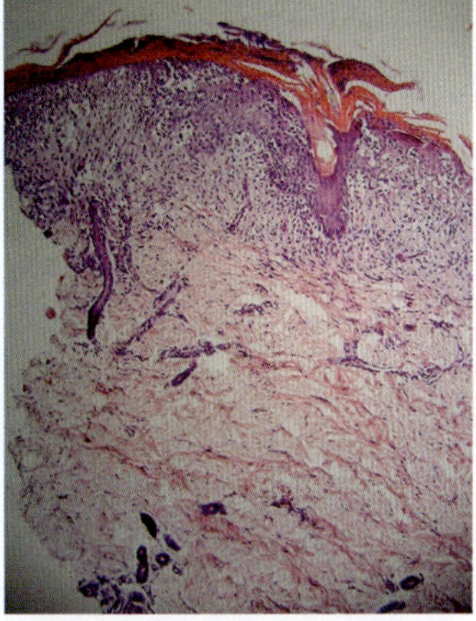

FIG. 5: Lichenoid infiltrate in papillary dermis. Also, cells are seen in the epidermis in pagetoid pattern.

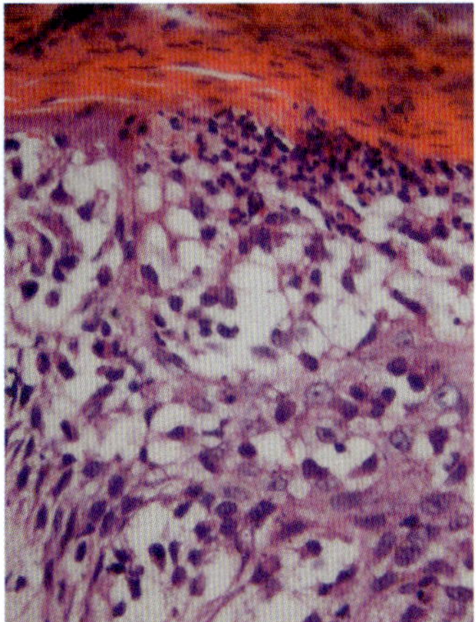

FIG. 6: Epidermotropism of Langerhans cells.

In xanthomatous pattern of LCH, admixture of foamy cells with Langerhans cells and eosinophils is seen in dermis.

On electron microscopy, rod-shaped or "tennis-racket" cytoplasmic organelles known as Birbeck granules are seen. Langerhans cells are positive for immunohistochemical markers like CD1a (Fig. 9) (specific marker) and S-100 (Fig. 10).

X-ray of bones may show osteolytic lesions. Chest X-ray in cases with pulmonary involvement shows nodular or interstitial infiltrates. In some cases, honeycomb appearance is seen. Magnetic resonance imaging and computed tomography scans may show infiltration in sella turcica. Assessment of endocrine function and bone marrow biopsy are needed to determine the extent and severity of disease.

## Treatment

Treatment is planned according to the extent of disease. For solitary skin or bone lesion excision, intralesional steroids, or

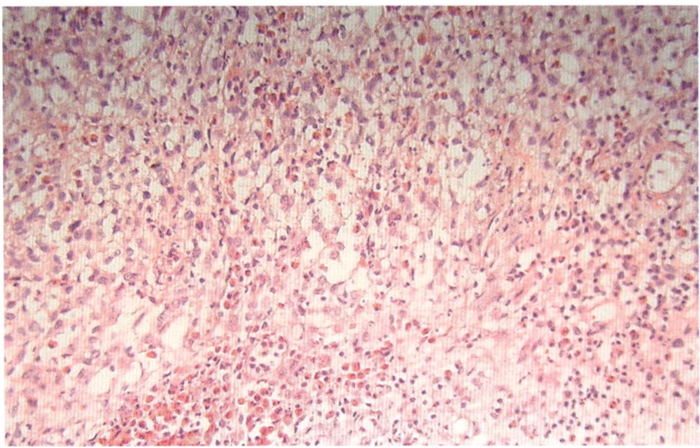

FIG. 7: Diffuse and dense infiltrate of Langerhans cells with many eosinophils.

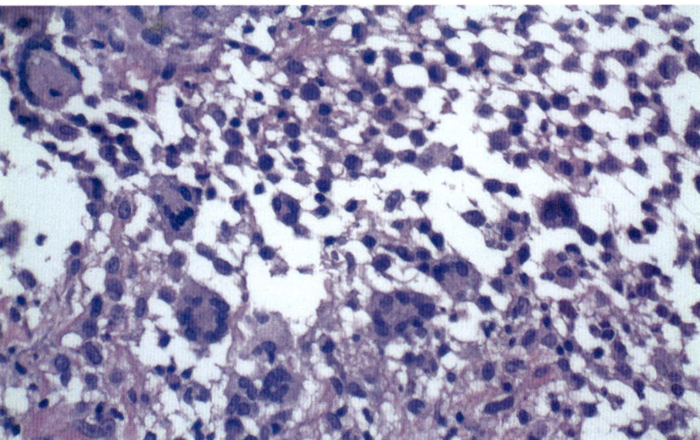

FIG. 8: Langerhans cells forming multinucleated giant cells giving granulomatous appearance.

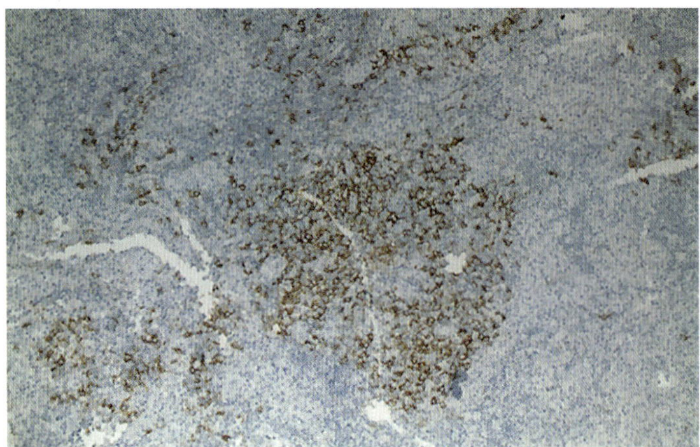

FIG. 9: Langerhans cells stained with CD1a stain.

radiation is used. For disease limited to skin, topical corticosteroids may be used. Visceral involvement often requires chemotherapy. Systemic steroids in combination with chemotherapeutic agents like methotrexate, etoposide, vinblastine, mercaptopurine, and cytarabine is effective. Bone marrow transplant may be helpful for cases with refractory LCH.

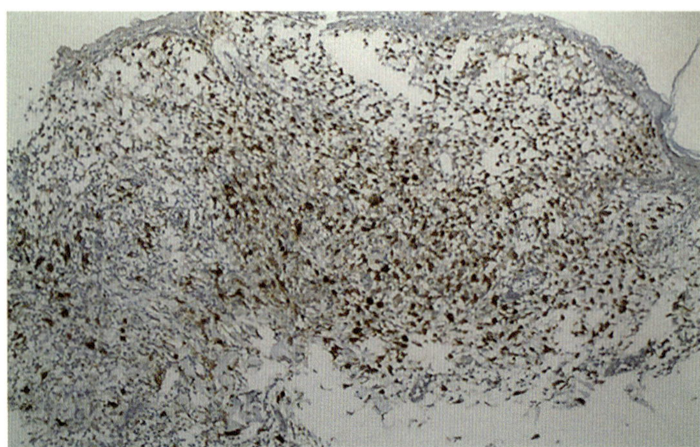

FIG. 10: Langerhans cells positive for S100 stain.

### Prognosis

Prognosis is excellent for cases with single focus of LCH. With multi focal disease, 60% have a chronic course, 30% achieve remission, and mortality is up to 10%. Bone marrow, extensive pulmonary involvement, liver and spleen involvement carry poor prognosis.

### Differential Diagnosis

Seborrheic dermatitis, juvenile xanthogranuloma, nodular scabies, xanthoma, and Darier disease.

## NON-LANGERHANS CELL HISTIOCYTOSIS

### Juvenile Xanthogranuloma

It is a benign and self-limiting non-Langerhans cell histiocytosis. It is the most common non-Langerhans cell disorder. JXG involves proliferation of a kind of histiocyte called dermal dendrocytes.

Juvenile xanthogranuloma mainly affects infants and small children with an average age of 2 years, although it can also occur in adults. In about 10–20% of cases, it is present since birth. It is more common in male children than in female children. Head and neck are the most common sites involved followed by trunk and extremities. Eighty percent of cases presents as single lesion. Asymptomatic, round to oval, firm, and reddish to yellowish nodules of size 0.5–1 cm are seen (small nodular form). Large nodular (1–2 cm) or giant-form (>2 cm) lesion has also been reported. Some cases may have both small and large nodular lesions. Spontaneous regression of skin lesions occurs over a period of few years in children but in adults, lesions usually persist; though uncommon extracutaneous lesions may occur along with skin lesions or as only visceral involvement. JXG can affect the eye, most commonly in young children with multiple skin lesions. Less commonly, JXG may involve locations such as the lung, liver, adrenal gland, appendix, bones, bone marrow, pituitary gland, central nervous system, kidney, heart, small and large intestines, and spleen. Oral lesions involving tongue, palate, and lips has been reported. Ocular lesions may lead to glaucoma and bleeding into anterior chamber so ocular screening is recommended for all children with multiple cutaneous lesions before the age of 2 years.

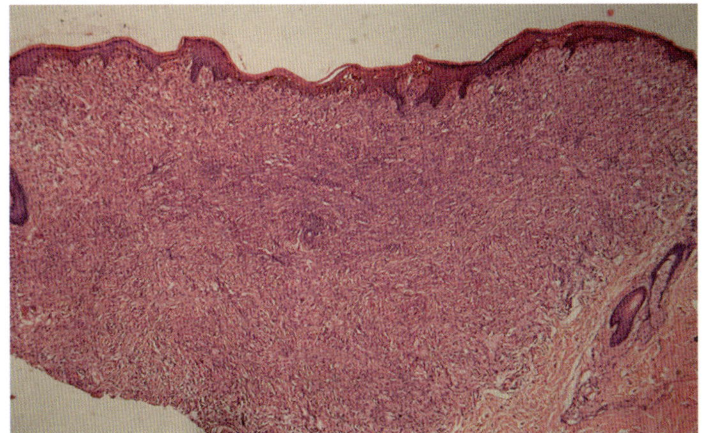

FIG. 11: Dense and diffuse infiltrate of pale histiocytes occupying papillary and reticular dermis.

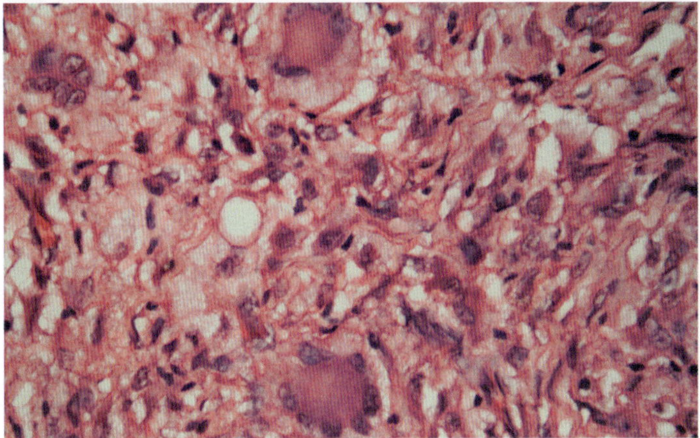

FIG. 12: Infiltrate composed of foamy macrophages and Touton giant cells (cells with wreath of nuclei and surrounding foamy cytoplasm).

Histopathological examination shows an elevated nodule with well-circumscribed infiltrate involving upper and reticular dermis (Fig. 11). At the periphery of lesion, epidermal collarette is seen. Infiltrate consists of macrophages, Touton giant cells, and foamy macrophages (Fig. 12). The infiltrate is usually negative for Langerhans cells markers (CD1a, S100) and do not show Birbeck granules on electron microscopy.

Juvenile xanthogranuloma may regress spontaneously. Solitary skin lesions can be excised surgically. In cases with multisystem involvement, chemotherapy regimens used to treat LCH may be effective.

Differential diagnosis for JXG includes benign cephalic histiocytosis, papular xanthoma, mastocytosis, and Spitz nevus.

## Benign Cephalic Histiocytosis

It is a rare condition with onset at age of 2 months to 3 years. The lesions first appear on the head followed by lesions on the neck and trunk. Asymptomatic, yellowish-to-brown colored papules or nodules appear which are few in number and relatively flat as compared to JXG. Mucosal and visceral involvement does not occur. Microscopic examination shows diffuse dermal infiltration of monomorphous macrophages in the upper dermis. Foamy cells are rare in infiltrate. S-100 and CD1a stains are negative. Lesions subside spontaneously in few years.

## Generalized Eruptive Histiocytosis (Generalized Eruptive Histiocytoma)

It is a rare variant of non-Langerhans cell histiocytosis, and mainly affects adults. It is rare in children. Clinically presents as widespread, symmetrical papules particularly involving the trunk and proximal extremities. New lesions may go on erupting for few years followed by spontaneous resolution. Mucosal lesions are rare and there is no visceral involvement.

Histologically dermal infiltrate of monomorphous vacuolated macrophages with absence of multinucleate giant cells is seen. S-100 and CD1a stains are negative. CD68 stain is positive.

The disease is self-limiting and does not produce systemic symptoms; therefore, there is no need for treatment. Psoralen and ultraviolet A therapy and isotretinoin have been reported to be useful in some cases. Though spontaneous resolution is known to occur, frequent monitoring is recommended due to case reports of patients who developed other severe forms of histiocytosis such as disseminated xanthoma.

## Indeterminate Cell Histiocytosis

Indeterminate cell histiocytosis is a rare neoplasm that is composed of cells with mixed characteristics of Langerhans cells and non-Langerhans cells. It can be seen in both children and adults. Multiple or solitary yellowish-to-brown colored papules, plaques or nodules occur. Visceral involvement of conjunctiva and bone are rare.

On light microscopy, monomorphous infiltrate of mononuclear cells, giant cells, and foamy cells is seen. Cells show positivity for S-100 and CD1a but do not have Birbeck granules on electron microscopic examination.

## Sea-blue Histiocytosis

It is a multisystemic infiltration by macrophages which contain a ceroid material within its cytoplasm. These histiocytes contain cytoplasmic granules that stain blue with May-Giemsa stain. These macrophages infiltrate the bone marrow, lung, liver, spleen, lymph nodes, and occasionally skin. Infiltration of the skin resulting in eyelid swelling and facial papules and nodules has been reported. Sea-blue histiocytosis has been described in patients with myeloid leukemia and adult Niemann-Pick disease type B.

## Xanthoma Disseminatum (Montgomery Syndrome)

Xanthoma disseminatum is a rare nonfamilial, non-Langerhans cell histiocytosis characterized by lipid deposition in skin and internal organs due to histiocytic cell proliferation. It predominantly affects males during childhood or at onset of adulthood. Numerous widely disseminated yellowish-to-brown papules and nodules appear which characteristically involve the popliteal fossa, cubital fossa, inguinal folds, and eyelids. Half of the cases have involvement of oral, oropharyngeal, laryngeal, conjunctival, and corneal mucosa. Other systemic complications that occur are diabetes insipidus, hypopituitarism, epilepsy, hydrocephalus, and ataxia. Three clinical variants have been proposed on the basis of disease progression and prognosis. A common persistent form, a less common progressive form with systemic involvement, and a rare form of self-limited disease. Patients with XD are usually normolipemic but mild hyperlipidemia is found in few cases.

Xanthoma disseminatum needs differentiation from planar xanthomas, papular xanthomas, malignant histiocytosis, and LCH.

Histopathology of early lesion shows predominantly scalloped macrophages while older lesions additionally show foamy cells, Touton giant cells, and other inflammatory cells like lymphocytes and neutrophils. On immunohistochemistry, cells are positive for CD68 and factor XIIIa.

Although the natural history of XD is usually benign, with spontaneous resolution of cutaneous lesions over years, lesions in certain anatomical locations may result in substantial morbidity and death. There is no consensus regarding curative therapy for XD. Response to any form of therapy in XD has been mostly unsatisfactory. Cyclophosphamide has been tried with some success in few patients.

## Reticulohistiocytosis

Reticulohistiocytosis is a rare form of histiocytosis that can affect the skin and other organs. Two distinct forms of reticulohistiocytosis have been described here:

- Reticulohistiocytoma
- Multicentric reticulohistiocytosis

  Both have similar histological features but different clinical presentation.

- *Reticulohistiocytoma*: Solitary, firm nodule occurs over head neck region or over upper part of trunk. Young adults and middle-aged are commonly affected. It has female preponderance. There is no systemic involvement, and prognosis is good. Lesion resolves spontaneously over few months to years
- *Multicentric reticulohistiocytosis*: This very rare and more aggressive multisystem disease is characterized by skin lesions, mucosal lesions, and arthritis. It usually arises in middle-aged persons around the age of 50 years and has female preponderance. Associated malignancies have been reported in 25% of cases. Multiple, firm, reddish-to-brown-colored papules and nodules of size 5–10 mm or larger occur on the fingers and hands. In some cases, papules may be arranged about the nailfold giving it coral-bead appearance. Other sites where lesions are commonly seen are arms, face, neck, and ears. Mucosal lesions in the oral cavity and on sclera occur in few cases. Skin lesions may cause destruction of cartilage around the ears and nose resulting in a disfigured appearance.

Joint involvement is common and presents as symmetric erosive polyarthritis mimicking rheumatoid arthritis. In half of the cases, arthritis precedes the appearance of skin lesion and in 30% cases, both occur simultaneously. Arthritis most commonly involves the fingers, hands, knees, and shoulders but any joint can be affected. In some cases, arthritis can be rapidly destructive leading to mutilations. Other organs like muscle, liver, lymph nodes, myocardium, pericardium, and pleura may be involved.

Histopathology of skin lesions shows mononuclear and multinucleated cells in the dermis (Fig. 13). Numerous multinucleate giant cells with an abundant smooth or slightly granular eosinophilic cytoplasm having "ground glass" appearance are characteristic (Fig. 14).

Systemic corticosteroids with steroid-sparing agents like hydroxychloroquine, methotrexate, and cyclophosphamide have been tried according to the severity of the disease. Disease may go into remission after a course of 8–10 years in many cases but may leave behind joint deformities.

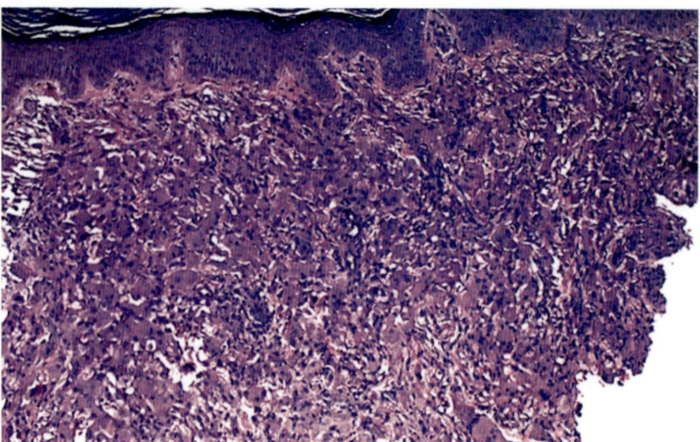

**FIG. 13:** Dense diffuse granulomatous infiltrate in the upper and mid dermis.

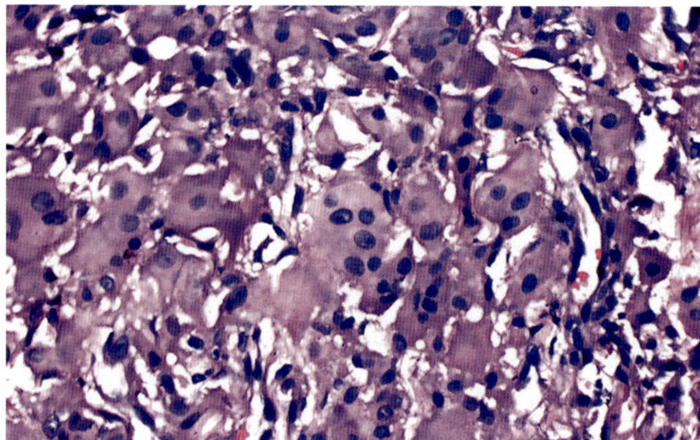

**FIG. 14:** Multinucleate giant cells with an abundant smooth or slightly granular eosinophilic cytoplasm having "ground glass".

## Rosai–Dorfman Disease

Rosai–Dorfman disease, also known as SHML, is a rare histiocytic disorder described by two pathologists, Juan Rosai and Ronald Dorfman, in 1969. It affects equal numbers of males and females. It is most commonly seen in the first 10 years of life, but it also occurs in adult patients.

Massive, painless, and usually bilateral cervical lymphadenopathy is the most common clinical presentation. It is usually associated with fever, night sweats, and weight loss. Extranodal involvement is common and skin is the most common extranodal site involved. Cutaneous involvement is seen as papules and nodules.

Skin lesion under light microscope shows infiltrate of lymphocytes and macrophages which gives appearance of lymph node in the skin. Multinucleated or foamy cells may be seen. Emperipolesis of lymphocytes is hallmark histological feature.

In most of the cases, disease may remit spontaneously. For symptomatic and persistent disease, surgical excision, radiotherapy, systemic steroids with or without chemotherapy may be tried.

## Papular Xanthoma

Papular xanthoma is a rare normolipemic non-Langerhans cell histiocytosis. Adults are usually affected but cases in children have been reported. Few or several generalized brown-to-yellowish papular lesions occur over the trunk and extremities. Lesions rarely can occur on the head. Morphologically, these lesions may mimic lesions of XD but the distribution pattern is different. Histologically, foamy macrophages with numerous Touton giant cells are seen in the dermis. In children, treatment is not required as the condition is self-limiting but in adults, the disease is progressive and there is no satisfactory treatment.

## Diffuse Normolipemic Plane Xanthoma

It is a rare kind of normolipemic xanthoma which can be considered as a paraneoplastic phenomenon. Yellowish papules or flat patches or plaques with barely palpable borders occur predominantly over face and trunk. On face, lesions occur in periorbital area resembling lesions of xanthelasma palpebrarum. Blood investigations show normal lipid levels. Some cases may be associated with malignancies, most commonly hematological which include gammopathies, cryoglobulinemia, and myeloproliferative disorders like leukemia, or lymphoma. Skin lesions may precede these conditions by several years.

Histologically, an infiltrate consisting of foamy macrophages in the papillary and mid-dermis with a perivascular localization is seen.

Lesions can be removed by excision, chemabrasion, dermabrasion, or abrasive laser therapy.

## Necrobiotic Xanthogranuloma

It is a rare disease which typically affects elderly adults. It manifests as yellowish plaques and nodules with atrophy, telangiectasia, and occasionally ulceration. The periorbital area is the commonest site of involvement followed by trunk and extremities. It is commonly associated with paraproteinemia, usually immunoglobulin G monoclonal gammopathy, and multiple myeloma.

Microscopically, areas of necrosis surrounded by palisade of granuloma occupying the dermis and subcutaneous tissue are seen. Cholesterol clefts and Touton giant cells, foreign body giant cells and plasma cells are seen.

Various treatment modalities used include chemotherapy, intralesional and systemic steroids, radiotherapy, and surgical excision.

## Verruciform Xanthoma

It is one of the normolipemic xanthoma which is rare and presents as solitary, asymptomatic, papillomatous or cauliflower like, hyperkeratotic nodule. Most common site of occurrence is oral cavity and genital area. In oral cavity, gingival or alveolar mucosa is commonly involved. Cutaneous extraoral lesions are usually associated with conditions like lymphedema, epidermal nevi, and congenital hemidysplasia with ichthyosiform erythroderma and limb defects (CHILD) syndrome.

On low power, histopathological features resemble a viral wart. Marked elongation of rete ridges is seen and elongated dermal papillae show foamy cells which may occasionally have granular appearance. Papillae also show dilated capillaries. Overlying epidermis shows parakeratosis. Surgical excision is the treatment of choice.

## SUGGESTED READINGS


1. Badalian-Very G, Vergilio JA, Degar BA, et al. Recurrent BRAF mutations in Langerhans cell histiocytosis. Blood. 2010;116:1919-23.
2. Blankenship DW, Zech L, Mirzabeigi M, et al. Verruciform xanthoma of the upper-extremity in the absence of chronic skin disease or syndrome: a case report and review of the literature. J Cutan Pathol. 2013;40:745-52.
3. Breier F, Zegler B, Reiter H, et al. Papular xanthoma; a clinicopathological study of 10 cases. J Cutan Pathol. 2002;29:200-6.
4. Chang MW, Frieden IJ, Good W. The risk intraocular juvenile xanthogranuloma: survey of current practices and assessment of risk. J Am Acad Dermatol. 1996;34:445-9.
5. Fang S, Chen AJ. Facial cutaneous Rosai–Dorfman disease: A case report and literature review. Exp Ther Med. 2015;9:1389-92.
6. Fichera G, Anastasio E, Capasso F, et al. Diffuse plane normolipemic xanthomatosis associated with Takayasu's disease and hyperhomocysteinemia: a case report. Indian J Dermatol Venereol Leprol. 2004;70:230-3.
7. Flaitz C, Allen C, Neville B, et al. Juvenile xanthogranuloma of the oral cavity in children: a clinicopathologic study. Oral Surg Oral Med Oral Pathol Oral Radiol Endod. 2002;94:345-52.
8. Haimovic A, Chernoff K, Hale CS, et al. Indeterminate cell histiocytosis that presented clinically as benign cephalic histiocytosis. Dermatol Online J. 2014:16;20.
9. Harris N, Jaffe E, Diebold J, et al. The World Health Organization classification of neoplastic diseases of the hematopoietic and lymphoid tissues. Report of the Clinical Advisory Committee meeting, Airlie House, Virginia, November, 1997. Ann Oncol. 1999;10:1419-32.
10. Histiocytosis Association. WHistiocytic Disorders. [online] Available from https://www.histio.org/page.aspx?pid=378#.WtcWbdRublU [Accessed April 2018].
11. James W, Berger T, Elston D. Macrophage /monocyte disorder. In: James W (Ed.). Andrews' Diseases of the Skin: Clinical Dermatology, 10th edition. Canada: Saunders Elsevier; 2006. p. 714.
12. Kesik V, Citak C, Kismet E, et al. Hematopoietic stem cell transplantation in Langerhans cell histiocytosis: case report and review of the literature. Pediatr Transplant. 2009;13:371-4.
13. Komp D, El Mahdi A, Starling K, et al. Quality of survival in Histiocytosis X: a Southwest Oncology Group study. Med Pediatr Oncol. 1980;8:35-40.
14. Liu ZQ, Liu R, Shi XD, et al. Juvenile xanthogranuloma: 3 cases report and literature review. 2011;32:614-7.
15. Longaker MA, Frieden IJ, LeBoit PE, et al. Congenital "self-healing" Langerhans cell histiocytosis: the need for long-term follow-up. J Am Acad Dermatol. 1994;31:910-6.
16. Repiso T, Roca-Miralles M, Kanitakis J, et al. Generalized eruptive histiocytoma evolving into xanthoma disseminatum in a 4-year-old boy. Br J Dermatol. 1995;132:978-82.
17. Samson JF, Libu GK, Philip M, et al. Benign cephalic histiocytosis. Indian Dermatol Online J. 2013;4:300-1.
18. Satter EK, High WA. Langerhans cell histiocytosis: a review of the current recommendations of the Histiocyte Society. Pediatr Dermatol. 2008;25:291-5.
19. Seaton ED, Pillai GJ, Chu AC. Treatment of xanthoma disseminatum with cyclophosphamide. Br J Dermatol. 2004;150:346-9.
20. Selmi C, Greenspan A, Huntley A, et al. Multicentric reticulohistiocytosis: a critical review. Curr Rheumatol Rep. 2015;17:511.
21. Sharath Kumar BC, Nandini AS, Niveditha SR, et al. Generalized eruptive histiocytosis mimicking leprosy. Indian J Dermatol Venereol Leprol. 2011;77:498-502.
22. US National Library of Medicine. MedlinePlus. Histiocytosis [Internet] [cited April 2018]. Available from: http://www.nlm.nih.gov/medlineplus/ency/article/000068.htm.
23. Wood AJ, Wagner MV, Abbott JJ, et al. Necrobiotic xanthogranuloma: a review of 17 cases with emphasis on clinical and pathologic correlation. Arch Dermatol. 2009;145:279-84.
24. Zak IT, Altinok D, Neilsen SS, et al. Xanthoma disseminatum of the central nervous system and cranium. AJNR Am J Neuroradiol. 2006;27:919-21.
25. Zina AM, Bundino S, Pippione M. Sea-blue histiocyte syndrome with cutaneous involvement. Case report with ultrastructural findings. Dermatologica. 1987;174:39-44.

# 37 CHAPTER Noninfectious Granulomatous Diseases of Skin

*Archana Singal, Deepashree Daulatabad*

## INTRODUCTION

Granulomatous disorders include a large number of diverse entities that are primarily characterized by granuloma formation on histopathology.

Following types of granulomatous reaction have been described:

- *Sarcoidal granuloma or naked granulomas:* Collection of epithelioid histiocytes and giant cells with a paucity of surrounding lymphocytes and plasma cells
- *Tuberculoid granuloma:* Collection of epithelioid histiocytes, Langhans as well as foreign body giant cells with a rim of lymphocytes and plasma cells. These granulomas tend to be confluent and caseation necrosis may develop
- *Necrobiotic granuloma:* Poorly formed granulomas that are characterized by the common feature of presence of necrobiosis. Inflammatory cells may be admixed with the necrobiosis or may palisade around it
- *Suppurative granuloma:* The cluster of epithelioid histiocytes and multinucleated giant cells have a collection of neutrophils at the center and chronic inflammatory cells at the periphery
- *Foreign body granuloma:* Collection of epithelioid histiocyte with foreign body giant cells and the inciting foreign body at center
- *Miscellaneous:* Have variable appearance.

Apart from this, granulomatous dermatitis can be classified as infectious granuloma and noninfectious granuloma. Conditions where these granulomas are found is mentioned in table 1.

## SARCOIDOSIS

Sarcoidosis is a multiorgan inflammatory disease characterized by the development of epithelioid cell granulomas without caseation in one or several organs including skin.

Sarcoidosis has a worldwide distribution with a rising prevalence. Prevalence is higher among females, mostly in 3$^{rd}$–4$^{th}$ decades, with a smaller peak beyond 50 years of age, in industrialized nations and the Afro-Caribbean races.

### Etiopathogenesis

The etiopathogenesis of sarcoidosis is largely elusive.

- *Genetic susceptibility*: Familial clustering and increase in the incidence among monozygotic twins than dizygotic twins have been observed.

Genes that have been found to play role in it are represented in flowchart 1

- *Human leukocyte antigen (HLA) associations*: Various HLAs have been found to be involved
    - HLAs associated with increased susceptibility are HLA-DR 11, 12, 14, 15, 17, HLA-DRB*1101, and HLA-DQB1
    - HLAs that are protective—HLA-DR1, DR4, and possibly HLA DQ*0202.
- *Non-HLA association*: Tumor necrosis factor-α (TNF-α), interleukin-1 (IL-1), vitamin D receptor, NRAMP-1, CCR2, ACE, and COX-2.

**TABLE 1: Different types of granulomatous reaction**

| Sarcoidal | Tuberculoid | Necrobiotic | Suppurative | Foreign body | Miscellaneous |
|---|---|---|---|---|---|
| • Sarcoidosis<br>• Reaction to foreign material | • Tuberculosis<br>• Tuberculids<br>• Leprosy<br>• Late syphilis<br>• Leishmaniasis<br>• Rosacea<br>• Crohn's disease | • Granuloma annulare<br>• Necrobiosis lipoidica<br>• Necrobiotic xanthogranuloma<br>• Rheumatoid nodule<br>• Rheumatic fever nodule<br>• Reaction to foreign material | • Fungal infection –(sporotrichosis, eumycetoma)<br>• Nontuberculous mycobacteria<br>• Cat-scratch disease<br>• Lymphogranuloma venereum<br>• Granulomatous variant of pyoderma gangrenosum<br>• Ruptured cyst or follicle | • Endogenous material<br>• Exogenous material | • Interstitial granulomatous dermatitis<br>• Interstitial granulomatous drug reaction<br>• Elastolytic granuloma<br>• Melkersson–Rosenthal syndrome<br>• Granulomas in immunodeficiency |

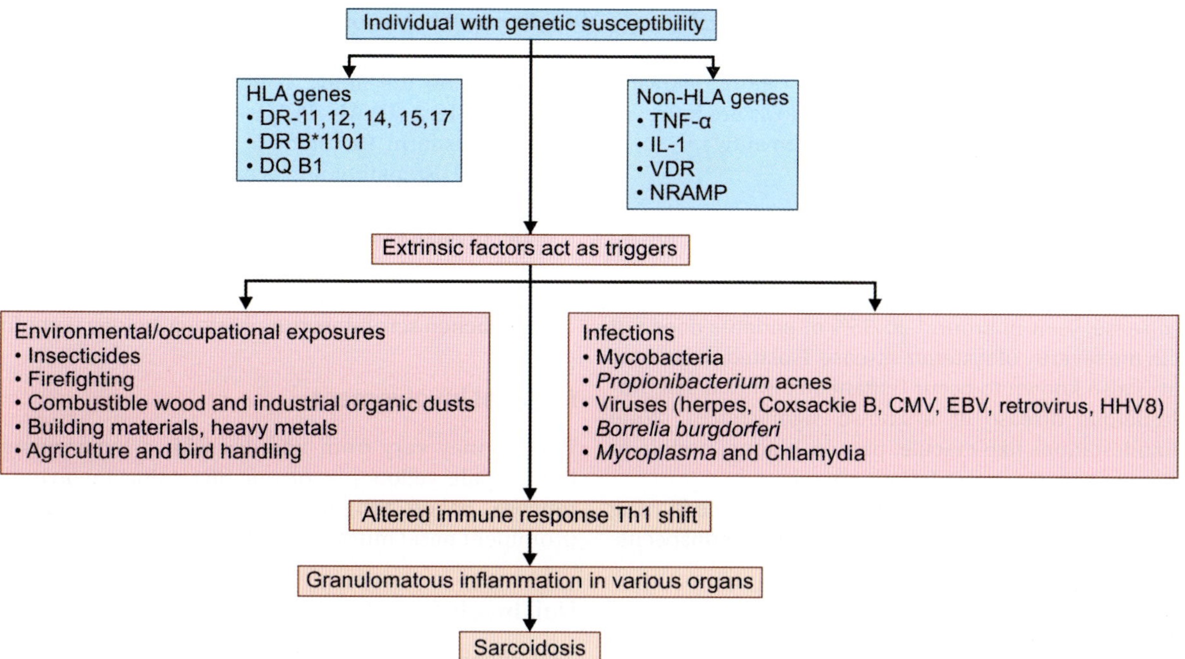


CMV, cytomegalovirus; TNF, tumor necrosis factor; IL, interleukin; HLA, human leukocyte antigen; EBV, Epstein–Barr virus; HHV, human herpes virus.

**FLOWCHART 1:** Etiological factors of sarcoidosis.

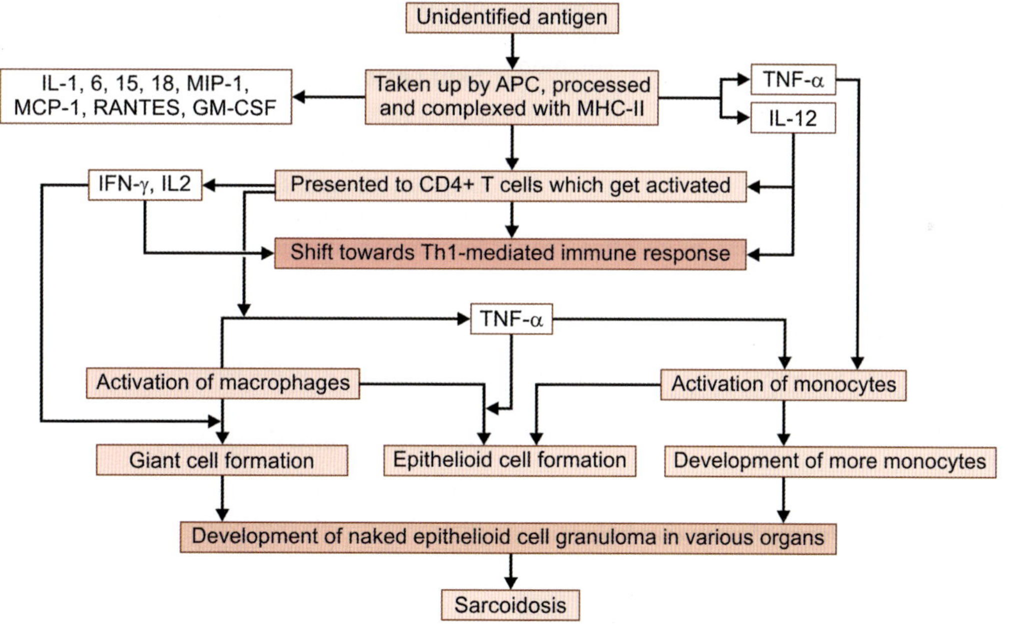


APC, antigen-presenting cell; MHC, major histocompatibility complex; TNF, tumor necrosis factor; IL: interleukin; IFN, interferon; MCP, monocyte chemoattractant protein; RANTES, regulated upon activation, normal T cell expressed, and secreted; GM-CSF, granulocyte-macrophage colony-stimulating factor.

**FLOWCHART 2:** Pathogenesis of sarcoidosis and role of cytokines.

- *Extrinsic antigen*: Occupational or environmental exposure or infectious agents might be the inciting agents (Flowchart 1)
- *Immunological factors*: Unidentified antigens are taken up by the antigen-presenting cells (APCs). Through formation of major histocompatibility complex (MHC)-peptide complexes, activated APCs secrete TNF-α, IL-1, IL-6, IL-12, IL-15, IL-18, MIP-1, MCP-1, RANTES, and GM-CSF. Whereas, the activated CD4 cells predominantly secrete IL-2 and interferon (INF)-γ, as well as enhance the TNF-α production from the activated macrophages. Th1 immune response is upregulated. Usually, the low virulence and persistence of the antigen perpetuates the immune response culminating in granuloma formation in various organs (Flowchart 2)
- *Immune paradox*: Peripheral immune response is suppressed as suggested by cutaneous anergy to tuberculin and peripheral blood T-cell lymphopenia. This is in contrast to the extensive upregulation of cellular immune response leading to granuloma formation in the target organs. This phenomenon of anergy of delayed type hypersensitivity in a setting of exuberant systemic granulomatous response is termed as "immune paradox". It has been suggested that global regulatory T-cells amplifications or attenuated dendritic cell

(DC) function are supposed to induce the peripheral anergy by inhibiting both IL-2 production and T-cell proliferation without any downregulation of local TNF-α allowing granuloma formation. Patients with sarcoidosis are however able to mount immune response to the Kveim antigen.

## Clinical Presentation

### Sarcoidosis of the Skin

Cutaneous disease, seen in around 20–35% of patients does not correlate with the severity of systemic disease. Isolated cutaneous involvement is also known to occur (cutaneous-limited sarcoid-like granulomatous disease of unknown significance). Wide variety of manifestations like macule, papule, plaque, nodule to ulcerative, or psoriasiform presentations are seen.

Cutaneous manifestations are categorized as specific (having epithelioid cell granulomas on histopathology) or nonspecific (Table 2).

### Classical Cutaneous Forms of Sarcoidosis (Table 3)

- *Scar sarcoidosis*: Sarcoidal granuloma over a pre-existing scar may be the only manifestation of sarcoidosis. Unlike keloid, this is asymptomatic (Figs 6 and 7)
- *Subcutaneous sarcoidosis*: It is a rare form that presents as tender or painless nodules on extremities. Systemic involvement is often present in these patients, most common being hilar adenopathy but usually not severe. Spontaneous resolution can occur.

### Unusual and Atypical Forms

- Alopecia—presents as scarring alopecia more often than nonscarring
- Atrophic forms—can be generalized or localized (legs) and often associated with ulceration
- Erythrodermic sarcoidosis—extremely rare and presents with erythematous scaly plaques that coalesce into larger infiltrated brownish-red sheets, associated with marked lymphadenopathy

**TABLE 2: Different morphological forms of cutaneous lesions in sarcoidosis**

| Classical forms | Unusual or atypical forms |
|---|---|
| • Lupus pernio<br>• Angiolupoid (Brocq–Pautrier)<br>• Erythematous and erythematopapular<br>• "Scar sarcoidosis"<br>• Papular ("small nodular")<br>• Nodular<br>• Annular (or circinate)<br>• Plaque<br>• Subcutaneous<br>• Erythema nodosum<br>• Erythrodermic (Schaumann) | • Alopecia<br>• Atrophic<br>• Erythrodermic sarcoidosis<br>• Hypopigmentation<br>• Ichthyosiform sarcoidosis<br>• Lichenoid forms<br>• Rare miscellaneous forms—pseudotumoral, psoriasiform and pruriginous varieties, lupus erythematosus-like and lupoid forms, polymorphous light eruption type, generalized perifollicular pustules and papules, keratotic palmar lesions |

- Hypopigmentation: Macular hypopigmentation or hypopigmented areas around a central indurated lesion occurring mainly on the limbs. It may respond to psoralen (P) plus ultraviolet A (UVA)—PUVA—but is resistant to corticosteroids
- Ichthyosiform sarcoidosis: Systemic involvement is always found. Histopathology reveals epidermal changes suggestive of ichthyosis vulgaris, whereas the dermis demonstrates the presence of noncaseating epithelioid cell granulomas suggestive of sarcoidosis
- *Lichenoid forms*: Clinically manifests similar to lichen planus and lichen scrofulosorum. Histopathology is confirmatory.

### Mucosal Involvement

Lesions may vary from nodules with a hyperpigmented halo, diffuse pale yellow plaques or ulceration involving the buccal mucosa, palate, tongue, or larynx. Lupus pernio may have a prominent nasal mucosal involvement.

### Nail Involvement

Nail changes are rare in sarcoidosis and often associated with systemic disease and bone cysts of the underlying phalanx. The changes include thickening, opacity, fragility, layering, convexity, longitudinal ridging, pitting, atrophy, nail loss, pterygium and red or brown discoloration of the nail beds.

### Skin Lesions in Children

Sarcoidosis in childhood is uncommon. The early onset disease usually begins before 5 years of age and the late onset develops between 10 and 15 years. The former presents with arthritis, uveitis, and skin disease, whereas the latter resembles the adult form mainly affecting the lungs, skin, and the reticuloendothelial system. The early onset form is known to be due to sporadic mutation in the *NOD2* gene. Blau syndrome is considered to be the same as early onset sarcoidosis with the same mutation, differing only in being familial.

### Sarcoidosis and Pregnancy

Sarcoidosis tends to improve in pregnancy, probably due to increased serum cortisol levels and tends to relapse postpartum. Thus, a chest X-ray within 6 months of delivery is often recommended. It does not affect fertility, or any risk of fetal or obstetrical complications in absence of significant cardio-pulmonary compromise.

### Sarcoidosis in Elderly

A second but smaller peak of sarcoidosis does occur after 50 years of age. Solid organ malignancies (lung, stomach, intestine, uterus) that may give rise to a granulomatous reaction in the draining lymph nodes should be ruled out. Corticosteroids or immunosuppressive adjuvants are relatively contraindicated.

## Systemic Involvement

In the stricter sense, the diagnosis of sarcoidosis requires the involvement of at least two organ systems. This frequently involves lungs, heart, central nervous system, and other organs

**TABLE 3: Overview of the characteristic features of the different classical lesions of sarcoidosis**

| Type | Site | Morphology | Course | Remarks |
|---|---|---|---|---|
| Angiolupoid (Fig. 1) | Near the medial canthus | Orange red or reddish brown colored soft hemispherical nodule, up to 2 in number, with marked telangiectasias | Persistent, subacute to chronic | Also named as Brocq–Pautrier angiolupoid |
| Annular form (circinate) (Fig. 2) | Forehead, face, and neck | Gyrate, yellowish red lesions, with mild scaling. Progress centrifugally with central healing, depigmentation, and slight atrophy | Subacute to chronic; persistent | Cardiac involvement |
| Erythema nodosum (Fig. 3) | Lower limbs or shins | Tender evanescent ill-defined nodules, resolve with hyperpigmentation | Acute and benign variety; spontaneous resolution | Most common nonspecific manifestation |
| Lupus pernio | Symmetrically on nose, cheeks, ears, fingers, hands, and toes | Soft, doughy or indurated dusky violaceous nodules and plaques, glistening surface, stretched epidermis and large pilosebaceous follicles. Involved ear lobes may become massive ("turkey ears") | Chronic; tends to persist | Warrants thorough systemic evaluation |
| Maculopapular and erythematous forms (Fig. 4) | Neck, trunk, extremities, and mucous membranes | Transient, diffuse, "prodromal" maculopapular eruptions | Acute and subacute; tends to resolve | Associated with acute organ involvement |
| Nodular forms | Proximal parts of the limbs, the trunk, and the face | Well circumscribed, yellowish-red at first, becoming violaceous, soft or firm, round lesions, telangiectatic marks, or pale atrophic patches | Subacute-chronic; tend to be indolent | Are nontender and noninflammatory |
| Papular sarcoid (small nodular type) (Fig. 5) | Face, especially around the eyelids and nasolabial folds and extensors of extremities | Apple jelly appearance of papules on diascopy | Acute and subacute; favorable prognosis | Most common specific manifestation of cutaneous sarcoidosis. |
| Plaque form | Limbs, shoulders, buttocks, and thighs | Large diffuse plaques and nodules | Chronic; tend to persist | May form annular lesions |

like kidney (Table 4). In addition, sarcoidosis might have following associations:

- *Infections*: Viral wart, invasive fungal infections
- *Immunologically mediated conditions*: Thyroid abnormalities and Addison's disease, chronic urticaria and connective tissue disorders
- Vasculitis
- *Malignancy*: Lymphoproliferative disease, carcinoma cervix, lung, testis, and uterus
- Necrobiosis lipoidica and granuloma annulare (GA)
- *Reproductive*: Uterus (menorrhagia), granulomas in ovaries or breast. Testes may be involved.

## Course and Prognosis

The prognosis of sarcoidosis is often difficult to predict. Progressive pulmonary disease, renal involvement and cardiac involvement (sudden cardiac deaths) are main causes of death. African-American, chronic and persistent forms of cutaneous sarcoidosis, and stage II and beyond pulmonary disease are considered poor prognostic indicators.

## Diagnosis

Sarcoidosis is a diagnosis of exclusion and can never be accomplished with certainty. Following parameters are essential for diagnosing sarcoidosis:

- Compatible clinicoradiographic findings
- Demonstration of granulomas on histopathology
- Careful exclusion of known causes of granulomatous disease
- Evidence of disease in at least two organs.

## Histopathology

The classic pathologic finding of sarcoidosis is well demarcated, compact islands of mononuclear phagocytes consisting of epithelioid cells and macrophages (Fig.8). Besides skin, various sites may reveal the granulomatous process characteristic of sarcoidosis like mucosa, conjunctiva, lower lip, lymph nodes like epitrochlear, or scalene lymph nodes. Other modalities for evaluation may include mediastinoscopy with mediastinal node biopsy, transbronchial lung biopsy, liver biopsy, gastrocnemius muscle biopsy (even without muscular complaints).

The T4 lymphocytes are present throughout the granuloma admixed with the epithelioid cells, whereas the T8 suppressor lymphocytes are restricted to the peripheral mantle.

Histologically, infective conditions like tuberculosis, atypical mycobacterial infections, some fungal infections, and noninfective conditions like rheumatoid nodules, foreign body reactions need to be differentiated. Special stains and polarization microscopy may be helpful. However, about one-fourth cases of sarcoidosis also demonstrate polarisable material. Sarcoidal granulomas differ from that of tubercular in being non-necrotizing or noncaseating and "naked", i.e., they lack or have very sparse peripheral rim of lymphocytes. The epithelioid cells may merge and form giant cells which are usually the Langhans type that contain the inclusions Schaumann's and asteroid bodies.

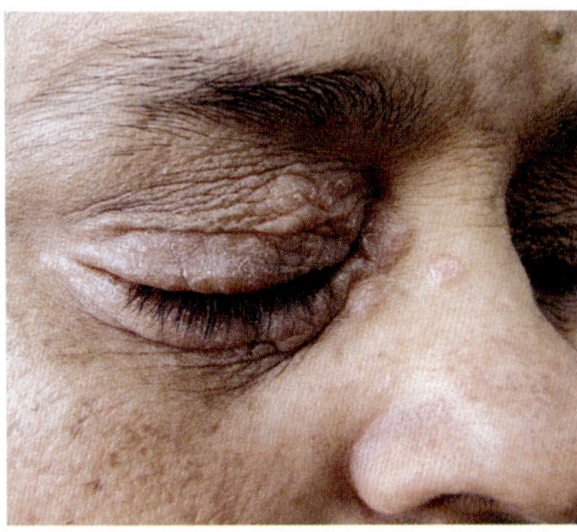

**FIG. 1:** Angiolupoid sarcoid lesions around right eye in a woman.

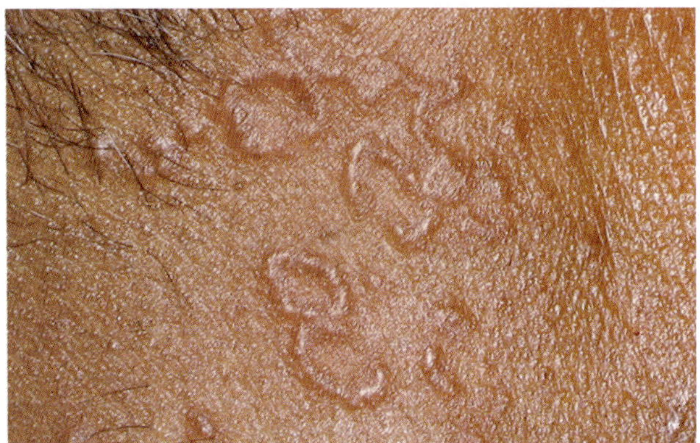

**FIG. 2:** Annular lesions of sarcoid on the nape of neck in a man.

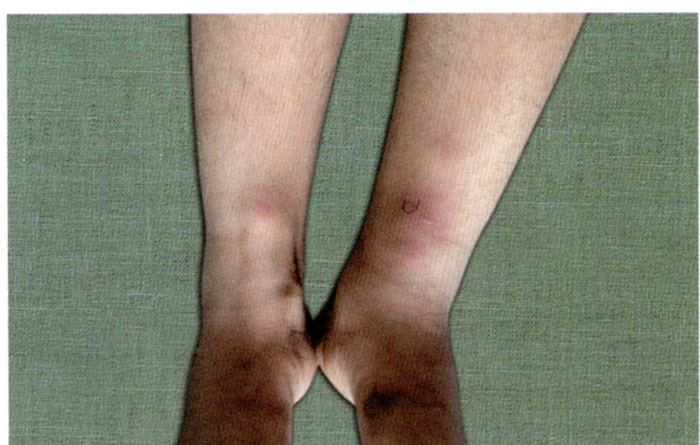

**FIG. 3:** Erythematous tender nodules of erythema nodosum over shins.

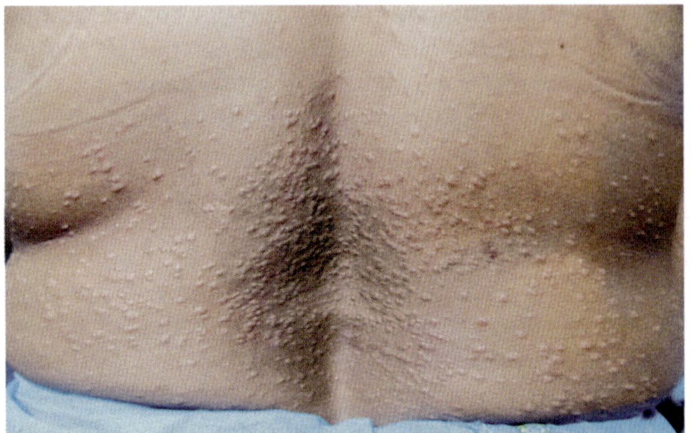

**FIG. 4:** Multiple erythematous papular sarcoidosis lesions over trunk in a woman.

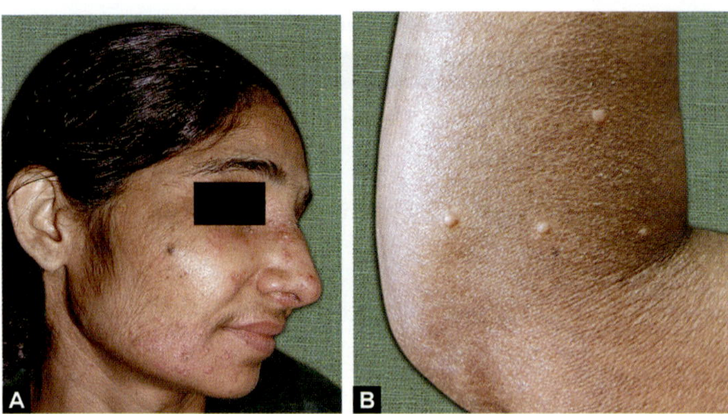

**FIG. 5:** Papular sarcoid lesion on face and arm.

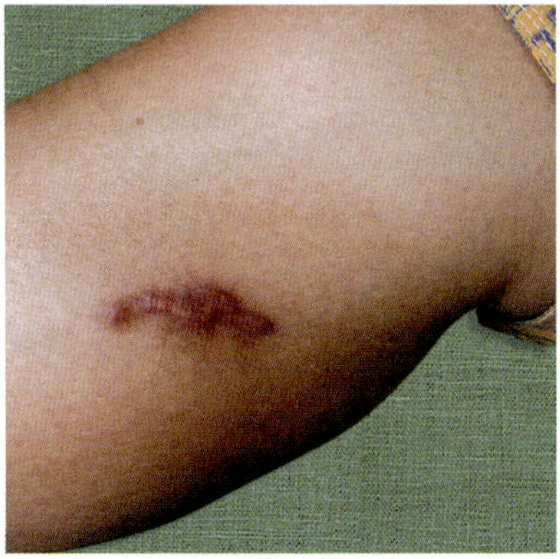

**FIG. 6:** Development of sarcoid lesion over traumatic scar in a young girl.

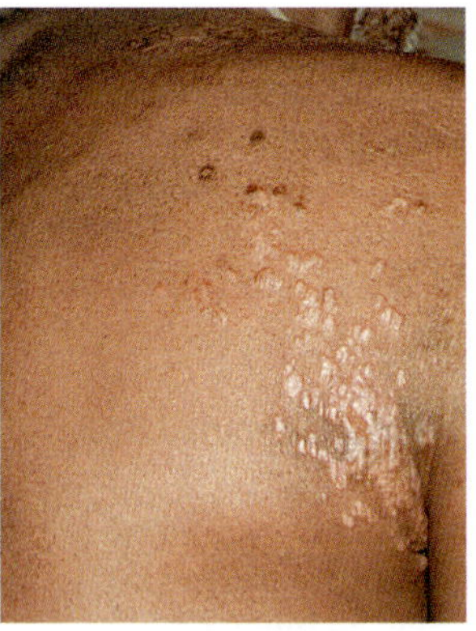

**FIG. 7:** Sarcoid lesions over healed herpes zoster of thoracic dermatome.

## Inclusions

*Schaumann's bodies (conchoidal bodies)*: Large, round to oval, concentrically lamellated, calcified structures, usually present within the cytoplasm of giant cells. These stain dark blue due to presence of calcium.

- *Asteroid bodies*: Common intracytoplasmic stellate inclusions within giant cells. Appear to have brown-red center with radiating blue spikes on staining with phosphotungstic acid-hematoxylin
- *Hamazaki–Wesenberg bodies (yellow bodies, spindle bodies, chromogenic bodies)*: Seen in the lymph nodes and represent giant extracellular and intracellular lysosomes. These are seen as yellow-brown, oval or spindle-shaped structures about

**TABLE 4: Systemic involvement and screening**

| System | Systemic manifestations |
|---|---|
| General | Fatigue, malaise, weight loss |
| Pulmonary | • Cough<br>• Dyspnea<br>• Chest pain<br>• Hilar and mediastinal lymphadenopathy, prominent bronchovascular bundles, nodules along bronchi, vessels, and subpleura, ground-glass opacification, parenchymal masses or consolidation, fibrosis in upper zone |
| Upper respiratory tract | • Nasal obstruction<br>• Crusting, epistaxis<br>• Nasal polyps<br>• Mucosal granulomas<br>• Coexistence with lupus pernio is common |
| Cardiac | • Conduction defects (atrioventricular block or bundle-branch blocks)<br>• Tachyarrhythmias<br>• Cardiomyopathy<br>• Congestive heart failure<br>• Sudden death, pericardial effusion |
| Central nervous system | • Cranial neuropathy<br>• Diabetes insipidus<br>• Hypopituitarism<br>• Seizures<br>• Meningoencephalopathy<br>• Hydrocephalus<br>• Myelopathy/radiculopathy<br>• Peripheral neuropathy |
| Ocular involvement | • Uveitis<br>• Lofgren's syndrome<br>• Heerfordt's syndrome<br>• Retinochoroiditis<br>• Conjunctivitis (millet seed nodules, near eyelid margins)<br>• Lacrimal gland enlargement, keratoconjunctivitis sicca, dacryocystitis<br>• Mikulicz's syndrome (bilateral swelling of the lacrimal and salivary glands)<br>• Retrobulbar optic neuritis<br>• Optic atrophy<br>• Orbital mass/proptosis<br>• Diplopia<br>• Glaucoma, cataract<br>• Raised intraocular pressure, papilledema |
| Reticulo-endothelial system | • Lymphadenopathy<br>• Hepatomegaly<br>• Splenomegaly |
| Musculoskeletal system | • Acute polyarthritis usually with erythema nodosum<br>• Chronic arthritis<br>• Diffuse granulomatous myositis |
| Renal involvement | • Hypercalciuria<br>• Hypercalcemia<br>• Granulomatous interstitial nephritis<br>• Glomerular disease<br>• Obstructive uropathy<br>• End-stage renal disease (rare) |

**BOX 1 Evaluation recommended in a patient with sarcoidosis**

- Rule out occupational/environmental exposure
- Complete physical examination
- Complete blood count with ESR
- Serum biochemistry—liver and kidney function tests, calcium, 1,25 dihydroxyvitamin D level
- *Urinalysis*: If H/o stones, then 24-hour urine calcium
- Pulmonary involvement –
  - *Chest X-ray*: Posteroanterior and lateral views
  - *Pulmonary function tests*: Spirometry and DLCO
  - If pulmonary involvement strongly suspected or above tests abnormal
    - HRCT
    - Transbronchial biopsy
- Cardiac involvement –
  - ECG
  - Echo
  - Holter monitor
  - If cardiac involvement strongly suspected/above tests abnormal
    - Positron emission tomography (PET) scanning
    - Cardiac magnetic resonance imaging (MRI)
    - Radionuclide scanning
- *Ophthalmological evaluation*: Slit-lamp examination, fundoscopy, conjunctival biopsy
- Serum ACE levels
- Rule out tuberculosis
  - Sputum AFB staining and culture
  - Tuberculin skin test
  - Interferon-γ release assays
- Thyroid function tests
- Vitamin D25, vitamin D1,25

DLCO, diffusing capacity of the lungs for carbon monoxide; ACE, angiotensin converting enzyme; ECG, electrocardiography; ESR, erythrocyte sedimentation rate; HRCT, high-resolution computed tomography; AFB, acid-fast bacillus.

0.5–0.8 μm in size on hematoxylin and eosin stains. These are periodic acid–Schiff (PAS) and Grocott–Methenamine silver positive, and often have budding yeast-like appearance, hence may be mistaken for fungal organism.

Erythema nodosum lesions show septal panniculitis as in the idiopathic form.

Once the cutaneous granulomas have been documented, it is imperative to look for systemic involvement to make a definitive diagnosis of sarcoidosis. A protocol for diagnosis of sarcoidosis is presented in box 1.

Some clinical presentations like Lofgren's syndrome (bilateral hilar adenopathy on chest radiography, erythema nodosum skin lesions, fever, and arthritis/arthralgias), Heerfordt syndrome (uveitis, parotitis, and fever) and asymptomatic bilateral hilar lymphadenopathy are highly suggestive of sarcoidosis, and in the absence of an alternative diagnosis (such as infection or lymphoma), the diagnosis of sarcoidosis can be accepted without a tissue biopsy confirmation.

## Other Investigations

Hand radiographs may show cystic changes only in chronic disease.

Angiotensin-converting enzyme (ACE) is produced by the epithelioid cells of the sarcoidal granuloma. An increase of 2–3 times the upper normal limit gives an idea about the burden of granulomas and is also helpful to monitor disease activity. This may be raised in other disorders (Table 5).

- *Gallium scan*: Gallium-67 accumulates in regions of hyperemia created by inflammatory process as well as in the macrophages. Hence, scans of gallium uptake can demonstrate the organs involved by the granulomatous process, although cutaneous involvement is not picked up. Two classical signs of sarcoidosis seen on gallium scans are:
    - *Panda sign*: Bilateral lacrimal and parotid glands uptake of gallium
    - *Lambda sign*: Bilateral hilar and right paratracheal uptake of gallium
- *Kveim test*: Intradermal injection of a crude homogenate of sarcoid tissue produced papules with characteristic epithelioid cell granulomas on histopathological examination. The test was further refined by use of particulate suspension of splenic tissue of patients with definite diagnosis of sarcoidosis. But, the test has been discontinued now due to the potential infective nature of the antigen source. Classically, 0.1–0.2 mL of the antigen is injected intradermally into the forearm and histopathological evaluation done around 6 weeks after injection.

### Markers of Disease Activity

Various clinical, biochemical as well as the radiological markers of increase in disease activity of sarcoidosis are described in table 5.

## Treatment (Flowchart 3 and Fig. 8)

It is important to weigh the effect of long-term immunosuppression against chances of spontaneous remission. A conservative approach is preferred whenever possible.

### Topical Therapy

1. Class I ultra-potent topical corticosteroids
2. Intralesional triamcinolone (3–10 mg/mL every 3–4 weeks)
3. Tacrolimus
4. The PUVA therapy has been used in hypopigmented sarcoid which is usually resistant to topical steroids. Can also be used in erythrodermic sarcoidosis
5. Cosmetic camouflage can be of help especially in severely disfiguring lupus pernio.

**TABLE 5: Markers of disease activity in sarcoidosis**

| Clinical markers | Biochemical markers | Imaging |
|---|---|---|
| Fever, uveitis, erythema nodosum, lupus pernio, changing scars, polyarthralgia, breathlessness, increase in lacrimal gland size | Serum angiotensin converting enzyme, hypercalcemia, lysozyme, β2-microglobulin, neopterin, collagenase, fibronectin, chitotriosidase, soluble interleukin-2 receptor (sIL-2R), Krebs Von den Lungen-6 (KL-6), YKL-40 (human cartilage glycoprotein 39), soluble intercellular adhesion molecule 1 (ICAM-1) | Worsening or new changes on chest radiographs, ground-glass attenuation on high-resolution computed tomography scan, positive 67-Ga uptake, bone cysts |

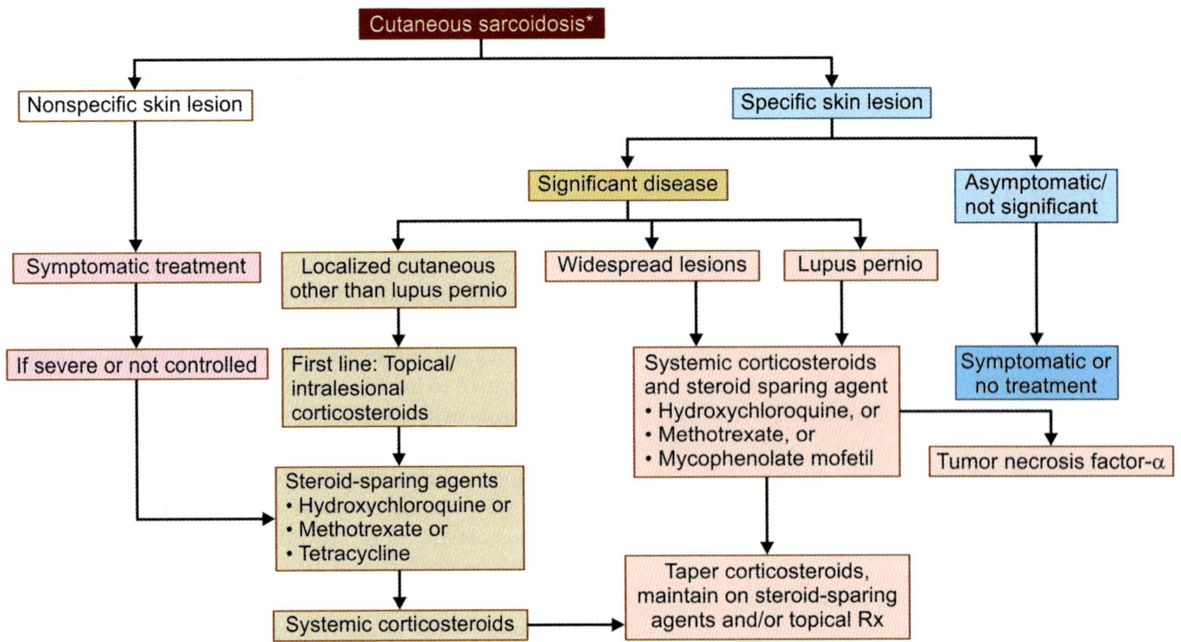


**FLOWCHART 3:** Approach to the management of sarcoidosis.

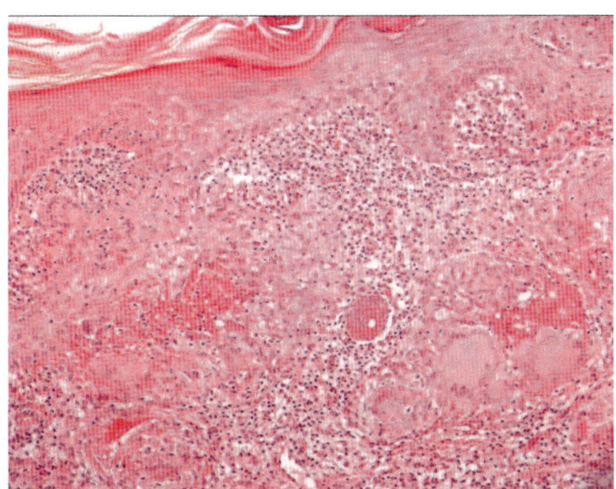

FIG. 8: Noncaseating, naked epithelioid cell sarcoidal granuloma with multiple Langhans giant cell.

**BOX 2 Indications for the initiation of systemic therapy**

- Persistent fever or weight loss
- Widespread cutaneous sarcoidosis or disfiguring skin disease like lupus pernio
- Persistent lymphadenopathy
- Evidence of symptomatic systemic involvement
  - Symptomatic or progressive pulmonary disease
  - Posterior ocular disease or anterior disease not responding to local steroids
  - Liver disease with significant dysfunction or hepatosplenomegaly, thrombocytopenia
  - Nervous system disease
  - Hypercalcemia
  - Myocardial disease
  - Myopathy or myositis
  - Renal involvement

## Systemic Therapy

Indications for systemic therapy are given in box 2. Frequent follow-ups should be ensured and the risk versus benefit ratio of the therapy be assessed.

The systemic treatment options include:

- *Corticosteroids*: They remain the mainstay of treatment in rapidly progressive and severely disfiguring cutaneous sarcoidosis. The treatment is initiated at the dose of 0.5–1 mg/kg/day (prednisolone equivalent) till a good clinical response is obtained, which usually takes 1–3 months. Subsequently, the dose is tapered to lowest maintenance dose, preferable 10 mg alternate days. It has been observed that cutaneous sarcoidosis improves at lower doses than normally used for pulmonary involvement, whereas neurological involvement calls for a higher dosage regimen
- *Hydroxychloroquine and chloroquine*: These are effective for skin and joint, sarcoid and hypercalcemia. A baseline ophthalmological evaluation is mandatory prior to initiation of therapy. The role of chloroquine is better established than hydroxychloroquine, but the latter has low risk of ocular toxicity
- Tetracycline derivatives like doxycycline and minocycline have been used in cutaneous sarcoidosis. These agents probably act via the immunomodulatory properties rather than antimicrobial activity. Minocycline monotherapy is advocated for 3 months in patients with mainly cutaneous sarcoidosis requiring systemic therapy. Patient may be started simultaneously on both hydroxychloroquine and minocycline
- *Methotrexate*: After corticosteroids, methotrexate is the next most studied agent. It is used predominantly for recalcitrant skin disease or as a corticosteroid-sparing agent. It is given at the dose of 7.5–25 mg/week with careful monitoring of the liver functions and the complete blood counts. Improvement is observed within a month but the maximal response takes 6 months
- Mycophenolate mofetil is another alternative, given at a dose of 30–45 mg/kg daily
- Azathioprine is another relatively safe steroid-sparing agent that has been used in sarcoidosis
- Cyclophosphamide is effective in many forms of sarcoidosis but the drug is often reserved for potentially life-threatening cases due to its potential toxicity
- TNF-α blockers have been evaluated in view of the role of TNF-α in pathogenesis of granuloma formation. Thalidomide has been used in recalcitrant skin lesions, especially lupus pernio. But, due to sedation, peripheral neuropathy and teratogenicity, the use is limited and biologics have been explored. Etanercept, infliximab, and adalimumab have shown good results in recalcitrant cases unresponsive to traditional therapeutic modalities. Therefore, TNF-α antagonists are recommended as the second-line therapy for corticosteroid-unresponsive lupus pernio. In fact, sarcoid-like granuloma formation has been reported with these biologics in patients with arthritis and other inflammatory diseases. Discontinuation of therapy leads to partial or complete regression.

Other therapeutic agents are allopurinol, isotretinoin, pentoxifylline, fumaric acid esters, and melatonin. PUVA light phototherapy, photodynamic therapy, pulsed-dye lasers, and $CO_2$ lasers. Reconstructive surgery for severely disfiguring lesions.

The response to cyclosporine is variable. Levamisole is not recommended.

Patients on treatment need to be followed up as per the recommendations for the particular drug therapy being used. Otherwise, an annual follow-up is recommended for all patients, which should include:

- Chest X-ray (posterior, anterior and lateral)

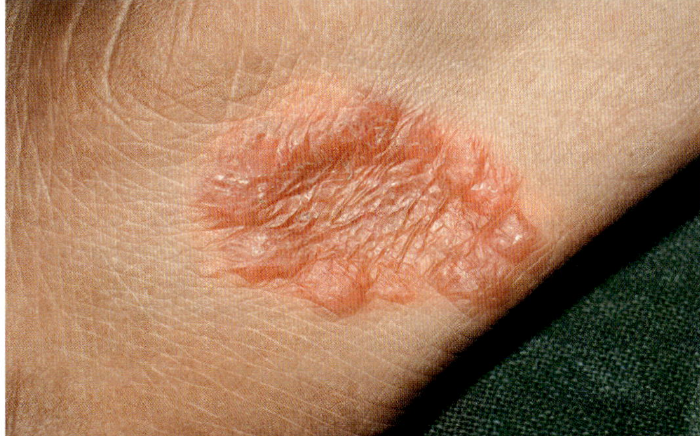

FIG. 9: Close up of annular plaque of closely set papules in localized granuloma annulare.

- Pulmonary function tests (spirometry and diffusion capacity for carbon monoxide)
- Ophthalmologic examination
- Complete blood count
- Comprehensive serum chemistries (including calcium, liver function tests, creatinine).

# NECROBIOTIC DISORDERS

## Granuloma Annulare

Granuloma annulare is a relatively common, benign inflammatory dermatosis that was first described by Colcott Fox in 1895. It belongs to the group of necrobiotic disorders that are characterized by foci of alteration of collagen, known as necrobiosis, surrounded by histiocytes and lymphocytes. GA in its classical form presents as erythematous, nonscaly annular lesions.

Granuloma annulare mostly develops within first three decades of life sparing early infancy and is twice as common in women, although it can affect any age group. Generalized GA has a later age of onset in $4^{th}$–$7^{th}$ decades.

### Etiopathogenesis

The exact etiopathogenesis of GA is not well understood. It is often considered as a reaction pattern occurring in response to various inciting factors, such as insect bites, vaccination trauma, viral infections [human papillomavirus, varicella zoster virus, Epstein-Barr virus (EBV), parvovirus B19, hepatitis C virus, and human immunodeficiency virus (HIV)].

A higher prevalence of HLA-Bw35 has been demonstrated in individuals with generalized GA, as compared with controls and those with localized lesions.

### Clinical Features

Classically, they present as localized, generalized, perforating and subcutaneous variants. Other less common forms include patch, linear, "follicular pustulous" GA and papular umbilicated forms.

- *Localized GA*: It is the most common form, and presents as single or multiple asymptomatic annular or arciform erythematous nonscaly plaques of closely set papules usually affecting the extremities (Fig. 9). The discrete papules are better visualized on stretching the skin
- *Generalized or disseminated GA*: It presents with numerous skin-colored erythematous papules or plaques, which are often annular in configuration, over a generalized distribution especially over trunk (Fig. 10) and extremities. There is relative sparing of the head and neck, palms, soles and the mucosa. It is a less common form which presents at a later age than localized form and is more common in the HIV-positive patients
- *Perforating GA*: In this variant, the patient presents with perforating lesions with transepidermal elimination of damaged collagen. The lesions are yellowish papules discharging clear fluid, which dries and forms crust, and lesions heal with scarring
- *Subcutaneous GA*: It is a rare form that presents with single or multiple painless subcutaneous nodules over scalp or pretibial region, especially in children. These are also known as benign rheumatoid nodules, pseudorheumatoid nodules, deep GA, and subcutaneous palisading granuloma.

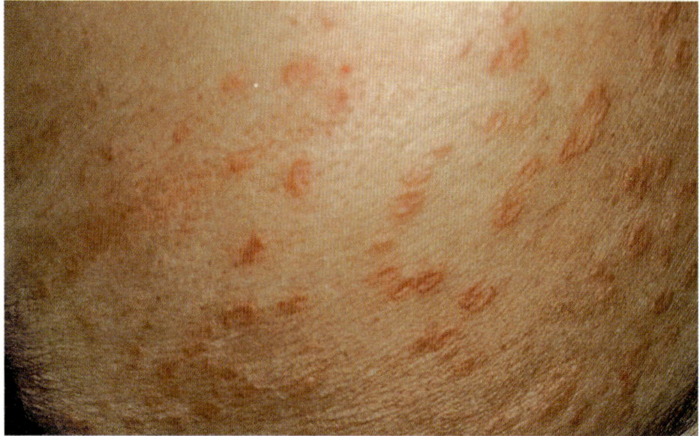

*Note:* Annular morphology is maintained in most lesions.

**FIG. 10:** Multiple eruptive lesions of granuloma annulare on trunk.

Granuloma annulare has been reportedly found to be associated with diabetes mellitus, dyslipidemia, malignancies (atypical GA), autoimmune thyroiditis, toxic adenoma of the thyroid (Plummer's disease), uveitis, temporal arteritis, morphoea, necrobiosis lipoidica, and sarcoidosis.

Both type I and type II DM have been reported with GA, although the association with type I is stronger. Hematological malignancies are more often associated with GA rather than solid organ malignancies. Of these, Hodgkin's and non-Hodgkin's lymphomas, mycosis fungoides, B-cell lymphomas have been reported. Moreover, the skin lesions arising from the lymphoma may mimic GA, and it may be difficult to distinguish even histopathologically.

### Histopathology

The histopathology of GA is characterized by three main features: foci of degeneration of collagen or necrobiosis, lymphohistiocytic infiltrate and prominent deposition of mucin. The foci of necrobiosis are seen as eosinophilic homogeneous mass of degenerated collagen (H and E). Special stains like alcian blue or colloidal iron help identify the mucin. Three patterns have been recognized, necrobiotic palisading granulomas, an interstitial form, and granulomas of sarcoidal or tuberculoid type. Of these, the interstitial pattern is the most common and occurs in approximately 70% of cases, the second most common pattern being the palisading pattern seen in about 25% of biopsies.

- *Interstitial pattern*: Necrobiosis is less defined. Lymphohistiocytic infiltrate is seen perivascularly and between the collagen bundles. Basophilic mucin is seen infiltrating between collagen bundles in the mid and upper dermis with separation and incomplete degeneration of collagen fibers. Interstitial pattern is more common in localized GA compared to generalized GA and is also associated with patch type GA. In the interstitial pattern, there are no formed areas of necrobiosis, histiocytes and lymphocytes are present around blood vessels and between collagen bundles, and collagen fibers are separated by mucin
- Palisading pattern is characterized by central foci of necrobiosis in mid to upper dermis, surrounded by lympho-

**TABLE 6: Differential diagnosis of granuloma annulare (GA)**

| Localized GA | Generalized GA | Perforating GA | Subcutaneous GA |
|---|---|---|---|
| • Tinea corporis<br>• Annular lichen planus<br>• Erythema annulare centrifugum<br>• Erythema multiforme<br>• Erythema migrans<br>• Tuberculides<br>• Tertiary syphilis<br>• Sarcoidosis<br>• Annular elastolytic giant cell granuloma | • Secondary syphilis<br>• Arthropod bites<br>• Id eruption<br>• Eruptive xanthoma<br>• Eruptive syringoma<br>• Eruptive histiocytoma | • Molluscum contagiosum<br>• Perforating collagenosis<br>• Acquired perforating dermatosis<br>• Perforating sarcoidosis<br>• Papulonecrotic tuberculid<br>• Elastosis perforans serpiginosa | • Trauma<br>• Deep fungal infection<br>• Tumors<br>• Sarcoidosis<br>• Rheumatoid nodule |

histiocytic inflammatory infiltrates that palisade around this foci. This pattern is common in both localized and generalized GA and also observed in subcutaneous GA. Perforating GA is characterized by transepidermal elimination of mucinous, degenerating collagen fibers surrounded by palisading granulomas
- Sarcoidal or tuberculoid type granuloma is rare. Epithelioid histiocytic nodules that resemble the sarcoidal or tuberculoid granulomas are present.

Eosinophils may also be present and the presence of mucin and eosinophils can help distinguish GA from sarcoidosis.

## Immunohistochemistry

Intense expression of CD68/PGM1 is reported along with a fainter detection of CD68/KP-1 and a variable detection of lysozyme in the lymphocytic infiltrate.

## Differential Diagnosis

Differential diagnosis of GA are mentioned in table 6.

## Treatment

The localized form of GA if not cosmetically disfiguring can be left as such. Topical or intralesional corticosteroids form the first line of therapy. Various treatment options are summarized in table 7.

**TABLE 7: Treatment options for granuloma annulare (GA)**

| Localized GA | Generalized GA |
|---|---|
| First-line therapy<br>• Potent topical corticosteroids with or without occlusion<br>• Intralesional corticosteroids—2.5–10 mg/cc triamcinolone acetonide | First-line therapy<br>• Topical and/or intralesional corticosteroids<br>• Topical calcineurin inhibitors—tacrolimus and pimecrolimus<br>• Ultraviolet A1, psoralen ultraviolet A, narrowband ultraviolet B phototherapy<br>• Systemic drugs—hydroxychloroquine, dapsone, isotretinoin, cyclosporine |
| Other therapeutic modalities<br>• Cryotherapy<br>• Interferon-γ<br>• Photodynamic therapy<br>• Pulsed-dye laser<br>• Tacrolimus<br>• Imiquimod | Other therapeutic modalities (case reports/series)<br>• Nicotinamide<br>• Infliximab, adalimumab, etanercept<br>• Pentoxifylline<br>• Clofazimine<br>• Hydroxyurea, chlorambucil<br>• Fumaric acid esters<br>• Doxycycline<br>• Combination of rifampin, ofloxacin, and minocycline |

# Necrobiosis Lipoidica

Necrobiosis lipoidica is a disorder of necrobiosis accompanied by granulomatous reaction, blood vessel wall thickening and cutaneous lipid deposition, clinically characterized by sharply demarcated plaques of atrophic yellowish skin, which may ulcerate. Necrobiosis lipoidica is common in young women. Earlier age of onset is seen in insulin-dependent diabetics.

The etiology is poorly understood, but a strong association with diabetes points toward role of microangiopathy and immunoglobulin deposition in development of the lesions.

The lesions begin as erythematous papules that slowly extend peripherally with an indurated edge. Over time, larger area may be involved and the plaques develop a yellowish hue with prominent telangiectasias and a shiny atrophic surface. Ulcerations may develop. They typically develop on shins and are bilaterally distributed. Other rarer sites are scalp, face and extremities or trunk. Hypoesthesia or anesthesia, and hypohidrosis may be present and are correlated with the observation of decreased cutaneous nerves found on histopathology.

## Histopathology

Histopathologically, necrobiosis lipoidica resembles GA but differ in being a deeper process that involves the subcutaneous tissue and dermis with extensive areas of necrobiosis. The epidermis is typically spared in GA, whereas it may be atrophic or even absent (if ulcerated) in case of necrobiosis lipoidica. At low magnification, a characteristic tier-like or layered arrangement of the granulomas is visible along with areas of collagen degeneration. Another differentiating feature is the thickening of the blood vessel walls caused by immune-reactant deposition (immunoglobulin M, immunoglobulin A, C3 and fibrinogen) which can be picked up on direct immuno-fluorescence. Demonstration of lipids with the help of special stains and relative scarcity of mucin also aid in diagnosis. Superficial blood vessels may be dilated and increased in number, responsible for the visible telangiectasias.

### Treatment

Atrophy tends to persist. The treatment is on similar lines as that of GA. Additionally, split-thickness autografting or excision and grafting are other viable options. Aspirin and dipyridamole have been used.

## Granuloma Multiforme

Granuloma multiforme was first described by Leiker in patients from Nigeria. The condition is endemic to certain villages of eastern Nigeria where it is called as "Ununo Enyi" (meaning elephant ringworm in the local Ibo language). Although prevalent in Africa, it is also often reported from Indonesia and India.

### Clinical Features

It predominantly affects women over 40 years of age and presents as skin-colored papules to plaques which often coalesce-forming annular or arciform morphology. The lesions usually develop over photoexposed areas. Clinically, the lesions may be mistaken for that of leprosy, but intact lesional sensation and sweating can help differentiate this entity.

### Histopathology

The histopathology shows focal areas of necrobiosis, with loss of elastic tissue, surrounded by histiocytes. Multinucleated giant cells, perivascular lymphocytic infiltrate, plasma cells and eosinophils may be seen. Lack of acid-fast bacilli and no neural involvement further help in ruling out leprosy, especially in endemic zones.

### Differential Diagnosis

Granuloma annulare, tuberculoid leprosy, actinic granuloma, and annular sarcoidosis.

### Treatment

These lesions tend to persist for months or years altogether and usually are highly resistant to any form of treatment. A trial of topical steroids may be given.

## Necrobiotic Xanthogranuloma

Necrobiotic xanthogranuloma is characterized clinically by presence of xanthomatous lesions, histopathologically by presence of necrobiosis and their association with paraproteinemias. It was recognized as a distinct entity by Kossard et al. in 1980.

### Clinical Features

Classically, reddish-yellowish xanthomatous nodules or plaques are present in a periorbital distribution in 80% of the cases. Other sites of predilection include extremities and the trunk. There may be atrophy and ulceration, especially in lesions over the trunk. Ocular involvement in the form of conjunctivitis, keratitis, uveitis, proptosis and even blindness has been reported. Systemic symptoms like fatigue, nausea, vomiting, Raynaud's phenomenon, pulmonary and cardiac involvement have all been reported. Up to 80% of the patients have associated monoclonal gammopathy, immunoglobulin G type with $\kappa$ or $\lambda$ light chains.

### Pathogenesis

It is speculated that the abnormal paraproteins become complexed with circulating lipids and get deposited in the skin. These deposits then elicit a foreign body granulomatous reaction characterized by proliferation of macrophages.

### Histopathology

Necrobiotic xanthogranuloma is characterized by sheets or nodules of granuloma formation involving the dermis and subcutaneous tissue. The granulomas consist of various types of multinucleated giant cells like Touton giant cells and bizarre angulated giant cells. Areas of necrobiosis are seen surrounding the granulomas along with cholesterol clefts which give a foamy appearance.

### Differential Diagnosis

Granuloma annulare, necrobiosis lipoidica.

### Treatment

Treatment is primarily directed at the associated paraproteinemia and involves use of cytotoxics like melphalan, chlorambucil, INF-$\alpha$2b, nitrogen mustard, cyclophosphamide, methotrexate, azathioprine, high-dose steroids, and thalidomide. Plasmapheresis has been used in cases not responding to cytotoxics, to reduce the levels of circulating immunoglobulins.

## Palisaded Neutrophilic and Granulomatous Dermatitis

Palisaded neutrophilic and granulomatous dermatitis (PNGD) is a rare heterogeneous entity that is often associated with multiple underlying diseases; the most prominent association being connective tissue disorders, such as lupus erythematosus and rheumatoid arthritis or even drugs like methotrexate and TNF-$\alpha$ inhibitors.

### Clinical Features

The lesions present as papulonodular lesions with smooth, ulcerated, or umbilicated surfaces and are usually symmetrically distributed over the extremities. In interstitial granulomatous dermatitis, considered to be a variant of PNGD, the patients may present with plaques or subcutaneous cords which may be linear or arciform, ("rope sign") typically on the trunk.

### Histopathology

There are three histologic patterns of PNGD depending on the stage of the lesion:

1. Early lesion resembles leukocytoclastic vasculitis with strands of amorphous basophilic material

2. Fully developed lesion resembles GA but differ in containing a prominent neutrophilic infiltrate with thin degenerated collagen bundles, fibrin and mucin
3. Final stage resembles necrobiosis lipoidica.

### Treatment

Palisaded neutrophilic and granulomatous dermatitis has a variable course and may persist for years altogether. Treatment of choice seems to be oral glucocorticoids. Other options include colchicine, cyclosporine, cyclophosphamide, hydroxychloroquine, nonsteroidal anti-inflammatory drugs, and dapsone.

## Rheumatoid Nodules

Rheumatoid nodules are classically associated with rheumatoid arthritis (rheumatoid factor in high titer) and develop in nearly 20% of the patients.

### Clinical Features

Rheumatoid nodules present as deeply seated firm nodules or masses, most commonly over the proximal ulna and the olecranon process. Other less commonly affected sites include the metacarpophalangeal and proximal interphalangeal joints, over amputation stumps, knees, scapulae, buttocks, sacrum, and ear. Extracutaneous involvement in the form of pulmonary or cardiac nodules are also reported.

These lesions may be single or multiple and vary in size from a few millimeters to 5 cm. Sometimes, they precede the development of rheumatoid arthritis. The term rheumatoid nodulosis is used for the patients who present with multiple nodules over extremities with intermittent arthralgias but no evidence of rheumatoid arthritis.

### Histopathology

Rheumatoid nodules are located in the deep dermis to subcutaneous tissue. There is central focus of necrobiosis, seen as a homogeneous pink staining area with fibrinoid degeneration of collagen. Nuclear fragments and basophilic material may be present but mucin is minimal or absent. These foci are surrounded by palisading histiocytes. Surrounding these histiocytes are sparse inflammatory infiltrates and fibrosis.

# FOREIGN BODY GRANULOMATOUS REACTION

## Foreign Body Granuloma

Foreign substances in the skin can produce two kinds of reactions depending on the type of foreign body implanted and the host immune response:

- *Nonallergic foreign body reaction*: This is characterized by a granulomatous response comprised of histiocytes and foreign body giant cells which surround the foreign body and try to shield it. The detection of engulfed foreign body within the macrophages or giant cells helps clinch the diagnosis. The most common cause of such a reaction is a ruptured hair follicle or follicular cyst. Other endogenous substances which can be responsible are urates in gout, ruptured pilomatricoma or epidermoid cysts. Exogenous sources include silk and nylon sutures, paraffin, silicone gel, talc, surgical glove starch powder, cactus spines, etc. Polarizing microscopy can help identify these foreign bodies, as many of these are doubly refractile, e.g., nylon sutures, wood, talc, surgical glove starch powder, and sea urchin spines
- *Allergic foreign body reaction*: This develops in individuals who are specifically sensitized to the foreign body. Histopathologically, these show a sarcoidal or tuberculoid pattern. Phagocytosis of the foreign substance is minimal and not prominent. The common causes include zirconium, beryllium, and certain dyes used in tattoos.

The different foreign body reactions have been elaborated in table 8. Many of these foreign bodies can be detected by X-ray spectrometry or radiographic analysis.

## Tattoo-induced Granulomatous Reaction

Most of the reactions to tattoos develop due to the red dyes containing mercuric sulfide, such as cinnabar. Red pigment like ferric hydrate (sienna or red ocher), cadmium selenide (cadmium red), and organic dyes are somewhat safer. Reactions have been

**TABLE 8: Foreign body reactions with the respective clinical scenarios and associated histological features**

| Foreign body | Source and clinical scenario | Histopathology |
|---|---|---|
| Paraffinoma | Cosmetic injections of oily substances (paraffin) into the breasts, genitalia, or scalp | • "Swiss cheese" appearance (ovoid/round cavities occupied by the oil). Multinucleated foreign-body giant cells. Variable fibrosis and eosinophils<br>• Special stains on frozen sections—orange with sudan IV or oil red O |
| Silicone granuloma | Leakage or rupture of silicone gel from breast implants | • "Swiss cheese" appearance (ovoid/round cavities occupied by the oil). Multinucleated foreign-body giant cells<br>• Variable fibrosis and eosinophils |
| Talc granuloma | Accidental contamination of wound with magnesium silicate | • Histiocytes and multinucleated giant cells, which may contain visible talc particles. Talc crystals—needle shaped with yellow-brown or blue-green hue. In polarized light—white birefringent particles |
| Starch granuloma | Contamination of wounds with surgical gloves powdered with corn starch | • Histiocytes and multinucleated giant cells. Starch granules—seen as ill-defined ovoid basophilic structures (10–20 μm diameter) within foreign-body giant cells<br>• Periodic acid–Schiff and methenamine silver positive. In polarized light—characteristic birefringence, showing a Maltese cross configuration |

Continued

*Continued*

| Foreign body | Source and clinical scenario | Histopathology |
|---|---|---|
| Silica granuloma | Silica (silicon dioxide) present in rocks, soil, sand, and glass may contaminate wounds | • Epithelioid histiocytes with sparse lymphocytic infiltrate, multinucleate giant cells with silica crystals (up to 100 μm in length). In polarized light—doubly refractile particles seen<br>• Sarcoid like granulomas in case of development of delayed hypersensitivity |
| Zirconium granuloma | Deodorant sticks containing zirconium lactate and creams containing zirconium oxide | • Allergic granulomatous reaction with multiple epithelioid cells and few giant cells and a sparse to dense lymphocytic infiltrate (simulates sarcoidosis). Zirconium not visualized under polarized light due to small size |
| Titanium granuloma | Rare, may occur after body piercing | • Histiocytes, lymphocytes, and plasma cells. Macrophages may contain minute brown-black particles |
| Zinc-induced granuloma | Zinc containing insulin preparations may rarely lead to granulomatous reaction. Initially presents as sterile furunculoid lesions with later fibrosis | • Early furunculoid lesion—dense neutrophilic infiltrate with multiple birefringent rhomboidal crystals of zinc insulin. Later, fibrosis and granulomatous inflammation |
| Beryllium granuloma | • No longer seen now. Beryllium-containing compounds were used in manufacture of fluorescent light tubes<br>• These presented as incomplete healing of the laceration, followed by swelling, induration, tenderness and central ulceration | • Cutaneous granulomas of systemic berylliosis—similar to those of sarcoidosis. Purely local granulomas—show central necrosis, dense infiltrate of lymphocytes may be present. Epidermis shows acanthosis and possibly ulceration<br>• Beryllium particles are not seen in histologic sections |

reported with chrome green, cobalt blue, purple manganese salts, yellow cadmium sulfide, and iron oxide. The reaction can be lichenoid, eczematous, pseudoepitheliomatous, photoallergic,or granulomatous.

### Histopathology

The tattoo granules are scattered throughout the infiltrate. As discussed in the section on foreign body granulomas, the reaction may be either of the sarcoidal type or the foreign-body type depending on the histopathological picture.

## INTERSTITIAL GRANULOMATOUS DRUG REACTION

### Clinical Features

Interstitial granulomatous drug reaction is an uncommon pattern of drug reaction that presents with annular to solid erythematous plaques on the proximal extremities and intertriginous areas. Various agents have been implicated like calcium channel blockers, ACE inhibitors, lipid-lowering agents, antihistamines, diuretics, anticonvulsants, antidepressants, allopurinol, thalidomide, anti-TNF agents and even herbal medications. Reaction generally completely subsides once the offending drug is withdrawn.

### Histopathology

There is an interstitial infiltrate of lymphocytes and histiocytes within collagen bundles along with slight fragmentation of collagen fibers. A variable number of eosinophils and neutrophils may also be observed along with vacuolar interface change.

### Differential Diagnosis

Granuloma annulare and PNGD: Vacuolar interface in histopathology helps differentiate the interstitial granulomatous drug reaction from these entities.

## SUGGESTED READINGS


1. Adams DO. The granulomatous inflammatory response. Am J Pathol. 1976:84:163-92.
2. Ali MM, Atwan AA, Gonzalez ML. Cutaneous sarcoidosis: updates in the pathogenesis. J Eur Acad Dermatol Venereol. 2010;24:747-55.
3. Atzori L, Pilloni L, Pinna AL. Interstitial granulomatous drug reaction due to febuxostat. Indian J Dermatol Venereol Leprol. 2014;80:182-4.
4. Baughman RP, Lower EE, Du Bois R. Sarcoidosis. Lancet. 2003;361:1111-8.
5. Brecher A palisaded neutrophilic and granulomatous dermatitis. Dermatol Online J. 2003;9:1.
6. El Sayed F, Torbey G, Chababi M. Childhood sarcoidosis: diagnostic issues. Dermatol Online J. 2013;19:20037.
7. Haimovic A, Sanchez M, Judson MA, et al. Sarcoidosis: a comprehensive review and update for the dermatologist: part I. Cutaneous disease. J Am Acad Dermatol. 2012;66:699.e1-18.
8. Hanna WM, Moreno-Merlo F, Andrighetti L. Granuloma annulare: an elastic tissue disease? Case report and literature review. Ultrastruct Pathol. 1999;23:33.
9. He Y, Maverakis E, Ramirez-Maverakis D, et al. Combination therapy with intralesional triamcinolone and oral dapsone for management of palisaded neutrophilic and granulomatous dermatitis. Dermatol Online J. 2013;19(2):17.
10. Kim MS, Lee JH, Park K, et al. Allopurinol-induced: DRESS syndrome with a histologic pattern consistent with interstitial granulomatous drug reaction. Am J Dermatopathol. 2014;36:193-6.
11. King TE. Clinical manifestations and diagnosis of sarcoidosis In: Post TW (Ed). UpToDate. Waltham, MA: UpToDate; 2011.
12. Kumari R, Thappa DM, Chougule A, et al. Granuloma multiforme: a report from India. Indian J Dermatol Venereol Leprol. 2009;75:296-9.
13. Marcoval J, Mana J, Moreno A, et al. Subcutaneous sarcoidosis-clinicopathological study of 10 cases. Br J Dermatol. 2005;153:790-4.
14. Mathew S, Bauer KL, Fischoeder A, et al. The anergic state in sarcoidosis is associated with diminished dendritic cell function. J Immunol. 2008;181:746-55.

15. Miyara M, Amoura Z, Parizot C, et al. The immune paradox of sarcoidosis and regulatory T cells. J Exp Med. 2006;203:359-70.
16. Momen SE, Al-Niaimmi F. Sarcoid and the nail: review of the literature. Clin Exp Dermatol. 2013;38:119-24.
17. Pandhi D, Sonthalia S, Singal A. Mortimer's Malady revisited: a case ofpolymorphic cutaneous and systemic sarcoidosis. Indian J Dermatol Venereol Leprol. 2010;76:448.
18. Reed J, deShazo RD, Houle TT, et al. Clinical features of sarcoid rhinosinusitis. Am J Med. 2010;123:856.
19. Rose BD, Rizzato G. Renal disease in sarcoidosis. In: Post TW (Ed). UpToDate. Waltham, MA: UpToDate; 2012.
20. Sequeira W, Aggarwal R. Sarcoid arthropathy. In: Post TW (Ed). UpToDate. Waltham, MA: UpToDate; 2012.
21. Singal A, Vij A, Pandhi D. Post herpes-zoster scar sarcoidosis with pulmonary involvement. Indian Dermatol Online J. 2014;5:77-9.
22. Statement on sarcoidosis: joint statement of the American Thoracic Society (ATS), the European Respiratory Society (ERS) and the World Association of Sarcoidosis and Other Granulomatous Disorders (WASOG) adopted by the ATS Board of Directors and by the ERS Executive Committee, February 1999. Am J Respir Crit Care Med. 1999;160:736-55.
23. Stefanaki K, Tsivitanidou-Kakourou T, Stefanaki C, et al. Histological and immunohistochemical study of granuloma annulare and subcutaneous granuloma annulare in children. J Cutan Pathol. 2007;34:392-6.
24. Stephenson SR, Campbell SM, Drew GS, et al. Palisaded neutrophilic and granulomatous dermatitis in a patient with rheumatoid arthritis on adalimumab. J Cutan Pathol. 2011;38:644-8.
25. Wahlstrom J, Katchar K, Wigzell H, et al. Analysis of intracellular cytokines in CD4+ and CD8+ lung and blood T cells in sarcoidosis. Am J Respir Crit Care Med. 2001;163:115-21.
26. Wanat KA, Rosenbach M. A practical approach to cutaneous sarcoidosis. Am J Clin Dermatol. 2014;15:283-97.
27. Wouters CH, Maes A, Foley KP, Bertin J, Rose CD. Blau Syndrome, the prototypic auto-inflammatory granulomatous disease. Pediatr Rheumatol Online J. 2014; 12:33.

# 13 SECTION Vascular Disorders

# 38 CHAPTER Cutaneous Vascular Abnormalities (Malformations and Tumors)

Nilendu Sarma, Sayantani Chakraborty

## INTRODUCTION

Vascular anomalies represent a spectrum of disorders from a simple "birthmark" to life-threatening entities.

Hamartomas arise from defective embryologic development resulting in miscellaneous collection of abnormally arranged but indigenous tissues. Malformations also develop from aberration in embryological development. However these are different from hamartoma. There is no evidence of tissue proliferation, a feature that differentiates it from benign and malignant neoplasias. These may progress along with the child's overall body growth.

Cutaneous vascular abnormalities present in versatile manner and classification of these conditions is associated with too many controversies. Accurate diagnosis is important for appropriate evaluation and management and it often requires multidisciplinary specialists. The earliest classification of these disorders was done by Virchow which was purely a pathological classification. The other attempts to classify this disorder were by World Health Organization.

The seminal classification by Mulliken and Glowacki formed the basis of classification of vascular abnormalities. Most updated classification by International Society for the Study of Vascular Anomalies (ISSVA), approved in 2014 during the Melbourne Meeting provides a more clinically relevant and flexible knowledge including new genetic and histologic information.

According to the most widely used classification system of ISSVA, cutaneous vascular abnormalities have been divided into two subtypes:

- Vascular malformations
- Vascular tumors

Some abnormalities like verrucous hemangioma, multifocal lymphangioendotheliomatosis with thrombocytopenia/cutaneovisceral angiomatosis with thrombocytopenia (MLT/CAT), Kaposiform lymphangiomatosis (KLA) and PTEN (type) hamartoma of soft tissue/"angiomatosis" of soft tissue are still mentioned as "unclassified" entities.

## VASCULAR MALFORMATIONS

Vascular malformations have been classified into various types based on the structure involved, like capillary, venous, arterial, lymphatic, and combined anomalies. Another very commonly used terms are "slow-flow" (capillary, venous, lymphatic, or a combination of them) and "high-flow" (arteriovenous) vascular malformations.

Malformation may result in alteration in function as in nevus anemicus where malformation is characterized by hyperfunctioning tissue. Various vascular malformations have been described below.

Vascular malformations have been recently classified by ISSVA. Based on the involved vessel type, following types of malformation are found:

- Capillary malformations (CMs)
- Lymphatic malformations (LMs)
- Venous malformations (VMs)
- Arteriovenous malformations (AVMs)
- Arteriovenous fistula (AVF).

Each of this may be present as isolated abnormality (simple) or two or more these may be simultaneously present (combined), e.g., CVM (capillary-venous malformation) or CLAVM (capillary-lymphatic-arteriovenous malformations). Malformation can affect major vessel and also be associated with other anomalies (syndromes).

## CLASSIFICATION

International Society for the Study of Vascular Anomalies has recommended a classification of all types of vascular anomaly. Some of the dermatologically important parts are mentioned below.

Capillary malformations can be the isolated abnormality (simple) or a part of multiple other abnormalities. Common examples of simple CMs are Nevus simplex (Salmon patch/"angel kiss", "stork bite"), Cutaneous and/or mucosal CM [port wine stain (PWS)]. CM are known to be associated with bone and/or soft tissue overgrowth, central nervous system (CNS) and/or ocular anomalies as in Sturge-Weber syndrome, with AVM (CM-AVM), in a syndrome called microcephaly-capillary malformation (MICCAP), megalencephaly-capillary malformation-polymicrogyria (MCAP), hereditary hemorrhagic telangiectasia (HHT) (different types) and cutis marmorata telangiectatica congenita (CMTC).

Most common type of LM has been named as common/cystic type. LM has been classified into various subtypes based on sizes like macrocystic, microcystic, and mixed cystic LM, associated anomaly/syndrome (e.g., LM in Gorham-Stout disease), and distribution [generalized lymphatic anomaly (GLA)], morphology (channel type LM). Different types of primary lymphedema have also been included in this classification.

Venous malformation has been classified as common, familial VM cutaneomucosal (VMCM), blue rubber bleb nevus (Bean) syndrome, glomuvenous malformation (GVM) and different types of cerebral cavernous malformation (CCM) (different types).

## Salmon Patch

Salmon patch is an extremely common vascular abnormality, seen in about 30–40% of the neonates, presenting with irregular, pink or red macular lesions with or without fine telangiectasia. The most common sites are the nape of the neck, forehead, upper eyelids and less commonly, the sacral region and most of the lesions, especially those on the face fade within the first year of life while those on the neck and trunk may be more persistent. The sacral lesions may be associated with occult spinal dysraphism. Histopathologically, the lesions consist of ectatic superficial dermal capillaries (Fig. 1).

## Port Wine Stain (Nevus Flammeus)

Port wine stains are vascular nevi/malformation characterized by ectasia of vessels usually involving capillaries (30–300 µm diameter) and postcapillary venules in the papillary and mid-reticular dermis. These appear at birth and are noted in about 0.3–0.5% of infants. They persist throughout the life. These are generally sporadic but familial cases (autosomal dominant with low penetrance) may occur.

### Clinical Features

Initially the lesions appear as macular telangiectatic pale pink patch commonly on the facial region along the distribution of the trigeminal nerve, limbs, and mucosa. With age, the color darkens and there may be some elevations on the surface forming papulo-nodular lesion with soft tissue overgrowth.

Soft tissue swelling or a bony overgrowth may develop under a PWS especially over the face and there may be unilateral limb hypertrophy and lymphatic abnormality. There may be ocular complications like choroidal granuloma, and glaucoma.

Sometimes, PWS may be seen in syndromes having other forms of vascular anomaly, and often noted over LMs like in Klippel–Trénaunay syndrome, Parkes-Weber syndrome and Sturge-Weber syndrome.

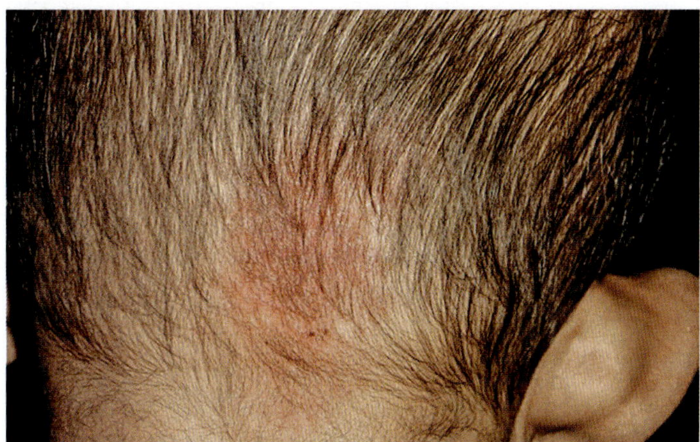

**FIG. 1:** Salmon patch.

### Etiopathogenesis

Etiopathogenesis of this condition may be linked to abnormal neural regulation (deficiency of sympathetic innervation) of the capillaries leading to dilatation. Genetic analysis of the familial PWS cases has located CMC1-locus for susceptibility of PWS on chromosome 5q.

### Treatment

The treatment of choice is pulsed tunable dye laser (PDL) which reduces number and size of red cells in the vessels by selective photothermolysis. However many cases are resistant to PDL.

## Cutis Marmorata Telangiectatica Congenita

It is an uncommon, congenital, localized or generalized vascular malformation that resembles physiological cutis marmorata in neonates. Clinically it appears as fixed reticular erythema that produce marbling of the skin. But this marbling is fixed and does not disappear after warming. There are distinctive depressed lines that occur due to atrophy of the skin and subcutaneous tissues, a feature not seen in physiologic cutis marmorata.

The most common sites of involvement are the limbs or the hemi-trunk. There is a distinct demarcation line between the affected and the normal skin. Sometimes the surface is ulcerated. The color lightens with age.

This may be associated with numerous other congenital anomalies; aplasia cutis, cleft palate, limb hypoplasia/hyperplasia, macrocephaly, macrosomia, segmental overgrowth, CNS malformations, pigmented nevus, widespread Mongolian spot, syndactyly, hypothyroidism, anogenital anomalies, glaucoma and developmental delay.

CMTC is an important feature in Adams-Oliver syndrome.

## Nevus Syndromes

There are many syndromes that have associated vascular nevi. Capillary nevi or PWS may be associated with many other disorders as mentioned in box 1.

## Sturge–Weber syndrome

This syndrome comprises of congenital facial PWS along with ipsilateral CNS vascular malformation (leptomeningeal angiomatosis). The latter is mostly present over the posterior parietal and occipital lobe of the cerebral cortex and vascular malformation of the choroid of the eye leading to glaucoma.

### Pathogenesis

Somatic mutation during early embryogenesis in the anterior neural fold results in SWS.

### Clinical Features

Port wine stains in this condition involve the upper eyelid but may sometimes involve the lower eyelid. Rarely it may extend

**BOX 1 Syndromes associated with port wine stains**

- Sturge–Weber syndrome (SWS)
- Klippel–Trénaunay syndrome (KTS)
- Parkes-Weber syndrome
- Phakomatosis pigmentovascularis
- Cobb syndrome
- Wyburn-Mason syndrome
- Proteus syndrome
- Roberts syndrome
- Beckwith–Wiedemann syndrome
- TAR syndrome
- Rubinstein-Taybi syndrome
- Coat's disease

TAR, thrombocytopenia-absent radius.

to the mucosal surfaces and leads to concomitant gingival hypertrophy. Association of SWS with Klippel-Trenaunay syndrome has been reported. Epileptic seizure and mental retardation is common. Hemiplegia is noted in approximately 30% of cases.

Choroidal angiomas lead to mechanical obstruction at the angle of the anterior chamber as well as increased production of aqueous humor results in the development of glaucoma. Ophthalmological examination from early life is recommended in children with CMs of eyelids to detect glaucoma at the earliest. Hypertrophy may occur on the affected part (Figs 2 and 3).

## Investigations

Plain X-ray shows sinuous "tramline/railroad-track calcification" of the cerebral cortex. Both MRI and CT scans may be used to detect the cerebral and ocular defects. Gadolinium enhanced MRI scan helps in earlier detection of the cerebral vascular lesions. PET scan will help to view areas of ischemia.

## Management

The management of the condition aims at control of seizure, glaucoma, and laser therapy should be attempted for PWS.

# Klippel–Trénaunay Syndrome

It is characterized by PWS, varicosity, soft tissue, and bony overgrowth. Not all patients have all these three features.

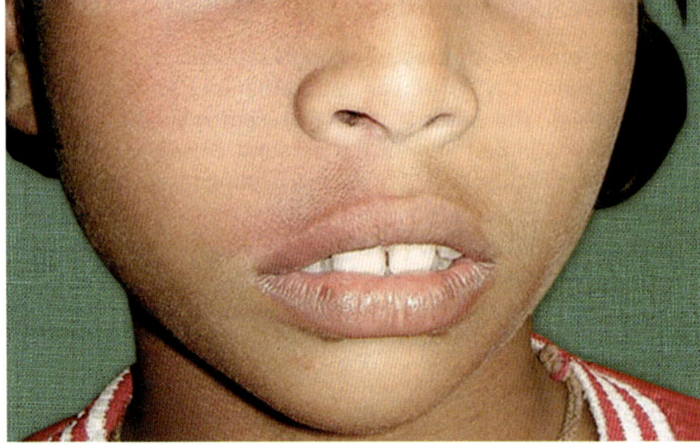

**FIG. 2:** Large unilateral port wine stains and asymmetrical facial hypertrophy of the affected side in Sturge–Weber syndrome.

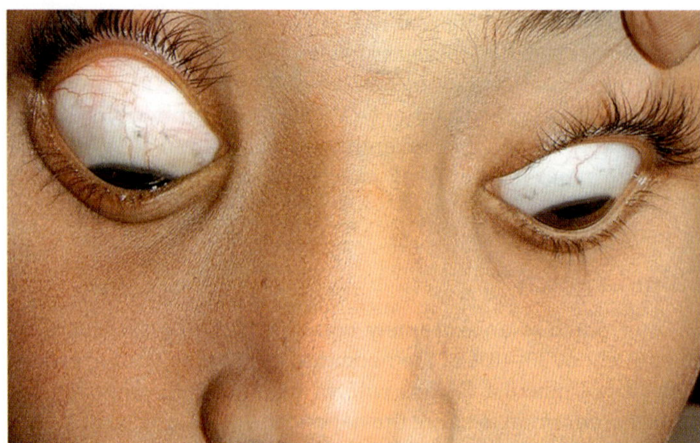

**FIG. 3:** Port wine stains with capillary proliferation in bulbal conjunctiva in Sturge–Weber syndrome.

## Pathogenesis

Exact pathogenesis of KTS is unknown. It occurs sporadically but may occasionally be inherited. Happle proposed paradominant inheritance and role of acquired mutation during embryogenesis causing loss of heterozygosity and manifestation of the disease. Proposed theories suggest role of genetic abnormality. Genomic mutation has been detected in E133K that causes upregulation of VG5Q which is an important angiogenic factor located on chromosome 5q13.3 leading to increased angiogenesis.

## Clinical Features

Port wine stain manifests at birth and involvement of lower limb is commoner than other areas. It may involve both upper and lower limb; both limb involvement is usually ipsilateral. Geographical shaped large lesions often involve the adjacent trunk. Presence of geographical PWS may predict occurrence of more severe disease or development of lymphatic abnormalities.

During late infancy and adolescence venous varicosities usually develop involving both superficial and deep veins. Differentiation should be made from other disorders like Parkes-Weber syndrome, Servelle-Martorell syndrome, Proteus syndrome, hemihyperplasia and lipomata syndrome. All of these syndromes feature PWS and limb overgrowth, except Servelle-Martorell syndrome, which shows limb undergrowth, capillary stains and varicose veins. Parkes-Weber syndrome has arteriovenous shunt with fast flow malformation whereas KTS has a slow flow malformation.

## Diagnosis

X-ray of the limbs show bony overgrowth and can be done to compare and assess the bony overgrowth. Echo/Doppler and duplex scans are useful for diagnosis and evaluation of vascular abnormality. MRI may be used to detect soft tissue overgrowth, bony and lymphatic anomalies.

## Management

Superficial and deep venous dilatation may be managed conservatively with compression bandage. Superficial dilatation may be surgically removed if indicated. PWS can be treated with pulse dye laser. Bony overgrowth may be managed in consultation with a pediatric orthopedic surgeon.

## SYNDROMES WITH VENOUS MALFORMATION

### Maffucci Syndrome

This condition starts manifesting in early childhood as superficial and deep VMs in skin and subcutaneous tissue appearing as soft, bluish, exophytic, and tender nodules. The cutaneous lesions are composed of thick and thin-walled vascular spaces with single endothelial lining.

Enchondromas, usually affecting the phalanges and long bones are present. There may be oral and intra-abdominal venous and lymphatic anomalies. Most significant complication is development of malignancy of the affected bone, most common being chondrosarcoma. Vascular tumors like spindle-cell hemangioendothelioma have been reported. Tumors of breast, ovary, pancreas, parathyroid, and pituitary gland have also been found.

### Blue Rubber Bleb Nevus Syndrome

This is a rare disorder characterized by VMs of the skin and gastrointestinal tract and occasionally of other systems like CNS, orbit, muscle and genitourinary tract. This syndrome usually appears to be sporadic but familial cases have been reported.

#### Clinical Features

Lesions appear at or just after birth but may appear/become apparent late as deep-blue, soft, rubber-like vascular compressible nodule (bleb). It commonly affects palms, soles, and trunk but any area may be affected including scalp and mucosa. Large lesions may lead to bony deformities, even fracture from direct compressive effect.

Gastrointestinal (GI) tract lesions may cause pain due to intussusception and bleeding.

GI tract hemorrhage is a very serious complication. It may give rise to soft tissue hematomas. Hemorrhage may be subclinical or features of consumptive coagulopathy which may occur even in infancy.

#### Diagnosis

Differential diagnosis includes Maffucci syndrome and isolated venous malformation. MRI and CT scan may assist in identification of visceral lesions.

#### Treatment

Interferon-α, systemic steroids, carbon dioxide laser, sclerotherapy, subcutaneous octreotide and surgical removal have been used. Anti-androgen sirolimus has also been used. Argon or Nd:YAG laser ablation have been used for management for symptomatic gastrointestinal VMs.

## VASCULAR TUMORS

Vascular tumors/neoplasms are characterized by proliferation of endothelial cells. Comprehensive classification of vascular tumors has been published by ISSVA. They have classified all vascular tumors into three types:

1. Benign
2. Locally aggressive or borderline vascular tumors and
3. Malignant vascular tumors.

- Benign vascular tumors has been further subdivided into following subtypes:
  - Infantile hemangioma (IH)
  - Congenital hemangioma
  - Tufted angioma
  - Spindle-cell hemangioma
  - Epithelioid hemangioma
  - Pyogenic granuloma.
- Locally aggressive vascular tumors have been classified into retiform hemangioendothelioma, papillary intralymphatic angioendothelioma (PILA), Dabska tumor, Kaposi sarcoma, composite hemangioendothelioma and some other types
- Angiosarcoma, epithelioid hemangioendothelioma are the two main proposed subtypes of malignant vascular tumors.

### Infantile Hemangioma

Infantile hemangioma is a form of benign vascular tumor and is the most common form of vascular tumor in children. This is characterized by onset during first month of life, rapid proliferation, followed by a slower phase of involution. Previously, this was also known as "strawberry hemangioma" and "capillary hemangioma" are currently not in use.

#### Pathogenesis

Infantile hemangioma develops due to the imbalance of the angiogenic and antiangiogenic factors resulting in unregulated proliferation of endothelial cells.

Role of insulin-like growth factor 2, interferon, endothelial expression of the integrins-3, 51 and 3, vascular endothelial growth factor (VGEF 1 and 2), basic fibroblastic growth factor, Tie-2 and angiopoietin-2 has been proposed in the proliferation phase.

Involution phase shows increased expression of metalloproteinase-1 and other apoptosis-associated proteins.

Myeloid markers like CD14, CD15, CD32, and CD83 have been demonstrated in IH indicating the possible role of myeloid cells in its pathogenesis.

Presently GLUT-1 is known to play an important role in differentiation of difficult vascular lesions. This marker is present in all cases of infantile hemangioma at every stage and is negative in malformations.

Usually IH occurs sporadically with only infrequent report of inherited cases. Specific genetic mutation has not been identified. Functional mosaicism of X chromosome (nonrandom inactivation) has been demonstrated in some patients. In familial cases, linkage to the locus 5q31-33 in the candidate genes *FGFR4*, *PDG-FRB*, and *FLT4* has been detected.

Vasculogenesis (the formation of primitive blood vessels from angioblasts) rather than angiogenesis (the growth of new vessels from existing vessels) has been implicated.

#### Clinical Features

Infantile hemangioma starts as a flat relatively hypopigmented area on the skin, sometimes with telangiectatic vessels across

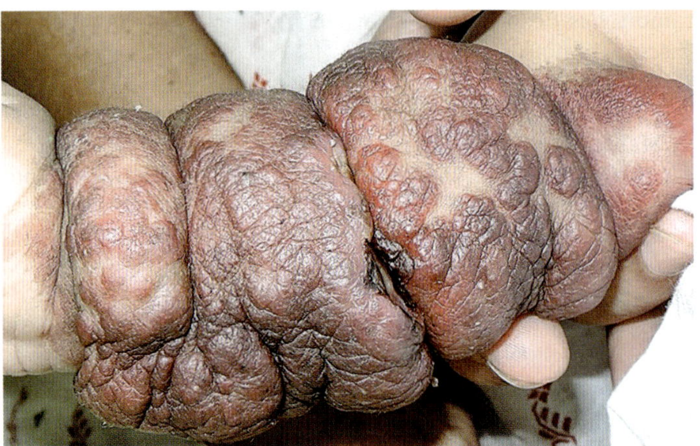

FIG. 4: Large infantile hemangioma.

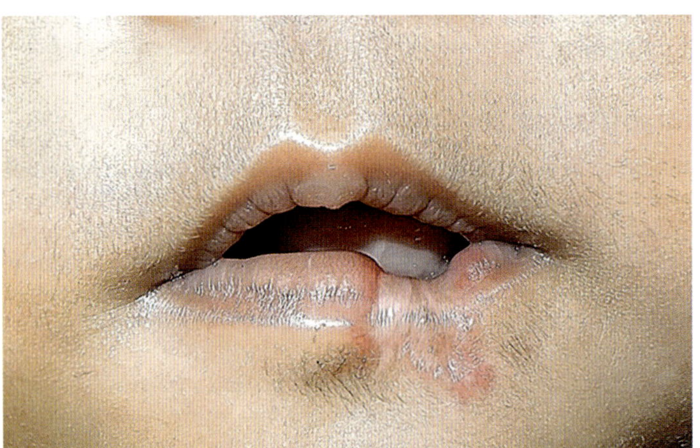

FIG. 5: Atrophy following healing of infantile hemangioma.

it. Soon scarlet red swelling with lobulated surface develops. When there is a deeper component, it may appear as warm, compressible, bluish mass having a "bag of worms" feeling. Girls and premature infants have higher prevalence (Fig. 4).

Proliferative phase lasts till 1 year of age when spontaneous regression starts that continues till 7–8 years of age. After resolution, atrophy or telangiectasia or loose skin persists (Fig. 5). IH can be categorized into the following types:

- Focal
- Segmental, higher rate of underlying structural anomalies
- Indeterminate
- Multifocal, associated with higher occurrence of visceral hemangiomas
- Multiple IH and segmental hemangiomas have poorer prognosis, because of higher chances of complications.

Infantile hemangioma occurring in certain locations are of prognostic and therapeutic importance as these may be associated with certain location specific complications.

Prognosis and complication depends on site, number, size, speed of growth, and few other factors. Periorbital hemangiomas may lead to blindness, compressive optic neuropathy and exposure keratopathy (Fig. 6).

Subglottic hemangioma, large parotid gland hemangiomas are also associated with high rates of complication.

Lumbosacral hemangiomatosis often associated with underlying anomalies like imperforate anus, tethered spinal cord, renal, and genital defects.

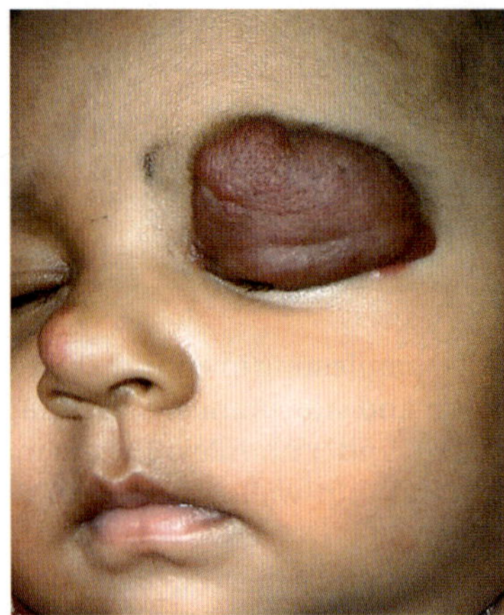

FIG. 6: Infantile hemangioma over upper eyelid is an indication for necessity of aggressive management.

Neonatal hemangiomatosis is a condition where large number (few to hundred) of small cutaneous hemangiomas occur at birth. This condition is also known as benign neonatal hemangiomatosis. The lesions show increase in size for the first few months and thereafter involution occurs with complete resolution within first 2–3 years.

Multifocal/diffuse neonatal hemangiomatosis is characterized by multiple cutaneous and visceral hemangiomas involving liver, gastrointestinal tract, lungs, and brain. The most common complications are cardiac failure, hemorrhage, and multiorgan failure.

## Systemic Involvement

Any patient with more than five cutaneous IH has high risk of liver involvement. Hepatic hemangiomas is frequently associated with hypothyroidism in children due to production of substances with 3-iodothyronine deiodinase activity.

## Complications

### Ulceration

*Infection*: *S. aureus*, group A β-hemolytic streptococci and *Enterobacteriaceae* are the common pathogens or it may be polymicrobial.

### Localized Bleeding

*Rapid growth*: This may occur due to rapid growth during proliferative phase or intralesional bleeding.

## Cosmetic Disfigurement

*Airway obstruction*: It is now well-established that Kasabach-Merritt syndrome is not a complication of IH.

## Management

Small IH not causing or not having the potential for any medical complication or significant disfigurement is best left untreated with regular follow-up. Close monitoring is necessary for the following hemangioma.

- Rapidly proliferative

**BOX 2 Indications of active management of infantile hemangioma**

- Rapid growth/internal hemorrhage
- Precarious location
- Involvement of ulceration and infection prone sites
- Syndrome-associated hemangioma
- Disseminated hemangiomatosis
- Cosmetic deformity

- Large hemangiomas with risk of hemorrhage, obstruction of vital organs, or functional impairment
- Hemangiomas with deeper component
- Hemangiomas with segmental and indeterminate morphology.

Most severe IHs are best treated early in the proliferative phase to prevent sequelae (Box 2).

Depending upon the indications, therapeutic options for IH are topical or systemic.

Topical drugs are effective in superficial hemangioma. Potent topical corticosteroid, it enhances vasoconstriction and inhibits angiogenesis. This is used primarily for thin and superficial lesions (e.g., periocular lesions).

Imiquimod 5% cream acts through activation IFN-γ which has antiangiogenic effect.

Topical tacrolimus and pimecrolimus, topical beta-blocker (Timololmaleate gel, 0.5%) and topical becaplermin gel (0.01%) (recombinant platelet derived growth factor) are all considered safe and effective treatment. The latter is however painful with higher risk of secondary infection. Patient may need to be hospitalized. This has been used in perineal hemangioma with ulceration.

Intralesional triamcinolone acetonide and bleomycin are effective in reducing size of hemangioma.

### Systemic Therapy

Various systemic agents used for the treatment of IH are:

- Corticosteroid
- Interferon α-2a
- Vincristine
- Cyclophosphamide
- Propranolol.

*Corticosteroids*: Systemic corticosteroid is the first line of treatment for all rapidly progressive IH associated with mechanical obstruction due to large size and is considered a life-saving management. It can effectively halt the proliferation.

The starting dose of prednisolone is 2–3 mg/kg/day as single morning dose during the proliferative phase.

Systemic CS enhances vasoconstriction and inhibits angiogenesis. Upregulation of the mitochondrial enzyme cytochrome-b, clusterin/ApoJ (possible markers of apoptosis) is also suggested. Systemic CS is slowly tapered and stopped before the age of 1 year.

*Propranolol*: It is a nonselective beta-blocker. It arrests the growth of proliferating hemangiomas and shows excellent response in the management of periorbital, subglottic, parotid gland hemangioma, and ulcerated IH.

Treatment is best performed in hospitalized patients. Usual dose is 0.5 mg/kg/day in three divided doses. This dose has to be escalated every week till it is 2 mg/kg/day. Withdrawal should also be cautiously done with gradual dose reduction. Cardiac complications may happen in up to 2 weeks (maximum within 4–8 days) after stopping the drug.

*Interferon α-2a*: This is potent immunomodulator with additional antiangiogenic effect, antifibroblastic effect, and antiendothelial cell and antismooth muscle activity. It is used to treat life-threatening IH, which have failed to respond to steroid therapy; administered subcutaneously in a dose of 1–3 million U/m$^2$ of body surface area daily. Adverse effects like spastic diplegia can occur. Hence, its use should be limited only in the treatment of life threatening cases nonresponsive to systemic steroids.

*Vincristine*: In large endangering hemangiomas vincristine may be effective when steroids fail to control. The dose is 0.05 mg/kg, to a maximum of 2 mg (in children weighing ≤10 kg) or 1–2 mg/m$^2$ (in children weighing ≥10 kg or having body surface area ≥1 m$^2$). It is administered intravenously on a weekly basis.

*Cyclophosphamide*: Cyclophosphamide has been used in the management of life-threatening cases (e.g., hemangiomatosis with heart failure) which are refractory to treatment with oral corticosteroids.

### Other Treatment Modalities

Intermittent pneumatic and continuous compression has been used to treat symptomatic hemangiomas especially for the lesions over extremities. Its mechanism of action is not known. Bisphosphonates have antiangiogenic effect and local delivery of bisphosphonates as a potential treatment of hemangiomas is under research. Large periocular hemangiomas, refractory ulcerated hemangiomas, and nasal-tip hemangiomas are indications for surgical management. If surgery is planned, excision before school age is the best time.

## Congenital Hemangioma

Congenital hemangioma is a vascular tumor present at birth. There is no postnatal proliferative phase in these tumors. Depending upon the biological behavior these are categorized into:

- Rapidly involuting congenital hemangioma (RICH)
- Noninvoluting congenital hemangioma (NICH)
- Partially involuting congenital hemangiomas (PICH).

The former type behaves similarly as IH but show involution more rapidly often within the first year of life. NICH lesions grow maximally in the intrauterine phase and do not show much sign of regression in postnatal period.

This condition shows equal sex distribution. Classical presentation is that of solitary lesion overhead, limbs, or near joints which may appear as bluish/purple plaque or tumor with peripheral pale zone and overlying telangiectasia. On Doppler examination NICH lesions show fast flow and are often confused with AVMs while the RICH lesions show uniform hyperechoic masses and centrilobular draining vessels.

### Histopathology

Rapidly involuting congenital hemangioma lesions show lobules comprised of plump endothelial cells. Thickened basement membrane zone indicates involution phase. NICH lesions show large lobules catered by small vessels with intervening fibrosis and dermal arteriovenous microfistulae. GLUT-1 is negative in both the types.

### Treatment

Surgical excision is the treatment of choice in NICH.

## Tufted Angioma

Tufted angioma or angioblastoma is rare, benign vascular neoplasm of the skin and subcutaneous tissue. It presents as ill-defined, slow progressive, dull red/brownish/purple, tender, angiomatous papules and plaques with a mottled surface on the upper trunk, neck, and proximal parts of the limbs between the ages of 1–5 years. But congenital lesions or adult onset is also noted. Rarely scalp, perianal skin and oral mucosa are involved. Annular lesions have been reported occasionally. Spontaneous regression is rare. Exceptionally, it has been found to appear during pregnancy and regress after parturition.

Histopathologically, there are irregularly distributed vascular tufts in the dermis and subcutis, composed of plump endothelial cells and spindle-shaped pericytes. The endothelial cells stain positively for CD31 and CD34, and strongly label for smooth muscle actin.

Rarely, the course may be complicated with Kasabach–Merritt syndrome. Malignant transformation has not been reported.

Treatment consists of excision, soft X-ray therapy, pulsed-dye laser, potent topical corticosteroids and interferon-$\gamma$.

## Verrucous Hemangioma

This is a variant of hemangioma appearing at birth as PWS which gradually deepens in color and the surface gradually becomes verrucous. Lower limb is the common site. There may be recurrent bleeding and infection. Spontaneous involution rarely occurs. Histopathological features are hyperkeratosis, acanthosis, papillomatosis with underlying capillary hemangioma. Surgical excision is the treatment of choice.

## Kaposiform Hemangioendothelioma

This rare vascular tumor usually involves retroperitoneum and skin. This appears in childhood and shows rapid growth. Spontaneous regression may occur rarely. Bleeding and Kasabach-Merritt phenomenon, especially in retroperitoneal lesion may lead to death. Histopathology shows deeply infiltrated tightly packed lobules and sheets of rounded and spindled shaped endothelial cells and pericytes reaching upto the subcutis and even muscles. Excision is the treatment of choice to avoid complication.

## SUGGESTED READINGS


1. Al Dhaybi R, Powell J, McCuaig C, et al. Differentiation of vascular tumors from vascular malformations by expression of Wilms tumor 1 gene: evaluation of 126 cases. J Am Acad Dermatol. 2010;63(6):1052-7.
2. Bastarrika G, Redondo P, Sierra A, et al. New techniques for the evaluation and therapeutic planning of patients with Klippele Tre'naunay syndrome. J Am Acad Dermatol. 2007;56:242-9.
3. Batta K, Goodyear HM, Moss C, et al. Randomised controlled study of early pulsed dye laser treatment of uncomplicated childhood haemangiomas: results of a 1-year analysis. Lancet. 2002;360:521-7.
4. Chakraborty S, Gharami RC, Das NK, et al. Annular tufted angioma: a rare entity. Int J Dermatol. 2009;48(6):614-6.
5. Chiller KG, Passaro D, Frieden IJ. Hemangiomas of infancy: clinical characteristics, morphologic subtypes, and their relationship to race, ethnicity, and sex. Arch Dermatol. 2002;138:1567-76.
6. Devillers AC, de Waard-van der Spek FB, Oranje AP. Cutis marmorata telangiectatica congenita. Clinical features in 35 cases. Arch Dermatol. 1999;135:34-8.
7. Enjolras O, Soupre V, Picard A. Classification of superficial vascular anomalies. Presse Med. 2010;39(4):457-64.
8. Enjolras O, Wassef M, Mazoyer E, et al. Infants with Kasabach-Merritt syndrome do not have "true" hemangiomas. J Pediatr. 1997;130:631-40.
9. Fawcett SL, Grant I, Hall PN, et al. Vincristine as a treatment for a large haemangioma threatening vital functions. Br J Plast Surg. 2004;57:168-71.
10. Garzon MC, Enjolras O, Frieden IJ. Vascular tumours and vascular malformations: evidence for an association. J Am Acad Dermatol. 2000;42:275-9.
11. Garzon MC, Lucky AW, Hawrot A, et al. Ultrapotent topical corticosteroid treatment of hemangiomas of infancy. J Am Acad Dermatol. 2005;52:281-6.
12. Hofhuis WJ, Oranje AP, Bouquet J, et al. Blue rubber bleb nevus syndrome: report of a case with consumption coagulopathy complicated by manifest thrombosis. Eur J Pediatr. 1990;149:526-8.
13. International Society for the Study of Vascular Anomalies. ISSVA Classification of Vascular Anomalies, 2014. Milwaukee: ISSVA; 2014.
14. Lee NH, Choi EH, Choi WK, et al. Maffucci's syndrome with oral and intestinal haemangioma. Br J Dermatol. 1999;140:968-9.
15. Mattassi R. Differential diagnosis in congenital vascular-bone syndromes. Semin Vasc Surg. 1993;6:233-44.
16. Michaud AP, Bauman NM, Burke DK, et al. Spastic diplegia and other motor disturbances in infants receiving interferon-alpha. Laryngoscope. 2004;114:1231-6.
17. Neri I, Balestri R, Patrizi A. Hemangiomas: new insight and medical treatment. Dermatol Ther. 2012;25:322-34.
18. Nguyen VA, Furhapter C, Romani N, et al. Infantile hemangioma is a proliferation of beta 4-negative endothelial cells adjacent to HLA-DR-positive cells with dendritic cell morphology. Hum Pathol. 2004;35:739-44.
19. Sangueza OP, Kasper RC, LeBoit P, et al. Vascular tumors. In: LeBoit PE, Burg G, Weedon D, Sarasain A (Eds). Pathology and Genetics of Skin Tumors: World Health Organization Classification of Tumours. Lyon, France: IARC Press; 2006. pp. 233-46.
20. Sarma N, Chakraborty S. Birthmarks or clinical significance. In. Sarkar R, Inamadar AC, Palit A. Eds: Advances in Pediatric Dermatology - 2: Neonatal Dermatology. Jaypee Brothers Medical Publishers (P) Ltd. New Delhi. 2014,198-221
21. Sarma N, Chakraborty S. Nevi and nevoid disorders. In: Inamader AC, Palit A, Rghunatha S. Eds. Textbook of pediatric dermatology, (2nd ed). Jaypee Brothers Medical Publishers (P) Ltd. New Delhi. 2014,460-494
22. Sarma N, Das S, Roy AK. Annular tufted angioma. Indian J Dermatol Venereol Leprol. 2007;73(6):435-6.
23. Viljoen D, Saxe N, Pearn J, et al. The cutaneous manifestations of the Klippel-Trenaunay-Weber syndrome. Clin Exp Dermatol. 1987;12:12-7.
24. Walter JW, North PE, Waner M, et al. Somatic mutation of vascular endothelial growth factor receptors in juvenile hemangioma. Genes Chromosomes Cancer. 2002;33:295-303.
25. Wassef M, Blei F, Adams D, et al. Vascular Anomalies classification: recommendations from the International Society for the Study of Vascular Anomalies. Pediatrics. 2015;136:e203-14.
26. Yuksekkaya H, Ozbek O, Keser M, et al. Blue rubber bleb nevus syndrome: successful treatment with sirolimus. Pediatrics. 2012;129(4):e1080-4.
27. Zhang L, Chen Q, Li D, et al. Evaluation of the role of serum vascular endothelial growth factor and urinary basic fibroblast growth factor in differential diagnosis of vascular anomalies. Zhonghua Yi Xue Za Zhi. 2011;91:1092-5.

# 39 CHAPTER Cutaneous Vasculitis

*Brijesh Nair, Nilendu Sarma*

## INTRODUCTION

Cutaneous vasculitis comprises a group of disease entities that are characterized by predominant skin involvement and varying degrees of systemic manifestations. They can be primary or secondary to other underlying diseases. The morphology of cutaneous lesions depends on vessel size, the anatomical site affected, and the stage of development of the lesion. The progress of vasculitis to involve systemic organ systems is determined by genetic predisposition, host responses, local conditions, and exposure to trigger factors. Systemic and localized vasculitis often affects the skin and subcutis, due to its vascularity, hemodynamic factors, and its propensity to be exposed to the vagaries of the external environmental influences.

## HISTORICAL PERSPECTIVE

It was as early as 1866 that Kussmaul and Maier reported the first case of systemic vasculitis (periarteritis nodosa). Zeek put forth a classification system for vasculitis differentiating patients mostly on organ system involvement. This initial scheme eventuated into the American College of Rheumatology's (ACR) classification system. The most widely adopted vasculitis classification system is that of the Chapel Hill Consensus Conference (CHCC). It was later revised in 2012 with a significant remark that it is a nomenclature (nosological) system and does not set out to delineate diagnostic disease criteria.

## EPIDEMIOLOGY

All ages, the females more than males and adults more than children can develop cutaneous vasculitis. The prevalence of cutaneous small vessel vasculitis (CSVV) is 15 cases per million. Henoch-Schönlein purpura (HSP) occurs mostly in less than 10 years of age and is the most common childhood vasculitis at incidence of 10–20 cases per 100,000 children per year. Urticarial vasculitis occurs mostly in females in fifth decade with hypocomplementemic vasculitis almost exclusively in females. Cryoglobulinemic vasculitis is rare at 4.8 cases per million.

## CLASSIFICATION

The Chapel Hill revised classification system (2012) is the main system of classification which is much utilized in classifying the vasculitides. The same is depicted in box 1. CHCC addresses noninfective vasculitis caused by direct vessel invasion by pathogens but fails to identify many patients with Wegener's granulomatosis (WG) and microscopic polyangiitis (MPA). Classic polyarteritis nodosa (PAN) is likely to be diagnosed less frequently as per CHCC as compared to ACR criteria, due to differences in interpretation. There is substantial overlap with respect to arterial involvement and vessel size (variable vessel vasculitis in the revised Chapel Hill Consensus).

Chapel Hill revised classification system has classified vasculitides into seven types: (1) large vessel vasculitis (Takayasu arteritis, giant cell arteritis); (2) medium vessel vasculitis (polyarteritis nodosa, Kawasaki disease); (3) small vessel vasculitis; (4) variable vessel vasculitis (Behçet's disease, Cogan's syndrome); (5) single-organ vasculitis [cutaneous leukocytoclastic angiitis (CLA), cutaneous arteritis, primary central nervous system (CNS) vasculitis, isolated aortitis]; (6) vasculitis associated with systemic disease (lupus vasculitis, rheumatoid vasculitis, sarcoid vasculitis); and (7) vasculitis associated with probable etiologies like vasculitis-associated with hepatitis C virus (cryoglobulinemic vasculitis), hepatitis B, syphilis, drugs [immune complex vasculitis, antineutrophil

**BOX 1 Types of vasculitides***

- Large-vessel vasculitis, e.g., Takayasu arteritis
- Medium-vessel vasculitis, e.g., polyarteritis nodosa
- Small-vessel vasculitis
  - Antineutrophil cytoplasmic antibody (ANCA)-associated vasculitis, e.g., microscopic polyangiitis
  - Immune complex, e.g., cryoglobulinemic vasculitis, immunoglobulin A vasculitis, hypocomplementemic urticarial vasculitis
- Variable vessel vasculitis, e.g., Behçet's disease
- Single-organ vasculitis, e.g., cutaneous leukocytoclastic angiitis
- Vasculitis associated with systemic disease, e.g., connective tissue diseases
- Vasculitis associated with probable etiology, e.g., vasculitis associated with hepatitis C virus (cryoglobulinemic), hepatitis B virus, drugs (immune complex)

*Prepared on the basis of Chapel Hill Consensus Conference 2012 revised nomenclature system of the vasculitides (Jennette JC, Falk RJ, Bacon PA, et al. 2012 revised International Chapel Hill Consensus Conference Nomenclature of Vasculitides. Arthritis Rheum. 2013;65:1-11.)

**BOX 2 Histological classification of vasculitis**

**Neutrophilic (immune complex mediated)**
- Cutaneous leukocytoclastic vasculitis
- IgA vasculitis
- Acute infantile hemorrhagic edema
- Urticarial vasculitis
- Cryoglobulinemic vasculitis
- Septic vasculitis
- Cutaneous polyarteritis nodosa*
- Nodular vasculitis (erythema induratum)*

**Lymphocytic**
- Vasculitis in lichenoid dermatoses—pityriasis lichenoides et varioliformis acuta
- Vasculitis in T-cell lymphomas and lymphomatoid papulosis
- Connective tissue diseases
- Graft-versus-host disease
- Behçet's disease†
- Degos' disease†
- Kawasaki disease*

**Eosinophilic vasculitis**
- Hypereosinophilic syndrome
- Connective tissue diseases

**Granulomatous**

Granuloma with dermal fibrosis:
- Erythema elevatum diutinum
- Granuloma faciale

ANCA-associated/ pauci-immune [direct immunofluorescence (DIF)-ve]:
- Wegener's granulomatosis
- Microscopic polyangiitis (microscopic polyarteritis nodosa)
- Churg-Strauss syndrome
- Drug-induced ANCA-associated vasculitis

IgA, immunoglobulin A; ANCA, antineutrophil cytoplasmic antibody.

*Note:* Overall, only vasculitis involving small vessels are included. Vasculitis having additional involvement of medium-sized vessels† are also included. Some types of vasculitis that spare small vessels and involve large vessel* are also included here as these conditions often present with cutaneous manifestations.

**BOX 3 Secondary vasculitis**

- Drug induced—penicillin, sulfas, minocycline, NSAIDs, penicillamine, allopurinol, hydralazine, thiazides, hydantoins, vaccines, radiocontrast, tumor necrosis factor inhibitors, bortezomib, granulocyte colony-stimulating factor
- Connective tissue diseases—systemic lupus erythematosus (SLE), rheumatoid arthritis, Sjögren's syndrome
- Malignancy—hematologic, lymphoproliferative, solid organ tumors
- Gastrointestinal diseases—Crohn's disease, Primary biliary cirrhosis, bowel bypass disease
- Infection—hepatitis C virus, hepatitis B virus, HIV, mycoses, *Streptococcus, Meningococcus,* syphilis, Hansen's disease, *Staphylococcus, Gonococcus, Rickettsia,* infective endocarditis
- Periodic fevers
- Miscellaneous—antiphospholipid antibody (APLA) syndrome, Goodpasture's disease, cystic fibrosis

NSAIDs, nonsteroidal anti-inflammatorydrugs.

cytoplasmic antibody (ANCA)-associated vasculitis] and cancer (Box 1). CSVV can eventuate into a medium vessel vasculitic entity or a systemic vasculitis over a period of time. The large vessel vasculitides like Takayasu arteritis, giant cell arteritis, and Kawasaki disease are not usually associated with cutaneous small and medium vessel vasculitis. To date, no ideal system of classification exists for vasculitis. Classification based on histological features has also been proposed (Box 2).

## SECONDARY VASCULITIS

According to revised CHCC 2012 classification, vasculitis associated with systemic diseases and the category associated with probable etiologies (Box 1) often are considered to be secondary vasculitides (Box 3) whereas the other categories have been considered primary (or idiopathic) vasculitides. The name of a secondary vasculitic entity should carry a prefix term specifying the systemic disease (e.g., rheumatoid vasculitis, lupus vasculitis, sarcoidosis vasculitis, relapsing polychondritis).

## CUTANEOUS PSEUDOVASCULITIS

A large group of disorders exist which may be confused for vasculitis, making diagnosis a tedious task. A classification scheme of these mimics of vasculitis is delineated in box 4. Histologically, pseudovasculitis lacks vessel damage that defines vasculitis. Thus, they are also known as vasculopathy.

**BOX 4 Classification of cutaneous pseudovasculitis**

- Infectious disease—bacterial endocarditis, disseminated gonococcal infection, pulmonary histoplasmosis, coccidioidomycosis, syphilis, Lyme disease
- Drug-induced vasospasm among other causes—cocaine, levamisole, amphetamines, ergot alkaloids, methysergide, arsenic, heparin/warfarin necrosis
- Coagulopathies/thrombotic microangiopathies
  - Idiopathic thrombocytopenic purpura
  - Antiphospholipid antibody syndrome, protein C/S deficiency, hyperhomocysteinemia, MTHFR mutations, factor V Leiden, antithrombin III deficiency
  - Livedoid vasculopathy
  - Thrombotic thrombocytopenic purpura
  - Purpura fulminans
  - Disseminated intravascular coagulation
  - Monoclonal gammopathy (type 1 cryoglobulinemia)
  - Sickle cell disease
- Blood vessel incompetence
  - Scurvy
  - Solar/senile purpura
  - Pigmented purpuric dermatitis
- Neoplasms
  - Atrial myxoma
  - Lymphoma
  - Carcinomatosis
- Atheroembolic disease
  - Cholesterol embolus
  - Fat embolism
- Miscellaneous—calciphylaxis, amyloidosis, cryofibrinogenemia, radiation arteriopathy, primary hyperoxaluria

MTHFR, methylenetetrahydrofolate reductase.

## CLINICAL PRESENTATION

The cutaneous vasculitides are characterized by protean manifestations with considerable overlap in the symptomatology that depend on the predominant type of vascular involvement (Table 1). Typically a maculopapular rash is the initial presentation that may be followed by more classical lesions like palpable

**TABLE 1: Clinical manifestations based on predominant vessel size**

| | Small | Medium |
|---|---|---|
| Skin | Palpable purpura, splinter hemorrhages, urticaria, vesiculobullous lesions | Nodules, ulcers, livedo reticularis, pitted digital scars, digital gangrene |
| Systemic | Glomerulonephritis, pulmonary hemorrhages, gastrointestinal colic, scleritis, episcleritis, uveitis | Mononeuritis multiplex, aneurysms, infarct, hypertension (renal artery) |

purpura. Other skin lesions, such as nonpalpable macules and patches, urticaria, bullous lesions, vesicles, pustules, splinter hemorrhages, nodules, ulcerations, or nonspecific changes may also be observed in various combinations. Because of increased hydrostatic pressure, skin lesions are more common on the legs and buttocks. Nodules and ulceration indicate medium-sized vessel involvement. Fever, weight loss, malaise, arthralgias, and arthritis are common to both cutaneous and systemic but more common in the latter type. Involvement of sites other than the lower limbs and livedo reticularis are indications of vasculitis with systemic involvement, but exceptions are common. Larger vessel involvement is typically manifested with limb claudication, asymmetric blood pressure, absence of pulses, aortic dilation, bruits.

## PATHOGENESIS

The pathogenesis of vasculitis involves the complex interplay of antigens (often cryptic), inflammatory cells, vascular endothelium, and resultant cytokine milieu. Specifically, vasculitis can be pathogenically termed (1) allergic vasculitis, (2) antibody-mediated vasculitis, (3) immune complex-mediated vasculitis, and (4) T-cell-mediated hypersensitivity vasculitis. Other immunopathologic mechanisms, such as antibody neutralization, T-cell-mediated cytotoxic reactions and granulomatous infiltration resulting from nonimmune mechanisms, and may also certain vasculitides. The pathogenetic mechanisms of some vasculitic conditions are depicted in table 2. A proposed algorithm of pathogenesis of cutaneous vasculitis is depicted in flowchart 1. All CSVV and some mixed and medium vessel diseases are mediated by immune complex deposition in presence of antigen excess. These complexes deposit in postcapillary venules and initiate the disease process. The postcapillary venules are the epicenter of immune deposits due to low oxygen content, slow rheological characteristics and stasis. Cytokine-mediated, proinflammatory changes in the expression and function of adhesion molecules team up with abnormal leukocyte activation and endothelial cell activation which may be the main causes of vessel damage. Langerhans cells and other dendritic cells are key assisting factors in the pathogenesis. The membrane attack complex (complement C5–C9) plays a very important role in disease pathogenesis by direct insertion into endothelial cell membrane, and subsequent release of growth factors and cytokines.

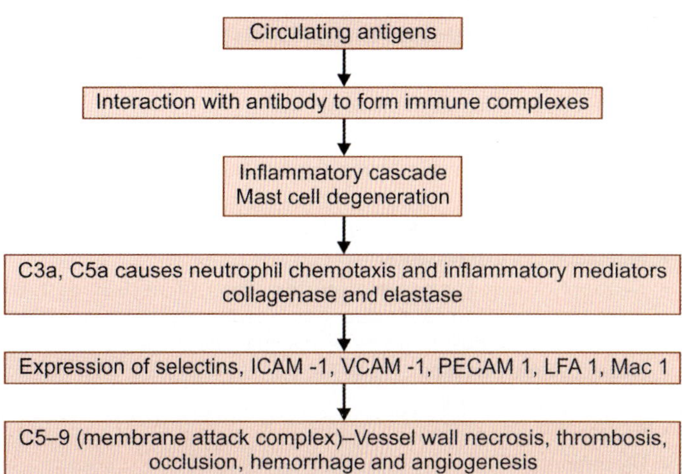


**FLOWCHART 1:** Pathogenesis of vasculitides.

**TABLE 2: Pathogenetic mechanisms and resultant representative vasculitis**

| Pathogenetic mechanism | Vasculitic syndrome |
|---|---|
| Direct infection | Rickettsial infections |
| Type I anaphylactic | Eosinophilic vasculitis, Churg–Strauss syndrome |
| Type II cytotoxic–cytolytic antibody | Wegener's granulomatosis, microscopic polyangiitis |
| Type III immune complex | Henoch–Schönlein purpura, cutaneous leukocytoclastic angiitis, cryoglobulinemic vasculitis, polyarteritis nodosa |
| Type IV delayed hypersensitivity | Giant cell arteritis, chronic graft versus host disease, Sneddon syndrome |

Antineutrophil cytoplasmic antibodies are primarily directed against intracellular neutrophilic proteins [proteinase 3, myeloperoxidase (MPO)], which translocate to cell surface and these neutrophils which express ANCA on cell surface have the capability of initiating vascular damage without immune complex deposition. Hence, ANCA-associated vasculitides are broadly classified as "pauci-immune". Persistent inflammation leads to development of ANCA which perpetuates inflammation by activating neutrophils and endothelial cells, which forms a kind of self-feeding loop of vascular annihilation. This vascular phenomenon manifest itself systemically by eliciting diffuse endothelial dysfunction by release of tumor necrosis factor (TNF) and C-reactive protein (CRP) directly into the bloodstream.

## PATTERNS OF VASCULITIC EVOLUTION

Three patterns of disease evolution occur in cutaneous vasculitis: (1) single acute, self-limited episode (resolving in <6 months) due to drug or infectious trigger (60%); (2) relapsing disease with symptom-free interregnum usually (e.g., HSP and connective tissue vasculitis—20%); and (3) a chronic, unremitting disease characterized by repeated conflagrations and troughs (e.g., cryoglobulinemia and malignancy—20%).

## HISTOPATHOLOGICAL CRITERIA

Vasculitis is primarily a histological diagnosis. Small-sized blood vessel cutaneous vasculitis generally includes capillaries, postcapillary venules, and nonmuscular arterioles which are found mainly within the superficial papillary dermis. Medium-sized blood vessels have muscular walls and are found in the deep reticular dermis, near dermal-subcuticular junction. Larger vessels are not found within the skin.

**BOX 5 Histopathological criteria for diagnosis of vasculitis**

*Two of the three pathognomonic criteria must be met*:
1. Inflammatory infiltrate in the vessel wall
2. Disruption and damage of vessel wall by inflammatory infiltrate
3. Intramural/intraluminal fibrin deposition and/or endothelial necrosis

*Clues to diagnosis of vasculitis (not pathognomonic)*:
- Red blood cell extravasation
- Neutrophils and karyorrhexis (nuclear dust) (If nuclear dust is abundant, the most likely diagnosis is leukocytoclastic vasculitis (LCV). If nuclear dust is absent or minimal and there are thrombi, suspect septic vasculitis
- Eccrine gland necrosis
- Endothelial cell swelling
- Ulceration
- Necrosis/infarct
- Thrombosis

*Sequelae*:
- Lamination (onion skinning) of vessel wall
- Endarteritis obliterans
- Neovascularization of adventitia

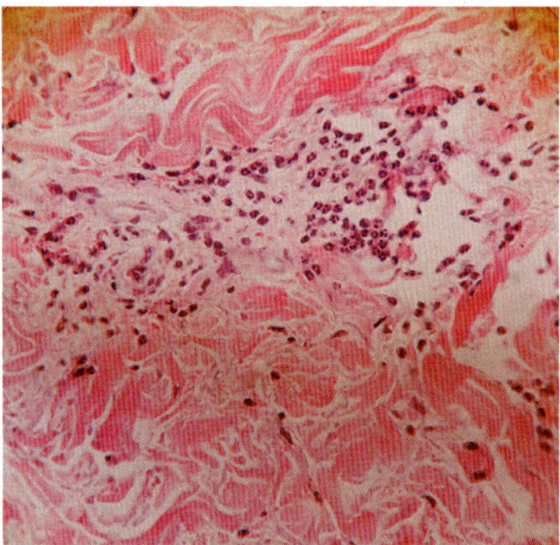

**FIG. 1:** Vasculitis. Dermis shows multiple vessels surrounded and infiltrated by dense inflammatory infiltrate.

Definitive diagnosis of vasculitis requires presence of leukocytoclastic vasculitis (LCV) and signs of vessel damage (Box 5). Histopathology is characterized by inflammatory infiltrates within and around the walls of vessels accompanied by fibrin deposition (fibrinoid necrosis), necrotic endothelial and inflammatory cells like neutrophils, and immune deposits. Signs of endothelial damage are endothelial swelling, shrinkage, or sloughing. Extravasation of red blood cells (RBCs), necrosis, and ulceration are also observed. Neovascularization, lamination of the adventitia, media, and/or intima of vessels (onion skinning), perivascular nuclear dust (LCV), loss of the elastic lamina in muscular vessels, and vessel wall areas affected by inflammatory infiltrate are also findings under the microscope (Figs 1 and 2).

## INVESTIGATIONS AND WORKUP

A complete medical history and a thorough physical examination are crucial for diagnosis. Examinations of skin, eye, cardiovascular system, joints and entheses, and respiratory, digestive and nervous systems are important. Complete blood counts, urine for proteins and casts, an electrocardiogram, skiagram of the chest are

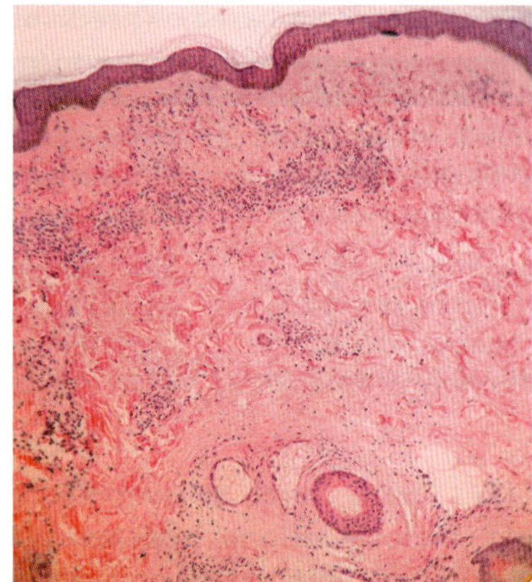

**FIG. 2:** Vasculitis. Fibrinoid changes in a small vessel along with predominantly neutrophilic infiltrate in the vessel wall and perivascular areas.

mandatory basic investigations. Depending on the characteristics of the underlying pathology, antinuclear antibodies (ANAs), ANCA, rheumatoid factor, cryoglobulins, total complement and its fractions, antistreptolysin O titers (ASO), immunoelectrophoresis (IPEP) of proteins should also be performed. Pseudovasculitis should be ruled out (see earlier section).

A definitive diagnosis of vasculitis has to be histopathological as few vasculitic syndromes have pathognomonic clinical, radiographic, and/or laboratory findings. The biopsy should be taken from fresh lesions preferably less than 48 hours old. Size of the vessels involved as well as the presence/absence of either extravascular granulomas [suggestive of Churg–Strauss syndrome (CSS) or WG] or a lymphocyte-rich infiltrate [suggestive of an associated connective tissue disease (CTD)] dermal eosinophilia or neutrophilia, vacuolar interface dermatitis [systemic lupus erythematosus (SLE)], or dermal fibrosis [e.g., erythema elevatum diutinem (EED)] should be evaluated. ANCA-associated vasculitis (AAV) is associated with extravascular "blue" granulomas in granulomatosis with polyangiitis (GPA) and "red" granulomas in eosinophilic granulomatosis with polyangiitis (EGPA).

Direct immunofluorescence (DIF) should also be done on lesional skin biopsies preferably within the first 48 hours. Presence of immunoglobulin A (IgA) on DIF can be helpful in providing a diagnosis of HSP whereas immunoglobulin M (IgM) can be of prognostic significance and signifies systemic involvement. A suggested scheme of investigations is represented in box 6.

## TREATMENT

The therapeutic option in cutaneous vasculitis is dependent upon size of vessel involved, whether disease is involving skin alone or has systemic involvement and also on degree of systemic involvement and organ systems involved. Removal of causative agent is important. CSVV is often self-limiting. Bed rest, leg elevation, avoiding tight clothing, gradient support stockings, antihistaminics, and nonsteroidal anti-inflammatory drugs (NSAIDs) are commonly used. Chronic CSVV may require more aggressive systemic therapy. Generally, CSVV is treated with drugs like dapsone, colchicine, pentoxifylline, thalidomide and hydroxychloroquine; medium vessel vasculitis with corticosteroids, cyclophosphamide, steroid-sparing immunosuppressant drugs like azathioprine, methotrexate and rituximab; and large-vessel vasculitis with systemic corticosteroids. A therapeutic ladder is proposed in table 3. Detailed treatment guideline for specific conditions can be seen

**BOX 6 Diagnostic scheme for cutaneous vasculitides**

1. *Skin biopsy (3 specimens)*: (1) 4–6 mm punch or excisional biopsy extending to the subcutis for routine histologic examination; (2) 4 mm punch biopsy for direct immunofluorescence; (3) 4 mm punch biopsy for tissue culture and sensitivity
2. *Routine panel*:
   - Complete blood cell count with differential
   - Erythrocyte sedimentation rate, C-reactive protein
   - Bilirubin, aminotransferases, alkaline phosphatase
   - Albumin
   - Creatinine, blood-urea nitrogen
   - Serum electrolytes
   - Urine analysis—hematuria, proteinuria, casts
   - Stool guaiac
   - HBV/HCV/HIV serologies
3. Imaging—chest X-ray, ultrasound abdomen
4. Antineutrophil cytoplasmic antibody (ANCA), antinuclear antibody (ANA), rheumatoid factor, antidouble-stranded DNA, precipitins (Ro, La, RNP, Sm)
5. Cryoglobulins, complement levels (CH50, C3, C4)—a negative test should be based on normal results drawn during active flares on at least three different occasions
6. *Search for antigen*:
   - Culture sinuses, throat, any sputum, urine, vulva, cervix, stool, gluteal cleft
   - Culture any pustule that shows up
   - Panorex view of all teeth to rule out periapical abscess
   - Stool for ova and parasite (O&P)
   - KOH of feet/groin
7. *Paraproteinemia screens (optional)*: Serum protein electrophoresis, serum protein immunofixation, serum immunoglobulins, and random urine protein immunofixation
8. Circulating immune complexes
9. Venereal Disease Research Laboratory (VDRL)
10. Clotting (thrombosis) panel—factor V Leiden, prothrombin *G20210A* gene mutation, homocysteine level, antiphospholipid antibodies (including lupus anticoagulant, cardiolipin, and phosphatidylserine antibodies), factor VII activity level, antithrombin III, protein C activity level, protein S antigen level, methylenetetrahydrofolate reductase (*MTHFR*) mutation, fibrinogen and fibrinogen degradation products
11. If the patient is febrile and has a heart murmur, then blood cultures and echocardiography should be performed
12. Children with lesions suspected to be cutaneous polyarteritis nodosa (CPAN) should have antistreptolysin O titers evaluated because of the common role of streptococci in this setting
13. *Endothelial cell activation markers (research purposes)*: Soluble interleukin-2 receptor levels, soluble adhesion molecules [e.g., soluble intercellular adhesion molecule-1 (sICAM-1), soluble vascular adhesion molecule-1 (sVCAM-1)], von Willebrand factor, thrombomodulin, and antiendothelial cell antibodies (AECAs)

**TABLE 3: Therapeutic ladder of vasculitis**

| Nature of vasculitis | First-line therapy | Second-line therapy | Third-line therapy |
|---|---|---|---|
| Cutaneous small vessel vasculitis | • Discontinue culprit drugs<br>• Supportive care<br>• Treat infections/neoplasms<br>• Nonsteroidal anti-inflammatory drugs (NSAIDs)<br>• Antihistamines | • Colchicine 0.6 mg bid-tid; Max 3 mg/day<br>• Dapsone 50–200 mg/day<br>• Corticosteroids<br>• Hydroxychloroquine 200–400 mg/day<br>• Pentoxifylline 800–1,200 mg/day | • Azathioprine<br>• Methotrexate (MTX)<br>• Intravenous immunoglobulin (IVIg)<br>• Cyclosporine<br>• Cyclophosphamide<br>• Plasma exchange |
| Henoch–Schönlein [immunoglobulin A-associated vasculitis (IgAV)] | • Supportive care | • Colchicine 0.6 mg bid-tid; Max 3 mg/day<br>• Dapsone 50–200 mg/day<br>• Corticosteroids<br>• Azathioprine + Corticosteroid<br>• Cyclophosphamide + Corticosteroid<br>• Antihistamines | • IVIg<br>• Rituximab<br>• Mycophenolate<br>• Corticosteroid + Tacrolimus<br>• Aminocaproic acid<br>• Plasma exchange<br>• Factor XIII |
| Acute hemorrhagic edema of infancy | • Supportive care | | • Corticosteroids |
| Erythema elevatum diutinum | • NSAIDs<br>• Intralesional triamcinolone<br>• Dapsone | • Colchicine<br>• Hydroxychloroquine<br>• Tetracyclines | |
| Urticarial Vasculitis | • Antihistamines<br>• Indomethacin<br>• Dapsone<br>• Pentoxifylline<br>• Corticosteroid | • Colchicine<br>• Hydroxychloroquine<br>• Azathioprine<br>• MTX | • IVIg<br>• Rituximab<br>• Mycophenolate<br>• Cyclosporine<br>• Plasma exchange |

Continued

*Continued*

| Nature of vasculitis | First-line therapy | Second-line therapy | Third-line therapy |
|---|---|---|---|
| Cryoglobulinemic vasculitis | • Interferon (IFN) + Ribavirin<br>• Telaprevir, boceprevir<br>• Corticosteroids | • Corticosteroids + Cyclophosphamide | • IVIg<br>• Rituximab ± HCV therapy<br>• Plasma exchange |
| Cutaneous polyarteritis nodosa | • Treat HBV<br>• Discontinue culprit drugs<br>• NSAIDs<br>• Corticosteroids<br>• Penicillin | • MTX 7.5–15 mg/week<br>• Dapsone/sulfapyridine<br>• IVIg<br>• Pentoxifylline<br>• Mizoribine | • Colchicine<br>• Azathioprine<br>• Mycophenolate<br>• Tamoxifen<br>• Infliximab<br>• Tonsillectomy<br>• Warfarin |
| Classic PAN | • Corticosteroids + Lamivudine + IFN<br>• Plasma exchange | • Corticosteroids + Cyclophosphamide | • IVIg |
| ANCA-associated vasculitis [Wegener's granulomatosis (WG), Churg–Strauss syndrome (CSS), microscopic polyangiitis (MPA)] | • Corticosteroids + Cyclophosphamide<br>• Rituximab + Corticosteroids | • MTX<br>• Azathioprine<br>• MTX + Corticosteroids | • Trimethoprim-sulfamethoxazole (TMP-SMX) + Corticosteroids<br>• Plasma exchange<br>• IVIg<br>• Infliximab<br>• Alemtuzumab<br>• T-cell depletion<br>• Leflunomide<br>• Mycophenolate |

later in this chapter or other referral books. Patients with ulcerative or progressive skin disease may also require short courses of oral corticosteroids, which may be tapered in 4–6 weeks. Recurrence warrants addition of steroid-sparing drugs.

## PROGNOSTIC FACTORS

Patient prognosis is guided mainly by the presence systemic extension of disease like renal involvement (seen in about 43% of all CSVV). LCV usually has a chronic course (average 28 months). The identification of cryoglobulins, arthralgia and secondary vasculitis has been found to be risk factors for chronic disease. The presence of ulcers as the predominant feature along with paresthesia, fever, and absence of painful lesions are also pointers toward chronicity of the entity. In patients with HSP, a history of recent infection, fever, and the purpuric involvement of the trunk predict for renal involvement. The histopathological pointers to systemic vasculitic progression include the presence of cutaneous necrosis, the severity of vascular injury, and deep vasculitis. The presence of lesional IgA deposits, nephrotic syndrome, hypertension, decreased factor XIII activity, and renal failure on presentation are predictors of complex and protracted disease course. The clues to systemic vasculitis in association with or as a continuum of cutaneous vasculitis are shown in box 7.

**BOX 7 Clues to suspect systemic vasculitis**

- Fever of unknown origin
- Unexplained migratory polyarthritis
- Mononeuritis multiplex
- Rapidly progressive glomerulonephritis
- Palpable purpura
- Diffuse alveolar hemorrhage
- Unexplained infarction in multiple vascular territories
- Unexplained multisystem disease

## SPECIFIC FORMS OF VASCULITIS

### Leukocytoclastic Vasculitis (Cutaneous Leukocytoclastic Angiitis, Hypersensitivity Vasculitis, Cutaneous Necrotizing Venulitis)

This entity falls under the category of single-organ vasculitis in the revised CHCC 2012. This entity is almost synonymous with leukocytoclastic angiitis (CHCC 1994) and hypersensitivity vasculitis (ACR 1990) with one significant difference. Unlike all previous classifications, this has been mentioned as isolated cutaneous disease without any systemic involvement. Thus, most of the hypersensitivity vasculitis will not fall under this new category due to the more restricted classification criteria. Any subsequent development of systemic involvement will also eventually necessitate reclassification.

The ACR proposed the following criteria: (1) age more than 16 years at onset; (2) medications precipitating event; (3) palpable purpura; (4) cutaneous eruption; and (5) positive biopsy result (3/5 criteria required).

This is idiopathic in most cases. Infections (mostly upper respiratory tract infections) and drugs are most common specific etiologies. Beta-lactam antibiotics, NSAIDs, anticonvulsants and allopurinol are common precipitants. This starts abruptly after a gap of 1–3 weeks after the drug exposure.

Characteristic skin lesion is palpable purpura indicating involvement of small vessel. Urticarial vasculitis is also seen. More severe disease may show vesicles, bullae or pustules are uncommonly noticed (Fig. 3). Nodular lesions (medium vessel), ulcers (larger vessels), livedo (classically a sign of occlusive vasculopathy) are rare.

### Septic Vasculitis

One important scheme of classification of vasculitis is division into infective and noninfective vasculitis. Only primarily noninfective

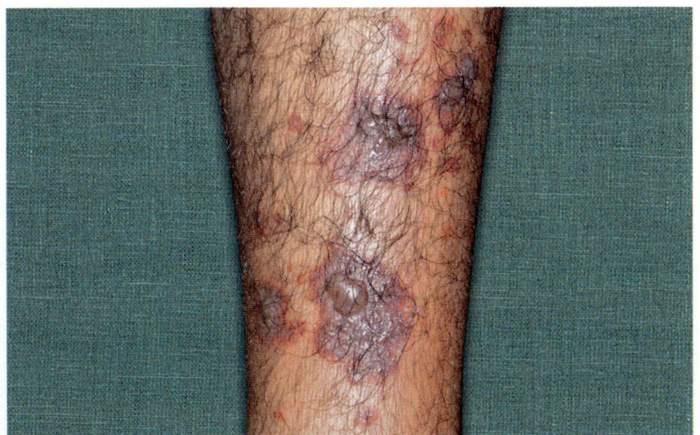

**FIG. 3:** Large purpuric lesions, and pustular eruptions in leukocytoclastic vasculitis.

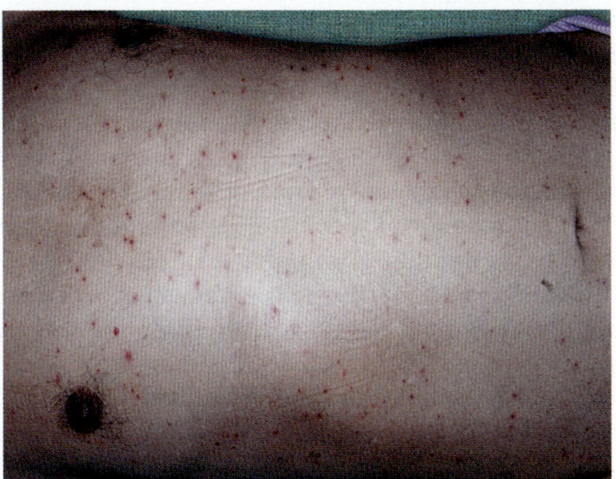

**FIG. 4:** Widespread purpuric eruptions in septic vasculitis.

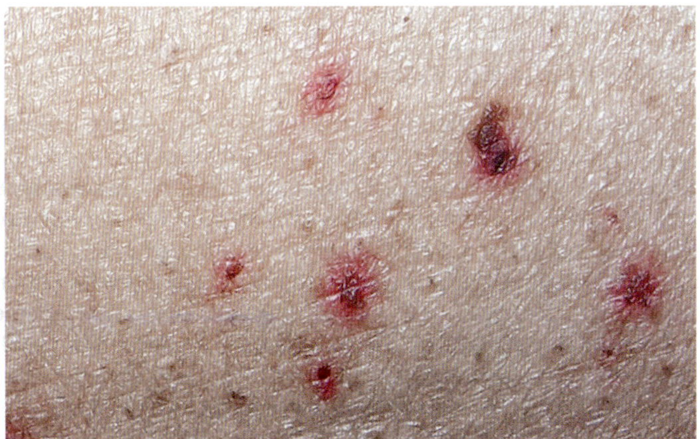

**FIG. 5:** Close-up view of septic vasculitis showing purpura, necrotic and pustular eruptions.

vasculitis has been addressed in the latest classification system (CHCC 2012). However, infection can indirectly lead to various vasculitis through immunological or other mechanisms.

Septic vasculitis is associated with septicemia due to *Neisseria meningitidis*, *Neisseria gonorrhoeae*, *Haemophilus influenzae*, *Streptococcus*, *Rickettsia*, *Candida*, infective endocarditis *Pseudomonas*, *Staphylococcus aureus*, syphilitic aortitis and *Aspergillus* species.

This manifests with systemic features like fever, arthralgia, and vesiculopustular or purpuric skin lesions (Figs 4 and 5).

Microorganisms are rarely found by Gram's stain in septic vasculitis with the exception of acute meningococcal septicemia in which large numbers of gram-negative diplococci are visualized in endothelial cells and polymorphonuclear leukocytes. Blood cultures can confirm the diagnosis. Immediate treatment with anti-infective agents is essential.

Treatment with systemic corticosteroids can lead to severe complications and are best avoided.

## Urticarial Vasculitis

Urticarial vasculitis is characterized by wheals lasting more than 24 hours with associated burning and pain and appears in crops, and resolves with purpura and hyperpigmentation. Angioedema is commonly associated.

Immunoglobulin G (IgG) antibody against C1q precipitin (C1q-p) are formed and vasculitis is caused by antigen–antibody complex deposition in the small vessels. Hypocomplementemia (low C1q) as observed in 35–64% of the patients has poorer prognosis than patients with normal complement level. IgG antibody against C1q is also sometimes seen in SLE. There may be some etiological link between these two conditions. Viral infections (hepatitis B and infectious mononucleosis), serum sickness, drug reactions, and hematologic disorders, and even solid tumors are considered possible etiologies. No recognizable etiology is identified in normocomplementemic urticarial vasculitis but can be associated with monoclonal gammopathy, neoplasia and cold exposure.

In general, patients with urticarial vasculitis have a chronic but benign course with a female preponderance. Systemic signs and symptoms like low-grade fever, migratory arthralgias, and abdominal pain are associated. Lymphadenopathy, splenomegaly, hematuria and microscopic proteinuria (glomerulonephritis), ocular involvement and obstructive pulmonary disease are observed.

Diagnosis is confirmed with presence of vasculitis (vessel damage or LCV). Neutrophilic vasculitis is classical but not found in earlier stages. In the normocomplementemic vasculitis, there may be lymphocytic and accompanied by a variable number of eosinophils.

## Immunoglobulin A Vasculitis (Henoch–Schönlein Purpura)

Henoch-Schönlein purpura is the most common vasculitis in children and an infrequent condition in adults in whom the disease is more severe than the former. It is associated with predominantly IgA deposits and affects skin, joints, glomeruli, and gastrointestinal (GI) tract. The term IgA vasculitis is now preferred over the eponym HSP.

Immunoglobulin G antibodies against abnormal IgA1 (abnormal glycosylation) form immune complex and are deposited tissue and in vessel wall inducing inflammation. This can occur as a single-organ vasculitis (IgA nephropathy, cutaneous IgA vasculitis) at least initially.

Upper respiratory tract (30–50%) or GI infection, diseases like liver disease, inflammatory bowel disease, ankylosing spondylitis, genetic and environmental factors food-related components can cause immunoglobulin A-associated vasculitis (IgAV). *Helicobacter pylori* and streptococci have been implicated too.

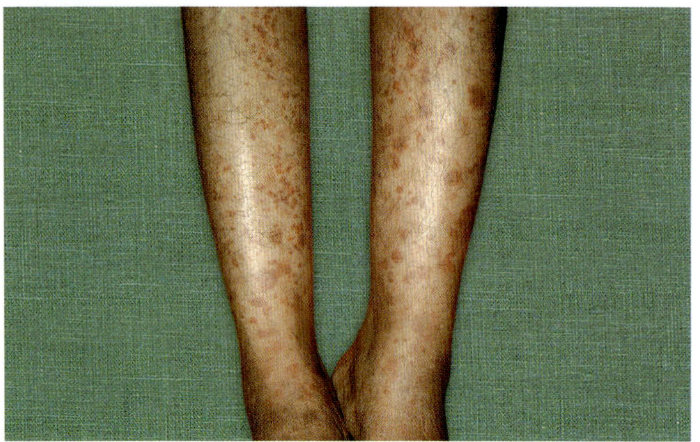

FIG. 6: Palpable purpura in IgA vasculitis.

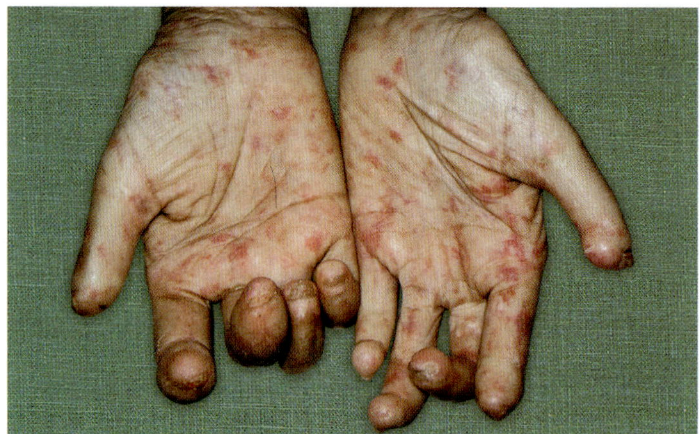

FIG. 7: Vasculitic eruptions on the hand in rheumatoid arthritis.

It is characterized by "classic pentad" of palpable purpura (100%), arthralgias (82%), abdominal pain (63%), renal disease-nephritis (40%), and GI bleed (33%). ACR criteria are (2/4 required for diagnosis): (1) palpable purpura; (2) age at onset less than 20 years; (3) bowel angina; and (4) vessel wall neutrophils on biopsy (Fig. 6).

Palpable purpura is the classical lesion. These appear in crops. Vesiculobullous eruptions, necrosis, gangrene, ulcers, erythema multiforme (EM)-like lesions are also seen. Orogenital mucosal purpura is also noted. GI system can be affected with colicky abdominal pain and vomiting and may be associated with underlying GI infarction, perforation, intussusception, pancreatitis, and cholecystitis. Any segment of the GI tract can be affected, but small bowel involvement is most common. CNS, respiratory system can also be involved. Scrotal vessel vasculitis can lead to severe pain.

The CHCC mandates that HSP can only be diagnosed only by the demonstration of IgA deposition within and around vessels in the superficial dermis. Proteinuria greater than 1 g/day during follow-up, hypertension, male sex, the involvement of 50% glomeruli with crescents, tubulointerstitial changes, and acute exacerbations were indicators to a poor outcome. Purpura above waist, recent history of infection, pyrexia, CRP/erythrocyte sedimentation rate (ESR) elevation are also indicators of renal involvement. Less than 20% patients observed over a period of 20 years develop chronic kidney disease. Urinalysis has to be repeated for 6 months as up to 40% relapse within 3–18 months after initial episode.

Overall, prognosis is favorable. Symptomatic treatment and NSAIDs are generally effective. Systemic corticosteroids, azathioprine, and cyclophosphamide are often used only in severe disease of joint, intestine, scrotum and progressive renal involvement. However, some studies have not confirmed long-term beneficial role of systemic corticosteroid (oral prednisone, 2 mg/kg/day) on preventing renal involvement and acute GI complications.

## Connective Tissue Disease Vasculitis

Connective tissue disease vasculitis (CTD) is an uncommon but important manifestation of CTD, frequently occurring in SLE, rheumatoid arthritis, and systemic sclerosis, and less commonly in dermatomyositis, and relapsing polychondritis. Compared to primary systemic vasculitis, more widespread organ involvement is found. The vascular size involved shows more variation in CTD vasculitis. Medium-vessel involvement in the skin is associated with cutaneous ulcers, nodules, digital gangrene, livedo reticularis, or pyoderma gangrenosum-like lesions. Histologically, it is characterized by lymphocytic vasculitis, and in case of SLE it is associated with basement membrane thickening and interface dermatitis. Compared to SLE patients without vasculitis, the presence of vasculitis patients have longer disease duration, are of younger age group, are more frequently male, and can be associated with cryoglobulinemia.

Rheumatoid vasculitis demonstrates acute painful punched-out ulcers affecting the pretibial and lateral malleolar regions (62%), hemorrhages (56%), nail fold infarcts called by the eponymous term Bywaters lesion (41%), gangrene, erythematous papulonodules, hemorrhagic vesicles, atrophie blanche and EED (Fig. 7).

## Cryoglobulinemic Vasculitis

Cryoglobulinemic vasculitis is characterized by elevated serum cryoglobulins and is linked with cryoglobulin deposits inside the vascular walls. The presence of rheumatoid factor-synthesizing B cells (the hallmark of mixed cryoglobulinemia) in combination with rheumatoid factor activity and cold-induced precipitation are key factors in pathogenesis. Cryoglobulins present are of two types: (1) monoclonal and (2) mixed. Monoclonal IgG or IgM cryoglobulins do not show positive rheumatoid factor activity (type I cryoglobulins—cause hyaline thrombi rather than vasculitis). Most patients with this variant have an underlying hematologic disorder (e.g., multiple myeloma, Waldenstrom macroglobulinemia). It presents as purpura, acral cyanosis, ulcers, or livedo reticularis. Mixed cryoglobulinemia can be polyclonal admixed with monoclonal antibodies (type II cryoglobulins) or polyclonal IgG and IgM molecules with rheumatoid factor activity (type III cryoglobulins). Hepatitis C infection, CTD, such as Sjögren's syndrome, and lymphoproliferative diseases are associated with mixed cryoglobulinemia. Many cases are idiopathic and are otherwise named essential mixed cryoglobulinemia.

Patients with cryoglobulinemic vasculitis are characterized by the clinical triad of purpura, arthralgias, and weakness (asthenia) (Fig. 8). Peripheral neuropathy and subclinical lymphocytic

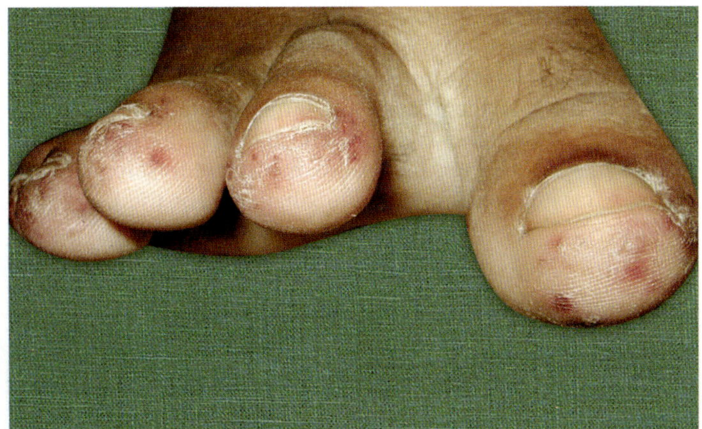

FIG. 8: Purpuric eruptions in cryoglobulinemia.

alveolitis are commonly observed. Renal complications, Raynaud phenomenon, and other systemic involvements have been described in less than 40% of the cases. Most patients report worsening of symptoms with exposure to cold.

Cryoglobulin serum level estimation is fraught with the risk of false-negatives due to the influence of the ambient temperature on their solubility and the possible decline during disease remissions. The term cryoglobulinemic syndrome is only used to describe symptomatic cases and not asymptomatic people incidentally detected to have cryoglobulinemia. Presence of renal involvement, or a concomitant tumor, and hepatitis C virus-induced mixed cryoglobulinemia (in many cases asymptomatic) are poor prognostic factors. A subset of patients with low serum C4 levels and high titers of rheumatoid factor have more renal and nervous system involvement.

A diagnostic criteria involving three out of four major criteria (mixed cryoglobulins, low C4 complement, LCV, purpura) and two out of seven minor criteria (rheumatoid factor positivity, hepatitis C virus, hepatitis B virus, clonal marrow/liver infiltrates of B cells, chronic hepatitis, membranoproliferative glomerulonephritis, peripheral neuropathy and cutaneous ulcers) has been proposed but not validated.

## Drug-induced Vasculitis

The drugs to be most frequently associated with vasculitis are propylthiouracil, hydralazine, granulocyte colony-stimulating factor (G-CSF), D-penicillamine, phenytoin, isotretinoin, allopurinol, cefaclor, minocycline, and methotrexate, respectively. Manifestations of drug-induced vasculitis are protean and range from small vessel vasculitis to systemic medium vessel vasculitis. The entity is associated with varied grades of severity up to fatality. The temporal connection for drug-induced vasculitis can be extremely variable leading to misdiagnoses. The difficulties are compounded by the lack of significant differences in clinical presentation, serologic abnormalities, and pathologic findings compared to idiopathic vasculitis. A high index of suspicion and cessation of culprit drug alone brings about prompt resolution. Severe life-endangering drug-induced vasculitis may warrant aggressive therapeutic modalities like steroids, cyclophosphamide, plasmapheresis, or hemodialysis. Tissue eosinophilia is a valuable histological pointer toward drug-induced vasculitis.

## Cutaneous Polyarteritis Nodosa

Cutaneous polyarteritis nodosa (CPAN) is characterized by necrotizing vasculitis of medium sized or small arteries without renal affectation. A clue to the presence of CPAN is the finding of nodules confined to the lower extremities associated with livedo. The disease is associated with negative ANA, rheumatoid factor estimation, cryoglobulins, and normocomplementemia. In two series of CPAN, 81% of patients had subcutaneous nodules, 69% had livedo reticularis, 44% had ulcers, 24% had peripheral neuropathy, and 1% had gangrene (Fig. 9). Gangrene is seen mostly in children (Fig. 10). Healed nodules appear as pigmented patch, reticulate pigmentation or white atrophic scar (Fig. 11).

Making the patient stand up for a few minutes to make the lesions more readily palpable can help decide the optimal site for biopsy. Deep biopsies are often necessary to see neutrophilic medium-sized vasculitis occurring in the reticular dermis and the subcutis. Serial sections may also be necessary to demonstrate the vasculitis, particularly when involvement is segmental and focal.

Long-term follow-up is necessary for CPAN because progression to systemic involvement can take as long as 18 years. The disease can be classified into three classes: (1) class I mild CPAN—nodular skin lesions, livedo reticularis, and/or mild polyneuropathy; (2) class II severe CPAN—prominent livedo,

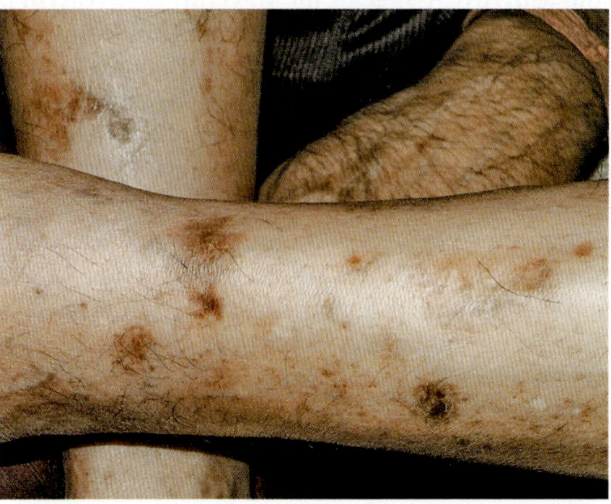

FIG. 9: Livedoid pigmentation and healed ulcer in cutaneous polyarteritis nodosa.

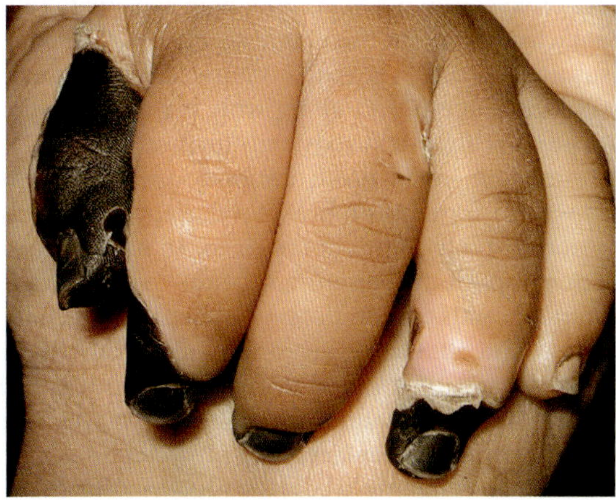

FIG. 10: Digital gangrene in cutaneous polyarteritis nodosa in a child.

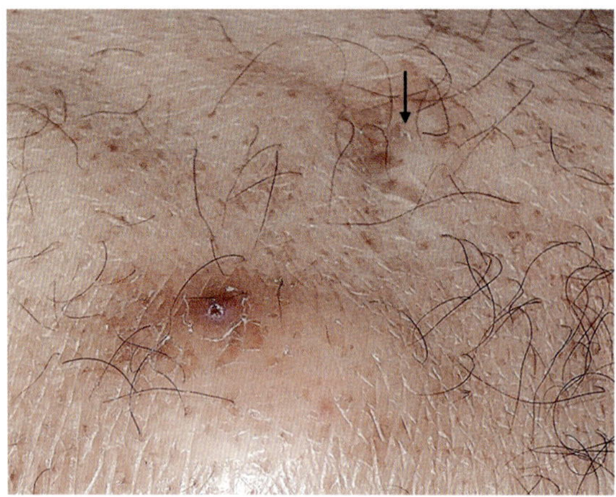

FIG. 11: Atrophic scar (arrow) in cutaneous polyarteritis nodosa.

ulcers, pain, polyneuropathy, and constitutional symptoms of fever, malaise, arthralgias; and (3) class III progressive systemic CPAN—necrosis with livedo, acral gangrene, musculoskeletal involvement, positive autoimmune tests, and increased visceral involvement.

## ANCA-associated Vasculitis

As described in earlier section, recent classification system recognizes AAV as necrotizing vasculitis involving small vessels associated with ANCA-specific for MPO (MPO-ANCA) or proteinase 3 (PR3-ANCA). There is few or no immune complex deposit in vessel wall. This is now understood that ANCA specificity identifies distinct categories of disease. AAV is subdivided further into MPA, granulomatosis with polyangiitis (WG/GPA), and eosinophilic granulomatosis with polyangiitis (EGPA/CSS) and ANCA-negative vasculitis.

Antineutrophil cytoplasmic antibody is typically absent in patients with PAN. P-ANCA is less specific for AAV and can be seen in CTD and other nonvasculitic entities. A positive ANCA test result should be interpreted with caution because the presence of ANCA is also associated with malaria, human immunodeficiency virus (HIV), GI diseases (inflammatory bowel disease, autoimmune hepatitis, primary biliary cirrhosis), and even in apparently healthy individuals. They can manifest as palpable purpura, pulmonary hemorrhage, mononeuritis, glomerulonephritis or thromboembolic events with most fatalities due to cardiac involvement.

Detection of serum c-ANCA has a high sensitivity (80%) and high specificity (100%) for the diagnosis of GPA. The concurrent demonstration of deficiency of immune deposits on indirect immunofluorescence (IDIF) along with the ANCA estimations increases the specificity and sensitivity further.

Antineutrophil cytoplasmic antibody-associated vasculitis responds well to immunosuppressive therapy but relapses are prone to occur in one-fourth of the cases. In AAV management, azathioprine was found to be more efficacious than mycophenolate in maintaining remission of disease. Cyclophosphamide pulses are preferred and should be given for 3–6 months till lifetime cumulative dosage of 25 g. Primary induction is achieved with steroids in combination with either cyclophosphamide or rituximab with early replacement of cyclophosphamide by methotrexate (up to 25 mg/week), azathioprine (2 mg/kg/day) or mycophenolate (up to 3 g/day). Adjuvant plasma exchange is also useful. Patients in continual remission for 1 year may be considered for steroid stoppage. Rituximab 375 mg/m$^2$/week for 4 weeks was found to be noninferior to cyclophosphamide 2 mg/kg/day in the management of AAV in a randomized controlled trial (RCT). Rituximab is most effective for management of refractory AAV. In relapsing disease, methylprednisolone pulses, course of cyclophosphamide or rituximab may be tried.

## Granulomatous Polyangiitis with Arteritis (Wegener's Granulomatosis)

Granulomatous polyangiitis with arteritis is characterized by granulomatous inflammation involving upper and lower respiratory tract, and necrotizing small to medium vessel vasculitis, with glomerulonephritis. Eye involvement, pulmonary bleeds and gingival hyperplasia are frequent.

The presence of cutaneous manifestations is variable and is associated with renal and joint involvement. Three categories of cutaneous disease exist in WG: (1) palpable or nonpalpable purpura due to small-vessel neutrophilic vasculitis; (2) subcutaneous nodules, ulcers, and digital infarcts (gangrene) secondary to medium vessel vasculitis; and (3) polymorphic lesions consisting of papules and nodules, pyoderma gangrenosum-like ulcers (also called malignant pyoderma), and gingival hyperplasia (strawberry gingivitis) (Figs 12 and 13).

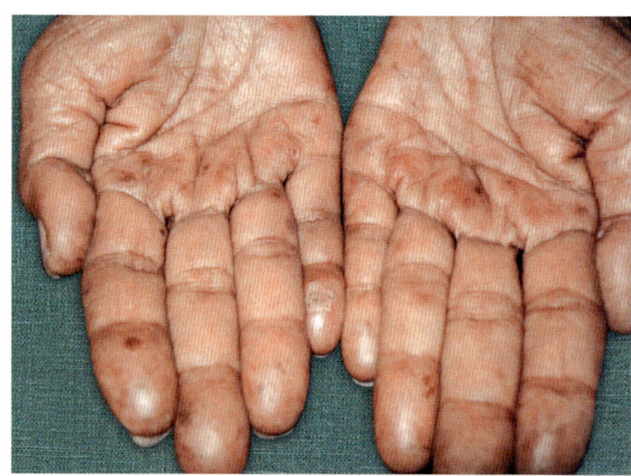

FIG. 12: Multiple purpuric lesions and ulcer on the palms and fingers in granulomatous polyangiitis with arteritis.

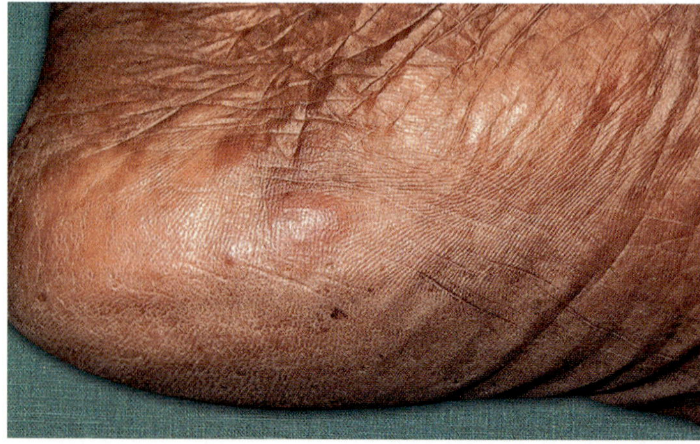

FIG. 13: Nodules on the side of sole in granulomatous polyangiitis with arteritis.

The most common histopathological finding in lesional skin biopsies is a neutrophilic vasculitis of the small- and medium-sized vessels. A triad comprising vasculitis, necrotic areas, and granulomatous inflammation is characteristic.

The following criteria have been proposed for the diagnosis of WG: (1) granulomatous inflammation of the respiratory tract or detection of infiltrates and cavities on imaging; (2) biopsy-verified necrotizing vasculitis in small- to medium-sized vessels or biopsy/positivity for glomerulonephritis or demonstration of proteinuria and hematuria (red cell casts), with positive c-ANCA; and (3) lack of eosinophilia in blood and biopsy samples. The presence of two criteria has a sensitivity of 88% and a specificity of 92%. The presence of sinusitis, urinary sediments pulmonary disease and c-ANCA positivity by enzyme-linked immunosorbent assay (ELISA) and IDIF exceeds 90% predictive value and precludes tissue diagnosis.

Limited (localized or initial phase) WG is defined as disease with no or minimal renal dysfunction, limited lung involvement, and no critical organ involvement (GI, CNS, eye) and is amenable to therapy with methotrexate.

## Eosinophilic Granulomatosis with Polyangiitis (Churg–Strauss Syndrome)

Eosinophilic granulomatosis with polyangiitis is associated with asthma and eosinophilia and eosinophil-rich granulomatous inflammation often involving the respiratory tract with/without cutaneous small to medium vessel vasculitis. ANCA positivity is more frequent when glomerulonephritis is present. Nongranulomatous eosinophil-rich inflammation of lungs, myocardium, and GI tract are common.

Onset is usually between ages 30 years and 50 years with respiratory symptoms ranging from allergic rhinitis, nasal polyposis, pansinusitis to treatment resistant asthma. Triggering factors include vaccines, and abrupt withdrawal of corticosteroid treatment. EGPA may evolve in several clinical stages: the first stage with persistent asthma, atopic diatheses and peripheral eosinophilia; the second stage characterized by tissue eosinophilia affecting one or more organs (e.g., eosinophilic pneumonia); the third and final phase is systemic vasculitis. Compared to WG and MPA, EGPA has less renal disease and more cutaneous, nerve, and cardiac diseases.

Skin involvement occurs in about 50% of patients, and manifests as lower limb purpuric macules or papules and nodules (which may progress to ulceration) on the scalp and the distal limbs. There can also be petechiae, ecchymoses and/or hemorrhagic bullae, urticaria or livedo reticularis.

Pathologic examination can reveal small and medium vessel LCV, tissue eosinophilia, and an extravascular granulomatous inflammatory infiltrate composed of a large number of eosinophils. Hematology analysis shows intense eosinophilia, which is accompanied by increased IgE during disease flares. Up to 50% test positive for p-ANCA, but c-ANCA can be found in 10–20% cases. Experimental therapies include leukotriene receptor antagonist therapy or monoclonal anti-IgE antibodies, such as omalizumab.

## Microscopic Polyangiitis

Microscopic polyangiitis is characterized by pauci-immune vasculitis involving superficial and medium-sized vasculature and manifests as a pulmonary-renal syndrome. There is no granulomatous inflammation, asthma, and eosinophilia.

The skin is involved and antibodies to p-ANCA are demonstrable in approximately 80%. Compared to WG and EGPA, MPA has a poorer prognosis with a 5-year overall survival of 45%. Skin involvement is seen in 65% or less of all MPA. Skin involvement of MPA resembles that in CLA and HSP. The following criteria for diagnosis have been proposed: (1) lack of biopsy markers of granulomatous inflammation; (2) biopsy confirmation of neutrophilic small vessel vasculitis and/or glomerulonephritis with few or no immune deposits; and (3) involvement of more than one organ system documented by biopsy or surrogate marker, such as proteinuria, hematuria for glomerulonephritis.

## Nodular Vasculitis (Erythema Induratum)

Nodular vasculitis (lobular panniculitis with vasculitis) was originally defined as erythema induratum (red, indurated plaques on the calf) associated with tuberculosis. There are two varieties of nodular vasculitis: (1) focal panniculitis (type I) with central neutrophilic muscular vasculitis and (2) diffuse panniculitis (type II) with multiple foci of neutrophilic small and muscular vessel vasculitis, with varying degrees of caseous necrosis and granulomas. Lobular panniculitis can be difficult to distinguish from CPAN; extravascular tuberculoid granulomas identified in the surrounding tissue can be a pointer to the diagnosis of erythema induratum.

## Lymphocytic Vasculitis

The broad classification under the head of lymphocytic vasculitis includes: lymphocytic endovasculitis, lymphocytic lichenoid vasculitis, and angiocentric/angiodestructive lymphocytic vasculitis. The third variant (angiocentric) is seen in cutaneous lymphomas, such as mycosis fungoides, lymphomatoid papulosis, angiocentric T-cell lymphoma and chronic lymphocytic leukemia (CLL) as also in CTD vasculitis. Lichenoid lymphocytic vasculitis is observed in herpetic dermatitis, chilblains lupus, lichenoid drug eruptions, pityriasis lichenoides (Mucha–Habermann disease), graft versus host disease, perniosis, and Degos' disease. In Kawasaki disease, lymphocytes mediate a panvasculitis that can lead to aneurysm formation and rupture in addition to luminal occlusion and infarction.

# CONCLUSION

Cutaneous vasculitides are a set of disorders which are having overlapping features which lead to a surfeit of dermatological misdiagnoses and difficulty in diagnosis. The vasculitides are also characterized by remissions and relapses which may be potentially fatal and might confuse the clinical dermatologist. The therapies currently available do not address the underlying mechanistic reasons for the disease and emphasize the requirement for basic research in the pathogenetic pathways of disease, thereby initiating interest in specific targets leading to a more personalized approach to vasculitis therapy.

# SUGGESTED READINGS

1. Bosco L, Peroni A, Schena D, et al. Cutaneous manifestations of Churg-Strauss syndrome: report of two cases and review of the literature. Clin Rheumatol. 2011;30:573-80.

2. Callen JP. Cutaneous vasculitis: what have we learned in the past 20 years? Arch Dermatol. 1998;134:355-7.
3. Carlson JA, Cavaliere LF, Grant-Kels JM. Cutaneous vasculitis: diagnosis and management. Clin Dermatol. 2006;24:414-29.
4. Carlson JA, Ng BT, Chen KR. Cutaneous vasculitis update: diagnostic criteria, classification, epidemiology, etiology, pathogenesis, evaluation and prognosis. Am J Dermatopathol. 2005;27:504-28.
5. Daoud MS, Hutton KP, Gibson LE. Cutaneous periarteritis nodosa: a clinicopathological study of 79 cases. Br J Dermatol. 1997;136:706-13.
6. Fries JF, Hunder GG, Bloch DA, et al. The American College of Rheumatology 1990 criteria for the classification of vasculitis. Summary. Arthritis Rheum. 1990;33:1135-6.
7. Gonzalez-Gay MA, Garcia-Porrua C, Salvarani C, et al. Cutaneous vasculitis: a diagnostic approach. Clin Exp Rheumatol. 2003;21(Suppl 32):S85-8.
8. Hernandez-Rodriguez J, Hoffman GS. Updating single-organ vasculitis. Curr Opin Rheumatol. 2012;24:38-45.
9. Hiemstra TF, Walsh M, Mahr A, et al. Mycophenolate mofetil vs azathioprine for remission maintenance in antineutrophil cytoplasmic antibody-associated vasculitis: a randomized controlled trial. JAMA. 2010;304:2381-8.
10. Huber AM, King J, McLaine P, et al. A randomized, placebo-controlled trial of prednisone in early Henoch-Schönlein purpura. BMC Med. 2004;2:7.
11. Jennette JC, Falk RJ, Bacon PA, et al. 2012 revised International Chapel Hill consensus conference nomenclature of vasculitides. Arthritis Rheum. 2013;65:1-11.
12. Kawakami T. New algorithm (KAWAKAMI algorithm) to diagnose primary cutaneous vasculitis. J Dermatol. 2010;37:113-24.
13. Knight GB, Gao L, Gragnani L, et al. Detection of WA B cells in hepatitis C virus infection: a potential prognostic marker for cryoglobulinemic vasculitis and B cell malignancies. Arthritis Rheum. 2010;62:2152-9.
14. Lie JT. Illustrated histopathologic classification criteria for selected vasculitis syndromes. American College of Rheumatology Subcommittee on Classification of Vasculitis. Arthritis Rheum. 1990;33:1074-87.
15. Luqmani RA, Bacon PA, Moots RJ, et al. Birmingham Vasculitis Activity Score (BVAS) in systemic necrotizing vasculitis. QJM. 1994;87:671-8.
16. Luqmani RA, Pathare S, Kwok-Fai TL. How to diagnose and treat secondary forms of vasculitis. Best Pract Res Clin Rheumatol. 2005;19:321-36.
17. Ntatsaki E, Carruthers D, Chakravarty K. BSR and BHPR guideline for the management of adults with ANCA-associated vasculitis. Rheumatology. 2014;262: 1-4.
18. Sorensen SF, Slot O, Tvede N, et al. A prospective study of vasculitis patients collected in a five year period: evaluation of the Chapel Hill nomenclature. Ann Rheum Dis. 2000;59:478-82.
19. Takeuchi S, Soma Y, Kawakami T. IgM in lesional skin of adults with Henoch-Schönlein purpura is an indication of renal involvement. J Am Acad Dermatol. 2010;63:1026-9.

40

CHAPTER

# Peripheral Vascular Disease

*Reena Rai, Pradeep Balasubramanian*

## INTRODUCTION

Many diseases lead to occlusion of smaller vessels. Many of these conditions manifest in the skin with ulcer, livedo, or in other ways. This chapter will focus on these disorders.

## LIVEDO RETICULARIS

Livid (bluish-red), reticulate (net-like) vascular pattern that results from alteration in the blood flow through the cutaneous microvasculature.

### Etiopathogenesis

Any process that reduces the blood flow to the skin or reduces the drainage of blood out of the skin will result in the accumulation of deoxygenated blood in the venous system thus resulting in livedo reticularis. The pallor corresponds to the base of the cone (arterial dominance) and livid color in the intervening areas corresponds to the areas of venous dominance (Figs 1 and 2).

### Classification

1. Congenital
2. Acquired

- Physiological
- Primary livedo without systemic association (idiopathic)
- Livedo secondary to systemic diseases.

*Physiological livedo/cutis marmorata*: It occurs in response to cold and disappears on rewarming. It is commonly seen in neonates, infants, and young children.

*Primary (idiopathic) livedo reticularis*: It is persistent and does not disappear on rewarming. It occurs due to the following causes:

- *Due to intraluminal pathology*:
  - *Increased blood components*: Thrombocythemia, polycythemia vera
  - *Abnormal proteins*: Paraproteinemia, cryoglobulinemia and cryofibrinogenemia
  - *Hypercoagulable states*: Antiphospholipid antibody (APLA), protein C/S deficiency, hyperhomocysteinemia, and factor V mutation
  - *Emboli*: Cholesterol, septic, and atrial myxoma
- *Vessel wall pathology*:
  - Vasculitis (small and medium vessels)
  - Sneddon's syndrome.

### Biopsy

To establish the etiology, the arteriole must be included in the biopsy. For this, a moderately large elliptical biopsy form the center of the net pattern must be done.

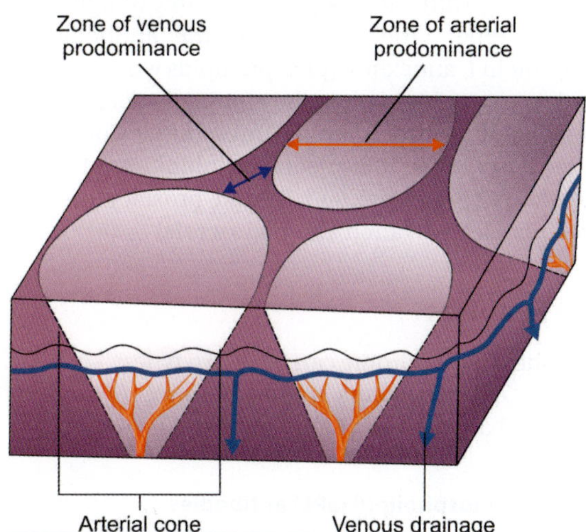


**FIG. 1:** Pathogenesis of livedo reticularis.

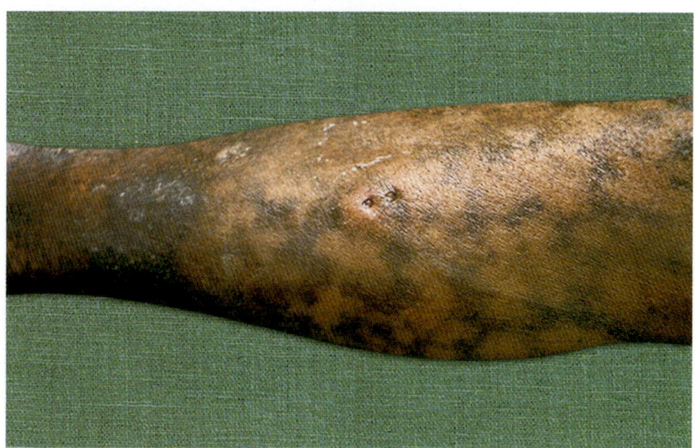

**FIG. 2:** Livedo reticularis secondary to hyperhomocysteinemia.

## Treatment

Livedo reticularis is a clinical sign and does not require treatment. It is unresponsive to medications and lasers. Underlying cause needs identification and treatment.

# LIVEDO RACEMOSA

It differs from livedo reticularis in the following aspects:
- The reticulate pattern is broken
- It is broader and larger than livedo reticularis.

*It occurs in*: APLA syndrome and Sneddon's syndrome.

# ANTIPHOSPHOLIPID ANTIBODY/LUPUS ANTICOAGULANT SYNDROME

Antiphospholipid syndrome (APS) is the association of antiphospholipid (aPL) antibodies with hypercoagulability resulting in arterial and/or venous thrombosis, and pregnancy morbidity/obstetric complications. The aPL antibodies include the antibodies that have the ability to bind to phospholipids (Table 1).

## Paradox in Antiphospholipid Syndrome

Antiphospholipid antibodies cause thrombosis *in vivo* whereas prolongation of clotting *in vitro*. This is because *in vitro*, the antibodies bind to phospholipids (clotting factors) in blood thus interfering with the coagulation pathway thus prolonging the clotting time. Whereas *in vivo*, the antibodies bind to β2-glycoprotein I, annexin V (phospholipids which line the vessel wall) with greater affinity than the clotting factors thus initiating the coagulation cascade causing thrombosis. Coagulation also results because of the aPL-mediated inhibition of endogenous anticoagulants (protein C and S) and prostacyclin. Antibody-mediated platelet activation also plays a role.

## Clinical Features

Antiphospholipid syndrome can be of two types:
- *Primary APS*: It occurs in the absence of underlying or associated diseases
- *Secondary APS*: It occurs in association with other autoimmune diseases namely systemic lupus erythematosus (SLE), rheumatoid arthritis, Sjögren's syndrome, etc.

**TABLE 1: Antiphospholipid (aPL) antibodies**

| Type of aPL antibody | Method of detection | Antiphospholipid antibodies |
|---|---|---|
| Functional antibodies (detected by clotting tests) | • Dilute Russell's viper venom time<br>• Kaolin clotting time<br>• Activated partial thromboplastin time | Lupus anticoagulant |
| Antibodies that are detected by tests that measure the levels of antibodies | Immunoassays (ELISA) | • Antibodies against<br>• Cardiolipin<br>• β2-glycoprotein I<br>• Prothrombin<br>• Annexin V (a phospholipid binding plasma protein) |

ELISA, enzyme-linked immunosorbent assay.

This can also occur in healthy individuals. Thus, they are considered significant only in the presence of clinical features suggestive of APS. The clinical features of both primary and secondary APS are identical. Skin manifestations occur in 40% of APS patients which may be the first clue to diagnose this syndrome. Thus, it is essential to be aware of the cutaneous features related to venous or arterial thrombosis or microthrombosis (Box 1). APS can cause various systemic complications. Pregnancy-related complications are most important and occur due to the placental infarcts mediated by aPL antibodies (Box 2).

## Diagnosis

Clinical and laboratory criteria for diagnosis have been published (Box 3).

Of the above aPL antibodies, anticardiolipin antibody detection has the maximum sensitivity and lupus anticoagulant antibody has the maximum specificity.

## Management of Antiphospholipid Syndrome

### Primary Prophylaxis

Low-dose aspirin is instituted in patients with aPL and no thrombotic events. Hydroxychloroquine reduced the formation of aPL-β2GPI complexes thus can be used for thromboprophylaxis in APS.

**BOX 1 Cutaneous findings in antiphospholipid syndrome (APS)**

- Livedo reticularis
- Livedo racemosa
- Superficial thrombophlebitis migrans
- Leg ulcers secondary (Fig. 3)
- Digital gangrene or infarct
- Retiform purpura or retiform infarct
- Widespread cutaneous necrosis (catastrophic APS)
- Splinter hemorrhage
- Raynaud's phenomenon
- Atrophie blanche
- Pseudo-Kaposi's sarcoma
- Pyoderma gangrenosum-like ulcer
- Vasculitis-like lesions
- Anetoderma-like lesions with thrombosis
- Degos (malignant atrophic papulosis)-like lesions
- Sneddon's syndrome

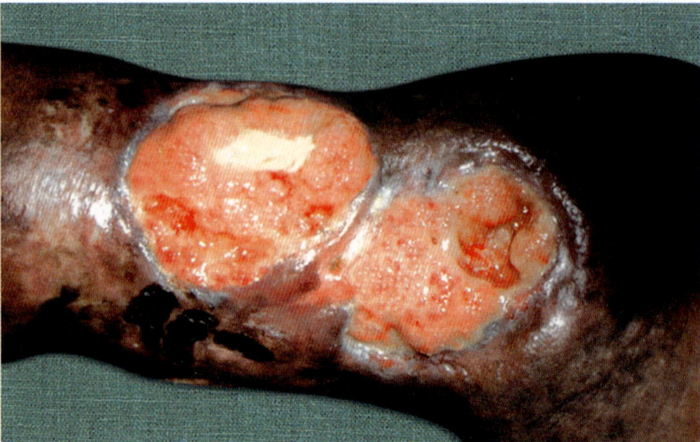

**FIG. 3:** Antiphospholipid syndrome with leg ulcers.

**BOX 2 Noncutaneous features of antiphospholipid syndrome**

- Deep vein thrombosis
- Pulmonary embolism
- Stroke and transient ischemic attacks
- Central retinal artery and vein occlusion
- Thrombocytopenia and hemolytic anemia
- Heart valve disease

**Pregnancy-related complications:**

- Recurrent spontaneous abortions
- Premature birth
- Pre-eclampsia
- Eclampsia
- Placental insufficiency

**BOX 3 Classification criteria for detection of antiphospholipid syndrome (APS)**

**Clinical criteria**

- *Vascular thrombosis*: One or more clinical episodes of arterial, venous, or small vessel thrombosis in any tissue or organ confirmed by objectively validated criteria (imaging or Doppler studies or histopathology), with the exception of superficial venous thrombosis
- *Pregnancy morbidity*:
  - One or more unexplained deaths of a morphologically normal fetus at or beyond the 10th week of gestation, with normal fetal morphology documented by ultrasound or by direct examination of the fetus, or
  - One or more premature births of a morphologically normal neonate at or before the 34th week of gestation because of severe pre-eclampsia or eclampsia or severe placental insufficiency, or
  - Three or more unexplained consecutive spontaneous abortions before the 10th week of gestation, with maternal anatomic or hormonal abnormalities and paternal and maternal chromosomal causes excluded

**Laboratory criteria**

- Lupus anticoagulant presents in plasma, on two or more occasions, at least 12 weeks apart, detected according to the guidelines of the International Society on Thrombosis and Hemostasis (Subcommittee on Lupus Anticoagulants/Antiphospholipid Antibodies)
- Anticardiolipin antibody of immunoglobulin G (IgG) and/or immunoglobulin M (IgM) isotype in serum or plasma, presents in medium or high titer on two or more occasions, at least 12 weeks apart, measured by a standardized ELISA
- Anti-β2-glycoprotein I of IgG and/or IgM isotype in serum or plasma (titer >99th percentile) on two or more occasions, at least 12 weeks apart, measured by a standardized ELISA according to recommended procedures

Definitive diagnosis of APS is made if one clinical and one laboratory criteria are satisfied 12 weeks apart.

## Secondary Prophylaxis

It refers to the treatment initiated after the occurrence of thrombotic events to prevent further attacks. Low-molecular-weight heparin has been used in the initial phase followed by warfarin in the management of APS. The target international normalized ratio (INR) in the patients on warfarin therapy is 2.0–3.0.

Recently intravenous immunoglobulin and plasmapheresis have also been used successfully in patients with APS.

# MALIGNANT ATROPHIC PAPULOSIS (DEGOS DISEASE)

The lesions of Degos disease represent thrombo-occlusive vasculopathy which can occur in two settings namely:

- Idiopathic (classical Degos disease and benign variant)
- Associated with other connective tissue disease namely APLA, lupus erythematosus, systemic sclerosis, and dermatomyositis (secondary Degos or Degos-like lesions).

## Classic Degos Disease

The cutaneous lesions precede the onset of systemic involvement.

### Systemic involvement

- Gastrointestinal (GI) tract—abdominal pain, diarrhea, melena, bowel perforation, peritonitis
- Central nervous system (CNS)—hemorrhagic or ischemic stroke.

## Benign Degos Disease

Cutaneous involvement occurs without visceral manifestations.

### Cutaneous Lesions

Lesions occur in crops.

Stages of evolution of the lesions:

Rose-colored macules

↓

Round dome-shaped papules

↓

Display central umbilication or necrosis

↓

Porcelain white atrophic papule with a rim of erythema or telangiectasia (Fig. 4)

↓

The rim resolves leaving varicelliform scars.

The lesions are localized on the trunk and limbs. Face, scalp, palms, and soles are usually spared.

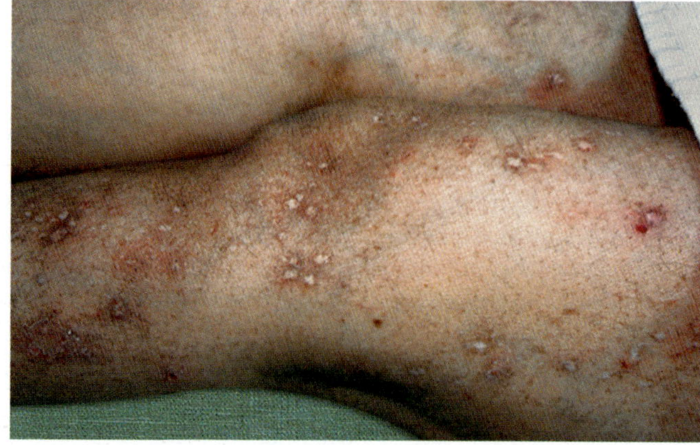

**FIG. 4:** Degos-like lesion in antiphospholipid antibody syndrome.

## Histopathology

Wedge-shaped area of dermal necrosis extending from papillary dermis to deep reticular dermis associated with mucin deposition and dermal edema.

At the base of the lesion, the vessel shows the following features: thrombosis, endothelial proliferation, vessel wall thickening, and sparse or absent perivascular infiltrates.

## Investigations

Antinuclear antibody (ANA) profile, anticardiolipin antibody, and lupus anticoagulant need to be done to rule out secondary Degos disease.

## Complications

- Gastrointestinal—GI perforation, peritonitis, GI hemorrhage, obstruction and fistulae
- Nervous system—cerebral or spinal cord infarcts
- Occasionally respiratory failure and myocardial infarction can happen.

## Management of Degos Disease

- *First line—antiplatelet agents*: Aspirin, clopidogrel and dipyridamole
- *Second line*: Heparin or other anticoagulants
- *Adjunctive measures*: Control of cardiovascular risk factors, pentoxifylline.

# SNEDDON'S SYNDROME

It is characterized by generalized livedo racemosa or livedo reticularis associated with cerebrovascular lesions. It is twice as common in women as in men. Typically it occurs in 4th or 5th decade. Livedo racemosa is usually the first manifestation, initially affecting the lower trunk and proximal part of legs.

## Neurological Lesions

Nonspecific neurological prodrome—headache, migraine, vertigo, dizziness

↓

Focal neurological deficits (sensory or motor) or cognitive changes.

## Investigations

Antinuclear antibody and aPL antibodies can occasionally be positive in whom the infarct commonly happens in the territory of main cerebral artery whereas those with negative infarct are prone to develop small lacunar infarcts. Biopsy from the center of livedo shows thrombotic occlusion or endarteritis of dermal arteriole.

## Treatment

Avoidance of risk factors (smoking, oral contraceptives, treatment of hypertension and dyslipidemia).

Anticoagulants in patients with positive aPL antibodies to maintain INR between 2 and 3.

# HEPARIN-INDUCED THROMBOCYTOPENIA AND SKIN NECROSIS

It is a paradoxical response to heparin more commonly seen in female. Unfractionated heparin (bovine more than porcine) is three times more likely to be associated with heparin-induced thrombocytopenia (HIT) than low-molecular-weight heparin. The risk is highest in postsurgical patients followed by medical patients and least with obstetric patients.

## Pathogenesis

Heparin binds to platelet factor 4 (PF4)

↓

Induces a conformational change to PF4

↓

Antibodies formed against heparin-PF4

↓

Causes platelet aggregation leading to thrombus formation and vaso-occlusion.

## Clinical Features

Patients with HIT develop absolute or relative thrombocytopenia (90%) followed by venous or arterial thrombosis or skin necrosis. Commonly develop in the initial 2 weeks following initiation of heparin, can develop later too (delayed-onset HIT). Skin lesions are commonly located at the site of subcutaneous injection, but can occur elsewhere also (Fig. 5).

## Treatment

Heparin should be stopped immediately. Low-molecular weight heparin and Coumadin are also contraindicated. The anticoagulants currently used to treat HIT include danaparoid (heparinoid), lepirudin, or argatroban.

# COUMADIN (COUMARIN, WARFARIN)-INDUCED SKIN NECROSIS

This commonly occurs within 3–5 days of Coumadin initiation. It is due to protein C inhibition which happens earlier than clotting factors, thus leading to unopposed action of clotting factors resulting in thrombosis and skin necrosis. Coumadin necrosis

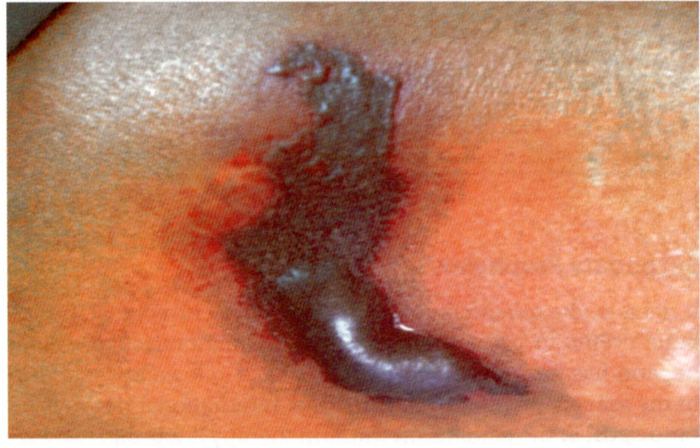

**FIG. 5:** Cutaneous necrosis due to heparin induced thrombocytopenia at the site of subcutaneous heparin injection.

commonly involves areas with abundant fatty tissue namely breast, hip, buttocks, and thigh. The peak incidence is in 6$^{th}$ and 7$^{th}$ decade and is four times more common in female. Restoration of protein C activity can be accomplished through protein C concentrates or fresh frozen plasma.

## SEPSIS-RELATED PURPURA FULMINANS WITH DIC: ACQUIRED SEVERE PROTEIN C DEFICIENCY

This occurs days to weeks after some preceding infection which includes pneumococcus, meningococcus, *Haemophilus,* and *Streptococcus* (α and β hemolytic). It presents as noninflammatory hemorrhage usually with a retiform, stellate or branching configuration with transition to necrosis and eschar. In patients with sepsis, disseminated intravascular coagulation (DIC) and retiform purpura, it seems reasonable to assume severe protein C deficiency and to administer protein C concentrates or fresh frozen plasma.

## POSTINFECTIOUS PURPURA FULMINANS DUE TO ACQUIRED SEVERE PROTEIN S DEFICIENCY

It occurs following varicella and streptococcal infection commonly in children, days to weeks after a febrile illness. It is due to the antibodies formed against protein S. Thus, replacement of protein S is not very effective since it is not due to simple clearing of protein S.

## ECTHYMA GANGRENOSUM

It is commonly caused by *Pseudomonas* more often in immunocompromised patients, characterized by erythematous papules or plaques that progress to bullous lesions, followed by hemorrhage and necrosis with retiform extension from margins. It occurs due to direct vaso-invasion induced by the causative organism. Anogenital area is the frequent site, but can occur elsewhere too. Ecthyma gangrenosum-like lesions are caused by gram-negative bacteria (*Escherichia coli, Klebsiella, Proteus,* and *Vibrio*) and vaso invasive fungi (*Aspergillus, Mucor, Fusarium,* and *Rhizopus*).

## INTRAVASCULAR LYMPHOMA

It is a lymphoma due to intraluminal proliferation of B-lymphocytes. CNS manifestations are the most common followed by the cutaneous manifestations namely infiltrated nodule or plaque, peau d'orange lesion, ulcer. The proximal extremities, lower abdomen and submammary areas are the common sites to be involved. Diagnosis is confirmed by skin biopsy which shows large B cells demonstrating monoclonality which fills the vascular lumen. Chemotherapy is the treatment.

## LEG ULCER

An ulcer is a breech in skin surface. Leg is the most common body site for development of ulcer. Although the distinction of acute versus chronic ulcer is not properly defined, ulcer persisting beyond 12 weeks is generally called as chronic ulcer. There are many unique anatomical and structural characteristics in leg that predispose it for development of ulcer as well as delay in healing even with treatment.

### Etiology

Venous insufficiency constitutes roughly about 70%, arterial disease 10%, and mixed etiology 15% of leg ulcers. The remaining 5% of leg ulcers result from other pathophysiological causes. Causes may be local or systemic (Box 4).

**BOX 4 Causes of leg ulcers**

- Venous
- Arterial—thromboangiitis obliterans, hypertension
- Infective
- Microvascular occlusion (Box 5)
- Hematologic—hemoglobinopathies
- Connective tissue disease (RA)
- Vasculitis
- Trauma
- Neuropathic
- Drug-induced—hydroxyurea
- Miscellaneous dermatoses—pyoderma gangrenosum, necrobiosis lipoidica, panniculitis, and calciphylaxis

RA, rheumatoid arthritis.

**BOX 5 Causes of microvascular occlusion**

**Microvascular Occlusion Disorders**

- Occlusion due to platelet plugs
  - Heparin-induced thrombocytopenia
  - Myeloproliferative disorders
  - Paroxysmal nocturnal hemoglobinuria
  - Thrombotic thrombocytopenic purpura/hemolytic-uremic syndrome
- Occlusion due to cryogelling
  - Cryoglobulinemia
  - Cryofibrinogenemia
  - Cold-agglutinin-related occlusion
- Occlusion due to vessel-invasive organisms
  - Ecthyma gangrenosum
  - Lucio's phenomenon
  - Vessel-invasive fungi
  - Disseminated strongyloidiasis
- Occlusion due to embolus
  - Cholesterol embolus
  - Oxalate crystal embolus
  - Atrial myxoma
  - Cardiac sterile thrombi
  - Septic emboli
  - Fat emboli
- Occlusion due to systemic coagulopathies with cutaneous manifestations
  - Protein C/S/thrombomodulin pathway anomalies
    - Neonatal purpura fulminans
    - Coumadin necrosis
    - Sepsis-related purpura fulminans
    - Postinfectious purpura fulminans
- Antiphospholipid antibody syndrome
- Occlusion due to vascular coagulopathies
  - Sneddon's syndrome
  - Livedoid vasculopathy/atrophie blanche
  - Malignant atrophic papulosis
- Occlusion due to reticulocyte occlusion
  - Sickle cell disease
  - Other severe hemolytic anemias

## Approach to Diagnosis in a Leg Ulcer

As the etiology of the leg ulcer can be too many, diagnosis is often difficult.

A detailed history is very important. Nature of initial lesions, history of recurrence, exposure to any precipitating event, speed of progression, presence and intensity of pain, conditions that aggravate and improve pain especially relation with walking and details of past treatment are important.

Clinical examination has to be meticulous to evaluate the site, margin, surface, surrounding skin, associated varicosity, number of ulcers, tenderness, signs of neuropathy, presence of skin and other diseases that might be of importance should be meticulously examined.

Proper investigations have to be carried out in detail to identify the etiology because management depends on exact etiology. Systemic diseases, presence of secondary contact sensitization and infection need to be identified (Box 6).

*Ankle-brachial pressure index (ABPI)*: A noninvasive test using the handheld Doppler ultrasound which identifies peripheral arterial disease in the leg. Systolic blood pressure (BP) is measured at the brachial artery and at the ankle level.

$$\text{ABPI} = \frac{\text{Highest systolic foot pressure (dorsalis pedis/posterior tibial artery)}}{\text{Highest systolic brachial BP}}$$

- *ABPI*: 0.8–1.2—indicative of good arterial flow. Suggestive of venous etiology if ulcer is present
- *ABPI*: Less than 0.8 with clinical picture of arterial disease—arterial insufficiency
- *ABPI*: More than 1.2—suggestive of possible arterial calcification.

*Duplex ultrasound*: A noninvasive test which combines ultrasound with Doppler ultrasonography. Blood flow through arteries and veins can be investigated to reveal any obstructions. It allows direct visualization of veins, identifies flow through valves and can map both superficial and deep veins.

*Photoplethysmography*: A noninvasive test which measures venous refill time. This determines the efficiency of the calf muscle pump and the presence of any abnormal venous reflux. Patients with problems in superficial or deep veins usually have poor emptying of the veins and abnormally rapid refilling (<25 s).

*Pulse oximetry*: It measures oxygen saturation of blood in a digit.

*Histopathology*: Wound biopsy only if malignancy or other etiology is suspected.

**BOX 6 Suggested laboratory investigations in leg ulcer**

- Complete blood count—to rule out infection, anemia, and polycythemia
- Blood sugars, HbA1c for diabetic status
- Serum albumin
- Iron—to rule out nutritional deficiency
- Serum homocysteine levels—increased in vitamin B6, B12 and folate deficiency
- Screening for lupus anticoagulant, anticardiolipin antibodies
- Protein C, protein S, and antithrombin III, factor V Leiden
- Wound swabs for bacterial culture and sensitivities
- Patch testing—common allergens are neomycin, lanolin, bacitracin, formaldehyde, and parabens
- Duplex ultrasound
- Ankle-brachial pressure index
- Photoplethysmography
- Pulse oximetry
- Histopathology

# VENOUS LEG ULCER

Venous ulcers are the most common cause of leg ulcer.

## Pathophysiology

Normal system of venous drainage of blood from the lower limbs is hampered in cases of deep vein thrombosis, perforator insufficiency, superficial and deep vein insufficiencies, arterio-venous fistulas and neuromuscular dysfunction. These lead to increased pressure in the distal veins of the leg which is responsible for venous hypertension. Thus, venous incompetence and calf muscle pump insufficiency are the two initial factors which are responsible for the main pathophysiological factor namely venous hypertension.

There are three major theories of how ulceration develops:

1. *Fibrin cuff theory*: Fibrinogen leaks from dilated capillaries of the epidermis forming a pericapillary fibrin cuff resulting in reduced diffusion of oxygenated blood to the tissues resulting in ulceration
2. *Leukocyte entrapment theory*: Sluggish movement of the blood within these capillaries leads to entrapment of leukocytes and releases of inflammatory mediators [intercellular adhesion molecule-1 (ICAM-1), vascular cell adhesion molecule-1 (VCAM-1)] and reactive oxygen species resulting in vasospasm of functioning capillary loops aggravating ischemia thereby resulting in ulceration
3. *Microangiopathy theory*: Occasionally capillaries in patients with venous leg ulcers are occluded by microthrombi due to intracapillary stasis.

## Clinical Examination

Ninety-five percent of venous ulceration is in the gaiter area of the leg, e.g., area around the malleoli. The ulcer bed is often covered with a fibrinous layer mixed with granulation tissue, surrounded by an irregular, gently sloping edge. Pitting edema, lipodermatosclerosis and atrophie blanche may be present (Fig. 6).

## Management of Venous Leg Ulcer

### Dressings

Maintaining a moist environment thus accelerating wound healing. This can be accomplished by frequent application of saline dressings over the wound which helps to keep the wound surface moist, debrides the wound and removes the surface bacteria.

A wide range of dressings are available, including hydrocolloids (e.g., DuoDerm), foams, hydrogels, pastes, and

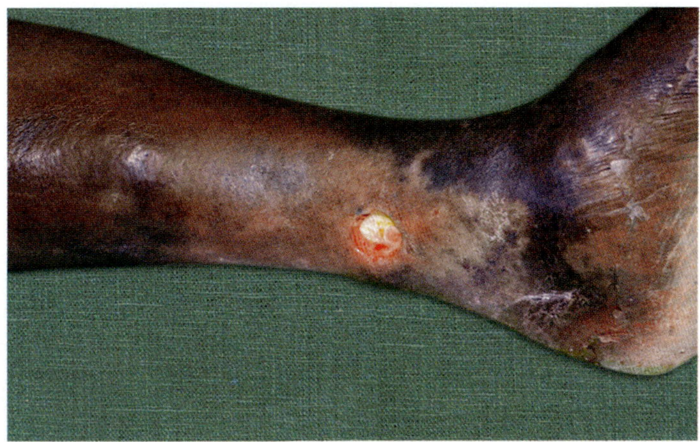

FIG. 6: Venous ulcer with surrounding lipodermatosclerosis.

simple nonadherent dressings. There is no significant difference among dressing types.

### Topical Antibiotics and Antiseptics

Wound healing is impaired when bacterial colonization exceeds 105 organisms per gram of tissue. As systemic antibiotics are reserved only for patients with evidence of infection, topical antiseptics and antibiotics have been used to reduce the wound bioburden.

The various preparations used include:

- Iodine containing preparations
  - Povidone-iodine
  - Silver compounds
  - Iodosorb (cadexomer iodine)—for controlled release of iodine.
- Metronidazole gel provides good anaerobic coverage
- Retapamulin, used as a topical antibiotic, is effective against gram-positive bacteria including methicillin-resistant *Staphylococcus aureus* (MRSA)
- Mupirocin ointment is effective against gram-negative organisms including MRSA
- Modified Dakin's solution (hypochlorite) at a concentration of 0.025% elicits antimicrobial effects.

Neomycin and bacitracin are avoided because of their potential to cause allergic sensitization.

*Periwound protection*: The skin surrounding the ulcer can be damaged due to excess moisture, wound fluid proteases. Barrier creams and ointments are available which protect the skin around the ulcer. These include: petroleum jelly, Unna's paste.

## Systemic Treatment

### Fibrinolytics

- Stanozolol, an anabolic steroid in the dose of 2 mg twice daily reduces the pain and dermal thickness in acute lipodermatosclerosis
- Pentoxifylline, substituted xanthine in a dose of 400 mg thrice a day also has fibrinolytic properties. It acts by decreasing blood viscosity, increases red blood cell deformability, inhibits platelet aggregation and production of proinflammatory cytokines.

Other drugs which can be used as adjuvant to compression therapy are:

- Oral enteric coated aspirin (300 mg) which causes inhibition of platelet activation and reduction of pain and inflammation
- Micronized purified flavonoid fraction which reduces leukocyte adhesion, free radical formation, decreasing venous wall permeability, increasing venous tone, and protecting cells from effects of hypoxia
- *Calcium dobesilate*: A synthetic venoactive drug thought to have antioxidant property, reduces capillary permeability, increases venous tone and reduces inflammation.

## Compression Therapy

Compression therapy is the standard of care for venous ulcers and chronic venous insufficiency. Reviews including one recent Cochrane review found that venous ulcers heal more quickly with compression therapy than without. Methods include inelastic, elastic, and intermittent pneumatic compression. Compression therapy reduces edema, improves venous reflux, enhances healing of ulcers, and reduces pain. Contraindications to compression therapy include clinically significant arterial disease and uncompensated heart failure.

*Elastic stockings*: It offers sustained compression during both rest and activity. Compression stockings are graded, with the higher pressure at the ankle and gradually decreasing pressure toward the knee and thigh. Compression stockings are removed at night and should be replaced at regular interval (Table 2).

Elastic bandages are alternatives to compression stockings. In addition, high compression has been proven more effective than low compression, and multilayer bandages are more effective than single layer. The disadvantage of multilayer compression bandages is that they require skilled application in the physician's office once per week, depending on drainage.

*Intermittent pneumatic compression*: This therapy comprises a pump that delivers air to inflatable and deflatable sleeves that embrace extremities, providing intermittent compression. It is generally reserved for bedridden patients who cannot tolerate continuous compression therapy.

**TABLE 2: Graduated compression stockings**

| Class of stockings | Pressure offered at the ankle level | Conditions in which it is used |
|---|---|---|
| Class I | 18–21 mm Hg | • Mild varicosity<br>• Early varicosity in pregnancy<br>• Heaviness of legs |
| Class II | 23–32 mm Hg | • Moderate varicose veins<br>• Moderate edema<br>• Pronounced varicosis in pregnancy<br>• Posthealing minor ulcerations<br>• Superficial thrombophlebitis and postsclerotherapy |
| Class III | 34–46 mm Hg | • Severe chronic venous insufficiency<br>• Marked edema and induration of skin |

*Four-layered bandaging*: High compression bandage system (sub-bandage pressure of 35–40 mm Hg at the ankle) that incorporates elastic layers to achieve sustained compression.

- Layer 1 is orthopedic wool
- Layer 2 is a cotton crepe bandage
- Layer 3 is an elastic compression bandage (maintains low level of pressure up to 20 mm Hg at the ankle)
- Layer 4 is a cohesive compression bandage and it retains the bandage in position (maintains a pressure of 30 mm Hg at the ankle).

*Intermittent pneumatic compression*: Used in those who do not respond to stockings or compression bandages.

### Other Treatments

Other treatments for venous ulcers include:

- Electric stimulation
- Hyperbaric oxygen
- Vacuum-assisted closure therapy, also known as negative pressure wound therapy, employs negative pressure to improve the blood flow, decreasse local tissue edema, and removes the excessive fluid from the ulcer bed. This is supposed to assist the formation of healthy granulation tissue and also removes the bacterial load from the wound bed
- Lasers in venous ulcers are used in two different ways. One way is to use the laser beam externally over the affected area on the leg and the other way is to pass the laser fiber into the lumen of the affected vein and use the laser beam endovenously. Hypotheses that have been postulated are improved metabolism of the affected tissue, stimulation of the tissue repair and increased collagen synthesis.

## ARTERIAL ULCERS

Arterial ulceration is due to a reduced arterial blood supply to the lower limb. The most common cause is atherosclerotic disease of the medium and large sized arteries. Other causes include diabetes, thromboangiitis, vasculitis, pyoderma gangrenosum, thalassemia, and sickle cell disease, some of which may predispose to the formation of atheroma. Further damage to the arterial system occurs with concurrent hypertension through damage of the intimal layer of the artery. The reduction in arterial blood supply results in tissue hypoxia and tissue damage. Thrombotic and atheroembolic episodes may contribute to tissue damage and ulcer formation.

### Clinical Examination

Arterial ulceration occurs over the toes, heels, and bony prominences of the foot. The ulcer appears "punched out", with well-demarcated edges and a pale, nongranulating, often necrotic base (Fig. 7). The surrounding skin may exhibit dusky erythema and may be cool to touch, hairless, thin, and brittle, with a shiny texture. The toe nails thicken and become opaque and may be lost. Gangrene of the extremities may also occur. Examination of the arterial system may show a decreased or absent pulse in the dorsalis pedis and posterior tibial arteries. There may be bruits in the proximal leg arteries, indicating the presence of atherosclerosis.

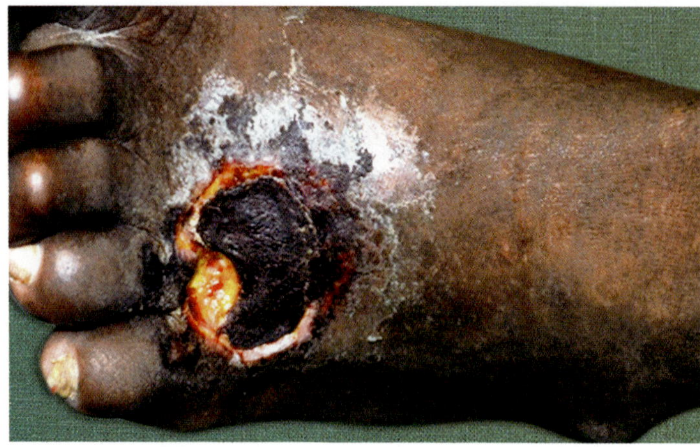

**FIG. 7:** Arterial ulcer.

### Management

If the leg affected by the venous leg ulcer is complicated by significant arterial insufficiency, consultation with a vascular surgeon is recommended. Any wound, acute or chronic, affected by ischemia as a result of severe arterial insufficiency, will not heal no matter what local measures are employed. If the arterial disease is considered uncorrectable or if the patient's general health precludes surgery, management becomes palliative and expectations of healing should be abandoned.

## SUGGESTED READINGS


1. Baker C, Kelly R. Other vascular disorders. In: Bolognia JL (Ed). Dermatology, 2nd edition. Philadelphia: Mosby Elsevier; 2008. pp. 1615-8.
2. Casey G. Causes and management of leg and foot ulcers. Nursing Standard. 2004;18(45):57-8.
3. Cox NH, Piette WW. Purpura and microvascular occlusion. In: Burns T (Ed). Rook's Textbook of Dermatology, 8th edition. Philadelphia: Wiley-Blackwell; 2010. pp. 26-46.
4. Dogra S, Rai R. Venous leg ulcer: topical treatment, dressings and surgical debridement. Indian Dermatol Online J. 2014;5:371-3.
5. Fletcher A, Cullum N, Sheldon TA. A systematic review of compression treatment for venous leg ulcers. BMJ. 1997;315(7108):576-80.
6. Lipsker D. Malignant atrophic papulosis (Degos disease). In: Goldsmith LA (Ed). Fitzpatrick's Dermatology in General Medicine, 8th edition. New York, NY: McGraw-Hill; 2012. pp. 2072-6.
7. Majid I. Venous leg ulcers: other treatments. Indian Dermatol Online J. 2014;5: 383-5.
8. Nair B. Venous leg ulcer: systemic therapy. Indian Dermatol Online J. 2014;5:374-7.
9. O'Meara S, Cullum NA, Nelson EA. Compression for venous leg ulcers. Cochrane Database Syst Rev. 2009;(1):CD000265.
10. Palfreyman S, Nelson EA, Michaels JA. Dressings for venous leg ulcers: systematic review and meta-analysis. BMJ. 2007;335(7613):244.
11. Rai R, Sekar CS, Kumaresan M. Antiphospholipid syndrome in dermatology: an update. Indian J Dermatol Venereol Leprol. 2010;76(2):116-24.
12. Vasudevan B. Venous leg ulcers: pathophysiology and classification. Indian Dermatol Online J. 2014;5:366-7.

# 41 CHAPTER Kawasaki Disease

*Nilendu Sarma*

## INTRODUCTION

Kawasaki disease (KD) is a self-limiting, acute febrile illness, mostly affecting the infants and young children. This was first described by Tomisaku Kawasaki of Japan in l967.

## EPIDEMIOLOGY

This is more common among boys. About 77% of the patients are below 5 years. There is a seasonal variation with more cases seen during winter and early spring. Blacks, Asians, children of Japanese ancestry, Americans of Asian, and Pacific Island descent suffer more commonly, possibly due to genetic susceptibility. However, this is also known to occur in other countries and in Asia. Older children often have higher prevalence of cardiovascular complications possibly due to late diagnosis.

## ETIOLOGY

Presence of fever, rash, enanthem, conjunctival injection, cervical lymphadenopathy, seasonal aggravation, self-limited course, and apparent endemic waves strongly suggest some role of infection in causation of KD. Immunological response to different microbial agents as well as superantigens possibly play role. Other possible factors/mediators are genetic predisposition, role of CD68+ monocyte/macrophages, CD8+ (cytotoxic) lymphocytes, and oligoclonal IgA plasma cells.

Respiratory illness, carpet cleaning fluids, eczema and humidifier are reported to be associated with increased chance of KD.

Proposed mechanisms for damage of the coronary vessel are activation of matrix metalloproteinases enzymes, vascular endothelial growth factor (VEGF), monocyte chemotactic and activating factor (MCAF or MCP-1), and tumor necrosis factor-$\alpha$ (TNF-$\alpha$).

## CLINICAL FEATURES

Kawasaki disease is defined by Centre for Disease Control as an illness in a patient with fever of five or more days duration (or fever until the date of administration of intravenous immunoglobulin if it is given before the 5$^{th}$ day of fever), and the presence of at least four of the five clinical signs given in box 1.

Cases with fever and coronary artery abnormalities but lacking case definition are classified as "incomplete" KD, a term that is now preferred over "atypical KD". This is more common in child of less than 6 months of age or in adolescent. Echocardiography is thus mandatory investigations in such situation.

**BOX 1 Clinical diagnosis of Kawasaki disease**

- Fever for 5 days or more
- Principal clinical features (minimum four required for a diagnosis of Kawasaki disease):
  - Rashes
  - Cervical lymphadenopathy (≥ one lymph node, at least 1.5 cm in diameter)
  - Bilateral conjunctival injection
  - Oral mucosal changes
  - Peripheral extremity changes

Remittent fever with high spike often reaching 102–104°F. Untreated, fever persists for average 11 days or even longer. Successful treatment may shorten the duration. Fever is an indicator of ongoing active vasculitic process thus a determinant of coronary aneurysm.

Skin rash, involves trunk and limbs, starts within 5 days of fever, is frequently polymorphic and nonspecific. These range from diffuse maculopapular eruption (most common), urticarial, scarlatiniform, erythroderma, and erythema-multiforme-like or a fine micropustular (acute generalized exanthematous pustulosis like) eruption. Bullous and vesicular rash are not seen. Rash may be accentuated over perineal region and early desquamation may be characteristically present in this area. Distinctive involvement of other folds like elbow is also seen. Eye lid involvement is occasionally seen (Figs 1 and 2).

Other important features are erythema of palms, soles and edema of hands, feet (acute stage), (Figs 3 and 4) periungual peeling of fingers toes in 2$^{nd}$ to 3$^{rd}$ weeks (subacute stage), dry, cracked lips, diffuse nonexudative oropharyngeal inflammation without any ulcer and strawberry tongue, unilateral cervical lymphadenopathy bilateral painless (unless complicated with mild iridocyclitis or anterior uveiitis) bulbar nonexudative conjunctivitis, conjunctival edema, or corneal ulceration.

## SYSTEMIC FEATURES

There are many systemic features that may be seen in KD. Polyarthritis, acute abdomen, diarrhea, vomiting, abdominal pain, and acute acalculous distension of the gallbladder (hydrops) are found (Box 2).

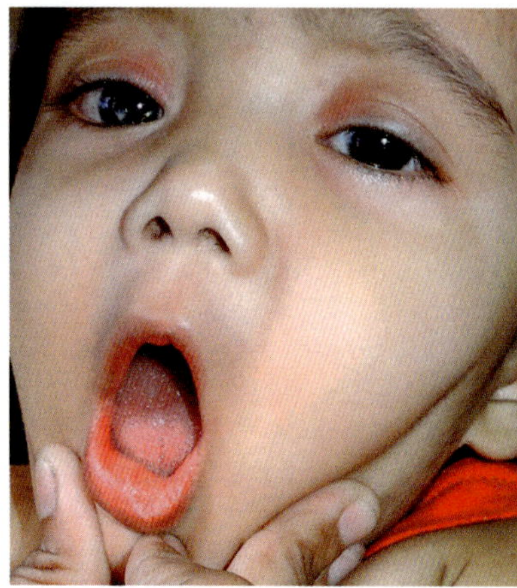

**FIG. 1:** Inflamed lips and bilateral nonexudative bulbar conjunctivitis in Kawasaki disease.

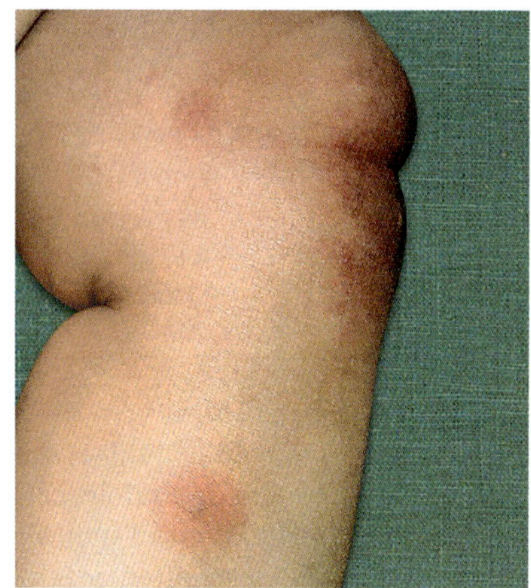

**FIG. 2:** Urticarial eruptions (knee) and target lesion in Kawasaki disease.

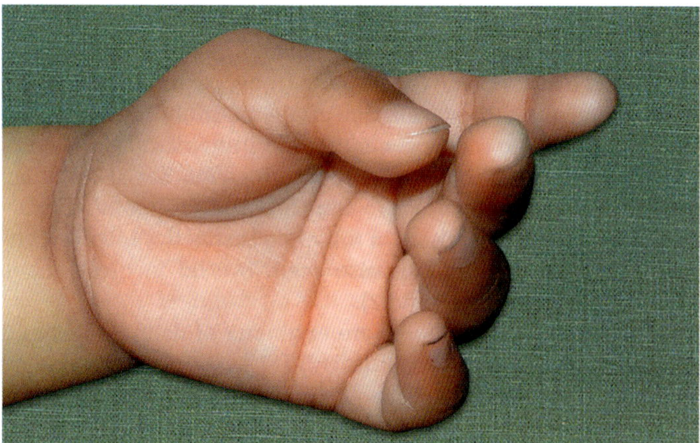

**FIG. 3:** Palmar erythema and edema in Kawasaki disease.

Kawasaki disease is a systemic vasculitis. There is frequent involvement of pericardium, myocardium, endocardium, valves, and coronary arteries.

Involvement of coronary artery may lead to development of aneurysms, ectasia and also myocardial infarction, ischemic heart diseases or sudden death. Aneurysm may develop in even up to 25% of cases. This rarely develops before 10 days of illness but early suspicion of this complication is possible with 2D echocardiography (2D echo) or coronary angiography. Perivascular brightness, ectasia, and lack of tapering of the coronary arteries are known to be highly suggestive in the early stages.

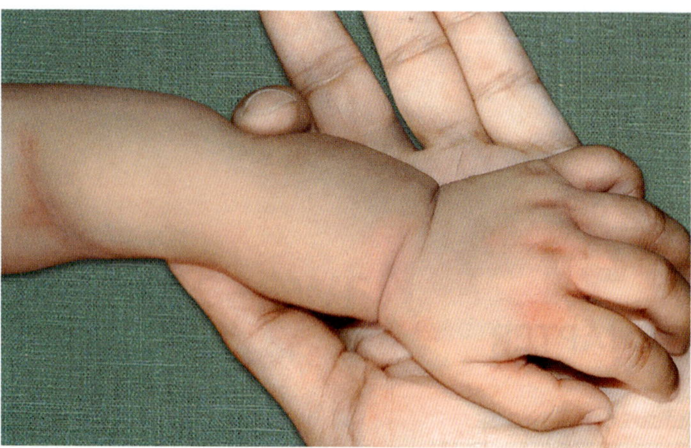

**FIG. 4:** Edema of the dorsum of the hand and flexural inflammation in Kawasaki disease.

**BOX 2 Systemic involvement in Kawasaki disease**

- Cardiovascular findings
  - Congestive heart failure, myocarditis, pericarditis, valvular regurgitation
  - Coronary artery abnormalities
  - Aneurysms of medium-size noncoronary arteries
  - Raynaud's phenomenon
  - Peripheral gangrene
- Musculoskeletal system
  - Arthritis, arthralgia
- Gastrointestinal tract
  - Diarrhea, vomiting, abdominal pain
  - Hepatic dysfunction
  - Hydrops of gallbladder
- Central nervous system
  - Extreme irritability
  - Aseptic meningitis
  - Sensorineural hearing loss
- Genitourinary system
  - Urethritis/meatitis
- Other findings
  - Erythema, induration at Bacillus Calmette–Guérin inoculation site
  - Anterior uveitis (mild)
  - Desquamating rash in groin

**BOX 3 Laboratory findings in acute Kawasaki disease**

- Leukocytosis with neutrophilia and immature forms
- Elevated erythrocyte sedimentation rate
- Elevated C-reactive protein
- Anemia
- Abnormal plasma lipids
- Hypoalbuminemia
- Hyponatremia
- Thrombocytosis after week 1
- Sterile pyuria
- Elevated serum transaminases
- Elevated serum gamma glutamyl transpeptidase
- Pleocytosis of cerebrospinal fluid
- Leukocytosis in synovial fluid
- Arrhythmia, prolonged PR interval, or nonspecific ST and T wave changes

## LABORATORY DIAGNOSIS

Diagnosis is essentially clinical based on laboratory investigations are usually suggestive (Box 3). Leukocytosis, often with anemia, elevated erythrocyte sedimentation rate (ESR), C-reactive protein (CRP) and thrombocytosis (2nd to 3rd week) is detected. Lower platelet count may indicate disseminated intravascular coagulation thus is risk factor for subsequent coronary aneurysms. Treatment with intravenous immunoglobulin (IVIG) may sometimes lead to hemolysis. However, clinical criteria may miss some cases. Use of laboratory investigations especially, echocardiography is increasing being considered as an important diagnostic tool in cases that fail clinical criteria but are otherwise suspicious.

Coronary arterial dilatation can be measured much early (*Z* score) before actual ectasia develops. A value of more than or equal to 2.5, measured in either proximal right coronary artery (RCA) or left anterior descending coronary artery (LAD) is unusual without KD.

## TREATMENT

Diagnosis of KD requires a minimum of 4 days of fever. Thus treatment specific for KD can be started on 4th day of disease.

Aspirin is usually the first drug to be used in KD. It has important anti-inflammatory (at high doses) and antiplatelet (at low doses) properties. However, it does not reduce the chance of development of coronary abnormalities.

*Dose at early acute stage*: 80–100 mg/kg/day in four doses. This can be used till day 14 of illness or till 48–72 hours after fever subsides. This high dose should be followed by low dose therapy (3–5 mg/kg/day) and continued till at least 6–8 weeks if no coronary involvement is detected. If coronary abnormality is detected, aspirin may be continued indefinitely. Ibuprofen should not be used with aspirin as it antagonizes the irreversible platelet inhibitory function of aspirin.

Aspirin can cause Reye syndrome in children after infection with varicella or influenza.

Intravenous immunoglobulin has anti-inflammatory property and modulates cytokine production, inhibits superantigens and stimulates T-cell suppressor activity. It is used in the dose of 2 g/kg in a single infusion together with aspirin. It should be started within the first 10 days of fever (preferably within 7 days of illness)

When children present (or diagnosed) after 10 day, IVIG also should be used if

- Fever persist
- Aneurysms detected
- Signs of ongoing systemic inflammation (high ESR, CRP).

Cases that show persistent or relapse of fever after more than or equal to 36 hours after IVIG therapy, this can be repeated (2 g/kg).

Measles and varicella immunizations need to be postponed for 11 months after IVIG therapy.

### Other Drugs

Cases that failed to respond to two doses of IVIG may be given methylprednisolone, (30 mg/kg, once daily for 1–3 days, infused over 3 hours). However, there is lack of recommendation in use of systemic corticosteroid in KD.

*Other therapeutic agents tried are*: Pentoxifylline (TNF-$\alpha$ inhibitor), plasma exchange, ulinastatin (human trypsin inhibitor), Abciximab (platelet glycoprotein IIb/IIIa receptor inhibitor), infliximab, and cyclophosphamide often in conjunction with oral steroids.

## SUGGESTED READINGS

1. Newburger JW, Takahashi M, Gerber MA, et al. Committee on Rheumatic Fever, Endocarditis and Kawasaki Disease; Council on Cardiovascular Disease in the Young; American Heart Association; American Academy of Pediatrics. Diagnosis, treatment, and long-term management of Kawasaki disease: a statement for health professionals from the Committee on Rheumatic Fever, Endocarditis and Kawasaki Disease, Council on Cardiovascular Disease in the Young, American Heart Association. Circulation. 2004;110:2747-71.
2. Bayers S, Shulman ST, Paller AS. Kawasaki disease: part I. Diagnosis, clinical features, and pathogenesis. J Am Acad Dermatol. 2013;69(4):501.e1-11
3. Galeotti C, Kaveri SV, Cimaz R, et al. Predisposing factors, pathogenesis and therapeutic intervention of Kawasaki disease. Drug Discov Today. 2016;piiS1359-6446(16)30291-4.
4. Newburger JW, Takahashi M, Burns JC. Kawasaki disease. J Am Coll Cardiol. 2016.
5. Rigante D, Andreozzi L, Fastiggi M, et al. Critical overview of the risk scoring systems to predict non-responsiveness to intravenous immunoglobulin in kawasaki syndrome. Int J Mol Sci. 2016;17(3):278.

# 14 SECTION Disorders of Connective Tissues

# 42 CHAPTER Ectodermal Dysplasia

*Indrashis Podder, Nilendu Sarma*

## INTRODUCTION

Ectodermal dysplasias (EDs) refer to a group of heterogeneous genetic disorders characterized by congenital, inherited, structural, and/or functional abnormalities (dysplasia) in classical or major ectodermal structures (hair, teeth, nails, and sweat glands, mentioned according to decreasing order of frequency) with or without involvement of other ectodermal structures. Involvement of nonectodermal structures is seen in ectodermal dysplasia syndromes.

Defining the condition is the most crucial primary step for the classification. About 186 diseases may fit into the list of ED. Many of these diseases are commonly listed under different disease category. Pachyonychia congenita, Keratitis-ichthyosis-deafness (KID) syndrome, dermatopathia pigmentosa reticularis, and hypomelanosis of Ito are just few examples of such conditions which are by definition a type of ED but commonly discussed elsewhere. With upgradation of knowledge and many previously described ED are found to be same disease and many new disease entities are incorporated in the list.

Pure ectodermal dysplasias are defined as ED where only ectodermal derivatives are affected without any associated abnormalities of derivatives of any other embryonic layers. In contrast, ED involving additionally mesoderm or derivatives of other embryonic organs is called "ectodermal dysplasia syndromes".

## CLASSIFICATION OF ECTODERMAL DYSPLASIA

Traditional system of classification of ED is based on clinical signs and symptoms (Freire-Maia). This is more practical for helpful easy diagnosis and classification. With identification of more and more molecular level information including involved genes, there are proposals for an updated and newer classification based on molecular defect. Although additional information on genetic defect in the existing clinical classification is important, exclusive molecular classification is difficult and incomplete at this moment as only few ED have a known genetic defect.

Most accepted system of classification divides ED into two groups, group A and B. Group A, ED is classified when two or more of the classical ectodermal (major) structures are involved (hair, teeth, nails, and sweat glands, numbered in that order). Thus, there are many subgroups based on wide range of combinations possible (e.g. 1-2-3-4, 2-3-4, 1-3-4, 1-2, 3-4, etc.) making the list of diseases very long. In group B, only one classical ectodermal structure is involved that is mentioned with a number 5 (e.g., 1-5. 2-5, 3-5, 4-5). There is involvement of some other ectodermal organs like mammary glands, central nervous system, thyroid, thymus, anterior pituitary, adrenal medulla, melanocytes, external ear, cornea, conjunctiva, lacrimal gland or duct, and meibomian glands.

## PATHOGENESIS

Ectodermal dysplasia is genetic disease due to different mutations that are inherited in various mode—X-linked recessive, autosomal recessive, and dominant. There are many genes identified. It has been found that mutation in different genes can lead to one ED and mutation in one gene can lead to different ED phenotype.

Pathogenesis of ED involves defect at various molecular levels leading to defect in cell stability, developmental regulation or epithelial-mesenchymal interaction, cell-to-cell communication and signaling, adhesion, development, and cytoskeleton maintenance.

## HYPOHIDROTIC ECTODERMAL DYSPLASIA OR ANHIDROTIC ECTODERMAL DYSPLASIA OR CHRIST-SIEMENS-TOURAINE SYNDROME (X-LINKED)

Hypohidrotic ectodermal dysplasia (HED) is characterized by the triad of hypotrichosis, anodontia or hypodontia, and anhidrosis or hypohidrosis. This is the most common (80%) of all EDs with an incidence of about 1 in 100,000 live boys. There is no racial predilection. This form of ED is characterized by inability to sweat adequately. Recently, a subtype has been discovered which is associated with immune defects (hyper IgM) [Hypohidrotic ectodermal dysplasia with immune deficiency (HED-ID)]; occurring due to mutations in the *NEMO* gene (responsible for incontinentia pigmenti).

### Pathogenesis

This is an X-linked recessive disease but autosomal dominant and recessive transmission can also occur. X-linked HED occurs due to mutations in *EDA* (Xq12q13.1) that encodes the epithelial morphogen ectodysplasin A [tumor necrosis factor (TNF) family ligand]. Autosomal recessive HED occurs due to *EDAR* (2q13) that encodes the ectodysplasin A receptor (TNF receptor) and autosomal dominant HED due to *EDARADD* (1q42.3) that encodes EDAR-associated death domain (EDARADD) protein. These TNF ligands and its receptor are important molecules for ectodermal appendage formation and organogenesis through regulating epithelial-mesenchymal interactions and signaling pathways. Other mutations like *WNT10A*, *TRAF6*, *NFKBIA* or *EDA2R* may also be responsible. Recently, the affected component of this pathway has been described, called SHARPIN. *IKBKG* (Xq28) mutations are responsible for the syndrome HED with immunodeficiency.

## Clinical Features

Males are affected as this is X-linked disease. However, females may show mild and partial manifestation like oligodontia, conical incisors, hypotrichosis, and hypohidrosis that may be manifested in blaschkoid pattern due to Lyonization. In autosomal forms, females and males are equally affected.

Hypohidrotic ectodermal dysplasia usually has a typical facies characterized by frontal bossing and hypoplastic mandible, flat nasal bridge with depressed nasal tip, periorbital hyperpigmentation with wrinkles, sparse eyebrows and eyelashes, full lips, and sebaceous hyperplasia which may resemble milia.

Scalp, eyebrow, eyelashes, and body hair are sparse to absent; when present is usually blonde (Figs 1 and 2). Both primary and secondary dentition are affected. Altered shape (peg-shaped) and number is seen (Fig. 3). Delayed dentition is often the first clue to diagnosis. Some patients may be completely edentulous.

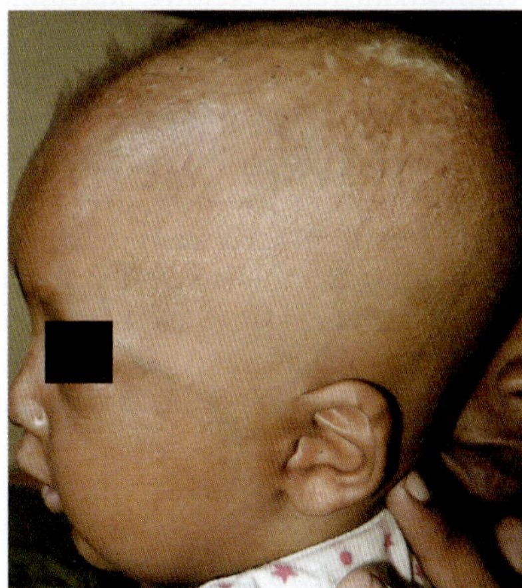

FIG. 1: Sparse hair and frontal bossing in hypohidrotic ectodermal dysplasia.

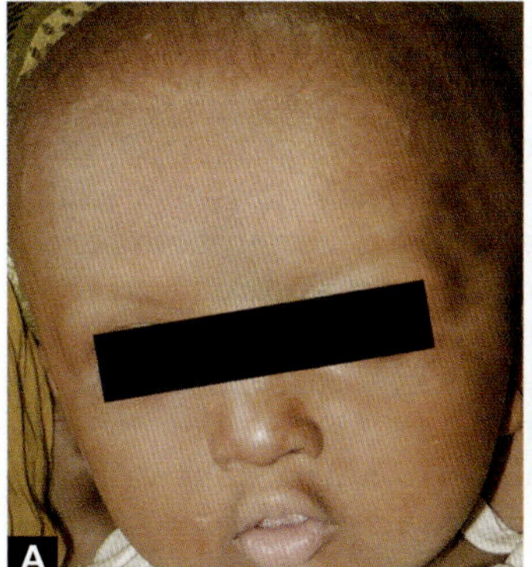

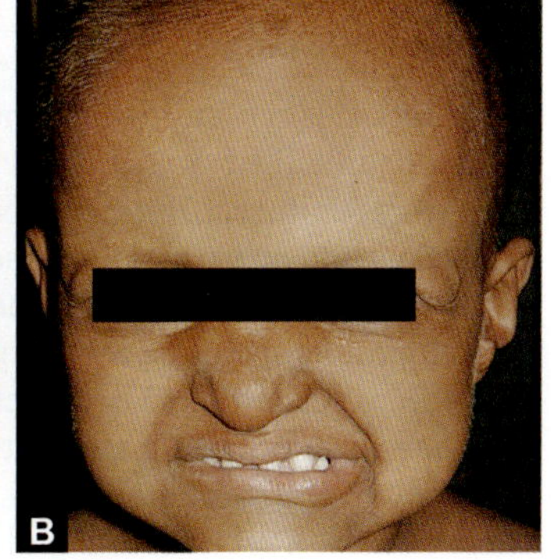

FIG. 2: Typical facial appearance in hypohidrotic ectodermal dysplasia.

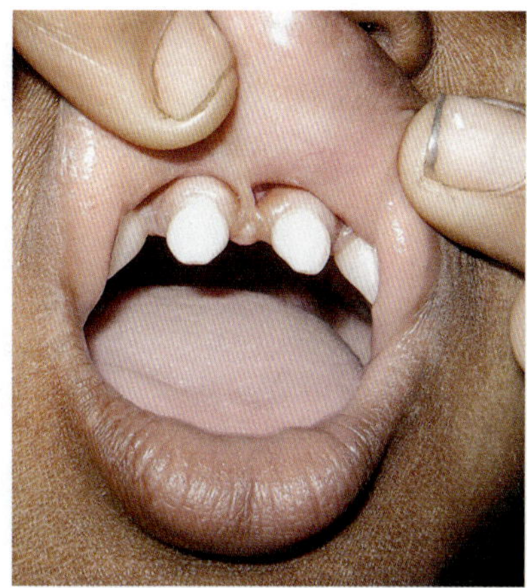

FIG. 3: Conical teeth in ectodermal dysplasia.

Nasal secretions are extremely thick; may lead to atrophic rhinitis. There is an increased occurrence of upper respiratory tract infection (URTI) and lower respiratory tract infection (LRTI).

Nails are normal in most cases. Mild nail dystrophy is noticed in some cases. Nail growth is usually slow. Split nail is common. Toenails are generally unaffected.

Most affected patients are unable to sweat properly (hypohidrosis). As a result, there is increased core body temperature (hyperpyrexia) which may even lead to heat stroke. This can cause brain damage at early life in undiagnosed cases. The skin is thin, dry, and smooth. Neonatal scaling is often a clue to diagnosis. Dermatoglyphics may be lost. Eczema may be a major problem due to dry skin. There may be localized hyperkeratosis. Dryness also involves eye and most patients suffer from nasopharyngeal dryness and dry eyes and its complications like chronic conjunctivitis and blepharitis.

## Laboratory Diagnosis

Lack of sweating test can be confirmed with pilocarpine-induced sweat production. Skin biopsy shows atrophic epidermis and eccrine sweat glands incompletely developed or absent. Confirmation can be done with molecular diagnostic techniques. Diagnosis of fetal disease can be done with chorionic villus biopsy or fetal skin biopsy through fetoscopy.

## Treatment

Maintaining ambient temperature to prevent hyperthermia and its complications, external cooling methods are most crucial. Dermatologic treatment for eczema, infections, dry skin, and other supportive treatment is also done. Treatment of complications (URTI, LRTI, and atrophic rhinitis) is also needed. Genetic counseling is important especially for carrier females.

# HIDROTIC ECTODERMAL DYSPLASIA OR CLOUSTON SYNDROME

This is a relatively rare disorder. Unlike HED, hidrotic ectodermal dysplasia lacks a characteristic facies and sweating abnormality. There are two varieties: Clouston syndrome and Christianson-Fourie type (rare).

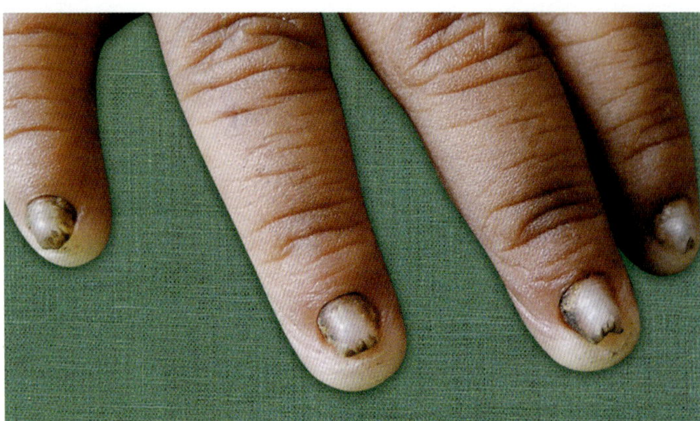

**FIG. 4:** Nail changes in hidrotic ectodermal dysplasia.

## Pathogenesis

This is inherited as autosomal dominant disease. An extremely rare autosomal recessive form has also been identified. There is mutation in the *GJB6* gene that encodes connexin 30.

## Clinical Features

It presents with sparse, brittle, pale scalp and body hair, absent or scanty eyebrow or eyelashes, and characteristic yet variable changes in nail. Nail plates are often appear white or yellow, grow slowly, thick, and short. Skin is dry, rough, scaly, and pigmented (Fig. 4).

A form of reticulate hyperpigmentation, involving knees, elbows, and fingers, is described. Palmoplantar keratoderma is seen. Other features are conjunctivitis, occasional strabismus, mental retardation, cataract, myopia, and short stature.

The teeth are usually normal. There may be hypo or anodontia and tendency for early decay.

## Laboratory Investigations

No specific laboratory investigation; high index of clinical suspicion is must, and genetic analysis (confirmatory).

## Treatment

Emollients to keep the skin, palms, and soles moist and smooth; avoidance of infections.

# ANKYLOBLEPHARON-ECTODERMAL DYSPLASIA-CLEFT SYNDROME (HAY–WELLS SYNDROME)

This is an extremely rare syndrome which shows autosomal dominant inheritance of variable expressivity.

## Pathogenesis

This syndrome occurs due to a missense mutation affecting the sterile alpha motif (SAM) domain of the *TP73L* (p63) gene that is considered crucial for development of craniofacial structures and extremities and skin differentiation. Mutations in *TP63* leads to development of Hay-Wells syndrome and Rapp-Hodgkin syndrome and also four more different EDs: Acro-dermato-ungual-lacrimal-tooth (ADULT) syndrome, ectrodactyly-ectodermal dysplasia-cleft 3 (EEC3), limb-mammary syndrome, and split hand or foot malformation 4 (a B group ED).

## Clinical Features

Congenital adhesion of the upper and lower eyelid margins by fibrous bands (ankyloblepharon filiforme adnatum) is a distinctive feature. Cleft palate is common but cleft lip is uncommon. Neonatal erythroderma is seen in almost 75% of cases. Collodion membrane, severe, recurrent scalp erosions and infections are typical features. Nasal bridge is broad with a hypoplastic maxilla. The scalp hair is wiry, coarse, and sparse. Eyebrows, eyelashes, body and pubic hair may be sparse or absent. There is hypodontia, discolored conical teeth, and nails show variable degrees of abnormalities with thick and hyperconvex plates. Nails may be completely absent. Hypohydrosis is mild. There may be heat intolerance but never hyperpyrexia. Despite involvement of same gene, severe abnormalities like limb abnormalities that are seen in EEC and that occur due to involvement of "other" ectodermal organs, is not seen in Hay-Wells patients. Other features are lacrimal gland abnormality or atresia and supernumerary nipples.

## Laboratory Investigations

Nothing specific; confirmation can be done by genetic analysis.

## Treatment

Emollients for symptomatic relief; clefting, ankyloblepharon, etc. need surgical correction.

# ECTRODACTYLY-ECTODERMAL DYSPLASIA-CLEFT SYNDROME

This is an extremely rare disorder with barely 150 cases being reported till date. It shows an autosomal dominant inheritance of low penetrance and variable expressivity. Previously, EEC was classified into three subtypes. EEC2 and EEC3 are now considered to be a single disease and called EEC3. EEC3 is the most common subtype (90%).

## Pathogenesis

Ectrodactyly-ectodermal dysplasia-cleft 3 is caused by mutation in *TP63* gene.

## Clinical Features

Although this is an ectodermal dysplasia, associated manifestations like limb abnormality and cleft lip or palate are more prominent features. There is lobster claw deformity of the hands and feet that are caused by ectrodactyly with tetramelic 3–4 syndactyly. Metacarpal and metatarsal are often hypoplastic. Scalp hair is light, coarse, and dry. Eyebrows, eyelashes, and body and pubic hair may also be affected.

There is hypodontia, premature loss, and nails show variable degrees of abnormalities with transverse ridges and pitting. There is mild hypohydrosis and can cause occasional heat intolerance.

Skin appears dry, scaly especially on the lower limbs and palmoplantar hyperkeratosis.

Other defects are structural anomalies of the genitourinary tract, megaureter, renal agenesis, urethral atresia, hydronephrosis, lacrimal gland abnormalities or atresia, blepharophimosis, strabismus, deafness, choanal atresia, and mammary gland or nipple hypoplasia.

### Laboratory Investigations

X-ray of hand or foot deformities show missing or hypoplastic metacarpal or metatarsal bones; confirmation by genetic analysis.

### Treatment

Emollients for symptomatic relief; clefting and ectrodactyly need surgical correction.

## RAPP–HODGKIN SYNDROME

This syndrome is also transmitted in an autosomal dominant fashion; very rare in occurrence.

### Pathogenesis

This syndrome occurs due to mutation affecting the SAM domain of the *TP63* gene. Now it is known that this and Hay-Wells syndrome occur due to same mutation. So, many consider these two as same disease.

### Clinical Features

The scalp hair is light, coarse, and sparse, often with steel-wool texture. Hair structural defects like pili torti or pili canaliculi may be seen. Other hair may be affected. Similar to some other ED syndrome, recalcitrant, inflammatory scalp dermatitis with secondary scarring alopecia is also seen. There is often a typical facies characterized by high forehead, narrow nose, cleft lip or palate, and maxillary hyperplasia. Hypodontia, discolored conical teeth, variable degrees of nail abnormalities with ridging and pitting, and brittle nails are seen.

Sweating is decreased. Other features are clefting of lip or palate and hypospadias in males.

### Laboratory Investigations

Nothing specific; confirmation by genetic analysis.

### Treatment

Emollients for symptomatic relief; Clefting and hypospadias need surgical correction.

Recently, a new condition has been described called the ectodermal dysplasia skin fragility (EDSF) syndrome which, according to many is a suprabasal form of epidermolysis bullosa simplex. This occurs due to loss-of-function mutations of the *PKP1* gene encoding plakophilin 1. This condition is clinically characterized by the presence of skin erosions and crusting, notably with perioral fissuring, palmoplantar hyperkeratosis, growth delay, hypotrichosis or alopecia, and nail dystrophy. No cardiac anomalies have been reported.

## SUGGESTED READINGS


1. Freire Maia N. Ectodermal dysplasias revisited. Acta Genet Med Gemellol. 1977;26:121-31.
2. Freire Maia N. Ectodermal dysplasias. Hum Hered. 1971;21:309-12.
3. Itin PH, Fistarol SK. Ectodermal dysplasias. Am J Med Genet C Semin Med Genet. 2004;131C:45-51.
4. Lamartine J. Towards a new classification of ectodermal dysplasias. Clin Exp Dermatol. 2003;28:351-5.
5. Laurikkala J, Mikkola M, Mustonen T, et al. TNF signaling via the ligand-receptor pair ectodysplasin and edar controls the function of epithelial signaling centers and is regulated by Wnt and Activin during tooth organogenesis. Dev Biol. 2001;229:443-55.
6. McGrath JA, Duijf PH, Doetsch V, et al. Hay–Wells syndrome is caused by heterozygous missense mutations in the SAM domain of p63. Hum Mol Genet. 2001;10:221-9.
7. Priolo M, Lagan AC. Ectodermal dysplasias: a new clinical-genetic classification. J Med Genet. 2001;38:579-85.
8. Priolo M, Silengo M, Lerone M, et al. Ectodermal dysplasias: not only 'skin' deep. Clin Genet. 2000;58:415-30.
9. Visinoni AF, Lisboa-Costa T, Pagnan NA, et al. Ectodermal dysplasias: clinical and molecular review. Am J Med Genet Part A. 2009;149A:1980-2002.
10. Zarnegar BJ, Webster DE, Lopez-Pajares V, et al. Genomic profiling of a human organotypic model of AEC syndrome reveals ZNF750 as an essential downstream target of mutant TP63. Am J Hum Genet. 2012;91:435-43.

# 43 CHAPTER Disorders of Collagen and Related Skin Disorders

*Nilendu Sarma, Indrashis Podder, Somodyuti Chandra*

## EHLERS–DANLOS SYNDROME (CUTIS HYPERELASTICA)

### Introduction

Ehlers-Danlos syndrome (EDS), a group of relatively rare genetic disorder affecting collagen, the most important structural component of connective tissue of skin, bones, and blood vessels. Collagen defect results in weakness of the connective tissues of these organs. Distinguishing manifestation of EDS involves skin and joint leading to hyperextensible skin and joints. However, additional organ involvement (major blood vessel, intestine, and uterus) that leads to tearing of these organs is characteristic of different subtypes of EDS.

### Classification

Classification of EDS has been repeatedly revised. The original "Berlin Nosology" (1988) had 11 subtypes. With expanding knowledge on biochemical and molecular aspect, it was reclassified in 1998 and this is popularly known as "Villefranche Nosology," and recognized six subtypes. Since then, many novel subtypes have been published. Genetic defects have been identified with the help of next-generation sequencing (NGS).

A newer classification has been proposed in 2017. This classification has proposed 13 subtypes and suggested that with the exception of hypermobile EDS for which no genetic locus has been identified, diagnosis of EDS should be confirmed with mutation analysis. When genetic confirmation is unavailable or not possible, the diagnosis should be mentioned as "provisional clinical diagnosis".

Similar to earlier system, major and minor criteria have been proposed for clinical diagnosis of the subtypes.

Occipital horn syndrome, fibronectin-deficient (EDS X), familial articular hypermobility (EDS XI), X-linked EDS with muscle hematoma (EDS V), X-L filamin A related EDS with periventricular nodular heterotopia are no longer considered as EDS (Table 1).

**TABLE 1: Classification of Ehlers–Danlos syndrome (EDS)**

| New names (2017) | Older name (Villefranche Nomenclature in bracket) | Inheritance pattern | Genes (involved proteins in bracket) |
|---|---|---|---|
| Classical EDS (eEDS) | Gravis/EDS I (Classical type)<br>Mitis/EDS II (Classical type) | AD | Major: *COL5A1*, *COL5A2* (Type V collagen)<br>Minor: *COL1A1* (Type I collagen) |
| Classical-like EDS (clEDS) | – | AR | *TNXB* (Tenascin XB) |
| Cardiac-valvular (cvEDS) | Human dermatosparaxis EDS VIIC/Cardiac-valvular EDS (Dermatosparaxis type) | AR | *COL1A2* (Type I collagen) |
| Vascular EDS (vEDS) | Arterial-ecchymotic EDS/ EDS IV (Vascular type) | AD | Major: *COL3A1* (Type III collagen)<br>Rare: *COL1A1* (Type I collagen) |
| Hypermobile EDS (hEDS) | Hypermobile, EDS III (Hypermobility type) | AD | Unknown |
| Arthrochalasia EDS (aEDS) | Arthrochalasis multiplex congenita, EDS VIIA, EDS VIIB (Arthrochalasia type) | AD | *COL1A1*, *COL1A2* (Type I collagen) |
| Dermatosparaxis EDS (dEDS) | Human dermatosparaxis, EDS VIIC, Cardiac-valvular EDS (Dermatosparaxis type) | AR | *ADAMTS2* (*ADAMTS-2*) |
| Kyphoscoliotic EDS (kEDS) | Ocular-scoliotic EDS, EDS VI, EDS VIA (Kyphoscoliosis type) | – | *PLOD1*<br>*FKBP14* |
| Brittle cornea syndrome (BCS) | Brittle cornea syndrome | AR | *ZNF469*<br>*PRDM5* |

*Continued*

*Continued*

| New names (2017) | Older name (Villefranche Nomenclature in bracket) | Inheritance pattern | Genes (involved proteins in bracket) |
|---|---|---|---|
| Spondylodysplastic EDS (spEDS) | EDS progeroid (EDS progeroid type), EDS progeroid type 2, (EDS progeroid type 1) spondylocheirodysplastic EDS | AR | *B4GALT7*<br>*B3GALT6*<br>*SLC39A13* |
| Musculocontractural EDS (mcEDS) | Adducted thumb-clubfoot syndrome, EDS Kosho type, EDS musculocontractural type | AR | *CHST14*<br>*DSE* |
| Myopathic EDS (mEDS) | – | AD or AR | *COL12A1* |
| Periodontal EDS (pEDS) | EDS VIII (EDS periodontitis) | AD | *C1R*<br>*C1S* |

AD, autosomal dominant; AR, autosomal recessive.

## Pathogenesis

Ehlers–Danlos Syndrome is caused by a defect in collagen synthesis of components of collagen and proper assembling. The collagen lacks the natural strength. Most of the types are inherited as autosomal dominant or recessive disorders while some rare subtypes are transmitted as X-linked recessive disorders. The affected genes like *COL1A1*, *COL1A2*, *COL3A1*, *COL5A1*, and *COL5A2* are involved in synthesis of different types of collagen and other genes like *ADAMTS2*, *PLOD1*, and *TNXB* are necessary for synthesis of vital proteins that bind to collagen for its normal functioning. Defective collagen results in weakness in the connective tissues like skin, bones, cartilage, and ligaments.

## Classical Ehlers–Danlos Syndrome

This is inherited as autosomal dominant disorder. A heterozygous mutation in *COL5A1* or *COL5A2* is found in more than 90% cases. *COL5A1* gene is mapped on the chromosome 9 (9q34.2q34.3), and *COL5A2* gene located on chromosome 2 (2q31).

Skin is soft, lax, fragile, and stretchable that extends easily and snaps back on release. There is easy tearing and bruising. Abnormal and delayed wound healing forming broad, widened, atrophic and "cigarette paper" scars.

There are molluscoid pseudotumors that are basically herniations of subcutaneous fat through atrophic dermal scars. They appear as blue-grey, spongy, 1–2 cm nodules over easily trauma-prone sites such as the shin, forearm, and Achilles tendon.

Subcutaneous spheroids are subcutaneous nodules those are hard, calcified, and develop due to fat necrosis. Livedo reticularis is also seen.

Patients may have typical facies characterized by broad nasal bridge, thin lips; pinched nose; large eyes with epicanthic folds, hollow cheeks and tight, lobeless ears. In addition, there is premature ageing of hands and feet (acrogeria).

Apart from skin, other organs are also affected in different subtypes of EDS. Muscle tone is poor. Major vessels may rupture. Valvular heart damage is also seen. Other abnormalities are hiatal hernia, collapsed lung, platelet aggregation failure, peripartum bleeding, cervical, uterine rupture, carpal tunnel syndrome, Arnold–Chiari malformation and sleep apnea.

Excessive extensibility of most of the joints leads to easy dislocation, poor muscle tone, and delayed physical milestones. Joints develop osteoarthritis and permanent deformity. Joint deformity like kyphoscoliosis and flat foot are also noted. Increased curvature deformity of the spinal bones may cause respiratory difficulty.

### Diagnosis

*Major diagnostic criteria*:
- Skin hyperextensibility and atrophic scarring and
- Generalized joint hypermobility (GJH) (evaluated according to the Beighton score).

*Minor criteria*:
- Easy bruising
- Soft, doughy skin
- Skin fragility (or traumatic splitting)
- Molluscoid pseudotumors
- Subcutaneous spheroids
- Hernia (presence or history of)
- Epicanthal folds
- Complications of joint hypermobility (e.g., sprains, luxation etc.)
- Presence of clinical signs in first degree relative.

Minimum clinical diagnostic criteria include either two major criteria or one major criteria and/or three minor criteria. Confirmation of diagnosis requires detection of the mutation.

## Classical-like Ehlers–Danlos Syndrome

This has three major criteria:
1. Hyperextensible skin, velvety skin texture, and no atrophic scarring
2. The GJH with or without recurrent dislocations (shoulder and ankle or other)
3. Easy bruisability.

*Minor criteria*:
- Foot deformity (broad/plump forefoot, brachydactyly with excessive skin, pes planus, etc.)
- Unexplained pedal edema, muscle weakness, atrophy of muscles in hands and feet, axonal polyneuropathy, acrogeric hands, clinodactyly, brachydactyly, and prolapse of vagina, rectum, uterus.

## Hypermobility Ehlers–Danlos Syndrome

This is a genetically heterogeneous disease and there is yet no confirmed mutation. This is a less severe form of EDS and is also dominantly inherited.

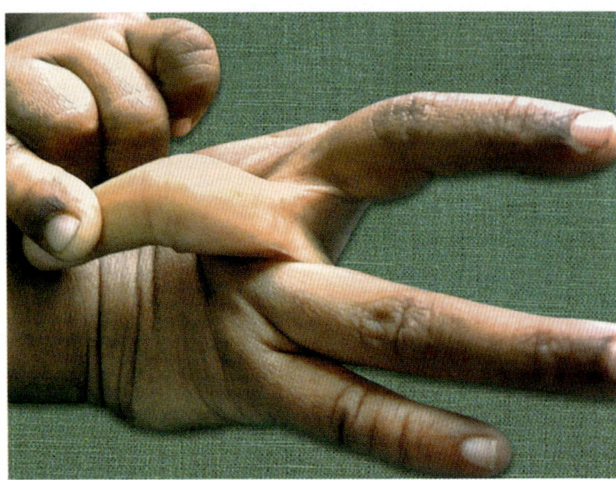

FIG. 1: Excessive mobility of finger joints in Ehlers-Danlos syndrome.

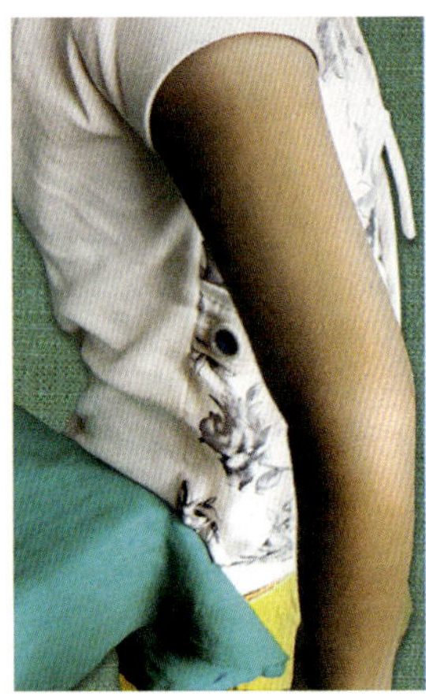

FIG. 2: Ehlers–Danlos syndrome showing hyperextension of elbow joint.

Skin is smooth and hyperextensibe and minimally affected. Hypermobility involving large and small joint and spine leading to frequent joint dislocations of shoulder, patella, or the temporomandibular joint are seen (Figs 1 and 2). Various other disorders presenting with hypermobility of the joints may be mimicked.

Generalized joint hypermobility is the most important clinical criterion of this condition. This is assessed by Beighton score. As per the proposal of the committee on behalf of the International Consortium on the Ehlers–Danlos Syndromes, a diagnosis of hEDS requires age-wise scoring (≥6 for prepubertal children and adolescents, ≥5 for pubertal men and women up for 50 years or less and ≥4 for more than 50 years of age).

Persistent joint pain may resemble fibromyalgia. Autonomic dysfunction like postural orthostatic tachycardia syndrome (POTS), postural acrocyanosis and syncope can occur. Resistance to local anesthetic drugs and opioids has been reported.

Skin extensibility is of variable degree. Atrophic scaring is an important clue.

Diagnosis is clinical and requires presence of specific combinations of clinical features. Readers are suggested to read the original publication.

## Vascular Ehlers–Danlos Syndrome

Inherited as autosomal dominant disorder, this is a potentially life-threatening form of EDS and is caused by mutations in *COL3A1* gene that is located on the long arm of chromosome 2 (2q31).

This is characterized by spontaneous vascular or visceral rupture and the absence of large joint hyperextensibility and skin hyperextensibility. Joint hyperextensibility is present only in digits. Arterial rupture may involve the iliac, splenic, or renal arteries or dissection of aortic aneurysm. There is significant risk for spontaneous rupture of internal organs (such as the intestine and gravid uterus) and muscles. Acute abdominal pain is a classical and common presentation.

Major and minor diagnostic criteria have been proposed (Revised Nosology, Villefranche, 1997). Thin, translucent skin, arterial/intestinal/uterine fragility/rupture, bruising, and typical facies are four major criteria. Presence of two of the four major criteria proposed by is highly suggestive of the diagnosis.

Other features that are considered minor criteria are acrogeria, hypermobility of small joints, tendon and muscle rupture, clubfoot, early-onset varicose veins, arteriovenous fistula, pneumothorax/pneumohemothorax, gingival recession, positive family history, sudden death in close relative.

Loss of facial fat results in typical facial appearance. Fat loss may be more extensive leading to a premature ageing appearance and prominence of veins on the chest.

Two phenotypic forms occur. Acrogeric type is characterized by thin, translucent skin of distal extremities, prominent eyes, peaked nose, giving an aged look. Ecchymotic type is characterized by easy bruisability. This may falsely appear as signs of child abuse.

Lifespan is shortened with a median age of death of 48 years.

## Kyphoscoliosis Ehlers–Danlos Syndrome

This is recessively inherited and is most often serious. This is caused by mutation in *PLOD1* gene. Diagnosis may be done with presence of all the proposed major criteria in an infant. These are generalized joint laxity, severe muscle hypotonia at birth, scoliosis at birth, progressive, scleral fragility, and rupture of the ocular globe.

Severe hypotonia in the early life manifests as floppy baby. Thus, this condition needs to be differentiated in all floppy infants. Disease becomes crippling with increasing age due to muscle hypotonia and joint laxity.

There are other minor features that suggest the diagnosis like atrophic scaring, early-onset and severe hypotonia at birth or in early life, marfanoid habitus, increased tissue fragility and easy bruising, arterial rupture, microcornea, osteopenia, and positive family history.

Apart from microcornea, there may be scleral fragility, keratoconus, retinal detachment, and glaucoma. Joint hypermobility may result in dislocations.

## Arthrochalasia Ehlers–Danlos Syndrome

### *Classical Features*

- Congenital hip dislocation
- Hypermobile joints with recurrent subluxations and dislocations affecting both large and small joints
- Thoracolumbar scoliosis
- Short stature
- Muscle hypotonia
- Caused by *COL1A1* gene or the *COL1A2* gene mutation.

### Dermatosparaxis Ehlers–Danlos Syndrome

#### *Classical Features*

- Severe skin fragility, sagging redundant skin
- Large hernias
- Easy bruising
- Blue sclerae can be present
- Mutation in *ADAMTS2* gene.

## Diagnosis of Ehlers–Danlos Syndrome

The diagnosis is generally made clinically. As mentioned earlier, confirmation is now mandatory with genetic analysis except for Hypermobile EDS (hEDS). Severity of the disease may be assessed with available scoring method.

Biochemical defects may be done for some types. Vascular type may require suitable imaging system. However, some special diagnostic modalities may be employed for certain subtypes like immunofluorescence staining of fibroblast for procollagen III (type IV EDS), assessing the ratio of urinary lysyl pyridinoline to hydroxyl lysyl pyridinoline (type VI EDS) (the mean value of this ratio in kyphoscoliosis EDS is about 6.0, compared with 0.2 in normal individuals). Genetic analysis and DNA sequencing to identify the mutant gene serves as the confirmatory test. Prenatal diagnosis can be done by chorionic villus sampling to terminate affected pregnancies, if desired. Electron microscopy may be done if available.

## Differential Diagnosis

Ehlers–Danlos syndrome must be differentiated from other disorders having hypermobile joints ± hyperextensible skin like Marfan syndrome (disproportionate tall stature, lens dislocation, pectus carinatum, and progressive aortic dilatation), cutis laxa [loose, redundant skin which only slowly returns from distension (normal recoil in EDS)], osteogenesis imperfecta (OI), Loeys-Dietz syndrome, Larsen syndrome (specific craniofacial features), and Stickler syndrome (high myopia, hearing loss, specific craniofacial features).

## Treatment

There is no specific treatment; genetic counseling and monitoring for complications must be done for all types. Cardiology assessment with echocardiogram, regular follow-up, physiotherapy and occupational therapy, and shin pads to reduce injury especially in childhood are few basic stapes that should be followed in all.

Some patients of type VI EDS (kyphoscoliotic EDS) respond to oral ascorbic acid; vascular EDS (vEDS) patients are advised to avoid pregnancy, strenuous exercises or sport that might raise intracranial tension.

# EHLERS-DANLOS SYNDROME RELATED DISORDERS

## Occipital Horn Syndrome (X-linked Cutis Laxa/Ehlers–Danlos Syndrome Type IX)

### Introduction

This is a very rare disorder. Earlier, it was classified as EDS type IX. Now it has been removed from EDS group of diseases. It affects only males with the manifestations appearing within the first decade of life. Three diseases—Menkes disease, occipital horn syndrome (OHS), and *ATP7A*-related distal motor neuropathy (DMN) are caused by the same genetic defect.

### Pathogenesis

It is an X-linked recessive disorder caused by a mutation in the *ATP7A* gene; coding for copper transporting ATPase. There is defective collagen cross-linking.

Activity of copper dependent enzymes such as dopamine beta hydroxylase (DBH) and lysyl oxidase is reduced. There is defective intestinal copper absorption, accumulation of copper in other tissues. Thus, both OHS and Menkes disease (and not *ATP7A*-related DMN) are characterized by low copper concentrations in some tissues.

### Clinical Features

This disorder is characterized by presence of loose, lax, wrinkled, hyperextensible skin (cutis laxa), bony overgrowth at the occipital area (at the sites of attachment of the trapezius muscle and the sternocleidomastoid muscle to the occipital bone), and hyperextensible and hypermobile digits; but larger joints of elbow and knee show only limited extension.

Occipital horn may be palpable or detected in X-ray. Affected individuals have short stature, low normal intelligence to mild mental retardation. They often have premature aged appearance and short clavicle.

Other important features are vascular aneurysm, bladder diverticula, ureteric and gastrointestinal (GI) diverticula, inguinal hernias, emphysema, and inguinal hernia. Affected individuals usually have normal or slightly reduced intelligence.

### Diagnosis

Low levels of serum copper and ceruloplasmin is a constant finding, lysyl oxidase activity in cultured cells and skin samples is also reduced. Skeletal X-rays, voiding cystourethrogram and angiogram are other investigations which may aid in diagnosis. Identification of the genetic defect can confirm the diagnosis.

### Treatment

There is no specific treatment for underlying disorder. However, genetic counseling and monitoring for complications is essential. Parenteral copper administration does not correct the low lysyl oxidase activity.

## Osteogenesis Imperfecta

### Introduction

Osteogenesis imperfecta, also known as brittle bone disease, is a clinically and genetically heterogeneous group of heritable connective tissue disorder. Markedly reduced strength of the bones with resulting increased tendency for fracture and deformity is the classical finding in OI. The estimated incidence of this disorder is approximately 1 in 15–20,000 births; occurring in all races and ethnic groups with no sex predilection.

## Pathogenesis

This is a collagen-related disorder. Most common types, type I to IV in the original Sillence classification comprises more than 80% of all cases. These are caused by mutation in genes coding for α1 and α2 chains of type I collagen (*COL1A1* and *COL1A2*) and are mediated as autosomal dominant disorders. Newer subtypes have been detected where mutations involve proteins that are not collagen but are necessary for post-translational modification of type I collagen. Mostly these are autosomal recessive. Some occasional unclassified cases are reported to occur due to involvement of other proteins.

There are cases that occur due to mosaicism involving germ-line cells of one of the parent who are clinically normal.

As type I collagen is an important structural protein for bone, tendon, ligament, skin, and sclerae, the physeal and periosteal osteoblasts are unable to form sufficient osteoid, thus hampering bone remodeling.

## Classification

David Sillence (1979) originally classified OI into four types. Later many other types have been added with identification of different phenotypic features and also newer genetic defects. At one point, subdivision of OI included I to XI subtypes.

To avoid confusions, a revised classification, known as 2010 Nosology was published by the International Nomenclature group for Constitutional Disorders ICHG of the Skeleton (INCDS). They classified OI into five groups (one additional group over the original Sillence classification) (Table 2).

It is important to understand that this new classification is based on phenotypic characteristics. Type 1, 4, and 5 have mild to moderate severity in contrast to the progressively deforming and perinatally lethal variants, type 2 and 3.

## Clinical Features

Easy fractures throughout life are the most important criteria (Fig. 3). Other associated features of OI are blue sclera, hearing loss, hypermobile joints, dentinogenesis imperfecta (DI), valvular dysfunction of the heart, aortic root dilatation, short stature, and progressive skeletal deformity.

Clinical manifestations of OI vary from mild (type 1) to very severe diseases that may be fatal in-utero or in perinatal period. It is characterized by soft, fragile, easily fractured bones, blue or grey sclera, early onset deafness and teeth deformities (known as DI).

**TABLE 2: Classification and clinical features of osteogenesis imperfecta (OI)**

| Type and inheritance | Genes | Severity | Clinical features |
|---|---|---|---|
| Osteogenesis imperfecta, OI (type 1), AD | *COL1A1, COL1A2* | Non-deforming form | Increased bone fragility, blue sclerae, conductive hearing loss commencing in adolescence, DI |
| Osteogenesis imperfecta (OI type 2), AD, AR | *COL1A1*<br>*COL1A2*<br>*CRTAP, LEPRE1, PPIB* | Perinatal lethal form | Extremely severe involvement of skeletal, joint, and extraskeletal system |
| Osteogenesis imperfecta, (OI type 3), AD, AR | *COL1A1*<br>*COL1A2*<br>*CRTAP*<br>*LEPRE1*<br>*PPIB*<br>*SERPINH1*<br>*BMP1*<br>*FKBP10*<br>*PLOD2*<br>*SERPINF1*<br>*SP7*<br>*WNT1*<br>*TMEM*<br>*CREB3L1 SEC24D* | Progressively deforming type | Bone fragility and multiple fractures at new born or infantile age leading to progressive deformity of the skeleton. Blue sclera may be present at early life but improves slowly. Usually no hearing impairment |
| Osteogenesis imperfecta, (OI type 4), AD, AR | *COL1A1*<br>*COL1A2*<br>*CRTAP*<br>*PPIB*<br>*FKBP10*<br>*SERPINF1*<br>*WNT1*<br>*SP7* | Moderate severity | Fragile bones, osteoporosis, and variable degrees of deformity of long bones and spine, normal sclera and no hearing impairment |
| Osteogenesis imperfecta with calcification of the interosseous membranes and/or hypertrophic callus (OI type 5), AD | *IFITM5* | Moderate severity | Interosseous membranes in the forearm and legs develop progressive calcification, normal sclera, no DI |

AD, autosomal dominant; AR, autosomal recessive; DI, dentinogenesis imperfecta.

*Source*: Bonafe L, Cormier-Daire V, Hall C, et al. Nosology and classification of genetic skeletal disorders: 2015 revision. Am J Med Genet A. 2015;167A:2869-92.

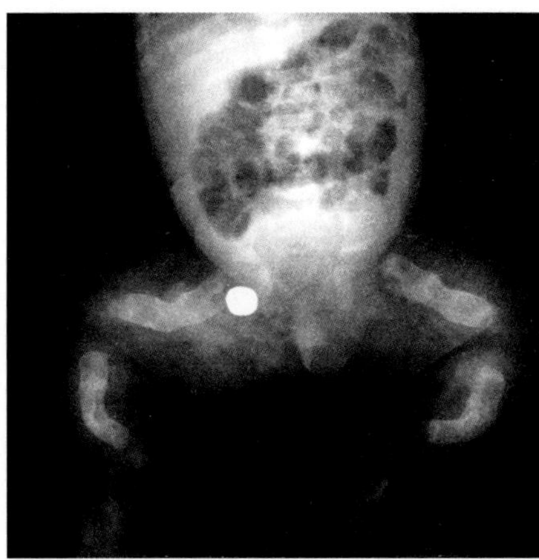

**FIG. 3:** Bone fragility and multiple fracture leading to gross deformity in osteogenesis imperfecta.

*Courtesy:* Dr Sohini Sengupta, Associate Professor, Department of Radiology, Dr B C Roy Post Graduate Institute of Pediatric Science, West Bengal.

Blue sclera occurs due to thinned sclera. Initially it was thought to be a disease defining feature. Now it is known that its presence is not present in all cases of even type-I, which has highest prevalence of this feature. Type III and IV may also have this feature. Recessive variants generally show white sclera but type V and VI may feature a light blue sclera. Although, blue sclera is traditionally known to be due to thinness of the sclera, no difference in thickness has been proved. Presence of increased electron dense granular material between scleral collagen fibers has been reported.

Although as many as 10% of patients with OI type 1 may not experience a fracture in their long bones during their childhood, sophisticated investigations like dual energy X-ray absorptiometry (DEXA) of the skeleton and peripheral quantitative computerized tomography (pQCT) have confirmed reduced bone density. Osteoporosis that develops in the majority of patients with OI also contributes to the bone fragility. Poorly ossified bones progressively give rise to deformities like bowing of long bones and kyphoscoliosis as the child grows older. The long bones frequently appear osteoporotic on radiography, with hypertrophic calluses in the areas subjected to repeated trauma. Rhizomelia or shortening of proximal segment of limbs is a distinguishing feature of autosomal recessive variants (VII, VIII). The most common cause or morbidity and mortality in these patients is respiratory insufficiency.

Short stature is a distinguishing feature in OI. This occurs due to repeated fracture, deficiency of some growth regulating proteins or due to unknown mechanisms. Growth retardation mostly occurs during the 1-5 years of age. Lower limb shortening is most prominent.

## Diagnosis

Diagnosis is based on family history coupled with typical clinical features and supported by characteristic radiographic imaging and DEXA scan. Plain radiography is very helpful.

Typical findings on bone histological examination of bone may give a clue to the type of OI—e.g., "mesh-like" appearance of the lamellae are found in type V, while "fish-scale" pattern is seen in type VI. Genetic study and collagen analysis are helpful for establishing the diagnosis.

## Differential Diagnosis

This condition must be differentiated from other similar phenotypic conditions like rickets, osteomalacia, idiopathic juvenile osteoporosis, skeletal syndromes like achondroplasia and child abuse.

Intrauterine fetus suffering from OI often feature large head and short limbs. This has to be differentiated from thanatophoric dysplasia, achondrogenesis type I, and campomelic dysplasia. Infantile hypophosphatasia that present with osteoporosis, short limbs, low serum alkaline phosphatase (ALP), increased inorganic pyrophosphate can be differentiated from OI that shows normal to increased ALP.

## Treatment

There is no curative treatment. Goals of therapy are to reduce fracture rates, prevent long-bone deformities, and maximize mobility and other functional capabilities. A multidisciplinary approach is most beneficial consisting of physical, medical and orthopedic support. Physical therapy is mandatory in the form of muscle and bone strengthening exercises, supportive braces and casts. Surgical interventions may be needed for correcting fractures and deformities, wherever needed. A few systemic medications have been found to be beneficial like.

Bisphosphonates (increase bone density in OI by inhibiting osteoclast activity). The lowest effective dose has to be used. Use is beneficial but there are risks too. Specialists should be consulted before use. Cyclic intravenous pamidronate (bisphosphonate) is very helpful even in severe types like type 3. This may reduce fracture frequency, achieve normal bone density, and near normal growth velocity. However, this does not help in more severe type 2.

Denosumab (monoclonal Ab to RANKL) is reported to be more effective than bisphosphonates.

Growth hormones are useful but are still under research. Another investigational drug are neutralizing sclerostin antibody. Gene therapy is a promising treatment option for the years to come.

## SUGGESTED READINGS


1. Barnes AM, Carter EM, Cabral WA, et al. Lack of cyclophilin B in osteogenesis imperfecta with normal collagen folding. New Engl J Med. 2010;362:521-8.
2. Beighton P, de Paepe A, Danks D, et al. International nosology of heritable disorders of connective tissue, Berlin, 1986. Am J Med Genet. 1988;29:581-94.
3. Beighton P, De Paepe A, Steinmann B, et al. Ehlers-Danlos syndromes: revised nosology, Villefranche, 1997. Ehlers Danlos National Foundation (USA) and Ehlers Danlos Support Group (UK). Am J Med Genet. 1998;77:31-7.
4. Bonafe L, Cormier-Daire V, Hall C, et al. Nosology and classification of genetic skeletal disorders: 2015 revision. Am J Med Genet Part A. 2015;167A:2869-92.
5. Fassier FR. Osteogenesis imperfecta. In: Pediatric Lower Limb Deformities. Switzerland: Springer International Publishing; 2016. pp. 255-65.
6. Forlino A, Cabral WA, Barnes AM, et al. New perspectives on osteogenesis imperfecta. Nat Rev Endocrinol. 2011;7(9): 540-57.
7. Guo D, Regalado ES, Gong L, et al. LOX mutations predispose to thoracic aortic aneurysms and dissections. Circ Res. 2016;118(6):928-34.
8. Henkin S, Negrotto SM, Tweet MS, et al. Spontaneous coronary artery dissection and its association with heritable connective tissue disorders. Heart. 2016;102(11):876-81.
9. Lawrence EJ. The clinical presentation of Ehlers Danlos syndrome. Adv Neonat Care. 2005;5 (6): 301-14.

10. Legros L, Revencu N, Nassogne MC, et al. Multiple bladder diverticula caused by occipital horn syndrome. Archives de pediatrie: organe officiel de la Societe francaise de pediatrie. 2015;22:1147-50.
11. Levy HP. Ehlers-Danlos Syndrome, Hypermobility Type. In: Pagon RA, Adam MP, Ardinger HH (Eds). Seattle (WA): University of Washington, Seattle; 2016.
12. Malfait F, Francomano C, Byers P, et al. The 2017 international classification of the Ehlers-Danlos syndromes. Am J Med Genet C Semin Med Genet. 2017;175:8-26.
13. Marini J, Smith SM. Osteogenesis Imperfecta. In: De Groot LJ, Beck-Peccoz P, Chrousos G, Dungan K, Grossman A, Hershman JM, Koch C, McLachlan R, New M, Rebar R, Singer F, Vinik A, Weickert MO (Eds). South Dartmouth (MA): MDText.com, Inc.; 2015.
14. Marini JC, Cabral WA, Barnes AM, et al. Components of the collagen prolyl 3-hydroxylation complex are crucial for normal bone development. Cell Cycle. 2007;6:1675-81.
15. Thomas IH, DiMeglio LA. Advances in the Classification and Treatment of Osteogenesis Imperfecta. Curr Osteopor Rep. 2016;14:1-9.
16. Tsukahara M, Imaizumi K, Kawai S, et al. Occipital horn syndrome: report of a patient and review of the literature. Clin Genet. 1994;45:32-5.
17. Van Damme T, Syx D, Coucke P, et al. Genetics of the Ehlers–Danlos syndrome: more than collagen disorders. Expert Opin Orphan Drugs. 2015;3:379-92.
18. Van Dijk FS, Nesbitt IM, Zwikstra EH, et al. PPIB mutations cause severe osteogenesis imperfecta. Am J Hum Genet. 2009;85:521-7.

# 44 CHAPTER Pachydermoperiostosis and Relapsing Polychondritis

*Somodyuti Chandra, Indrashis Podder, Nilendu Sarma*

## PACHYDERMOPERIOSTOSIS

It is a rare benign genetic disorder, first described by Solente and Gole in 1935. It is characterized by pachydermia (thickening of facial skin or scalp), periostosis (hypertrophic osteoarthropathy or thickening of bones), and digital clubbing.

### Etiopathogenesis

This is an autosomal dominant disorder with incomplete penetrance. Recently, autosomal recessive forms having mutation in *HPGD* gene (coding for NAD dependent 15-hydroxyprostaglandin dehydrogenase) have been demonstrated. Recently mutation in a new gene called the solute carrier organic anion transporter family, member 2A1 (SLCO2A1) has been reported. Though exact cause is yet to be elucidated, there is abnormal peripheral microvascular blood flow resulting in endothelial cell activation and release of platelet derived growth factor (PDGF) which in turn leads to soft tissue overgrowth, clubbing and periostosis.

### Types

It may occur in three forms:

1. *Complete form*: With all three features of pachydermia, periostosis, and digital clubbing
2. *Incomplete form*: Without skin involvement
3. *Forme fruste*: Clubbing and pachydermia are present with no bony involvement.

### Clinical Features

This disorder usually arises after puberty.

- Skin of the face and scalp gets thickened and is thrown into folds (cutis verticis gyrata). The skin of hands and feet also becomes coarse and thickened. Apart from these seborrhea, acne, folliculitis and palmoplantar hyperhidrosis have been reported
- Skeletal involvement includes clubbing or bulbous deformities of fingers and toes, thickening and widening of phalanges and distal part of long bones producing spade-like hands and feet and arthritis with joint effusion.

Other rare associations include hypertrophic gastropathy, peptic ulcers, gynecomastia, acro-osteolysis of fingers and toes, bladder cancer, Crohn's disease, bone marrow failure due to myelofibrosis and undifferentiated arthritis.

### Histopathology

The epidermis shows hyperkeratosis and acanthosis. Dermis demonstrates increase in dermal collagen and mucin deposition along with sebaceous and eccrine gland hyperplasia.

### Differential Diagnosis

This condition has to be differentiated from acromegaly, lepromatous leprosy, scleromyxedema, thyroid acropachy, and other secondary causes of hypertrophic osteoarthropathy like lung abscess, carcinoma lung, congenital cyanotic heart disease, infective endocarditis, etc.

### Treatment

The therapy is mainly symptomatic. Isotretinoin in a dosage of 1 mg/kg/day (upto a cumulative dosage of 8 g) is beneficial for treatment of seborrhea. About 20% aluminum hexachlorohydrate and BTX-A injection are used for treating hyperhidrosis. Nonsteroidal anti-inflammatory drugs (NSAIDs) and colchicine can be given to attain symptomatic relief in joint pain. Bisphosphonates especially risedronate, pamidronate, or alendronate with adequate vitamin D and calcium supplementation may also be given. Infliximab has been tried with unsatisfying results. A recent study has shown etoricoxib to be effective in the treatment of this condition.

## RELAPSING POLYCHONDRITIS/ ATROPHIC POLYCHONDRITIS/SYSTEMIC CHONDROMALACIA

It is an uncommon, multisystemic inflammatory and potentially destructive disease characterized by recurrent episodes of inflammation of the cartilage of various tissues of the body. Dermatological manifestations are often the presenting sign; and hence early diagnosis and prompt intervention can prevent complications.

This disorder may affect all races but is more common in Caucasians; the usual age of onset is between 40 years and 60 years, though childhood cases have been described. There is no sexual predilection.

## Etiopathogenesis

The exact etiology is unknown; multiple precipitating factors have been implicated. HLA-DR4 may play an important role. This disorder is frequently associated with other autoimmune diseases like systemic lupus erythematosus (SLE), rheumatoid arthritis, Hashimoto's disease, Behcet's disease, etc. The key pathogenic mechanism is the development of autoimmunity against cartilage components including types II, IX, and XI collagens as well as other constituent proteins such as matrilin-1. Also, at a cellular level, it is likely that Th1 cells play a major role, as evidenced by levels of interferon-$\gamma$, interleukin-12, and interleukin-2 correlating with disease activity.

## Clinical Manifestations

Skin lesions are found in 17–39% of patients and consist of erythema and edema overlying inflamed cartilage. Nonspecific skin lesions include aphthous ulcers, subcutaneous nodules, palpable purpura, livedo reticularis, leg ulcers, urticarial vasculitis, and Sweet syndrome. Auricular chondritis is the hallmark clinical feature characterized by sudden pain, swelling, and redness develop involving one or both ears but sparing the ear lobes (Fig. 1). Calcification and nodules are common sequel. Nonerosive seronegative inflammatory polyarthritis affecting the ankles, elbow, wrists, proximal interphalangeal joints, metacarpophalangeal joints, and metatarsophalangeal joints are often present. Apart from these features; nasal chondritis (pain, nasal fullness, epistaxis, saddle nose deformity), ocular inflammation (recurrent episodes of episcleritis, scleritis, uveitis, chorioretinitis) (Fig. 2), respiratory tract chondritis (wheezing, dyspnea, cough, stridor, hoarseness, respiratory obstruction and recurrent pneumonia), audiovestibular chondritis (sudden hearing loss, which is usually permanent, while tinnitus, nausea, vomiting, nystagmus, and vertigo may subside), cardiovascular involvement (involvement of heart valves, aortitis, pericarditis, conduction defects, and even myocardial infarction) have been reported in varying number of cases. Cerebral vasculitis and glomerulonephritis have also been rarely reported.

## Diagnosis

A criterion has been laid down for the accurate diagnosis of this condition as this is primarily a clinical diagnosis.

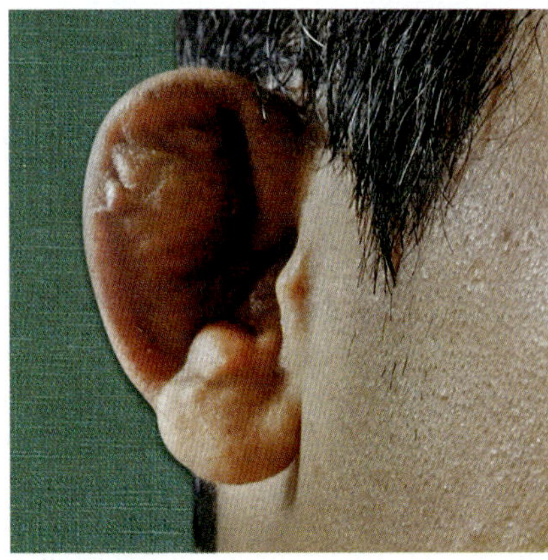

**FIG. 1:** Auricular chondritis in relapsing polychondritis.

*Courtesy*: Dr Sherina Laskar, Resident Physician, Department of Dermatology, Gauhati Medical College, Guwahati, Assam.

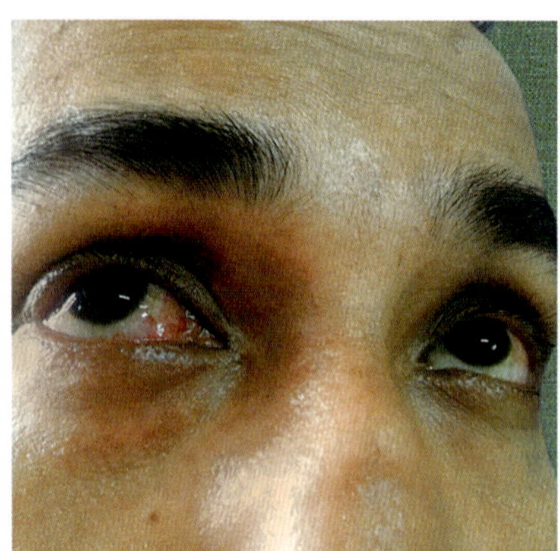

**FIG. 2:** Ocular inflammation and saddle nose deformity in relapsing polychondritis.

*Courtesy*: Dr Sherina Laskar, Resident Physician, Department of Dermatology, Gauhati Medical College, Guwahati, Assam.

### McAdam et al. Criteria (3 of 6 Clinical Features Necessary for Diagnosis)

1. Bilateral auricular chondritis
2. Nonerosive seronegative inflammatory polyarthritis
3. Nasal chondritis
4. Ocular inflammation
5. Respiratory tract chondritis
6. Audiovestibular damage.

Recently, imaging techniques are being employed like MRI, CT scan to assess the extent and severity of this condition. Pulmonary function tests can indicate the degree of respiratory system involvement.

## Treatment

Therapy depends upon severity and extent of disease. Acute episode is controlled with systemic corticosteroid (0.5–1.0 mg/kg/day) or "pulse" methylprednisolone (1,000 mg/day); while for localized disease NSAIDs is effective. Alternatively, dapsone with/without steroids can induce remission. Second-line steroid-sparing agents that can be used are cyclophosphamide, azathioprine, methotrexate, cyclosporine, colchicine, and chlorambucil. Newer drugs like infliximab, etanercept, adalimumab, and abatacept are currently being investigated. Surgical reconstruction of nose and larynx may be required in difficult cases not responding to conservative management.

## SUGGESTED READINGS

1. Burrows NP, Lovell CR. Disorders of Connective Tissue. In: Burns T, Breathnach S, Cox N (Eds). Rook's Textbook of Dermatology, 8th edition. West Sussex: Wiley-Blackwell Publisher (P) Ltd; 2010. p. 45.41-42.
2. Lee JH, Hong SP, Ko JK, et al. A case of pachydermoperiostosis combined with undifferentiated arthritis. J Rheumat Dis. 2015;22:256-9.
3. Li ZT, Wang D, Wang S. Successful treatment of pachydermoperiostosis with etoricoxib in a patient with a homozygous splice-site mutation in the SLCO2A1 gene. Br J Dermatol. 2016.
4. Minakawa S, Kaneko T, Niizeki H, et al. Case of pachydermoperiostosis with solute carrier organic anion transporter family, member 2A1 (SLCO2A1) mutations. J Dermatol. 2015;42:908-10.
5. Sainz-de-la-Maza M, Molina N, Gonzalez-Gonzalez LA, et al. Scleritis associated with relapsing polychondritis. Br J Ophthalmol. 2016;100(9):1290-4.
6. Usuba A, Yamashiro T, Handa H, et al. Quantitative computed tomography measurement of tracheal cross-sectional areas in relapsing polychondritis: correlations with spirometric values. Respiration. 2015;90:468-73.
7. Vitale A, Sota J, Rigante D, et al. Relapsing polychondritis: an update on pathogenesis, clinical features, diagnostic tools, and therapeutic perspectives. Curr Rheumatol Rep. 2016;18:1-3.

# 45 CHAPTER Disorders of Elastic Tissue and Related Disorders

Indrashis Podder, Nilendu Sarma, Somodyuti Chandra

## PSEUDOXANTHOMA ELASTICUM (GRÖNBLAD–STRANDBERG SYNDROME/ SYSTEMATIZED ELASTORRHEXIS)

### Introduction

Pseudoxanthoma elasticum is an autosomal recessive, inherited disorder affecting the elastic tissue in the dermis, blood vessels and Brusch's membrane of the eye. This disorder is characterized by generalized fragmentation and distortion of elastic tissue associated with its progressive calcification.

### History

- The French dermatologist Balzer first described the skin manifestations of this condition, and linked it with elastic tissue degeneration in 1884
- Darier coined the term "pseudoxanthome elastique", to differentiate it from xanthoma in 1896
- In 1920, Grönblad and Strandberg recognized the association of this condition with cyclic vomiting syndrome (CVS) disorders and angioid streaks
- In 2000, genetic defect was localized to the *ABCC6* gene coding for a ATP-binding cassette (ABC) transporter.

### Epidemiology

This is rare autosomal recessive disorder (1 in 25,000 to 1 in 100,000) live births, which shows slight female preponderance without any racial predisposition. Skin changes are usually absent at birth developing during childhood.

### Etiology and Pathogenesis

This disorder occurs due to loss-of-function mutation of the *ABCC6* gene present on chromosome 16p leading to production of altered *MRP6* (transmembrane ATP-binding cassette transporter) protein. It is yet unclear about the exact mechanism of this defect, the pseudoxanthoma elasticum (PXE). Possibly, faulty or aberrant expression of MRP6 leads to clumping, distortion, and calcification of elastic fibers in target organs (skin, blood vessels, and retina) with subsequent calcium deposition.

### Clinical Features

Disease shows a progressive course. Severity varies widely with some types having mild manifestations and some having severe disease. Some occasional patients have generalized skin involvement.

#### Cutaneous Features

Discreet, small (1–3 mm), yellowish papules are considered primary lesions in PXE. These usually start during the end of first decade and progress gradually with newer lesions that coalesce in a linear or reticular pattern to form plaques. Typically, it has a cobblestone or "plucked chicken skin" or "Moroccan leather" appearance. Initial sites are side of neck and then it involves medial neck and flexural areas like axilla during the teenage period. Other flexural areas are also affected (Fig. 1). Nonflexural areas like anterior wrists, umbilicus, or lumbar skin area affected less commonly.

The affected skin is soft, lax, and slightly wrinkled may hang in folds especially in the aged. Most severely affected areas, there is loss elasticity leading to sagging and redundant skin mimicking cutis laxa. Occasionally there may be spontaneous perforating lesions (perforating PXE). The mucosa (soft palate and inner aspect of lower lips) may also be affected with a cobblestone appearance. Lebwohl et al. have shown in study that affected individuals under the age of 30 years have increased horizontal and oblique mental creases. This can serve as important diagnostic clue as this is very rare in normal individual.

#### Cardiovascular Features

Calcification and narrowing of blood vessels may result in intermittent claudication, diminished peripheral pulses, and hypertension. Hypertension and mitral valve prolapse is commonly seen.

#### Ocular Features

Angioid streaks are the most common ocular finding characterized by slate-gray, poorly defined streaks radiating from the optic disc (retina). This occurs due to fissuring of the Bruch membrane of the retina.

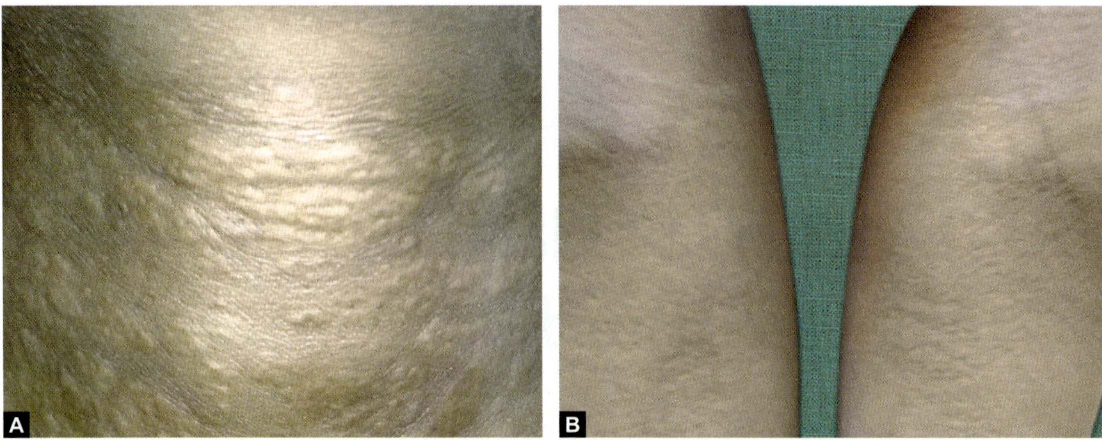

**FIG. 1: A,** Yellowish plaques on the neck in PXE; **B,** Plucked chicken appearance in elbow.
*Courtesy*: Dr Atasi Samanta, Consultant Dermatologist, Kolkata.

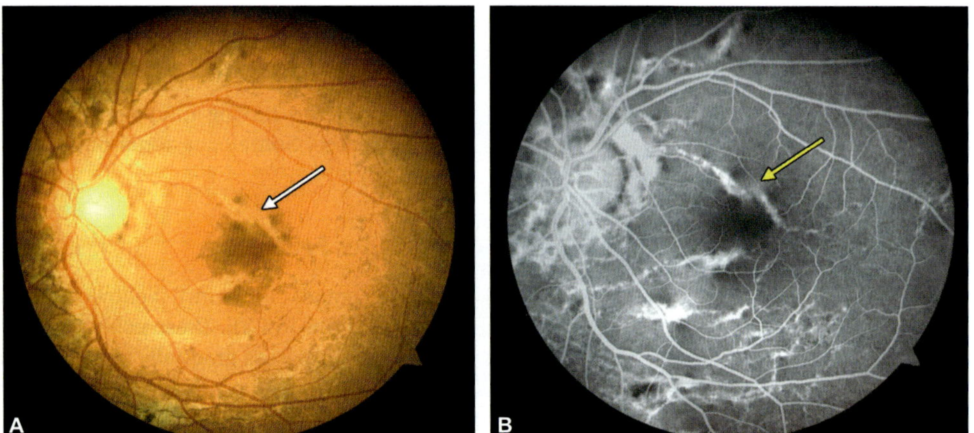

**FIG. 2: A,** Angioid streaks in the left eye in PXE (white arrow); **B,** Angioid streaks as seen with fluorescein angiogram.
*Courtesy*: Dr Debdulal Chakraborty, Senior Consultant, Department of Vireoretina Services, Disha Eye Hospitals, Kolkata.

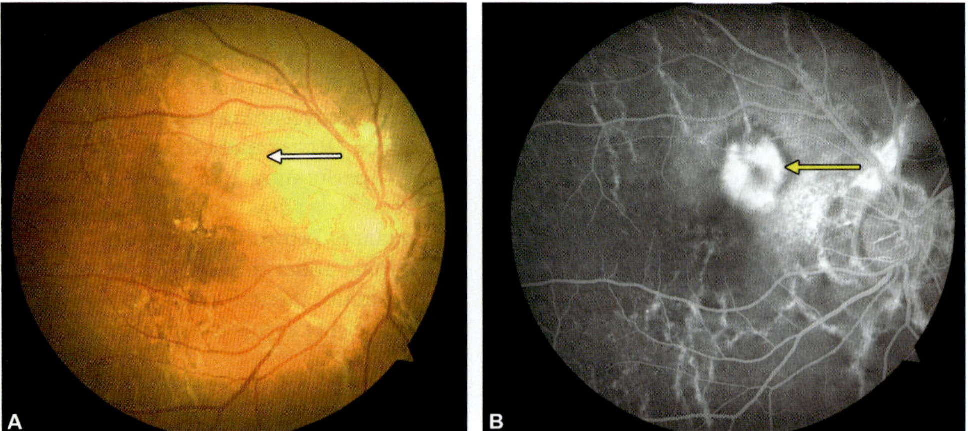

**FIG. 3: A,** Choroidal neovascularisation in the right eye of the same patient; **B,** Choroidal neovascularisation as seen with fluorescein angiogram.
*Courtesy*: Dr Debdulal Chakraborty, Senior Consultant, Department of Vireoretina Services, Disha Eye Hospitals, Kolkata.

They are one of the most distinctive features of PXE. Although they are not vessel, their radiating distribution pattern around the disc or peripapillary area mimics vascular structure. They are readily visualized by—fluorescein fundus angiography and indocyanine green angiography are best technique for their identification but routine ophthalmoscopy is sufficient for their diagnosis (Fig. 2).

Other ocular findings include drusen, "leopard spotting" (speckled yellowish mottling at the posterior pole), small, round pigmented dots spread over macula and optic disc (string of pearls), neovascularization, and retinal hemorrhage (Fig. 3). Vision may be severely impaired.

Gastrointestinal hemorrhage may occur in some cases (about 5% of cases) during adolescence.

Interestingly, pregnancy remains mostly uncomplicated. Associated abnormalities of vitamin D metabolism, nephrocalcinosis, systemic sclerosis, β-thalassemia, Marfan syndrome, and vitamin K deficiency have also been reported.

## Histopathology

The epidermis is usually normal. The dermis shows clumped, distorted, fragmented, and swollen elastic fibers are present in the mid and deep reticular dermis. In advanced lesions calcium deposits may be detected on these altered elastic fibers (purple clumps on H and E staining). Similar changes may be seen in the connective tissue of the media and, intima of the blood vessels, Bruch's membrane of the eye, and in the endocardium and pericardium (heart). Advanced cases may present with calcification involving any organ. Typical histological features of aberrant clumped and fragmented, and calcified elastic fibers in the dermis may be seen even in clinically normal appearing skin.

## Diagnosis

Diagnostic criteria of PXE were proposed long back in 1994. Clinical skin involvement showing presence of yellow cobblestone lesions in flexural locations, histopathologic features showing elastic tissue and calcium or von Kossa stains in the affected areas, and ocular disease (angioid streaks, peau d'orange, or maculopathy) in adults older than 20 years of age were considered major features. Additional minor criteria were histopathologic signs of elastic tissue and calcium or von Kossa stains in the unaffected skin and family history of PXE in first-degree relatives.

However, diagnosis is not straightforward. Not all features develop simultaneously. Ocular changes like angioid streaks take time to develop. So, this should not be used in children for diagnosis of PXE. Thus, based on variable presence of the criteria among affected peoples, PXA was classified into five categories.

1. Category I: All three major criteria
2. Category IIa: One major (angioid streaks) and two minor
3. Category IIb: One major (angioid streaks) and one minor (Elastic fiber calcification non-lesional skin)
4. Category IIc: One major (angioid streaks) and one minor (family history of PXE in first-degree relatives)
5. Category III: Two minor.

### Current Minimal Criteria for the Clinical Diagnosis of PXE

Since this original criterion was published, causative mutation of PXE has been identified in the *ABCC6* gene. This has increased the diagnostic accuracy. It has been found that that clinical manifestation may be partially or completely absent in cases with underlying mutation of PXE. Mutation analysis tests are not available in most of the centers. Thus, mutation involving *ABCC6* gene, although is confirmatory, has not been included in the minimum diagnostic criteria that comprise presence of angioid streaks and dermal elastorrhexia (with or without clinically visible typical skin changes). Presence of mutation is considered a presumptive diagnosis and is useful in children. Absence of a positive family history or symptomatic atheromatosis does not exclude the diagnosis.

## Differential Diagnosis

### Mimickers of Skin Findings

- Acquired pseudo PXE related to hemoglobinopathy (β-thalassemia, this can also have systemic findings)
- Papular elastorrhexis
- Elastosis perforans serpiginosa
- Perforating periumbilical PXE
- Buschke-Ollendorff syndrome
- Aging—normal chronological ageing or solar elastosis
- Fibroelastolytic papulosis
- Late onset focal dermal elastosis
- Cutis laxa
- Ehlers-Danlos syndromes
- *Individuals with mutations in gamma-glutamyl carboxylase*: Cutis laxa like features and similar HPE findings. Additionally, they show deficiency of vitamin K-dependent clotting factors
- D-penicillamine treatment.

### Mimickers of Cardiovascular Changes

Generalized arterial calcification of infancy.

### Mimickers of Eye Changes

- Late stages of macular degeneration
- Sickle thalassemia and β-thalassemia
- Paget's disease
- Elastosis perforans serpiginosa
- Paget's disease of bone
- Phosphatemia
- Marfan syndrome
- Sickle cell anemia
- Lead poisoning.

## Treatment

There is no definitive therapy. Proper genetic counseling and prenatal diagnosis is needed to avoid this disorder. Early detection helps to avoid complications and other organ involvement. Complications should be treated at the earliest [e.g., ocular complications, chorionic villus sampling (CVS) complications, etc.] mandating prompt referral. Dietary modification in the form of low calcium, antioxidants rich diets may be tried.

Aspirin, nonsteroidal anti-inflammatory drugs, or other hypocoagulant drugs should be avoided.

Recently, ranibizumab has been reported to be effective in the treatment of PXE induced choroidal neovascularization.

# MARFAN SYNDROME

## Introduction

Marfan syndrome is an autosomal dominant inherited disorder of the connective tissue primarily involving the elastic fibers characterized by cardiovascular, ocular, and skeletal abnormalities.

## Epidemiology

Marfan's syndrome is a relatively rare disorder with a prevalence of about 1 in 5,000–10,000 live births. Both familial and sporadic cases have been reported.

## Etiology and Pathogenesis

This is an autosomal dominant disorder; occurring due to loss-of-function mutation of the *fibrillin-1 (FBN1)* gene, located on chromosome 15q. Reduced levels of fibrillin leads to abnormal elastin-associated microtubules in the skin, eyes, and joints, etc. thus resulting in the clinical manifestations. Recent reports have implicated mutations in TGF-ß receptor genes also.

## Clinical Features

This syndrome primarily affects the cardiovascular, ocular, and skeletal systems along with some cutaneous features; the target being the elastic fibers. Skeletal features include exceptionally tall height in most of the cases, abnormal skeletal proportions, arachnodactyly, dolichocephalic skull, kyphoscoliosis, high arched palate and hyperextensible joints. Ocular features include ectopia lentis (usually upward), myopia, retinal detachment, blue sclera, and heterochromia iridis. Aneurysmal dilatation of the ascending aorta (most common), aortic and mitral incompetence constitute the cardiovascular features. Recently pulmonary artery aneurysm and pulmonary artery hypertension has also been reported. Cutaneous features include stria, scars, elastosis perforans serpiginosa, cutaneous hyperextensibility (may be associated with Ehlers-Danlos syndrome), and decreased subcutaneous fat on extremities.

## Diagnosis

Diagnostic criteria of Marfan syndrome have been revised in 2010. This is called revised Ghent nosology as it replaced the earlier criteria known as Ghent nosology that was introduced in 1996.

In the revised nosology, more diagnostic weightage has been put on aortic root aneurysm or dissection and ectopia lentis, more importance on molecular genetic test, removal of some clinical criteria, e.g., dilatation of the main pulmonary artery, dilatation or dissection of the descending thoracic or abdominal aorta, increased axial length of the globe, and abnormally flat cornea, joint hypermobility, and spondylolisthesis.

A few screening tests have been recommended in suspected individuals, which include:

- Positive thumb sign (the thumb when completely opposed in the clenched hand projects beyond the ulnar border)
- Positive wrist sign (the thumb and little finger overlap when wrapped around the opposite wrist)
- Lower segment (pubic ramus to floor): Upper segment (height minus lower segment) ratio less than one.

Joint hypermobility should be assessed in all patients.

## Differential Diagnoses

This disorder should be differentiated from other similar disorders like homocystinuria (blood levels of methionine and homocysteine are raised), multiple endocrine neoplasia syndrome, congenital contractural arachnodactyly (no CVS complications, mainly joint involvement), and Loeys-Dietz syndrome.

## Treatment

There is no specific treatment, proper counseling forms the mainstay in these patients. However, recent studies have shown health-related quality of life is unimpaired in children and adolescents with Marfan syndrome despite its distinctive phenotype. Complications in the form of systemic involvement must be treated promptly using multidisciplinary approach. Recently, Losartan (angiotensin receptor blocker having anti-TGF-β action) is being tried in this condition. Joint and bony deformities in advanced stages may need surgical correction. Aortic aneurysms may also be corrected by cardiothoracic surgery.

# ATROPHODERMA

## Follicular Atrophoderma

It is a rare, benign disorder of follicular dermal atrophy, characterized by dimple-like follicular pits without hair over the extensor aspect of hands, forearms, elbows, and feet. Some cases are associated with scrotal tongue.

Follicular atrophoderma may occur as a part of X-linked dominant chondrodysplasia punctata, and palmoplantar hyperkeratosis and hyperhidrosis and Bazex syndrome (Bazex Dupré-Christol syndrome). The latter is characterized by follicular atrophoderma, multiple milia, multiple basal cell carcinoma, hypotrichosis in males. This is different from acrokeratosis neoplasia, which is also known as Bazex syndrome and is a form of paraneoplastic syndrome.

## Idiopathic Atrophoderma of Pasini and Pierini

This is a form of dermal atrophy due to disorder of collagen, first described by Pasini in 1923, and later by Argentina, Pierini, and Vivoli in 1936.

### Etiology

The exact cause is unknown. Few familial cases have been reported. However, several authors have implicated infection with *Borrelia burgdorferi* as the triggering agent. Some considers this to be abortive variant of morphea. However, skin glycosaminoglycans differed between these two conditions.

### Clinical Manifestations

Most common age of onset is during second or third decade, with a female preponderance (F:M = 6:1). However, much early and late onset, even few cases of congenital onset is reported.

Single or multiple, sharply demarcated, smooth, round or oval lesions occur predominantly over trunk, and sometimes over lower extremities. Involvement of face, hand, and feet is considered rare. These usually start insidiously. When multiple lesions are present, they show a characteristic tendency for coalescing leading to a moth-eaten appearance. Distribution may be scattered or linear, zosteriform and size may be small (few centimeter) to large patches. Well-developed lesion has a typical depressed border (cliff drop or footprints in the snow appearance

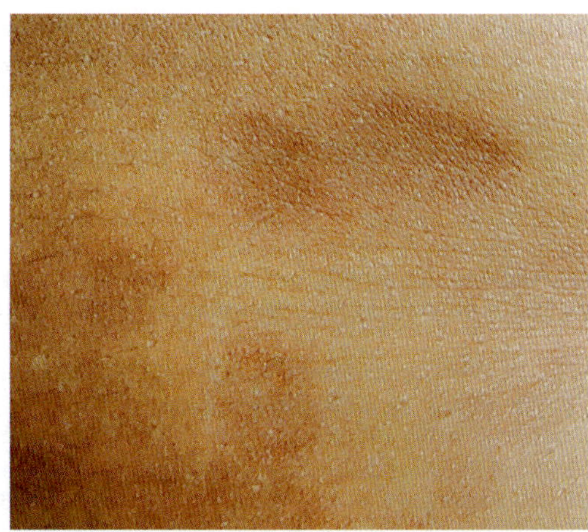

FIG. 4: Idiopathic atrophoderma of Pasini and Pierini in a young adult.

that is best seen with tangential lighting). These commonly appears hyperpigmented but may be hypopigmented or skin colored. Surface is smooth and otherwise unremarkable and is of normal consistency as that normal skin without any signs of stiffness unlike morphea (Fig. 4).

Although, inflammatory changes are noted in some, most cases are not associated with any erythema. This again differentiates from morphea that has a typical lilac border indicating inflammation. Despite these differences, morphea may be associated with this indicating some relationship.

Linear lesions are often called "linear atrophoderma of Moulin (LAM)". They are distributed along Blaschko's lines and are possibly caused by mosaicism. Apart from the linear Blaschkoid distribution, clinical and histological features are similar to generalized lesions.

Diagnostic criteria of LAM have been proposed on the basis of following features:

1. Childhood or adolescence onset
2. Hyperpigmented, slightly atrophic, and unilateral lesions along Blaschko lines on the trunk or limbs
3. No signs of preceding inflammation and subsequent induration
4. No progression or remission
5. Histologically, basal layer hyperpigmentation, normal dermis, connective tissue, and elastic fibers.

## Histopathology

Histopathological changes are often nondiagnostic. Mild epidermal atrophy may be present with increased basal layer pigmentation. Dermal thickness is usually found to be reduced. There is varying amount of homogenization and clumping of collagen bundles. Mild perivascular lymphohistiocytic infiltrate may be present. Elastic fibers are unaffected. Sparing of appendageal structures is characteristic and helps in differentiation form morphea.

## Treatment

Idiopathic atrophoderma of Pasini and Pierini and LAM is nonprogressive. Thus unlike morphea, which is progressive and may lead to significant morbidity especially the linear variety, these conditions may not require aggressive therapy with toxic drugs. Overall, efficacy of the available treatment is limited.

Cases associated with positive *B. burgdorferi* antibody titer, may respond to doxycycline (200 mg/day) for 6 weeks.

Oral and systemic steroids, antimalarials, and psoralen and ultraviolet A may be tried.

The hyperpigmentation that improves spontaneously to some extent have been found to improve with repeated sessions of Q-switched Alexandrite laser (755 nm).

LAM is reported to be improved with treatment like methotrexate.

# Atrophoderma Vermiculata

Atrophoderma vermiculata, also known as folliculitis ulerythematosa reticulata is a rare benign disorder characterized by inflammatory follicular, atrophy predominantly affecting children. It is now regarded as a type of keratosis pilaris atrophicans.

## Etiology

Majority of the cases are sporadic. Few familial cases with autosomal dominant inheritance have been described.

Abnormal keratinization of pilosebaceous unit appears to be the main pathological defect.

## Clinical Manifestations

The lesions usually begin in childhood with erythematous follicular papules symmetrically distributed over cheeks. With time these progress to develop 1–3 mm, round or oval shaped, closely placed shallow pits producing the hallmark "worm-eaten" or "honey-combed" reticular atrophy of the skin. Rarely, other sites like ears, forehead, upper lip, and extensor aspect of arms and legs may be involved (Fig. 5).

It may be associated with cataract, seizure, neurofibromatosis, Down syndrome, etc.

## Treatment

Treatment is challenging and often unsatisfactory. Topical and systemic retinoids, keratolytics, and dermabrasion may be effective.

Pulsed carbon dioxide laser and pulsed dye laser (585 nm) are also found to improve the erythema and appearance.

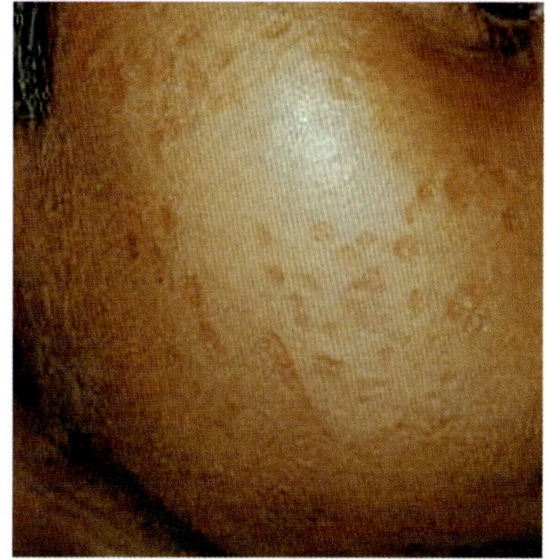

FIG. 5: Atrophic scar in atrophoderma vermiculatum on face.

## SUGGESTED READINGS


1. Ahmad AE, Papadopoulos N, Risteski P, et al. Early- and long-term outcomes after aortic surgery in patients with Marfan syndrome. Thorac cardiovasc Surg. 2016;64(S01):OP199.
2. Chassaing N, Martin L, Calvas P, et al. Pseudoxanthoma elasticum: a clinical, pathophysiological and genetic update including 11 novel ABCC6 mutations. J Med Genet. 2005;42(12):881-92.
3. Chiu P, Irons M, van de Rijn M, et al. Giant pulmonary artery aneurysm in a patient with Marfan syndrome and pulmonary hypertension. Circulation. 2016;133:1218-21.
4. Christen-Zäch S, Huber M, Struk B, et al. Pseudoxanthoma elasticum: evaluation of diagnostic criteria based on molecular data. Br J Dermatol. 2006;155(1):89-93.
5. Finger RP, Charbel Issa P, Hendig D, et al. Monthly ranibizumab for choroidal neovascularizations secondary to angioid streaks inpseudoxanthoma elasticum: a one-year prospective study. Am J Ophthalmol. 2011;152:695-703.
6. Garg A, Kumar P. Atrophoderma of Pasini and Pierini. Indian Dermatol Online J. 2011;2:126-8.
7. Lebwohl M, Neldner K, Pope FM, et al. Classification of pseudoxanthoma elasticum: report of a consensus conference. J Am Acad Dermatol. 1994;30:103-7.
8. Loeys BL, Dietz HC, Braverman AC, et al. The revised Ghent nosology for the Marfan syndrome. J Med Genet. 2010;47:476-85
9. Lopez N, Gallardo MA, Mendiola M, et al. A case of linear atrophoderma of Moulin. Actas Dermosifiliogr. 2008;99:165-7.
10. Pitcher A, Emberson J, Lacro RV, et al. Design and rationale of a prospective, collaborative meta-analysis of all randomized controlled trials of angiotensin receptor antagonists in Marfan syndrome, based on individual patient data: a report from the Marfan Treatment Trialists' Collaboration. Am Heart J. 2015;169:605-12.
11. Tan SK, Tay YK. Linear atrophoderma of Moulin. JAAD Case Rep. 2016;2:10-2.
12. Terry SF, Bercovitch L. Pseudoxanthoma Elasticum. In: Pagon RA, Adam MP, Ardinger HH (Eds). Seattle (WA): University of Washington, Seattle; 2016.
13. von Kodolitsch Y, De Backer J, Schüler H, et al. Perspectives on the revised Ghent criteria for the diagnosis of Marfan syndrome. Appl Clin Genet. 2015;8:137-55
14. Zahedi Niaki O, Sissons W, Nguyen VH, et al. Linear atrophoderma of Moulin: an underrecognized entity. Pediatr Rheumatol Online J. 2015;13:39.

# 46 CHAPTER Perforating Dermatoses and Striae Distensae

*Indrashis Podder, Nilendu Sarma, Somodyuti Chandra*

## PERFORATING DERMATOSES

### INTRODUCTION

The perforating dermatoses constitute a group of cutaneous disorders characterized by transepidermal elimination of collagen, elastic tissue or necrotic connective tissue from the dermis to exterior with little or no disruption of the surrounding structures. This group of disorders is usually characterized by the formation of papules or nodules with keratotic plugs. Various substances are extruded in the process of transepidermal elimination. This is classified based on the substance eliminated (Table 1).

### CLASSIFICATION

The different types of perforating disorders can be classified under the following heads:

A. *According to pathogenesis*:
   1. Primary perforating disorders
   2. Secondary perforating disorders
B. *According to the mode of occurrence*:
   1. Familial/inherited
   2. Acquired perforating dermatoses
C. According to the nature of eliminated substance.

### Primary Perforating Disorders

The perforating disorders which occur due to intrinsic defects in the epidermal keratinocytes, hair follicles, collagen or elastic tissue, with transepidermal elimination being the final common pathway. There are mainly four disorders under this category:

1. Reactive perforating collagenosis (RPC)
2. Elastosis perforans serpiginosa (EPS)
3. Perforating folliculitis
4. Acquired perforating dermatoses/Kyrle's disease.

**TABLE 1: Types of perforating diseases based on the nature of eliminated substance**

| Eliminated substance | Type of the perforating disorder |
|---|---|
| Collagen | Reactive perforating collagenosis (RPC) (inherited) |
| Elastic tissue | Elastosis perforans serpiginosa (EPS) |
| Necrotic material | Perforating folliculitis |
| Necrotic material, collagen, etc. | Acquired perforating dermatoses viz. Kyrle's disease, acquired RPC, etc. |
| Calcified elastic tissue | Perforating periumbilical calcific elastosis |

### Secondary Perforating Disorders

These groups of perforating disorders occur due to some underlying cutaneous disorder. There are several cutaneous disorders which may result in secondary perforating disorders. Some of the important ones are mentioned here:

- *Perforation of endogenous substances*:
  - Chondrodermatitis nodularis helicis
  - Hematomas
  - Perforating pseudoxanthoma elasticum (PXE)
  - Gout
  - Perforating calcinosis
- *Perforation of exogenous foreign materials*:
  - Silica
  - Wood splinters
  - Caustic drilling fluids (petrochemical industry)
- *Due to infectious diseases/organisms*:
  - Chromoblastomycosis
  - Botryomycosis
- *Extrusion of neoplastic cells*:
  - Melanoma
  - Paget's disease
  - Mycosis fungoides.

### Familial/Inherited Perforating Disorders

This group of disorders is often inherited and present during childhood ages. The familial perforating disorders are given here:

- RPC
- EPS
- Perforating folliculitis.

### Acquired Perforating Dermatoses

These disorders generally result secondary to many underlying systemic diseases and manifest in the adulthood. Following conditions are known to induce acquired perforating diseases.

- Long-standing diabetes mellitus
- Chronic renal failure patients undergoing dialysis
- Chronic liver disease (rare).

## Reactive Perforating Collagenosis

Reactive perforating collagenosis is a rare inherited form of perforating dermatosis in which collagen is extruded through the epidermis. These lesions are usually precipitated by cold temperature and trauma.

### *Epidemiology*

Being familial, this disorder commonly presents in the childhood. No sexual or racial predisposition has been observed.

### *Etiology and Pathogenesis*

Although the exact pathogenesis is not clear, it has been proposed that there is a basic defect that is mediated genetically or acquired in the underlying collagen. Altered collagen is extruded owing to necrolysis of the overlying epidermis.

Several other pathomechanisms have been proposed viz. altered vitamin A and/or D metabolism, alteration of vascular flow, deposition of substances like uric acid, hydroxyapatite, silicon, etc.; although these claims are yet to be substantiated.

### *Clinical Features*

- This disorder usually starts in the childhood as small keratotic papules
- Most common sites—extensor surface of the hands, elbows, knees
- Each papule reaches a size of about 4–6 mm over the following 3–4 weeks; then becomes umbilicated with a keratinous plug
- The lesions usually regress spontaneously over 6–8 weeks to leave behind a hypopigmented, atrophic small scar
- Koebner phenomenon may be positive.

### *Histology*

Histopathology shows localized area of hyperkeratosis (keratotic plug), variable parakeratosis, and presence of keratotic debris. In the dermis, there is localized collection of altered collagen in the papillary dermis, which is surrounded and engulfed by focal epidermal proliferation; these materials extend through the epidermis into the crusted plaque (transepidermal elimination). Neutrophilic infiltration is seen in the early stages that turn to lymphocytic later. The surrounding dermis appears to be unremarkable.

Tissue stained with Verhoeff-Van Gieson (VVG) stain can be used to delineate the collagen abnormality.

### *Differential Diagnosis*

The following conditions may closely mimic RPC. Some of the important ones are given here:

- Molluscum contagiosum
- Prurigo nodularis
- Perforating folliculitis
- EPS
- Perforating granuloma annulare
- Kyrle's disease.

### *Treatment*

- *General measures*: Avoidance of cold, trauma
- *Topical*: Retinoids (tretinoin, tazarotene), topical steroids under occlusion, emollients
- *Systemic*: Oral isotretinoin, methotrexate, systemic corticosteroids, antibiotics (doxycycline, clindamycin, tetracycline)
- *Others*: The PUVA, NBUVB, cryotherapy, laser ablation, electrosurgery.

## Verrucous Perforating Collagenoma

This is a rare, nonfamilial variant of RPC in which severe trauma leads to the formation of verrucous papules and nodules; which show transepidermal elimination of collagen.

## Elastosis Perforans Serpiginosa

Elastosis perforans serpiginosa is a rare inherited form of perforating dermatosis in which the material extruded through the epidermis is derived from elastic fibers in the upper dermis.

### *Epidemiology*

This disorder usually presents in the childhood; isolated EPS may have an autosomal dominant inheritance. Males are affected nearly four times compared to females.

### *Etiology and Pathogenesis*

The precise mechanism is not known, however genetically determined defect of elastic tissue may be involved (copper deficiency may play an additional role). The altered elastic tissue may provoke a cellular response that ultimately leads to extrusion of the abnormal elastic tissue.

Almost 40% cases are associated with connective tissue disorders viz. PXE, Ehlers-Danlos syndrome (EDS), Marfan syndrome (MFS), and osteogenesis imperfecta (OI).

Association with Down syndrome, mental deficiency, penicillamine (drug), moyamoya disease, and scabies is reported.

### *Clinical Features*

Usual age of onset is first to second decade and males are more commonly affected than females. Typical presentation is small, keratotic, umbilicated papules characteristically arranged in linear, circular or serpiginous patterns. Most common sites are neck (back, sides), cheeks, arms, thighs; occasionally bilaterally symmetrical.

Rings may reach a diameter of 15–20 cm over time. Lesions may heal spontaneously after several years; residual atrophic scars.

Histopathology sows localized area of hyperkeratosis (keratotic plug), variable parakeratosis, acanthosis and presence of keratotic debris. In the dermis, there is localized collection of altered elastic tissue in the papillary dermis (circumscribed plug), surrounded and engulfed by focal epidermal proliferation; these materials extend through the epidermis into the crusted plaque (transepidermal elimination) through a direct channel. The plug consists of horny material in its upper third and amorphous debris derived from elastin in its lower two-thirds. The dermis surrounding the plug shows basophilic cells and foreign body type giant cells.

Special stain like VVG stain may be used to show the alterations in elastic fibers (black).

In penicillamine induced cases of EPS, elastic fibers may have a characteristic bramble-bush or lumpy-bumpy appearance.

### *Differential Diagnoses*

Some of the important differential diagnoses are:

- Porokeratosis of Mibelli

- RPC
- Perforating granuloma annulare
- Tinea corporis
- Annular sarcoidosis.

### *Treatment*

- *Topical:* Retinoids, topical steroids under occlusion, imiquimod, and emollients
- *Systemic:* Oral isotretinoin and systemic corticosteroids
- *Others:* Cello tape stripping of surface keratinous material, cryotherapy, laser ablation, electrosurgery (curettage), Aminolevulinic acid-photodynamic therapy (effective treatment of d-penicillamine induced EPS).

Discontinuation of penicillamine if implicated as the causative agent.

## Acquired Reactive Perforating Dermatoses and Kyrle's Disease

Acquired reactive perforating dermatoses refer to an umbrella term encompassing all perforating disorders arising in adults. Some people use the eponym Kyrle's disease as a synonym; while others prefer to define it as the excoriated hyperplastic nodules seen at the end-stage of folliculitis.

### *Etiology*

The important systemic conditions which may lead to the development of acquired perforating dermatoses is given here:

- Long-standing diabetes mellitus; diabetic foot
- Chronic renal failure patients on dialysis
- Chronic liver disease (rare)
- Internal malignancies (rare)
- Rarely, caustic fluids used in petrochemical industries, calcium containing drilling fluids, intradermal injection can cause this.

### *Types*

Based on the histologic findings, the acquired perforating dermatoses can be of the following types:

- Acquired RPC (most common)
- Acquired EPS
- Perforating PXE
- Perforating periumbilical calcific elastosis.

### *Clinical Features*

Typically, these appear as keratotic, umbilicated papules and nodules, with a central crust (Fig. 1). Leg is commonly affected. This may also be generalized. Recently, Blaschkoid distribution of generalized Kyrle's disease has been reported.

Very rarely, periumbilical, keratotic papules and plaques are described in black, multiparous women. This is called perforating periumbilical calcific elastosis.

### *Histopathology*

Discussed earlier in relevant sections (RPC/EPS).

### *Complication*

Recently, few authors have reported the development of squamous cell carcinoma on Kyrle's disease scar.

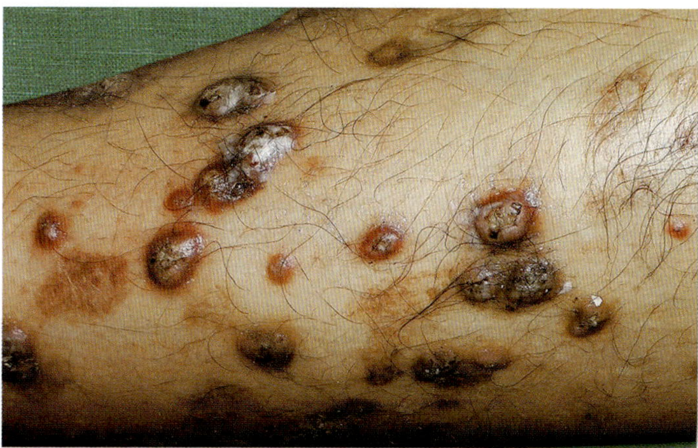

**FIG. 1:** Acquired perforating dermatoses.

### *Treatment*

- Phototherapy (PUVA, NBUVB, BBUVB) is most effective
- Treatment of underlying condition (e.g., control of diabetes mellitus, renal transplantation, etc.)
- *Other*: Retinoids, corticosteroids, emollients.

## Perforating Folliculitis

Perforating folliculitis is a relatively common acquired perforating disorder. However, some authors consider it as ordinary folliculitis with follicular rupture, i.e., not a part of perforating disease spectrum.

### *Epidemiology*

Most commonly occurs in young adults, slight female preponderance.

### *Etiology*

Most commonly associated with dialysis in chronic renal failure. Recently it has been reported to be associated with anti-synthetase syndrome, lenalidomide, sorafenib, and nilotinib. A role of C-kit receptor is being investigated.

### *Clinical Features*

- Multiple itchy, follicular papules
- Overlying scale/crust may be present
- Most common sites are trunk and extremities.

### *Differential Diagnosis*

- EPS
- RPC
- Prurigo nodularis
- Molluscum contagiosum
- Kyrle's disease (some authors consider it to be synonymous).

### *Histopathology*

These are focal hyperkeratosis, acanthosis, plugged follicular orifice, suppurative folliculitis, necrotic debri, and acute inflammatory cells around distorted follicles; penetrating collagen and elastic fibers into the follicular space.

Special stains (VVG) may be used for detection of collagen and elastic tissue.

### *Treatment*

Treatment of the underlying condition (renal transplantation, control of diabetes) is very important.

- *Topical:* Retinoids, topical, and intralesional corticosteroids
- *Systemic:* Retinoids, corticosteroids, methotrexate
- *Others:* Phototherapy (PUVA), electrosurgery, laser ablation.

# STRIAE DISTENSAE (STRETCH MARKS)

## INTRODUCTION

Striae are common skin lesions characterized by localized dermal scarring. These do not cause any medical problem, however they are a source of significant psychological distress to the patient.

## ETIOPATHOGENESIS

Etiology is multifactorial. The possible pathogenetic mechanisms are as follows:

Mechanical effect of stretching that may occur during pregnancy, obesity, weight lifting, or even normal pubertal growth spurt lead to rupture of connective tissue framework. Systemic corticosteroid in the form of iatrogenic use or disease (Cushing's syndrome) predisposes to development of striae. Other conditions that may increase the chance of striae are immunosuppression and sudden weight loss as may occur in tuberculosis, typhoid, HIV, antiretroviral therapy (ART) (Indinavir), anorexia nervosa, and also chronic liver disease. Patients of Ehlers–Danlos syndrome do not develop striae during pregnancy.

## CLINICAL MANIFESTATIONS

These are long, few mm wide, slightly concave, irregularly linear lesions that usually run almost parallel to the skin tension lines. Early lesions are slightly raised and pink colored (known as striae rubra) and gradually become greyish white and atopic (known as striae alba) overtime. The common sites are outer aspect of thigh and lumbosacral region in boys and thighs, upper arms, buttocks and breast in girls (Fig. 2). Striae in Cushing syndrome and those induced by corticosteroids are larger and more widely distributed.

## HISTOPATHOLOGY

Histology of striae simulates that of a scar. Epidermis is atopic, thin, flat with loss of rete ridges. Dermis shows densely packed collagen parallel to the skin surface. Inflammatory changes and dermal edema predominate in early lesions.

## DIFFERENTIAL DIAGNOSIS

Linear focal elastosis—characterized by raised, yellow linear bands arranged horizontally over lower back.

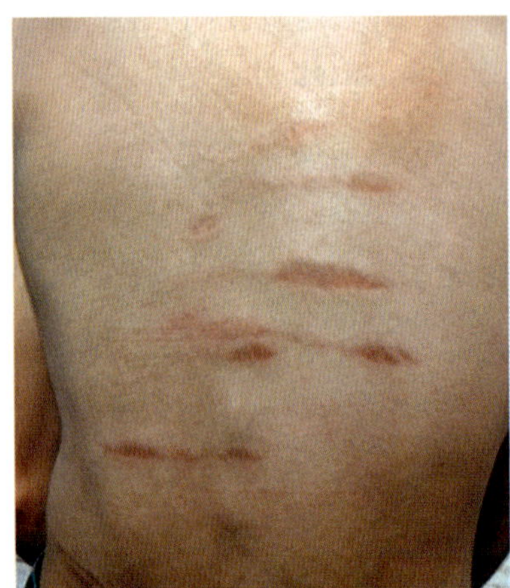

**FIG. 2:** Atrophic striae on the back of a young male.

*Courtesy*: Dr Sayantani Chakraborty, Assistant Professor Department of Dermatology, RG Kar Medical College, West Bengal.

## TREATMENT

Several treatment modalities have been proposed, yet none is consistently effective. Treatment must be instituted during active state before scarring process is complete. Topical tretinoin (0.1%), pulsed dye laser (585 nm) and nonablative fractional photothermolysis using the 1550 nm laser can be used in mature striae.

## SUGGESTED READINGS


1. Al-Himdani S, Ud-Din S, Gilmore S, et al. Striae distensae: a comprehensive review and evidence-based evaluation of prophylaxis and treatment. Br J Dermatol. 2014;170(3):527-47.
2. Batalla A, Menéndez L, Blay P, et al. Delayed onset perforating folliculitis associated with sorafenib. Australas J Dermatol. 2014;55:233-5.
3. Bodman M, Ehredt D Jr, Barker R, et al. Kyrle disease a rare dermatologic condition associated with the diabetic foot. J Am Pediatr Med Assoc. 2015;105:451-5.
4. Cerio R, Calnan CD, Wilson-Jones E. A clinico-pathological study of reactive perforating collagenosis: report of 10 cases. Br J Dermatol .1987;117 (Suppl 32):16-7.
5. Espinosa PS, Baumann RJ, Vaishnav AG. Elastosis perforans serpiginosa, Down syndrome, and moyamoya disease. Pediatr Neurol. 2008;38:287-8.
6. Kassardjian M, Frederickson J, Griffith J, et al. Elastosis perforans serpiginosa in association with scabies mite. J Clin Aesthet Dermatol. 2013;6:36-40.
7. Kuiper EM, Kardaun SH. Late onset perforating folliculitis induced by lenalidomide: a case report. Br J Dermatol. 2015;173:618-20.
8. Llamas-Velasco M, Steegmann JL, Carrascosa R, et al. Perforating folliculitis in a patient treated with nilotinib: a further evidence of C-kit involvement. Am J Dermatopathol. 2014;36:592-3.
9. Podder I. Perforating Dermatoses. In: Vasudevan B (Ed). Clinical Correlation with Diagnostic Implications in Dermatology, 1st edition. New Delhi: Jaypee Brothers Medical Publishers (P) Ltd; 2017: p 286-289
10. Rallis E, Stavropoulos PG, Papafragkaki DK, et al. Squamous cell carcinoma developed on Kyrle's disease scar. J Buon. 2014;19:317-8.
11. Saldanha LF, Gonick HC, Rodriguez HJ, et al. Silicon-related syndrome in dialysis patients. Nephron. 1997;77:48-56.
12. Shaw KC, Kaley JR, Darling MD, et al. A case of perforating folliculitis in association with antisynthetase syndrome. J Biol Regul Homeost Agents. 2015;29:95-8.
13. Verma R, Vasudevan B, Kakkar S, et al. Kyrle's disease presenting in an extensive distribution along lines of Blaschko. Indian J Dermatol. 2015;60:423.
14. Wang D, Liang J, Xu J, et al. Effective treatment of d-penicillamine induced elastosis perforans serpiginosa with ALA-PDT. Photodiagnosis Photodyn Ther. 2015;12:140-2.

# 47 CHAPTER Disorders of Dermal Connective Tissues

*Smita Nagpal*

## INTRODUCTION

The dermis and subcutaneous tissue hold and support the epidermis. The dermis is organized into papillary and reticular regions. It is a dense, interwoven collagen, and elastic matrix. Beneath the epidermis is a narrow zone called papillary dermis, which includes an even narrower subepidermal connective tissue band beneath the basal lamina. The reticular dermis has superficial intermediate and deep reticular zones. The organization of the fibrous connective tissue helps distinguish each region. In this chapter, the alterations in the dermal tissue that have been recognized ultrastructurally in skin from patients with connective tissue diseases are discussed.

## FIBROMATOSES

The fibromatoses represents a group of disease processes defined by the proliferation of generally mature fibroblasts associated with mature collagen. Some are present at birth or develop in early childhood (e.g., juvenile fibromatoses) and some may appear in adulthood.

The lesions of fibromatoses are benign but they tend to infiltrate and recur when removed and usually do not metastasize.

They all have similar histologic appearance containing spindle-shaped myofibroblastic cells, dense deposits of intercellular collagen fibers, variable amounts of extracellular myxoid matrix, and compressed and elongated vessels.

The fibromatoses can be classified as follows:

1. Superficial fibromatoses (fascial fibromatoses)—low aggressive
   a. Palmar (Dupuytren's)
   b. Plantar
   c. Penile (Peyronie's)
   d. Knuckle pads
   e. Nodular fasciitis
   f. Elastofibroma
   g. Fibrous papule of the face
2. Deep fibromatoses (nonmetastasizing fibrosarcoma/desmoid tumors)—highly aggressive
3. Fibrous proliferation of infancy and childhood.

### Superficial Fibromatoses

Superficial fibromatoses are fibroblastic proliferations arising in the palmar or plantar soft tissues. The tumors consist of small nodules that infiltrate the aponeurosis and subcutaneous fat. Histologically, they are characterized by plump, immature-appearing spindle shaped cells, moderate amounts of collagen, and elongated vessels. Older lesions are less cellular and more densely collagenous (Table 1).

A Dupuytren contracture (or palmar fibromatoses) is the most common of superficial fibromatoses characterized by presence of firm nodules on the palmar surface of the hand with coalescing cords of soft tissue on the webs and digits. It is progressive

**TABLE 1: Characteristics of superficial and deep fibromatoses**

| | Superficial fibromatoses | | | Deep fibromatoses | |
|---|---|---|---|---|---|
| Characteristics | Palmar | Plantar | Abdominal wall | Intra-abdominal (mesenteric) | Extra-abdominal |
| Recurrence rate | 30–40% | 20–40% | 15–30% | 23% overall (90% Gardeners) | 19–77% |
| Age | Often >65 years of age | 3–5$^{th}$ decade | 20–30 years of age | Average 41 years of age | Peak 25–30 years-of-age |
| Sex | 80% male | 66% male | 87% female | 55% male | Female predilection |
| Incidence | 1–2% of population | 0.23% of population | 49% of deep fibromatoses | 8% of deep fibromatoses | 43% of deep fibromatoses |
| Association with Gardners | No | No | Yes | Yes with mesenteric subtype | Yes |

condition that causes shortening and thickening of the fibrous tissue of the palmar fascia and leads to with contractures that draw one or more fingers into flexion at the metacarpophalangeal (MCP) joint or proximal interphalangeal (PIP) joint. It affects 1–2% of the population.

Pathologically, Dupuytren's contracture is characterized by fibroblastic proliferation and disorderly collagen deposition with fascial thickening.

### Treatment

Medically, it can be treated with intralesional triamcinolone and lidocaine. Radiation therapy and a relatively new medicine called collagenase clostridium histolyticum can also be used. These are generally most effective if used before the condition becomes severe. Surgical release of palmar fascia is indicated in patients with severe functional impairment and neurovascular deficit in a finger.

## Plantar Fibromatoses

Plantar fibromatoses is a group of conditions with the common characteristics of plantar location and histologic features of mature collagen and fibroblasts with no malignant cytologic features.

The term plantar fibromatoses is used for different conditions, as follows:

- *Ledderhose disease (plantar equivalent of palmar Dupuytren contracture)*: Repeated trauma, long-term alcohol consumption, chronic liver disease, diabetes, and epilepsy have been reported to be associated. Often, patients also have other fibrosing conditions such as Dupuytren contracture, knuckle pads, or Peyronie disease. Heredity is also a clear factor in many patients.

  Clinically, one or more small, asymptomatic, round, or flattened hard nodules that are generally located on the medial side of the sole. Flexion deformities usually do not occur in opposition to Dupuytren contracture
- *A more uncommon plantar, and superficial fibromatoses*: Superficial plantar fibromatoses appear as one or more asymptomatic, flat nodules of fibrous consistency and variable size. They are most commonly located on the plantar aspect of the anteromedial portion of the heel pad. This is seen in children and young adults.

### Diagnosis

All types of plantar fibromatoses have a dense fibrocellular tissue with mature collagen and fibrocytes in various stages of maturation, but they do not have prominent atypical features or abnormal mitotic activity. The overlying epidermis and superficial dermal tissue are usually normal.

The myofibroblast is the key proliferative cell in some so-called fibromatoses; therefore, these might be better named myofibromatoses. In these fibromatoses, results of tests for cytologic markers in muscle cells are positive.

Osseous metaplasia and distinct multinucleate giant cells have been reported in Ledderhose disease.

### Treatment

Medical treatment like anti-inflammatory medication, and intralesional corticosteroids are not effective in plantar fibromatoses.

For Ledderhose disease, fasciectomy and excision of the fibrous tissue are the only possible treatments. Ledderhose disease has a favorable prognosis, although slow progression is not uncommon.

For the other forms of plantar fibromatoses, surgery is the only therapeutic alternative.

## Peyronie's Disease (Penile Fibromatoses)

Peyronie's disease is caused by scar tissue, called plaque, which forms along the length of the penis in the corpora cavernosa. This plaque is not visible, and depending on the severity of the condition, the plaque can cause the penis to bend, making sexual intercourse difficult and occasionally painful. The cause of Peyronie's disease is unclear.

## Knuckle Pads

Knuckle pads are benign, asymptomatic, well-circumscribed, smooth, firm, skin-colored papules, nodules, or plaques, located in the skin over the dorsal aspects of the MCP and IP joints. A history of repetitive trauma related to sports or occupation is often present (Fig. 1).

Neither medical nor surgical interventions for knuckle pads are very effective. Applications of keratolytics, such as salicylic acid or urea, have helped to soften and even reduce the lesions. Surgical intervention may be indicated if knuckle pads cause a functional problem.

## Pachydermodactyly

Pachydermodactyly is a rare, benign form of digital fibromatosis and this is characterized by asymptomatic soft tissue swelling that affects the lateral aspects of the PIP joints of the fingers. The possibility of repetitive minor trauma by habitual or compulsive habits of interlacing the fingers or rubbing of the fingers has been suggested.

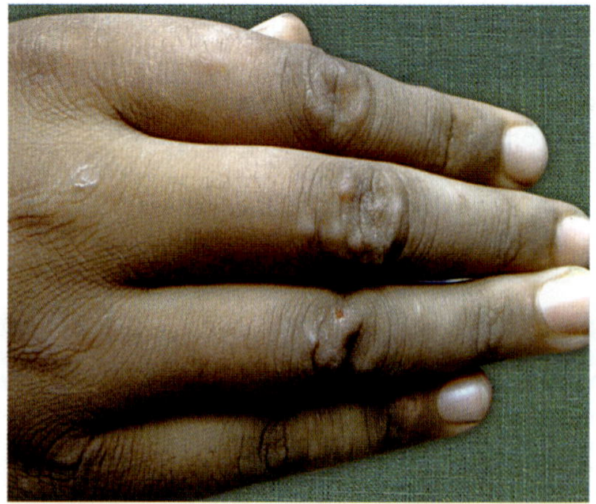

**FIG. 1:** Knuckle pads.

*Courtesy:* Dr Nilendu Sarma, Associate Professor and Head, Department of Dermatology, Dr BC Roy Post Graduate Institute of Pediatric Sciences, West Bengal.

## Infantile Digital Fibromatoses

Infantile digital fibromatoses (IDF) (synonyms: Reye's tumor, recurrent digital fibrous tumor of childhood, multiple hyaline fibromatosis, IDF, and juvenile dermatofibroma) is a benign asymptomatic nodular proliferation of fibrous tissue occurring almost exclusively on the dorsal and lateral aspects of the fingers or the toes. It appears as smooth, round, single, or confluent nodules (<2 cm) developing in early months of life, rarely later.

Unique histologic features are diagnostic of IDF. Interlacing fascicles of uniform spindle-shaped cells and collagen bundles are seen in the dermis or subcutis. Mitotic figures are not found. A characteristic feature is the presence of distinctive, perinuclear, and eosinophilic cytoplasmic inclusion bodies. This finding has suggested a possible role of viral infection that has not yet been confirmed. Masson trichrome stains these characteristic perinuclear inclusion bodies deep red. Immunohistochemical stains are positive for vimentin, cytokeratin, desmin, calponin, and alpha-smooth muscle actin but negative for keratin and muscle actin. Ultrastructurally, they are found to be myofibroblast.

There is definite chance of spontaneous resolution. On the other hand, even, wide local surgical excision is associated recurrence in up to 60% of cases.

## Acrokeratoelastoidosis

Acrokeratoelastoidosis (AKE) is a rare genodermatosis. In AKE, there are small, firm papules, or plaques on the sides of the hands and feet. An abnormality in the secretion or excretion of elastic material by fibroblasts in the dermis may cause these nodules.It was first described by Costa in 1953.

It can be autosomal dominant or sporadic. It usually is seen during puberty, or sometimes later, and then remains stable. It is usually not congenital. In most of the cases no treatment is necessary. AKE usually differs from keratoelastoidosis marginalis and focal acral hyperkeratosis on histology.

## Acrochordon (Skin Tags)

An acrochordon is a small, soft, common, benign, and usually pedunculated neoplasm that is found particularly in persons who are obese. It is usually skin colored or hyperpigmented, and it may appear as surface nodules or papillomas on healthy skin (Fig. 2). Most acrochordons vary in size from 2 to 5 mm in diameter, although larger acrochordons up to 5 cm in diameter are sometimes evident. The most frequent localizations are the neck and the axillae, but any skin fold, including the groin, may be affected.

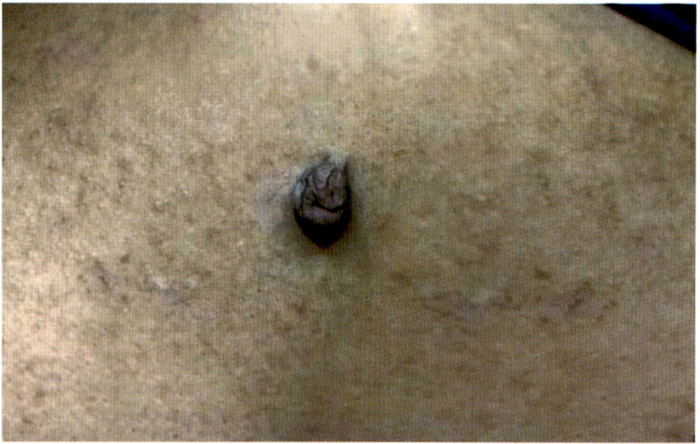

**FIG. 2:** Skin tag on thigh.
*Courtesy:* Dr Sayantani Chakraborty, Assistant Professor Department of Dermatology, RG Kar Medical College, West Bengal.

### Treatment

As tags are benign, treatment is unnecessary unless the tags become frequently irritated or present a cosmetic concern. If removal is desired, it can be done using cauterization, cryosurgery, excision, or surgical ligation.

#### *Nodular Fasciitis*

This is a benign, solitary subcutaneous nodule of less than 5 cm, generally showing a rapid growth, sometimes tender, generally seen in young adults (first three decades of life). Head, neck, upper extremities, and trunk are the most common sites. Previous history of trauma may be present. Clinically and histologically, nodular fasciitis may be mistaken for a sarcoma.

There is reactive (non-neoplastic) proliferation of mitotically active spindle cell in the subcutaneous tissue and the deep fascia and less commonly in the muscle in dermis. Its characteristic infiltrative nature is highly mimicker of neoplastic sarcoma.

In histology, immature spindle shaped fibroblasts and myofibroblasts with many mitoses are present haphazardly in a loose myxoid stroma with plenty of vascular components (capillary, slit-like spaces, and extravasated red blood cells) and with giant cells. Based on predominant cell types, histologically, nodular fasciitis has been classified into three subtypes—myxoid, cellular, and fibrotic (more collagen).

Immunohistochemically, smooth muscle actin and vimentin are detected.

Surgical excision is the treatment of choice and recurrence is rare.

## Digital Papular Calcific Elastosis

Digital papular calcific elastosis (DPCE) is an acquired papular acrokeratoderma. It predominantly affects the radial side of the index finger, first web space, and ulnar side of the thumb. It usually occurs in the middle-aged and elderly. Burks et al. first described the clinical and histological features in five cases of DPCE, which they termed degenerative collagenous plaques of the hands in 1960. The condition was named DPCE in 1990 after a comprehensive study of 20 patients showed that this was a more accurate, descriptive term for the clinical and histological features.

## Desmoid Tumors

Desmoid tumors are fibrous neoplasms originating from the musculoaponeurotic structures throughout the body. The term desmoid, coined by Muller in 1838, is derived from the Greek word desmos, which means tendon-like.

Desmoid tumors are infiltrative, usually well-differentiated, firm overgrowths of fibrous tissue, and are locally aggressive with no known potential for metastasis or dedifferentiation. They are also called aggressive fibromatoses for marked cellularity and aggressive local behavior. This course and the tendency for recurrence make the treatment of these relatively rare fibrous tumors challenging.

Desmoid tumors are rare, they account for about 0.03% of all neoplasms and less than 3% of all soft tissue tumors. The estimated incidence in the general population is 2–4 per million population per year.

## Pathophysiology

Desmoid tumors most commonly arise from the rectus abdominis muscle in postpartum women and in scars due to abdominal surgery. They may arise in any skeletal muscle. The myofibroblast is the cell considered to be responsible for the development of desmoid tumors.

A minority of desmoid tumors are caused by mutations in a gene called familial adenomatous polyposis (FAP or Gardner syndrome).

It has been proposed that, excess beta-catenin, whether caused by *CTNNB1* or *APC* gene mutations, promotes uncontrolled growth and division of cells, allowing the formation of desmoid tumors. In Ledderhose disease and other superficial fibromatoses, cytoplasmic, and nuclear accumulation of beta-catenin accumulation has been reported though there are no mutations in either exon 3 of beta-catenin or in *APC*.

## Clinical Features

Although desmoid tumors can arise in any skeletal muscle, they most commonly develop in the anterior abdominal wall and shoulder girdle. Retroperitoneal neoplasms are more common in familial polyposis coli and Gardner syndrome after abdominal surgery than in other conditions.

Peripheral desmoid tumors are firm, smooth, and mobile. They often adhere to surrounding structures. The overlying skin is usually unaffected. The presence of such a soft tissue growth should alert the clinician to delve more deeply into the family history for evidence of familial polyposis coli and Gardner syndrome. Extra-abdominal desmoid tumors are rare and may be first evident as gradually increasing leg swelling. Desmoid tumors may rarely appear on the foot.

## Diagnosis

To diagnose the tumors immunostaining with vimentin, alpha smooth muscle actin, muscle actin, and desmin can be done. Performing an APC mutational analysis is usually the most diagnostic. Esophagogastroduodenoscopy and colonoscopy can also be done.

Computed tomography (CT) scanning and magnetic resonance imaging (MRI) are used for the diagnosis and follow-up of desmoid tumors. They can help determine the extent of the tumor and its relationship to nearby structures, especially prior to surgical removal. MRI is superior to CT scanning in defining the pattern and the extent of involvement as well as in determining if recurrence has occurred after surgery.

## Treatment

Surgical excision with negative surgical margins is the most successful primary treatment modality for desmoid tumors. There is a high risk for recurrence if there are positive margins after surgery.

Other options of treatment for patients who are not surgical candidates or who refuse surgery are:

- Radiation therapy (postoperatively, preoperatively, or as the sole treatment)
- Antiestrogens and prostaglandin inhibitors may also be used
- Chemotherapy with doxorubicin, dacarbazine, and carboplatin may be used in cases of recurrent extra-abdominal desmoid tumors in which surgery is contraindicated or in cases of recurrence
- Systemic doxorubicin, and ifosfamide is effective for intra-abdominal desmoid tumors (Gardner syndrome).

# Fibromatoses in Children

The benign fibromatoses of childhood can be classified as follows:

- Those with a generally indolent course
  - Myofibroma/myofibromatosis
  - Fibromatosis colli
  - Fibrous hamartoma of infancy
  - Nodular fasciitis
- Those with potential for a locally aggressive course
  - Infantile (desmoid type) fibromatosis
  - Plantar-palmar fibromatosis
  - Gingival fibromatosis
  - Digital (inclusion body) fibromatosis
  - Calcifying aponeurotic fibroma
  - Giant cell fibroblastoma.

# Stiff Skin Syndrome (Congenital Fascial Dystrophy)

This is a rare hereditary connective tissue disorder with its onset at birth or early childhood characterized by stony-hard skin, firmly bound to underlying tissues, and contracture with limitation of joint mobility, especially of the large joints.

Hard skin may be smooth or nodular and is prominent in areas with abundant fascia such as the thighs, buttocks, trunk, shoulder, and upper arm. Joints commonly showing restricted movement are knee, hip, lumbar spine, and shoulder leading to bizarre posture and gait.

This shows an insidious progress. Absence of any systemic organ involvement is very typical. Most cases have a good prognosis, but in severe cases patients may incur growth retardation and restrictive pulmonary changes due to cutaneous stiffness. Hypertrichosis is sometimes associated.

Management is supportive. Rehabilitation exercises should start at an early age and be continued throughout life to prevent contractures and restrictive pulmonary changes.

# Infantile Restrictive Dermopathy

It is a rare autosomal recessive disorder caused by a single mutation in the *ZMPSTE24* gene. It presents at birth with taut shiny skin, open mouth, micrognathia, low set ears, small nose, and widely spaced cranial sutures.

# Infantile Systemic Hyalinosis and Juvenile Hyaline Fibromatosis

Infantile systemic hyalinosis (ISH) is a rare familial autosomal recessive disease of unknown etiology. Juvenile hyaline fibromatosis the allelic variants of ISH and involves the same gene.

The clinical features are evident either at birth or within 6 months of life. The presentation is painful progressive joint contractures, thickened skin with reddish-blue or hyperpigmentation over bony prominences, small pearly facial papules, and gingival hypertrophy, fleshy nodules in the perianal region, diarrhea, increased susceptibility to bone fractures, infections, and failure to thrive.

This is a progressive disorder that may lead to death within the first 2 years of life, mostly due to recurrent chest infection and diarrhea. Debulking of hypertrophic gingiva and excision of some symptomatic skin masses in these patients are indicated for comfort and smooth nursing care of the patients and to allow better rehabilitation.

### Winchester Syndrome

Winchester syndrome is a syndrome of pathologic changes consisting of dwarfism (resulting from disturbances of the skeletal-articular system), corneal opacities, coarsening of facial features, leathery skin, and hypertrichosis. It is one of the inherited osteolyses, or "vanishing bone" syndromes.

## OTHER DISORDERS WITH DIFFUSE FIBROSIS

### Nephrogenic Systemic Fibrosis

Nephrogenic systemic fibrosis (NSF) is a fibrosing disorder seen only in patients with kidney failure. It is characterized by two primary features—thickening and hardening of the skin overlying the extremities and trunk and marked expansion and fibrosis of the dermis in association with CD34-positive fibrocytes.

Some patients can have fibrosis of deeper structures, including muscle, fascia, lungs, and heart. NSF has also been called dialysis-associated systemic fibrosis. However, this term is too narrow since the disease is not limited to patients on dialysis.

The number of cases has declined dramatically since initial reports, most certainly due to the avoidance of gadolinium containing agents among at-risk patients.

The skin disease presents with plaques, papules, and/or nodules, with the affected skin becoming thickened and firm with a peau d' orange (orange peel-like) appearance. Manifestations of systemic involvement may include muscle induration, joint contracture, and fibrosis of the lungs, pleura, diaphragm, myocardium, pericardium, and dura mater.

#### Treatment

There is no proven medical therapy for NSF other than recovery of renal function. Several treatments and combinations of treatments have been evaluated, but none has shown consistent benefit.

### GEMSS Syndrome

It is an autosomal dominant condition comprising of GEMSS (Glaucoma, Ectopia, Microspherophakia, Stiff joints, Short stature)"pseudoathletic" build. Cutaneous sclerosis of the upper back and limbs is seen.

### POEMS Syndrome

It includes polyneuropathy, organomegaly (liver, spleen, or lymph nodes), endocrinopathy, M protein (a monoclonal gammopathy), and skin lesions. The cause of POEMS syndrome is unknown, although chronic overproduction of proinflammatory and other cytokines appears to be a major feature of this disorder. Cutaneous findings include hyperpigmentation, hyperhidrosis, hypertrichosis, and diffuse thickening resembling scleroderma. Rarely, angiomas, white fingernails, and alopecia are seen. It appears to be a rare variant of myelomatosis.

### Environmental and Drug-induced Scleroderma

Environmental trigger factors can induce a scleroderma-like reaction in a genetically susceptible host. Exposure to vinyl chloride monomer in workers involved in polyvinyl chloride production, silica dust, and organic solvents like trichloroethylene and perchlorethylene, epoxy resins, and various drugs like penicillamine, sodium valproate, carbidopa, bleomycin, appetite suppressants, and diltiazem can produce cutaneous fibrosis. Toxic oil syndrome is a multisystem illness associated with acute fever, pulmonary edema, myalgia, and pruritic exanthema followed by widespread cutaneous sclerosis. Eosinophilia is often present. Aniline denaturant mixed in rapeseed oil is implicated.

### Colloid Milium

In colloid milium, there are multiple, dome-shaped, and amber- or flesh-colored papules usually in sun exposed sites. Dermal colloid is seen under light microscopy.

The four variants of colloid milium are:

1. Adult-onset
2. A nodular form (nodular colloid degeneration)
3. A juvenile form
4. A pigmented form, due to excess use of hydroquinone.

Colloid milium is a degenerative condition linked to excessive sun exposure and possibly exposure to petroleum products and hydroquinone. The origin of the colloid deposition in the dermis is not certain, but it is thought to be due to degeneration of elastic fibers in the adult form and due to degeneration of UV-transformed keratin.

Dermabrasion, cryotherapy, and diathermy have been tried with limited success. Advice about sunscreen use may also be helpful. Systemic ascorbic acid and exfoliating agents have also been tried with variable results. The Er:YAG laser and photodynamic therapy using methyl-aminolevulinate cream as a photosensitizer have also been tried.

### White Fibrous Papulosis of the Neck

Clinically, this condition is characterized by asymptomatic white papules that appear mainly around the neck in elderly persons. The papules are approximately 2–3 mm in diameter, round to oval, clearly marginated, and unrelated to the hair follicles. The major pathologic change revealed by light microscopic examination is a relatively circumscribed area of thickened collagen bundles in the papillary to mid-dermis.

## Heberden Nodes and Bouchard Nodes

Heberden's nodes are hard or bony swellings that can develop in the distal interphalangeal joints. They are a sign of osteoarthritis and are caused by formation of osteophytes (calcific spurs) of the articular (joint) cartilage in response to repeated trauma at the joint. They are named after William Heberden.

Heberden's nodes typically develop in middle age, beginning either with a chronic swelling of the affected joints or the sudden painful onset of redness, numbness, and loss of manual dexterity. This initial inflammation and pain eventually subsides, and the patient is left with a permanent bony outgrowth that often skews the fingertip sideways.

Heberden's nodes are more common in women than in men, and there seems to be a genetic component involved in predisposition to the condition.

Bouchard's nodes are similar bony growths in the PIP joints, and are also associated with osteoarthritis.

## Hypertrophic Scars and Keloids

Keloids are the result of an overgrowth of dense fibrous tissue that usually develops after healing of a skin injury (Figs 3 and 4). The tissue extends beyond the borders of the original wound, does not usually regress spontaneously, and tends to recur after excision.

They occur due to trauma to the skin, both physical (e.g., earlobe piercing, surgery) and pathological (e.g., acne, chickenpox). The susceptibility increases due to presence of foreign material, infection, hematoma, or increased skin tension.

In hypertrophic scars, there are erythematous, pruritic, and raised fibrous lesions. It usually does not expand beyond the boundaries of the initial injury and can spontaneously partially resolve. They are more common after injuries that involve the deep dermis and after thermal injuries.

### Pathophysiology

Hypertrophic scars and keloids are formed due to variations of typical wound healing. During the normal wound healing process, anabolic, and catabolic processes equilibrium is achieved in approximately 6–8 weeks after the injury. After this, the strength of the wound is around 30–40% of healthy skin.

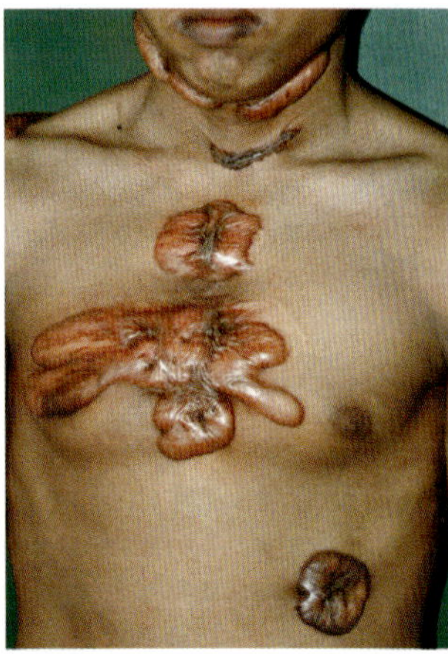

**FIG. 3:** Keloid on chest.

*Courtesy:* Dr Somesh Gupta, Department of Dermatology & Venereology, All India Institute of Medical Sciences, New Delhi.

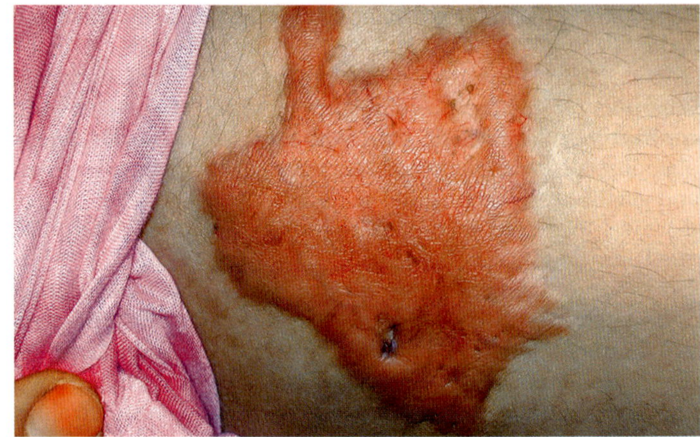

**FIG. 4:** Postburn keloid on abdomen.

*Courtesy:* Dr Somesh Gupta, Department of Dermatology & Venereology, All India Institute of Medical Sciences, New Delhi.

During the process of scar maturation cross-linking of collagen fibers occurs and the scar improves. The scar becomes hyperemic and thickened. It can subside gradually over months and become flat, white, stretched, and mature scar.

If there is an imbalance between the anabolic and catabolic phase and more collagen is produced, scar grows and becomes elevated above the skin.

The identifying structural unit of hypertrophic scars and keloids is the collagen nodule. It is made up of a high density of fibroblasts and unidirectional collagen fibrils which are arranged in highly organized orientation. They also have rich vasculature, thickened epidermal cell layer, and high mesenchymal cell density.

Keloids and hypertrophic scars are difficult to differentiate in the early phases of formation. Histologically, there is presence of broad, dull, and pink bundles of collagen (hyalinized bundles of collagen) in keloids, which are not present in hypertrophic scars.

### Pathogenesis

This is unknown. Ethnic factor are possibly important pigmented race, individuals of African, Asian, and Hispanic are prone to develop keloid.

### Treatment

Keloids and hypertrophic scars may be asymptomatic. They may also be tender, painful, or pruritic or they may cause a burning sensation. In addition to symptomatic relief, cosmetic concern is the primary reason patients seek medical intervention.

The treatment of keloids depend on the location, size, and depth of the lesion; patients age; and response to treatment.

The treatment options for hypertrophic scars and keloids are intralesional corticosteroid injections, occlusive dressings, compression therapy, cryosurgery, excision, radiation therapy, laser therapy, interferon therapy, 5-fluorouracil (5-FU), doxorubicin, bleomycin, verapamil, retinoic acid, imiquimod 5% cream, tamoxifen, tacrolimus, and botulinum toxin. One double blind control trial among 40 patients showed 5-FU was significantly more effective than intralesional steroids in the treatment of KD.

The other promising therapies include antiangiogenic factors, including vascular endothelial growth factor inhibitors (e.g., bevacizumab), phototherapy (photodynamic therapy, UVA-1 therapy, narrowband UVB therapy), transforming growth factor β3, tumor necrosis factor-α inhibitors (etanercept), and recombinant human interleukin-10, which are directed at decreasing collagen synthesis.

## SUGGESTED READINGS


1. DeBrule MB, Mott RC, Funk C, et al. Osseous metaplasia in plantar fibromatosis: a case report. J Foot Ankle Surg. 2004;43(6):430-2.
2. Evans HL. Multinucleated giant cells in plantar fibromatosis. Am J Surg Pathol. 2002;26(2):244-8.
3. McPoil TG, Martin RL, Cornwall MW, et al. Heel pain--plantar fasciitis: clinical practice guildelines linked to the international classification of function, disability, and health from the orthopaedic section of the American Physical Therapy Association. J Orthop Sports PhysTher. 2008;38(4):A1-8.
4. Montgomery E, Lee JH, Abraham SC, et al. Superficial fibromatoses are genetically distinct from deep fibromatoses. Mod Pathol. 2001;14(7):695-701.
5. Reitamo JJ, Häyry P, Nykyri E, et al. The desmoid tumor. I. Incidence, sex, age- and anatomical distribution in the Finnish population. Am J Clin Pathol. 1982;77:665.
6. Wiedemann HR, Burgio GR, Aldenhoff P, et al. The proteus syndrome. Partial gigantism of the hands and/or feet, nevi, hemihypertrophy, subcutaneous tumors, macrocephaly or other skull anomalies and possible accelerated growth and visceral affections. Eur J Pediatr. 1983;140(1):5-12.
7. Wu C, Amini-Nik S, Nadesan P, et al. Aggressive fibromatosis (desmoid tumor) is derived from mesenchymal progenitor cells. Cancer Res. 2010;70(19):7690-8.

# 48 CHAPTER Connective Tissue Disorders

*Rajesh Kumar, Parasar Ghosh*

## INTRODUCTION

Connective tissue disorders (CTDs) are a group of autoimmune multisystem diseases of unknown etiology characterized by autoantibodies directed against cellular component and clinically have varied and distinctive features. The diseases under this category have many common clinical and serological markers and often, there is an overlap. The common diseases under this group are lupus erythematosus [systemic lupus erythematosus (SLE) and discoid lupus erythematosus (DLE)], systemic sclerosis, morphea (localized and generalized), dermatomyositis (DM), and mixed connective tissue diseases (MCTDs). Previously, these entities were grouped under either collagen diseases or collagen vascular diseases. These terminologies are incorrect as there are no enough evidences to suggest that collagen is primarily at fault.

These diseases are also called autoimmune diseases as the circulating specific antibodies bind self-protein and attack organ-specific system. These disease-specific antibodies are serologic markers of specific CTDs.

## LUPUS ERYTHEMATOSUS

Lupus erythematosus is a group of heterogeneous illnesses as a result of autoantibodies against own deoxyribonucleic acid (DNA). The disease has varied presentation with involvement of skin only at one end to several organs at the other end. The skin lesions may be typical of lupus erythematosus and called lupus-specific skin lesions or lesions may be seen in other diseases (nonspecific lupus erythematosus lesions). The lupus specific skin lesions are categorized into acute cutaneous lupus erythematosus (ACLE), subacute cutaneous lupus erythematosus (SCLE) or chronic cutaneous lupus erythematosus (CCLE) (Flowchart 1). The nonspecific lesions are nonscarring alopecia, mouth ulcer, photosensitivity, and Raynaud's phenomenon. It is more predominant in females (male to female ratio—1:9).

### Acute Cutaneous Lupus Erythematosus

The ACLE has a typical onset of malar rash (butterfly rash) (Fig. 1) and is usually associated with visceral involvement. The erythema is confined to malar area, bridge of the nose, and characteristically spares the nasolabial folds. The erythema is invariably associated with some amount of edema. In few cases, the forehead, chin and V area of neck may be involved and give an overall appearance of swollen face. In rare occurrence, the morbilliform rash may be generalized (generalized ACLE) and typically involves arms and hands. The knuckles of the hand are invariably spared. The cutaneous lesions of ACLE are often precipitated by ultraviolet (UV) rays or sun exposure. The lesions may last for weeks to months depending upon the underlying disease activity and sun exposure. The malar rash may heal with pigmentation or may persist as persistent erythema. ACLE lesions may be associated with SCLE skin lesions but rarely has CCLE (discoid) lesions.

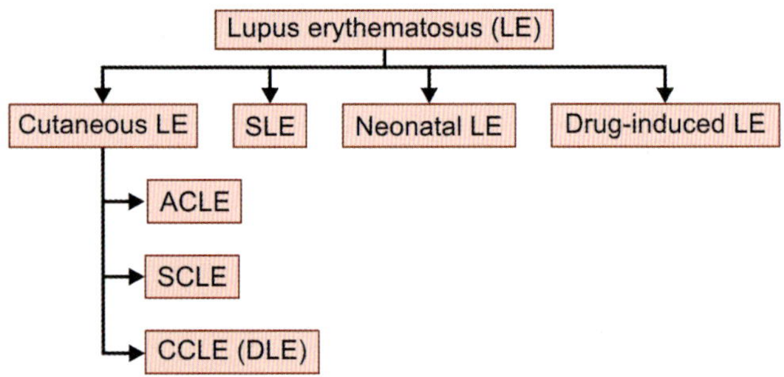


SLE, systemic lupus erythematosus; ACLE, acute cutaneous lupus erythematosus; SCLE, subacute cutaneous lupus erythematosus; CCLE, chronic cutaneous lupus erythematosus; DLE, discoid lupus erythematosus.

**FLOWCHART 1:** Types of lupus erythematosus

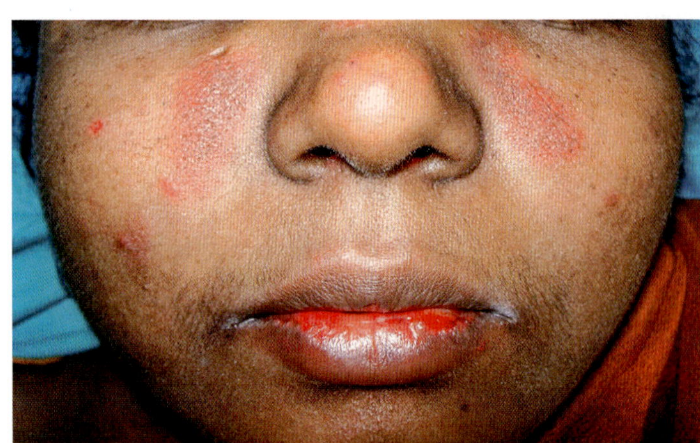

**FIG. 1:** Malar (butterfly) rash.

**BOX 1 Clinical type of subacute cutaneous lupus erythematosus**

- Polymorphous light eruption type lesions
- Annular lesions
- Papulosquamous (psoriasiform) lesions
- Neonatal lupus erythematosus
- Drug-induced lupus erythematosus

**BOX 2 Type of chronic cutaneous lupus erythematosus [discoid lupus erythematosus (DLE)]**

- Classic DLE (either localized or generalized)
- Hypertrophic or verrucous DLE
- Lupus panniculitis/profundus
- Mucosal DLE (oral or conjunctival)
- Lichenoid DLE (lupus erythematosus/lichen planus overlap)
- Tumid DLE

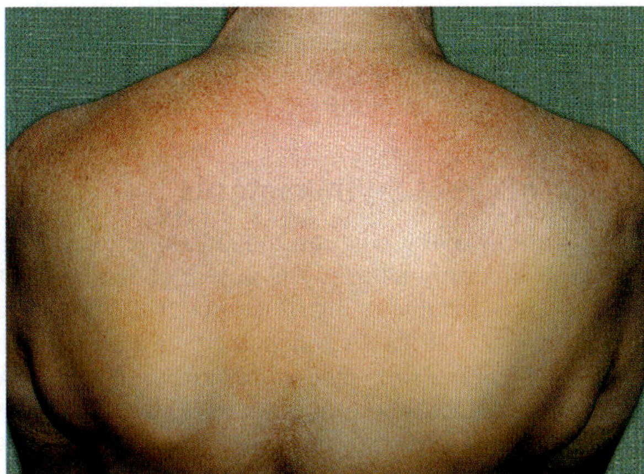

**FIG. 2:** Acute cutaneous lupus erythematosus.
*Courtesy*: Dr Saurabh Singh, Associate Professor, AIIMS , Jodhpur, Rajasthan.

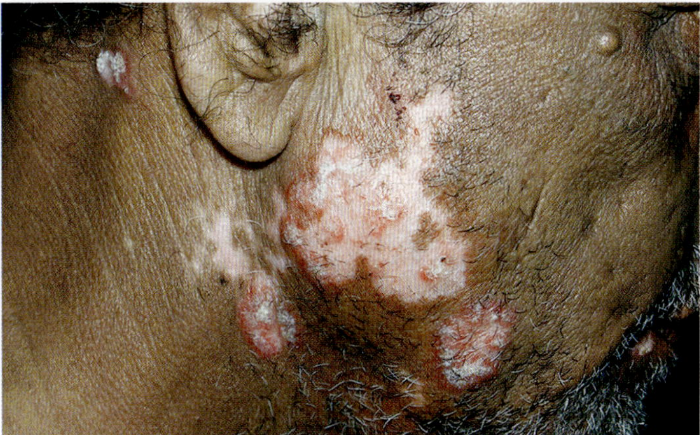

**FIG. 3:** Chronic cutaneous lupus erythematosus discoid lupus erythematosus.

## Subacute Cutaneous Lupus Erythematosus (Box 1)

This variant of lupus erythematosus has distinct clinicopathological features characterized by erythematous to papulosquamous (psoriasiform) and annular lesions predominantly over sun-exposed areas (Fig. 2). The lesions are precipitated by and sensitive to sunlight. Invariably these patients have circulating antibodies to the Ro/SSA nucleoprotein. The lesions are long-lasting and heal with vitiligo-like lesions. Approximately 15–20% of cases may be either associated with ACLE or few DLE like lesions. The basic difference from ACLE is that these lesions are long lasting, little thicker and heal with hypo- to depigmentation whereas the lesions of ACLE are edematous and heal without pigmentation. Approximately 10–15% cases of ACLE may develop into severe SLE involving inner organs [kidney and central nervous system (CNS)]. Neonatal lupus erythematosus (NLE) and drug-induced lupus erythematosus (DILE) have features of SCLE.

## Chronic Cutaneous Lupus Erythematosus

Chronic cutaneous lupus erythematosus most commonly referred as DLE has several subtypes. They may be localized as confined to face and neck or generalized with lesions involving below neck. Less common forms are hypertrophic and wart like lesions on palms and soles (painful), oral DLE, lupus tumidus, and lupus panniculitis (Box 2). The classical CCLE (DLE) lesion is coin-shaped lesion with prominent hyperpigmented margin (Fig. 3). The overall appearance is like a mixture of erythema, depigmentation, scaling and atrophy (Box 3). They may take different shape and sizes. The hair follicles within the lesions are prominent and dilated. They are often occupied by the keratin of overlying scales. When one removes the scale the portion occupying the hair follicle came out as spike or carpet tack (the famous "carpet tack" sign).

**BOX 3 Clinical feature of discoid lupus erythematosus**

Chronic cutaneous lupus erythematosus
- Well-defined margin with hyperpigmentation
- Central atrophy with telangiectasias
- Carpet tack sign
- Face, scalp, ear

**BOX 4 Lupus erythematosus, nonspecific skin lesions**

- Vasculopathy (urticarial, vasculitic and livedo reticularis type of lesions)
- Mucosal lesions
- Nonscarring alopecia (lupus hair)
- Bullous lupus erythematosus

## Systemic Lupus Erythematosus

In SLE, apart from systemic involvement the patient may develop one or more skin manifestations. The skin findings are specific to lupus erythematosus or nonspecific which may occur in other CTDs (Box 4). The lupus erythematosus-specific skin lesions are malar or discoid rash (Fig. 1), photosensitivity to exposed areas, oral ulcers (Fig. 4) and in advanced case lupus hair. Sometimes, there may be erythema multiforme (EM)-like lesions (Rowell's syndrome), annular lesions (SCLE), intense reaction to sun exposure (edema of the face or bullous lesions). In nonspecific lesions, there are reticulate telangiectatic erythema on palms (both thenar and hypothenar eminences), palmar aspect of fingers, urticarial lesions (nonpruritic and fixed in position) and Raynaud's phenomenon.

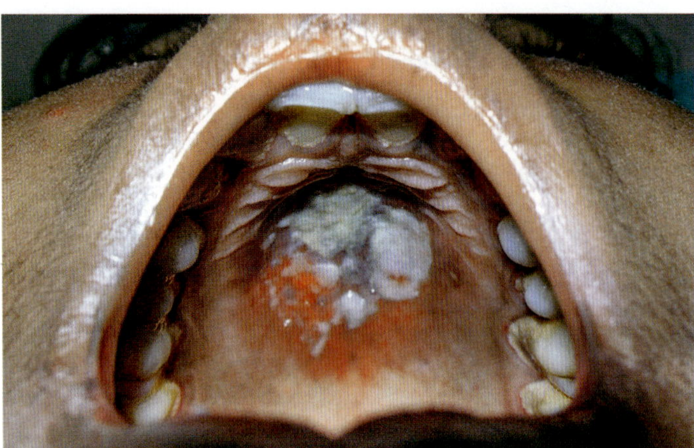

**FIG. 4:** Oral ulcer with superadded *Candida* infection in a patient with systemic lupus erythematosus.

**BOX 5 Features of drug-induced lupus erythematosus**

- *Features are those of SCLE*: Annular or psoriasiform plaque
- Definitive history and temporal association of drug intake
- Fever, serositis, hepatosplenomegaly
- Older age of onset
- Absence of malar rash, oral ulcers
- Arthralgia and arthritis are prominent features

SCLE, subacute cutaneous lupus erythematosus.

**BOX 6 Drug-induced lupus erythematosus**

- *Definite (well-controlled studies)*: Hydralazine, procainamide, isoniazid, chlorpromazine
- *Possible*: Carbamazepine, phenytoin, penicillamine, beta-blockers
- *Probable*: Tetracycline, penicillin, griseofulvin, psoralen plus ultraviolet A (PUVA) therapy
- *Recently documented*: Terbinafine , calcium channel blockers, efalizumab, leflunomide, docetaxel

## Drug-induced Lupus Erythematosus

Drug-induced lupus erythematosus manifests similarly as SLE in milder form. The clinical features are more like a SCLE (Box 5). The patients may develop the lesions after 3 weeks to 2 years after intake of suspected drugs. As compared to SLE, the age of onset is older and has no history of prior SLE. Invariably, the only symptoms are arthritis or arthralgia (90% of the cases). Other systemic involvements like fever, serositis (pleurisy and pericarditis) and hepatosplenomegaly and also skin manifestations. The typical skin manifestations of SLE (butterfly rash, alopecia, discoid lesions, and oral ulcers) are missing in DILE. The clinical features are those of SCLE (annular or papulosquamous). The drugs commonly implicated in inducing DILE are procainamide, hydralazine, isoniazid, hydrochlorothiazides, calcium channel blockers (diltiazem, nifedipine), biologics (etanercept, infliximab), and a growing list of newer drugs (Box 6). The lesions and serological markers [antinuclear antibody (ANA) and anti-Ro] start decreasing after withdrawal of the offending drugs.

## Neonatal Lupus Erythematosus

Neonatal lupus erythematosus may be due to transplacental passage of maternal autoantibodies to the fetus. The most characteristics clinical features of NLE are skin lesions and congenital heart block. The skin lesions either present at birth or appear within a month. The lesions characteristically involve face particularly around eyes. The typical lesions are scaly erythematous plaques with central atrophy. Around eye, they give an appearance of raccoon's eye, owl eye or eye mask. These infants may have transient hemolytic anemia, thrombocytopenia, leukopenia, and hepatosplenomegaly. The mother of the affected infant may have an active disease of SLE or Sjögren's syndrome with anti-Ro or anti-La antibody positivity.

## Evaluation of Lupus Erythematosus

The diagnosis essentially is a combination of clinical findings supported by laboratory tests. The essential laboratory tests are skin biopsy, complete blood count (CBC), erythrocyte sedimentation rate (ESR), ANA and anticytoplasmic antibodies.

Table 1 depicts the simplified version of the latest Systemic Lupus International Collaborating Clinics (SLICC) classification criteria for SLE. Readers are requested to read the original publication.

### Antinuclear Antibodies

The ANA test is a nonspecific test and titer below 1:16 is considered negative and the titer above 1:64 is significant. Almost all type of patterns (peripheral, homogeneous, speckled and nucleolar) except anticentromere (positive in CREST syndrome) are common in SLE. The ANA positivity is highest (approximately 100 %) in SLE and drug induced lupus. In SCLE, ANA positivity is around 70% and NLE its 30%. The ANA is negative in CCLE (DLE). However, ANA negative SLE has been reported.

**TABLE 1: Diagnosing systemic lupus erythematosus (2012 SLICC SLE criteria)**

*Requirements*: More than or equal to four criteria (at least 1 clinical and 1 laboratory criteria) or biopsy proven lupus nephritis with positive antinuclear antibody or anti-DNA

| Clinical criteria | Immunological criteria |
|---|---|
| • Acute cutaneous lupus<br>• Chronic cutaneous lupus<br>• Oral or nasal ulcers<br>• Nonscarring alopecia<br>• Arthritis<br>• Serositis<br>• Renal<br>• Neurologic<br>• Hemolytic anemia<br>• Leukopenia<br>• Thrombocytopenia (<100,000/mm$^3$) | • Antinuclear antibody<br>• Anti-DNA<br>• Anti-Sm<br>• Antiphospholipid Ab<br>• Low complement (C3, C4, CH50)<br>• Direct Coombs test (do not count in presence of hemolytic anemia) |

Ab, antibodies; DNA, deoxyribonucleic acid; SLICC, Systemic Lupus International Collaborating Clinics.

*With permission from*: Petri M, Orbai AM, Alarcón GS, et al. Derivation and validation of the Systemic Lupus International Collaborating Clinics classification criteria for systemic lupus erythematosus. Arthritis Rheum. 2012;64(8):2677-86.

### Anti-double Stranded DNA Antibodies

Serum anti-double stranded DNA (anti-dsDNA) antibodies are specific for SLE or ACLE. The levels of anti-dsDNA antibodies may be helpful in monitoring the diseases. These antibodies are positive in 20–30% cases of Sjögren's syndrome or MCTDs. Occasionally (<5%), it is positive in systemic sclerosis and CCLE (DLE).

### Antibodies to Extractable Nuclear Antigens

In this group of autoantibodies, the SS-A (Ro) and SS-B (La) are positive in NLE and in 60% cases SS-A (Ro) is positive in SCLE. The Sm antibodies (against Smith antigen) are highly specific for LE. Antihistone antibodies are specific for DILE.

### Skin Biopsy (Histopathology)

The histopathological findings of different subset of lupus erythematosus are summarized in table 2.

## Treatment of Lupus Erythematosus

Various options and a step-ladder for the management are mentioned in table 3.

**TABLE 2: Histopathology of different lupus erythematosus lesions**

| Histopathology findings | ACLE | SCLE | CCLE(DLE) |
|---|---|---|---|
| Follicular plugging | 0 | 0 | +++ |
| Hyperkeratosis | + | ++ | +++ |
| Thickened basement membrane | 0 | + | +++ |
| Lichenoid infiltrate | + | ++ | +++ |
| Periappendageal inflammation | 0 | + | +++ |

0, absent; +, mild; ++, moderate; +++, heavy.
ACLE, acute cutaneous lupus erythematosus; SCLE, subacute cutaneous lupus erythematosus; CCLE, chronic cutaneous lupus erythematosus; DLE, discoid lupus erythematosus.

1. *Photoprotection*: As the lesions of lupus erythematosus are initiated and aggravated by exposure to sunlight. Strict photoprotection is must in patients with lupus erythematosus.
   - Avoidance of peak hour (noon) sunlight between 10 AM and 3 PM
   - Use of broad-spectrum sunscreen: Apply 20–30 minutes before going out and should be repeated at an interval of 3–4 hours
   - Broad-brimmed hat, full sleeve tightly woven clothes.
2. *Corticosteroids*:
   - Topical either in form of cream, ointment and lotion depending upon the site and severity of skin lesions
   - Intralesional, in case of hypertrophic DLE or lesions not responding to topical
   - Systemic, in case of SLE, the dose and duration varies according to severity of the disease.
3. *Antimalarials*: They play an important role in treating cutaneous lupus erythematosus. How it acts is unknown, but may be via photoprotection and immunomodulation.
   - Chloroquine: 4 mg/kg/day
   - Hydroxychloroquine: 6.5 mg/kg/day, 200–400 mg/day.

   Ophthalmological examination (at baseline and then yearly) is must to monitor the ocular toxicity of the antimalarials.
4. *Biologicals*: Recently, different biologics have been used in the treatment of SLE notable among are rituximab, abatacept and belimumab. Out of these only belimumab is approved for ANA positive SLE. Belimumab, fully humanized monoclonal antibody inhibiting B-lymphocyte stimulator action. It is given as 10 mg/kg intravenously once in 2 weeks for 6 weeks (3 doses at an interval of 2 weeks) then 4 weeks.

## DERMATOMYOSITIS

Dermatomyositis combines inflammatory myopathy along with skin lesions. Bohan and Peter suggested the criteria to diagnose DM (Box 7).

**TABLE 3: Treatment options of lupus erythematosus**

| Treatment | | |
|---|---|---|
| First line | Topical corticosteroids | Potent class 1 corticosteroids for 2 weeks then switch to mid-potent class 4 |
| | Topical calcineurin inhibitor | Either tacrolimus 0.1% bid or pimecrolimus 1% bid |
| | Interalesional steroids | 2.5–10 mg/cc |
| Second line | Aminoquinolines [chloroquine, hydroxychloroquine (HCQ), quinacrine] | HCQ: 6.5 mg/kg/day(start with 400 mg/day for initial 2 months then reduce it to 200 mg/day for rest of life)<br>Chloroquine: 3.5 mg/kg/day<br>Quinacrine (add only when monotherapy with HCQ or chloroquine failed) 100 mg daily |
| | Prednisolone | 1–2 mg/kg body weight per day depending upon the severity of the disease |
| | Thalidomide | 50–200 mg/day, monitor sensory neuropathy |
| Third line | Azathioprine | 1.5–2.5 mg/kg/day |
| | Mycophenolate mofetil | 2.5–3.5 mg/kg/day |
| | Methotrexate | 7.5–25 mg/week |
| | Dapsone | 50–200 mg/day |
| | Isotretinoin | 0.5–2 mg/kg/day |
| | Acitretin | 10–50 mg/day |

**BOX 7 Bohan and Peter (modified) criteria of diagnosing dermatomyositis (DM)**

*Major criteria:*
- Typical skin rash
- Proximal muscle weakness (symmetric)
- Abnormal muscle biopsy
- Elevation of skeletal muscle enzymes [creatine phosphokinase, aldolase, serum glutamic oxaloacetic transaminase]
- Electromyographic evidence of myopathy

*Criteria for diagnosing DM:*
- *Definitive*: Skin rash and three major criteria
- *Probable*: Skin rash and two major criteria
- *Possible*: Skin rash and one major criteria

**BOX 8 Types of inflammatory myopathies**

- Dermatomyositis (DM)
  - Adult-onset
    - Classic DM
    - DM with malignancy
    - DM overlap with SLE or MCTD
    - Amyopathic DM (DM sine myositis)
  - Juvenile-onset (JDMS)
    - Classic DM
    - Amyopathic JDMS
- Polymyositis
- Inclusion body myositis

MCTD, mixed connective tissue disease; SLE, systemic lupus erythematosus; JDMS, juvenile dermatomyositis

**TABLE 4: Difference between adult-onset dermatomyositis and juvenile dermatomyositis**

| Clinical feature | Adult-onset DM | Juvenile DM |
|---|---|---|
| Malignancy | +++ | + |
| Interstitial lung disease | +++ | 0 |
| Calcinosis cutis and ulceration | + | +++ |

0, absent; +, mild; ++, moderate; +++, heavy.
DM, dermatomyositis.

The idiopathic inflammatory myopathies (Box 8) may be of three types but DM per se is clinically divided into two types: (1) childhood-onset and (2) adult-onset DM (Table 4).

- *Childhood-onset (juvenile DM)*: It has better prognosis compared to adult-onset disease
- *Adult-onset*: It has prolonged and progressive course unless treated and may be either preceded or followed by malignancy.

Average age of disease onset in childhood is 6.9 years while adult variant is seen between 40 and 60 years with a female to male ratio of 2.3:1.

## Etiology

Exact etiopathogenesis is not known. Inflammatory changes may start by interaction of genetic predisposition with antigen stimulation and other environmental agents leading to disease manifestations.

Infective agents like Coxsackie B virus and group A streptococci are frequently associated with onset as well as disease flares. Environmental factors like excessive sun exposure may precipitate the disease.

*Drug-induced DM*: There are drugs known to cause DM are hydroxyurea, penicillamine, quinidine, phenylbutazone, and statins.

## Clinical Features

*Skin manifestations*: In 50% patients, rash is often the first symptom mainly starting in sun-exposed areas.

- *Heliotrope rash*: The characteristic periorbital violaceous erythema (heliotrope) may cross the bridge of nose in a mask like distribution and involve the ears also (Fig. 5)
- *Gottron's papules*: Papules over joints especially the metacarpophalangeal, proximal phalangeal, and distal phalangeal joints of hand (Fig. 6)
- *Gottron's sign*: Symmetrical lilac erythema with edema over interphalangeal or metacarpophalangeal joints, elbows and knees
- Nailfold telangiectasias, malar erythema, and poikiloderma
- *Shawl sign*: It is a symmetric confluent violaceous erythema extending from dorsum of hands, forearms, and arms to shoulder and neck (Fig. 7)
- *Calcinosis cutis*: Hard calcium deposits in the skin seen especially in juvenile variants; some times with ulcerations (Fig. 8)
- *Mechanic hands*: Development of symmetric hyperkeratosis over ulnar side of thumbs and radial side of fingers
- *Proximal myopathy*: Weakness of proximal muscles result in difficulty in getting up from bed, climbing stairs or combing hair. Gowers' sign (climbing up the body) is positive
- Hoarseness of voice and dysphagia are serious manifestations and require immediate hospitalization and require aggressive treatment
- *Other manifestations*:
  - Cardiomyopathy
  - Raynaud's phenomenon
  - Arthralgia
  - Malignancy (especially adult DM).

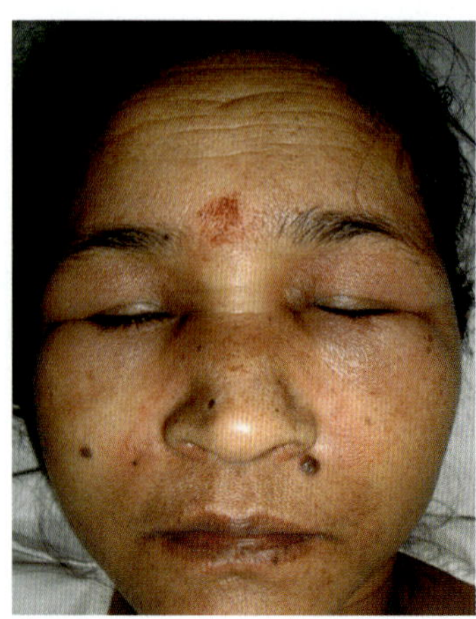

**FIG. 5:** Heliotrope rash.
*Courtesy*: Dr Saurabh Singh, Associate Professor, AIIMS, Jodhpur, Rajasthan.

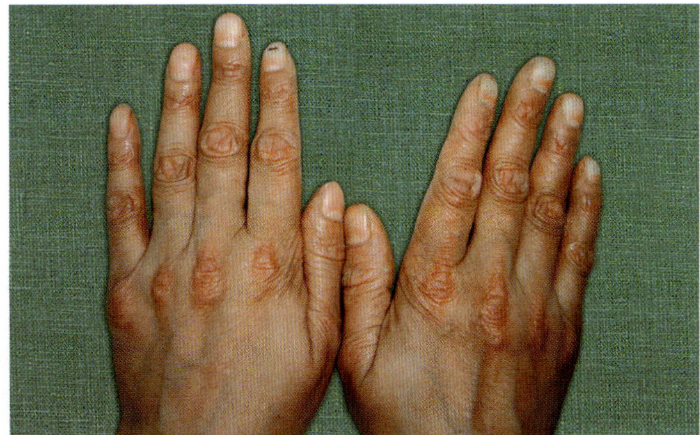

**FIG. 6:** Gottron's papules.
*Courtesy*: Dr Saurabh Singh, Associate Professor, AIIMS , Jodhpur, Rajasthan.

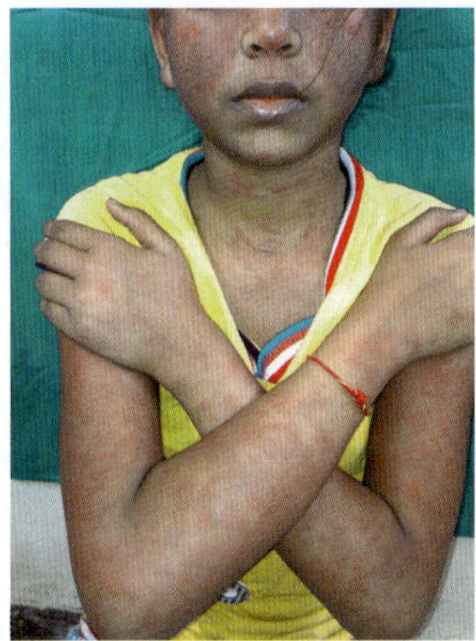

**FIG. 7:** Shawl sign.
*Courtesy*: Dr Saurabh Singh, Associate Professor, AIIMS , Jodhpur, Rajasthan.

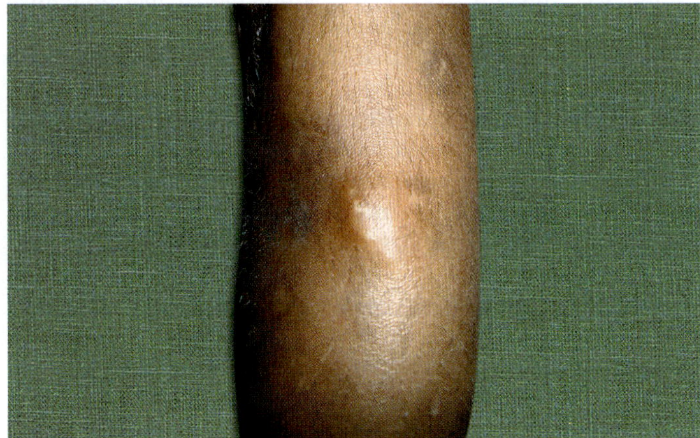

**FIG. 8:** Calcinosis cutis.
*Courtesy*: Dr Saurabh Singh, Associate Professor, AIIMS , Jodhpur, Rajasthan.

## Evaluation of Dermatomyositis

Protocol for evaluation of dermatomyositis/polymyositis is presented in box 9. The skin rash of DM may sometimes be confused with SLE rash (Table 5).

**BOX 9 Evaluation of the patient with dermatomyositis**

- *History*:
  - Previous malignancy
  - Associated symptoms
  - History of toxins, infections, travel, vaccination, or drug intake
- *Physical examination*:
  - Dermatological evaluation
  - *ENT evaluation*: To exclude nasopharyngeal carcinoma
  - *Women*: To rule out pelvic and breast cancer
  - *Men*: To rule out colorectal and prostate cancer
- *Evaluation of muscle disease*:
  - *Muscle enzymes*: CPK, LDH, aldolase EMG
  - *MRI*: Espcially preferred in childern in whom EMG (being painful) is usually avoided
  - *Muscle biopsy*: Espcially in cases of polymyositis
- *Skin disease evaluation*:
  - Lesional biopsy for routine histopathology evaluation
  - Immunofluorescence in selected patient
- *Routine studies*:
  - Complete blood count
  - Comprehensive metabolic panel and urine analysis
  - Thyroid function tests
  - Stool occult blood tests
  - Electrocardiography
  - Women: Pap smear, CA-125
  - Gastrointestinal endoscopy
  - Fasting glucose and lipid profile (in children)
- *Radiographic*:
  - Chest X-ray, high-resolution computed tomography
  - CT scan chest/abdomen
  - *Women*: Pelvic ultrasound, pelvic CT scan, mammography
- Pulmonary function tests (with diffusions studies)

ENT, ear nose throat; CPK, creatine phosphokinase; LDH, lactate dehydrogenase; EMG, electromyography; MRI, magnetic resonance imaging; CT, computed tomography.

**TABLE 5: Differential diagnosis dermatomyositis with systemic lupus erythematosus**

| Systemic lupus erythematosus | Dermatomyositis |
|---|---|
| Malar rash | Periorbital heliotrope rash |
| No Gottron's papule | Gottron's papule seen |
| Preferential involvement of skin between the joints (joints spared) | Joints are involved (interphalangeal joints and metacarpophalangeal joints) |
| Proximal muscle may involve | Proximal muscle prominent |
| Pruritus may be | Pruritus is a prominent feature |
| • *Laboratory*:<br>○ ANA ++<br>○ Anti-Ro (SSA) +<br>○ Anti-ds DNA ++<br>○ Anti-Sm ++ | • *Laboratory*:<br>○ ANA ++<br>○ Anti-Jo-1 ++<br>○ Anti-SRP antibody (signal recognition particle)<br>○ Anti-Mi-2 |
| *Malignancy*: Nil | Malignancy associated in 20–30% |

ANA, antinuclear antibody; DNA, deoxyribonucleic acid; SSA, Sjögren's-syndrome-related antigen A.

## Treatment of Dermatomyositis

1. *General measures*: Sun protection, use of moisturizers, and antihistaminics
2. *Immunosuppressive therapy*: Steroids are mainstay of therapy to reduce the inflammation and control the disease. They can be given as oral prednisolone 1–2 mg/kg/day. The treatment is usually given for at least 2–3 years after achievement of remission. However, many patients require lifelong treatment.

   Steroid may cause proximal myopathy in itself. To differentiate idiopathic myositis from drug-induced myopathy, we need to take a good drug history. If the treatment seems to be inadequate, then to increase the dose of corticosteroids. If weakness improves then it was due to disease; if it worsens, it is steroid-induced.

   Other immunosuppressive drugs used are weekly methotrexate (15–20 mg/$m^2$/week), azathioprine (1–2 mg/kg/day), and cyclosporine (3 mg/kg/day)
3. Physical and occupational therapy.

# SCLERODERMA

Scleroderma is a chronic disease of unknown cause and includes a spectrum of disorders caused by fibrosis affecting the dermis. Peak age is 30–50 years with female to male ratio of 4:1.

## Etiopathogenesis

The exact cause is unknown, but it appears to be due to injury to vascular endothelium. Autoimmune process plays an important role in pathogenesis with presence of ANAs specific for topoisomerase I (Scl-70) and centromere. Rarely, it occurs due to exposure to polyvinyl chloride, bleomycin, and pentazocine. Graft- versus-host reaction may cause sclerosis of the skin.

## Classification

Classification of scleroderma has been shown in box 10.

**BOX 10 Classification of scleroderma**

- Localized scleroderma:
  - Morphea (plaque, guttate or subcutaneous)
  - Generalized morphea
  - Linear scleroderma (en coup de sabre)
- Systemic sclerosis:
  - Limited (no truncal involvement)
  - Diffuse (widespread skin involvement)
  - CREST syndrome (both limited and diffuse may manifest)

## Clinical Features

- *Raynaud phenomenon*: It is the earliest and most frequent symptom induced by cold and sometimes stress. It affects fingers, toes, ears and tip of nose. The episodes occur due to arterial spasm and typical sequence of color changes occur in form of whitening, cyanosis and hyperemia. Frequent and prolonged episodes eventually lead to sclerodactyly, fingertip ulcerations, or even gangrene
- *Skin changes*: It starts as edematous phase lasting for several months with edema of hands, feet and sometimes face. Gradually and progressively edema decreases followed by skin tightening which spreads proximally. There is a typical facies which comprises of smoothening of facial lines, breaking nose, thinning of lips, difficulty in opening mouth, radial furrowing around mouth (purse string). The atrophic skin becomes shiny and waxy with ulcers over pressure points like elbows. The patient may develop widespread hyperpigmentation that simulates Addison's disease, more commonly there is a patchy, often follicular hypo- or hyperpigmentation (salt and pepper appearance). Telangiectasia may occur on face, chest, lips, and fingertips
- *Pulmonary diseases*: It occurs due to arterial and interstitial involvement resulting in exertion dyspnea, decreased diffusion capacity, pulmonary hypertension and right-sided heart failure
- *Renal involvement*: It causes renovascular hypertension
- *Other systems*: Esophageal involvement may lead to dysphagia
- The CREST syndrome is an acronym for clinical manifestations found in both localized and diffuse systemic sclerosis and characterized by:
  - **C**alcinosis
  - **R**aynaud's phenomenon
  - **E**sophageal dysmotility
  - **S**clerodactyly
  - **T**elangiectasias.

## Evaluation of Scleroderma

Patient frequently gives history of Raynaud's phenomenon. Skin changes typical of scleroderma are helpful for clinical diagnosis. Serological markers like ANA, anticentromere antibody, antitopoisomerase antibodies (formerly Scl-70) are often necessary. Pulmonary function tests, echocardiography, barium meal swallow are done to evaluate the extent of systemic involvement.

Criteria have been devised for diagnosis. One major and two minor criteria are required for diagnosis. Please refer to the original publication for detailed discussion on the criteria.

The criteria are not applicable to patients with skin thickening sparing the finger or to patients who have scleroderma-like disorder that better explains their manifestations (e.g., nephrogenic sclerosing fibrosis, generalized morphea, eosinophilic fasciitis, scleroderma diabeticorum, scleromyxedema, erythromelalgia, porphyria, lichen sclerosus, graft-versus-host disease, diabetic cheiroarthropathy)

The total score is determined by adding the maximum weight (score) in each category.

Patients with a total score of more than or equal to nine are classified as definite scleroderma. This has a sensitivity of 91% and specificity of 92%.

## Treatment

No specific treatment is available.

1. Avoidance of cold, wearing socks and gloves, and using warm water

2. Immunosuppressive agents like corticosteroids and methotrexate for skin tighetening. Mycophenolate, cyclophosphamide and recently rituximab for lung involvement. Phosphodiesterase inhibitors and endothelin receptor antagonists for pulmonary artery hypertension
3. Parenteral prostaglandins for ischemic digits, calcium channel blockers, and topical vasodilators like nitroglycerin paste can be used
4. Physical and occupational therapy.

## LOCALIZED SCLERODERMA (MORPHEA)

This is strictly a cutaneous disorder with no systemic involvement. Most common presentation is solitary or multiple circumscribed patches of erythema that gradually changes to sclerotic atrophic plaques. There is lesional loss of sweating and reduced hair. Most common sites involved are upper trunk, abdomen, buttocks, legs, and face.

### Variants

- *Linear morphea:* Linear indurated plaque most commonly on extremities but when confined to frontal scalp, mid-face and forehead it is called "en coup de sabre"
- *Generalized morphea*: Widespread involvement, multiple plaques (4 or more lesions, and individual lesions may be larger than 3 cm) and with no systemic features
- *Morphea profunda*: It is a type of subcutaneous morphea/deep morphea characterized by fibrotic bands over shoulder, back and neck. The overlying skin is either hyper- or hypopigmente
- *Pansclerotic morphea*: A rare form of mutilating morphea affecting skin, subcutaneous fat, fascia, muscles, and even bone
- *Parry–Romberg syndrome (progressive hemifacial atrophy)*: Loss of tissue on one side of the face that may involve dermis, subcutaneous tissue, muscle, and bone. The overlying skin is mobile.

### Diagnosis

- *Skin biopsy*: It is showing dermal sclerosis with apparent pulling up of appendages
- Antinuclear antibodies are infrequent.

### Treatment

Topical corticosteroids, calcipotriene, and ultraviolet A (UVA) therapy are effective modalities of treatment.

## MIXED CONNECTIVE TISSUE DISEASE

Mixed connective tissue disease or overlap syndrome is a rare autoimmune disorder that has features of three other CTDs (SLE, scleroderma, and polymyositis). It is more common in female of 40–60 years age group.

### Etiology

The exact cause is not known.

**BOX 11 Features of mixed connective tissue disease**

- An overlap symptoms and signs of SLE, scleroderma and DM
- High concentration of ENA (anti-U1 RNP)
- Speckled ANA
- Swollen hands and digits (sausage like)
- Raynaud's phenomenon

ANA, antinuclear antibody; DM, dermatomyositis; ENA, erythrocytes nuclear alteration; RNP, ribonucleo protein; SLE, systemic lupus erythematosus.

**BOX 12 Alarcon–Segovia diagnostic criteria for mixed connective tissue disease (MCTD)**

- *Serological criteria*: Positive anti-U1 RNP at hemagglutination titer >1:1,600
- *Clinical criteria*:
  - Edema of hands
  - Synovitis
  - Myositis
  - Raynaud´s
  - Acrosclerosis
- *Requirements*:
  - Serological
  - At least three clinical features
  - Association of hand edema, Raynaud´s and acrosclerosis requires at least one other feature

RNP, ribonucleo protein.

### Clinical Features

Apart from nonspecific symptoms like fatigue, muscle pain, joint pain,and low-grade fever, the patient may have classic symptoms of MCTD like Raynaud's phenomenon, swollen sausage-like fingers, inflamed joints and muscle, and pulmonary hypertension (Box 11).

### Diagnosis

Diagnosis in case of MCTD is a difficult to make and often delayed as it has a feature of three common CTDs like SLE, DM, and scleroderma which may be evolving. However, a few features are typical of MCTD like high concentration of specific erythrocytes nuclear alterations (ENAs) (anti-U1 RNP), puffy fingers and trigeminal neuropathy. The kidneys and CNS is not commonly involved or if involved it is usually. The arthritis is usually severe unlike SLE. All patients of MCTD have positive ANA with speckled pattern. Different diagnostic criteria are available; one of them is Alarcon–Segovia diagnostic criteria (Box 12).

### Treatment

The treatment may be tailored in a given patient according to clinical presentation and severity.

- Mild form of MCTD only requires nonsteroidal anti-inflammatory drugs (NSAIDs) for arthritis fever and myalgia
- Antimalarials and systemic steroids (low dose) as and when required to treat the inflammation
- Severe MCTD requires high dose of systemic corticosteroids and other immunosuppressant (methotrexate or cyclosporine)

- Pulmonary hypertension is a prominent feature of MCTD and it should be treated with appropriate antihypertensive medications.

## SUGGESTED READINGS


1. Alarcon-Segovia D, Cardiel MH. Comparison between 3 diagnostic criteria for mixed connective tissue disease. Study of 593 patients. J Rheumatol. 1989;16:328-34.
2. Auriemma M, Capo A, Meogrossi G, et al. Cutaneous signs of classical dermatomyositis. G Ital Dermatol Venereol. 2014;149(5):505-17.
3. Bailey EE, Fiorentino DF. Amyopathic dermatomyositis: definitions, diagnosis, and management. Curr Rheumatol Rep. 2014;16(12):465.
4. Bossini-Castillo L, López-Isac E, Mayes MD, et al. Genetics of systemic sclerosis. Semin Immunopathol. 2015;37(5):443-51.
5. Brugos B, Sebestyen L, Tarr T, et al. Use of cyclophosphamide and other immunosuppressive drugs in the treatment of patients with lupus nephritis. Pharmazie. 2014;69:442-4.
6. Careta MF, Romiti R. Localized scleroderma: clinical spectrum and therapeutic update. An Bras Dermatol. 2015;90(1):62-73.
7. Carvalho JC, Costa TN, De Moura HH, et al. Scleredema Adultorum of Buschke. Skinmed. 2014;12(6):337-40.
8. Condie D, Grabell D, Jacobe H. Comparison of outcomes in adults with pediatric-onset morphea and those with adult-onset morphea: a cross-sectional study from the morphea in adults and children cohort. Arthritis Rheumatol. 2014;66:3496-504.
9. Ding HJ, Gordon C. New biologic therapy for systemic lupus erythematosus. Curr Opin Pharmacol. 2013;13:405-12.
10. Elhai M, Avouac J, Kahan A, et al. Systemic sclerosis: recent insights. Joint Bone Spine. 2015;82(3):148-53.
11. Fraticelli P, Gabrielli B, Pomponio G, et al. Imatinib in Scleroderma Italian Study Group. Low dose oral imatinib in the treatment of systemic sclerosis interstitial lung disease unresponsive to cyclophosphamide: a phase II pilot study. Arthritis Res Ther. 2014;16:R144.
12. Freites-Martinez A, Aguado-Lobo M, Calderón-Komaromy A, et al. Mucocutaneous presentation of systemic lupus erythematosus. J Pediatr. 2014;165:631.
13. Hui-Yuen JS, Li XQ, Askanase AD. Belimumab in systemic lupus erythematosus: a perspective review. Ther Adv Musculoskelet Dis. 2015;7:115-21.
14. Iaccarino L, Ghirardello A, Bettio S, et al. The clinical features, diagnosis and classification of dermatomyositis. J Autoimmun. 2014;48-49:122-7.
15. Kavian N, Batteux F. Macro- and microvascular disease in systemic sclerosis. Vascul Pharmacol. 2015;71:16-23.
16. McQueen FM, Solanki K. Rituximab in diffuse cutaneous systemic sclerosis: should we be using it today? Rheumatology (Oxford). 2015;54(5):757-67.
17. Merrill JT, Buyon JP, Utset T. A 2014 update on the management of patients with systemic lupus erythematosus. Semin Arthritis Rheum. 2014;44(2):e1-2.
18. Muro Y, Sugiura K, Akiyama M. Cutaneous manifestations in dermatomyositis: key clinical and serological features-a comprehensive review. Clin Rev Allergy Immunol. 2016;51(3):293-302.
19. Naffaa ME, Bishara R, Braun-Moscovici Y, et al. Unusual sequelae of adult-onset dermatomyositis. BMJ Case Reports. 2014.
20. Nico MM, Bologna SB, Lourenço SV. The lip in lupus erythematosus. Clin Exp Dermatol. 2014;39:563-9.
21. Ortigosa LC, Reis VM. Dermatomyositis: analysis of 109 patients surveyed at the Hospital das Clínicas (HCFMUSP), São Paulo, Brazil. An Bras Dermatol. 2014;89(5):719-27.
22. Parodi A, Cozzani E. Cutaneous manifestations of lupus erythematosus. G Ital Dermatol Venereol. 2014;149:549-54.
23. Petri M, Orbai AM, Alarcón GS, et al. Derivation and validation of the Systemic Lupus International Collaborating Clinics classification criteria for systemic lupus erythematosus. Arthritis Rheum. 2012;64(8):2677-86.
24. Ponte C, Clark KE, Orteu C, et al. Exuberant skin involvement in Systemic Lupus Erythematosus: a clinical case report. Acta Reumatol Port. 2014;39:277-8.
25. Quinn N, MacMahon J, Irvine AD, et al. Sweet syndrome revealing systemic lupus erythematosus. Ir Med J. 2015;108(2):59-60.
26. Singalavanija S, Limpongsanurak W, Aoongern S. Neonatal lupus erythematosus: a 20-year retrospective study. J Med Assoc Thai. 2014;97 Suppl 6:S74-82.
27. Troyanov Y, Targoff IN, Payette MP, et al. Redefining dermatomyositis: a description of new diagnostic criteria that differentiate pure dermatomyositis from overlap myositis with dermatomyositis features. Medicine (Baltimore). 2014;93(24):318-32.
28. van den Hoogen F, Khanna D, Fransen J, et al. 2013 classification criteria for systemic sclerosis: an American College of Rheumatology/European League Against Rheumatism collaborative initiative. Ann Rheum Dis. 2013;72(11):1747-55.

# 49 CHAPTER Disorders of Subcutaneous Fat

Saumya Panda, Aparajita Ghosh

## INTRODUCTION

The subcutaneous fat or the panniculus forms the insulating layer of the skin just beneath the dermis. It is a metabolically active tissue composed of adipocytes or fat cells. It is compartmentalized into lobules by fibrous septae which provide structural integrity and serve as conduits for the vasculature. The microlobule which is comprised of a small number of adipocytes supplied by a single blood vessel forms the basic functional unit of the panniculus.

## PANNICULITIS

Panniculitis refers to an inflammation of the subcutaneous tissue or panniculus. A diverse group of cutaneous or systemic disorders may result in such an inflammation, but in spite of the varied etiology, the presentation is usually similar with erythematous nodules or induration, mostly located at the lower extremities.

Panniculitis is classified for diagnostic purpose based on the predominant pattern of inflammation (septal or lobular), the presence or absence of vasculitis, the predominant type of infiltrate, and other specific histopathological features, if any (Table 1).

Large excision or incision biopsy with adequate depth is necessary with examination of serial sections of the specimen for proper diagnosis. The nature and distribution of the inflammatory infiltrate change with time, and hence it is preferable to sample newer lesions as older ones may show nonspecific findings.

Some of the common types of panniculitis are discussed below.

### Erythema Nodosum

It is one of the most common forms of panniculitis.

#### Etiopathogenesis

It is a cutaneous reaction pattern to a wide variety of etiologic factors. Some of the most common causes are infections (streptococcal and mycobacterial), pregnancy, drugs [oral contraceptive pills (OCPs), sulphonamides, etc.], vaccination, autoimmune

**TABLE 1: Classification of panniculitis**

| Predominantly septal | Predominantly lobular |
|---|---|
| • Without vasculitis<br>○ Lymphocytes and plasma cells<br>– Necrobiosis lipoidica (granulomatous)<br>– Deep morphea<br>○ Histiocytes (mostly)<br>– Subcutaneous granuloma annulare<br>– Rheumatoid nodule<br>– Necrobiotic xanthogranuloma<br>– Erythema nodosum | • Without vasculitis<br>○ *Few inflammatory cells*:<br>– Sclerosing panniculitis, calciphylaxis (vascular calcification), and sclerema neonatorum (needle shaped crystals in adipocytes)<br>○ *Lymphocytes*:<br>– Cold panniculitis and lupus panniculitis<br>○ *Neutrophils*:<br>– Pancreatic panniculitis (extensive fat necrosis with saponification)<br>– Alpha-1 antitrypsin deficiency panniculitis<br>– Infective panniculitis<br>○ *Granulomatous*:<br>– Subcutaneous sarcoidosis, traumatic panniculitis, and lipomembranous fat necrosis<br>– Subcutaneous fat necrosis of newborn,<br>– Post steroid panniculitis (crystals in adipocytes)<br>– Cytophagic histiocytic panniculitis—panniculitis like subcutaneous lymphoma<br>– Sclerosing postradiation panniculitis (sclerosis of septa) |
| • With vasculitis<br>○ Superficial thrombophlebitis(veins)<br>○ Cutaneous polyarteritis nodosa | • *With vasculitis*:<br>– Erythema nodosum leprosum and Lucio phenomenon<br>– Nodular vasculitis (erythema induratum of Bazin) |

disorders [rheumatoid arthritis, systemic lupus erythematosus (SLE), and Sjögren's syndrome], sarcoidosis, inflammatory bowel disease, malignancies (lymphoma, leukemia, malignancy of gastrointestinal (GI) tract, etc.), Behcet's disease, Sweet's syndrome, etc.

It is a delayed hypersensitivity type reaction due to immune complex deposition in venules. A possible genetic predisposition has been implicated.

## Clinical Features

The condition is more common in females. It may occur at any age but is commoner in the third decade of life. It presents with erythematous tender nodules and plaques mostly involving the extensors of the lower extremities (Fig. 1), which resolve spontaneously without ulceration, scarring or atrophy over a period of 3–6 weeks. Lesions may be recurrent.

## Histopathology

It is a predominantly septal panniculitis with no vasculitis. Early lesions show presence of neutrophils while lymphocytes, histiocytes, and multinucleated giant cells appear in later stages. Miescher's radial granulomas (small well-defined collections of histiocytes around a central cleft) are considered to be pathognomonic.

## Investigations

Necessary investigations are listed in box 1.

## Treatment

It is aimed at correcting the underlying condition where possible. Nonsteroidal anti-inflammatory drugs (NSAIDs) can be given for symptomatic relief. Potassium iodide (2–10 drops TID), colchicine (0.6–1.2 mg BD), hydroxychloroquine (200 mg BD), etc. have been found to be effective. Rarely systemic corticosteroids may be required in severe cases without underlying infection.

A few of the more important panniculitic entities have been summarized in table 2 (Figs 2 to 9).

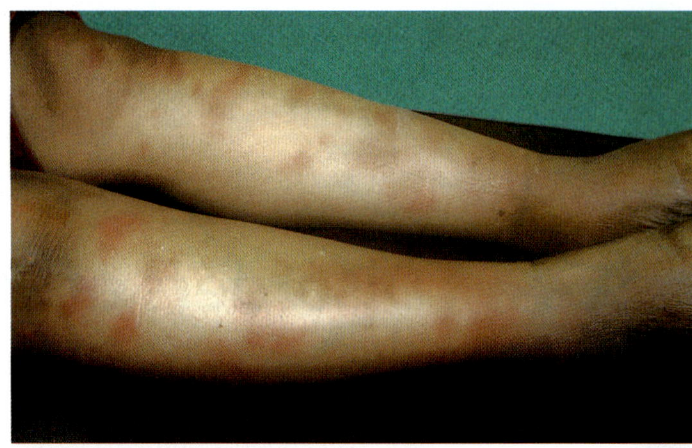

**FIG. 1:** Erythema nodosum.

**BOX 1 Investigations in erythema nodosum**

- Complete blood count (slightly raised WBC counts and raised ESR)
- ASO titer (changing titer—s/o recent streptococcal infection)
- Throat swab culture
- Mantoux test
- Chest X-ray (may show features of TB or hilar lymphadenopathy—s/o sarcoidosis)

WBC, white blood cell; ESR, erythrocyte sedimentation rate; ASO, antistreptolysin O; TB, tuberculosis.

**TABLE 2: Important panniculitides**

| Type of panniculitis | Etiopathogenesis | Clinical feature | HPE feature | Lab tests and treatment |
|---|---|---|---|---|
| Erythema induratum of Bazin | Possibly a tuberculid | In young and middle aged females. Nontender violaceous nodules on legs (calves and anterolateral aspect) with ulceration | Lobular panniculitis with granulomatous inflammation ± necrosis ± vasculitis | • Mantoux—strongly positive, chest X-ray, CBC<br>• Antitubercular drugs, potassium iodide, dapsone, colchicines, antimalarials, and tetracyclines |
| Erythema nodosum leprosum | Leprosy type II reaction. Arthus phenomenon with immune complex deposition | Evanescent erythematous nodules mostly on flexural aspect of forearms, medial thighs, and face. Systemic symptoms like fever, arthralgia, etc. may be present | Lobular and septal neutrophilic panniculitis with vasculitis. Neutrophilic infiltration of dermis with dermal edema. Background HP changes s/o leprosy may be present | Treatment—Symptomatic with NSAIDs in mild cases. Clofazimine, oral prednisolone, and thalidomide |
| Alpha-1-antitrypsin deficiency | Tissue damage due to uncontrolled activation lymphocytes, macrophages, neutrophils, complement pathway, and lack of inhibition of serum proteases | Erythematous nodules and plaques over large areas on arms, thighs, trunk, and face with ulceration and drainage of oily fluid | • Mixed (septal + lobular) panniculitis + lobular necrosis ± vasculitis<br>• Neutrophilic infiltrate in early stages, histiocytes, and lipophages later. Dystrophic calcification | Decreased levels of α-1 antitrypsin in plasma |



*Continued*

*Continued*

| Type of panniculitis | Etiopathogenesis | Clinical feature | HPE feature | Lab tests and treatment |
|---|---|---|---|---|
| Lupus panniculitis | Autoimmune, may be the only manifestation of LE or may be associated with DLE or SLE | F >M, tender deep-seated nodules, often in crops over proximal extremities, arms, shoulders, buttocks, trunk, breast (lupus mastitis), and face. Heals leaving depressed atrophic area | • Predominantly lobular or mixed (septal + lobular) panniculitis. Lymphocytic infiltrate + hyaline fat necrosis. Mucin deposition and calcification ± changes s/o DLE in epidermis and dermis<br>• DIF—IgG, IgM, and C3 at the D-E junction, IgG around adipocytes | • ANA (sometimes positive, anti dsDNA may be positive), CBC, and C4 levels (might be decreased, especially in children)<br>• Treated with antimalarials, oral corticosteroids, other immunosuppressants (cyclophosphamide, azathioprine, and MM), and thalidomide. Sunscreen recommended. Fat grafts and fillers for cosmetic improvement only in patients in long remission |
| Pancreatic panniculitis | Background of pancreatic disease. Fat necrosis due to release of pancreatic enzymes—lipases, trypsin, amylase, etc. | Lesions located mostly in distal part of lower extremities, around ankle, and knees. Thighs, buttocks, arms, abdomen, chest, and scalp. Nodules may ulcerate to discharge oily fluid | Predominantly lobular panniculitis without vasculitis. Saponification of fat with dystrophic calcification. Coagulative necrosis of adipocytes with "ghost adipocyte" formation. Infiltrate—neutrophilic in early stages and granulomatous with foamy histiocytes, giant cells in late stages | • Increased serum lipase, amylase, or trypsin<br>• CBC—increased TLC with eosinophilia<br>• Increased tumor marker levels (CEA and Ca 19.9)<br>• USG and CT scan to demonstrate the pancreas and its disease<br>• Treatment; supportive measures and treatment of underlying pancreatic disease |
| Traumatic panniculitis | Due to physical or chemical trauma. Includes "factitial panniculitis" | Distribution depends on the cause. Often seen on the breast | Nonspecific lobular or mixed panniculitis. Inflammatory infiltrate may consist of neutrophils, lymphocytes, and macrophages (may contain refractile foreign material). Fibrosis in later stages | Treatment—symptomatic. May require debridement. May require psychiatric support for cases of factitial panniculitis |
| Cold panniculitis | Type of traumatic panniculitis. More common in infants and children (greater percentage of saturated fatty acids). May occur in adults exposed to extreme cold. "equestrian panniculitis" (EP), "subcutaneous fat necrosis of newborn" (SFNN), "sclerema neonatorum (SN)", "chilblains", and "frostbite" | In children—cheeks and submental area. EP—anterolateral thighs. SFNN—thighs, buttocks, cheeks, and back, arms. SN—diffuse, ascending board like rigidity. Chilblain and frostbite—mostly acral | Predominantly lobular panniculitis. Inflammation maximum at the junction of dermis and subcutis. Infiltrate—lymphohistiocytic, giants cells may be present. SFNN—needle shaped clefts in adipocytes and giant cells. SN—needle shaped clefts in adipocytes in radial array. Sparse inflammation. Chilblains—lymphocytic vasculitis with subepidermal edema. Frostbite—dermal edema, subepidermal bulla, and keratinocyte necrosis | SN—usually fatal. Other cold induced panniculitis are usually self resolving in 2–3 weeks. Preventive measures are recommended |
| Sclerosing panniculitis | Also called "lipodermatosclerosis". Background of venous insufficiency, thrombophlebitis with stasis, and lymphedema | Affects lower legs mostly above ankle. In well-developed lesions there is marked induration with woody consistency, and fibrosis leading to "inverted champagne bottle" appearance | Thickening and fibrosis of septa with atrophy of the lobules. Lipophagic granuloma may be present at the periphery, lymphohistiocytic infiltrate with foamy macrophages. RBC extravasation and hemosiderin deposition in the dermis | • Doppler study of blood vessels of lower extremities<br>• Treatment—correction of venous stasis. Surgery, compression stockings, etc. Stanozolol can show some improvement due to fibrinolytic activity. Pentoxifylline and tocopherol may be useful |



*Continued*

*Continued*

| Type of panniculitis | Etiopathogenesis | Clinical feature | HPE feature | Lab tests and treatment |
|---|---|---|---|---|
| Calciphylaxis | • Background of renal disease, especially in patients undergoing dialysis and secondary hyperparathyroidism. Obesity and diabetes may predispose<br>• Dysregulation of calcium and phosphate metabolism resulting in elevated calcium or phosphorus product and cutaneous vascular calcification | Painful indurated violaceous plaques, surrounded by reticulate purpura. Deep irregular or stellate ulcers with eschar formation, mostly on medial thighs, buttocks, and lower abdomen | Septal and lobular panniculitis. Calcification of small and medium sized blood vessels with intimal hyperplasia and thrombosis. Epidermal ulceration and necrosis of dermis and subcutis. Perivascular neutrophilic and lymphohistiocytic infiltrate | • Serum PTH, calcium, and phosphate levels (they may often but not always be elevated)<br>• Treatment—adjusting serum calcium and phosphate levels with dietary modifications, phosphate binders, and bisphosphonates. Sodium thiosulphate (as calcium chelator for improving vascular calcium load). Parathyroidectomy is controversial. Cinacalcet is calcimimetic has been used as an alternative to parathyroidectomy<br>• Still general prognosis is poor |

CBC, complete blood count; NSAID, nonsteroidal anti-inflammatory drug; ANA, antinuclear antibody; dsDNA, double-stranded deoxyribonucleic acid; LE, lupus erythematosus; DLE, discoid lupus erythematosus; SLE, systemic lupus erythematosus; DIF, direct immunofluorescence; IgG, immunoglobulin G; IgM, immunoglobulin M; TLC, total leukocyte count; CEA, carcinoembryonic antigen; USG, ultrasonography; CT, computed tomography; RBC, red blood cell; PTH, parathyroid hormone; HPE, histopathological examination; F, female; M, male; and MM, mycophenolate mofetil.

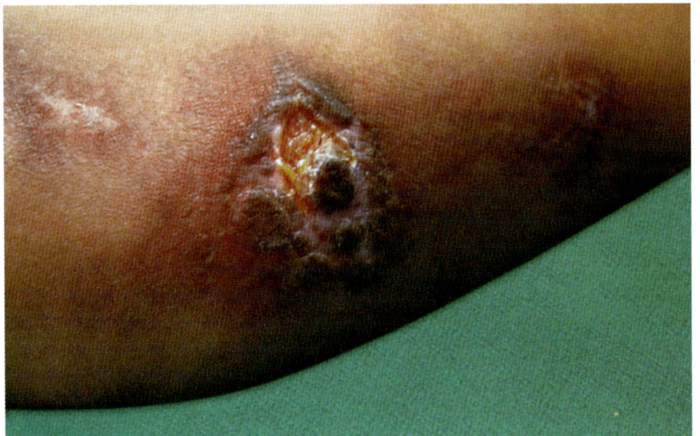

**FIG. 2:** Lupus panniculitis presenting with ulceration on elbow.

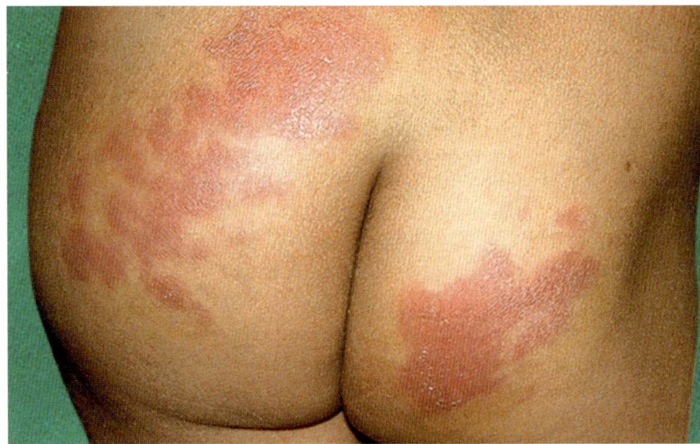

**FIG. 4:** Lupus panniculitis on the buttocks of a 4-year old child presenting with confluent erythematous tender plaques.

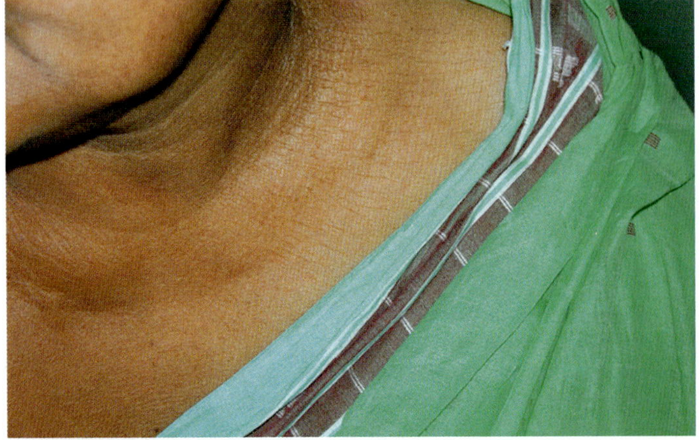

**FIG. 3:** Lupus panniculitis presenting as unilateral atrophoderma of neck.

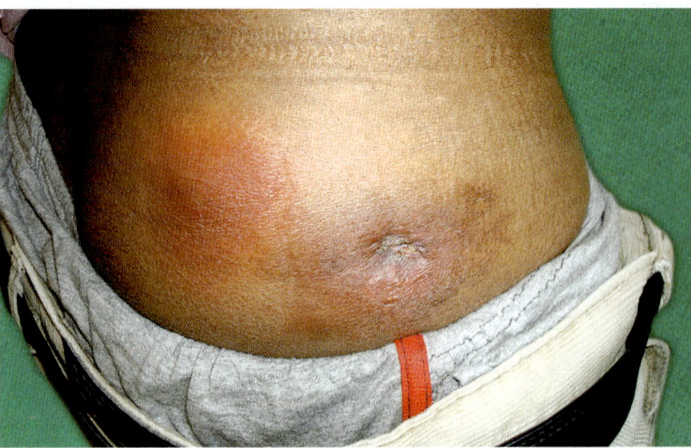

**FIG. 5:** Postinjection panniculitis.

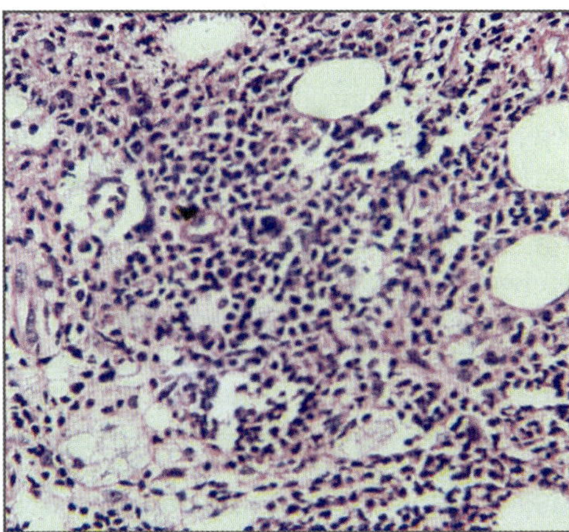

**FIG. 6:** Lupus panniculitis featuring lobular panniculitis, lymphocytic infiltrate, hyaline fat necrosis, and mucin deposition (H&E, 400x).

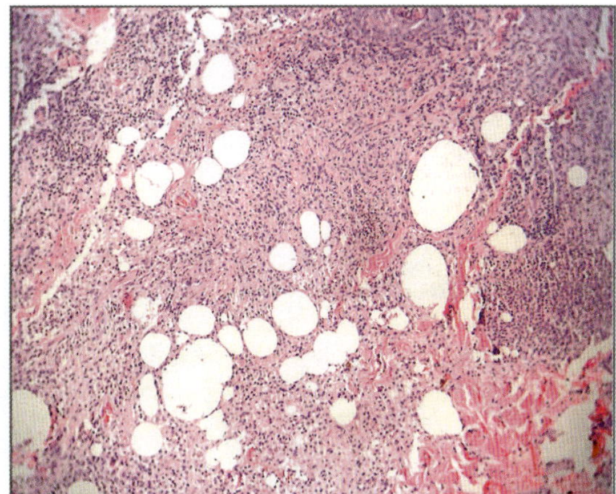

**FIG. 8:** Foreign body induced granulomatous panniculitis (H&E, 100x).

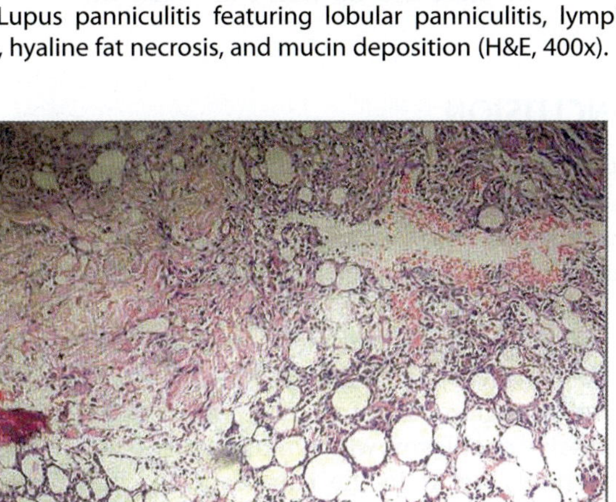

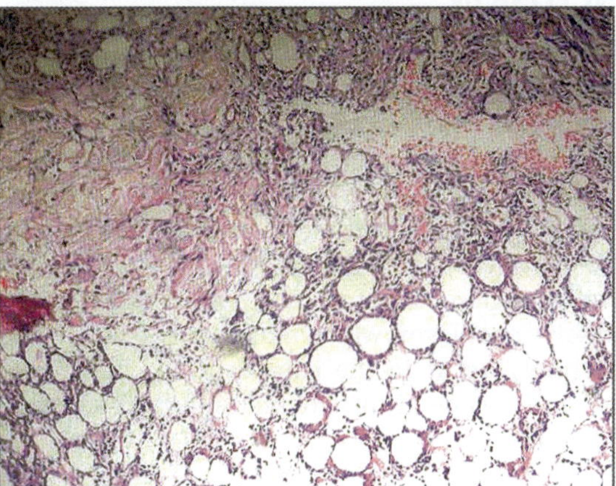

**FIG. 7:** Lobular panniculitis in Weber–Christian disease (idiopathic panniculitis with no other systemic feature or association) (H&E, 400x).

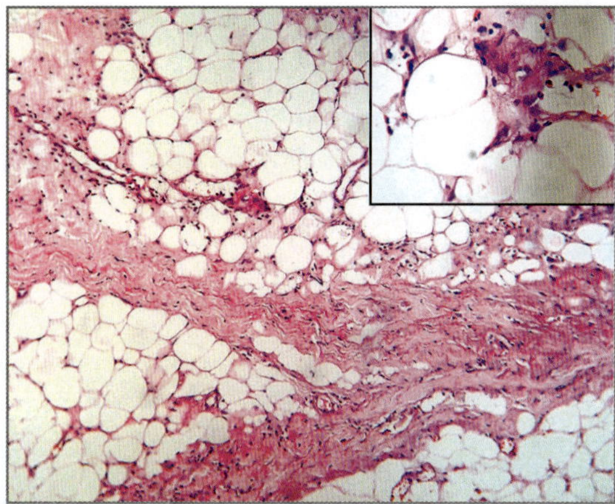

**FIG. 9:** Eosinophilic panniculitis—showing prominent eosinophilic (inset) septal and lobular infiltration ( H&E, 400x).

## LIPODYSTROPHY

This is defined as localized or generalized selective loss of adipose tissue. The extent of loss of fat can be partial or complete. Ectopic fat deposition in internal organs mostly muscle and liver and systemic complications in the form of insulin resistance, hypertriglyceridemia, and often accompany this group of conditions. A relative leptin deficiency is supposed to play an important role in the pathogenesis.

Lipodystrophies are broadly classified into two types—familial or inherited and acquired (Table 3).

**TABLE 3: Classification of lipodystrophy**

| Familial or inherited lipodystrophies | Acquired lipodystrophies |
|---|---|
| • Congenital generalized LD<br>  ○ Types 1, 2, 3, and 4<br>• Familial partial LD<br>  ○ Types 1, 2, 3, 4, and 5<br>• Mandibuloacral dysplasia associated LD<br>  ○ Types A and B<br>• Mandibular hypoplasia, deafness, and progeroid features associated LD<br>• Autoinflammatory LD<br>• Neonatal progeroid syndrome | • Acquired generalized LD (Lawrence syndrome)<br>• Acquired partial LD (Barraquer–Simons syndrome)<br>• HAART-induced LD (due to protease inhibitor)<br>• Localized LD |

LD, lipodystrophy; HAART, highly active antiretroviral therapy.

### Investigations

Diagnosis is mostly clinical (Fig. 10). Blood glucose and insulin levels, lipid profile, liver function test, and ultrasonography (USG) to detect hepatic steatosis may be performed. Skiagram for detecting skeletal defect in congenital varieties. Genotyping is done for research purposes only.

### Treatment

Dietary modification and increased physical activity are advised. Metformin, other oral hypoglycemics, insulin, and lipid lowering drugs may be used as required for control of underlying metabolic abnormalities. Treatment with injectable metreleptin (a recombinant analog of human leptin) has shown promise especially in cases with severe metabolic abnormalities but there is a chance of developing neutralizing antibodies and lymphoma.

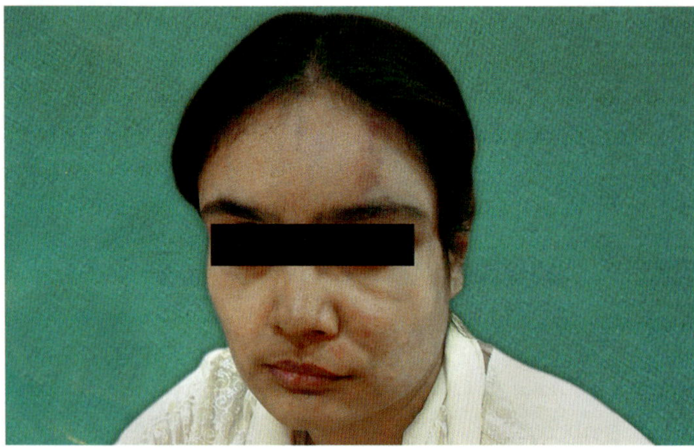

**FIG. 10:** Acquired localized facial lipodystrophy.

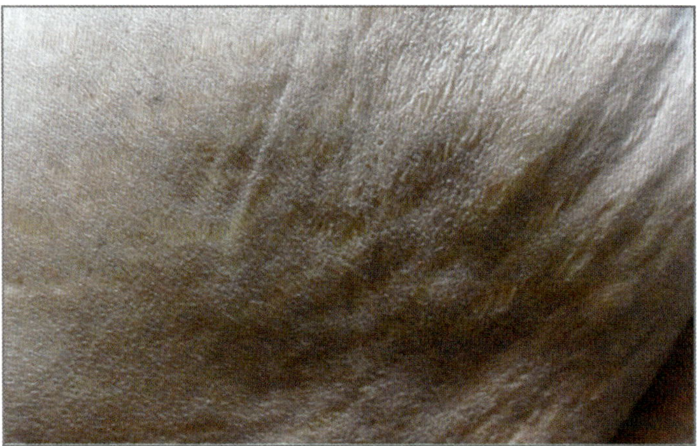

**FIG. 11:** Cellulite in a woman in her fifth decade.

**BOX 2 Grades of cellulite**

- Grade 1—No clinical features but early histopathological changes (increased thickness of areolar layer and increased capillary permeability)
- Grade 2—Pallor, decreased elasticity and temperature on skin compression or muscle contraction. No pain and changes not evident at rest
- Grade 3—Changes of grade 2 + orange peel appearance evident even at rest, increasing on skin compression or muscle contraction. Presence of nodules on palpation
- Grade 4—Changes of grade 3 with larger and more painful nodules adherent to deeper tissues.

## CELLULITE

It is a degenerative condition of the subcutaneous tissue, which results in a padded or orange peel appearance of the overlying skin. The condition is found predominantly in women and has a predilection for affecting the thighs, pelvic area, and lower abdomen (Fig. 11). Estrogen plays an important role in its formation. Other predisposing factors are race (more common in Caucasians) and obesity, though it is also seen in lean individuals. The clinical grading of cellulite is described in box 2.

### Treatment

Control of aggravating factors through weight reduction, regular exercise, dietary modification, etc. is important. Physical methods like iontophoresis, extra corporeal shock wave therapy, thermotherapy, massage to stimulate lymphatic drainage, electrolipophoresis, unipolar or bipolar radiofrequency, laser-induced lipolysis, and infrared therapy have been tried with varying success. Certain pharmacologic agents in topical and systemic formulations like methylxanthines (aminophylline, theophylline, and caffeine), β-agonists (isoproterenol and adrenaline), and α-antagonists (yohimbine and phentolamine) have demonstrated benefits due to their lipolytic effects. Botanicals like asiatic centella, gingko biloba extracts, etc. have been tried but there are no well-controlled trials to evaluate their benefits.

## CONCLUSION

Disorders of the subcutaneous tissue are common and often disfiguring or painful. They may sometimes occur as part of systemic diseases. Histopathology and appropriate investigations are crucial to diagnosing these wide variety of conditions with surprisingly similar presentations.

Proliferation of adipose tissue may also occur as part of hamartomas, nevi or other tumours like lipomas, angiolipomas, myolipomas, angiomyolipomas, and fibrolipomas. Liposarcomas are aggressive neoplasms which mostly arise from deeper tissues but may rarely occur in the subcutaneous fat. Such entities are outside the scope of this chapter and hence have not been dicussed here.

## SUGGESTED READINGS


1. Acosta KA, Haver MC, Kelly B. Etiology and therapeutic management of erythema nodosum during pregnancy: an update. Am J Clin Dermatol. 2013;14(3):215-22.
2. Barton SJ, Heymann WR. Potassium iodide in dermatology: a 19th century drug for the 21st century—uses, pharmacology, adverse effects, and contraindications. J Am Acad Dermatol. 2000;43(4):691-7.
3. Blake T, Manahan M, Rodins K. Erythema Nodosum–A Review of an Uncommon Panniculitis. Dermatol Online J. 2014;20(4):22376.
4. Bunyamin K, Onat AM, Pehlivan Y. Multiclinical experiences in erythema nodosum: rheumatology clinics versus dermatology and infection diseases clinics. Rheumatol Int. 2013;33(2):315-8.
5. Chan JL, Lutz K, Cochran E, et al. Clinical effects of long-term metreleptin treatment in patients with lipodystrophy. Endocr Pract. 2011;17(6):922-32.
6. Cohen PR. Combined Reduced-Antigen Content Tetanus, Diphtheria, and Acellular Pertussis (Tdap) Vaccine-Related Erythema Nodosum: Case Report and Review of Vaccine-Associated Erythema Nodosum. Dermatol Ther. 2013;3(2):191-7.
7. De la Casa Almeida M, Suarez Serrano C, Rebollo Roldán J, et al. Cellulite's aetiology: a review. J Eur Acad Dermatol Venereol, 2013;27(3):273-8.
8. Garg A. Clinical review: Lipodystrophies: genetic and acquired body fat disorders. J Clin Endocrinol Metab. 2011;96(11):3313-25.
9. Gilchrist H, Patterson JW. Erythema nodosum and erythema induratum (nodular vasculitis): diagnosis and management. Dermatol Ther. 2010;23(4):320-7.
10. Goldman A, Gotkin RH, Sarnoff DS, et al. Cellulite: a new treatment approach combining subdermal Nd: YAG laser lipolysis and autologous fat transplantation. Aesthet Surg J. 2008;28(6):656-62.
11. Knobloch K, Kraemer R. Extracorporeal shock wave therapy (ESWT) for the treatment of cellulite–A current metaanalysis. Int J Surg. 2015;24(Pt 4):210-7.
12. McNutt NS, Moreno A, Contreras F. Inflammatory diseases of the subcutaneous fat. In: Elder DE, Elenitsas R, Johnson Jr BL, Murphy GF, Xu X (Eds). Lever's histopathology of the skin, 10th edition. Philadelphia: Lippincott Williams & Wilkins; 2009. pp. 511-5.

13. Merlen JF, Curri SB. Anatomico-pathological causes of cellulite. Journal des maladies vasculaires, 1984;9(Suppl A):53-4.
14. Mert A, Kumbasar H, Ozaras R, et al. Erythema nodosum: an evaluation of 100 cases. Clin Exp Rheumatol. 2007;25(4):563-70.
15. Rawlings AV. Cellulite and its treatment. Int J Cosmet Sci. 2006;28(3):175-90.
16. Requena L, Sánchez Yus E. Panniculitis. Part II. Mostly lobular panniculitis. J Am Acad Dermatol. 2001;45(3):325-64.
17. Requena L, Yus ES. Erythema nodosum. Dermatol Clin. 2008;26(4):425-38.
18. Requena L, Yus ES. Panniculitis. Part I. Mostly septal panniculitis. J Am Acad Dermatol. 2001;45(2):163-86.
19. Rossi AM, Katz BE. A modern approach to the treatment of cellulite. Dermatol Clin. 2014;32(1):51-9.
20. Simha V. Metreleptin for metabolic disorders associated with generalized or partial lipodystrophy. Expert Rev Endocrinol Metab. 2014;9(3):205-12.
21. Ter Poorten MC, Thiers BH. Panniculitis. Dermatol Clin. 2002;20(3):421-33.
22. Wasson S, Govindarajan G, Folzenlogen D. Concurrent occurrence of Sweet's syndrome and erythema nodosum: an overlap in the spectrum of reactive dermatoses. Clin Rheumatol. 2006;25(2):268-72.
23. Yosipovitch G, DeVore A, Dawn A. Obesity and the skin: skin physiology and skin manifestations of obesity. J Am Acad Dermatol. 2007;56(6):901-6.

# 15 SECTION Nutritional and Metabolic Disorders

# 50 CHAPTER Nutrition and Skin Disease

*Tanmay Padhi, Swetalina Pradhan*

## INTRODUCTION

All living organisms consume macronutrients and micronutrients for growth and homeostasis. Whereas carbohydrates, proteins, and lipids are the macronutrients, micronutrients comprise of vitamins and minerals. Imbalance in nutritional equilibrium is reflected in skin as various dermatological disorders.

## PROTEIN–ENERGY MALNUTRITION

Protein–energy malnutrition is a spectrum of related disease that includes marasmus, kwashiorkor and marasmic-kwashiorkor. Marasmus represents deficiency of both protein and calories and is diagnosed in children who are below 60% of their ideal body weight without edema. Kwashiorkor occurs with protein deficiency alone and is diagnosed in children between 60% and 80% of their ideal body weight. Marasmic-kwashiorkor shows features of both conditions (Box 1).

### Clinical Features of Protein–Energy Malnutrition

Patients of kwashiorkor present with edema and a generalized eczematous dermatitis which is known as "flaking enamel paint dermatoses". The skin lesions present as hyperpigmented plaques raised above the skin surface usually over bony prominences. There occurs exfoliation and fissuring of skin in a "crazy pavement" pattern over the flexures. Pigmentary changes are prominent and include both hypo- and hyperpigmentation. Perioral pallor and hypopigmentation over the legs are commonly seen. The pigmentary changes seen in kwashiorkor are believed to be due to associated zinc deficiency.

The hair is thin and brittle. Alternate bands of light and dark color within the hair shaft observed in kwashiorkor have been referred to as the "flag sign". The hair grown during periods of poor nutrition is pale whereas that during normal nutrition is pigmented. Mucosal involvement in the form of cheilosis, glossitis, xerophthalmia, and vulvovaginitis is also seen in this condition.

The clinical findings of marasmus include dry wrinkled skin, thin, brittle hairs, and dystrophy of nails. A characteristic Monkey facies may be seen with loss of buccal pad of fat. Follicular hyperkeratosis is seen particularly in adults. Marasmic children often have delayed wound healing. Increased growth of lanugo hairs is occasionally found in marasmus.

Adults can also have protein–energy malnutrition and when they suffer from protein deficiency, they usually present with xerosis, acquired ichthyosis, perioral and periorbital hyperpigmentation, and diffuse telogen effluvium.

**BOX 1 Proteins**

- *Biological functions*: Major functional and structural component of keratin, collagen, hair, nails, and intracellular matrix precursors for many coenzymes, hormones, nucleic acids
- *RDA*: 46–56 g/day
- *Dietary sources*:
  - Animal sources—meat, poultry, fish, eggs, milk, cheese, and yogurt
  - Plant sources—legumes, grains, nuts, seeds, and vegetables
- *Deficiency states*: Inadequate diet, ignorance of proper infant-rearing practices, feeding with over diluted milk, and failure or abandonment of breastfeeding

RDA, recommended dietary allowances.

### Diagnosis

A protein-deficient diet confirmed by history, and presence of edema, fissuring of skin, and dyspigmentation often make the diagnosis easy. Complete blood count, total serum protein, serum albumin, and albumin-globulin ratio are the investigations of choice to confirm the clinical findings.

### Treatment

Treatment consists of animal protein supplementation, correction of electrolyte and zinc deficiency and institution of appropriate nutrient-rich diet. Treatment of associated skin infections with appropriate oral and topical antibacterial agents and moisturizers is warranted in such cases.

## ESSENTIAL FATTY ACIDS

Essential fatty acids (EFAs) represent a group of 18-, 20-, or 22-carbon polyunsaturated fatty acids that cannot be synthesized *de novo* by the human body. Major EFAs of clinical significance are linoleic acid and its products, linolenic acid, and arachidonic acid (Box 2).

**BOX 2 Essential fatty acids**

- *Biological functions*: Lamellar granule formation, integral part of epidermal ceramides, maintenance of epidermal barrier, nerve growth and development, act as precursor of eicosanoids
- *AI*: 1.1–1.6 g/day
- *Dietary sources*: Soybean oil, canola oil, flaxseed oil, fish oils, fatty fish, meats, and eggs
- *Deficiency states*: Low birth weight babies, infants with gastro-intestinal anomalies or inflammatory bowel disease and exclusive skimmed milk feeding, pancreatic failure, cystic fibrosis, alcoholism, malabsorption, intestinal surgery, and prolonged total parenteral nutrition

AI, adequate intake level.

## Clinical Features of EFA Deficiency

Dermatological manifestations of EFA deficiency include a dry scaly skin with occasional non-healing ulcers and superficial erosions, periorificial and intertriginous dermatitis, traumatic purpura secondary to capillary fragility, diffuse alopecia, and impaired growth of nails. The dermatitis seen in EFA deficiency is similar to that in zinc and biotin deficiency, but is more widespread with less periorificial involvement. Abnormal EFA metabolism has been associated with a variety of cutaneous disorders such as psoriasis, atopic dermatitis, phrynoderma, and acne.

### Diagnosis

A ratio of eicosatrienoic acid to arachidonic acid of more than 0.4 is diagnostic of EFA deficiency.

### Treatment and Prevention

Diet rich in EFA with at least 1–2% of daily calorie intake from it should be advised to those at risk of EFA deficiency. Intravenous lipid infusion is the definitive therapy. Topical safflower or soybean oil may be tried in those developing pancreatitis as an adverse effect of intravenous lipid infusion.

# FAT-SOLUBLE VITAMINS

## Vitamin A

Vitamin A (retinol) is a cyclic polyene alcohol. It is present in diet as the vitamin itself or as its precursor β-carotene. It is essential for the reproductive system, bone formation, and vision (Box 3).

**BOX 3 Vitamin A**

- *Biological functions*: Helps in differentiation and proliferation of epidermal and mesenchymal cells, antioxidant action, influence sebaceous gland activity, and important for rhodopsin synthesis required for normal vision. It also has role in gene expression, reproduction, embryonic development, growth, and immune function
- *RDA*: 700–900 µg/day
- *Dietary sources*: Fruits, carrots, yellow and green vegetables, egg yolk, butter, liver, and fish oils
- *Deficiency states*: Inadequate intake, liver diseases and fat malabsorption states such as bowel bypass surgery, pancreatic insufficiency, Crohn's disease, celiac disease and cystic fibrosis, and zinc deficiency

RDA, recommended dietary allowances.

### Clinical Features of Vitamin A Deficiency

The cutaneous findings of vitamin A deficiency are results of abnormal keratinization. Deficiency of vitamin A typically manifests as a diffuse xerosis of skin with prominence of hair follicles. Phrynoderma or "toad skin" (Fig. 1) refers to presence of crateriform papules with a central keratotic plug seen over lateral aspects of arms and thigh, extensor forearms and legs, buttocks, and occasionally the face. Individual lesions are firm, pigmented papules containing a central intrafollicular keratotic plug. It is not specific to vitamin A deficiency and is also seen in deficiencies of vitamin B complex, vitamin E, vitamin C, and EFAs. Other features of vitamin A deficiency are perforating folliculitis and thin, broken hairs.

### Diagnosis

Diagnosis of vitamin A deficiency is made when blood levels are less than 20 µg/dL and an improvement in clinical signs occur after vitamin A supplementation.

### Treatment

The treatment is oral vitamin A supplementation 100,000 IU/day along with a diet rich in vitamin A until symptoms resolve and serum levels normalize. The cutaneous lesions of phrynoderma also respond to keratolytics such as salicylic acid ointment.

## Vitamin A Intoxication

Vitamin A toxicity is the result of excess intake of vitamin A usually more than 20 times the recommended dietary allowances (RDA) in a child or 100 times the RDA in an adult. It can occur in a chronic form in those with moderately excess intake for months to years. It can be iatrogenic when deficiency states are treated with excessive amounts of vitamin A or drugs like isotretinoin used in the management of acne.

### Clinical Features of Vitamin A Excess

The signs of vitamin A excess include dryness of skin and lips, peeling of palms and soles, follicular hyperkeratosis, dryness and loss of scalp hairs and erosions of the angle of mouth.

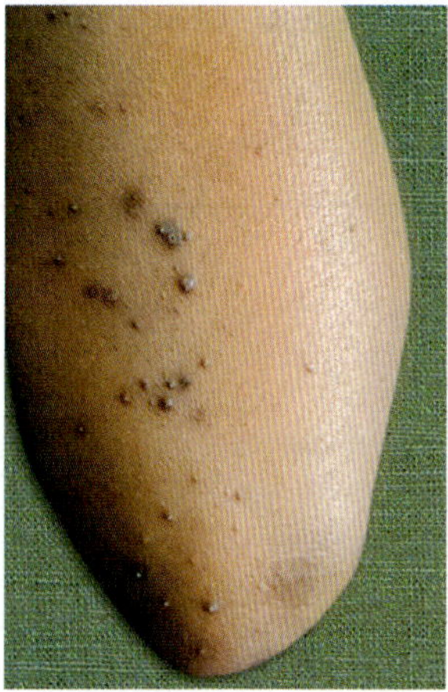

**FIG. 1:** Phrynoderma.

## Carotenoderma

Beta-carotene is the natural provitamin of vitamin A. Carotenes cannot be synthesized by the body and are obtained through intake of carotene rich foods. A high intake of food containing carotene, especially carrots, causes carotenemia (increased carotene in plasma) and may induce carotenoderma.

### Clinical Findings

The carotene is excreted by sebaceous glands and in sweat, so the yellow pigmentation appears first on the face, predominantly in the nasolabial folds and forehead, and then progresses to manifest diffusely, especially on the palms and soles. Carotenoderma, in contrast to jaundice, spares mucous membranes, like the sclera.

### Treatment

Treatment involves discontinuation of excessive carotene intake, and carotenoderma typically fades as the intake of carotene decreases.

## Vitamin E (Tocopherol)

They are a group of chemicals containing tocopherols and tocotrienols out of which D-α-tocopherol is the most biologically active form. Fat soluble vitamin E is located in stratum corneum and has a possible role in protecting it from various exogenous assaults (Box 4).

### Clinical Features of Vitamin E Deficiency

Features of peripheral neuritis can be seen in tocopherol deficiency. Cutaneous manifestations of vitamin E deficiency include erythema with dry, scaly skin and exfoliation, yellowish scaling with crusting over the scalp.

### Diagnosis

Plasma tocopherol level less than 3 mg/L indicates a deficient state.

### Treatment

A daily intake of 0.8 mg of vitamin E per gram of essential fatty acid should be taken. In adults about 100–400 mg can be given as a therapeutic dose.

**BOX 4 Vitamin E**

- *Biological functions*: Antioxidation, protective effect on cellular membranes
- *RDA*: 15 mg/day
- *Dietary sources*: Various vegetable oils, palm oil, corn, whole wheat flour, nuts, and some meats
- *Deficiency states*: Premature babies, genetic abnormalities of vitamin E metabolism, fat malabsorption syndromes or protein-energy malnutrition, chronic alcoholism with erythrodermic psoriasis, thalassemia, sickle cell anemia, and oral contraceptive use

RDA, recommended dietary allowances.

## Vitamin K

It naturally occurs in two forms. Vitamin K1 or phylloquinone is found in plant products such as vegetables, fruits, and vitamin K2 or menaquinone is synthesized by intestinal bacterial flora (Box 5).

### Clinical Features of Vitamin K Deficiency

Dermatological manifestation of vitamin K deficiency in neonates is ecchymoses and it can also present with bleeding from internal organs.

Purpura, ecchymoses, and gingival bleeding is found in older children and adults with vitamin K deficiency.

### Diagnosis

A deficiency of vitamin K is suggested by elevations in both prothrombin time and activated partial thromboplastin time.

### Treatment

Neonatal prophylaxis is achieved by a single intramuscular dose of 0.5–1 mg of vitamin K. Management of vitamin K deficiency constitutes intramuscular injection of vitamin K with supportive measures like infusion of fresh frozen plasma and other specific coagulation factors.

## Vitamin D

There are two forms of vitamin D: (1) vitamin D2 or ergocalciferol, and (2) vitamin D3 or cholecalciferol. Vitamin D2 is found in many plant and animal sources and can be consumed through diet. The epidermis contains 7-dehydrocholesterol which on exposure to UV radiation gets converted to vitamin D3 (Box 6).

**BOX 5 Vitamin K**

- *Biological functions*: Carboxylation of glutamate residues on coagulation factors II, VII, IX, X, and proteins C and S
- *RDA*: Infants 10–20 μg/day, children 15–100 μg/day, and adults 90–120 μg/day
- *Dietary sources*: Green, leafy vegetables, legumes, soybeans, cereals, and liver
- *Deficiency states*: Neonates—poor transplacental transfer, low dietary intake, maternal intake of anticoagulant drugs or phenytoin, and exclusive breast feeding; adults—liver diseases and intake of drugs like coumarin, salicylates, and cholestyramine

RDA, recommended dietary allowances.

**BOX 6 Vitamin D**

- *Biological functions*: Regulation of calcium and phosphorus absorption and deposition, maintenance of serum level of enzyme alkaline phosphatase
- *RDA*: 15 μg/day
- *Dietary sources*: Cod-liver oil, butter, eggs, and liver
- *Deficiency states*: Inadequate synthesis in elderly people, limited exposure to sunshine, regular use of sunscreens, anticonvulsants, fat malabsorption, high cereal diet and exclusive breast feeding without vitamin D supplementation

RDA, recommended dietary allowances.

### Clinical Features of Vitamin D Deficiency

Association of vitamin D deficiency has been reported in patients of atopic dermatitis, vitiligo, and alopecia areata.

### Diagnosis

Serum 25(OH) vitamin D3 level less than 5 ng/mL indicates deficiency.

### Treatment

Vitamin D3 supplementation of 400–800 IU/day should be recommended along with exposure to morning sunlight.

## Vitamin D Intoxication

Vitamin D intoxication occurs with long-continued administration of more than 100,000 IU daily.

### Clinical Features

Anorexia, vomiting, headache, diarrhea, hypercalcemia and hypercalciuria with osteoporosis, resembling the action of parathyroid hormone.

### Treatment

Withdrawal of vitamin D, a low-calcium diet and systemic corticosteroids are the mainstay of treatment of vitamin D excess.

## Vitamin B Complex

The vitamins of the B complex are of great clinical significance. Isolated deficiencies of certain B vitamins are uncommon. Mostly combined deficiencies of the vitamins belonging to the group are involved, often occurring as a result of insufficient supply of protein and other essential nutrients (zinc, essential fatty acids). The vitamin B group includes:

- Aneurin (thiamine) (vitamin B1)
- Riboflavin (vitamin B2)
- Niacin (nicotinic acid) (B3)
- Pyridoxine (vitamin B6)
- Cyanocobalamin (vitamin B12)
- Folic acid
- Pantothenic acid
- Biotin (vitamin H).

## Vitamin B1 (Thiamine)

The important function of thiamine is to help in the metabolism of carbohydrates in the body (Box 7).

### Clinical Features of Vitamin B1 Deficiency

The classical form of vitamin B1 deficiency is beriberi, characterized by anorexia, weakness, constipation, symmetrical progressive polyneuritis, cardiac insufficiency with edema, and wasting of musculature. Foot drop and wrist drop are seen in severe cases.

**BOX 7 Vitamin B1**

- *Biological functions*: Involved in carbohydrate metabolism, growth processes and in the function of the nervous system
- *RDA*: 1.1–1.2 mg/day
- *Dietary sources*: Yeast, cereals, liver, meat, potato, fish, eggs, vegetables, wheat germ, etc.
- *Deficiency states*: Consuming polished rice as the staple food, chronic alcoholism, pregnancy, lactation, chronic dialysis, diabetes mellitus, ulcerative colitis, celiac disease, achlorhydria, and myxedema

RDA, recommended dietary allowances.

Skin manifestations in this vitamin deficiency are edema and red tongue with burning sensation. Besides not much other skin lesions are noted.

### Diagnosis

Diagnosis of vitamin B1 deficiency is made by estimation of erythrocyte thiamine transketolase activity before and after thiamine pyrophosphate stimulation. An increase in transketolase activity by more than 30% after addition of thiamine pyrophosphate is diagnostic of beriberi.

### Treatment

Treatment of this condition consists of vitamin B1 supplementation in the form of 2–3 mg three times daily till serum levels are normalized.

## Vitamin B2 (Riboflavin)

Riboflavin is a d-ribitolisoalloxazine derivative that is widely distributed in plant and animal tissues (Box 8).

### Clinical Features of Vitamin B2 Deficiency

The classic findings are the oral-ocular-genital syndrome. Angular cheilitis also known as perleche, (Fig. 2) xerosis and fissuring of lips, atrophic glossitis, (Fig. 3) a dermatitis resembling seborrheic dermatitis. Swollen magenta-colored tongue, scrotal dermatitis with scaling, crusting with lichenification and intertriginous inflammation of the inguinal region are the major characteristic features of this condition. Infants usually have the dermatitis in the inguinal area whereas adults tend to have it over facial creases, wrinkles, and perianal region. The scrotal dermatitis characteristically spares the midline and ranges from erythema and minimal scaling to confluent red papules, fissuring and massive swelling. Balanitis and acquired phimosis are occasionally seen.

**BOX 8 Vitamin B2**

- *Biological functions*: Oxidation-reduction reactions in cellular respiration and oxidative phosphorylation and vitamin B6 metabolism
- *RDA*: 1.1–1.3 mg/day
- *Dietary sources*: Dairy products, nuts, meat, eggs, whole grain and enriched bread products, fatty fish, and green leafy vegetables
- *Deficiency states*: Alcoholism, phototherapy in neonatal jaundice, zinc deficiency, hypothyroidism, and drugs like chlorpromazine

RDA, recommended dietary allowances.

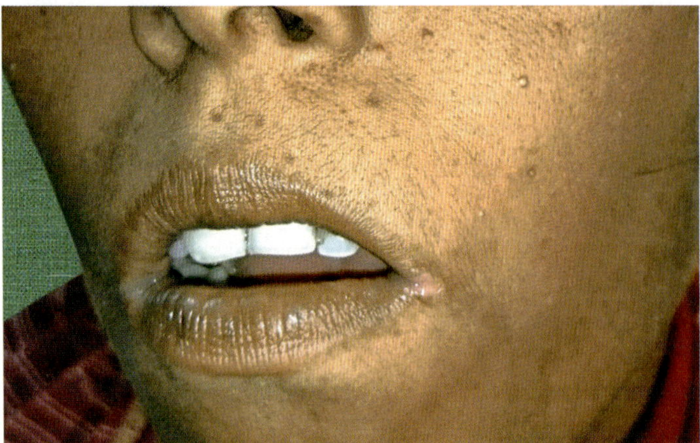

FIG. 2: Angular stomatitis.

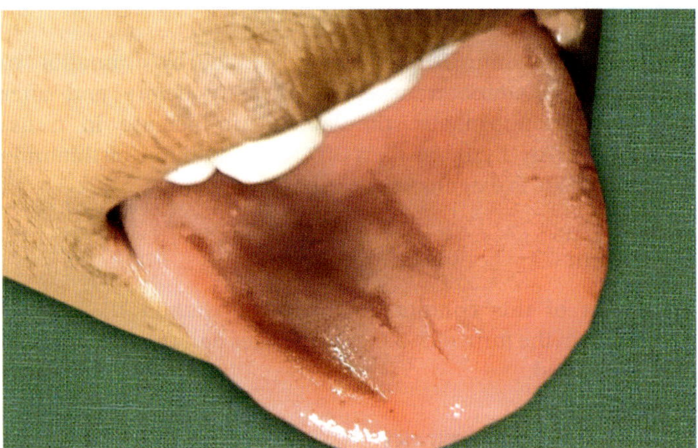

FIG. 3: Atrophic glossitis.

### Diagnosis

Altered erythrocyte glutathione reductase activity combined with a positive outcome on trial of riboflavin supplementation is often diagnostic of the condition.

### Treatment

Treatment consists of supplementation of 5–15 mg riboflavin 2–3 times daily for 2 weeks along with a diet rich in riboflavin.

## Vitamin B3 (Niacin)

It is otherwise known as nicotinic acid or niacinamide and is obtainable from various dietary sources. It also can be synthesized in the human body from tryptophan. People whose staple diet is maize or jowar and those with protein deficiency are prone to develop niacin deficiency (Box 9).

**BOX 9 Niacin**

- *Biological functions*: Component of nicotinamide adenine dinucleotide and nicotinamide adenine dinucleotide phosphate, which donate or accept hydrogen in various biochemical reactions. Help biosynthesis of ceramides and other stratum corneum lipids
- *RDA*: 14–16 mg/day
- *Dietary sources*: Dairy products, eggs, enriched breads and cereals, fish, lean meats, legumes, nuts, and poultry products
- *Deficiency states*: Inadequate dietary intake, alcoholism, carcinoid tumors, Hartnup disease, anorexia nervosa, Crohn's disease and gastrointestinal surgery, prolonged intravenous supplementation, drugs like isoniazid, azathioprine, 5-fluorouracil, ethionamide, protionamide, and pyrazinamide, antiepileptics like phenytoin and carbamazepine

RDA, recommended dietary allowances.

## Pellagra

### Clinical Features

It is an eczematous photosensitive dermatitis. It presents as sharply demarcated, keratotic, and hyperpigmented eczematous lesion. The eruption, in its acute stage, can be vesicular or bullous. Involvement of Dorsum of hands, and feet gives rise to "Boot and Gauntlet" appearance. There may be rash over butterfly area over face and upper central area of chest and neck (Casal's necklace) are the most commonly affected sites.

The cutaneous changes seen in pellagra occur more slowly than typical in sunburn and also take longer to recover. They usually present symmetrically but asymmetrical lesions are also seen particularly over the sites of eczema, injury, or stasis.

A seborrheic dermatitis like eruption over the nose with yellow, powdery scales over the follicular orifices also known as "sulfur flakes" is commonly seen in pellagra. Mucosal lesions consist of dry and fissured lips, atrophy or erythema and ulceration of tongue and buccal mucosa otherwise known as scarlet glossitis. There may be vulvovaginitis and scrotal dermatitis.

### Diagnosis

Diagnosis is made from suggestive clinical features and a rapid response to vitamin supplementation. Measurement of niacin metabolites such as N-methylnicontinamide and pyridine in urine is used in doubtful cases.

### Treatment

Oral niacinamide 0.5 mg/day is the treatment of choice. In severe cases, however, intravenous niacin is administered to reverse the cellular effects of niacin deficiency. Topical therapy includes emollients, sunscreens, and antibiotic creams.

## Vitamin B6 (Pyridoxine)

Pyridoxine is a pyridine derivative. Vitamin B6 describes three interchangeable molecules: (1) pyridoxine, (2) pyridoxamine, and (3) pyridoxal. The most common form existing is pyridoxal-5-phosphate (Box 10).

**BOX 10 Vitamin B6**

- *Biological functions*: Decarboxylation and transamination of amino acids, gluconeogenesis, and conversion of tryptophan to niacin, sphingolipid synthesis, prostaglandin synthesis, and neurotransmitter synthesis
- *RDA*: 1.3 mg/day
- *Dietary sources*: Meats, whole grains, vegetables, and nuts
- *Deficiency states*: Alcoholism, small bowel disorders (Crohn's disease and celiac disease), medications like isoniazid, hydralazine, penicillamine, and oral contraceptives

RDA, recommended dietary allowances.

### Clinical Features of Vitamin B6 Deficiency

Skin changes include a seborrheic dermatitis-like eruption, atrophic glossitis with ulceration, angular cheilitis, conjunctivitis, and intertrigo. Occasionally, a pellagra-like eruption may occur.

### Diagnosis

Vitamin B6 can be evaluated by mean measurement of plasma pyridoxal-5-phosphate. Low levels of plasma pyridoxal-5-phosphate indicate deficiency.

### Treatment

Deficiency is treated by discontinuation of suspected drugs and pyridoxine supplementation 100 mg/day.

## Vitamin B9 (Folate)

Folic acid is a compound consisting of pteridine, p-aminobenzoic acid, and glutamic acid (Box 11).

### Clinical Features of Folic Acid Deficiency

Mucocutaneous findings include glossitis with atrophy of the filiform papillae, angular cheilitis, mucosal ulceration, seborrheic dermatitis, and diffuse brown hyperpigmentation in the palmar creases and flexures.

### Diagnosis

Macrocytic and megaloblastic anemia with hypersegmentation of neutrophils in peripheral blood picture along with reduced serum and erythrocyte folate levels are suggestive of folate deficiency.

### Treatment

Folic acid supplementation (1–5 mg/day) and discontinuation of antifolate medications is recommended.

## Vitamin B12 (Cyanocobalamin)

### Clinical Features of Vitamin B12 Deficiency

Atrophic glossitis, generalized and Addisonian hyperpigmentation, vitiligo, and canities are the main dermatologic manifestations. Flexures, palmar creases, soles and knuckles, and pressure points like terminal digits are predominantly affected in hyperpigmentation associated with vitamin B12 deficiency.

**BOX 11 Folic acid**

- *Biological functions*: Transport of single-carbon units and role in growth and erythrocyte production, DNA and RNA synthesis
- *RDA*: 400 µg/day
- *Dietary sources*: Liver, wheat bran, beans, and green leafy vegetables
- *Deficiency states*: Alcoholism, malabsorption syndromes, and antifolate drugs such as methotrexate, trimethoprim, oral contraceptives, and pyrimethamine and antiepileptics

RDA, recommended dietary allowances.

**BOX 12 Vitamin B12**

- *Biological functions*: Acts as coenzyme for methionine synthesis used in DNA, protein, and lipid metabolism and succinyl-CoA synthesis used in fat and carbohydrate metabolism
- *RDA*: 2.4 µg/day
- *Dietary sources*: Liver, eggs, milk, beef, and other meats
- *Deficiency states*: Gastrointestinal abnormalities, such as a deficiency of intrinsic factor, achlorhydria, ileal diseases, and malabsorption syndromes, metformin administration, and long-term antacid ingestion

RDA, recommended dietary allowances.

The tongue is bright red, sore with atrophy of the filiform papillae, otherwise known as Hunter's glossitis. Early vitamin B12 deficiency presents as a linear form of glossitis. Melanonychia and premature graying of hair are other important features (Box 12).

### Diagnosis

Low serum cobalamin levels, i.e., less than 200 pg/mL is diagnostic of vitamin B12 deficiency.

### Treatment

Vitamin B12 supplementation both via parenteral and oral route is often curative for the dermatological abnormalities. Intramuscular injections of 1 mg/week for 1 month and then 1 mg/month usually reverse the pigmentary changes.

## Vitamin C (Ascorbic Acid)

Vitamin C is a relatively strong organic acid, chemically related to the carbohydrates. Only the laevo form is biologically active. In ascorbic acid deficiency, collagen and ground-substance synthesis are depressed, which results in various mucocutaneous changes (Box 13).

### Clinical Features of Vitamin C Deficiency

Petechiae and ecchymoses around the hair follicles are also a common finding of scurvy. There may be bleeding gums and painful bruises over areas prone to trauma.

Enlargement of hair follicles with keratotic plugging over the back, posterior thighs, buttocks, and shin is the earliest cutaneous

**BOX 13 Vitamin C**

- *Biological functions*: Vitamin C plays an important role in collagen and ground substance formation by intracellular hydroxylation of peptide-bound proline, metabolism of amino acids like phenylalanine and tyrosine, reduction of folic acid to folinic acid, prostaglandin metabolism, and transport of fatty acids
- *RDA*: 75–90 mg/day
- *Dietary sources*: Cabbage, potatoes, green vegetables, and fruits
- *Deficiency states*: Inadequate dietary consumption, smoking and alcoholism, dietary restriction in ulcerative colitis, Whipple disease, peptic ulcers and gastroesophageal reflux, parenteral nutrition and drugs like aspirin, indomethacin, tetracycline, oral contraceptives and corticosteroids

RDA, recommended dietary allowances.

sign of vitamin C deficiency. The hairs within these plugged follicles become curled, resulting in corkscrew hairs Woody edema with discoloration occurs over the ankles particularly in cases of chronic vitamin C deficiency. Impaired wound healing may occasionally be found.

### Diagnosis

Clinical features consistent with scurvy with leukocyte ascorbate level less than 75 mg/L is suggestive of vitamin C deficiency.

### Treatment

Deficiency state is treated with oral vitamin C supplementation along with a diet rich in protein.

## BIOTIN

Biotin is a water-soluble, sulfur-containing, and heterocyclic carboxylic acid involved in bacterial metabolism and possibly functioning as a coenzyme in decarboxylation and other enzymatic processes (Box 14).

### Clinical Features of Biotin Deficiency

Cutaneous manifestations of biotin deficiency include seborrheic dermatitis, periorificial erythema and scaling around the eyes, nose and anal region, glossitis, thinning of hair with patchy or diffuse alopecia, and dystrophy of nails. The periorificial dermatitis may resemble acrodermatitis enteropathica.

### Diagnosis

The diagnosis of the inherited forms is made by detecting organic aminoaciduria of 3-hydroxyisovaleric acid. Measurement of serum biotinidase can distinguish biotinidase deficiency from holocarboxylase deficiency.

### Treatment

Treatment of biotin deficiency consists of oral supplementation in the form of 10–60 mg/day.

## ZINC

It is an important trace element which is a part of numerous enzymes required for metabolism of fat, protein, and nucleic acid. The zinc supply depends largely on protein content in the food and protein energy malnutrition is usually associated with zinc deficiency (Box 15).

**BOX 14 Biotin**

- *Biological functions*: It is a cofactor for fatty acid synthesis and lipogenesis, gluconeogenesis, and amino acid catabolism
- *RDA*: 30 µg/day
- *Dietary sources*: Eggs, liver, milk, peanuts, mushrooms, chocolates, and hazelnuts
- *Deficiency states*: Prolonged diarrhea, raw egg white intake, parenteral nutrition, long-term antibiotics, and anticonvulsant use

RDA, Recommended dietary allowances

**BOX 15 Zinc**

- *Biological functions*: Helps in protein and nucleic acid synthesis; essential component of many metalloenzymes involved in cellular and metabolic functions; role in cell division and growth, fetal and brain development
- *RDA*: 8–11 mg/day
- *Dietary sources*: Shellfish, legumes, nuts, whole grain, and green leafy vegetables
- *Deficiency states*: Intestinal malabsorption syndromes, alcoholism, liver disease, burns, and prolonged parenteral nutrition

RDA, recommended dietary allowances

The dermatitis found in all forms of zinc deficiency is pustular and bullous with an acral and periorificial distribution.

### Acrodermatitis Enteropathica

It is a rare autosomal recessive disorder where impaired zinc absorption occurs because of a defect in an intestinal zinc transporter, the human ZIP4 protein encoded on the *SLC39A4* gene. Mutations in this gene prevent appropriate enteral zinc absorption. It is usually seen when an infant is weaned off breastfeeding.

#### Clinical Features

An eczematous erosive dermatitis over the hands and feet and around the orifices is the hallmark of this condition. Vesicles, bullae, pustules, erosions, and crusting are seen over the affected areas. Over time, the lesions develop a crusted border. Vitiligo like depigmented patches have also been reported in acrodermatitis enteropathica. The affected children usually have thinning of nail plate, periungual bullae, paronychia, gray and lusterless hairs, and nonscarring alopecia. The patients are more susceptible to infection by *Candida albicans* and *Staphylococcus aureus*. Chronic lesions may be more psoriasiform in morphology.

### Acquired Zinc Deficiency

It can occur in all age groups and present in acute or chronic form. The acute form is characterized by vesiculobullous lesions over the palmar creases, sole, and perioral and perianal region. The perioral lesions characteristically spare the vermillion border.

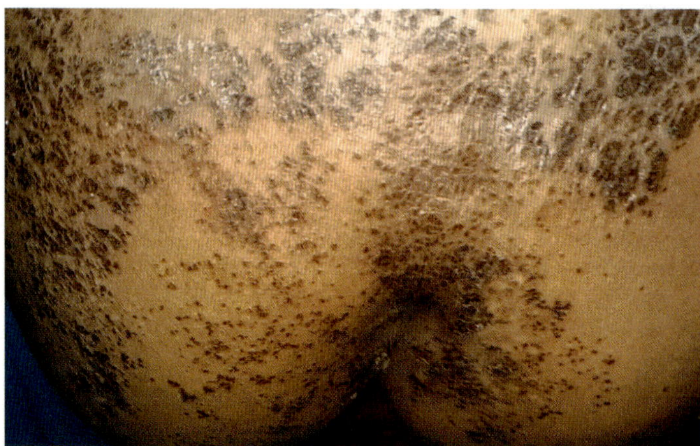

**FIG. 4:** Zinc deficiency in an adult.

There are usually features of acute paronychia and angular stomatitis. Hyperpigmented, hyperkeratotic psoriasiform lesions over bony prominences such as elbows, knees, knuckles, and ankles are the most prominent cutaneous signs of chronic zinc deficiency. Seborrheic dermatitis like lesions, acneifrom eruptions and xerosis of skin (Fig. 4) are other reported features. Hair changes include diffuse thinning and patchy alopecia, pigmentary changes and nails show prominent transverse depressions or Beau's lines. Impaired development of secondary sexual characters with gonadal atrophy can also be seen in chronic zinc deficiency.

### Diagnosis

The diagnosis can be confirmed by low serum zinc levels and low serum alkaline phosphatase levels.

### Treatment

Zinc sulfate 2–3 mg/kg/day is the treatment of choice. The treatment should be continued well into adulthood in acrodermatitis enteropathica.

## COPPER

### Clinical Findings of Copper Deficiency

Cutaneous manifestations of copper deficiency include reduced pigmentation of hair and skin and progressive and symmetric sensory loss and motor weakness of both upper and lower extremities (Box 16).

### Menkes Disease

Menkes disease, also known as kinky hair disease is a rare X-linked recessive disorder where mutation in the so called Menkes gene results in decreased concentrations of copper because of impaired intestinal absorption. The affected child has a cherubic face with depigmented, lustureless hair that becomes twisted around their long axes. Pili torti, monilethrix, and trichorrhexis nodosa are other hair shaft abnormalities.

#### Diagnosis

Low serum copper levels, microcytic anemia and neutropenia are suggestive.

**BOX 16 Copper**

- *Biological functions*: Essential component of several metalloenzymes, including tyrosinase and lysyl oxidase involved in melanin biosynthesis and collagen cross-linking
- Also involved in free radical detoxification and oxidation-reduction reactions
- *RDA*: 900 µg/day
- *Dietary sources*: Fish, oysters, whole grains, beef and pork liver, chocolate, eggs, and raisins
- *Deficiency states*: Malnutrition, malabsorptive states like celiac disease, cystic fibrosis, gastric bypass surgery, and short bowel syndrome, parenteral nutrition, infants with a strictly cow's milk diet, and excessive intake of antacids, zinc, iron, or vitamin C

RDA, recommended dietary allowances.

#### Treatment

It consists of dietary supplementation of copper in the diet.

## IRON

### Clinical Features

Mucocutaneous findings of iron deficiency include atrophic glossitis, angular stomatitis, xerosis of skin, and generalized pruritus. Thinning and spoon shaped convexity of nail plates also known as koilonychias are seen. Brittle lusterless hairs with alternate bands of hypo- and hyperpigmentation have also been described (Box 17).

### Diagnosis

Microcytic anemia and low levels of serum iron, ferritin, total iron binding capacity and transferrin saturation.

### Treatment

It consists of iron sulfate supplementation, 325 mg three times a day.

## SELENIUM

Selenium is found across all organs of the body and it works in close association with vitamin E in protecting the body against oxidative stress (Box 18).

### Clinical Features of Selenium Deficiency

Manifestations in children include hypopigmentation of the skin and hair (pseudoalbinism). Leukonychia and Terry-like nails have been reported. Elevated glutathione level in selenium deficiency probably interferes with melanin synthesis. Serum selenium levels are of prognostic value in the follow-up of malignant melanoma and cutaneous T-cell lymphoma.

**BOX 17 Iron**

- *Biological functions*: Involved in heme synthesis, oxidation-reduction reactions, collagen synthesis, and as a cofactor for various enzymes
- *RDA*: 8–18 mg/day
- *Dietary sources*: Red meats, egg yolks, dried beans, nuts, dried fruits, green leafy vegetables, and enriched grain products
- *Deficiency states*: Inadequate dietary intake or chronic blood loss as in menstrual disorders, GI bleeding, and malignancies

RDA, recommended dietary allowances; GI, gastrointestinal.

**BOX 18 Selenium**

- *Biological functions*: Essential component of the antioxidant glutathione peroxidase, important role in tissue repair
- *RDA*: 55 µg/day
- *Dietary sources*: Seafood, red meat, egg yolks, grain product, and chicken
- *Deficiency states*: Restricted protein diets, unsupplemented parenteral nutrition, and malabsorption states and persons living in areas with low soil selenium level

RDA, recommended dietary allowances.

## Diagnosis

Diagnosis of selenium deficiency is suggested by low plasma selenium levels and glutathione peroxidase activity.

## Treatment

It consists of supplementation of selenium in doses of 2 mg/kg/day.

## SUGGESTED READINGS


1. Aksu Cerman A, Sarikaya Solak S, Kivanc Altunay I. Vitamin D deficiency in alopecia areata. Br J Dermatol. 2014;170(6):1299-304.
2. Al-Dabagh A, Davis SA, Kinney MA, et al. The effect of folate supplementation on methotrexate efficacy and toxicity in psoriasis patients and folic acid use by dermatologists in the USA. Am J Clin Dermatol. 2013;14(3):155-61.
3. Alhaj E, Alhaj N, Alhaj NE. Diffuse alopecia in a child due to dietary zinc deficiency. Skin Med. 2007;6(4):199-200.
4. Aspuru K, Villa C, López SG. Optimal management of iron deficiency anemia due to poor dietary intake. Int J Gen Med. 2011;4:741-50.
5. Baek JH, Shin YH, Chung IH, et al. The link between serum vitamin D level, sensitization to food allergens, and the severity of atopic dermatitis in infancy. J Pediatr. 2014;165(4):849-54.
6. Battat R, Kopylov U, Szilagyi A, et al. Vitamin B12 deficiency in inflammatory bowel disease: prevalence, risk factors, evaluation, and management. Inflamm Bowel Dis. 2014;20(6):1120-8.
7. Bermejo F, Algaba A, Guerra I, et al. Response to letter: folate deficiency in Crohn's disease. Scand J Gastroenterol. 2014;49(2):255-6.
8. Bruno MC, Vilela MA, Oliveira CA. Study on dermatoses and their prevalence in groups of confirmed alcoholic individuals in comparison to a non-alcoholic group of individuals. An Bras Dermatol. 2013;88(3):368-75.
9. Chue CD, Rajpar SF, Bhat J. An acrodermatitis enteropathica-like eruption secondary to acquired zinc deficiency in an exclusively breast-fed premature infant. Int J Dermatol. 2008;47:372-3.
10. Cox JA, Beachkofsky T, Dominguez A. Flaky paint dermatosis. Kwashiorkor. JAMA Dermatol. 2014;150(1):85-6.
11. Demir N, Koc A, Üstyol L, et al. Clinical and neurological findings of severe vitamin B12 deficiency in infancy and importance of early diagnosis and treatment. J Paediatr Child Health. 2013;49(10):820-4.
12. Etani Y, Nishimoto Y, Kawamoto K, et al. Selenium deficiency in children and adolescents nourished by parenteral nutrition and/or selenium-deficient enteral formula. J Trace Elem Med Biol. 2014;pii:S0946-672X(14)00170-9.
13. Fei GQ, Zhong C, Jin L, et al. Clinical characteristics and MR imaging features of nonalcoholic Wernicke encephalopathy. Am J Neuroradiol. 2008;29(1):164-9.
14. Guevara Pacheco G, Chávez Cortés E, Castillo-Durán C. Micronutrient deficiencies and celiac disease in Pediatrics. Arch Argent Pediatr. 2014;112(5):457-63.
15. Huang SC, Wei JC, Lin PT, et al. Plasma pyridoxal 5'-phosphate is not associated with inflammatory and immune responses after adjusting for serum albumin in patients with rheumatoid arthritis: a preliminary study. Ann Nutr Metab. 2012;60(2):83-9.
16. Kilic M, Taskesen M, Coskun T, et al. A zinc sulphate-resistant acrodermatitis enteropathica patient with a novel mutation in SLC39A4 Gene. JIMD Rep. 2012; 2:25-8.
17. Kismul H, Van den Broeck J, Lunde TM. Diet and kwashiorkor: a prospective study from rural DR Congo. Peer J. 2014;2:e350.
18. Kotilea K, Quennery S, Decroës V, et al. Successful sublingual cobalamin treatment in a child with short-bowel syndrome. J Pediatr Pharmacol Ther. 2014;19(1):60-3.
19. Koul PA, Ahmad SH, Ahmad F, et al. Vitamin d toxicity in adults: a case series from an area with endemic hypovitaminosis D. Oman Med J. 2011;26(3):201-4.
20. Kuloğlu Z, Kirsaçlioğlu CT, Kansu A, et al. Celiac disease: presentation of 109 children. Yonsei Med J. 2009;50(5):617-23.
21. Kumar N, Ahlskog JE, Gross JB Jr. Acquired hypocupremia after gastric surgery. Clin Gastroenterol Hepatol. 2004;2:1074-9.
22. Kumar V, Kumar M, Yadav M. Alopecia in vitamin D-dependent rickets type II responding to 1$\alpha$-hydroxycholecalciferol.Ann Trop Paediatr 2010;30(4):329-33.
23. Léger D. Scurvy: reemergence of nutritional deficiencies. Can Fam Physician. 2008;54(10):1403-6.
24. Mahamid M, Abu-Elhija O, Samamra M, et al. Association between vitamin D levels and alopecia areata. Isr Med Assoc J. 2014;16(6):367-70.
25. Manzo G, De Gennaro A, Cozzolino A, et al. MR imaging findings in alcoholic and nonalcoholic acute Wernicke's encephalopathy: a review. Biomed Res Int. 2014;2014:503-96.
26. Maqbool A, Schall JI, Gallagher PRet al. Relation between dietary fat intake type and serum fatty acid status in children with cystic fibrosis. J Pediatr Gastroenterol Nutr. 2012;55(5):605-11.
27. Minns AB, Ghafouri N, Clark RF. Isoniazid-induced status epilepticus in a pediatric patient after inadequate pyridoxine therapy. Pediatr Emerg Care. 2010;26(5):380-1
28. Moulin P, Cinq-Frais C, Gangloff C, et al. Thiamine deficiency in infants: a case report. Arch Pediatr. 2014;21(4):392-5.
29. Mukhopadhyay D, Das MK, Dhar S, et al. Multiple carboxylase deficiency (late onset) due to deficiency of biotinidase. Indian J Dermatol. 2014;59(5):502-4.
30. Ong J, Randhawa R. Scurvy in an alcoholic patient treated with intravenous vitamins. BMJ Case Rep. 2014;pii: bcr2013009479.
31. Park KK, Brodell RT, Helms SE. Angular Cheilitis, Part 2: Nutritional, Systemic, and Drug-Related Causes and Treatment. Cutis. 2011;88:27-32.
32. Prakasha SR, Mustafa AS, Baikunje S, et al. "Dry" and "wet" beriberi mimicking critical illness polyneuropathy. Ann Indian Acad Neurol. 2013;16(4):687-9.
33. Prousky JE. Pellagra may be a rare secondary complication of anorexia nervosa: a systematic review of the literature. Altern Med Rev. 2003;8(2):180-5.
34. Ragunatha S, Kumar VJ, Murugesh SB. A clinical study of 125 patients with phrynoderma. Indian J Dermatol. 2011;56(4):389-92.
35. Singh AK, Kumar A, Karmakar D, et al. Association of B12 deficiency and clinical neuropathy with metformin use in type 2 diabetes patients. J Postgrad Med. 2013;59(4):253-7.
36. Stratigos AJ, Antoniou C, Papathanakou E, et al. Spectrum of idiopathic photodermatoses in a Mediterranean country. Int J Dermatol. 2003;42(6):449-54.
37. Subramanian VS, Subramanya SB, Ghosal A, et al. Chronic alcohol feeding inhibits physiological and molecular parameters of intestinal and renal riboflavin transport. Am J Physiol Cell Physiol. 2013;305(5):C539-46.
38. Wan P, Moat S, Anstey A. Pellagra: a review with emphasis on photosensitivity.Br J Dermatol. 2011;164(6):1188-200.
39. Wang AH, Still C. Old world meets modern: a case report of scurvy. Nutr Clin Pract. 2007;22(4):445-8.
40. Wilson HO, Datta DB. Complications from micronutrient deficiency following bariatric surgery. Ann Clin Biochem. 2014;51(Pt 6):705-9.

# 51 CHAPTER Porphyria and Other Amino Acid Metabolic Disorders

Saurav Kundu, Kumar Satya Prakash

## PORPHYRIA AND HEME METABOLISM

### INTRODUCTION

Porphyrias are metabolic disorders of heme biosynthesis resulting from a predominantly hereditary catalytic deficiency of the 2nd–8th enzyme involved in the porphyrin-heme biosynthetic pathway. They are inherited as autosomal dominant, autosomal recessive, or X-linked traits, with the exception of the most common type, porphyria cutanea tarda (PCT), which usually is sporadic.

### HEME BIOSYNTHESIS

Heme is required for a variety of hemoproteins like hemoglobin, myoglobin, respiratory cytochromes, and cytochrome P450 enzymes. Synthesis of hemoglobin in erythroid precursor cells contributes about 85% of daily heme synthesis in humans. Most of the rest are used by hepatocytes for the synthesis of cytochrome P450 enzymes.

The conversion of glycine and succinyl coenzyme A to heme involves eight enzymatic steps. The first and last three enzymes in the pathway are located in the mitochondrion, whereas remaining four are in the cytosol. These eight enzymes are encoded by nine genes.

- Glycine + Succinyl CoA
  ↓ALA synthetase
- Delta-aminolevulinic acid
  ↓ALA dehydratase: ALA dehydratase deficiency porphyria
- Porphobilinogen (PBG)
  ↓PBG deaminase: Acute intermittent porphyria
- Hydroxymethylbilane
  ↓Uroporphyrinogen III cosynthetase: Congenital erythropoietic porphyria
- Uroporphyrinogen III
  ↓Uroporphyrinogen decarboxylase: Porphyria cutanea tarda
- Coproporphyrinogen III
  ↓Coproporphyrinogen oxidase: Hereditary coproporphyria
- Protoporphyrinogen IX
  ↓Protoporphyrinogen oxidase: Variegate porphyria
- Protoporphyrin IX
  ↓Ferrochelatase: Erythropoietic protoporphyria
- Heme.

### CLASSIFICATION

Porphyria may be classified as erythropoietic and hepatic forms according to the major site of enzyme deficiency leading to overproduction and accumulation of porphyrin precursors or porphyrins.

From a dermatologist's perspective, the porphyria may be classified as cutaneous and noncutaneous forms. It may be also classified as acute and nonacute forms, thereby primarily considering the risk of life-threatening acute neurological attacks.

For simplicity eight major porphyrias may be classified into three groups:

1. Acute hepatic porphyria—four
2. Hepatic cutaneous porphyria PCT—one
3. Erythropoietic cutaneous porphyria—three.

#### Acute Porphyria

- Acute intermittent porphyria (AIP)
- Variegate porphyria (VP)
- Hereditary coproporphyria (HCP)
- ALA-D deficiency porphyria (ALA-D).

#### Nonacute Porphyria

- Porphyria cutanea tarda
- Erythropoietic protoporphyria
- Congenital erythropoietic porphyria
- Hepatoerythropoietic porphyria.

### ACUTE PORPHYRIA

This group includes three autosomal dominant (AIP, VP, HCP) and one autosomal recessive (ALA-D) porphyria. AIP is most common and ALA-D is rare (<10 patient till date). Life-threatening acute neurologic attacks, typically seen after puberty. Abdominal pain, the most common symptom is usually colicky, steady, and poorly localized. Others are constipation, distension, and decreased bowel sounds. Other common manifestations include seizures, mental symptoms, muscles weakness, sensory loss, tremors, sweating, dysuria, bladder distension, paraplegia, tetraplegia, and variety of other neurological and psychiatric signs.

VP and HCP can also present with cutaneous symptoms like increased photosensitivity, blistering, erosions, scars, and postinflammatory hyperpigmentation on the sun-exposed areas. Thus VP and HCP also referred to as neurocutaneous porphyria.

Acute porphyric attack can be precipitated by a variety of factors, including porphyrinogenic drugs, alcohol, hormonal changes, recurrent or chronic infection, and reduced caloric intake.

## NONACUTE PORPHYRIA

### Porphyria Cutanea Tarda

Most common porphyria, it is of two types: (1) sporadic or acquired (type 1)—deficiency of enzyme in liver; (2) familial or hereditary (type 2)—autosomal dominant and deficiency of enzyme in all tissues.

This usually presents in adults with increased photosensitivity, skin fragility, blistering, erosions, crust, and milia formation on the sun-exposed areas. Hyperpigmentation, hypertrichosis, sclerodermoid changes, and scarring alopecia may be seen.

On histopathological examination, subepidermal cell-poor blister with festooned dermal papilla (due to deposition of PAS-positive glycoprotein in and around vessels wall of upper dermis) is seen.

Direct immunofluorescence shows immunoglobulin G, complement and fibrinogen at the dermo-epidermal junction and around blood vessel of papillary dermis.

### Erythropoietic Protoporphyria

This is the most common erythropoietic porphyria and also most common porphyria of children.

This is transmitted as autosomal dominant disorder. Erythropoietic protoporphyria (EPP) presents with cutaneous photosensitivity which begins in early childhood. EPP may associated with cholestasis and severe liver disease.

The acute episode includes burning pain, stinging, and pruritus in sun-exposed skin mainly of nose, cheeks, and dorsum of hands. Subsequently, erythema and edema develops. Vesicular lesions are rare. Skin symptoms usually develops within minutes of sun exposure, often starting in early spring, continue through summer and diminishing in fall and winter. Chronic skin changes include lichenification and wax-like scarring mainly of nose. Hyperpigmentation, hirsutism, and severe scarring are rare.

Histological examination shows vacuolization of epidermal cells. Later intercellular edema, vacuolization and lysis of endothelial cells of superficial dermal vessels occurs. Finally, PAS-positive hyaline material deposited in capillary basement membranes causing its thickening and degeneration.

### Congenital Erythropoietic Porphyria

It is an autosomal recessive disorder and is extremely rare. It manifests shortly after birth or may be recognised in utero as a cause of nonimmune hydrops fetalis.

Presents with severe cutaneous photosensitivity leading to blistering, erosions, ulceration, excoriation, scarring, deformities, and mutilation (Fig. 1 ).

Other findings like erythrodontia, hemolytic anemia, and splenomegaly can be seen.

### Hepatoerythropoietic Porphyria

It is an autosomal recessive variant of hereditary PCT. This is rare, mostly reported in USA and Europe.

This usually presents in early childhood. Dark urine in the diaper is most common and often the first sign. Later, severe cutaneous photosensitivity develops and presents with blister, pruritus, hyperpigmentation, hypertrichosis and sclerodermatous changes.

## DIAGNOSIS

Clinical presentation is important. Histopathological examination many be suggestive.

Biochemical changes are often required for confirmation of diagnosis:

- *Porphyria cutanea tarda*: Increased excretion of uroporphyrin, 7-carboxyl porphyrins and coproporphyrins in urine and isocoproporphyrin in feces. Plasma porphyrins are also

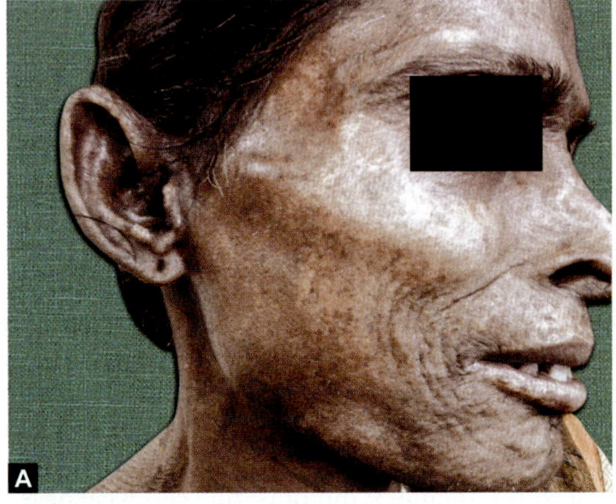


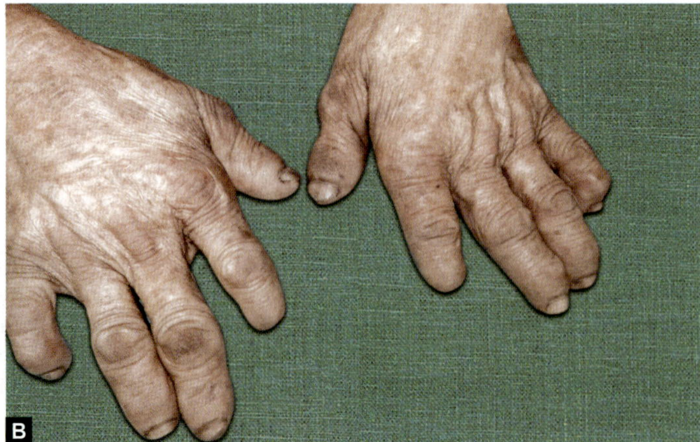


**FIG. 1: A,** and **B,** Congenital erythropoietic porphyria.

*Courtesy*: Dr Sayantani Chakraborty, Assistant Professor, Department of Dermatology, RG Kar Medical College, West Bengal.

increased. URO-decarboxylase activity is half in type 2 PCT and normal in type 1
- *Erythropoietic protoporphyria*: Free protoporphyrin is increased in erythrocytes, plasma, feces, and some other tissues like liver but normal in urine
- *Congenital erythropoietic porphyria (CEP)*: Increased excretion of uroporphyrin-I and coproporphyrin-I in urine and coproporphyrin-I in stool. URO-synthetase activity is markedly decreased
- *Hepatoerythropoietic porphyria (HEP)*: Increased excretion of uroporphyrin, hepta-carboxylated porphyrins in urine and coproporphyrin, isocoproporphyrin in stool. Level of zinc-chelated protoporphyrin is increased in erythrocytes
- *Acute porphyria*: Diagnosis is based on C/F and biochemical changes of urine and stool.

## TREATMENT

### Nonacute Porphyria

- Photoprotection and avoidance of sunlight exposure and trauma
- PCT: Avoid alcohol, stop estrogen and iron therapy, phlebotomy (400–500 mL every 2 weeks for 3–6 months), low-dose chloroquine (125 mg twice weekly till porphyrin excretion become normal)
- EPP: Oral β-carotene usually given from February to October in dose of 30–90 mg/day in children and 60–180 mg/day in adult, desirable maximum plasma level is 600–800 μg/dL. For hepatic complications, cholestyramine, charcoal, intravenous hemin, plasmapheresis, and liver transplant are options
- CEP: Change day-night rhythm, splenectomy, bone-marrow transplantation, and cord blood transplantation
- HEP: Change day-night rhythm.

### Acute Porphyria

Treatment of cutaneous manifestations similar to that of nonacute porphyria and for systemic symptoms patients referred to the concerned specialists.

# DISORDERS OF AMINO ACID METABOLISM

## INTRODUCTION

Inborn errors of amino acid metabolism are a group of rare and diverse disorders in which the synthesis and/or degradation of amino acids is impaired. It has many clinical phenotypes depending on the enzyme defect. The clinical presentation can range from asymptomatic to life-threatening metabolic crisis at neonatal age as well as mental retardation at later age.

## INCIDENCE AND MODE OF TRANSMISSION

Most of these are autosomal recessive disorders. Incidence of metabolic disorders affecting amino acids was found to be approximately 24 children per 100,000 live birth in a study conducted in British Columbia, Canada. No Indian data are available till date.

## CLASSIFICATION AND OVERVIEW OF AMINO ACID METABOLIC DISORDERS

Twenty amino acids both essential and nonessential are involved in metabolism. Each amino acids is further broken down into ammonia, $CO_2$, and water. Disorders of amino acid metabolism can be categorized into four groups:

1. Disorders of amino acid break down
2. Urea cycle defect
3. Disorders of amino acid transport
4. Organic acidemia.

### Disorders of Amino Acid Break Down

- Phenylketonuria
- Tyrosinemia
- Alkaptonuria
- Homocystinuria
- Nonketotic hyperglycinemia.

### Urea Cycle Defect

- N-acetyl glutamate synthase deficiency
- Carbamoyl phosphate synthetase deficiency
- Citrullinemia
- Argininosuccinic aciduria.

### Disorders of Amino Acid Transport

- Cystinuria
- Hartnup disease.

### Organic Acidemia

- Propionic acidemia
- Methylmalonic acidemia
- Maple syrup urine disease.

Most of the amino acid metabolic diseases have certain common features, such as poor feeding, lethargy, hypotonia, vomiting, dehydration, and failure to thrive. Cutaneous lesions resembling acrodermatitis enteropathica with diffuse alopecia and brittle hair is also fairly common. The distinctive features of the individual diseases are outlined here. Most of the diseases are autosomal recessively inherited.

### Phenylketonuria

*Enzyme deficient:* Phenylalanine hydroxylase.

#### Clinical Features

Patients with phenylketonuria presents with blond hair, blue eyes, fair skin, eczematous skin changes, sclerodermatous skin changes, and mental retardation. Seizures may be seen. There are also increased deep tendon reflexes.

### Tyrosinemia

Three types are recognized clinically:

1. *Type-I (hepatorenal)*: Caused by deficiency of fumaryl acetoacetate hydrolase

2. *Type-II (oculocutaneous)*: Caused by deficiency of tyrosine amino transferase
3. *Neonatal*: Seen in preterm infants.

### Clinical Features

- *Type I*: Fever, jaundice, edema, liver disease, and resultant hepatic failure
- *Type II*: Painful blisters and erosion over palm and sole that later become hyperkeratotic, mainly affecting thenar, hypothenar prominences and tips of digits.

Other findings are herpetiform corneal ulcer and mental retardation.

## Alkaptonuria

*Enzyme deficient*: Homogentisic acid oxidase.

### Clinical Features

Urine is dark and becomes black on standing. Deposition of pigmentation in the connective tissue leads to brown to black sclera and ear cartilage. Involvement of articular cartilages leads to arthritis.

Internal organ involvement, such as cardiac valves, trachea, and larynx. Urolithiasis may develop.

## Urea Cycle Defect

### Clinical Features

This is characterized by neurological manifestation such as mental retardation, seizures, episodic lethargy, ataxia, and hepatomegaly. Friable and brittle hair mimic trichorrhexis nodosa.

## Cystinuria

Defective transepithelial transport of cysteine and diabasic amino acid.

### Clinical Features

Persistent kidney stones and resultant obstructive uropathy.

## Hartnup Disease

Defective amino acid transport in the kidney and intestine and increased excretion of tryptophan metabolites.

### Clinical Features

Typically, pellagra-like skin lesions, photosensitivity, intermittent ataxia and tremor are seen.

## Organic Acidemia

### Clinical Features

This is characterized by neurological damage, developmental delay, hyperammonemia, ketoacidosis and hypoglycemia.

## Homocystinuria

*Enzyme deficient:* Cystathionine-β-synthase

### Clinical Features

Classical features are flushing, marfanoid habitus, mental retardation and seizure and ocular symptoms like glaucoma, ectopia lentis, and myopia.

# DIAGNOSIS

Congenital metabolic diseases can be detected by newborn screening tests as these tests help in earlier diagnosis and treatment, and results in better outcome with lesser chances of metabolic complications.

Prenatal diagnosis is possible in suspected cases by:

- Chorionic villus sampling/amniocentesis
- Measurement of the relevant metabolites/enzyme levels depending on the suspected disorders
- DNA analysis.

Common screening tests used in the diagnosis of congenital amino acid metabolism disorders are:

- *Ferric chloride tests*: To detect elevated phenylalanine levels in phenylketonuria
- *Ninhydrin paper chromatography*: To detect elevated/deficient amino acid levels in blood/urine
- *Guthrie bacterial inhibition assay*: To detect the levels of phenylalanine in plasma and the ratio of phenylalanine and tyrosine which is elevated in phenylketonuria. The quantitative assessment is done by tandem mass spectrometry and results are confirmed by specific tests
- *Liquid ion exchange chromatography*: To detect abnormal amino acid pattern and quantitative analysis
- *Gas chromatography/mass spectrometry*: To detect urine organic acid level in organic acidemia
- Plasma acylcarnitine analysis by mass spectrometry in organic acidemias.

## Specific Diagnostic Test

- *Tissue biopsy*: Mainly liver, muscle, brain, and bone marrow
- Skin biopsy and fibroblast cultivation for specific enzyme testing
- Specific DNA testing.

# TREATMENT

Disorders of amino acid metabolism can be managed under the following heading.

## Treatment of the Underlying Enzyme Deficiency and its Consequences

### Dietary Restriction

- Low tyrosine, low phenylalanine diet in tyrosinemia
- Low phenylalanine diet in phenylketonuria
- Low protein, low tyrosine, low phenylalanine diet in alkaptonuria.

## Dietary Supplementation

- Fish oil, tyrosine, and large amino acid supplementation in phenylketonuria
- Amino acid based formula promote growth and anabolism in patients of organic aciduria.

## Vitamin Supplementation

- Tetrahydrobiopterin supplementation increase phenylalanine hydroxylase activity in phenylketonuria
- Vitamin C supplementation prevent oxidation of homogentisic acid in patients of alkaptonuria.

## Dialysis

- To treat episodic hyperammnonemia in children with inborn error of urea synthesis
- Enzyme replacement
- Gene therapy
- Bone marrow and organ transplantation.

## Treatment of Complications

- Ocular, neurological, musculoskeletal, and other systemic complication to be managed by corresponding specialists
- Palmoplantar keratoderma of tyrosinemia type II can be managed by systemic etretinate.

# SUGGESTED READINGS


1. Abadie V, Berthelot J, Feillet F, et al. Neonatal screening and long term follow up of phenylketonuria. The French Database. Early Hum Dev. 2006;26:149-58.
2. Applegarth DA, Toone JR, Lowry RB. Incidence of inborn errors of metabolism in British Columbia 1969–1996. Pediatrics. 2000;105(1):e10.
3. Camp KM, Lloyd Puryear MA, Huntington KC. Nutritional treatment for inborn errors of metabolism: indications, regulations and availability of medicinal foods and dietary supplements using phenylkeyonuria as an example. Mol Genet Metab. 2012;107(1-2):3-9.
4. Cox TM. Erythropoietic protoporphyria. J Inherit Metab Dis. 1997;20:258-69.
5. Doss M, von Tiepermann R, Schneider J, et al. New type of hepatic porphyria with porphobilinogen synthase defect and intermittent acute clinical manifestation. Klin Wochenschr. 1979;57:1123-7.
6. Dupuis-Girod S, Akkari V, Ged C, et al. Successful match-unrelated donor bone marrow transplantation for congenital erythropoietic porphyria( Gunther disease). Eur J Pediatr. 2005;164(2):104-7
7. Fontanellas A, Mazurier F, Landry M, et al. Reversion of hepatobiliary alterations by bone marrow transplantation in a murine model of erythropoietic protoporphyria. Hepatology. 2000;32(1):73-81.
8. Fritsch C, Bolsen K, Ruzicka T, et al. Congenital erythropoietic porphyria. J Am Acad Dermatol. 1997;36(4):594-610.
9. Haim S, Gilhar A, Cohen A. Cutaneous manifestation associated with aminoaciduria: a report of 2 cases. Dermatologica. 1978;156:244-50.
10. Hanley WB. Adult Phenylketonuria. Am J Med. 2004;117:590-4.
11. Kleijer WJ, Garritsen VH, van der Sterre ML, et al. Prenatal diagnosis of citrullinemia and arginosuccinic aciduria: evidence for a transmission ratio distortion in citrullinemia. Prenat Diagn. 2006;26:242.
12. Kolanko E, Bickle K, Keehn C, et al. Subepidermal blistering disorders: a clinical and histopathologic review. Semin Cutan Med Surg. 2004;23:10-8.
13. Kontos AP, Ozog D, Bichakjian C, et al. Congenital erythropoietic porphyria associated with myelodysplasia presenting in 72 year- old man: report of a case and review of the literature. Br J Dermatol. 2003;148(1):160-4.
14. Layer G, Reichelt J, Jahn D, et al. Structure and function of enzymes in heme biosynthesis. Protein Sci. 2010;19(6):1137-61.
15. Lecha M. Erythropoietic protoporphyria. Photodermatol Photoimmunol Photomed. 2003;19:142-6.
16. Manisha B, Robert JD. The porphyrias: advances in diagnosis and treatment. Blood. 2012;120:19-27.
17. McGuire BM, Bonkovsky HL, Carithers RL Jr, et al. Liver transplantation for erythropoieticprotoporphyria liver disease. Liver Transpl. 2005;11(12):1590-6.
18. Moore MR, Hift RJ. Drugs in the acute porphyrias: toxicogenetic diseases. Cell Mol Biol. 1997;43:89-94.
19. Nova MP, Kaufman M, Halperin A. Scleroderma like skin induration in a child with phenylketonuria: a clinicopathological correlation and review of literature. J Am Acad Dermatol. 1992;26:329-33.
20. Poblete Gutiérrez P, Wiederholt T, Merk HF, et al. The porphyrias: clinical presentation, diagnosis and treatment. Eur J Dermatol. 2006;16(3):230-40.
21. Puy H, Gouya L, Deybach JC. Porphyrias. Lancet. 2010;375(9718):924-37.
22. Scott CR. The genetic tyrosinemias. Am J Med Genet C Semin Med Genet. 2006; 142C(2):121-6.
23. Smith W, Kishnani PS, Lee B, et al. Urea cycle disorders: clinical presentation outside new born period. Crit Care Clin. 2005;21(4):9-17.
24. Thunell S, Harper P. Porphyrins, porphyrin metabolism, porphyrias: III. Diagnosis, care and monitoring in porphyria cutanea tarda: suggestions for a handling programme. Scand J Clin Lab Invest. 2000;60(7):561-79.
25. Walter JH, MacDonald A. The use of amino acid supplements in inherited metabolic disease. J Inherit Metab Dis. 2006;29(2-3):279-80.

# 52 CHAPTER Deposition Disorders of Skin

*Nagaraju Donthula, Sendhil Kumaran M*

## INTRODUCTION

Cutaneous deposits are a varied group of substances which are usually not normal constituents of the skin. They are laid down, usually in the dermis, in a variety of different skin diseases.

There are basically five broad categories of deposits.

1. Calcium salts
2. Hyaline and mucin deposits
3. Pigments, heavy metals and drug pigment complexes
4. Cosmetic cutaneous implants such as collagen andsilicone which are used intradermally and subcutaneously
5. Other substances such as oxalate crystals and fiberglass.

Few of them evoke an inflammatory reaction with majority of them produce no response. The cutaneous deposition disorders of calcium are described here.

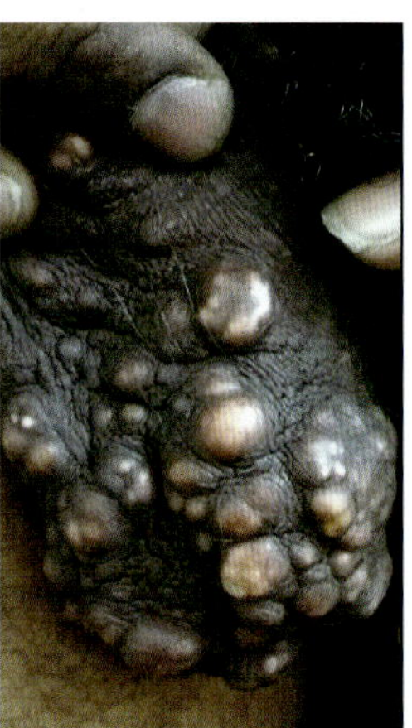

**FIG. 1:** Idiopathic scrotal calcinosis.

## CALCINOSIS CUTIS

It is divided into three types:

1. Dystrophic variety, when the calcium is deposited in damaged or degenerate tissue
2. Metastatic form associated with elevated serum levels of calcium or phosphate or both
3. Idiopathic calcification

In many cases, the pathogenesis is unknown and these belong to third idiopathic group. Sometimes, several mechanisms lead to the formation of the calcium deposits. Bone morphogenetic protein 4, β-catenin, osteopontin, osteonectin, and osteocalcin functional abnormalities may lead to idiopathic variety.

### Idiopathic Scrotal Calcinosis

Single or multiple lesions, up to 3 cm or more in diameter, develop in the scrotal skin usually in children or young adults. Sometimes, they may break down and discharge chalky material (Fig. 1). It was suggested that the lesions are dystrophic calcification of eccrine duct milia or of epidermal cysts, although this was being disputed. Scrotal calcinosis results from calcification of hair follicular or epidermal cysts, but this epithelium is not seen at the end of process. Calcification of degenerate dartoic muscle is suggested as a cause. A similar process involving the vulva and penis is reported.

### Dystrophic Calcification

Calcinosis cutis universalis, a type of dystrophic calcification is usually seen in dermatomyositis, lupus erythematosus and porphyria cutanea tarda . Calcinosis cutis universalis is also seen as an idiopathic phenomenon in the absence of any underlying disease or altered calcium/phosphate levels. Calcinosis circumscripta in which few minor deposits are seen is usually observed in scleroderma. Other dystrophic types are seen rarely, in burns scars, acne scars, trauma sites, venous ulcers, radiation sites, injection sites, at violin pressure point, keloids, and calcium gluconate injection sites (Fig. 2). Chronic kidney patients usually have higher tendency to develop dystrophic calcification due calcium containing heparin injection usage in them. It is also observed in industrial workers using calcium containing drilling fluids, in infants with herpes infection and acute leucamias as koebner phenomenon and in patients with genetic connective tissue disorders such as ehlers- Danlos syndrome and pseudoxanthoma elasticum. Extensive cutaneous calcification has been seen in pseudoxanthoma elasticum. Koebnerization is seen in infants, of acute leukemias along scratching. The dystrophic calcification of the CREST syndrome responded to treatment with intravenous immunoglobulin of underlying disorders (Fig. 3).

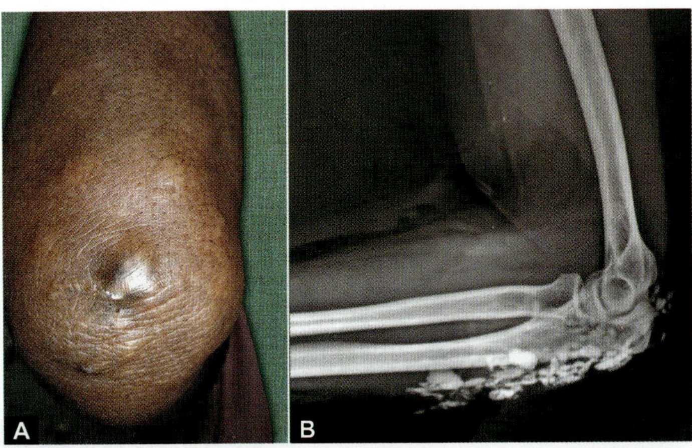


FIG. 2: **A,** Skin colored nodular lesion over left elbow; **B,** Calcium deposits in soft tissue around left elbow joint.

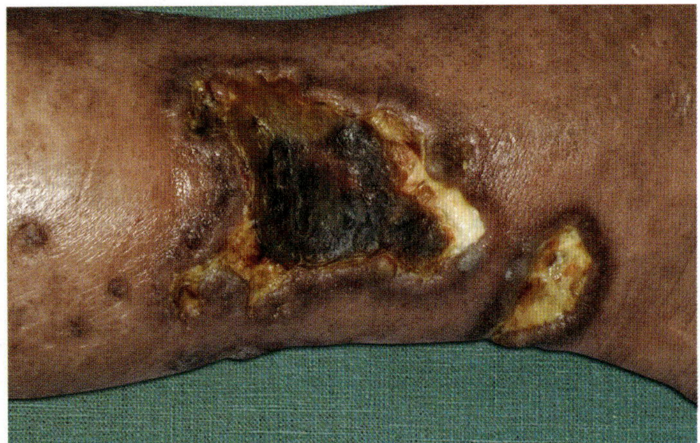

FIG. 4: Calciphylaxis.

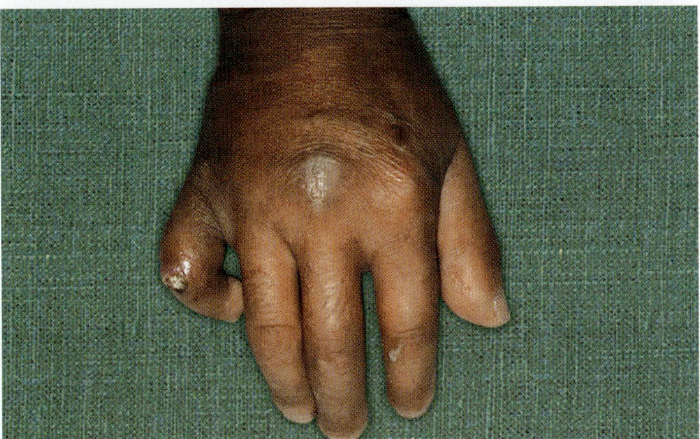

FIG. 3: CREST syndrome.

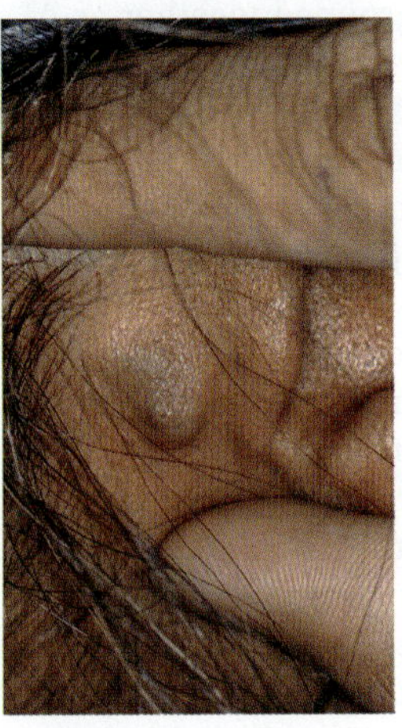

FIG. 5: Calcified sebaceous cyst.

## Metastatic Calcification

Cutaneous metastatic calcification is uncommon but can be observed in few cases of hyperparathyroidism, hypervitaminosis D, and in patients with destructive lesions of bone such multiple myoloma and in patients of chronic renal failure. Metastatic cutaneous calcification is seen in flexural areas such as groins, axillae and abdomen. These deposits are located in deep dermis and subcutaneous areas.

## Calciphylaxis (Calcific Uremic Arteriolopathy)

It is the rapid calcification of small and medium sized vessel walls. Its frequency is estimated about 4.1% in patients undergoing hemodialysis. It is commonly seen in elderly patients. It presents as painful livedo reticularis and tender erythematous plaques or nodules on the buttocks, abdomen, breasts, and the upper and lower extremities. The lesions become necrotic and ulcerate (Fig. 4). The penis is also rarely involved. Most cases are seen with end-stage renal failure with secondary hyperparathyroidism, but it is also seen with primary hyperparathyroidism, metastatic breast carcinoma, presumptive functional protein C and protein S deficiency induced by chemotherapy, alcoholic cirrhosis, warfarin therapy in a diabetic patient, and vitamin K therapy. An idiopathic variety is also seen very rarely. Obesity and systemic corticosteroids are risk factors for the development of calciphylaxis.

Recent studies implies the significance of NFkB role as inhibitors of RANKL-RANK-NFkB pathway such as bisphosphonates, recombinant osteoprotegrin and anti RANKL antibodies are shown helpful treatment modalities. Mortality rate of 60-80% has been shown due to secondary complications such as wound infection, sepsis and organ failure. Other treatment modalities tried in calicphylaxis are debridement, cinacalcet, bisphosphonates, sodium thiosulfate and low dose tissue plasminogen activator.

## Calcification of Cysts and Neoplasms

Calcification is usually seen in long standing benign and malignant neoplasms such as trichelemmal cysts, BCCs, hemangiomas, syringomas etc. They alter the texture and color of the neoplasms causing diagnostic difficulty. Calcification of sebaceous cysts is also seen causing bluish tinge to the cysts (Fig. 5). Nanobacteria species are postulated to be pathogenic factor in calcification of neoplasms although they are never detected.

# HYALINE DEPOSITS

Hyaline deposits are amorphous deposits usually seen in dermis. They are seen in metabolic disorders such as amyoloidosis, erythropoietic protoporphyrias, and lipoid proteinosis. Sometimes they are also crystalline type as in gouty tophi but they appear amorphous after dissolve in aqueous fixative. They are also seen in benign lesions such as colloid milium and after corticosteroid injection.

## Amyloidosis

Amyloidosis defined as the extracellular deposition of eosinophilic hyaline material of autologous origin. It has characteristic staining properties and unique fibrillar structure with origin from both skin and extracutaneous sites. 16 different fibril proteins have been found so far. Most of them are unrelated to the skin.

Six amyloid proteins are important in cutaneous amyloidosis: AA, ATTR, Aλ, Aκ, Aβ2M, and AK. Mixed amyloid deposits, containing two or more of these proteins are rare.

- AA (amyloid A protein) is seen in chronic inflammatory conditions, corresponding to secondary systemic amyloidosis
- ATTR (amyloid transthyretin protein) is seen in familial amyloidosis
- Aλ and Aκ are grouped together as AL (amyloid light chain protein). These proteins are seen in myeloproliferative diseases, such as multiple myeloma, or in idiopathic variety. Aλ is seen more than Aκ. It is usually seen in nodular cutaneous amyloidosis
- Aβ2M (amyloid β2-microglobulin protein) is usually seen in patients of long-term hemodialysis. It deposits mainly in the skeletal and articular system, but subcutaneous deposits are rarely seen. Improvements in hemodialysis have may lead to resolving of this type of amyloid
- AK (amyloid keratin protein) is seen in localized cutaneous amyloidosis, both lichen amyloidosis and macular amyloidosis. Proteins, such as amyloid P, apolipoprotein E, glycosaminoglycans, and immunoglobulins are seen non-specifically in cutaneous amyloidosis. Amyloid P, is a non-fibrillar glycoprotein which binds to all types of amyloid fibrils. In primary cutaneous amyloidosis, the amyloid is of keratinocyte origin, but how the keratin intermediate filaments transform into amyloid (AK) is to be elucidated. Apoptosis of keratinocytes may result in deposition of keratin as an abnormal protein. Another theory is that macrophages in the dermis process a normal alpha pattern of keratin into a beta-pleated sheet pattern. Active secretion of amyloid by basal keratinocytes is another theory. Several subclasses of keratin are found, in particular CK5. However, appendageal contribution to the amyloid deposits is favored by presence of CK7, CK17, and CK19 in some lesions. Suggested causative factors in the formation of this type of amyloid are prolonged friction, pruritus, genetic predisposition, Epstein-Barr virus (EBV), and environmental factors.

### Localized Cutaneous Amyloidosis

- Lichen, macular, and biphasic
- Nodular
- Poikilodermatous
- Anosacral
- Familial cutaneous.

### Lichen, Macular, and Biphasic Amyloidosis

Macular amyloidosis is usually seen in brownish to black skinned individuals such as Asians and Middle Eastern population. It presents as hyperpigmented patches involving extensors of arms and legs and high predilection for involvement on the back and interscapular regions. It is seen after prolonged rubbing or scratching and frequently pruritic. Uncommonly they involve the thighs, knees, or elbows. (Figs 6 to 8) The Q-switched Nd:YAG laser is used widely to reduce the pigmentation in patches of macular amyloidosis.

Lichen amyloidosis and macular amyloidosis are considered clinical variants of the same process as transformation from one to the other (biphasic form), are commonly seed. There is no systemic

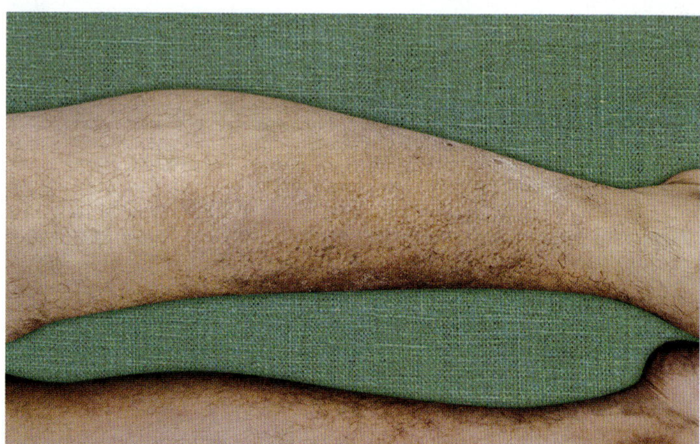

**FIG. 6:** Macular amyloidosis.

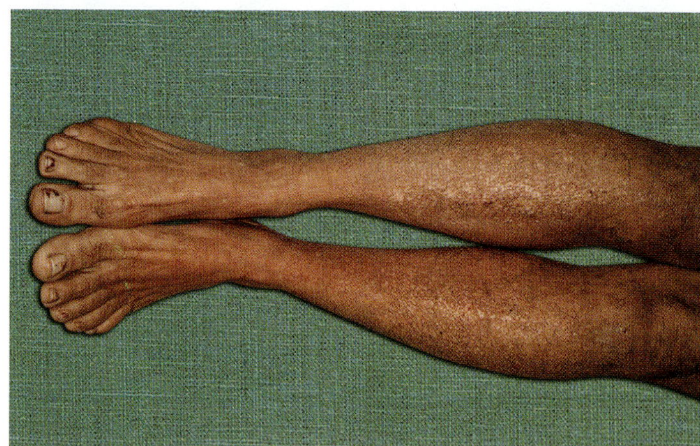

**FIG. 7:** Lichen amyloidosis.

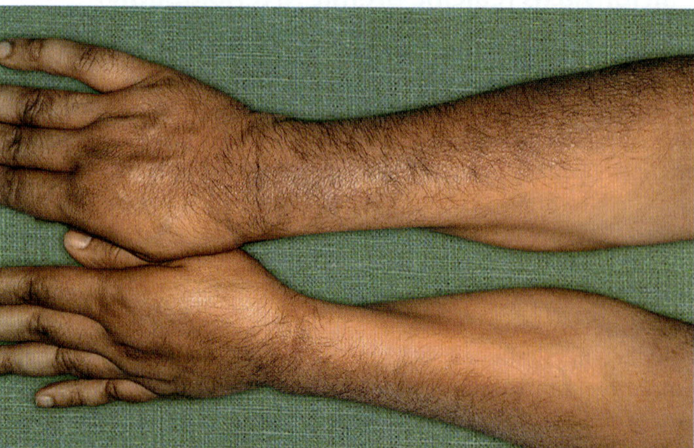

**FIG. 8:** Biphasic amyloidosis.

involvement in lichen amyloidosis or macular amyloidosis. An association with chronic pruritus and multiple endocrine neoplasia syndrome 2A, chronic EBV infection, Kimura's disease, and angiolymphoid hyperplasia with eosinophilia has been suggested. Its rare occurrence in human immunodeficiency virus (HIV)-associated papular pruritus and refractory atopic dermatitis lead to believe pruritus as etiological factor. A Brazilian family with localized cutaneous amyloidosis due to a mutation in the oncostatin M receptor-β (*OSMR*) gene is reported. Basic type amyloids keratins are commonly seen with predominance of keratin 5. Lichen amyloidosis presents as small, discrete, often pruritic, and waxy papules with a predilection for the extensor surfaces of the lower extremities. Rarely cold area involvement with sparing of high temperature areas, such as penis and groin is seen. Dermabrasion, combined bath PUVA photochemotherapy and oral acitretin, acitretin alone, hydrocolloid dressings, and the pulsed dye laser are tried in the treatment of lichen amyloidosis.

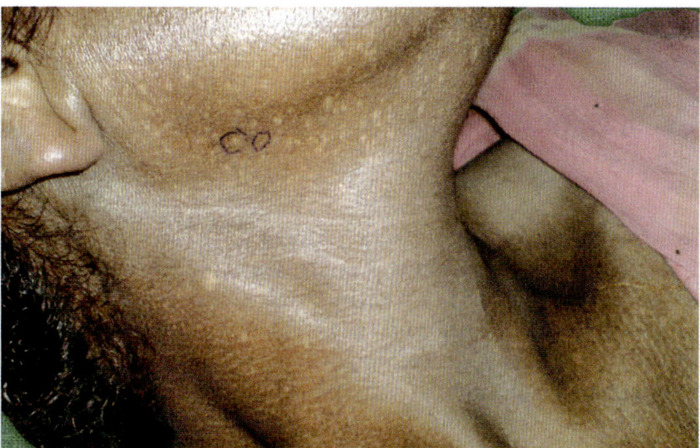


**FIG. 9:** Poikilodermatous amyloidosis.

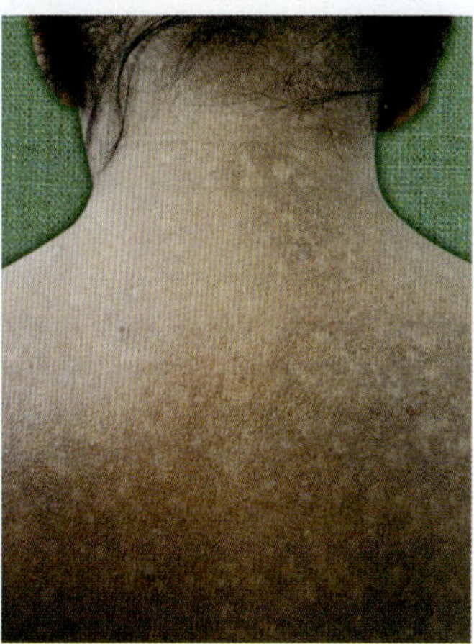

**FIG. 10:** Amyloidosis dyschromatosis.

## Nodular Amyloidosis

Primary cutaneous nodular amyloidosis is rarest morphological form of cutaneous amyloidosis presenting commonly as waxy skin colored to reddish yellow nodules or infiltrating plaques in acral areas, face, trunk, and genitalia of elderly patients with female sex predominance. Trauma is implicated as an etiological factor. Their size varies from few millimeters to few centimeters with overlying skin is atrophic. Occasionally nodular lesions may show hemorrhagic spots due to fragile vessels. They may present as bullae or tumor like masses rarely. It is associated with Sjögrens syndrome and diabetes mellitus. Primary localized cutaneous nodular amyloidosis sometimes can progress to systemic involvement in 7% of patients in a recent study in contrast to 50% of patients in prior studies. There is associated paraproteinemia in up to 40% patients which remained static in majority of patients except one who progressed to systemic involvement over 23-year follow-up in a study of 15 patients. Thus it requires long-term regular follow-up of patients. On histopathology AL, β2 microglobulin and rarely altered keratin are seen.

Treatment of nodular amyloidosis is individualized based on clinical presentation and availability of different modalities. It involves removal or destruction by shaving, excision, dermabration, $CO_2$ laser, and electrodessication with variable success rates. Recurrence is common after all the modalities even after surgical excision in which procuring hemostasis is difficult due to fragile vessels by surrounding amyloid deposits.

## Poikilodermatous Amyloidosis

Poikilodermatous lesions are very rare. A distinct subset of patients have short stature, early onset, light sensitivity, and sometimes palmoplantar keratoderma constitute the poikilodermatous cutaneous amyloidosis syndrome (Fig. 9). Amyloidosis cutis dyschromica (Fig. 10), characterized by reticulate hyperpigmentation with hypopigmented spots over much of the body is considered one of the poikilodermatous variant. It is thought to be a familial disorder.

## Primary Systemic Amyloidosis

Primary systemic amyloidosis is a rare disorder with reported incidence of 8 per 1 million persons per year. However, cutaneous involvement is commonly seen in this form of amyloidosis particularly myeloma-associated amyloidosis, with lesions in approximately one-third of patients. They present as nonpruritic, waxy papules on the scalp, face, and neck and sometimes the genitalia with a predilection for the periorbital areas. Plaque-like lesions sometimes develop on the hands and flexural areas. Hemorrhage into the lesions is commonly seen. Rarely, it may present as alopecia, occlusion of the external auditory canals, chronic paronychia, nail dystrophy, digital nodules, bullous lesions, condyloma-like lesions in the perianal region, muscle pseudohypertrophy, and elastolytic lesions (acquired cutis laxa).

The fibrillar protein is derived from light chains of immunoglobulin (AL), either λ or κ. The coexistence of β2-microglobulin has been seen. Lenalidomide is tried in the treatment of amyloidosis associated with multiple myeloma with higher cutaneous adverse reactions to this therapy. The median survival is about 13 months from diagnosis.

## Secondary Systemic Amyloidosis

Clinical involvement of the skin is very common in cases of secondary systemic amyloidosis with underlying chronic skin diseases, such as lepromatous leprosy, mycosis fungoides, hidradenitis suppurativa, arthropathic psoriasis, or dystrophic epidermolysis bullosa. Secondary amyloidosis may be seen in patients on hemodialysis with deposition of β2-microglobulin. In other secondary causes, the fibrillar component is AA protein. It is proposed that the presence of AL amyloidosis may lead to the development of AA amyloidosis secondary to chronic inflammation.

## Lipoid Proteinosis

Lipoid proteinosis, also known as Urbach-Wiethe disease, is a rare, autosomal recessive genodermatosis. It usually involves skin, oral cavity and larynx. Majority of the cases are reported from turkey and Africa although seen worldwide. Child usually presents with hoarseness of voice, recurrent cutaneous infections sometimes with vesicobullous lesions healing with atrophic pock like scars. Waxy, hyperkeratotic papules and plaques are seen on face scalp, neck and extremities (Fig. 11). When they are seen in eyelid margins they can cause blepharosis. Verrucous lesions on extensor areas such as knees and elbows are also seen. Localized form, limited to hyperkeratotic lesions on both hands and wrists has been reported. Organ dysfunction secondary to deposition is rare. Epilepsy may be seen with calcification of the hippocampus.

Lipoid proteinosis results from mutations in the gene (ECM1) encoding extracellular matrix protein 1 which is present in chromosome 1q21. History of consanguinity is observed in 20% cases. Although mechanism of ECM1 causing this amorphous hyaline deposition is unknown. It is postulated that ECM1 binds heparin sulfate and perlecan by acting as biological glue resulting in integrity of basement membrane and interstitial collagen fibril aseembly.

In the epidermis ECM1 plays a role in keratinocyte differentiation. The deposited materials include laminin and collagen of types IV and V and a relative low levels of collagen type I. Steroids, chloroquine, etretinate, and D-penicillamine have been tried with some success.

## Waldenström's Macroglobulinemia

Translucent papules, formed by deposits of monoclonal IgM, are rare manifestation of this disorder. The deposits surround blood vessels and hair follicles. Ultrastructurally, the deposits are composed of fibrillar and granular material.

## Mucinosis

The mucinosis results from the deposition of basophilic, finely granular and stringy material (mucin) in the connective tissues of the dermis (dermal mucinosis), in the pilosebaceous follicles (follicular mucinosis), or in the epidermis and tumors derived therefrom (epithelial mucinosis). Glycosaminoglycans are a major class of extracellular complex polysaccharides predominantly seen in dermal mucinosis.

There are four classes:

1. Heparin/heparan
2. Chondroitin/dermatan
3. Keratan
4. Hyaluronan (hyaluronic acid).

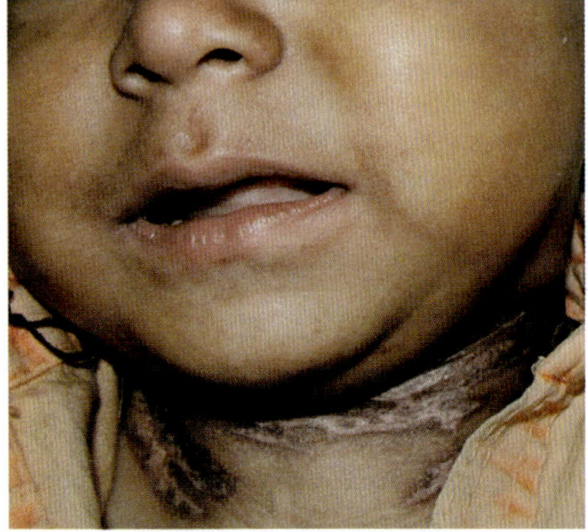

**FIG. 11:** Thickened, firm lips and tongue, waxy, thickened and hyperkeratotic plaques in the neck in a child with lipoid proteinosis.

## Generalized Myxedema

It is seen in patients of hypothyroidism. It involves the eyes, nose, and cheeks, often giving a characteristic facies, and also on the distal extremities. The skin is cold, dry, and pale with widespread xerosis, especially on the extensor surfaces. A diffuse, nonscarring alopecia is seen sometimes. Cutis verticis gyrata is a rare presentation. Palmoplantar keratoderma is an uncommon presentation of myxedema. Glycosaminoglycans remain deposited in the skin due to impaired degradation, rather than increased synthesis. Muscle weakness is sometimes present. Generalized and pretibial myxedema have been grouped together as "dysthyroidotic mucinoses".

## Pretibial Myxedema (Thyroid Dermopathy)

Pretibial myxedema (thyroid dermopathy) is seen in 1–4% of patients with Graves' disease, with exophthalmos. Rarely, it may be seen with nonthyrotoxic Graves' disease, Hashimoto's thyroiditis, ectopic, hyperplastic nodule arising in a thyroglossal duct residue, euthyroid patients with stasis dermatitis, and in patients with morbid obesity that have lower leg lymphedema (Fig. 12).

It usually presents as diffuse nonpitting edema with circumscribed nodular lesions and thick skin mimicking elephentiasis in long standing cases. Overlap of nodular lesions to diffuse lesions is observed. It is usually seen in anterior aspect of lower legs and dorsum of feet but rarely seen in face, neck and ears, hypertrichosis and hyperhidorsis is observed on lesions of the myxedema. Other features of hyperthyroidism such as proptosis and acropachy (digital clubbing and diaphyseal proliferation) are seen rarely. It resolves very slowly after the correction of underlying hyperthyroidism taking many years.

The precise pathogenesis of pretibial myxedema is unknown, but thought to be due to stimulation of fibroblasts secondary to circulating factor present in serum and also upregulation of IGF-1 receptors in fibroblasts presumably due to response from octreotide. Older theory of long-acting thyroid stimulating antibodies is no longer substantiated. There is no primary lymphatic abnormality. Hydrostatic forces appear to play a role in the localization of the pretibial mucinosis.

## Papular Mucinosis and Scleromyxedema

Papular mucinosis (lichen myxedematosus) is a rare cutaneous mucinosis in which multiple, asymptomatic, pale or waxy papules, 2–3 mm in diameter, develop on the hands, forearms, face, neck, and upper trunk (Fig. 13). Rarely, it is associated with hepatitis C, HIV infection, L-tryptophan-induced eosinophilia-myalgia syndrome, generalized morphea, subclinical hypo-

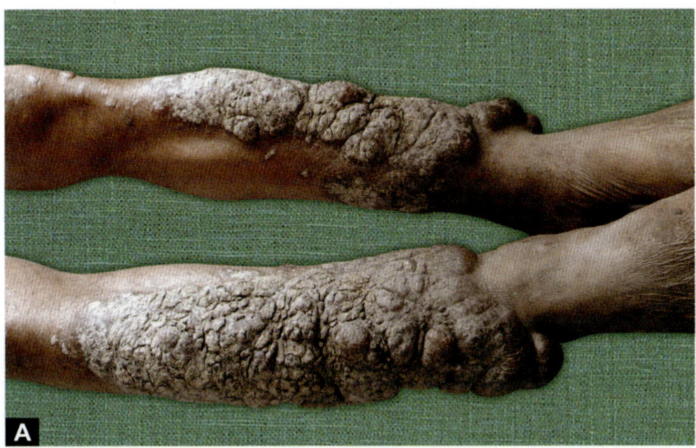

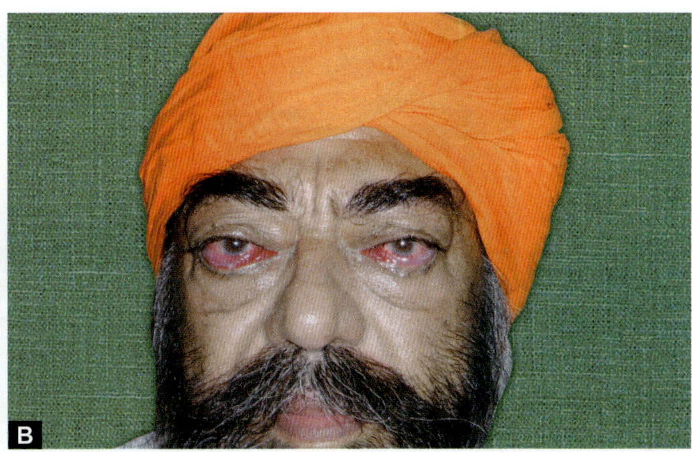

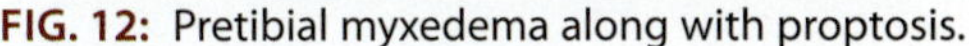

FIG. 12: Pretibial myxedema along with proptosis.

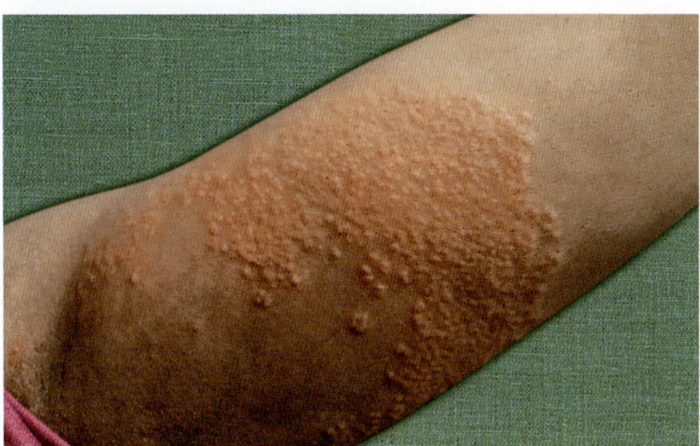

FIG. 13: Papular mucinosis.

thyroidism, and morbid obesity. It resolves spontaneously in some patients. Scleromyxedema is a variant in which lichenoid papules and plaques are accompanied by skin thickening involving almost the entire body with predominance of face, neck, hands, and forearms in adults of age 3$^{rd}$ to 5$^{th}$ decade. Glabellar region involvement leads to leonine appearance. Scleromyxedema has higher chancw of systemic association such as paraprotienemia, chronic hepatitis C, pachydermoperiostosis, dermatomyositis, scleroderma, multiple keratoacanthomas. Scleromyxedema is two types generalized and localized. Generalized varian is called scleromyxedema and localized variants are acral persistent popular mucinosis, self healing popular mucinosis, popular mucinosis of infancy and nodular lichen myxedematosus. Trestment modalities such as IVIG, interferon alfa, prednisolone, retinoids, thalidomide and melphalan etc have been tried in diffuse variants. The localized type can be treated with tacrolimus ointment.

## Reticular Erythematous Mucinosis

Reticular erythematous mucinosis (REM) presents as erythematous maculopapules and infiltrated plaques, often with a reticulated or netlike pattern, in the midline of the back or chest, sometimes spreading to the upper abdomen in young to middle aged females (Fig. 14). Rarely, the face, arms and gums are involved. Sunlight and hormonal influences may cause exacerbation. It can progress to cutaneous lupus erythematosus or subside in few years. Hyaluronan deposition occurs by dermal dendrocytes. Topical tacrolimus and UVA1 radiation are tried as a safe alternative to systemic antimalarials in the treatment of REM.

## Scleredema

Scleredema (scleredema adultorum of Buschke) is characterized by the development of nonpitting induration of the skin with a predilection for symmetrical involvement of the posterior neck, the shoulders, the upper trunk, and the face. Rarely thighs and periorbital region is seen. In cases of more widespread involvement, the upper part of the body is always involved much more than the lower part, and the feet are spared. The condition occurs at all ages, although nearly 50% of cases develop in children and adolescents. There is a predilection for females. Based on clinical scenario it is divided into five groups:

- *Group I*: It associated with acute febrile illness, streptococci, and HIV and scabies infections. Spontaneous resolution occurs in approximately one-third of the postinfectious patients after 6–18 months
- *Group II*: It has an insidious onset, without any predisposing illness, and a protracted course
- *Group III*: It is associated with uncontrolled insulin-dependent, maturity onset diabetes. Vascular complications of diabetes are common. It can also be associated with type II diabetes
- *Group IV*: It is associated with a monoclonal gammopathy. Extracorporeal photopheresis and chemotherapy are tried as treatment options
- *Group V*: Miscellaneous associations such as mechanical stress, carcinoma of the gallbladder, and rheumatoid arthritis.

Sceleredema has slow onset with prolonged course. It is usually associated with ECG changes, pericordial effusion, pleural effusion and skeletal muscle involvement. Sometimes cellulitis, skin abscesses can trigger scleredema. Usually it is plain skin thickening but sometimes erythema is seen rarely. (Fig. 15).

The etiology is unknown, but thought to be due to activated phenotype of fibroblasts producing glycosaminoglycans. Scleredema has been successfully treated with UVA1 phototherapy.

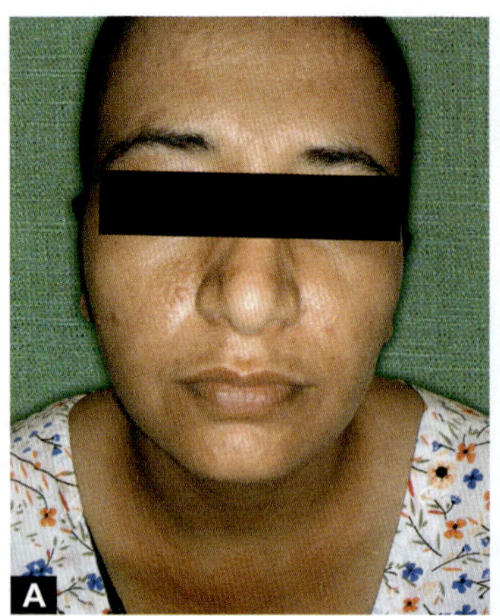


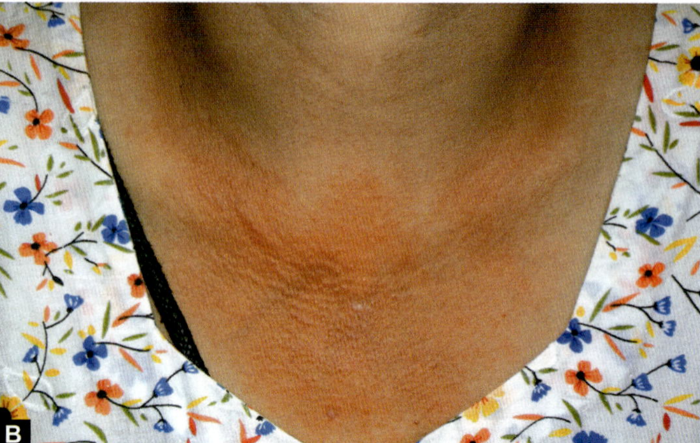


**FIG. 14:** Reticular erythematpus mucinosis.

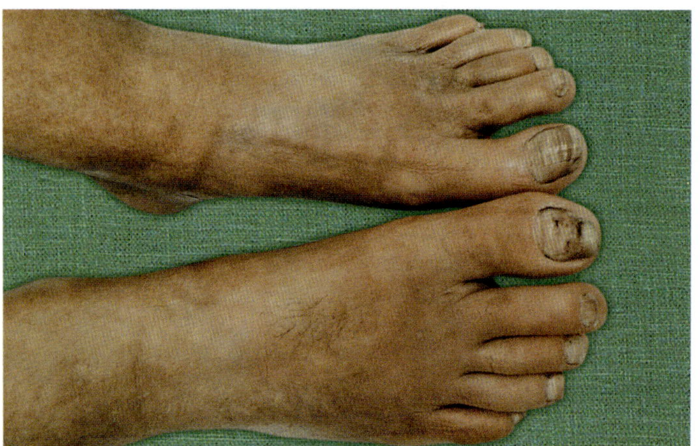

**FIG. 15:** Scleredema diabeticorum.

## Mucopolysaccharidoses

The mucopolysaccharidoses are a group of ten lysosomal storage diseases which result from the deficiency of specific lysosomal enzymes involved in the degradation of dermatan sulfate, heparan sulfate, or keratan sulfate, singly or in combination resulting in accumulation of mucopolysaccharides in various tissues and their excretion in urine. The specific enzyme defect can be identified using cultured fibroblasts, although in many instances a tentative diagnosis is possible on the clinical features alone. Prenatal diagnosis is possible on both cultured amniotic fluid cells and chorionic villus samples. Analysis of the urine for certain mucopolysaccharides will also assist in the diagnosis. The urine contains heparan sulfate in the Sanfilippo syndrome, keratan sulfate in the Morquio syndrome, dermatan sulfate in the Maroteaux–Lamy syndrome, and an excess of dermatan and heparan sulfates in varying proportions in the others.

The mucopolysaccharidoses share many clinical features.

- Skeletal abnormalities such as dysostosis multiplex are seen (except in Morquio's syndrome)
- Short stature (excluding Scheie's syndrome)
- Corneal clouding (except in the Hunter (MPS II) and Sanfilippo (MPS III) syndromes)
- Deafness, grotesque facies (gargoylism), hirsutism, premature arteriosclerosis, hepatosplenomegaly, and severe mental retardation (excluding MPS VI and MPS IS).

The best known of the mucopolysaccharidoses are:

- Hurler's syndrome , which has the worst prognosis and is due to a deficiency of α-L-iduronidase encoded by the IDUA gene at 4p16.3
- Hunter's syndrome, which results from a deficiency of iduronate-2-sulfate sulfatase. The only X-linked mucopolysaccharidosis with the gene defect located at Xq28
- Sanfilippo syndrome with gene defect is situated on chromosome 17q25.3. Numerous different mutations have been identified. Recently, the transmembrane protein 76 gene (TMEM76) has been identified as a possible cause of Sanfilippo syndrome type C, a disorder of heparan sulfate degradation due to a deficiency of the enzyme N-acetyltransferase.

Cutaneous manifestations of the mucopolysaccharidoses include:

- Excessive hair and dryness of the skin
- Mild thickening of skin. This is most marked in Hurler's syndrome where sclerodermoid thickening of the fingers and furrowing of the skin can occur
- Firm, flesh-colored to waxy papules and nodules are seen on the upper trunk, particularly in the scapular region giving rise to a characteristic cobblestone appearance, in Hunter's syndrome
- Extensive Mongolian spots are another manifestation of Hunter's syndrome.

Allogeneic bone marrow transplantation before the age of 2 years will halt disease progression in Hurler's syndrome. A recombinant human alpha-L-iduronidase has been tried.

## Colloid Milia

There are at least five distinct clinicopathological conditions that can be included under the umbrella term of "colloid milium and colloid degeneration".

The five variants are:

1. *Colloid milium*: Classic adult type
2. Juvenile colloid milium
3. Pigmented colloid milium (hydroquinone related)
4. Colloid degeneration (paracolloid)
5. Acral keratosis with eosinophilic dermal deposits.

### *Adult Type*

It develops in early to mid-adult life with numerous yellow-brown, semitranslucent, dome-shaped papules, 1–4 mm or more in diameter. They are discrete or clustered to form plaques involving the cheeks, ears, neck, and dorsum of the hands (Fig. 16). Verrucous lesions are rarely seen. Sometimes, it there is history of petroleum products application. The material in the dermis is thought to represent a degeneration product of elastic fibers induced by solar radiation (actinic elastoid).

#### *Juvenile Colloid Milium*

It is exceedingly rare. Papules or plaques develop, usually on the face and neck, prior to puberty. Conjunctival and gingival lesions are rarely seen. Recently it is proposed that juvenile colloid milium and ligneous conjunctivitis are different clinical phenotypes of severe type I plasminogen deficiency.

#### *Pigmented Colloid Milium*

It is found as gray to black clustered or confluent papules on the face, following the excessive use of hydroquinone bleaching creams.

#### *Colloid Degeneration (Paracolloid)*

It presents as nodular, plaque-like areas, usually in chronically sun-exposed skin, particularly the face (Fig. 17). This is probably a heterogeneous group as illustrated by the case occurring on penile skin.

#### *Acral Keratosis*

Acral keratosis with eosinophilic dermal deposits. It presents as agminated or solitary papules of the distal finger in elderly patients with amorphous eosinophilic deposits. They are slowly progressive.

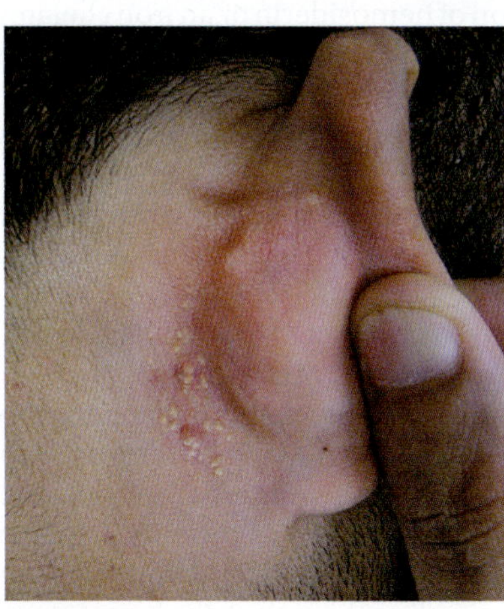

**FIG. 16:** Milia—adult type.

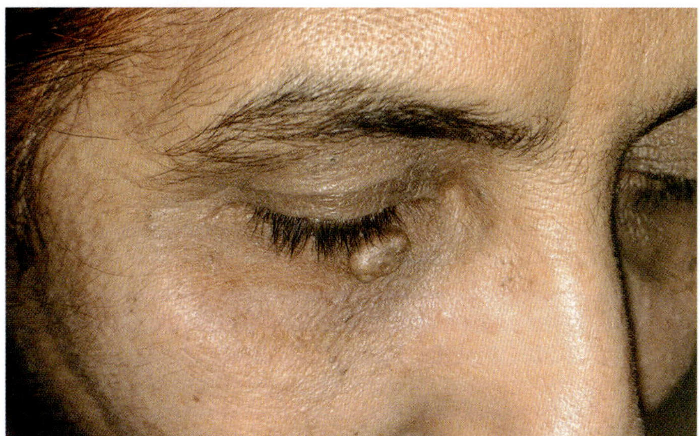

**FIG. 17:** Milia en plaque.

## PIGMENT AND RELATED DEPOSITS

Exogenous and endogenous pigmentary depositions are seen sometimes presenting as pigmentary deposition disorders at varying sites depending on the causative agents.

Iron, nickel and chromium deposition is seen after total elbow arthroplasty causing bluish grey pigmentation of forearm. Examples of such pigmentary deposition disorders are as follows.

### Ochronosis

Ochronosis refers to the yellow-brown or ocher pigment (homogentisic acid) deposited in collagen-containing tissues in alkaptonuria. Alkaptonuria is an autosomal recessive disorder with defect in hepatic and renal enzyme homogentisic acid oxidase. The term ochronosis is also used for the deposition of similar hydroquinone derivatives, phenol, picric acid used for various dermatological conditions. In alkaptonuria, there is bluish-black pigmentation of the face, neck, dorsum of the hands and palmoplantar region and bluish discoloration of the sclerae and of the cartilage of the ears and sometimes of the nose (Fig. 18). In hydroquinone-induced lesions, the face (particularly the malar areas), neck in areas of application of the cream, are involved. The dorsal aspect of the interphalangeal joints is frequently affected. There is hyperpigmentation, with variable development of finely papular and even colloid milium-like areas. Melanocytes are required for the pigmentation as melanin-hydroquinone combination products cause pigmentation.

### Hemochromatosis

Hemochromatosis is a multisystem disorder of iron metabolism in which cutaneous pigmentation is a manifestation in up to 90% of patients (bronzed diabetes). Bronze colored pigmentation involving all over the body with marked appearance on face. Slate gray colored pigmentation is also seen. The bronze color results from increased melanin in the basal layers of the epidermis and, to a lesser extent, some coexisting thinning of the epidermis. Slate-gray color results from hemosiderin deposits in the

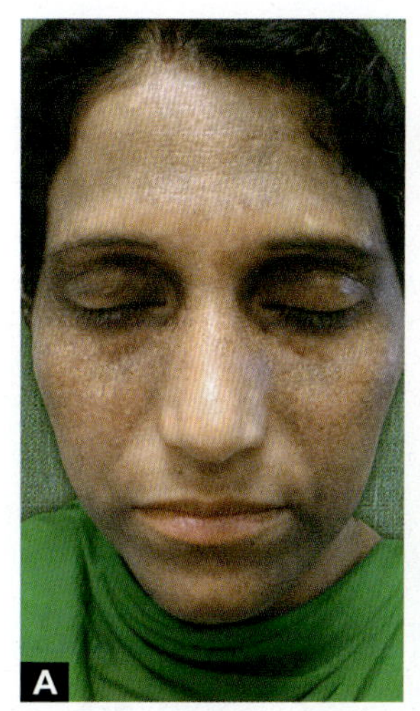


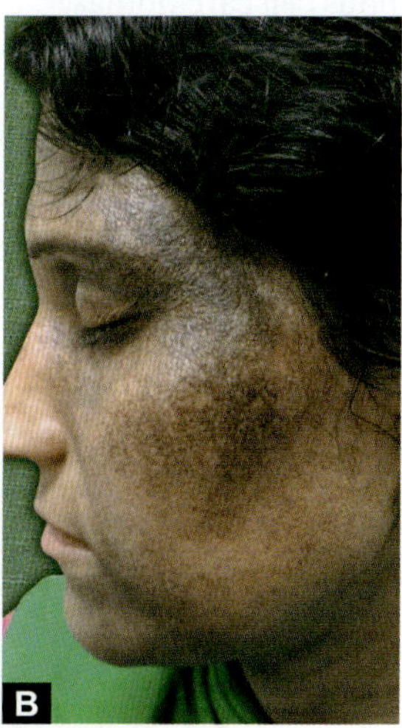


**FIG. 18:** Ochronosis.

epidermis as well as the dermis, and it is thought that epidermal hemosiderin contributes to the skin color in these patients. The absence of pigmentation in the vitiliginous areas of patients with both vitiligo and hemochromatosis indicates that hemosiderin in the usual dermal sites does not contribute significantly to the bronze color in patients with hemochromatosis. Epidermal and dermal deposition of hemosiderin gives slate grey hue to skin.

## Silver Deposition (Argyria)

Argyria, which refers to the systemic deposition of silver salts, is an iatrogenic disease resulting from the indiscriminate ingestion of silver containing compounds or their application to mucous membranes or burnt skin. They are seen as occupational hazards. Bizarre dietary fads and the availability of colloidal silver preparations as alternative health treatments have resulted in increased exposure in community. It causes permanent blue-gray pigmentation, resembling cyanosis, predominantly in sun-exposed areas. Azure blue colored lunula is seen sometimes. The photoactivated reduction of the absorbed silver salts to metallic silver may result in the pigmentation. It is also seen with prolonged topical application. Acupuncture needling and wearing silver ear rings.

## Gold Deposition (Chrysiasis)

Chrysiasis refers to the permanent blue-gray pigmentation of the skin, predominantly in sun-exposed areas resulting from the deposition of gold salts in the dermis, following gold injections for the treatment of rheumatoid arthritis and pemphigus. Its development is, in part, dose related, but light exposure and even laser therapy appear to favor its deposition. Gold also causes urticaria, lichenoid reaction, and pityriasis rosea like eruption.

## Arsenic

Chronic exposure to arsenic results in a diffuse, macular, bronze pigmentation, predominantly on the trunk with "raindrop" areas of normal or depigmented skin. The color is due to increased melanin in the basal layer and partly from the metal itself. Periungual pigmentation is also seen. Chronic arsenic ingestion sometimes cause thick hyperkeratotic palms and soles, and squamous cell carcinomas.

## Drugs

Cutaneous pigmentation sometimes is caused by drug deposition in epidermis and dermis forming varying complex substances or usually after lichenoid drug reaction or postinflammatory hyperpigmentation.

### Antimalarial Drugs

Antimalarial drugs cause several patterns of cutaneous pigmentation. Yellow pigmentation is sometimes seen with quinacrine (mepacrine), Small ochronosis like deposits are a rarely described. Slate gray to blue black pretibial pigmentation is more common. On histopathology, pigment granules staining for hemosiderin, melanins are seen in macrophages and extracellularly.

#### *Tetracycline*

Bluish pigmentation of cutaneous osteomas and bluish-green pigmentation in areas of trauma on the lower legs and acne scars is seen. Suprapharmological doses of tetracycline can cause diffuse pigmentation involving all over body.

#### *Minocycline (Fig. 19)*

Five different patterns of cutaneous pigmentation are seen during long-term therapy with minocycline:

- *Type I*: Bluish-black pigmentation of scars and old inflammatory foci, including sites of immunobullous diseases, due to deposition of hemosiderin or an iron chelate of minocycline
- *Type II*: Blue-gray circumscribed pigmentation of the lower legs and arms resulting from pigment which is probably a drug metabolite–protein complex chelated with iron and calcium
- *Type III*: A generalized muddy brown pigmentation due to increased melanin in the basal layer, and accentuated in sun-exposed areas
- *Type IV*: Blue gray pigmentation involving acne scar areas. It is thought to be variant of type I
- *Type V*: Blue black pigmentation involving lower extremities limited to subcutaneous plane on histopathology.

Combinations of these patterns are not uncommon. Blue colored sweating is seen in some patients. In patients with atopic dermatitis diffuse cutaneous pigmentation is seen in relatively short-term minocycline therapy, 3–28 days.

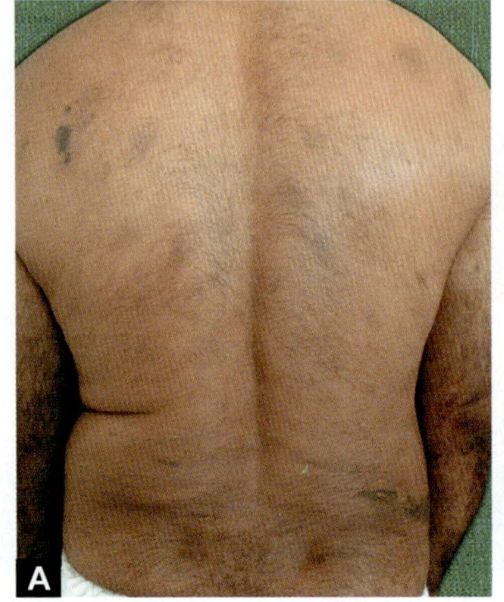


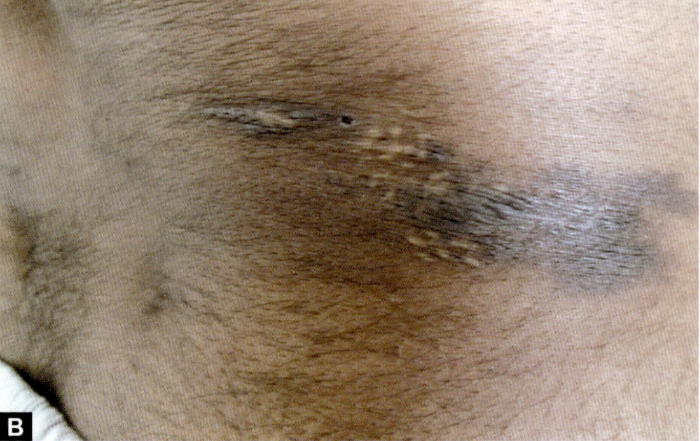


**FIG. 19:** Minocycline-induced pigmentation.

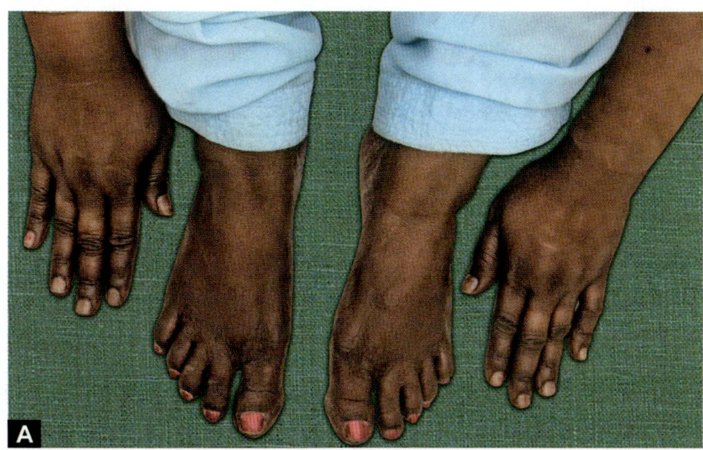


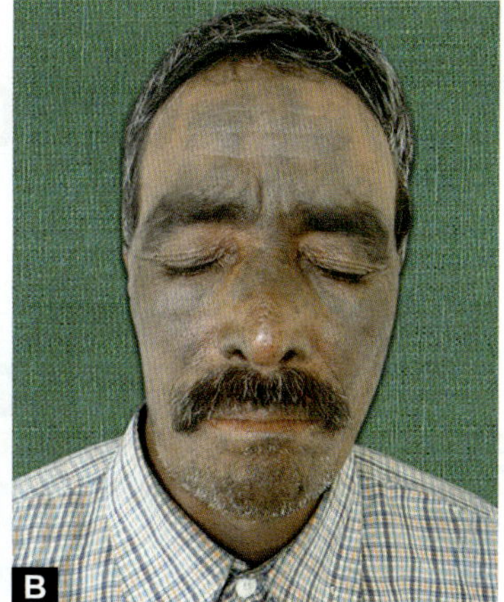


**FIG. 20:** Clofazamin-induced pigmentation.

## Clofazimine (Fig. 20)

The substituted phenazine dye clofazimine is used in the treatment of leprosy has uncommon side effect of the development of cutaneous and conjunctival pigmentation which has a reddish blue hue. Light microscopy of routine hematoxylin and eosin-stained sections fails to show the pigment but birefringent red clofazimine crystals are seen in fresh frozen sections. These deposits appear vivid red on fluorescence microscopy concentrating around blood vessels.

## ACKNOWLEDGMENTS

Thanking Dr Gitesh Sawatkar, Dr Vinay Keshvamurthy, and Dr Shraddha Uprety for picture contribution.

## SUGGESTED READINGS


1. Beers WH, Ince A, Moore TL. Scleredema adultorum of buschke: a case report and review of the literature. Semin Arthritis Rheum. 2006;35(6):355-9.
2. Borowicz J, Shama L, Miller R. Nodular cutaneous amyloidosis. Skin Med. 2011;9(5):316-8.
3. Celik O, Ipekci T, Kazimoglu H. Idiopathic scrotal calcinosis. Saudi Med J. 2013;34(12):1294-5.
4. Dubey S, Sharma R, Maheshwari V. Scrotal calcinosis: Idiopathic or dystrophic? Dermatol Online J. 2010;16(2):5.
5. Fatourechi V. Pretibial myxedema: pathophysiology and treatment options. Am J Clin Dermatol. 2005;6(5):295-309.
6. Fernandez-Flores A. Calcinosis cutis: critical review. Acta Dermatovenerologica Croat. 2011;19(1):43-50.
7. Fernandez-Flores A. Cutaneous amyloidosis: a concept review. Am J Dermatopathol. 2012;34(1):1-17.
8. Gutierrez A, Wetter DA. Calcinosis cutis in autoimmune connective tissue diseases. Dermatol Ther. 2012;25(2):195-206.
9. Hayashi M. Calciphylaxis: diagnosis and clinical features. Clin Exp Nephrol. 2013;17(4):498-503.
10. Ho MH, Chong LY. Poikiloderma-like cutaneous amyloidosis in an ethnic chinese girl. J Dermatol. 1998;25:730-4.
11. Jamaleddine FN, Salman SM, Shbaklo Z, et al. Idiopathic vulvar calcinosis: the counterpart of idiopathic scrotal calcinosis. Cutis. 1988;41(4):273-5.
12. Kim WB, Chang MC, Limacher JJ, Shaw JC. Nodular amyloidosis of the penis: A case demonstrating keratinocyte origin. JAMA Dermatol. 2015;151(8):910-12.
13. Kotwal V, Thakur A. Alkaptonuric ochronosis: A case report. Indian J Forensic Med Toxicol. 2012;6(2):10-2.
14. Loddenkemper K, Buttgereit F. Chrysiasis. Zeitschrift für Rheumatol. 2002;61(2): 173-4.
15. Mehrany K, Kist JM, Ahmed DDF, et al. Minocycline-induced cutaneous pigmentation. Int J Dermatol. 2003;42:551-2.
16. Qiao J, Fang H, Yao H. Amyloidosis cutis dyschromica. Orphanet J Rare Dis. 2012;7(1):1.
17. Saeed S, Sagatys E, Morgan MB. Acral keratosis with eosinophilic dermal deposits: a distinctive clinicopatholgic entity or colloid milium redux? J Cutan Pathol. 2006;33(10):679-85.
18. Sarkany RP, Breathnach SM, Morris AA, et al. Metabolic and Nutritional Disorders. In: Rook's Textbook of Dermatology. Oford: Wiley-Blackwell; 2010. pp. 1-103.
19. Stefanidou MP, Panayotides JG, Tosca AD. Milia en plaque: a case report and review of the literature. Dermatologic Surg. 2002;28(3):291-5.
20. Tan SK. Exogenous ochronosis - a diagnostic challenge. J Cosmet Dermatol. 2010;9(4):313-7.
21. Terushkin V, Boyd KP, Patel RR, et al. Primary localized cutaneous amyloidosis. Dermatol Online J. 2013;19(12):7.
22. Thareja S, Paghdal K, Lien MH, et al. Reticular erythematous mucinosis--a review. Int J Dermatol. 2012;51(8):903-9.
23. Wollina U, Konrad H, Schönlebe J. Lipoid proteinosis. Acta Dermatovenerologica Alp Pannonica Adriat. 2004;13(4):131-4.
24. Zembowicz A. Calciphylaxis: recognition and pathophysiological considerations. Pathol Case Rev. 2011;16(1):35-8.

# 16 SECTION Systemic Disorders

# 53 CHAPTER Systemic Diseases and Skin

Abhay Mani Martin, Lalit K Gupta

## INTRODUCTION

Skin is the largest organ of the body and acts as a mirror that often reflects the events occurring inside the body. It responds to these changes and thus is a sensitive indicator of alterations in the internal milieu of the various organ systems. Patients with internal disease may often be diagnosed initially by dermatologists on account of important clues they provide in the skin. Thus, skin diseases may not only be skin deep and the signs in skin may be early pointers to diagnose obscure internal diseases many of which may be serious and thus may help internist to manage them in time, thereby improving the overall prognosis of the patient. Classic examples of this may be rubor of polycythemia, icterus in hepatobiliary disease, intense itch of advanced renal or hepatic disease or Hodgkin's lymphoma and the diffuse hair loss seen in thyroid disorders. Likewise, candidal balanoposthitis is often the first clue that the patient may be a diabetic. Cutaneous manifestations of systemic disease can be specific or nonspecific. The cutaneous changes usually improve after the successful management of primary internal disease.

## ENDOCRINE SYSTEM AND THE SKIN

The physiology of epidermis, hair, nail, sebaceous glands, and melanocyte are under the profound influence of hormones. Deficiency or excess of hormones can alter the skin metabolism and their manifestations are recognized on the skin. These changes are brought about by the interaction of hormones with cell surface receptors.

## THYROID DISEASE AND THE SKIN

Subtle signs on the skin may be a presentation of thyroid disease. These effects are due to the effects of thyroid hormone on vascular network, keratinocyte, dermal stroma, sweat glands, hair metabolism, and on the nails. Deficiency and excess of thyroxine can cause distinctive skin manifestations that provide vital clues to diagnosis. The hormone exerts its effects via genes that regulate these target tissues.

### Hyperthyroidism

#### Causes

Excess thyroid hormone production may occur due to thyroiditis (including Graves' disease), solitary toxic nodule, toxic multinodular goiter, excessive thyroxine intake, iodine or iodine-containing drugs, such as amiodarone, or less commonly, a thyrotropin-secreting pituitary adenoma, molar pregnancy, struma ovarii, or metastatic follicular cancer.

#### Cutaneous Features

- *Warm, moist skin with facial flushing and palmar erythema*: These findings are as a result of vasodilatation due to increased sympathetic activity
- Generalized hyperhidrosis, especially involving the palms and soles occur due to increased sweat gland metabolism
- Addisonian type of hyperpigmentation usually sparing the buccal mucosa occurs and is due to increased adrenocorticotrophic hormone (ACTH) levels
- *Pretibial myxedema*: These are pink or skin colored nodules or plaques on the anterolateral aspects of lower limbs with prominent hair follicles giving a "peau d'orange" appearance. This occurs due to deposition of hyaluronic acid produced by fibroblasts and is considered a late manifestation of thyroid disease
- Soft and fine scalp hair with diffuse alopecia
- "*Plummer's nail*": Nails may show concave contour and distal onycholysis
- Graves' disease presents as a triad of exophthalmos, autoimmune thyroid disease (that manifests as thyromegaly) and pretibial myxedema.

### Hypothyroidism

#### Causes

Lowered thyroid levels are due to primary or idiopathic causes in the majority (95%) but may also occur secondary to other causes (5%), such as pituitary or hypothalamic dysfunction.

Congenital absence of thyroid tissue or congenital deficiency of thyroid hormone synthesizing enzymes are important causes of neonatal hypothyroidism. Severe iodine deficiency due to inadequate intake, especially in endemic areas intake of drugs (lithium, sulfonamides, bexarotene) and irradiation of the neck region causing tissue destruction are other causes of hypothyroidism.

The cutaneous features of hypothyroidism are:
- *Dry rough and coarse skin with puffy edema of hands, face, and eyelids*: This is presumed to be due to altered cutaneous hydration and lipid content with dermal deposition of acid mucopolysaccharides
- Cold and pale skin as a result of cutaneous vasoconstriction
- Yellowish discoloration of skin because of carotenemia
- Eruptive and tuberous xanthomas on elbows, knees, and buttocks due to altered lipid metabolism
- Pupura and ecchymoses occur due to fragile dermal vessels
- *Hertog's sign or madarosis*: Loss of lateral one-third of eyebrows
- Diffuse hair loss of scalp and body hair with dry coarse brittle hair.

### Diagnosis

The diagnosis of hypo- or hyperthyroidism is based on the values of thyroid stimulating hormone, triiodothyronine (T3), thyroxine (T4). However, free T3 and T4 are more sensitive markers than total values. Antithyroid peroxidase (anti-TPO) antibodies and antithyroglobulin antibodies are valuable in the diagnosis of autoimmune thyroiditis. Isotope scans may be needed to assess uptake of iodine like a functional adenoma, diffuse goiter and malignant thyroid nodule.

### Associations of Thyroid Disease

Thyroid diseases are known to be associated with various other disorders which may have coexisting skin manifestations. Some common associations are listed in table 1.

**TABLE 1: Skin manifestations associated with thyroid disease**

| Association with other autoimmune diseases | Association with bullous disease |
|---|---|
| • Alopecia areata<br>• Urticaria<br>• Vitiligo<br>• Psoriasis<br>• Lichen sclerosus<br>• Premature graying of hair<br>• Melasma | • Pemphigus foliaceus and vulgaris (Graves' disease)<br>• Bullous pemphigoid (Hashimoto's thyroiditis)<br>• Herpes gestationis (Graves' disease)<br>• Dermatitis herpetiformis (atrophic variant of Hashimoto's thyroiditis) |
| **Associated with endocrine diseases** | **Association with hematologic disorders** |
| • Diabetes mellitus<br>• Addison's disease<br>• Autoimmune polyglandular syndrome<br>• Insulin resistance syndromes<br>• Schmidt syndrome<br>(Idiopathic adrenal insufficiency, chronic lymphocytic thyroiditis, insulin-dependent diabetes mellitus, hypoparathyroidism, gonadal failure, pernicious anemia, mucocutaneous candidiasis, and thyrotoxicosis) | • Pernicious anemia<br>• Pure red cell aplasia<br>**Association with connective tissue disorders**<br>• Lupus erythematosus<br>• Dermatomyositis<br>• Systemic sclerosis<br>• Sjogren syndrome |

## SKIN IN ADRENAL DISEASE

### Disorders of Adrenal Hyperfunction

Adrenal hyperfunction resulting in cortisol, mineralocorticoid or sex steroid excess and attendant skin manifestations can occur in three settings—hypercortisolism, hyperaldosteronism, and congenital adrenal hyperplasia.

### Causes

Hypercortisolism is most often iatrogenic and occurs in the clinical setting due to prolonged systemic therapy or due to extensive topical steroid therapy. Other etiologies include ACTH production by pituitary adenoma, ectopic ACTH production from small cell lung cancer and bronchial carcinoids, direct hypersecretion of cortisols by adrenocortical adenomas and carcinomas and corticotropin-releasing hormone producing tumors of the hypothalamus.

**BOX 1 Clinical presentations of hypercortisolism (Fig. 1)**

- Truncal obesity (classically deposits of fat on clavicles and back of the neck, the "buffalo hump")
- "Moon facies" (facial fullness and plethora)
- Slender limbs
- Skin atrophy
- Poor wound healing
- Telangiectasia, easy bruising, and ecchymoses
- Striae (typically wide and red)
- Hirsutism
- Acneiform lesions (in contrast with acne vulgaris, the lesions are uniform, and comedones and cysts are absent)
- Propensity for fungal and bacterial infections
- Pigmentation (Addisonian type due to increased production of adrenocorticotrophic hormone and melanocyte-stimulating hormone)
- Male pattern baldness in women (also called FPHL or female pattern hair loss)

### Cutaneous Manifestations

Symptoms and signs are similar with both exogenous and endogenous causes. Adrenal disease may additionally induce androgenetic features due to production of sex steroids.

The common clinical features of hypercortisolism are summarized in box 1.

Hyperaldosteronism is not known to cause any skin manifestation.

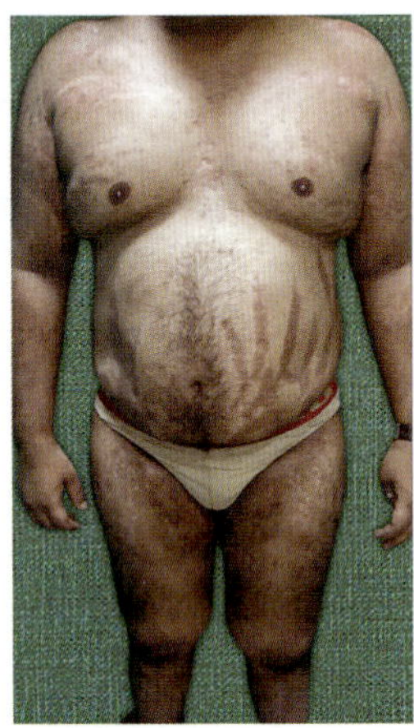

**FIG. 1:** Iatrogenic Cushing's disease.

Congenital adrenal hyperplasia is a result of deficiency of 21-hydroxylase enzyme due to defect in the *CYP21* gene. This results in failure of the body to convert 17-hydroxyprogesterone to cortisol.

This manifests with signs of virilization, acne, and hirsutism, as cortisol production is redirected to the androgen pathway. Some patients present with excess pigmentation especially of the lips, buccal mucosa, and genitalia due to compensatory increase of ACTH production. Short stature is a useful clue in the diagnosis of congenital adrenal hyperplasia, when differentiating from other causes of hirsutism like polycystic ovary disease or hyperinsulinemia.

### Diagnosis

Twenty-four hour urinary cortisol estimation and 1 mg overnight dexamethasone suppression test are useful screening tests.

### Treatment

Pituitary and adrenal adenomas are managed surgically. Such patients need lifelong replacement with glucocorticoids and mineralocorticoids.

Nelson's syndrome is a consequence of surgery and causes pituitary macroadenoma and cutaneous hyperpigmentation. This is treated by pituitary surgery.

Serotonin antagonists, dopamine or γ-aminobutyric acid agonists, somatostatin analogs act at the level of hypothalamic-pituitary axis. Corticosteroid receptors are the targets for mifepristone, a newer treatment modality. Metyrapone and aminoglutethimide act on the adrenal glands.

## Adrenal Insufficiency

This occurs due to a deficiency of cortisol production as a result of hypothalamic-pituitary, adrenal, or iatrogenic causes. Majority of cases are due to suppression of ACTH production by supraphysiologic doses of corticosteroids prescribed for inflammatory disorders. Primary adrenal insufficiency may occur as a result of autoimmune adrenalitis, infections (tuberculosis, meningococcemia, *pseudomonas*, and viral illnesses), malignancies (primary adrenal or metastatic adrenal disease), or hemorrhage into adrenals. Secondary adrenal insufficiency is due to hypothalamic or pituitary disease with decreased ACTH secretion.

### Clinical Features

- *General symptoms*: Wasting, fatigue, orthostatic hypotension, dizziness, anorexia, abdominal pain, and amenorrhea
- *Hyperpigmentation of the skin (Fig. 2)*: This is a classical cutaneous sign of adrenal insufficiency and has been attributed to the compensatory increase in ACTH production by the pituitary as well as probably intracutaneous ACTH production. It can present in varied patterns and sites. The sites of involvement are as listed below:
  - Light-exposed areas—face, dorsa of hands
  - Areas subject to friction—elbows, knees, and waistline
  - Areas of high pigmentation normally genital, perineum, axillae, areolae, and umbilicus
  - Palmar creases
  - Tongue and mucous membranes
  - Scars
  - Speckled skin pigmentation, and darkening of existing pigmented lesions
  - Nails—longitudinal melanonychia.
- Loss of axillary and pubic hair and improvement in acne in women are reported
- Autoimmune disease, especially vitiligo and alopecia areata are common associations. Diffuse hyperpigmentation along

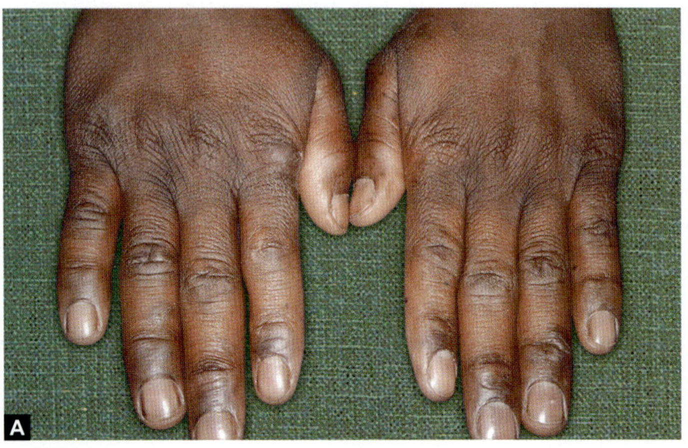



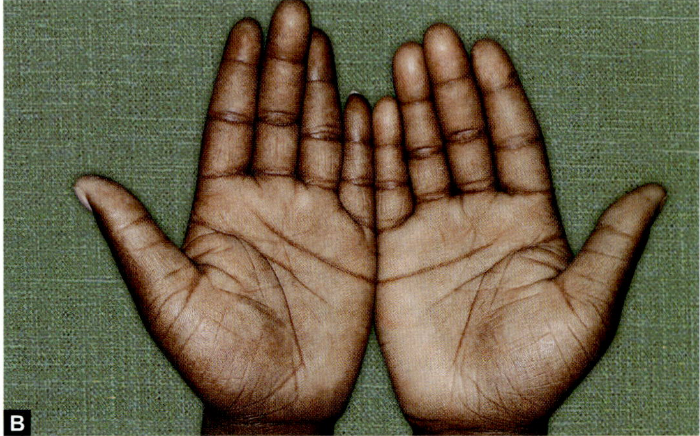



**FIG. 2: A,** Addisonian pigmentation dorsa; **B,** Addisonian pigmentation palm.
*Courtesy*: Dr Lalit Kumar Gupta, Senior Professor, Department of Dermatology, RNT Medical College, Udaipur, Rajasthan.

with the presence of these autoimmune skin disease should make one suspect autoimmune adrenalitis as a cause for adrenal insufficiency.

## Hyperandrogenism

Cutaneous hyperandrogenism is a distinctive manifestation of the effects of androgen or its derivatives on the skin. The main androgens exerting effects on the skin are dihydrotestosterone, dehydroepiandrosterone (DHEA), and androstenedione.
The causes of hyperandrogenism are listed in box 2.

### Clinical Features

The commonly encountered skin signs of cutaneous hyperandrogenism are seborrhea, acne, hirsutism, and androgenic alopecia or female pattern hair loss (FPHL). Presence of signs like clitoromegaly, deepening of voice and a male habitus suggests a possibility of virilism. Late onset adult acne and hirsutism are very common presentations of cutaneous hyperandrogenism in the recent times.

Hyperinsulinemia can present with signs of hyperandrogenism due to the effects of insulin levels on androgen synthesis. Hyperinsulinemia may have associated signs like skin tags and acanthosis nigricans in addition to acne, hirsutism, and androgenic alopecia or FPHL.

HAIR-AN syndrome (hirsutism, acne, insulin resistance, and acanthosis nigricans) and SAHA syndrome (seborrhea, acne, hirsutism, and androgenic alopecia) are distinctive phenotypic subsets of cutaneous hyperandrogenism.

### Diagnosis

Patients presenting with signs of cutaneous hyperandrogenism should be worked up with the following hormonal tests—luteinizing hormone, follicle stimulating hormone, DHEA or DHEA sulphate, serum testosterone, and prolactin levels.

**BOX 2 Causes of hyperandrogenism (Fig. 3)**

- *Adrenal*: Congenital adrenal hyperplasia, virilizing tumors of the adrenal
- *Ovarian*: Polycystic ovarian syndrome, virilizing ovarian tumors
- *Hypothalamic or pituitary*: Hyperprolactinemia, acromegaly, and Cushing's disease
- *Miscellaneous*: Exogenous intake of corticosteroids, anabolic steroids, and androgens

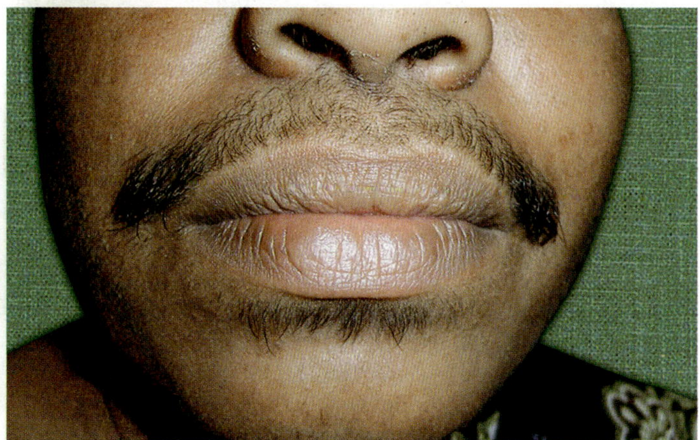

**FIG. 3:** Hirsutism in hypercortisolism.

### Treatment of Cutaneous Hyperandrogenism

Treatment is largely dependent on the etiology of the illness. The use of oral contraceptives, low-dose estrogens, and gonadotropin antagonist have been attempted with some success.

Metformin serves as an insulin sensitizer in hyperinsulinemic patients and polycystic ovary syndrome.

## SKIN MANIFESTATIONS OF DIABETES MELLITUS

Approximately 30% of patients with diabetes mellitus develop a skin disorder sometime during the course of disease. Many of these cutaneous changes are due to vascular and neuropathic changes associated with diabetes. Some are due to altered production of epidermal growth factors, accompanying metabolic disturbances, immune disturbances, and some hitherto unknown mechanisms. Some of the common presentations of diabetes based on their etiology is presented in table 2.

### Cutaneous Manifestations

The following is a brief overview of the specific cutaneous manifestations seen in diabetics:

- Acanthosis nigricans
- Skin tags
- HAIR-AN syndrome
- *Acral dry gangrene*: This occurs due to vaso-occlusive disease of the large vessels as well as atherosclerotic changes in the vessels
- *Acral erythema*: Erysipelas-like, well-demarcated areas of erythema on the hands and/or feet which may be due to small vessel occlusive disease with compensatory hyperemia. They are also presumed to be due to loss of vasomotor tone due to autonomic disturbances
- *Diabetic bullae (bullosis diabeticorum)*: This occurs in 0.5–2% of diabetic patients. They are tense, spontaneous, and noninflammatory bullae on the lower extremities with intra- or subepidermal separation without acantholysis. They may be solitary or multiple and are usually noted on the feet or legs. Trunk lesions have been reported. Lesions are spontaneous in onset and have no correlation to glycemic control in diabetics. They are self-limiting and do not need treatment. Large bullae may need to be ruptured if it causes inconvenience (e.g., sole or undersurface of toes). Secondary infection must be avoided
- *Diabetic cheiroarthropathy*: This is characterized by thickened skin and limited joint mobility of the hands and fingers, leading to flexion contractures (starting with the fifth digit and progressing radially) and an inability to approximate the palmar surfaces of the hands and fingers (prayer sign). It results from increased glycosylation of collagen in the skin and is associated with retinopathy, nephropathy, and duration (but not control) of the diabetes mellitus
- *Diabetic dermopathy*: Brown atrophic macules and patches on the shins, forearms, thighs, and over bony prominences possibly precipitated by trauma. Microangiopathy and neuropathy are involved in its pathogenesis

**TABLE 2: Clinical presentations of skin manifestations of diabetes mellitus (based on etiopathology)**

| A. Due to vascular changes | | |
|---|---|---|
| Microvascular injury | • Diabetic dermopathy<br>• Necrobiosis lipoidica diabeticorum<br>• Diabetic rubeosis | |
| Vaso-occlusive disease | • Diabetic ulcer<br>• Diabetic gangrene (wet and dry type) | • Atherosclerotic disease of the peripheral vessels<br>• Small vessel vasculopathy |
| **B. Due to neurologic injury** | | |
| Sensory neuropathy | Neurotrophic ulcer (Fig. 4) | |
| Motor neuropathy | Diabetic cheiroarthropathy, loss of small muscle integrity, joint deformity, and loss of far pads | |
| Autonomic neuropathy | Localized anhidrosis, dry skin, peripheral erythema, edema, and skin atrophy (Fig. 5) | |
| Diabetic foot | This occurs as a combination of sensorimotor and autonomic neuropathy | |
| **C. Due to metabolic derangements** | | |
| | • Acanthosis nigricans (Fig. 6)<br>• Xanthomas and xanthelasma (Fig. 7) | • Carotenemia<br>• Skin tags |
| **D. Due to treatment of diabetes** | | |
| | • Insulin lipodystrophy or lipoatrophy<br>• Allergy to insulin and oral hypoglycemic agents | |
| **E. Due to infections** | | |
| | • Bacterial—furuncles (Fig. 8), carbuncles, echthymas and pyodermas, Fournier's gangrene, and bullous impetigo in adults (Fig. 9)<br>• Viral—atypical and severe forms of herpes viruses (Fig. 10)<br>• Fungal—dermatophytic infections, intertrigo (Fig. 11), onychomycosis, candidal balanoposthitis (Fig. 12) and vulvovaginitis, oral candidiasis (Fig. 13)<br>• Systemic—fungal infections like mucormycosis<br>• Parasitic—more florid forms of scabies and pediculosis | |
| **F. Due to unknown mechanisms** | | |
| | Diabetic bullae (Fig. 14), Generalized pruritus (multiple mechanisms postulated) (Fig. 15) | |
| **G. Common associations of diabetes** | | |
| | Vitiligo, bullous pemphigoid, perforating disorders, disseminated granuloma annulare (Fig. 16), and acral erysipelas like erythema (elderly) (Fig. 17) | |

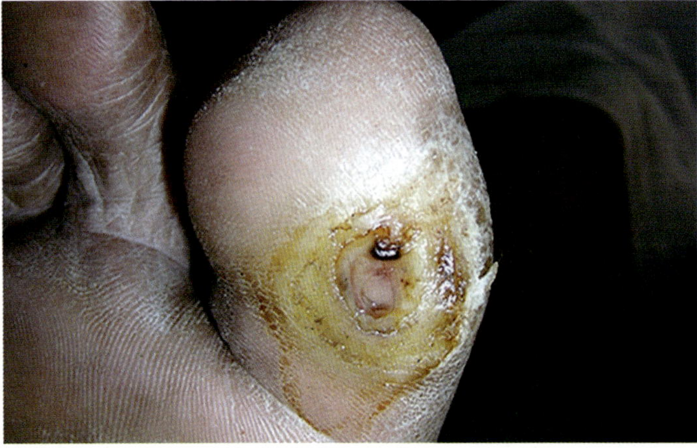

**FIG. 4:** Diabetic neuropathy with trophic ulceration.

- *Disseminated granuloma annulare*: Treatment of this condition is unsatisfactory. Disseminated granuloma annulare has been reported to respond to dapsone, isotretinoin, etretinate, hydroxychloroquine, niacinamide (1.5 g/day), fumaric acid esters, hydroxyurea, narrow-band ultraviolet B therapy, and psoralen and ultraviolet A therapy (PUVA). However, diabetics are known to have more recurrences and disseminated patterns that are resistant to treatment
- *Eruptive xanthomas*: Control of the diabetes mellitus results in a disappearance of the xanthomas
  - *Necrobiosis lipoidica diabeticorum (NLD)*: This is clinically characterized by well circumscribed, yellow brown patches with marked epidermal atrophy, most often on the shins. A red-brown rim may indicate activity at the border. Ulceration can occur and is often slow to heal. About one-third of patients with NLD have diabetes, one-third have impaired glucose tolerance and one-third have normal glucose tolerance. NLD may precede diabetes. Good control of diabetes does not result in improvement in manifestations of NLD.

The treatment of NLD is still elusive. Intralesional corticosteroid therapy has been tried to prevent expansion of lesions in early stages. Aspirin, dipyridamole, and pentoxifylline have been tried with partial success. Cyclosporine, tacrolimus ointment 0.1%, etanercept, mycophenolate mofetil, fumaric acid esters, photochemotherapy with topical PUVA, chloroquine (200 mg/day), hydroxychloroquine (400 mg/day), infliximab, and thalidomide (150 mg/day) are reported to be effective anecdotally. Ulcerated lesions have been treated with semipermeable dressings like

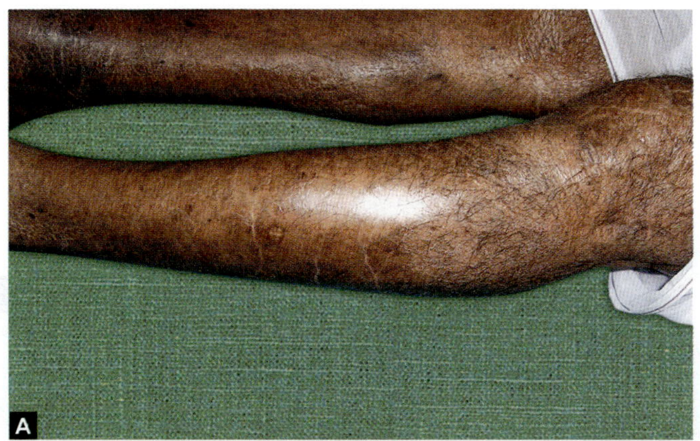

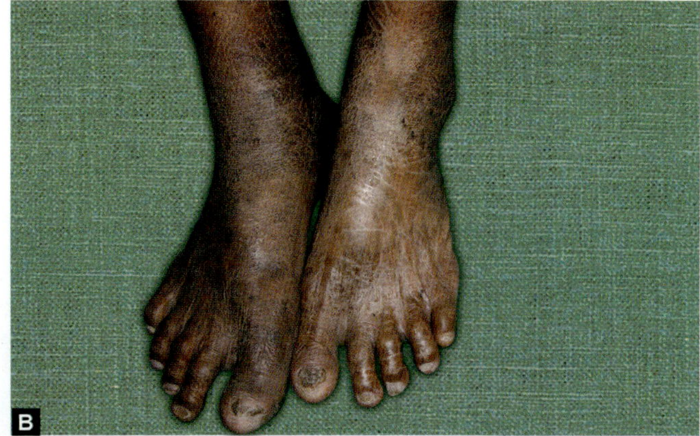

**FIG. 5: A,** Diabetic neuropathy with skin changes (atrophy, hair loss, and dryness); **B,** Diabetic neuropathic skin changes (atrophy and dryness).

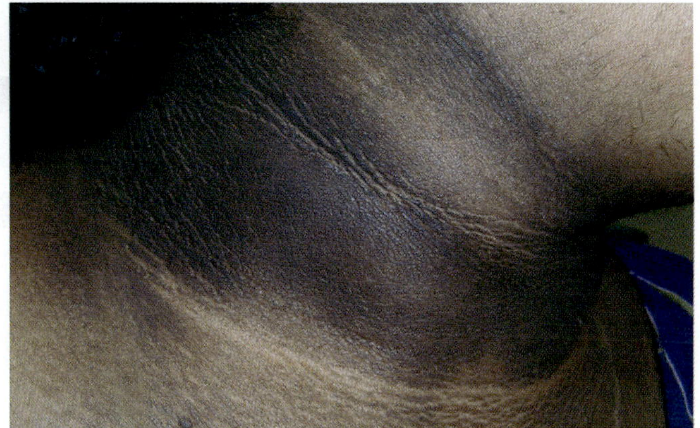

**FIG. 6:** Acanthosis nigricans as a marker of insulin resistance in diabetes.

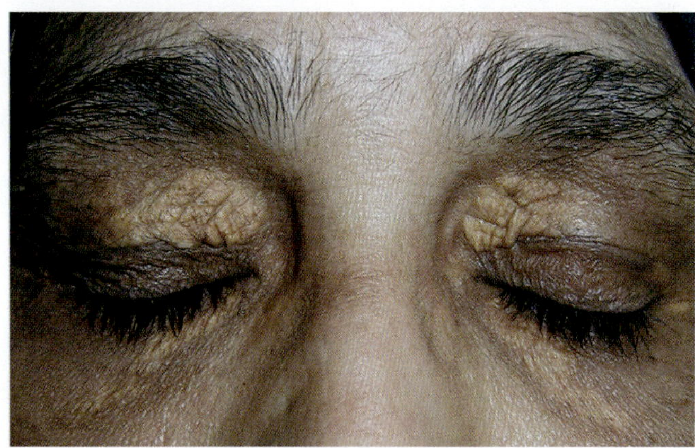

**FIG. 7:** Xanthelasma in diabetes.

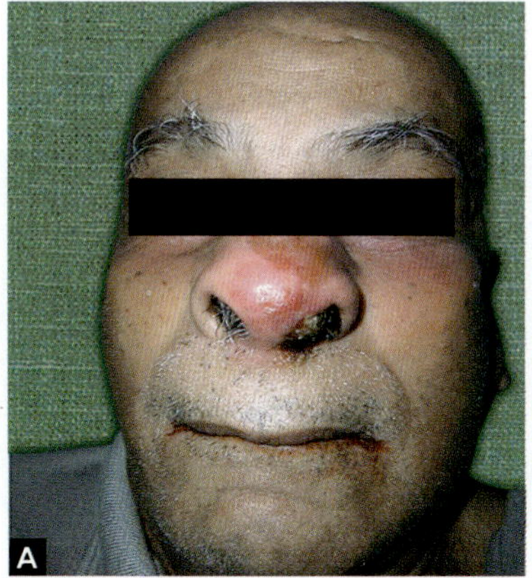

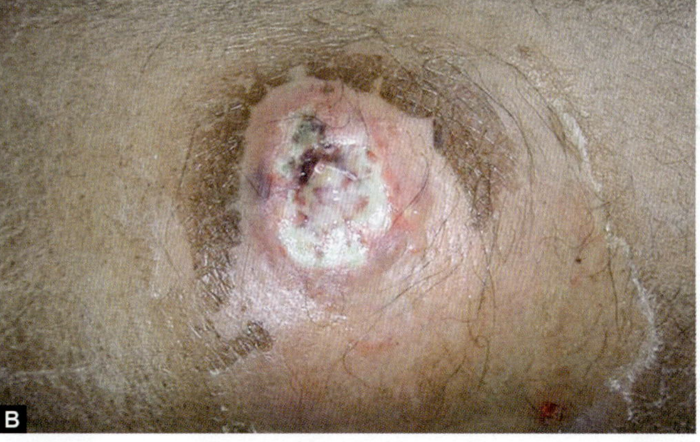

**FIG. 8: A,** Vestibulitis in diabetes; **B,** Furunculosis in diabetes.

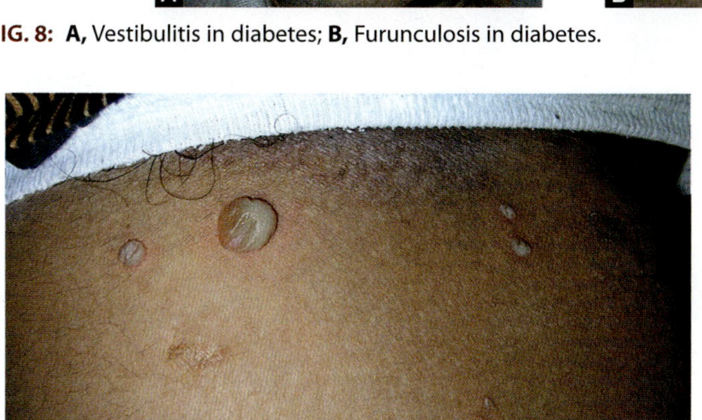

**FIG. 9:** Bullous impetigo in diabetes.

OpSite®, DuoDERM®. Skin grafting has been attempted for extensive ulcerated lesions.

- *Neuropathic leg ulcers*: Non-painful ulcerations at sites of pressure, most commonly on the foot, are a sign of severe sensory neuropathy. This is due to a combination of sensory and autonomic neuropathy, as well as vasculopathy of the vasa nervorum. The ulcers are characterized by a keratotic rim
- *Perforating disorders*: The cause is attributed to diabetic microangiopathy and lesions are due to minor injury, such as pressure or scratching
- *Rubeosis*: Chronic, flushed appearance of the face, neck, and upper extremities due to decreased vascular tone or microangiopathy. It is improved by dietary diabetic control

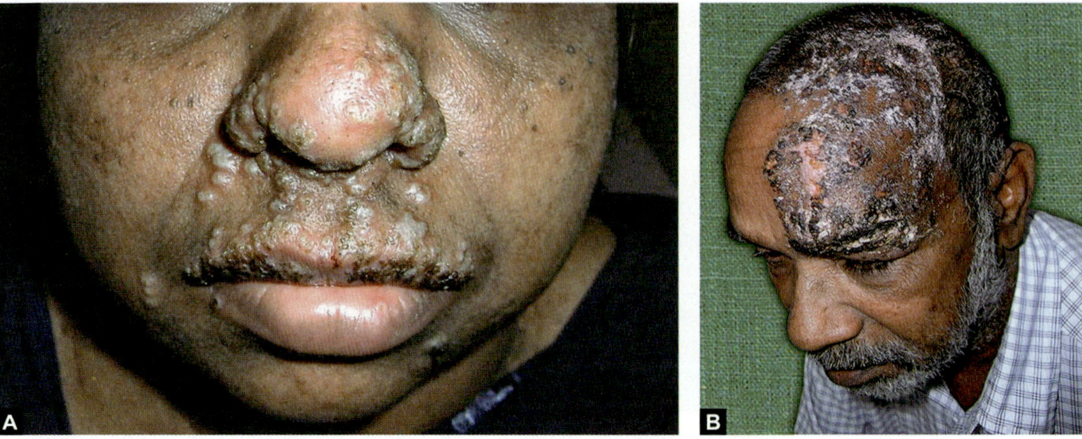


FIG. 10: **A,** Florid herpes simplex in diabetes; **B,** Florid necrotizing lesions of herpes zoster in diabetes.

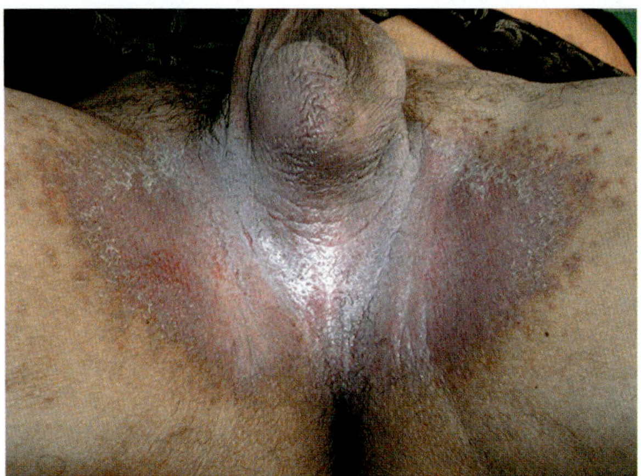

FIG. 11: Intertrigo with candidiasis in a male with poorly controlled diabetes.

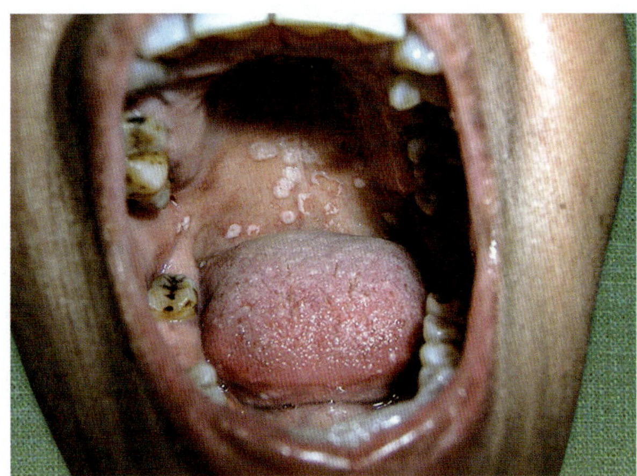

FIG. 13: Oral candidiasis in diabetes.

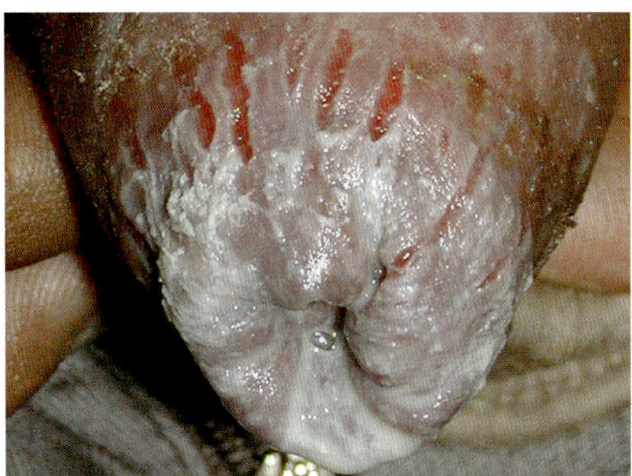

FIG. 12: Balanoposthitis in a male with uncontrolled diabetes.

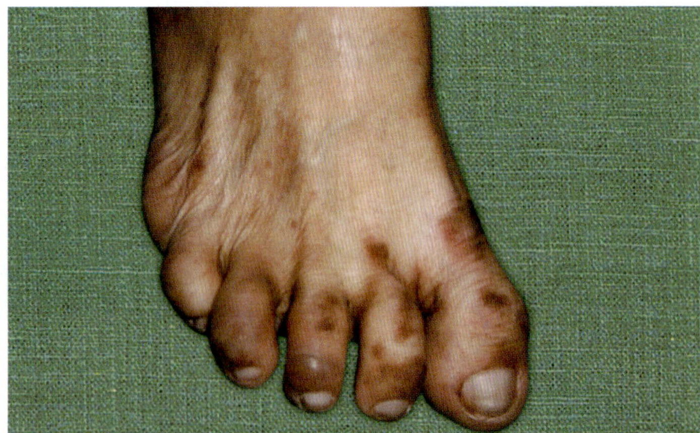

FIG. 14: Diabetic bullae.

- *Scleredema (adultorum of Buschke)*: Erythematous, woody, induration of the upper back and nape of neck with a peau d' orange appearance. Histologically it is characterized by increased deposition of collagen and mucin (acid mucopolysaccharides) due to excess insulin stimulation. It runs a very protracted course. Control of hyperglycemia does not improve scleredema.

## SKIN MANIFESTATIONS OF GASTROINTESTINAL DISEASES

### Oral Cavity Diseases

Many disease of the gastrointestinal tract can provide vital clue in the oral cavity. Aphthae, chronic ulcers, and pyostomatitis

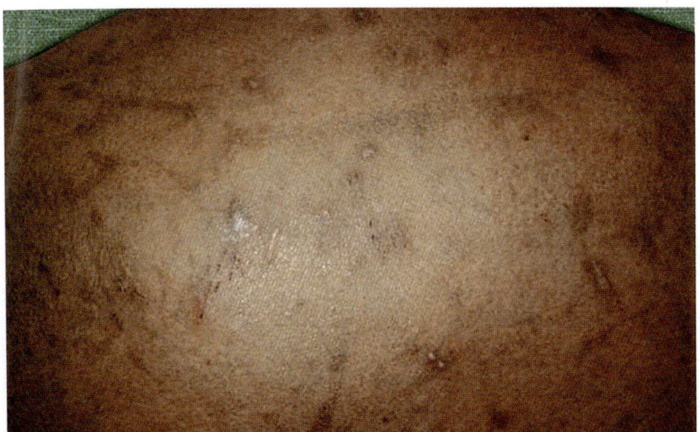

FIG. 15: Pruritus and excoriations of diabetes.

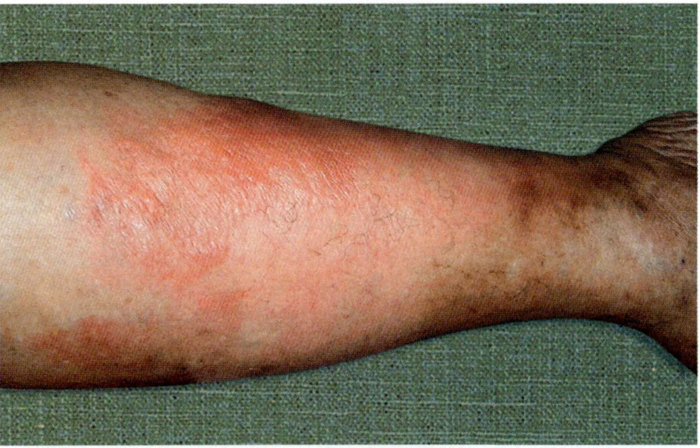

FIG. 17: Acral erysipelas-like erythema in diabetes.

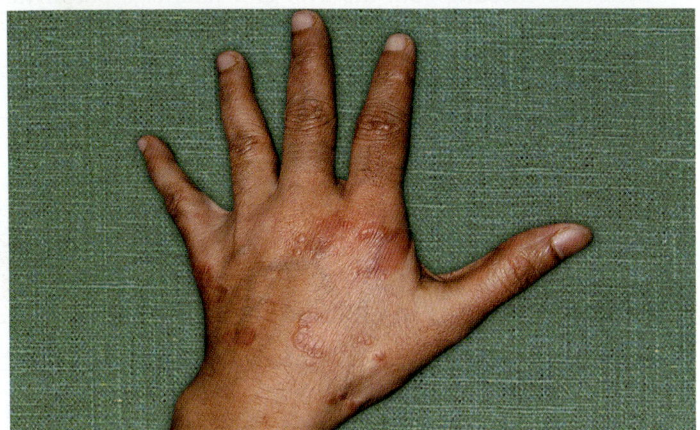

FIG. 16: Granuloma annulare in diabetes.

vegetans are features of ulcerative colitis whereas Crohn's disease presents as diffuse swelling, fissuring, cobblestoning, persistent ulcerations, polypoid lesions, angular cheilitis, granulomatous cheilitis or pyostomatitis vegetans. Recurrent oral ulceration may be the result of agranulocytosis, iron deficiency anemia, pernicious anemia, or nutritional deficiencies. It may also be a presentation of Behcet's disease, Reiter's disease, lupus erythematosus or systemic malignancy.

## Dysphagia

Systemic sclerosis presents as dysphagia. The presentations may vary from subtle signs of gastroesophageal reflux disease like heartburn or gaseous distension to frank esophageal obstruction depending on the severity of involvement.

Dermatomyositis may also present as esophageal dyskinesia due to skeletal muscle involvement of pharynx and upper third of esophageal musculature.

*Paterson-Brown-Kelly syndrome or Plummer-Vinson syndrome*, a presentation of severe iron deficiency anemia, presents with dysphagia besides angular cheilitis, atrophic glossitis, and brittle nails with or without koilonychia.

## Gastrointestinal Hemorrhage

Diseases of the gastrointestinal tract presenting with gastrointestinal hemorrhage may have cutaneous markers that serve as pointers to the possible etiology. The diseases and their possible cutaneous findings are listed in table 3.

## Polyposis Syndromes

Gastrointestinal polyposis syndromes have several cutaneous markers that may point toward the illness. The different polyposis syndromes and the relevant cutaneous markers are mentioned in table 4.

## Malabsorption

Malabsorption syndromes may have cutaneous manifestations that are distinctive of a particular disease, e.g., rash of acrodermatitis enteropathica and dermatitis herpetiformis. However, several diseases manifest on the skin as a secondary consequence

**TABLE 3: Skin manifestations of gastrointestinal diseases presenting as hemorrhage**

| Disease | Skin manifestation |
|---|---|
| Osler–Weber–Rendu syndrome (hereditary hemorrhagic telangiectasia) | Mucosal and cutaneous telangiectasia-tongue, lip, palate, nose, palms, and soles |
| Blue rubber bleb nevus syndrome | Cutaneous hemangiomas |
| Collagen vascular disorders | Cutaneous signs of systemic lupus erythematosus, scleroderma, dermatomyositis, etc. |
| Henoch–Schonlein purpura | Palpable purpura |
| Degos disease | Erythematous papules with umbilication that result in porcelain white macules |
| Pseudoxanthoma elasticum, Ehlers–Danlos syndrome | Plucked chicken skin appearance (yellowish papules) |

**TABLE 4: Gastrointestinal polyposis syndrome and their cutaneous markers**

| Polyposis | Skin marker |
|---|---|
| Gardner's syndrome | Large epidermoid cysts (on face, trunk, and scrotum) fibromas, lipomas, desmoids tumors, and osteomas |
| Peutz–Jeghers syndrome | Lentigines around lip, oral mucosa, and perianal areas |
| Cronkhite–Canada syndrome | Hyperpigmentation on hands arms, face and body folds, onychodystophy, loss of hair on the scalp eyebrows axillae and pubis |
| Muir–Torre syndrome | Multiple sebaceous gland neoplasms, keratoacanthomas, and basal cell carcinomas |
| Cowden's disease | Hamartomas |

of nutritional deficiencies, which in turn, is a result of the complications of the primary gastrointestinal diseases, e.g., celiac disease, and Whipple disease. A close search for the etiology of the nutritional deficiency would lead to the primary diagnosis.

Pigmentary changes may occur in diffuse, focal, Addisonian, pellagroid, and melasma-like patterns.

Acrodermatitis enteropathica presents with a distinctive scaly, erosive, or oozing rash with or without lichenification resembling an eczema. Lesions may also be papular, papulopustular or vesiculobullous. The lesions are distributed over the peristomal areas, namely perioral, perineal, and perianal regions. Alopecia, growth retardation, neuropsychiatric disorders, and recurrent infections are complications associated with the illness and worsen if unrecognized and not treated early. The disease may occur as a primary genetic disorder or as secondary to malabsorption or total parenteral nutrition. Supplementation of zinc in high doses is curative.

### Inflammatory Bowel Disease

Inflammatory bowel disease is a general term for a group of idiopathic chronic inflammatory diseases of the bowel. Ulcerative colitis and Crohn's disease are distinctive polygenic disorders that are part of this spectrum. Ulcerative colitis begins in the rectum and spreads proximally to involve the colon whereas Crohn's disease begins in the intestine and progresses to involve the entire gastrointestinal tract, often in a discontinuous fashion. The skin is an important site for extraintestinal signs and symptoms. Table 5 enlists the commonly associated skin presentation in inflammatory bowel disease.

## SKIN IN HEPATIC DISEASES

Hepatic diseases show several cutaneous stigmata. However, none of the cutaneous stigmata are specific to any disease including jaundice.

The cutaneous changes associated with hepatic diseases may be seen in the following settings:

- *Primary liver diseases with skin manifestations*: Cirrhosis, hemochromatosis, Wilson's disease, viral hepatitis, and primary biliary cirrhosis
- Disorders affecting both the liver and skin, e.g., porphyria cutanea tarda, erythropoietic porphyria, Gianotti–Crosti syndrome, syphilis, sarcoidosis, Gaucher's disease, Langerhans cell histiocytosis, systemic amyloidosis, etc.
- *Drug-induced hepatic disease with cutaneous changes*: Drug reaction with eosinophilia and systemic symptoms syndrome, Stevens–Johnson syndrome and toxic epidermal necrolysis, rifampicin, ketoconazole, minocycline, allopurinol and other hepatotoxic drugs.

### Cutaneous Changes in Chronic Liver Disease

Chronic liver disease is the endpoint of several diseases of the liver like cirrhosis (both alcoholic and non-alcoholic), infections like chronic hepatitis B and C, drugs and toxins, biliary obstruction (e.g., gallstones, carcinoma of the pancreas, and cystic fibrosis), metabolic diseases (hemochromatosis and Wilson's disease), and miscellaneous disorders like sarcoidosis, primary biliary cirrhosis. Several skin markers have been identified to point to a hepatic etiology. Jaundice is the most common of these manifestations. The commonly observed skin markers that have an association with hepatic disease are mentioned in table 6.

**TABLE 5: Cutaneous presentations of inflammatory bowel disease**

| Cutaneous sign | Features |
|---|---|
| Fissures and fistulae | • Most frequent complication of Crohn's disease<br>• Perianal fistulas occur in one-third of patients<br>• Fistulas may occur in peristomal areas and abdominal wall along with abscesses and fistulae |
| Metastatic Crohn's disease | Cutaneous granulomas |
| Mucosal lesions | Cobblestoning and ulcerations of oral cavity |
| Oral aphthosis | Associated with both ulcerative colitis and Crohn's disease in 6–8% cases. Frequently associated with active bowel inflammation |
| Pustular vasculitis (bowel associated dermatosis-arthritis syndrome) | Starts with a prodrome of fever chills and malaise followed by erythematous macules, indurated and painful papules, and sterile pustules |
| Pyoderma gangrenosum (PG) | • Occurs in 1–5% cases<br>• Presents as pustular lesions or chronic ulcers with a violaceous, undermined border |
| Erythema nodosum | • Occurs in 1–5% cases of inflammatory bowel disease<br>• Often accompanies inflammatory arthritis in Crohn's disease |
| Miscellaneous presentations | Sweet's syndrome, urticaria and urticarial vasculitis, erythema multiforme, epidermolysis bullosa acquisita, polyarteritis nodosa, and vitiligo |

**TABLE 6: Summary of skin manifestations of hepatic disease**

| | Skin manifestation | Features |
|---|---|---|
| Vascular phenomena | Spider nevi (nevus araneus) | • Central pulsatile arteriolar punctum with radiating branching blood vessels<br>• Seen in advanced cirrhosis<br>• Most often seen in the upper half of the body |
| | Telangiectasia | • Wiry telangiectasias are seen<br>• Mainly seen on photoexposed areas |
| | Palmar erythema (liver palms) | Diffuse or splotchy erythema of palms over thenar and hypothenar eminences and tips of fingers |
| | Petechiae, purpura, and easy bruisability | Due to coagulation defects, vitamin K deficiency, and prothrombin deficiency |
| | "Caput medusa" | • Dilated paraumbilical veins<br>• Seen in patients with portal hypertension owing to portal–systemic shunting |
| Pigmentary abnormalities | Jaundice | • Due to hyperbilirubinemia<br>• Hallmark of advanced liver disease but not specific (also seen in hemolysis and biliary disease) |
| | Diffuse hyperpigmentation | Occurs in advanced liver disease-alcoholic cirrhosis and primary biliary cirrhosis (PBC)<br>Due to increased melanin in the basal layer |
| – | Other patterns of pigmentation | • Blotchy areas of pigmentation initially focal and then generalized may be seen in PBC<br>• Accentuation of freckling and areolar pigmentation<br>• Pigmentation of palmar creases<br>• Chloasma-like pigmentation<br>• Yellowish or orange discoloration (xanthomas) |
| – | Bronze diabetes | • Seen in PBC<br>• Metallic brown pigmentation due to hemosiderin as well as melanin pigmentation |
| Pruritus | Moderate-to-severe itch<br>Excoriations | • Prominent feature of advanced liver disease, PBC, and biliary obstruction<br>• Pathogenesis unknown-presumed role for bile salts and endogenous opioid system<br>• Treatment—opioid antagonists (naloxone, naltrexone, and nalmefene)<br>• Cholestyramine, androgen |
| Nail changes | • Terry's nails<br>• Muehrcke's nails<br>• Clubbing<br>• Koilonychia<br>• Bluish or azure lunulae<br>• Splinter hemorrhages | • White nails<br>• Transverse white bands<br>• Spoon-shaped nails<br>• Seen in Wilson's disease |
| Hair changes | Sparse axillary, pubic, and body hair<br>Feminized pattern of pubic hair | Due to increased circulating estrogens |
| Hyperlipidemic skin changes | Xanthomas and xanthelasmas | – |
| Other changes | • Gynecomastia<br>• Testicular atrophy<br>• Loss of libido<br>• Oligospermia | Due to altered metabolism of sex hormones |
| | Nutritional disturbances | • Pellagrous changes—cause scaly pigmented changes on sun exposed areas and V of neck<br>• Knuckle pigmentation due to vitamin B12 deficiency<br>• "Flaky paint dermatosis" due to kwashiorkor in advanced nutritional deficiency |
| | Striae distensae, pseudo-Cushing's syndrome | • Found in lower abdomen, thighs, and buttocks<br>• Described with chronic alcoholism<br>• Moon face, truncal obesity, and proximal muscle wasting |
| | Fatigue, weight loss, anorexia, and vomiting | – |

*Continued*

*Continued*

| | Skin manifestation | Features |
|---|---|---|
| Associations | • Lichen planus | • Associated with PBC<br>• Associated with alcoholic cirrhosis |
| | • Xanthomas | • Associated more often with PBC |
| | • Vasculitis and pyoderma gangrenosum | • Associated with chronic viral hepatitis |
| | • Porphyria cutanea tarda | – |

**TABLE 7: Cutaneous manifestations in hepatitis infection**

| Disease | Manifestations | Remarks |
|---|---|---|
| Hepatitis A | • Jaundice<br>• Exanthematous rash<br>• Urticaria | Skin manifestations are rare in hepatitis A except for jaundice |
| Hepatitis B | • Urticaria<br>• Diffuse nonspecific erythema<br>• Serum sickness-like reactions | • Urticaria and serum sickness like reaction occurs in 20–30% of infected patients<br>• Immune complex-mediated immunologic reactions<br>• Histopathology reveals small vessel vasculitis<br>• Immunofluorescence (direct immunofluorescence) shows deposits of immunoglobulin G, immunoglobulin M, C3, and hepatitis B virus surface antigen |
| | • Erythema multiforme<br>• Erythema nodosum<br>• Vasculitis<br>• Cryoglobulinemia<br>• Pyoderma gangrenosum<br>• Henoch–Schonlein purpura<br>• Urticarial vasculitis<br>• Sweet's syndrome | A range of immune mediated responses are seen in association with hepatitis B |
| | Frequent association with polyarteritis nodosa | 20–30% associated with renal vasculitis without renal glomerulonephritis |
| | Gianotti Crosti syndrome | Presents with monomorphic papular eruptions over the knees, elbows, and buttocks. Now considered nonspecific as it is seen with multiple viral syndromes |
| Hepatitis C | • Essential mixed cryoglobulinemia<br>• Porphyria cutanea tarda<br>• Necrolytic acral erythema, polyarteritis nodosa<br>• Lichen planus<br>• General pruritus<br>• Urticarial vasculitis<br>• Serum sickness like syndrome | – |

## SKIN MANIFESTATIONS IN HEPATITIS

Acute hepatitis can occur with infections (hepatitis A, B, and C, cytomegalovirus, and Epstein Barr virus—infectious mononucleosis, rubella), drugs (dapsone, allopurinol, methotrexate, rifampicin, etc.), and toxins (alcohol, vinyl chloride, and intake of heavy metals).

The cutaneous markers of the common hepatitis infections are enumerated in table 7.

## SKIN MANIFESTATIONS OF RENAL DISEASE

Skin can be affected in diseases of renal system in a variety of ways:

- Cutaneous changes in renal failure; seen in almost all the patients
- Systemic diseases with prominent renal and cutaneous symptoms (e.g., Henoch-Schonlein purpura, Fabry's disease, systemic amyloidosis, nail-patella syndrome, tuberous sclerosis, Birt Hogg-Dubé syndrome)
- Diseases primarily affecting kidney where skin biopsy is helpful in making the diagnosis even when cutaneous findings are not prominent, like in primary systemic amyloidosis.

Heritable renocutaneous syndromes show cutaneous markers that are helpful in early diagnosis of the illness. It is important also to be aware of the possible renal complications in these diseases in order to intervene early, if necessary. Table 8 lists the diseases with the cutaneous findings and their prominent renal complications.

Diseases of cutaneous or systemic origin may present with features of renal and cutaneous involvement, e.g., systemic amyloidosis, Henoch-Schonlein purpura, systemic lupus

**TABLE 8: Renal and cutaneous findings in heritable renocutaneous syndromes**

| Disease | Cutaneous findings | Renal findings |
|---|---|---|
| Neurofibromatosis | Multiple neurofibromas, cafe au lait macules, and freckling | • Urinary outflow obstruction (impinging neurofibroma)<br>• Renal artery thrombosis<br>• Hypertension, which may also develop as a result of an associated pheochromocytoma or renal artery stenosis |
| Tuberous sclerosis | Shagreen patch, ash-leaf macule, facial angiofibromas, and periungual fibromas | Angiomyolipomas, renal cysts and malignant tumors, such as clear cell carcinoma |
| Nail–patella syndrome | • Nail dysplasia with triangular lunula<br>• Absent or small patella | • Proteinuria with or without hematuria<br>• End-stage renal disease |
| Birt–Hogg–Dube syndrome | Trichofolliculoma, trichodiscoma, and skin tags | Renal malignancies |
| von Hippel–Lindau disease | Hemangiomas and cafe au lait macules | Simple cyst or renal cell carcinoma |

erythematosus, scleroderma, systemic vasculitis, polyarteritis nodosa, and immunoglobulin A nephropathy.

## Cutaneous Findings in Chronic Renal Failure

- *Pigmentation*: Patients may present with a diffuse muddy brown pigmentation of the face and trunk as a result of retention of chromogens and deposition of melanin. Pigmentation may be confined to distal aspect of nails—"half-and-half nails". Anemia presents as pallor
- Generalized, severe pruritus is likely to be the result of slowly accumulated pruritogens of unknown nature. Pruritus may actually worsen after dialysis is begun. Lowering of magnesium concentration of dialysate, ultraviolet B radiation, oral cholestyramine, activated charcoal, erythropoietin, opioids, and gabapentin may be helpful in alleviating the renal pruritus
- *Perforating disorders*: Various perforating disorders including Kyrle's disease, reactive perforating collagenosis and perforating folliculitis collectively called as "acquired perforating dematoses of chronic renal failure" may be seen. They are keratotic, hyperpigmented, and pruritic papules up to 1 cm in diameter with a central keratinous plug that occur over extensor surfaces of limbs. Diabetes is often associated
- *Uremic frost*: Whitish deposition of crystallized urea over face, nostrils and neck, a rare finding these days
- *Calcification and calcific uremic arteriolopathy or calciphylaxis*: This is a serious life-threatening, thrombo-occlusive disease that occurs in the setting of renal failure. It shows a higher incidence in dialysis patients (4%) as compared to patients with chronic renal failure. It presents as papular or nodular cutaneous lesions around large joints or flexural sites. Metastatic calcification and thromboses in walls of small and medium-sized blood vessels in dermis and subcutis occur resulting in infarction of overlying skin. Painful hard plaques in livedoid pattern with necrotic ulceration (calciphylaxis) usually develop in the setting of chronic renal failure and secondary hyperparathyroidism.

Prominent differential diagnosis of calciphylaxis include cryoglobulinemia and cryofibrinogenemia, protein C and protein S deficiency, antiphospholipid syndrome, atherosclerotic peripheral vascular disease, cholesterol emboli, and disseminated intravascular coagulation. Coumarin necrosis also has a similar presentation and hence should be suspected when patients are on anticoagulants.

The workup should include erythrocyte sedimentation rate and C-reactive protein, coagulation profile-platelet count, protein C and protein S deficiency, serum calcium, phosphorus and parathyroid estimation (PTH), cryofibrinogen and cryoglobulin levels, antinuclear antibody, cytoplasmic anti-neutrophil cytoplasmic antibody and perinuclear anti-neutrophil cytoplasmic antibody (p-ANCA).

Treatment of calciphylaxis is largely supportive as the disease has a poor prognosis. The treatment that has shown good response so far is intravenous sodium thiosulfate. Cinacalcet, a calcimimetic agent that reduces PTH levels and a phosphate binder Sevelamer have shown modest benefit. Monitoring of calcium homeostasis is key to the response to treatment.

Stress should be on management of renal or hepatic failure. Death usually occurs due to septicemia and thromboembolism.

Uremic neuropathy of sensorimotor type, pseudoporphyria, gynecomastia and calcinosis cutis are the other cutaneous features that may develop in patients with renal failure.

# SKIN SIGNS OF HEMATOLOGICAL DISEASES

Skin is one of the predominantly involved organ in hematological disorders. The involvement may be specific, e.g., chloroma (in acute myelogenous purpura) or nonspecific as pallor and purpura in many hematological conditions of diverse etiologies.

- *Pallor*: Seen in anemia that can be a result of several causes like deficiency of iron, folate, and vitamin B12; hypoplasia or infiltration of bone marrow, hemoglobinopathies, and hemolysis. Erythema of palmar creases usually disappears if the hemoglobin falls below 7 g/dL and indicates severity of anemia
- *Rubor*: In polycythemia rubra that can be primary or secondary to chronic hypoxemia or excess erythropoietin secretion from renal tumors
- *Pruritus*: It can be seen in several conditions most notably in polycythemia rubra. Aquagenic pruritus may precede polycythemia vera by several years and may not necessarily abate following treatment. Generalized pruritus in elderly should warrant a search for underlying hematological malignancy, particularly lymphoma
- *Pigmentation*: Pigmentation of hands, feet, and face can be seen in deficiency of vitamin B12 and folate. It is also a striking feature of Fanconi's anemia. Pigmentation may also be seen as adverse reaction from chemotherapeutic agents used to treat hematological malignancies or from hemosiderosis resulting from multiple blood transfusion in patients with thalassemia

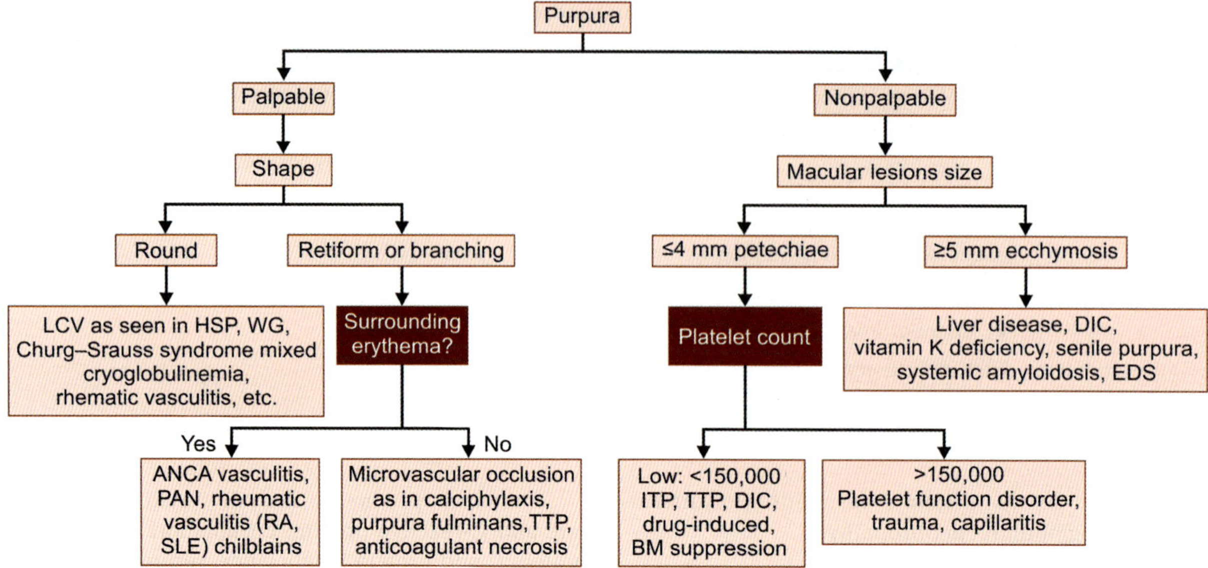


DIC, disseminated intravascular coagulation; EDS, Ehlers-Danlos syndrome; HSP, Henoch-Schonlein purpura; ITP, idiopathic thrombocytopenic purpura; LCV, leukocytoclastic vasculitis; RA, rheumatoid arthritis; SLE, systemic lupus erythematosus; TTP, thrombotic thrombocytopenic purpura; WG, Wegener's granulomatosis.

**FLOWCHART 1:** Evaluation of purpura.

- *Erythromelalgia*: Burning erythema of extremities usually the feet on warming (erythromelalgia) is usually seen in polycythemia, myelodysplasia, essential thrombocythemia and leukemia
- *Leg ulcerations*: Recurrent and recalcitrant leg ulcers, beginning since childhood can be an initial presentation of sickle cell disease and thalassemia
- *Paraneoplastic pemphigus*: Most commonly associated with B cell malignancies (lymphoma, chronic lymphatic leukemia, and Castleman's disease. An associated obliterative pneumonitis may be an important cause of mortality
- *Purpura*: Although not specific of hematological diseases, purpura is a common sign of these conditions seen in bleeding and clotting disorders, thrombocytopenias, thrombocythemias, thrombophilic disorders, multiple myeloma, leukemia, and myelodysplastic syndromes. Flowchart 1 depicts some causes of purpura with their essential features
- *Cutaneous infiltrates*: Infiltration of skin (leukemia cutis), though can occur in any type of leukemia, is commoner in acute monocytic and myelomonocytic leukemias. Cutaneous infiltrate can also occur in lymphomas and multiple myeloma
- *Miscellaneous cutaneous manifestations*: Acquired ichthyoses and erythroderma as in Hodgkin's lymphoma, Sweet syndrome, vasculitis, pyoderma gangrenosum, thrombophlebitis, and deep vein thrombosis can all be the features of hematological diseases.

## SUGGESTED READINGS

1. Ahn CS,,Yosipovitch G et al Diabetes and Skin Dermatological Signs Of Systemic Disease. In: Callen JP, Jorizzo JL, Zone JJ, Piette W, Rosenbach MA, Vleugels RA (Eds). Dermatological Signs of Systemic Disease, 5th edition. Philadelphia: Elsevier; 2016
2. Bourke J. Skin disorders in diabetes mellitus. In: Griffiths C, Barker J, Bleiker T, Chalmers R, Creamer D (Eds). Rooks Textbook of Dermatology, 9th edition. Oxford: Wiley Blackwell; 2016. pp. 64.1-7.
3. Johnston GA, Graham Brown RA. The Skin and Disorders of the Alimentary Tract, the Hepatobiliary System, Kidney, and Cardiopulmonary System. In: Wolff K, Goldsmith LA, Katz SI, Gilchrest BA, Paller AS, Leffell DJ (Eds). Fitzpatrick's Dermatology in General Medicine, 8th edition. New York: Mc Graw Hill; 1998. pp. 1446-61.
4. Molin S, Ruzicka T. The skin and the disorders of the kidney and urinary tract. In: Griffiths C, Barker J, Bleiker T, Chalmers R, Creamer D (Eds). Rooks Textbook of Dermatology, 9th edition. Oxford: Wiley Blackwell; 2016. pp. 153.1-6.

# 54 CHAPTER Psychocutaneous Disorders

*Amiya K Mukhopadhyay*

*"Skin is not just an envelope, but an organ."—Charles-Anne Lorry (1777)*

## INTRODUCTION

From the beginning of the history of cutaneous medicine, it has been repeatedly emphasized that the skin is not merely associated with some external disorders, but it is a canvas on which the pictures of many systemic diseases are also portrayed. In this regard the manifestation of various psychological disorders that affect the skin is worth mentioning. Apart from disease of the psyche, the skin acts as mirror on which the diverse colors of the emotion get reflected. It is the touch that gives a baby its first perception of sense.

It has been observed that patients suffering from various dermatological disorders suffer from sense of inferiority which may lead to depression. Many studies have shown that stress may play an important role in the pathogenesis of many skin diseases like chronic urticaria, recurrent herpes simplex, etc. Though patients with psychodermatological conditions should better be managed by a psychiatrist but as most of the patients either lack insight or are not comfortable to attend a psychiatric clinic in the beginning, a primary knowledge of various clinical manifestation of psychodermatological problems as far as the clinical manifestations, differential diagnoses and management is necessary for a dermatologist.

## EPIDEMIOLOGY

Psychiatric factors play an important role in the dermatological disorders. It has been estimated that significant psychiatric and psychosocial comorbidity is present in 30% of patients with skin diseases.

## PATHOGENESIS

The skin forms an interface where the outline of boundary of the "self" plays as body image of a person to himself/herself with which his inner sense confronts. Any disturbance in the balance of this interplay may affect the psyche that at times may lead to the psychocutaneous disorders.

Psychiatry mainly deals with the internal world or mind of the person whereas dermatology engages itself with the study of external disorders along with external manifestation of internal diseases. The interplay of psychodermatological disorder depends on the complex interaction between neuroendocrine and immune system which has been termed as neuro immuno-cutaneous system (NICS). This interaction depends on the release of mediators of inflammation from the NICS which is destabilized during inflammatory skin diseases and also psychological ailments.

Also a disturbed childhood with absence of positive upbringing may influence the future adult life and the person may develop disorders of body image, behavioral problem, etc. The other factors like psychosocial milieu, life events, personality of the concerned individual, etc. adds to the final outcome. Dysthymic condition, personality disturbance are often found in patients with some skin diseases like psoriasis, urticarial, etc. It has been reported that psychological stresses may cause disturbed barrier function of the skin that may lead to the various disorders of the skin.

## CLASSIFICATION

There are several classification systems which have been devised to describe psychocutaneous disorders, but till date none of them is universally accepted due to one or other limitations. The classification system prescribed by the DSM-TR (Diagnostic and Statistical Manual of Mental Disorders-Text Revision) may be very helpful for the psychiatrists but it appears cumbersome for the dermatologists. Hence considering all these aspects, a simple classification described by Lee and Koo seems suitable (Box 1).

**BOX 1 Classification of common psychocutaneous disorders**

- Psychophysiologic disorders
- Primary psychiatric disorders
- Secondary psychiatric disorders
- Cutaneous sensory disorders
- Nonpsychiatric cases where psychotropic agents are useful

# CLINICAL FEATURES OF COMMON PSYCHODERMATOLOGIC DISORDERS

The subject of psychodermatology is a vast ocean that itself may entail into a textbook, but such a detailed discussion is beyond the scope of this present treatise. Hence, a brief outline of the common disorders which are important in day-to-day practice is presented in the following sections.

## Delusion of Parasitosis (Synonym: Ekbom Syndrome)

**Key Points**

- Monosymptomatic hypochondriacal psychosis
- False and firm belief of infestation of the skin
- *Average age of onset*: 50–60 years
- *Sex incidence*: Below 50 years of age, male:female = 1:1; above 50 years of age, male:female = 1:2
- *Differential diagnoses*: Substance abuse (e.g., amphetamine, cocaine), dementia, cerebrovascular diseases, multiple sclerosis, malignancies, vitamin B12 deficiency, psychotic depression, depression with somatization, etc.
- *Treatment*: Pimozide, sulpiride, risperidone, olanzapine, etc.

Delusion of parasitosis is a primary psychiatric disorder where a patient has a fixed and firm belief of parasitic infestation in the absence of real such thing. Patients often suffer from sense of formication in the form of crawling, biting, or stinging. Younger patients should be enquired of their socioeconomic status and history of substance abuse. Sometimes, this type of delusion may be shared by another member of the family (Folie à deux) or may affect multiple members.

Patient usually presents with a history of formication and the severity of disturbance may even lead to the disturbances of normal daily activity including sleep. They also bring some material which they purportedly collected from their skin and place as an evidence of the alleged infesting creatures in an enclosed container or wrapped in a piece of paper (Fig. 1). They also develop secondary impetiginization of the scratched skin that has happened in attempts to catch the creatures.

Various substance abuse and some other disorders may mimic this ailment. Hence, a thorough search for a real infestation or presence of any other disorder should be done before making a diagnosis of delusion of parasitosis.

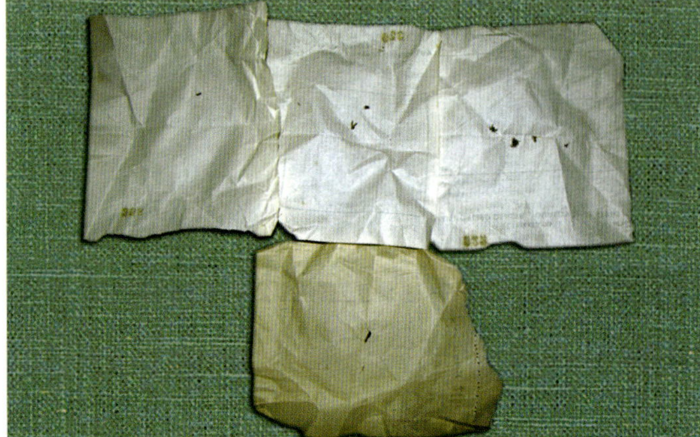

**FIG. 1:** Imaginary insects wrapped in paper pieces—brought by a patient with delusion of parasitosis.

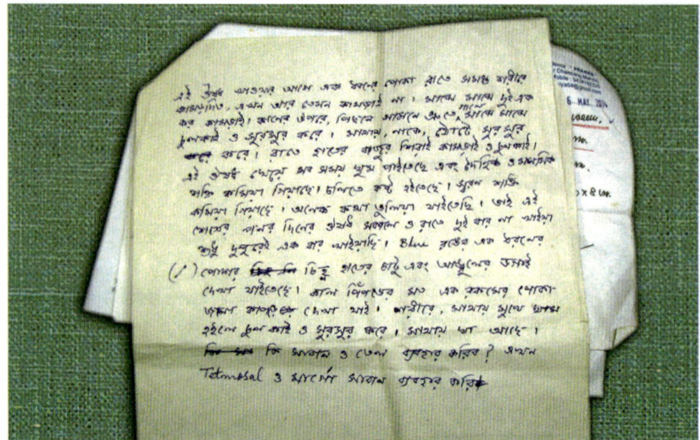

**FIG. 2:** Complaint written in Bengali by a patient with delusion of parasitosis during follow-up visit.

As far as the management is concerned the most important aspect is to form a rapport with the patient and to gain confidence. Most of the times patients are not convinced as the family members and the attending physicians have tried to persuade the patient about their false belief—which is not an appropriate way at least in the beginning. Some patients may bring their complaint in written form to gain attention which he hardly received in a busy dermatology clinic in his earlier consultations (Fig. 2).

Pharmacologic agents like pimozide, sulpiride, risperidone, olanzapine are very helpful. At times haloperidol may be needed.

## Dermatitis Artefacta (Factitial Dermatitis)

**Key Points**

- Rare disorder
- More common in women (male:female = 8:1)
- *Onset*: Adolescence or young adulthood
- Unusual and bizarre clinical picture, sharp cut border, geometric shape
- *Differential diagnoses*: Malingering, Munchausen's syndrome by proxy
- *Treatment*: Psychotherapy—antidepressant, antianxiety, antipsychotic medicines

Dermatitis artefacta is a psychocutaneous disorder where a patient injures his/her own skin in order to satisfy the psychological need. Patients are not always aware about their act. They develop this disorder as result of the maladaptive stress or may have borderline personality disorders.

The clinical manifestation of dermatitis artefacta can mimic any other diseases. The infliction may be caused by hands or any other instruments. It may be unilateral, bilateral, but the lesions are more prevalent in areas easy to reach. Sharp cut margins, difficult to corroborate with known clinical picture of other skin diseases should arouse suspicion (Fig. 3).

## Neurotic Excoriations

**Key Points**

- Common in middle aged ladies
- Repetitive irresistible desire to scratch, pick, or rub the skin
- Found in easily reachable body sites
- *Treatment*: Doxepin, topical and oral antipruritics, selective serotonin reuptake inhibitors

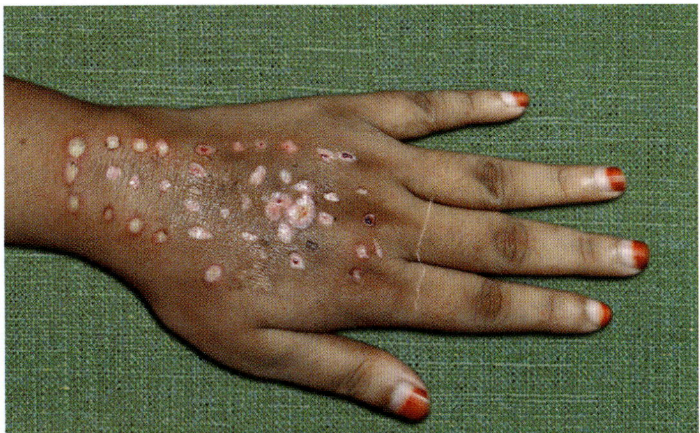

FIG. 3: Dermatitis artefacta—symmetric and arranged in an artistic manner.

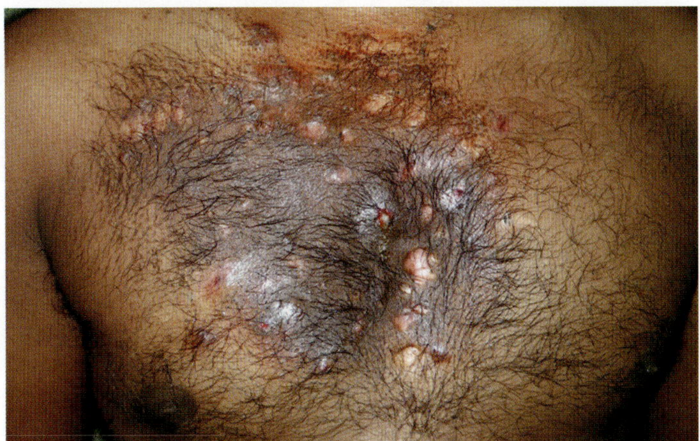

FIG. 4: Neurotic excoriation—excoriation and scar on a nevus.

In this disorder patient usually picks preexisting lesions like acne, keloids, sites of arthropod site etc. as repetitive, conscious and irresistible desire to pick, scratch, or rub the skin. The lesions are commonly located on the extensor surface of the forearms, scalp, upper back, and buttock but may affect other sites too (Fig. 4).

In children this may be a manifestation of the stress overlying an obsessive compulsive personality trait, but in adults frank psychiatric background of obsessive-compulsive disorders (OCD) may be present.

Treatment should include the management of pruritus, control of primary defects. Topical doxepin 5% cream, intralesional corticosteroids, oral doxepin and antihistaminic medicines are helpful.

## Acne Excoriée

### Key Points

- Common in older age group (mean age 30 years)
- More prevalent in females
- Marks of excoriation out of proportion to original acne lesion
- *Treatment*: Management of acne (oral isotretinoin, topical benzoyl peroxide, etc.), SSRIs, hypnosis, habit reversal therapy

SSRIs, serotonin reuptake inhibitors.

This psychodermatologic entity has been considered by many authorities as form of neurotic excoriation and often associated with OCD.

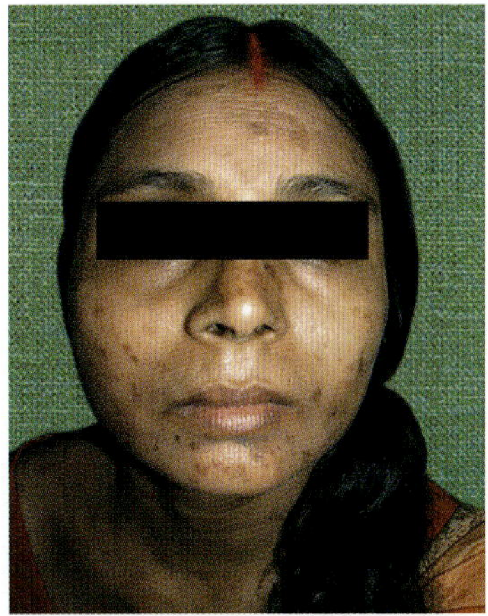

FIG. 5: Acne excoriée—scars with hyperpigmentation after habitual picking of acne.

Here the target lesion is preexisting acne. The severity of the excoriation is out of proportion to the acne lesions. The lesions are located in the preauricular region, chin, and forehead areas. Atrophy, scarring, and hyperpigmentation are common features (Fig. 5).

Management consists of control of acne, use of selective serotonin reuptake inhibitors (SSRIs) and psychotherapy.

## Trichotillomania

### Key Points

- Common in childhood
- Male:Female = 1:5
- Presence of short broken hairs (clinical) and pigmented hair casts (microscopic finding)
- *Differential diagnoses*: Alopecia areata, tinea capitis, pseudopelade
- *Treatment*: Behavior modification, positive reinforcement, SSRIs.

SSRIs, serotonin reuptake inhibitors.

Trichotillomania is a habitual self plucking of hairs which may be categorized a form of OCD. In a typical case most commonly scalp hair is pulled though hairs from the eye lashes, eye brows, pubis, and moustache are at times affected. Lesions are usually single in number but the size may be very big (Fig. 6). Some patient may chew and swallow the plucked hair that may lead to trichobezoar.

A common and important finding is the presence of broken hair. Microscopically, the presence of pigmented hair casts is diagnostic.

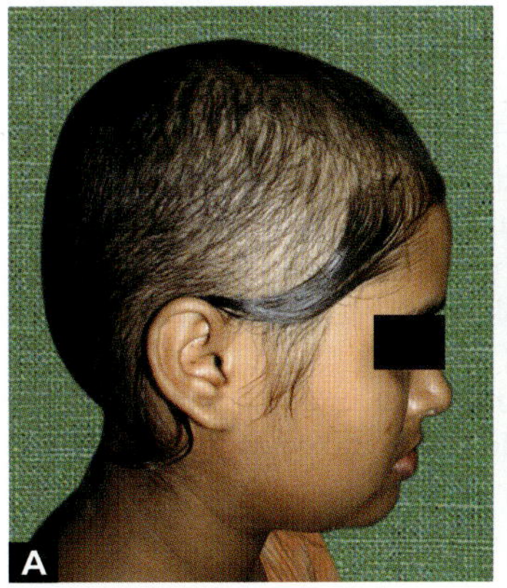



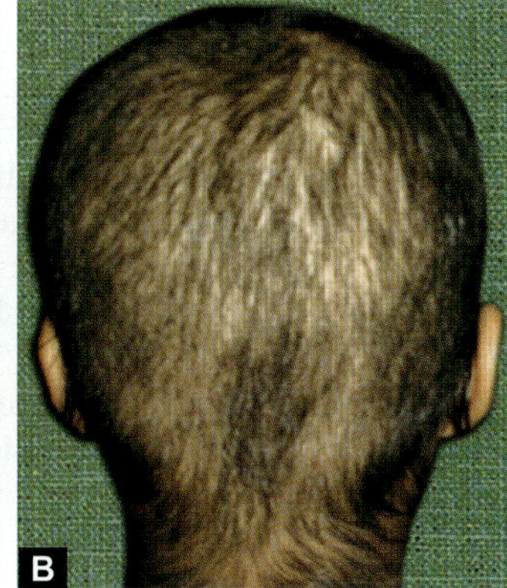



FIG. 6: Trichotillomania.

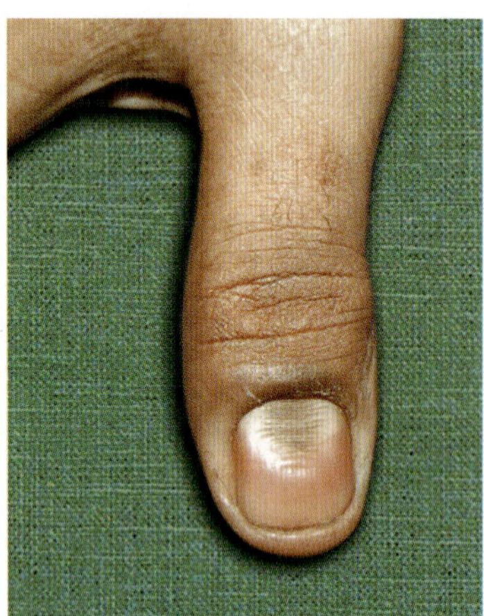

FIG. 7: Onychotillomania with habitual picking of the cuticle leading to damage of the nail plate.

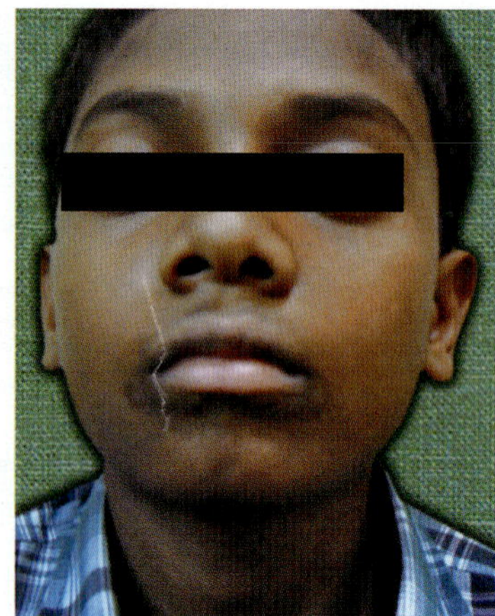

FIG. 8: Lip licking with perioral dermatitis.

Treatment includes behavior modification, positive reinforcement, etc. Pharmacotherapy with SSRIs is often rewarding.

### Onychotillomania and Onychophagia

These two entities are common in children and adolescents. These conditions reflect the underlying stress, or a psychological developmental problem or a manifestation of underlying depression.

Onychophagia usually affects finger nails. Onychotillomania on the other hand may involve any nails. This may lead to paronychia, nail dystrophy, and damage to the cuticle and nail plate (Fig. 7).

These disorders respond well to pimozide and clomipramine.

### Body Dysmorphic Disorders

Patients with body dysmorphic disorders have a basic defect in the perception of their own body image.

These patients are usually on the thirties, disturbed with the wrong perception of distortion of their body parts like face, hair, breasts, genitals, etc. They spend long hours before their mirrors obsessively. As the responsible psychiatric pathogenic factor may vary from OCD to delusion, the treatment also varies from SSRIs to antipsychotic medicines.

## OTHER LESS COMMON DISORDERS

Apart from the above mentioned psychocutaneous disorders, patients may present some times to the dermatologists with problems that have an underlying relation with psychiatric condition. Examples of these disorders include lip licking and perioral dermatitis (Fig. 8), knuckle biting (Fig. 9), prurigo nodularis (Fig. 10), psychogenic purpura, etc. Sometimes patient may come with injury to the skin as a features of suicidal or parasuicidal intent (Fig. 11).

These patients should be managed in an appropriate manner and help of a psychiatric professional should be sought whenever felt necessary.

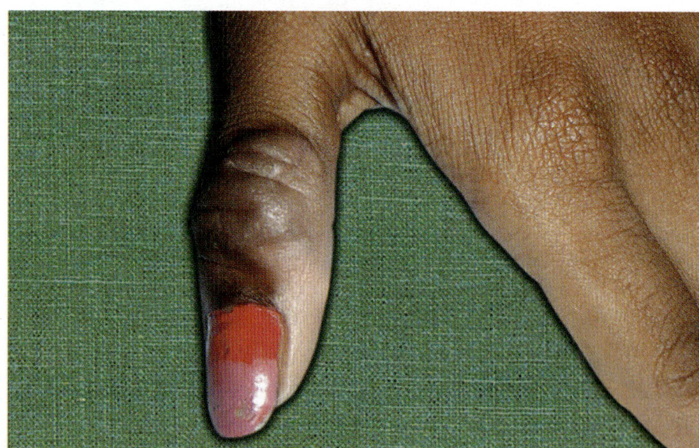

FIG. 9: Knuckle biting.

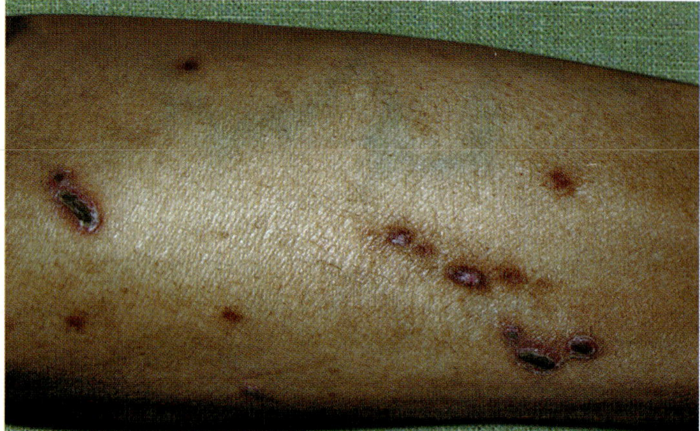

FIG. 10: Prurigo nodularis.

## DRUG AND PSYCHODERMATOLOGIC DISORDERS

As far as the drugs in psychodermatology are concerned, the topic may be viewed in the following ways:

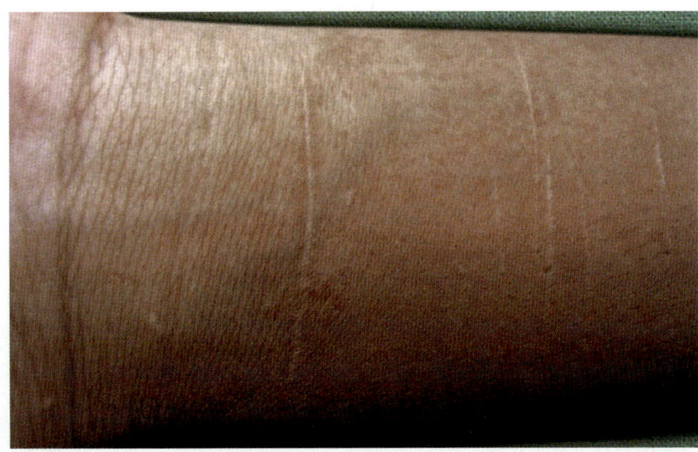

FIG. 11: Cut marks following self-injury on the flexor aspect of wrist caused by a failed attempt of suicide.

**TABLE 1: Commonly prescribed drugs in psychocutaneous diseases**

| Class | Drugs |
|---|---|
| Anxiolytic drugs | • Alprazolam<br>• Buspirone<br>• Paroxetine<br>• Venlafaxine |
| Antidepressant drugs | • Amitriptyline<br>• Doxepin<br>• Citalopram<br>• Escitalopram<br>• Fluoxetine<br>• Paroxetine<br>• Sertraline<br>• Venlafaxine |
| Antipsychotic drugs | • Olanzapine<br>• Pimozide<br>• Quetiapine<br>• Risperidone |
| Drugs used in obsessive-compulsive disorders | • Fluoxetine<br>• Paroxetine<br>• Sertraline |

- *Drugs needed to treat psychodermatologic disorders*: Various drugs are used in the management of the psychodermatologic disorders. Of these antipsychotic, antidepressant, anti-OCD and anxiolytic drugs are important (Table 1)
- Psychiatric side effects of the drugs used to treat dermatologic conditions.

There are many pharmacologic agents that are used to treat skin diseases may lead to psychiatric disturbances. The effects of systemic corticosteroids, dapsone, acyclovir, etc. in causing psychiatric symptoms are well known. Despite the fact that the association of isotretinoin with suicide is controversial, the topic generated much debate in the recent years.

## CONCLUSION

As almost every third patient attending dermatology clinic have some psychiatric comorbidity, therefore a fundamental knowledge of psychiatry is mandatory for any dermatologist. Many of the diseases require a specialized care from psychiatry professionals—hence the liaison between a dermatologist and a psychiatrist is complementary. It may be concluded that for assessing a patient with psychocutaneous complaint the sphere of enquiry should not only cover the basic dermatological difficulties but also the psychological aspects as well as drug history of the patient.

## SUGGESTED READINGS


1. Alder R, Cohen N, Felten D. Psychoneuroimmunology: interactions between the nervous system and immune system. Lancet. 1995;345(8942):99-103.
2. American Psychiatric Association. Diagnostic and Statistical Manual of Psychiatric Disorders, 4th edition (Text Revision). Washington, DC: American Psychiatric Association; 2000.
3. Amit Garg M, Chren M, Sands L, et al. Psychological stress perturbs epidermal barrier homeostasis. Arch Dermatol. 2001;137:53-9.
4. Bonneau RH. Stress induced modulation of the immune response to herpes simplex virus. In: Alder R (Ed). Psychoneroimmunology, 4th edition. New York: Elsevier, 2007. pp. 1077-97.
5. Cotteril JA. Dermatologic nondisease. Dermatol Clin. 1996;14:439-45.
6. Gupta MA, Gupta AK, Ellis CN, et al. Psychiatric evaluation of the dermatology patient. Dermatol Clin. 2005,23:591-9.
7. Hull PR, D'Arcy C. Acne, depression and suicide. Dermatol Clin. 2005;23:665-74.
8. Jafferani M. Psychodermatology: a guide to understanding common psychocutaneous disorders. J Clin Psychiatry. 2007;9(3):203-13.
9. Jerajani H, Jerajani R. Psychocutaneous disorders. Indian J Dermatol. 2006;51:5-7.
10. Koblenzer CS. Neurotic excoriations and dermatitis artefacta. Dermatol Clin. 1996;14:447-55.
11. Koo J, Lee CS. Psychocutaneou diseases. In: Bolognia JL, Jorizzo JL, Rapini RP (Eds). Dermatology, 2nd edition. New Delhi: Mosby- Elsevier; 2008. pp. 105-14.
12. Laihinen A. Psychosomatic aspects in dermatoses. Ann Clin Res. 1987;19:147-9.
13. Lee CS, Koo J. Psychopharmacologic therapies in dermatology: an update. Dermatol Clin. 200523:735-44.
14. Lee CS, Koo J. Psychotropic agents. In: Wolverton SE (Ed). Comprehensive dermatologic drug therapy, 2nd edition. Philadelphia: Saunders-Elsevier; 2007. pp. 437-58.
15. Marucha PT. Stress and wound healing. In: Alder R (Ed). Psychoneroimmunology, 4th edition. New York: Elsevier, 2007. pp. 825-37.
16. Millard LG, Millard J. Psychocutaneous disorders. In: Burns T, Breathnach S, Cox N (Eds). Rook's textbook of dermatology, 8th edition. Oxford: Wiley–Blackwell; 2010. pp. 64.1-55.
17. Mukhopadhyay AK, Dave JN, Vora NS, et al. Delusion of parasitosis. Guj Med J. 1994;41:99-100.
18. Poot F, Sampogna F, Onnis L. Basic knowledge in psychodermatology. J Euro Acad Dermatol Venereol. 2007;21:227-34.
19. Reider E, Tausk FA. Psychocutaneous skin disease. In: Goldsmith LA, Katz SI, Gichrist BA (Eds). Fitzpatrick's Dermatology in general medicine, 8th edition. New York: McGraw Hill; 2008. pp. 1158-65.
20. Sands GE. Three monosymptomatic hypochondriacal syndromes in dermatology. Dermatol Nurs. 1996;8:421-5.
21. Sneddon J, Sneddon I. Acne excorié; a protective device. Clin Exp Dermatol. 1983;8:65-8.
22. Zomer SF, DeWit RF, Van Bronswsijk, JE et al. Delusions of parasitosis. A psychiatric disorder to be treated by dermatologists? An analysis of 33 patients. Br J Dermatol 1998;138:1030-2.

# 55 CHAPTER Skin and Internal Malignancy

Sayantani Chakraborty, Anupam Das, Nilendu Sarma

## INTRODUCTION

Skin, the largest organ of the body often provides clues to diagnosis of internal malignancies. These clues, combined with a thorough clinical history, can play an important role in alerting the clinician to the presence of an underlying tumor. Although these dermatoses are rare and unusual, the recognition of some typical paraneoplastic dermatoses leads to the early diagnosis of a neoplasm and mandate a better prognosis.

The skin may be directly or indirectly involved in malignancies in the form of direct invasion or metastasis (e.g., leukemia cutis, cutaneous T-cell lymphoma, mammary Paget's disease).

The indirect effects that trigger the cutaneous signs or symptoms is caused by a variety of factors (inflammatory, proliferative, or metabolic factors) related to the neoplasia. Factors, such as polypeptides, hormones, cytokines, antibodies or growth factors act as mediators. In this case, there is no presence of neoplastic cells in the skin, and is considered a dermatological paraneoplastic syndrome (PNS).

Some genodermatoses predisposes the affected individual to various skin and internal neoplasia. In such cases, skin manifestations (often itself neoplastic) do not develop due to internal malignancy, but it should prompt searching for such internal malignancy.

## PARANEOPLASTIC SYNDROME

Paraneoplastic syndrome is defined as manifestation in other organs of some distant neoplasia. Skin and subcutaneous tissue is one important organ where PNS is expressed. PNS is caused by indirect mechanism that is yet to be explained and possibly mediated through biological mediators like hormones, peptides, or cytokines or due to some unknown metabolic disturbances induced by the neoplasia. There is no presence of any neoplastic cells in the skin.

By definition, classical PNS excludes the following:

- Manifestation caused by direct invasion or spread of the tumor (as in Paget's disease or metastasis)
- Manifestation caused secondary to the treatment of the malignancy
- When internal malignancy and the manifestation are both caused by a common precipitating condition like genetic predisposition.

**BOX 1 Curth's postulate**

- Both conditions of neoplasia and paraneoplasia begin simultaneously
- Develop a parallel course
- The skin lesion is not associated with a genetic syndrome
- A specific type of neoplasia is associated with a certain paraneoplastic syndrome
- The dermatosis is rare in the general population
- There is a statistically high frequency of association between both the conditions

Ideally, the association between the PNS and the neoplasia should be significant enough to prove the relation. The said skin manifestation should not be present unless the neoplasia is present and vice versa. In other words, the finding should not be seen in association with any non-neoplastic condition. But this is not found in most occasions in absolute terms. Neoplastic disorders may result in different PNS and the reverse is also true. However, it has to be remembered that to exclude simple chance coincidence, their association should not be very occasional.

Curth was the first one to propose criteria to define PNS (Box 1). Most of our current knowledge on PNS is based on his work.

## ASSOCIATION OF PARANEOPLASTIC SYNDROME AND INTERNAL MALIGNANCY

As already mentioned, the ideal PNS should indicate presence of some specific form of neoplasia. But, in reality, this is rare. Most of the dermatological PNS are also seen in many other non-neoplastic conditions. Most of these neoplasias also do not develop PNS always.

An exhaustive list of PNS with associated internal malignancy is mentioned in table 1.

Moreover, it is not unlikely to find different kind of PNS in a given neoplasia. Thus, strength of association between neoplasia and PNS varies significantly hampering a diagnostic reliability of these PNS (Box 2).

There are conditions that are well-known to be indicators of internal malignancy but the strength of association is weak. Some of examples of these are sign of Leser-Trélat, acquired ichthyosis, bullous pemphigoid, dermatitis herpetiformis, juvenile xanthogranulomas, necrobiotic xanthogranuloma, progressive systemic sclerosis, scleredema, and pruritus.

**TABLE 1: Association of paraneoplastic syndrome with internal malignancy**

| Dermatoses | Malignancies |
|---|---|
| • Bazex paraneoplastic acrokeratosis<br>• Malignant acanthosis nigricans<br>• Erythema gyratum repens<br>• Acquired hypertrichosis lanuginosa<br>• Necrolytic migratory erythema<br>• Paraneoplastic pemphigus<br>• Pityriasis rotunda<br>• Dermatomyositis<br>• Palmoplantar keratoderma<br>• Leser-Trélat sign<br>• Pyoderma gangrenosum<br>• Sweet syndrome | • Aerodigestive tract (oral cavity, larynx, pharynx, trachea, esophagus, and lung)<br>• Gastric malignancy<br>• Pulmonary, esophagus, and breast<br>• Colorectal carcinoma, pulmonary and breast carcinoma<br>• Glucagonoma<br>• Non–Hodgkin lymphoma, Castleman's disease, and thymoma<br>• Hepatocellular carcinoma<br>• Ovarian carcinoma<br>• Esophageal carcinoma<br>• Gastric and colorectal<br>• Myelodysplastic syndrome<br>• Acute myelogenous leukemia |

**BOX 2 Conditions having strong association with malignancy**

- Acquired hypertrichosis lanuginosa
- Acrokeratosis paraneoplastica of Bazex
- Erythema gyratum repens
- Necrolytic migratory erythema
- Paraneoplastic pemphigus
- Tripe palms
- Trousseau syndrome
- Hypertrophic osteoarthropathy
- Amyloidosis, primary systemic
- Scleromyxedema
- Carcinoid syndrome

## CLINICAL PRESENTATION

There can be diverse dermatological manifestations of PNS as mentioned below:

- PNS manifesting as non-inflamed superficial skin lesions like thickening, annular lesions
- PNS manifesting as inflamed lesions—erythema gyratum repens, necrolytic migratory erythema
- Specific manifestations—Sign of Leser–Trélat
- PNS manifesting as infiltrative plaques, nodules, and sclerosis
- PNS manifesting as connective tissue disease, endocrine disorders, and red swollen face
- PNS manifesting with blistering disease
- PNS manifesting as vasculitis, purpura, telangiectasia, ulcers and thromboembolic events, Raynoud's phenomena
- Other manifestations like pigmentation, acanthosis, lanugo hair, ichthyosis, urticaria, xanthomatous diseases, cold intolerance, pruritus, and flushing.

### Skin Thickening

Skin thickening and hardening may manifest as paraneoplastic disorder and may present as primary systemic amyloidosis, scleromyxedema, scleredema, and systemic sclerosis (Box 3).

**BOX 3 Paraneoplastic conditions involving skin thickening and hardening**

- Primary systemic amyloidosis
- Scleromyxedema
- Scleroderma
- Scleredema
- Pachydermoperiostosis

### Primary Systemic Amyloidosis

Amyloid light chain is associated with underlying malignancy, the most common one being multiple myeloma. Others include Hodgkin lymphoma and gastric, breast, and renal cell carcinoma.

Primary systemic amyloidosis frequently manifests with purpura, ecchymoses, spontaneously or with slight trauma, and even hemorrhagic blister over head and neck region. Racoon eye (bleeding around eye) is a known finding in this.

Soft, waxy papules, nodules and plaques are highly characteristic findings and develop on eye lids, behind ear, anogenital areas and other areas (Fig. 1). Amyloid infiltration results in development of macroglossia, a highly characteristic manifestation.

It may also present with patchy or diffuse alopecia, scleroderma-like (scleroderma amyloidosum) presentation in fingers, and myxedema-like skin lesions. Systemic infiltration also occurs in many organs like heart, blood vessels, kidney, liver, and gastrointestinal tract and can lead to complication. Nail dystrophy is also seen.

### Scleromyxedema

Scleromyxedema is characterized by deposition of excessive mucin in the dermis. This may be associated with monoclonal gammopathy in most of the cases. This clinically present with translucent waxy papules on an infiltrated and thickened skin base mostly affecting face and neck resulting into thickening of skin folds and giving rise to bull's face appearance (Figs 2 and 3).

Significant associations include paraproteinemias, multiple myeloma, Waldenström's macroglobulinemia, leukemia, Hodgkin lymphoma, non-Hodgkin lymphoma, and thymic carcinoma.

### Scleredema

Scleredema is characterized by stiffness of the skin. Clinically there may be peau-d' orange appearance on the skin. It is most commonly present on the face, upper back and always spares acral areas (Fig. 4).

This may develop after infections (often in children), in diabetes mellitus, or due to multiple myeloma or plasma cell dyscrasia. This has been reported after trauma and after drugs like infliximab, hyperparathyroidism, rheumatoid arthritis, Sjögren syndrome and carcinoid tumor. There is mucin deposition between thickened collagen bundles.

This may improve spontaneously. Internal condition need to be treated. Improvement with systemic steroids, cyclosporine, methotrexate, and UVA1 phototherapy is reported.

### Systemic Sclerosis

Systemic sclerosis, or systemic scleroderma, is a chronic inflammatory autoimmune condition characterized by vascular changes, fibrosis of the skin, and other organs.

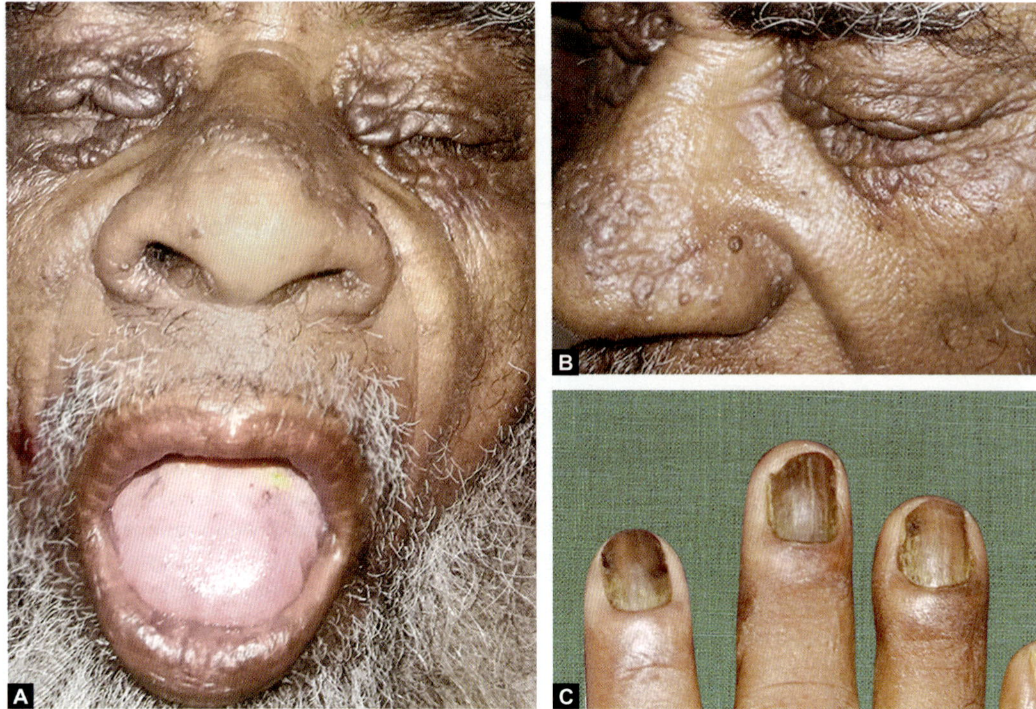

**FIG. 1: A,** Brownish, soft, waxy papules and plaques on the eye lids, nose and macroglossia in primary systemic amyloidosis; **B,** Lateral view of the same patient; **C,** Dark thickened finger nails with clubbing in the same patient.

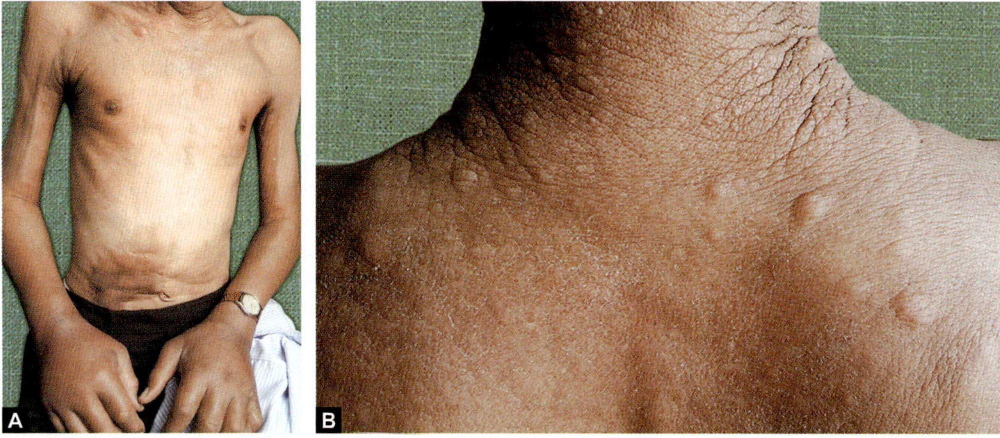

**FIG. 2: A,** Generalized skin thickening, nodular lesions, and bilateral nonpitting edema of acral regions in scleromyxedema; **B,** Indurated skin on back with nodular eruptions in same patient.

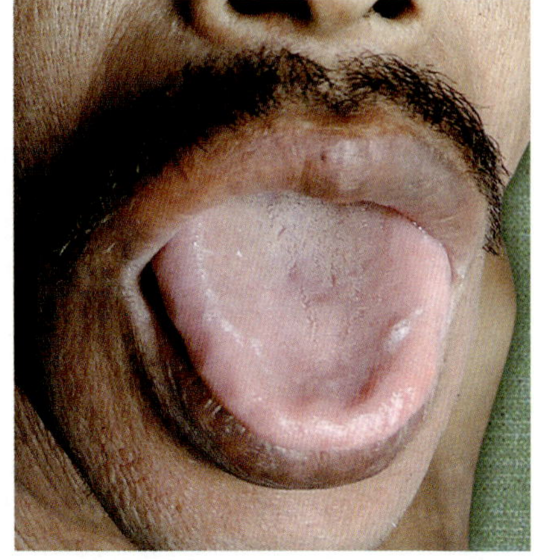

**FIG. 3:** Stiff and swollen tongue and lips in scleromyxedema.

**FIG. 4:** Scleredema in a patient with myeloma.

**BOX 4 Hyperpigmentation and internal malignancy**

- Ectopic adrenocorticotropic hormone syndrome
- Hemochromatosis
- Metastatic melanoma
- Malignant acanthosis nigricans
- Cronkhite–Canada syndrome
- Peutz–Jeghers syndrome
- Leukemia
- Hodgkin and non-Hodgkin lymphoma

Systemic sclerosis is associated with an increased risk of malignancy, in particular lung and breast cancer B-cell lymphoma. Altered B-cell function, which can give rise to lymphoid malignancies, has been implicated in the pathogenesis of this autoimmune disorder.

### Hypertrophic Osteoarthropathy

Secondary form of pachydermoperiostosis is associated with form is associated with the PNS in lung cancer, metastases to the lung, nasopharyngeal carcinoma, and other less common cancers.

## Hyperpigmentation

Hyperpigmentation as a sign of possible internal malignancy is seen in many conditions. Several malignancies may present with diffuse hyperpigmentation (Box 4).

Ectopic adrenocorticotropic hormone (ACTH) syndrome presents with diffuse hyperpigmentation over exposed areas (face, neck, back of hands), areas affected by trauma or subject to slight pressure and mucous membranes. There is increased production of the polypeptide lipotropin, which is capable of inducing the production of melanocyte-stimulating hormones (MSHs), which stimulate the production of melanocytes in the skin. This may be associated with small-cell lung carcinoma, medullary thyroid cancer, carcinoid tumor pheochromocytoma, and reproductive organ and pancreatic tumors. There may be elevated plasma cortisol and corticotrophin levels.

Diffuse hyperpigmentation is also a feature of hemochromatosis which is often associated with liver cancer.

Late-stage metastatic melanoma may be associated with diffuse melanosis, in rare cases which is characterized by a blue-gray color and believed to be caused by tumor lysis.

Hyperpigmentation in leukemia and Hodgkin and non-Hodgkin lymphoma is mediated via stimulation of melanin through secretion of factors from mast cells, fibroblasts, keratinocytes, endothelial cells, and lymphoid tumor cells.

Melanocytic macules and papules in the perianal and genital regions have been reported in association with lung adenocarcinoma.

Patients with periorificial melanotic macules, mostly present around the lips, nose, mucous membranes, and fingertips should be investigated for gastrointestinal polyposis and cancer as they may belong to the autosomal dominant disorder known as Peutz-Jeghar's syndrome.

## Inflammatory Disorders

The annular lesions associated with cutaneous malignancy are erythema gyratum repens, NME, erythema annulare centrifugum, reticular erythematous mucinosis, pityriasis rotunda, and subacute cutaneous lupus erythematosus.

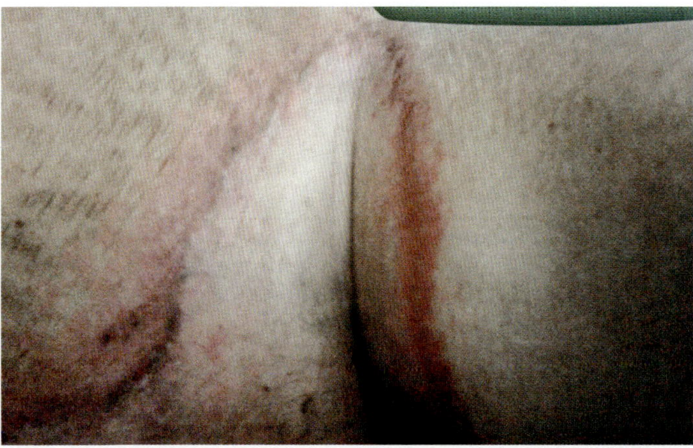

**FIG. 5:** Inflammatory lesions in the groin in necrolytic migratory erythema.

### Necrolytic Migratory Erythema

Necrolytic migratory erythema appears as erythematous scaly lesions with centrifugal growth. These are primarily distributed over the intertriginous areas (groin, perineum, buttocks, and lower abdomen), the central face (especially perioral) and distal extremities. This often mimics acrodermatitis enteropathica.

The lesions start as red-brown macules in perioral or inguinal regions and later necrotize and become covered with crusts (Fig. 5). Erythematous patches form plaques. Sometimes, there is formation of central bullae that rapidly rupture and eventually resolve. Active serpiginous margins also show presence of vesicles, erosions, and crusts.

Other features are sore tongue, sore mouth, cracked dry lips, and ridging of the nails.

There may be weight loss, malaise, intermittent diarrhea, hypokalemia, resistant diabetes mellitus, anemia, venous thrombosis, glossitis, diarrhea, steatorrhea, and psychiatric disorders.

Typically, this indicates presence of underlying glucagonoma. On histopathology, acute lesions show epidermal necrosis in stratum spinosum along with abundance of neutrophils and frank separation from the underlying intact epidermis. Chronic lesions show a psoriasiform pattern on biopsy.

For patients with glucagonoma, resection of the tumor is the only available therapeutic option.

### Erythema Gyratum Repens

Clinically, it presents as severely pruritic serpiginous band like patches arranged in concentric red swirls that progress very fast (in days). This is often referred to as a "wood-grain" appearance.

Common associations include malignancies of lung (32%), esophagus (8%), and breast (6%). This is a rare condition but the association with internal malignancies is very strong.

On rare occasions, erythema gyratum repens has also been observed in benign conditions, such as tuberculosis, calcinosis, and CREST (calcinosis, Raynaud's phenomenon, esophageal dysmotility, sclerodactyly, and telangiectasia) syndrome.
Treatment of the malignancy usually resolves the eruption.

## Annular Lesions

Annular lesions that may actually be PNS are mentioned in box 5.

| BOX 5 | Annular lesions |
|---|---|
| • Erythema annulare centrifugum<br>• Generalized granuloma annulare<br>• Reticular erythematous mucinosis<br>• Pityriasis rotunda<br>• Subacute cutaneous lupus erythematosus | |

Erythema annulare centrifugum is very rarely, seen in neoplastic disorders, such as lymphomas, leukemias, and malignant histiocytosis. Generalized granuloma annulare is a delayed hypersensitivity reaction to an unknown antigen.

There have also been rare reports of an association with Hodgkin lymphoma.

Pityriasis rotunda is a rare disease characterized by well-demarcated circular, scaling lesions. These may be lighter or darker than the surrounding skin. There is no associated inflammation or pruritus. Patients develop multiple lesions on the trunk that may coalesce. Malignancies associated include hepatocellular carcinoma, cancer of the stomach, esophagus, palate, and prostate and chronic lymphoid leukemia and multiple myeloma.

Reticular erythematous mucinosis is a primary cutaneous mucinosis characterized by reticular pruritic, erythematous lesions on the upper chest occurring in association with malignancies like cancer of the colon, breast, and lung.

## Keratoderma

### Tripe Palm or Acquired Pachydermatoglyphy

Also known as "acanthosis palmaris," tripe palms are characterized by thickened velvety palms similar to the rugose surface of the bovine stomach. Some authors suggest that it is a variant of acanthosis nigricans. It is often associated with malignant acanthosis nigricans and Leser–Trélat sign.

It presents with yellowish, velvety, diffuse palmar hyperkeratosis, with accentuated dermatoglyphic patterns, leading to a rough appearance that resembles the intestinal villosities, which explains the term tripe palms.

Neoplastic processes have been reported in 90% of cases, gastric and lung cancer accounting for 50% of tumors. Other neoplasms that have been correlated are breast and genitourinary tract cancers.

The role of TGF-α, melanocortin-1 and epidermal growth factor (EGF) has been postulated in the pathogenesis of these lesions.

Histological examination reveals acanthosis and hyperkeratosis, and perivascular deposition of mucin in the dermis may be observed.

### Acrokeratoses Paraneoplastica of Bazex

It presents with symmetric erythematous, scaling lesions that affect the hands, the feet, the elbows, and the knees. This may progress to palmoplantar keratoderma, marked nail dystrophy. Psoriasiform lesions of the ear and the trunk may occur. Histologically, it differs from psoriasis in the fact that there is focal parakeratosis, dyskeratotic keratinocytes and lymphocytic perivascular infiltrate. It is commonly associated malignancies are squamous cell carcinomas of the larynx, esophagus and lung.

Several factors have been implicated in the pathogenesis of acrokeratosis paraneoplastica of Bazex.

There may be antigen cross-reactivity between the tumor and the skin. Also production of a keratinocyte growth factor, vitamin A deficiency, and genetic susceptibility may play a role. Disseminated superficial porokeratosis may present as paraneoplastic manifestation in hematologic malignancies, hepatocellular carcinoma and cholangiocarcinoma.

Small plaque parapsoriasis is described in liposarcoma. Pityriasis rubra pilaris may be a cutaneous manifestation in Merkel cell carcinoma, hepatocellular carcinoma, breast, and lung carcinoma.

## Sign of Leser–Trélat

It primarily affects elderly individuals, without any gender or racial predilection. This is characterized by rapid appearance or growth of multiple pruritic seborrheic keratoses with or without inflammation (Fig. 6). Co-occurrence with other paraneoplastic dermatoses like acanthosis nigricans, and tripe palms are quite common.

The etiopathogenesis is not clear but elevated levels of TGF-alpha, EGF-α, IGF-1 and human EGF receptor 2/neu have been found. Adenocarcinomas of gastrointestinal tract account for the majority of malignancies described with the Leser-Trélat sign. Other significant associations include lymphoproliferative disorders like leukemias, lymphomas, Sézary syndrome and mycosis fungoides (21%). There are reports of association with transitional cell carcinoma of the bladder, kidney tumors, prostate, lung, ovary and kidney cancer, and melanoma.

All patients should be screened for neoplasms. Medical history, physical examination, complete blood count, serum biochemistry, chest radiography, mammography, Pap smear, PSA screening, upper digestive endoscopy and colonoscopy are mandatory. The prognosis is poor. Treatment is generally directed towards the underlying malignancy.

The keratotic lesions may respond to retinoids, trichloroacetic acid, cryosurgery, dermabrasion, lasers and shave excision.

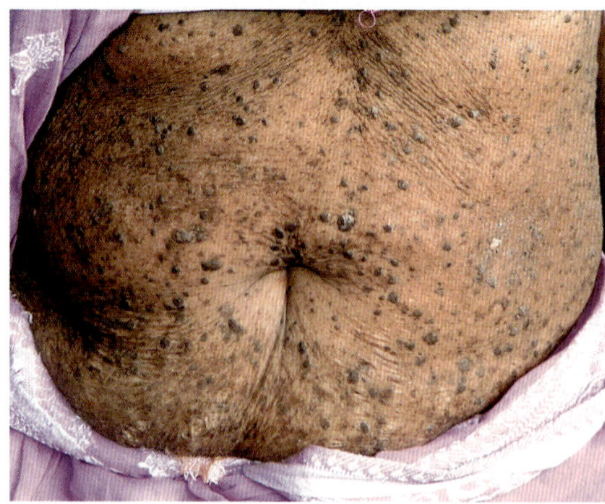

**FIG. 6:** Sudden appearance of many seborrheic keratosis in a middle-aged female who later diagnosed as having adenocarcinoma of colon (sign of Leser–Trélat).

## PNS manifesting as Autoimmune Connective Tissue Disease

### Dermatomyositis

Sudden onset of classical lesions of dermatomyositis (heliotrope rash, Gottron's papules, poikiloderma, dilated nail fold capillary loops and pruritic diffuse alopecia) should raise the suspicion of an underlying malignancy and the patients should be thoroughly investigated. Approximately 10–25% of cases are paraneoplastic.

Risk factors include elevated erythrocyte sedimentation rate, men over the age of 50 years, etc. Common associations include genitourinary malignancies, especially ovarian cancer and colon cancer. Other commonly seen malignancies include breast, lung, gastric, pancreatic, and lymphomas. Malignancies in cases of juvenile dermatomyositis is, however, extremely uncommon.

## Red Swollen Face

Episodic reddening of the face may be seen in endocrinal malignancies like carcinoid syndrome, pheochromocytoma, mastocytosis, dermatomyositis, SLE, mastocytosis, etc. Patients with neuroendocrine tumors present with carcinoid syndrome as a result of secretion of vasoactive substances, such as serotonin, histamine, bradykinin, and prostaglandins, characterized by repeated episodes of flushing, the severe cases may present with hyperpigmentation, pellagra-like lesions due to tryptophan depletion (hyperkeratosis, xerosis, scaling, glossitis), pachydermoperiostosis (with thickening of the skin) and digital clubbing, scleroderma-like lesions, brown orange plaques, pruritus, erythema annulare centrifugum, acrocyanosis, and pyoderma gangrenosum even. Diagnosis is confirmed by elevated levels of 5-hydroxyindoleacetic acid in a 24-hour urine test.

## Vascular Lesions

Vascular skin manifestations are quite nonspecific and include the entities listed in box 6. A detailed clinical history is required to establish a correlation with the underlying malignancy.

Clusters of telangiectasias on the anterior surface of the thorax may indicate breast cancer. Such telangiectasias may be present in subcutaneous metastasis, carcinoid syndrome, and hepatic adenocarcinoma.

Malignant angioendotheliomatosis may present with generalized telangiectasia which may be painful.

### Peripheral Ischemia

Peripheral ischemia occurs in paraneoplastic acral vascular syndrome, which is associated with stomach, small intestine, pancreatic, ovarian, and renal carcinoma and lymphoma. Patients with multiple myeloma, Waldenström macroglobulinemia and lymphoma may present with cryoglobulinemia and ischemia.

### Vasculitis

Vasculitis may occur in few cases of paraneoplastic disorders most of which are related to hematological malignancies like hairy cell leukemia, chronic lymphoid leukemia, myeloma, Hodgkin and non-Hodgkin lymphoma, acute myeloblastic leukemia, malignant histiocytosis, and myelodysplastic syndromes as cutaneous small vessel vasculitis and polyarteritis nodosa.

**BOX 6 Vascular lesions**

- Telangiectasia
- Vasculitis
- Peripheral ischemia
- Thrombophlebitis
- Livedo reticularis

The most common solid tumor associated with this paraneoplastic presentation is lung cancer, followed by gastrointestinal, renal, urinary, prostate, and breast cancer. More often they present as Henoch–Schönlein purpura.

It is hypothesized that there is formation of antigen-antibody immune complexes associated with the tumor, direct vascular damage to endothelial cells due to a cross reaction with antigens in the tumor cells, and a direct effect of leukemic cells (hairy cells) on the vascular.

Vasculitis can occur much earlier than the diagnosis of the primary tumor may be up to 2 years so a close suspicion and monitoring is required in at-risk patients who suffer from refractory and persistent vasculitis lesions.

### Thrombophlebitis

Patients with cancer have a considerably increased prevalence of deep vein thrombosis. Migratory thrombophlebitis (Trousseau syndrome), spontaneous, recurrent, multiple, superficial thrombophlebitis is found to occur in lymphomas, leukemia and cancers of prostrate, stomach, colon, and lung. This may be related to the general hypercoagulable state associated with the primary malignancy.

Thrombophlebitis of the subcutaneous veins of the anterolateral aspect of the chest and abdomen, known as Mondor disease, which is associated with breast carcinoma.

### Trousseau Syndrome

It is an acquired coagulopathy presenting as migratory thrombophlebitis, mostly in a background of an internal malignancy, commonly cancers of lung and pancreas. Certain characteristics of tumors (adenocarcinoma, metastatic progression, involvement of the gallbladder, gastrointestinal, pulmonary systems) have been shown to elevate the risk of development of Trousseau syndrome.

### Livedo Reticularis

Livedo reticularis is commonly associated with multiple myeloma cutaneous T-cell and B-cell lymphoma, angiotropic lymphoma, acute lymphoid leukemia, renal carcinoma, and inflammatory breast carcinoma.

### Palmar Erythema

Palmar erythema, an acral vascular syndrome is associated with lung cancer, Hodgkin lymphoma, myeloproliferative syndrome, gastric adenocarcinoma, and brain tumors.

### Purpura

Nonpalpable purpuric lesions and ecchymosis are commonly seen in multiple myeloma, Waldenström macroglobulinemia, lymphoma, chronic lymphoid leukemia, breast cancer, ovarian cancer, cervical cancer, prostate cancer, and undifferentiated

**BOX 7 Erosive and bullous lesions**

- Paraneoplastic pemphigus
- Pemphigus foliaceus
- Bullous pemphigoid
- Cicatricial pemphigoid
- Dermatitis herpetiformis
- Linear IgA dermatosis
- Epidermolysis bullosa acquisita

IgA, immunoglobulin A.

lung cancer which may be due to thrombocytopenia or idiopathic thrombocytopenic purpura.

Disseminated intravascular coagulation occurs in several malignant hematologic disorders and some solid tumors, such as pancreatic, gastrointestinal, and prostate cancer.

## Erosive and Bullous Lesions

Many internal neoplasias especially hematological and solid tumors may develop with bullous and erosive PNS (Box 7).

### Paraneoplastic Pemphigus

It is a paraneoplastic dermatosis characterized by pleomorphic lesions. It is characterized by intractable painful stomatitis and a polymorphous cutaneous eruption (pemphigus vulgaris-like, bullous pemphigoid like, erythema multiforme like, and lichen planus-like lesions).

Direct immunofluorescence shows deposition of IgG and C3 in the epidermal intercellular spaces, along with complement deposition along the basement membrane zone. Serum autoantibodies binding to the cell surface of skin and mucosae in a pattern typical for pemphigus, are typically observed. These serum autoantibodies usually identify desmogleins 1 and 3, desmoplakins, envoplakin, and periplakin.

This eruption is classically associated with non–Hodgkin lymphoma, chronic lymphocytic leukemia, Castleman's disease, retroperitoneal sarcoma, thymoma, Waldenstörm macroglobulinemia, and follicular dendritic cell sarcoma.

The underlying neoplasm is diagnosed before the onset of the disease in two-thirds of the cases. In rest one-third of the cases the neoplasm appears after the onset of the disease. So, it is important to screen cases with intractable and refractory course for the presence of any underlying malignancy.

The most commonly associated malignancies are non-Hodgkin lymphoma, chronic lymphoid leukemia, and Castleman disease, which is more common in children.

Less common malignancies are thymoma, Waldenström macroglobulinemia, lung adenocarcinoma, follicular lymphoma, retroperitoneal liposarcoma, and on occasions, hepatocellular carcinoma.

Histology shows combined features of blistering dermatosis and lichenoid infiltrate. The prognosis is poor. However, various agents which have been tried include systemic steroids, rituximab, daclizumab, cyclosporine, cyclophosphamide, mycophenolate mofetil, intravenous immunoglobulins, and plasmapheresis.

## Infiltrative Plaques and Nodules

Some paraneoplastic skin conditions are associated with inflammatory papules, plaques and nodules. Some of these conditions, like necrobiotic xanthogranuloma, multicentric reticulohistiocytosis, and Sweet syndrome, are strongly associated with underlying neoplasms. Erythema nodosum and sarcoidosis may also present with malignancies but are weakly associated.

### Necrobiotic Xanthogranuloma

The condition is associated with benign monoclonal gammopathy in 80% of cases. Associated malignancies include lymphoproliferative diseases, myeloma, chronic lymphoid leukemia, and Hodgkin and non-Hodgkin lymphoma. It presents as multiple yellowish plaques and subcutaneous nodules located in the periorbital region and on the head, the neck, the flexures of the extremities, and the trunk.

### Multicentric Reticulohistiocytosis

This is an important member of the group of non-Langerhans cell histiocytoses. Neoplasms like melanoma, hematologic malignancies, carcinomas of breast, colon, ovaries; though rare, have been reported in association with multicentric reticulohistiocytosis. It starts with skin-colored, pink, or brownish papules measuring between a few millimeters and 2 cm in diameter located on the dorsum of the fingers, around the nailfold (Fig. 7).

### Sweet Syndrome

Sweet syndrome is characterized by the sudden onset of multiple erythematous or violaceous papules, indurated plaques, and painful inflammatory nodules that are typically accompanied by fever, neutrophilia, and systemic alterations. Malignancy may be associated with sweet's syndrome in up to 40% cases and the commonly associated malignancies are acute myeloid leukemia and other hematological disorders, solid tumors like genitourinary, breast, lung, and gastrointestinal cancer.

### Pyoderma Gangrenosum

It manifests as painful pustules and rapid progression to deep ulcerations with undermined edges. Although pyoderma gangrenosum is usually not associated with malignancy, and presence of atypical features like hemorrhagic bullae, superficial lesions, rapid appearance, involvement of the upper extremities/hands, and scarring should raise the suspicion of internal cancers.

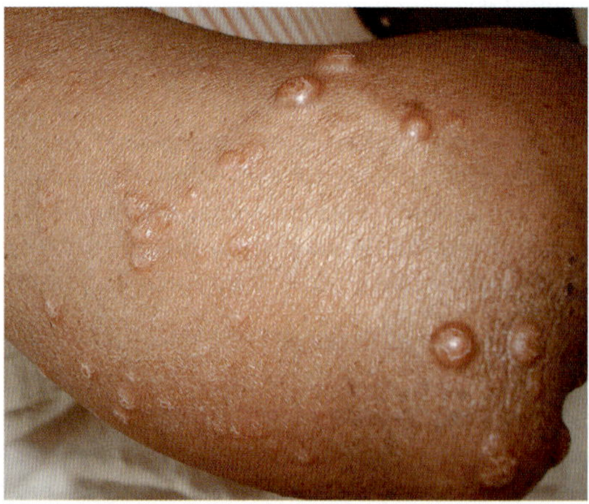

**FIG. 7:** Skin colored to slightly erythematous papulonodular eruption in multicentric reticulohistiocytosis.

Acute myelogenous leukemias, multiple myeloma and IgA paraproteinemias constitute the most important associations.

### Cutaneous Sarcoidosis

Cutaneous sarcoidosis presents with papules, plaques, nodules, lupus pernio, scar induration, ulceration, alopecia, hypopigmentation, lichenoid or psoriasiform lesions, and more rarely, nail dystrophy, or ichthyosiform lesions. The most common associated malignancies are hematological disorders.

## Miscellaneous Conditions

### Acanthosis Nigricans

Though mostly a benign disease but in rare situations, it may be a marker of an internal malignancy. It is characterized by gradual onset symmetric hyperpigmented, hyperkeratotic, verrucous and velvety plaques, commonly surrounded by acrochordons on the intertriginous skin. It may well affect mucosal surfaces and may sometimes be associated with pruritus. Malignancy associated acanthosis nigricans is characterized by sudden onset of the disease. The dermatosis in such cases is extensive, develops in elderly population, involves the mucosae and associated with tripe palms. This is mostly associated with intra-abdominal (gastric) malignancies. Its association is a strong predictor of the concerned malignancy. Approximately 25% of patients present with tripe palms (acquired pachydermatoglyphy) while in some patients sign of Leser-Trélat may be present.

The pathogenesis is not clear. It is believed that cytokines produced by neoplastic cells are involved, such as transforming growth factor alpha (TGF-$\alpha$), insulin growth factor-like (IGF-1), fibroblast growth factor and MSH.

Histopathology of acanthosis nigricans shows hyperkeratosis, papillomatosis and minimal acanthosis. Unfortunately, the onset of malignant acanthosis nigricans signifies terminal stage of the illness and the median survival is less than 24 months. Topical keratolytics, retinoids, oral metformin have been tried with debatable results. However, the treatment of the malignancy usually leads to resolution of the dermatosis.

### Pruritus and Prurigo

Pruritus is a common dermatological symptom which is commonly associated with malignancy like Hodgkin's lymphoma. This is often refractory to treatment and is observed with 25% of the patients with this cancer. It may also occur in breast cancer, carcinoid syndrome, cutaneous T-cell lymphoma, and gastrointestinal and hepatocellular carcinomas.

### Acquired Hypertrichosis Lanuginosa

It is a rare paraneoplastic dermatosis that was first described in 1865. Acquired hypertrichosis lanuginosa must be differentiated from hypertrichosis associated with endocrine or metabolic alterations (porphyria cutanea tarda and hyperthyroidism), and use of medications (cyclosporine, penicillamine, glucocorticoids, interferon, minoxidil, phenytoin, spironolactone, and cetuximab).

Women are more commonly affected. It presents with long, thin, soft, nonpigmented hair that affects the face and ears. It may involve the thorax and extremities, spreading in a craniocaudal manner. Palms, soles, scalp, and pubic areas are usually spared. Other cutaneous changes that may accompany this condition include painful glossitis, prominent fungiform papillae of tongue and angular cheilitis. Systemic associations include diarrhea, weight loss and lymphadenopathy. The condition is mostly associated with adenocarcinomas of the gastrointestinal tract, lung, breast, uterus, and leukemias.

Nonmalignant associations include hyperthyroidism, acquired immunodeficiency syndrome, porphyria cutanea tarda, anorexia nervosa, side effects of cyclosporine, phenytoin, penicillin, spironolactone, corticosteroids, and minoxidil.

The treatment is basically not satisfactory because by the time, these lesions appear; the underlying malignancy has progressed to its terminal stages. So, the management essentially relies upon treating the malignancy. For cosmetic reasons, the removal of hair may be tried using eflornithine cream, laser, mechanical, and chemical depilation agents.

### Acquired Ichthyosis

It is usually associated with hematological malignancies namely, lymphomas and leukemias. The sudden onset of ichthyotic lesions over the extensor aspects of extremities in an adult should raise the suspicion of an underlying malignancy.

Ichthyosis may be an early manifestation of selected systemic diseases (e.g., leprosy, hypothyroidism, lymphoma, and AIDS).

### Florid Cutaneous Papillomatosis

Onset of numerous lesions indistinguishable from common viral warts. The backs of the hands and the wrists are the initial sites, but eventually there is dissemination to the entire body and face. The lesions fail to show the presence of human papilloma virus.

Clinical associations include pruritus, acanthosis nigricans. The commonly occurring malignancy is gastric carcinoma. The onset of florid cutaneous papillomatosis preceded or occurred simultaneously with the diagnosis of malignancy in the majority of cases. The course of the skin lesions follows that of the internal malignancy.

## GENODERMATOSES WITH INCREASED CANCER RISK

Neoplasia, benign or malignant of skin and sometimes internal organs may be an important associated feature of some genodermatoses. Although the presence of neoplasia may not be a marker of any genodermatoses because neoplasia is more common and these genodermatoses are rarer, there may be other associated features that along with neoplasia may be strongly suggestive of these conditions. This constellation of features, when present should prompt meticulous, multidisciplinary approach to identify these genodermatoses.

There are some genodermatoses that are associated with malignant skin lesions and there are others that prominently feature benign skin tumors. Conditions in the first group are nevoid basal cell carcinoma syndrome, familial melanoma and xeroderma pigmentosum. Genodermatoses of the second group are mentioned in box 8.

**BOX 8 Genodermatoses associated with benign skin tumors**

- Tuberous sclerosis
- Neurofibromatoses 1 and 2
- Cowden's syndrome
- Muir–Torre syndrome
- Gardner syndrome

### Nevoid Basal Cell Carcinoma Syndrome

Also known as Gorlin syndrome, Gorlin-Goltz syndrome, this is an autosomal dominant disease and is characterized by multiple (>2) basal cell carcinoma (BCC), histology proven odontogenic keratocysts of the jaw, multiple (>2) palmoplantar pits, calcification of falx cerebri, bifid or prominently splayed ribs. These are considered major features. Other minor features are macrocephaly, cleft lip/ palate, skeletal abnormality, other neoplasia like ovarian fibroma and medulloblastoma.

### Muir–Torre Syndrome

This is clinically a closely similar condition to hereditary non-polyposis colon cancer (HNPCC). This is an autosomal dominant condition characterized mostly by internal cancer, most notably colorectal cancer present in about half of the cases. Cancers involving genitourinary tract, breast, head-neck, and small bowel are also seen. Multiple sebaceous gland tumors (sebaceous adenomas and carcinomas) and keratoacanthoma are less common but important feature of Muir–Torre syndrome.

### Cowden Syndrome

This is also known as multiple hamartoma syndrome. This is transmitted as autosomal dominant condition.

Benign mucocutaneous lesions are pathognomonic signs of this condition. Facial skin colored trichilemmoma, multiple oral papilloma/ fibroma on lips and buccal mucosa (cobblestone appearance) are the hallmark features. BCC, squamous cell carcinoma, melanoma and Merkel cell carcinoma are also seen but less commonly than benign tumors. In contrast, internal malignancies are prominent features forming many of the major diagnostic criteria. Breast cancers, follicular thyroid cancers, endometrial cancers, lung, and colon cancer are common and important internal cancers. Palmoplantar keratoses, structural abnormalities of urinary tract, gastrointestinal hamartoma, lipoma, mental retardation are important feature of the disease.

### Gardner Syndrome

Gardner syndrome, is characterized by the occurrence of large, multiple epidermal cysts, fibromas, leiomyomas, tricho-epitheliomas, and neurofibromas, is an autosomal dominant condition that can occur in association with colon cancer.

## OTHER CONDITIONS

Multiple leiomyomas is a band-like or segmental distribution and may be associated with renal cell tumors, forming part of a syndrome known as hereditary leiomyomatosis and renal cell cancer.

Familial atypical multiple mole melanoma syndrome is a relatively unknown genetic disorder associated with a high risk of melanoma and pancreatic cancer.

Fibrofolliculomas and trichodiscomas are seen in Birt-Hogg-Dubé syndrome which is an autosomal dominant disorder associated with an increased risk of lung and renal cell carcinoma.

Dermatologists can diagnose numerous systemic diseases because skin acts like a window to the internal milieu. Cutaneous PNS serve as vital clinical markers which can either precede, develop simultaneously or after the diagnosis of an underlying malignancy. A thorough knowledge of these conditions will prove beneficial in heralding the diagnosis and subsequent treatment of the much dreaded malignant conditions.

## CUTANEOUS METASTASIS

Any malignant neoplasm can metastasize to the skin. Cutaneous metastases from cancers of the lung, large intestine, and kidney are most prevalent in men; cancers of the breast and large intestine are most prevalent in women. The reported prevalence varies from 0.7 to 10% of all patients.

It is a dynamic and complex process resulting from autocrine activation of the motility factors by the cancer cells that stimulate their own tissue movement. There occurs increased expression of cadherins and integrins resulting to invasion and adhesion to the target tissue site. Cathepsins and matrix metalloproteinases also play important role in tissue matrix remodeling and adhesion. Angiogenic growth factors like vascular endothelial growth factor play an important role in angiogenesis that facilitate metastatic growth.

Patients presents with rapidly developing solitary or multiple subcutaneous nodules. These are round, oval rubbery in texture and variably mobile. They may have central umbilication. The malignancies that have more propensity to metastasize to skin are malignancies of breast, liver, kidney, gallbladder, colon/rectum, ovary, lung, endometrium, stomach, pancreas, etc. Patients with breast cancer may present variably with cutaneous metastasis in the form of carcinoma erysipeloides, carcinoma-en-cuirasse, peau-de-orange skin and inflammatory nodules.

## SUGGESTED READINGS

1. Bofek A, Rachowska R, Krajewska J, et al. Carcinoid syndrome with angioedema and urticaria. Arch Dermatol. 2008;144:691-2.
2. Boyce S, Harper J. Paraneoplastic dermatoses. Dermatol Clin. 2002;20:523-32.
3. Brinca A, Cardoso JC, Brites MM, et al. Florid cutaneous papillomatosis and acanthosis nigricans maligna revealing gastric adenocarcinoma. An Bras Dermatol. 2011;86:573-7.
4. Buggiani G, Krysenka A, Grazzini M, et al. Paraneoplastic vasculitis and paraneoplastic vascular syndromes. Dermatol Ther. 2010;23:597-605.
5. Cardoso Filho Fde A, Feitosa RG, Fechine CO, et al. Glucagonoma syndrome associated with necrolytic migratory erythema. Rev Assoc Med Bras. 2015;61(3):203-6.
6. Costa MC, Martinez NS, Belicha MG, et al. Acanthosis nigricans and "tripe palm" as paraneoplastic manifestations of metastatic tumor. An Bras Dermatol. 2012;87:498-500.
7. De La Torre-Lugo EM, Sanchez JL. Erythema gyratum repens. J Am Acad Dermatol. 2011;64:e89-90.
8. Dong Y, Wang M, Nong L, et. al. Clinical and laboratory characterization of 114 cases of Castleman disease patients from a single centre: paraneoplastic pemphigus is an unfavourable prognostic factor. Br J Haematol. 2015;169(6):834-42.
9. Ehst BD, Minzer-Conzetti K, Swerdlin A, et al. Cutaneous manifestations of internal malignancy. Curr Probl Surg. 2010;47:384-445.
10. El Tal AK, Tannous Z. Cutaneous vascular disorders associated with internal malignancy. Dermatol Clin. 2008;26:45-57.

11. Gaiser CA, Dhawan N. Paradoxical presentation of glucagonoma with delayed onset of necrolytic migratory erythema. Am J Med. 2015;128(2):e1-2.
12. González-Morán A, Román C, Galván C, et al. Acroqueratosis paraneoplásica de Bazex asociada a Carcinoma epidermoide oculto. Actas Dermosifilogr. 1993;841:63.
13. Jabbour SA. Skin manifestations of hormone-secreting tumors. Dermatol Ther. 2010;23:643-50.
14. Kelly S, Culican S, Silvestrini RA, et al. Comparative study of five serological assays for the diagnosis of paraneoplastic pemphigus. Pathology. 2015;47(1):58-61.
15. Krathen RA, Orengo IF, Rosen T. Cutaneous metastasis: a meta-analysis of data. South Med J. 2003:96:164-7.
16. Krawczyk M, Mykala-Ciesla J, Kolodziej-Jaskula A. Acanthosis nigricans as a paraneoplastic syndrome. Case reports and review of literature. Pol Arch Med Wewn. 2009;119:180-3.
17. Kurzydlo AM, Gillespie R. Paraneoplastic pityriasis rubra pilaris in association with bronchogenic carcinoma. Australas J Dermatol. 2004;45:130-2.
18. Ortega-Loayza AG, Ramos W, Gutierrez EL, et al. Cutaneous manifestations of internal malignancies in a tertiary health care hospital of a developing country. An Bras Dermatol. 2010;85:736-42.
19. Pelosof LC, Gerber DE. Paraneoplastic Syndromes: an approach to diagnosis and treatment. Mayo Clin Proc. 2010;85:838-54.
20. Pipkin CA, Lio PA. Cutaneous manifestations of internal malignancies: a review. Dermatol Clin. 2008;26:1-15.
21. Poszepczynska-Guigné E, Viguier M, Chosidow O, et al. Paraneoplastic acral vascular syndrome: epidemiologic features, clinical manifestations, and disease sequelae. J Am Acad Dermatol. 2002;47:47-52.
22. Ramos-E-Silva M, Carvalho JC, Carneiro SC. Cutaneous paraneoplasia. Clin Dermatol. 2011;29:541-7.
23. Reyes CM, Rudinskaya A, Kloss R, et al. Scleroderma-like illness as a presenting feature of multiple myeloma and amyloidosis. J Clin Rheumatol. 2008;14:161-5.
24. Russell P, Floridis J. Hypertrichosis lanuginosa acquisita: a rare dermatological disorder. Lancet. 2015:S0140-6736(15)00121-X.
25. Sariya D, Ruth K, Adams-McDonnell R, et al. Clinicopathologic correlation of cutaneous metastases: experience from a cancer center. Arch Dermatol. 2007:143: 613-20.
26. Schena D, Papagrigoraki A, Frigo A, et al. Eruptive disseminated porokeratosis associated with internal malignancies: a case report. Cutis. 2010;85:156-9.
27. Serrão V, Martins A, Ponte P, et al. Erythema gyratum repens as the initial manifestation of lung cancer. Eur J Dermatol. 2008;18:197-8.
28. Silva JA, Mesquita Kde C, Igreja AC, et al. Paraneoplastic cutaneous manifestations: concepts and updates. An Bras Dermatol. 2013;88(1):9-22.
29. Szekanecz E, Szamosi S, Gergely L, et al. Incidence of lymphoma in systemic sclerosis: a retrospective analysis of 218 Hungarian patients with systemic sclerosis. Clin Rheumatol. 2008;27:1163-6.
30. Sánchez NB, Canedo IF, García-Patos PE, et al. Paraneoplastic vasculitis associated with multiple myeloma. J Eur Acad Dermatol. 2004;18:731-5.
31. Tartaglia F, Blasi S, Sgueglia M, et al. Retroperitoneal liposarcoma associated with small plaque parapsoriasis. World J Surg Oncol. 2007;5:76.
32. Thiers BH, Sahn RE, Callen JP. Cutaneous manifestations of internal malignancy. CA Cancer J Clin. 2009;59:73-98.
33. Wong M, Grossman J, Hahn BH, et al. Cutaneous vasculitis in breast cancer treated with chemotherapy. Clin Immunol. 2008;129:3-9.
34. Worsnop F, Campalani E. Paraneoplastic hypertrichosis lanuginosa acquisita: a delayed presentation in quiescent chronic lymphocytic leukaemia. Clin Exp Dermatol. 2014;39(5):669-70.
35. Wu SL, Bai JG, Xu J, et al. Necrolytic migratory erythema as the first manifestation of pancreatic neuroendocrine tumor. World J Surg Oncol. 2014;12:220.
36. Yokokura H, Demitsu T, Kakurai M, et al. Paraneoplastic pemphigus mimicking erosive mucosal lichen planus associated with primary hepatocellular carcinoma. J Dermatol. 2006;33:842-5.
37. Yong AA, Tey HL. Paraneoplastic pemphigus. Australas J Dermatol. 2013; 54(4):241-50.

# 56 CHAPTER Dermatoses in Pregnancy

*Sayantani Chakraborty, Nilendu Sarma*

## INTRODUCTION

Skin changes in pregnancy can be classified as physiological skin changes, specific dermatoses of pregnancy and alteration in pre-existing skin diseases.

Pregnancy is also known to influence the course of pre-existing skin diseases in both positive and negative ways.

The specific dermatoses of pregnancy represent a heterogeneous group of pruritic skin diseases that have been recently reclassified and include pemphigoid (herpes) gestationis, polymorphic eruption of pregnancy (PEP) (syn. pruritic urticarial papules and plaques of pregnancy), intrahepatic cholestasis of pregnancy (ICP), and atopic eruption of pregnancy (AEP).

## PHYSIOLOGICAL CHANGES OF PREGNANCY

Physiologic skin changes in pregnancy include changes in pigmentation, alterations of the connective tissue, vascular system, and endocrine function as well as changes in hair and nails (Table 1). Hormonal, metabolic, and immunologic factors contribute to physiologic alterations in pigmentation, vessels, nevi, connective tissue, glands, hair, nails, and mucous membranes in pregnancy.

The most significant physiological skin change associated with pregnancy is pigmentation which manifests in the form of linea nigra, accentuated pigmentation around the axillae, genitalia, perineum, anus, areola, inner thighs, and neck. There may be darkening of pre-existing nevi lentigines and freckles. Melasma or chloasma also known as "mask of pregnancy" may affect up to 75% of pregnant females and is found to be more common in darker races.

The reasons for the changes in melanin concentration and distribution during pregnancy are not completely understood. Estrogen, progesterone, and melanocyte-stimulating hormone are known to stimulate melanocytes. Human placental lipids lead to increase in epidermal melanocytes and and upregulation of tyrosinase enzyme.

Striae distensae or striae gravidarum, also known as stretch marks, are commonly seen among pregnant women. They result when physical factors and hormones (relaxin, estrogen, and corticosteroids) cause thinning of elastin fibers and fibrillin microfibrils in the dermis, and there is shifting of the orientation of fiber from perpendicular to parallel relative to the dermal–epidermal junction.

Striae are most prominent on the abdomen, breast, and thighs, and may also appear on the lower back, buttocks, and upper arms.

Skin tags, known as molluscum fibrosum gravidarum, may form on the face, neck, axillae, chest, groin, or inframammary region, particularly during the second and third trimesters.

**TABLE 1: Physiological changes**

| | |
|---|---|
| Pigmentation | • Hyperpigmentation<br>• Linea nigra and accentuated pigmentation of nipple and areola<br>• Melasma |
| Connective tissue | • Striae distensae<br>• Molluscum fibrosum gravidarum<br>• Gynoid lipodystrophy<br>• Neurofibroma, dermatofibroma, and keloid |
| Vascular system | • Edema<br>• Varicosities/hemorrhoids<br>• Spider angiomas, telangiectasia<br>• Unilateral dermatomal nevoid telangiectasia<br>• Palmar erythema<br>• Gingiva hyperemia and hyperplasia<br>• Pyogenic granuloma |
| Hair | • Hypertrichosis<br>• Postpartum telogen effluvium<br>• Postpartum androgenetic alopecia |
| Nails | • Distal onycholysis<br>• Increased brittleness<br>• Subungual hyperkeratosis<br>• Transverse grooving |
| Glandular function | • Disturbed sebaceous gland function<br>• Acne gravidarum, montgomery glands<br>• Increased eccrine gland function—hyperhidrosis<br>• Decreased apocrine activity—Fox–Fordyce disease may get resolved |
| Pruritus | • Physiological<br>• Pathological |
| Mucosa | • Chadwick's sign<br>• Goodell's sign<br>• Nasal congestion<br>• Gum bleeding |

Neurofibromas may develop during gestation, while keloids, leiomyomas, dermatofibromas, and neurofibromas may enlarge.

Pruritus, common concern during pregnancy, may be part of a physiologic phenomenon, a pregnancy-related dermatosis, or may indicate underlying systemic disorder, such as liver, kidney, thyroid, or malignant disease. As many as 20% of pregnant patients are affected by pruritus with no detectable abnormality.

Spider angiomas often develop around second to fifth month of gestation, around the eyes or on the neck, face, upper chest, arms, or hands, appearing as red lesions with branches extending outward from a central puncta. High estrogen levels in pregnancy contribute to telangiectasias, blood vessel dilatation and proliferation. There may be unilateral dermatomal nevoid telangiectasia.

Various forms of vascular changes are commonly observed in pregnancy.

There may be varicosities over leg and vulvar region due to increase in venous pressure in pelvic, femoral veins. Subcutaneous hemangioendotheliomas, glomangiomas (glomus tumors), and pyogenic granulomas, which form on the gingiva or fingers may develop.

Disturbed sebaceous gland activity may lead to acne and there may be hyperhidrosis and miliaria due to eccrine gland hyperactivity.

Nails grow at an accelerated rate during pregnancy but may become soft, brittle, or dystrophic, with transverse grooves (Beau's lines), subungual hyperkeratosis, or onycholysis.

Hormonal change during pregnancy may lead to both increased and decreased hair growth. Due to slow shifting of anagen hairs to telogen, increased scalp hair density is noticed in most but there may also be mild frontoparietal androgenic alopecia in the third trimester that usually resolves later. There may be hirsutism due to increased ovarian and adrenal androgen.

Increased blood flow may cause a bluish-purple coloration of the vagina and cervix, is known as the Chadwick's sign and Goodell's sign, respectively. Gingival mucosa may show interdigital papillae that can cause pain, bleeding, or ulcerate. Hormonal changes in pregnancy are believed to contribute to hyperemia of the nasal mucosa and sinuses, causing nasal congestion.

## Pruritus in Pregnancy

Controversies exist in the diagnosis of itchy eruptions during pregnancy. This has resulted in frequent change in nomenclature of these conditions. These conditions are characterized by diverse kind of eruptions like urticaria, papules and plaques, erythema, eczema along with itching. Many suffer from atopic dermatitis and a large number of patients may develop atopic dermatitis for the first time in life during pregnancy. None of the lesions are specific for any conditions. However, they have some preference over other. Distribution, time of onset in relation to pregnancy, relapse in subsequent pregnancy, features of atopy and elevated immunoglobulin E (IgE) can be helpful in differentiation. As will be discussed, PEP, also known as pruritic urticarial papules and plaques of pregnancy (PUPPP), is typically characterized predominantly by urticarial lesions along striae, periumbilical sparing and onset in later pregnancy. But, when urticaria is absent in PEP or when eczematous lesions are predominant, a feature that may be seen in some cases can create diagnostic dilemma.

Conditions that are characterized by nonurticarial eruptions like nonspecific itchy papules, folliculitis-type lesions; erythema and eczematous eruption often pose the greatest challenge for diagnosis. Various names were in use for these conditions like prurigo gestationis of Besnier, prurigo of pregnancy and papular dermatitis of pregnancy.

Itching can be an important feature of ICP that is diagnosed with its definite laboratory alterations. Although ICP is a disease specific for pregnancy, may not be defined as true dermatoses.

# SPECIFIC DERMATOSES OF PREGNANCY

The specific dermatoses of pregnancy have undergone numerous changes in terminology and classification because of the lack of clarity regarding the pathogenesis and diagnosis of these conditions.

The most recent classification scheme was defined by Ambros-Rudolph et al. in 2006. Their classification involved four main categories. These are:

1. Pemphigoid gestationis
2. Polymorphic eruption of pregnancy
3. Intrahepatic cholestasis of pregnancy or obstetric cholestasis
4. Atopic eruption of pregnancy.

Among these, ICP and PG have risk for significant fetal complication if not managed properly. Fetus may suffer from prematurity, fetal distress, or even stillbirth. Impetigo herpetiformis (IH) is no longer considered as a specific pregnancy dermatoses as this is a form of pustular psoriasis that has flared up in pregnancy.

## Pemphigoid Gestationis

This is a rare autoimmune bullous disorder with an incidence of one in 50,000–60,000 pregnancies, pemphigoid gestationis (PG) presents mainly in the late pregnancy or immediate postpartum.

### Pathogenesis

It is associated with haplotypes HLA-DR3 and -DR4. It is more common in multigravid women in the third trimester, and it commonly recurs in subsequent pregnancies. The major target antigen in PG is the extracellular noncollagenous 16A (NC16A) domain of the transmembrane hemidesmosomal glycoprotein, collagen XVII (BP180), which consists of an intracellular N-terminal portion, a transmembrane region and a C-terminal ectodomain. This antigen is also present in the amniotic epithelium of placental tissues, the umbilical cord other than skin. When the placental antigen is presented to the maternal immune system by abnormally expressed HLA class II molecules, it triggers an immune response against the NC16A domain of collagen XVII (BP180). The NC16A antigen presents in the placental and umbilical cord epithelium cross-reacts with a cutaneous antigen resulting in cutaneous disease.

### Clinical Features

Clinical stage of the disease can be divided into two stages:

1. *Prebullous stage*: There is intense itching followed by appearance of erythematous urticarial papules and plaques typically starting from the abdomen and then spreading centrifugally to the rest of the body
2. *Bullous stage*: Following this, there is formation of tense bullae with usual sparing of the oral mucosa. The lesions

are predominant over the abdomen particularly around the umbilicus and below.

The lesions usually resolve within weeks to months following delivery, but may recur with menstruation and hormonal contraception and subsequent pregnancy. Very rarely (5%) a pregnancy may be passed over ("skip pregnancies"). Although there is an increase in the number of small-for-date babies, fetal prognosis is generally good. 10% of newborns may develop mild, transient skin lesions due to transfer of antibodies from the mother to the fetus, which resolve spontaneously within days to weeks.

## Diagnosis

*Skin biopsy for histopathological examination*: Histopathological findings from lesional skin depend on the stage and severity of the disease. Prebullous stage is characterized by edema of the upper and middle dermis accompanied by a predominantly perivascular inflammatory infiltrate, composed of lymphocytes, histiocytes, and a variable number of eosinophils.

The bullous stage reveals subepidermal separation that, ultrastructurally, may be located to the lamina lucida of the basement membrane zone.

*Immunofluorescence study*: The gold standard for diagnosis of PG is direct immunofluorescence from the perilesional skin which shows linear deposition of C3 along with IgG deposition in about 30% of the cases.

Circulating IgG antibodies is found in 30–100% cases which can be detected by indirect immunofluorescence.

Antibody levels may also be monitored using commercially available BP180-NC16a domain enzyme-linked immunoassay techniques that show a good correlation with disease activity that has similar specificity but increased sensitivity than indirect immunofluorescence.

## Treatment

Most cases are mild with good prognosis. Premature cesarean section is not indicated. This condition often improves after delivery with variable period of time.

During early pregnancy, oral antihistamines, topical steroids and emollients are used in case of mild disease. The systemic corticosteroids are the mainstay of treatment in patients with bullous eruption and extensive disease, in which cases, corticosteroids are used in the doses of 1–2 mg/kg. Dose adjustment needs to be done during delivery as there may be flare-ups. Postpartum, tetracyclines, nicotinamide, cyclophosphamide, ciclosporin, goserelin, azathioprine, dapsone, rituximab, plasmapheresis, or intravenous immunoglobulin may sometimes be considered for severe disease.

# Polymorphic Eruption of Pregnancy

This is also known as PUPPP. This is characterized by severely pruritic polymorphic eruptions usually occurring in a late stage of pregnancy.

There are many other names for this condition like toxemic rash of pregnancy, late-onset prurigo of pregnancy, and toxic erythema of pregnancy. PEP seems to be the most common specific dermatoses in pregnancy and its incidence appears as 1 in 200 pregnancies.

## Pathogenesis

Pathogenesis of this condition remains obscure. It usually affects primipara in their last trimester of pregnancy and immediate postpartum period. It is usually associated with excess maternal weight gain and conditions like twin pregnancy and polyhydramnios. It is thought that the rapid, late stretching of the abdominal wall causes damage to connective tissue in the striae and triggers the inflammatory response by unleashing antigenic character of the connective tissues within the striae.

Other factors that may contribute to PUPPP include elevated progesterone levels in multiple gestational pregnancies, increased vascularity, and then deposition of fetal DNA in skin containing damaged collagen.

## Clinical Presentation

Urticarial eruptions are most characteristic but nonurticarial lesions like erythema, eczema, papules are common. Tiny vesicles (that often are superimposed on urticarial lesion), purpuric, annular, and targetoid are seen les frequently but larger vesicles, and pustules are very rare (Figs 1 and 2).

Sometimes eczematous lesions may also be seen. It has a mean duration of persistence of 6–8 weeks, resolving in about 2 weeks following delivery. PUPPP tends not to recur with subsequent pregnancies.

Based on predominant lesional morphology, Aronson subdivided PEP into three subtypes: type 1 urticarial (predominantly), type 2 nonurticarial, and type 2-mixed. Predominantly nonurticarial lesions may have longer disease duration.

This starts in third trimester in most cases. It is generally short lived (mean 6 weeks) and improves after delivery. Recurrences in subsequent pregnancies, or precipitation after oral contraceptives or menstrual period is not common in PEP.

Distribution over the lower abdomen, upper thighs, involvement of striae distensae, periumbilical sparing, and occasional presence of perilesional halo are considered highly characteristic features. Absence of excoriation despite severe pruritus is also a typical feature. Face, palms, and soles are less commonly affected and mucosal involvement is not seen.

There is usually no risk to the mother or fetus and neonates born to mothers with PUPPP are not affected.

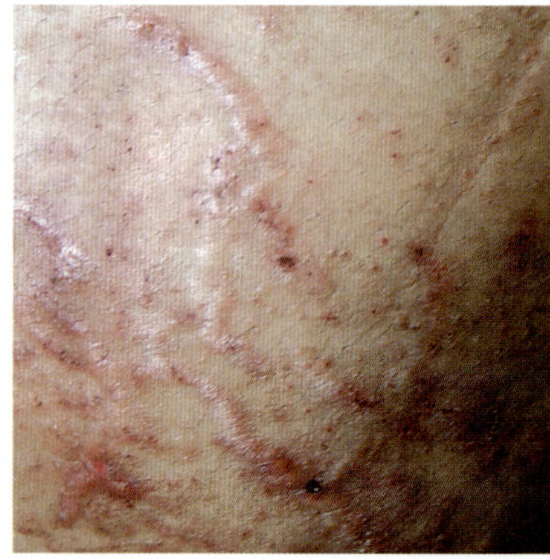

**FIG. 1:** Urticarial eruptions over striae in pruritic urticarial papules and plaques of pregnancy.

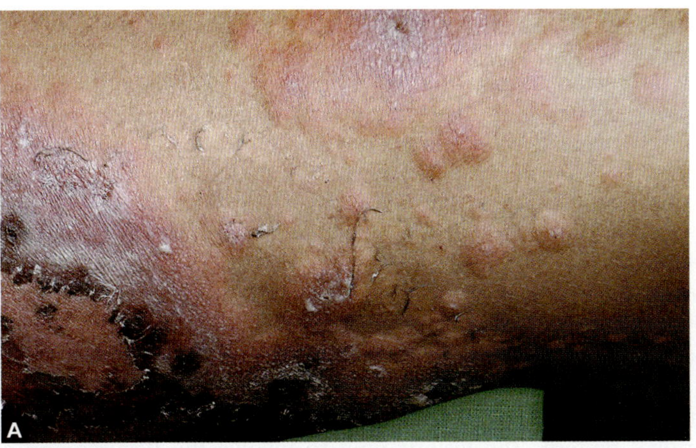


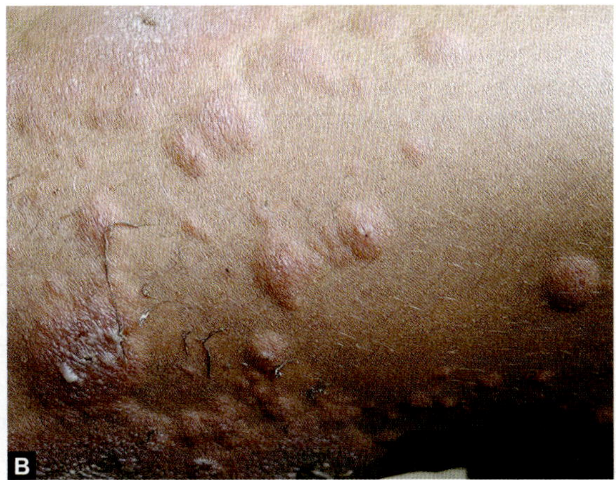


**FIG. 2:** More severe and polymorphous presentation in pruritic urticarial papules and plaques of pregnancy with urticarial eruptions, large purpuric patches, pustules, erosion and targetoid lesion.

### Laboratory Investigations

Urticarial lesions show presence of eosinophil in the dermal inflammatory infiltrate. Epidermis may show spongiosis, parakeratosis, and even exocytosis.

Direct and indirect immunofluorescence study is negative and such finding differentiates it from PG.

Considering the nondescriptive nature of most of the laboratory parameters, diagnosis is essentially clinical.

### Treatment

Treatment is mainly symptomatic aiming at relieving pruritus. In milder cases only antihistamines and soothing formulations like menthol, calamine are preferred. In moderately severe cases, topical potent corticosteroids alleviate symptoms effectively while cases not responding to topical corticosteroids, severe refractory cases with intractable pruritus may require systemic corticosteroids.

## Intrahepatic Cholestasis

Intrahepatic cholestasis of pregnancy, is a reversible form of hormonally triggered cholestasis that typically develops in genetically predisposed individuals in late pregnancy. It presents with pruritus and secondary skin lesions occur due to scratching.

It has a variable incidence and a geographical predisposition tending to occur at a greater frequencies in countries of South America like Chile. There is strong familial predisposition and a role of genetic factor is inevitable.

### Pathogenesis

Pregnancy is associated with cholestatic state due to the effect of hormones like estrogen and progesterone on the hepatic bile ducts. This leads to elevated bile acids in circulation of the mother and leads to pruritus. Recently, the role of genetic defect in bile acid secretion has been unraveled by endemic clustering and familial occurrence of the disease. Mutations of certain genes encoding for transport proteins necessary for bile excretion [e.g., the *ABCB4* (MDR 3) gene] have been identified in some ICP patients.

### Clinical Features

Intrahepatic cholestasis of pregnancy is not associated with primary skin lesions. It typically presents with sudden onset of severe pruritus that becomes generalized. The secondary skin lesions range from mild excoriation to severe prurigo nodularis like lesions. These usually affect the lower arms and legs but may also affect trunk and buttocks. These patients may present with jaundice in 10% of the cases typically within 2–4 weeks of onset of pruritus. These patients may also develop steatorrhea, malabsorption of fat-soluble vitamins and, in extreme cases, bleeding manifestation.

Fetal prognosis is a major concern in patients with ICP. It has been associated with an increased risk for prematurity, intrapartum fetal distress and stillbirths. Maternal prognosis is generally good except for the chances of intrapartum hemorrhage due to vitamin K deficiency in few cases. There is a 2.7-fold increased risk for gallstones in primigravidae with ICP as compared with pregnant women without cholestasis.

Subsequent pregnancies are at an increased risk for recurrence of ICP. Pregnancies occurring in first-degree relatives of patients with ICP are also at increased risk. Meconium staining is common in ICP and may indicate a poor fetal prognosis.

### Diagnosis

Intrahepatic cholestasis of pregnancy is suspected when bile acids in blood are raised more than 11 μmol/liter along with pruritus and particularly it has been correlated that outcome of pregnancy is poor when serum bile acids are more than 40 μmol/liter.

Other liver enzymes may also be raised. An abdominal ultrasound is recommended to exclude cholelithiasis if patient complains of abdominal pain.

### Treatment

Ursodeoxycholic acid (UDCA) helps in decreasing serum bile acid levels, reduces maternal pruritus and improves fetal outcome by decreasing the passage of bile acids to fetoplacental circulation. A dose of 15 mg/kg/day is administered either as a single or divided doses until delivery. However, UDCA is not licensed for use in pregnancy; thus, it requires special patient information.

Other drugs, including antihistamines, S-adenosyl-L-methionine, dexamethasone, and cholestyramine may be used. Risk of stillbirth increases as pregnancy progresses being highest after 38 weeks. Hence, delivery may be undertaken earlier to improve fetal outcome.

### Atopic Eruption of Pregnancy

Atopic eruption of pregnancy, said to be the most common dermatoses in pregnancy, is a benign pruritic disorder of pregnancy in patients with a personal and/or family history of atopy and/or elevated IgE levels after exclusion of the other dermatoses of pregnancy. The term was introduced into the literature by Ambros-Rudolph to encompass the clinical entities—eczema in pregnancy, prurigo of pregnancy, and pruritic folliculitis of pregnancy. It accounts for half of the patients and starts usually early, in 75% before the third trimester, and tends to recur in subsequent pregnancies due to the atopic background. Maternal and fetal prognosis is good.

#### Pathogenesis

The pathogenesis of AEP is thought to be triggered by a reduced cellular immunity and reduced production of Th1 cytokines [interleukin (IL)-2, interferon-γ, IL-12] in contrast to the dominant humoral immunity and increased secretion of Th2 cytokines (IL-4, IL-10).

#### Clinical Features

Eczema of pregnancy usually occurs in the third trimester. Clinically, it has been divided into two types: (1) E-type or the eczematous type in about two-third of the patients, and (2) the P-type or the papular type in about one-third of the patients. The E-type typically presents with eczematous lesions in flexural areas and the papular type usually represents with erythematous papules over the extremities.

Lesions in prurigo of pregnancy are characterized by erythematous papules and nodules on the extensor surface of the extremities resembling closely to prurigo nodularis.

Pruritic folliculitis of pregnancy, a rare dermatosis of pregnancy, occurs in about 1:3,000 pregnancies. It usually present in the second trimester of pregnancy with pruritic follicular, papular and pustular lesions over the trunk and the extremities.

#### Diagnosis

It is done mainly on clinical grounds and after exclusion of other pregnancy-associated dermatosis. Serum IgE may be raised in some cases, however, histopathology and immununofluorescence is unremarkable.

#### Treatment

In mild-to-moderate cases, antihistamines may be used to relieve symptoms. Narrowband ultraviolet B may be used in severe cases not responding to the first-line therapy. In severe and recalcitrant cases, use of short course systemic corticosteroid may be considered.

## PUSTULAR PSORIASIS OF PREGNANCY

Pustular psoriasis of pregnancy (PPP) is a rare variant of generalized pustular psoriasis occurring during pregnancy and needs special mention owing to the maternal and fetal morbidity. It is important to recognize the condition as early as possible and treat appropriately.

Historically, there has been controversy as to whether IH is a separate pregnancy-specific disease or a variant of generalized pustular psoriasis occurring in pregnancy; it is now considered by most to represent the latter.

Pustular psoriasis of pregnancy typically presents during the third trimester with symmetric erythematous plaques studded with sterile pustules at the margins of the plaques in a circinate pattern. The lesions tend to involve the flexures and spreads centrifugally. Subungual pustules may lead to onycholysis or rarely onychomadesis.

There is hypocalcemia, leukocytosis elevated erythrocyte sedimentation rate, low maternal serum calcium, phosphate, hypoalbuminemia and also low vitamin D because of hypoparathyroidism. Systemic symptoms like nausea, vomiting and diarrhea may occur.

### Laboratory Investigations

Histopathology demonstrates spongiform pustules with neutrophils. Psoriasiform hyperplasia and parakeratosis can also be seen. Immunofluorescence is negative in PPP.

### Treatment

- Systemic high dose corticosteroid like prednisolone is given in the doses of 60–80 mg/day with favorable outcome
- Cyclosporine is also advocated for the treatment of pustular psoriasis in pregnancy
- Narrowband ultraviolet B therapy may be instituted
- Early delivery may alleviate symptoms and avoid maternal complication and fetal risk.

## DERMATOSES ALTERED BY PREGNANCY

Myriad of pre-existing skin diseases are altered by pregnancy. Among them, the inflammatory diseases, rheumatic skin disease, infective diseases and skin tumors are affected either positively or negatively.

Inflammatory skin diseases can worsen or less often improve during pregnant state. Diseases that may develop or worsen in pregnancy are atopic dermatitis, urticaria, and erythema annulare centrifugum. There may be improvement in the plaques of psoriasis but worsening of pustular psoriasis may occur.

The complex immunological alterations occurring during gestation can affect the course of rheumatic skin disease sometimes resulting to flares. The diseases whose course may be affected are lupus erythematosus, rheumatoid arthritis, dermatomyositis, and scleroderma.

Since lupus erythematosus is mostly mediated through humoral immunity, it should logically follow that pregnancy induces flares in disease activity as humoral immunity is upregulated in pregnancy which may be about 2-3-fold rise in disease activity. The report of skin disease flares during pregnancy ranges from 21% to 90%. While the effect of pregnancy outcome by the disease shows variability. One in five pregnancies with systemic lupus erythematosus (SLE) may culminate into miscarriage or fetal death. The risk is highest in second trimester. The neonate may be affected manifesting disease at birth. Neonatal lupus erythematosus is a disease of newborn of mother suffering SLE and is related to transplacental passage of maternal anti-Ro/SSA, anti-LA or less commonly U1RNP antibodies to the fetus.

Approximately 75% of pregnant women with rheumatoid arthritis show improvement of their symptoms by second trimester. The possible cause is predicted to be due to the changes of the hormonal milieu causing downregulation of the regulatory T-cell activity. However, the diseases often flare up after pregnancy.

Most reports have suggested that pregnancy has little impact on the course of scleroderma. However, features like Raynaud's phenomenon shows improvement owing to pregnancy related vasodilatation. However, the disease itself may adversely affect the pregnancy outcome due its effects on vital systemic organs.

Patients with antiphospholipid syndrome may experience arterial and venous thrombosis, severe preeclampsia and eclampsia while there may be adverse outcome on pregnant woman with antiphospholipid syndrome resulting into miscarriage, stillbirth, intrauterine growth restriction (IUGR), etc.

Bacterial folliculitis may be encountered commonly during gestation so as vulvovaginal candidiasis. There may be exacerbation of leprosy during and within 6 months of lactation.

Herpes simplex virus may lead to disseminated disease during pregnancy while spontaneous abortion, prematurity, congenital/neonatal herpes, neurological complications to the fetus is common. Maternal varicella during pregnancy may lead to IUGR, low birth weight and congenital varicella syndrome.

Human papillomavirus infection during pregnancy may lead to genital wart in fetus, chorioretinitis, recurrent respiratory papillomatosis and preterm rupture of membranes.

Maternal rubella may lead to congenital rubella syndrome while measles during pregnancy leads to prematurity, spontaneous abortion, and neonatal measles.

The effects of sexually transmitted diseases during pregnancy are manifold having effect on both mother and baby. Syphilis leads to abortion, prematurity, infant death and early congenital syphilis and late syphilis in the newborn. *Chlamydia* infection leads to pelvic inflammatory disease, ectopic pregnancy, infertility, and postpartum endometritis while it causes neonatal conjunctivitis and pneumonia. Maternal gonorrhea leads to prematurity, IUGR, neonatal conjunctivitis, meningitis, scalp abscess, etc.

## SUGGESTED READINGS


1. Ahmadi D, Powell FC. Pruritic urticarial papules and plaques of pregnancy: current status. Australas J Dermatol. 2005;46:53-8.
2. Ambros-Rudolph CM, Glatz M, Trauner M, et al. The importance of serum bile acid level analysis and treatment with ursodeoxycholic acid in intrahepatic cholestasis of pregnancy, Arch Dermatol. 2007;143:757-62.
3. Ambros-Rudolph CM, Müllegger RR, Vaughn-Jones SA, et al. The specific dermatoses of pregnancy revisited and reclassified: results of a retrospective two center study on 505 pregnant patients. J Am Acad Dermatol. 2006;54: 395-404.
4. Ambros-Rudolph CM. Dermatoses of pregnancy – clues to diagnosis, fetal risk and therapy. Ann Dermatol. 2011;23 (3):265-75.
5. Aronson IK, Bond S, Fiedler VC, et al. Pruritic urticarial papules and plaques of pregnancy: clinical and immunopathologic observations in 57 patients. J Am Acad Dermatol. 1998;39:933-9.
6. Chang SE, Kim HH, Choi JH, et al. Impetigo herpetiformis followed by generalized pustular psoriasis: more evidence of same disease entity. Int J Dermatol. 2003;42:754-55.
7. Chappell LC, Gurung V, Seed PT, et al. Ursodeoxycholic acid versus placebo, and early term delivery versus expectant management, in women with intrahepatic cholestasis of pregnancy: semifactorial randomized clinical trial. BMJ. 2012;344:e3799.
8. Elling SV, Powell FC. Physiologic changes in the skin during pregnancy. Clin Dermatol. 1997;15:35-43.
9. Finch TM, Tan CY. Pustular psoriasis exacerbated by pregnancy and controlled by cyclosporin A. Br J Dermatol. 2000;142:582-4.
10. Garcia-Gonzalez E, Ahued-Ahued R, Arroyo E, et al. Immunology of the cutaneous disorders of pregnancy. Int J Dermatol. 1999;38:721-9.
11. Glantz A, Marschall HU, Mattson LA. Intrahepatic cholestasis of pregnancy: relationships between bile acid levels and fetal complication rates. Hepatology. 2004;40:467-74.
12. Holmes RC, Black MM. The specific dermatoses of pregnancy: a reappraisal with special emphasis on a proposed simplified clinical classification. Clin Exp Dermatol. 1982;7:65-73.
13. Koutroulis I, Papoutsis J, Kroumpouzos G. Atopic dermatitis in pregnancy: current status and shallenges. Obstet Gynecol Surv. 2011;66(10):654-63.
14. Kroumpouzos G, Cohen LM. Dermatoses of pregnancy. J Am Acad Dermatol. 2001;45:1-19.
15. Lehrhoff S, Pomeranz MK. Specific dermatoses of pregnancy and their treatment. Dermatol Ther. 2013;26(4):274-84.
16. Robinson A, Van Voorhees AS, Hsu S, et al. Treatment of pustular psoriasis: from the Medical Board of the National Psoriasis Foundation. J Am Acad Dermatol. 2012;67:279-88.
17. Ropponen A, Sund R, Riikionen S, et al. Intrahepatic cholestasis of pregnancy as an indicator of liver and biliary diseases: a population-based study. Hepatology. 2006;43:723-8.
18. Roth MM. Pregnancy dermatoses. Am J Clin Dermatol. 2011;12 (1):25-41.
19. Rudolf CM, Al Fares S, Vaughan-Jones SA, et al. Polymorphic eruption of pregnancy: clinicopathology and potential trigger factors in 181 patients. Br J Dermatol. 2006;154:54-60.
20. Shornick JK. Dermatoses of pregnancy. Semin Cutan Med Surg. 1998;17:172-81.
21. Soutou B, Aractingi S. Skin disease in pregnancy. Best Pract Res Clin Obstet Gynaecol. 2015;29(5):732-40.

# 17 SECTION Infections and Skin

# 57 CHAPTER Infective Exanthematous Disorders

Nilendu Sarma

## INTRODUCTION

Many viral and other infections in children are associated with skin rashes. This is called exanthem. Exanthems are often helpful in diagnosis of the conditions. However, there are overlaps and diagnosis may necessitate evaluation of many other features including laboratory confirmation. Viral infections are more common than bacterial or other infections (e.g., rickettsial infection). Traditionally, exanthematous disorders have been described numerically (Box 1). At present, many newer infections have been added to the list of infective exanthematous disorders.

Morphologically, exanthems have been described as erythematous, papular, vesicular, urticarial, pustular, and purpuric. In most occasions, disease present with a combination of these features. Thus, many prefer a more clinically oriented description as measles-like (morbilliform), or scarlet fever-like (scarlatiniform).

Some common exanthematous disorders have been discussed here.

## INFECTIOUS MONONUCLEOSIS

Infectious mononucleosis (IM) is not a rare condition. Adolescents are commonly affected as disease may be less symptomatic or even asymptomatic in younger children.

### Etiology

This is most commonly associated with Epstein–Barr virus (EBV). Less commonly, a similar condition is also seen with infection due to other agents like cytomegalovirus (CMV), hepatitis A, adenovirus, group A β-hemolytic *Streptococcus*, herpes virus 6 (HHV-6), rubella virus, HIV, *Toxoplasma gondii* and after some noninfective conditions like malignancy. Some drugs may also induce IM like rash. It should be remembered that IM is just one of the many manifestations of EBV that can also cause oral hairly leukoplakia, Gianotti–Crosti syndrome and many lymphoproliferative and neoplastic disorders.

**BOX 1 Classical childhood skin rashes**

- Measles
- Scarlet fever
- Rubella
- Dukes' disease
- Fifth disease (erythema infectiosum)
- Roseola

### Clinical Presentations

This is characterized by high and persistent fever, exudative tonsillopharyngitis and nontender lymphadenitis affecting mostly the cervical lymph nodes.

Skin rash is less commonly seen and is of variable pattern or rather nonspecific. Erythematous, urticarial, scarlatiniform, or even purpuric eruptions are commonly seen. However, a very characteristic maculopapular eruption may ensue in almost all patients about 1 week after ampicillin or amoxicillin and may be considered a diagnostic feature. Eyelid edema is an important feature. Other features are malaise, headache, hepatosplenomegaly, and jaundice.

This should be differentiated from scarlet fever (also present with pharyngitis).

### Investigations

Lymphocytosis, low platelet, neutropenia, elevated liver enzymes, alkaline phosphatase. Immunoglobulin M heterophile antibody is generally high from second week onward and is considered diagnostic. This may be negative in children under 4 years. Specific viral markers, EBV related proteins and DNA are now available and are confirmatory.

### Management

Supportive care is all that is required. Systemic corticosteroids are necessary in case of respiratory obstruction from massive tonsillar swelling, myocarditis, hemolysis, hemophagocytic syndrome, and massive splenomegaly.

## RUBELLA

Infection spreads through droplet but can also through conjunctiva. Infection can occur sporadically or as epidemic.

Incubation period is variable with a mean of 18 days. Virus may be present in nasopharyngeal secretions or in feces even 6–7 days before the onset of rash.

### Clinical Presentation

Prodromal features characterized by respiratory symptoms, fever, malaise, and headache may be absent in children.

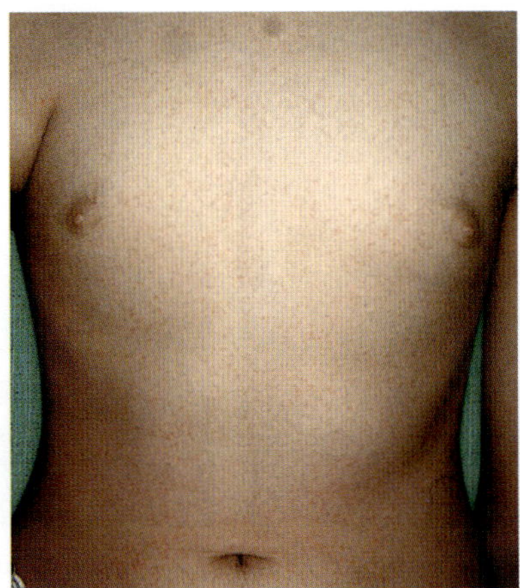

FIG. 1: Discrete papular eruptions in rubella in an adolescent.

Skin rash has typical presentation. This is pink or faintly erythematous, starts from face and rapidly involves trunks and extremities. Rash is short lasting. Rash on face may disappear by the time it reaches on extremities. It persists for about 3–5 days (average 3 days, so it was called 3-day measles). It remains discrete. Some lesions may occasionally coalesce on trunk (Fig. 1).

Unlike measles, rashes are less erythematous and usually improve without any pigmentation or scaling. Rarely cases may present with atypical skin rash, including morbilliform rash, scarlatiniform rash.

Three associated features need to be mentioned. Forchheimer spots (red spots on soft palate) may precede or accompany the skin rash in most cases but is not considered pathognomonic sign.

Arthralgia, mostly involving hand, wrist and knee starts almost simultaneously with skin rash. This is commoner in adults than children. Arthritis rarely persists more than 1 month.

Another feature is lymphadenopathy (usually involving posterior auricular, cervical, and suboccipital regions) that starts before the rash and persist for many weeks. Rarely, this may be absent.

Rubella does not cause any major complication. Occasionally encephalitis and purpura may be seen. Infection usually imparts lifelong immunity. Complication occurs when it affects pregnant mothers during first 16 weeks period. It can cause serious congenital infections.

Rubella can be mimicked by some other exanthematous disease like measles, scarlet fever, roseola. Occasionally, erythema infectiosum (parvovirus B19), infectious mononucleosis, and drug eruptions may also simulate this. Due to similar combination of features (fever, skin rash, and arthritis), differentiation from parvovirus infection may be difficult.

### Management

Rubella after birth is a mild self-limiting condition and requires only symptomatic treatment.

## MEASLES

This is a highly contagious disease (>90% secondary attack rate among exposed susceptible people). Mostly the children are affected.

### Etiology

This is caused by a paramyxovirus. It is transmitted through airborne droplets of respiratory or oral secretions. It is communicable many days before rash and persists till many days after rash develop. However, by the time rash desquamates, it becomes noncommunicable.

### Clinical Presentation

Incubation period is 1–2 weeks. Clinical symptoms of fever (often >40°C), headache, cough, coryza, red eyes (tarsal conjunctivitis), prostration, and periorbital edema develop during prodrome. Koplik's spots develop during prodrome. This looks like white sand surrounded by erythematous hallow. Eruptions are many and usually seen on the buccal mucosa beside 1$^{st}$ and 2$^{nd}$ upper molar. After 3–5 days of these symptoms, erythematous maculopapular skin rash develops on face (in front and behind the ear). Individual eruptions coalesce to appear as blotchy erythematous rash (Figs 2 and 3) This soon spread toward lower body areas and also on pals/soles. Desquamation starts early and leaves brown discoloration. Purpura may be seen in severe cases.

Severe disease may also lead to complications like pneumonia, bacterial superinfection, acute thrombocytopenic purpura, encephalitis, transient hepatitis, and subacute sclerosing panencephalitis.

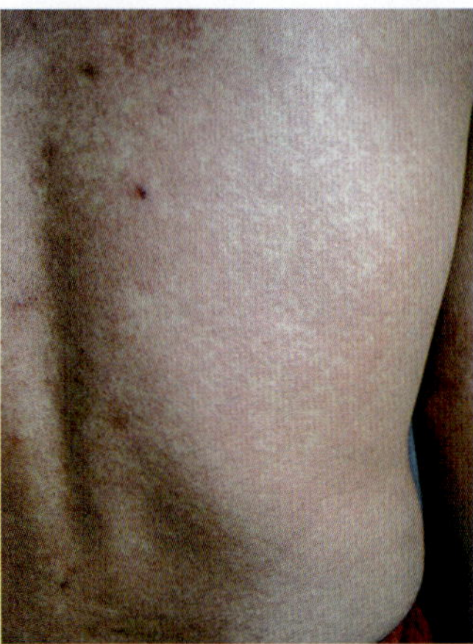

FIG. 2: Typical erythematous blotchy eruptions in measles.
*Courtesy*: Dr Vijay Zawar.

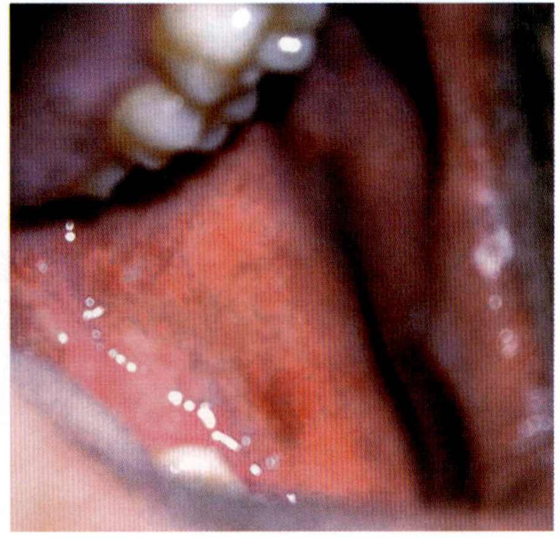

FIG. 3: Koplik's spot in measles.
*Courtesy*: Dr Vijay Zawar.

## Diagnosis

Clinical features are sufficient for diagnosis. Respiratory symptoms are more prominent than rubella. Rash is also darker and more brownish. Koplik's spot is very helpful in diagnosis. For research, other sophisticated modes of confirmation may be required like antibody detection or via viral culture or reverse transcription-polymerase chain reaction (PCR) of tissue fluids.

## Treatment

It should be supportive and vitamin A supplementation should be followed.

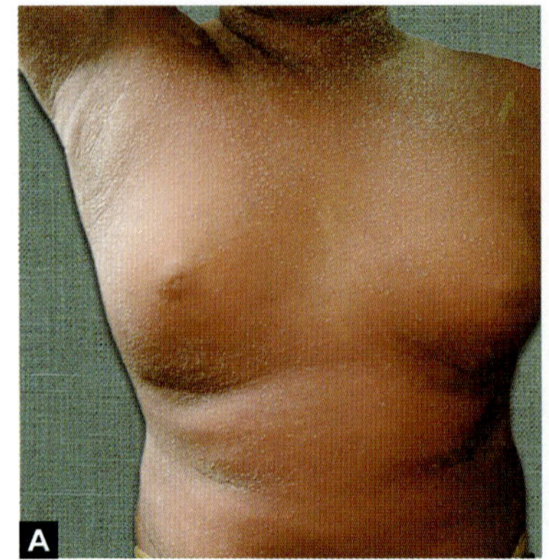

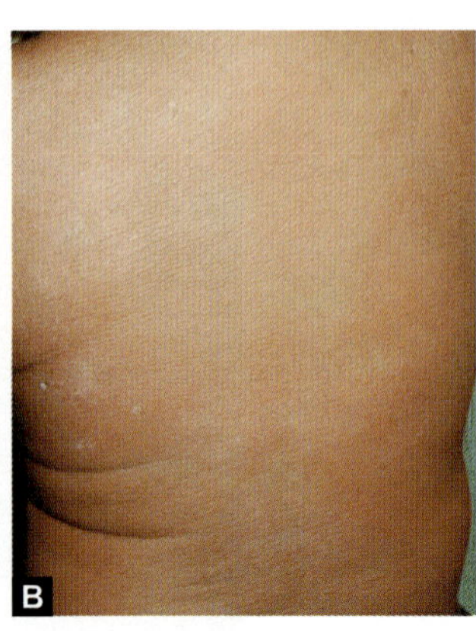

**FIG. 4: A,** Generalised erythroderma with extensive punctate papular eruptions with flexural intensification in scarlet fever; **B,** Diffuse erythema and fine papular eruptions in scarlet fever.

# SCARLET FEVER

## Etiology

This is caused by toxin released from group A *Streptococcus*, (*Streptococcus pyogenes*). Toxin induces a systemic disease along with skin rash. Primary focus of infection is generally purulent tonsillitis. Rarely, other primary focus like impetigo, toxins are produced when the *Streptococcus* are themselves infected by a virus called bacteriophage. It is important to know that not all group A *Streptococci* produce toxin and not all people are sensitive to it. Infection spread through droplets.

## Clinical Presentation

Children under the age of 10 years are primarily affected. There is high fever (101°F or more) that usually lasts for 3–5 days, typical skin rash, white followed by red tongue (strawberry tongue), painful throat infection, exudative tonsillitis, flushed face, and cervical lymphadenopathy.

Typical scarlet fever rash is confluent, macular erythema (scarlet) on neck and face with typical circumoral pallor. This looks like sunburn. Usually, this appears rough on palpation due to presence of extensive minute/punctuate eruptions (Fig. 4A). Blanching on slight pressure on the intense background erythema is a distinctive sign. (Fig. 4B). In the flexures, there are red/dark purpuric streaks (Pastia line). Rash usually improves on $6^{th}$ days of infection and is followed by distinctive scaling or desquamation (in sheets and flakes) especially in flexures and other areas including palms and soles. However, many febrile illnesses may show conspicuous exfoliation during healing (Fig. 5). Kawasaki disease is typically characterized by exfoliation of acral tips.

Strawberry tongue (red, bumpy) that follows a short phase of white coated tongue is a distinctive change in scarlet fever (Fig. 6). Strawberry tongue may also be found in Kawasaki disease, vitamin B 12 deficiency, toxic shock syndrome and allergic reaction to food and drugs. Cough and coryza are usually absent but headache, bodyache, abdominal pain nausea, and vomiting is not uncommon. Red tongue with swollen taste buds (appears white specs) appears as strawberry. Cases that start from impetigo do not have signs of painful throat infections. Sore throat usually improves in 5 days.

## Differential Diagnosis

Kawasaki disease and meningococcal disease (in 90% of cases, there is non-blanchable purpuric rash).

## Diagnosis

Group A *Streptococcus* can be identified from throat swab culture. However, presence of skin rash is mandatory. Outbreak if present usually helps in early diagnosis.

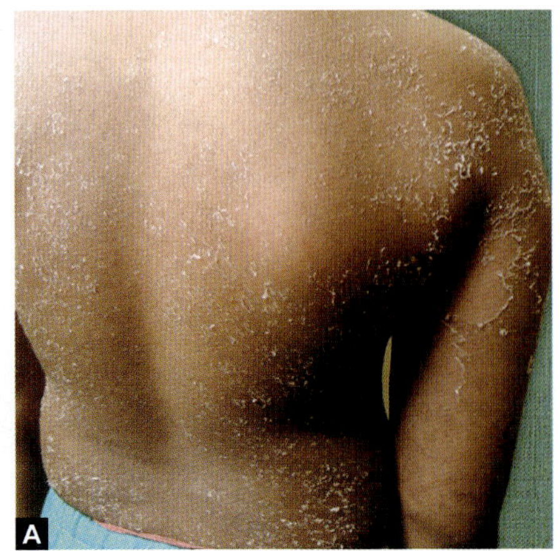

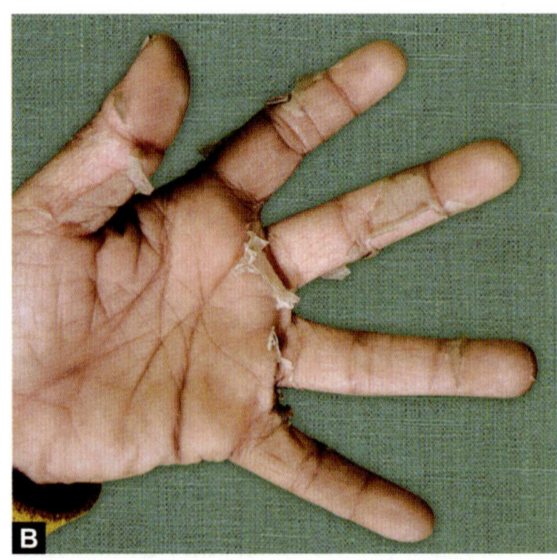

**FIG. 5: A,** Extensive exfoliation in scarlet fever; **B,** Thick exfoliation of hand in scarlet fever.

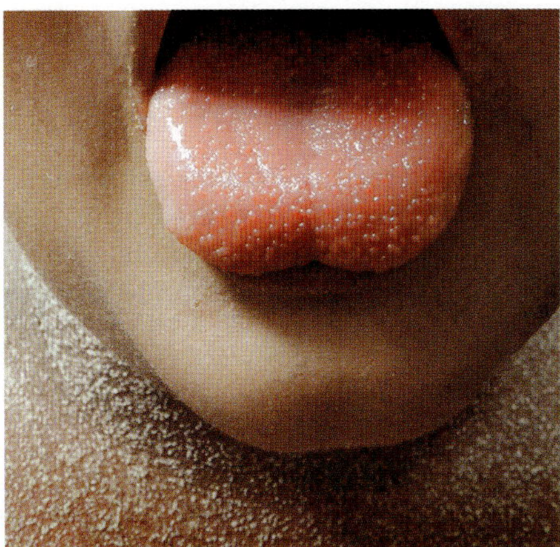

FIG. 6: Red toungue studded with prominent paillae (red strawberry tongue) in scarlet fever.

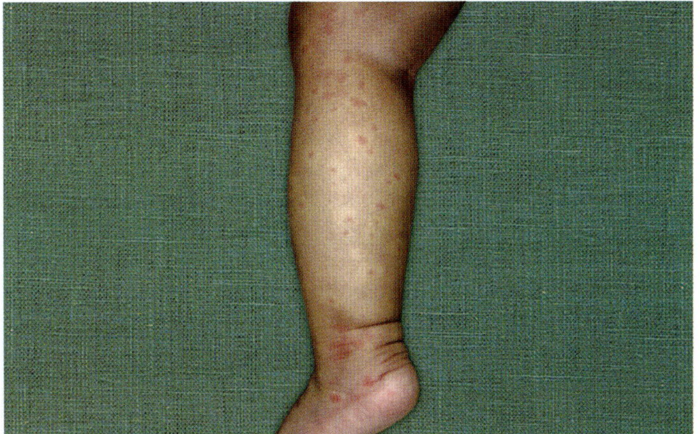

FIG. 7: Typical erythematous macules and papules with perilesional halo in roseola infantum.

## Complication

Infection may spread to involve other vital organs and can cause sinusitis, pneumonia, meningitis and septicemia. Fortunately, this is rare. There may be toxin mediated complications like glomerulonephritis, meningitis, rheumatic fever, and arthritis.

"Secondary malignant syndrome of scarlet fever" is relapse of fever and these complications about 18 days later in an untreated infection. This is very rare nowadays.

## Treatment

Penicillin (10 days course) is drug of choice and resistance is rare. Erythromycin can also be used but resistance to macrolides is now reported commonly. Some cases that develop rash of the disease after penicillin is started may be misdiagnosed as penicillin allergy. A proper evaluation is vital because true penicillin allergy is rare. This may avoid premature termination of treatment.

# ROSEOLA INFANTUM (SIXTH DISEASE)

This is also known as exanthema subitum. This is caused by HHV-6, 7. They can cause variety of condition. Roseola is one of these; the most distinctive one.

## Clinical Presentation

Classically this affects during the 6 month to 3 years age. Disease starts abruptly with irritability and high fever (101–106°F) sometimes associated with cough, diarrhea, and irritability. Fever subsides in 3–5 days. Typically skin rash starts after the fever is subsided. Characteristically, rash starts over trunk and then involves neck, face, and extremities. Typically, it takes 12 hours to completely develop and 2–3 days to fade.

The rash is known to be nondescript and is composed of blanchable erythematous macules and papules. Vasoconstriction leads to a halo around the erythematous macules or papules (perilesional halo) is very characteristic (Fig. 7). Many cases develop periorbital edema and cervical lymphadenopathy.

## Complications

Rarely complications like febrile seizure, pneumonitis, encephalopathy, encephalitis (during pre-exanthematous stage) may occur.

## Diagnosis

Skin rash may mimic the rash of rubella or measles. Cervical lymphadenopathy also mimics rubella. Eyelid edema and periorbital edema (Berliner's sign) is a classical finding that is present with fever. Some of the echovirus strain (subtype 16) may cause similar type of rash.

## Treatment

Treatment is supportive.

# ERYTHEMA INFECTIOSUM

This is a benign, self-limited disease with world-wide presence. This is also called fifth disease since its position in the classical childhood skin rashes that was used in past (Box 1).

## Etiology

This is caused by parvovirus B19 (human B19 erythrovirus), single-stranded DNA virus. Parvovirus B19 can cause many other diseases (Box 2). Infection spread through respiratory secretions like saliva and mucus and occasionally through blood.

## Clinical Presentation

This is seen commonly in school age children. One week of incubation period, short prodromal features like headache, low-grade fever, chill, symptoms of common cold (sore throat and coryza) starts. It last for about 3–4 days and is frequently unnoticed. Pruritus is common. This is followed by a symptom free period of

**BOX 2 Diseases caused by parvovirus B19**

- Erythema infectiosum
- Papular–purpuric gloves and stock syndrome
- Hematologic disorder
- Neurologic disorders
- Polyarthropathy
- Aplastic anemia (common in patients who already are already suffering from some forms of hemolytic disorders or immunodeficiency states).
- Hydrops fetalis (mother is infected in the first trimester)

about a week when prominent erythema develops on face (slapped-cheek appearance). This may extend over nose and perioral area.

This disappears within next 2–4 days. Subsequently, generalized symmetric erythematous maculopapular rash develops over arms, legs, and trunk. It soon develops a lace-like reticulate pattern with confluent normal appearing patches.

Immunoglobulin M antibody appears and viremia ends before rash appears, so rash stage is noninfective.

Rash shows relapse and remissions for many weeks often precipitated by exercise, irritation, stress, or overheating of the skin from sunlight or warm water bathing.

Apart from rash, other features of the disease are arthritis that is self-limited, nonerosive, and usually affects older people.

Transient, mild suppression of erythropoiesis may occur. This may progress to serious aplastic crisis in children with existing disorders of hemoglobin or other hemolytic disorders (sickle cell disease, hereditary spherocytosis, thalassemia, and glucose-6-phosphate dehydrogenase deficiency).

It can induce aplastic crisis in people who have existing hemolytic disorders. It may be fatal for the fetus when mother is infected in first trimester.

### Treatment

Symptomatic and supportive. Intravenous immunoglobulin may be helpful for immunocompromised children.

## PAPULAR-PURPURIC GLOVES AND SOCKS SYNDROME

Unlike many other exanthems, this is primarily seen in adolescents. Children are less commonly affected.

### Etiology

Most cases are caused by parvovirus B19 (human B19 erythrovirus). Cases due to hepatitis B (HBV), HHV6 and drugs like cotrimoxazole have been occasionally reported.

### Clinical Presentations

There is abrupt onset of erythematous and edematous changes symmetrically in the hand and feet, occasionally added with purpura. Rash is pruritic and has a sharp cutoff demarcation at wrist/ankle. Later on, vesicles may develop. A generalized papular rash and enanthem (erytherma/purpura/erosion) over oral mucosa (palate, tongue, and lips) may also develop.

Papular purpuric gloves and socks syndrome has to be differentiated from other conditions that has distinct involvement of the hands and feet and oral mucosa like hand-foot and mouth disease, rickettsial disease especially rocky-mountain spotted fever and also Kawasaki disease (palmar-plantar edema).

### Diagnosis

Viral serology or PCR.

### Management

Prevention of secondary spread to high-risk population like pregnant and people with hemolytic anemia is important.

## HAND, FOOT, AND MOUTH DISEASE

### Etiology

This is caused by enterovirus [coxsackievirus A16, enterovirus 71 (EV71)]. Occasional cases are caused by coxsackievirus A5, 7, 9,10, 16, B2, 5). Commonly this affects children. Transmission and spread occurs through fecal-oral route, direct contact with skin lesions, and oral secretions.

### Clinical Presentations

Prodrome is mild, short (3–6 days) and is characterized by fever, sore throat. This may be missed. Erythematous vesicular eruption that turns to painful ulcers develops on buccal mucosa, tongue, palate, gums, and lips (Fig. 8). Skin eruption develops almost simultaneously or 1–2 days later. Discrete, oval, erythematous papules and vesicles (2–10 mm), develop on hand and feet, perioral areas, buttocks, knees, and elbows (Fig. 9). Lesions on trunk and other areas are rare. Vesicles fluid turns to turbid rapidly.

Some cases can cause serious systemic illness involving neurological and cardiological systems. Aseptic meningitis, encephalitis, flaccid paralysis and death are reported.

There is high incidence of onychomadesis about 2 months following attack of hand, foot, and mouth disease (HFMD). This

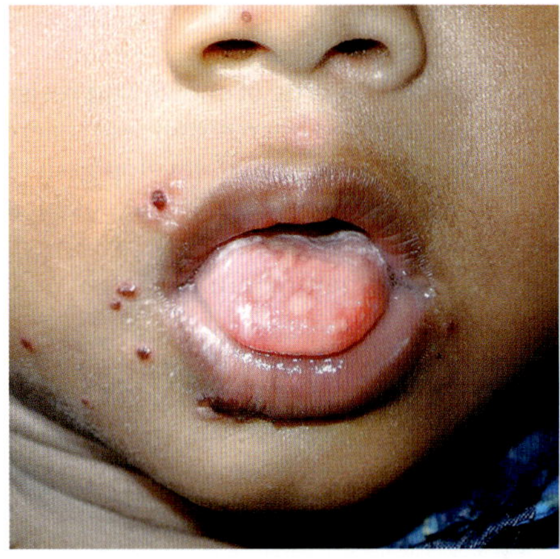

**FIG. 8:** Vesicular eruptions on tongue, lips and perioral areas in hand, foot, and mouth disease.

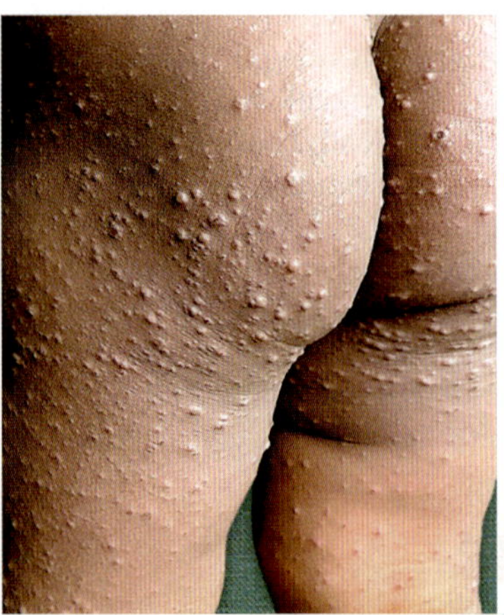

**FIG. 9:** Typical lesions of hand, foot, and mouth disease.

can be seen even among clinically unaffected siblings and parents of the affected children.

## Management

This is supportive. Prevention of disease spread to other is important.

# HERPANGINA

This is caused by Coxsackievirus A 1-10, 16, 22, B and rarely also by echovirus, end EV71.

Painful, erythematous, papulovesicular eruptions that rapidly turn to ulcers develop on palate and tonsillar area (Fig. 10). Typically, buccal mucosa and tongue is spared. Skin lesions are absent. Lymphadenopathy may be found. Neurological complications like aseptic meningitis, seizure, and myocarditis are rare. This has to be differentiated from HFMD and herpes simplex ulcers.

## Management

*Management* is symptomatic.

# PAPULAR ACRODERMATITIS OF CHILDHOOD/GIANOTTI CROSTI SYNDROME

This is also known as papulovesicular acrolocated syndrome. Children during age 1-6 years are commonly affected. Adult disease is very rare.

## Etiology

Suspected etiologies are viral infections (HBV, EBV, CMV, coxsackie virus, echovirus, poliovirus, respiratory syncytial virus, parainfluenza virus, hepatitis A, B, C, parvovirus B19, HIV, and HHV 6) or immunization.

## Clinical Presentations

A prodrome of fever, lymphadenopathy, cough, and cold may be present. Erythematous discrete, symmetrical, monomorphous papules, and papulovesicular eruptions develop over face, buttocks, and extensor surface of the extremities usually sparing the trunk (Figs 11 and 12). Eruptions are asymptomatic and nonitchy. Rarely purpura may be present. Extensive purpura is very rare but is reported. Skin rash heals in 3–4 weeks (almost always more than 10 days) and rarely in 6–8 weeks. Generally, recurrence is not seen. Mucosa is spared. Koebner's phenomena may be positive. Hepatomegaly and splenomegaly can occasionally be found.

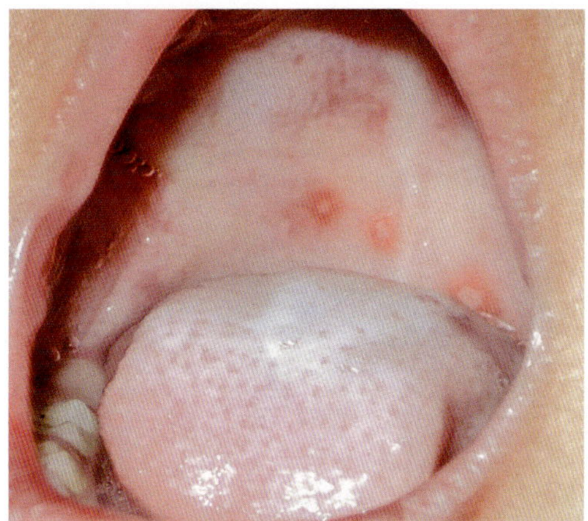

**FIG. 10** Erythematous, papulovesicular eruptions over soft palate, tonsillar pillar (not shown in the image) in herpangina.

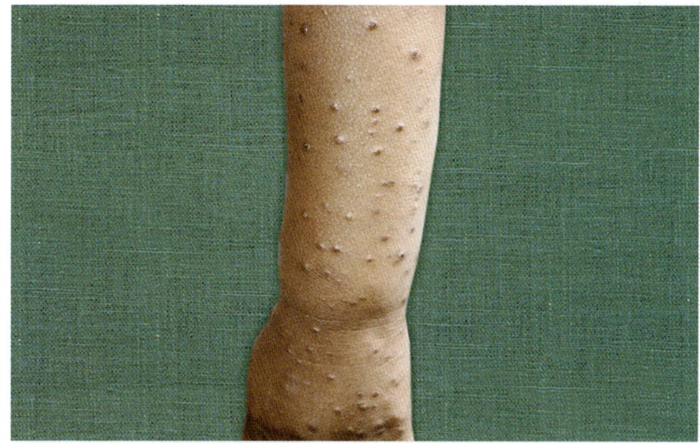

**FIG. 11** Monomorphic papules in papular acrodermatitis of childhood.

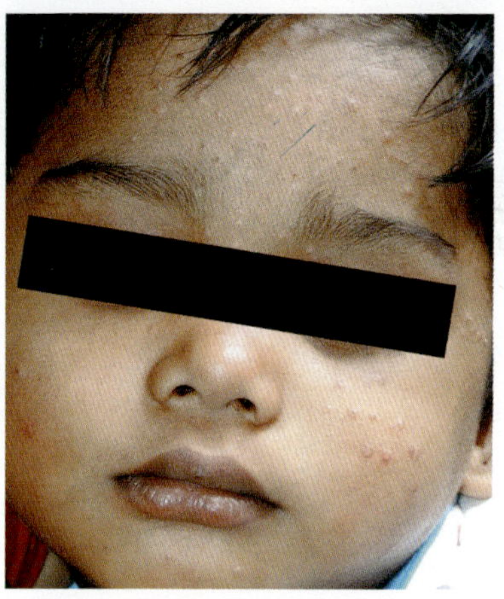

**FIG. 12** Papular eruptions on cheek in papular acrodermatitis of childhood.

## Management

Only supportive management is needed. Topical steroids are possibly not justifiable. Systemic corticosteroid (pulse therapy) has been used in severe cases. HBV vaccination has been reported to prevent this disease.

# UNILATERAL LATEROTHORACIC EXANTHEM (ASYMMETRIC PERIFLEXURAL EXANTHEM OF CHILDHOOD/SUPERIMPOSED LATERALIZED EXANTHEM OF CHILDHOOD

This is a rare exanthematous condition in children. Usually, the children aged 1–5 years are affected and majority occurs during winter and spring.

## Etiology

This is probably caused by virus infection. No etiologic agents have been confirmed so far.

## Clinical Presentation

Rash is itchy. This can be of various morphological patterns like erythematous macules, papules, scarlatiniform, morbilliform an even eczematous. Some may develop a lacy pattern. Most commonly, it starts unilaterally on one side of trunk and extend towards the axilla. It may extend further and may even become bilateral but initial side is always more severely affected. Rash desquamates with mild pigmentary changes. Healing is however slow and may take 3–8 weeks. Mild fever, diarrhea, and rhinitis are often associated supporting the viral pathogenesis.

## Diagnosis

Diagnosis is clinical. This has to be differentiated from allergic contact dermatitis, miliaria, other exanthems and atypical pityriasis rosea.

## Management

Symptomatic.

## SUGGESTED READINGS

1. Chuh A, Zawar V, Law M, et al. Gianotti-Crosti syndrome, pityriasis rosea, asymmetrical periflexural exanthem, unilateral mediothoracic exanthem, eruptive pseudoangiomatosis, and papular-purpuric gloves and socks syndrome: a brief review and arguments for diagnostic criteria. Infect Dis Rep. 2012;4(1):e12.
2. de Vries RD, Mesman AW, Geijtenbeek TB, et al. The pathogenesis of measles. Curr Opin Virol. 2012; 2:248-55.
3. González Saldaña N, Monroy Colín VA, Piña Ruiz G, et al. Clinical and laboratory characteristics of infectious mononucleosis by Epstein-Barr virus in Mexican children. BMC Res Notes. 2012;5:361.
4. Happle R, Nuñez-Giralda AI. Superimposed lateralized exanthema of childhood: a proposed explanation for an enigmatic disorder. Eur J Dermatol. 2012;22(4):542-4.
5. McCuaig CC, Russo P, Powell J, et al. Unilateral laterothoracic exanthem. A clinicopathologic study of forty-eight patients. J Am Acad Dermatol. 1996;34:979-84.
6. Niedermeier A, Pfützner W, Ruzicka T, et al. Superimposed lateralized exanthem of childhood: report of a case related to adenovirus infection. Clin Exp Dermatol. 2014;39(3):351-3.
7. Rostgaard K, Wohlfahrt J, Hjalgrim H. A genetic basis for infectious mononucleosis: evidence from a family study of hospitalized cases in Denmark. Clin Infect Dis. 2014;58(12):1684-9
8. Tse H, Bao JY, Davies MR, et al. Molecular characterization of the 2011 Hong Kong scarlet fever outbreak. J Infect Dis. 2012;206(3):341-51.

# 58 CHAPTER Bacterial Skin Infection

*Piyush Kumar, Nilay Kanti Das*

## INTRODUCTION

### Normal Skin Flora

Skin flora has significant role in preventing skin infection both by providing ecological competition for pathogenic bacteria and by hydrolyzing lipids of sebum to produce free fatty acids which are toxic to many bacteria. Aerobic cocci (*Staphylococcus aureus, Staphylococcus saprophyticus, Staphylococcus epidermidis,* and *Micrococcus* spp.) are the major constituents of normal skin flora and are found all over body while some organisms are localized to certain specific areas. For example, aerobic coryneform (*Corynebacterium minutissimum, Corynebacterium lipophilicus, Corynebacterium xerosis, Brevibacterium epidermidis,* etc.) predominate in moist intertriginous areas (e.g., axillae, groin, toe webs, body folds). Gram-negative bacteria (*Acinetobacter* spp.) are largely restricted to axillae, perineum, and antecubital fossa.

### Bacterial Skin and Soft Tissue Infections

When the skin barrier is breached by trauma or dermatoses, different bacteria, including the commensals (described earlier) might infect the skin and underlying soft tissues. Sometimes, the bacteria infect the internal organs first, and then spread to cause skin and soft tissue infections (SSTI). The SSTIs have variable clinical presentations and severity of the disease, and are common presentations to both out-patient departments and the emergency department. The approach to management of bacterial SSTIs has been summarized in box 1. As soon as sample is collected, antibiotic treatment is started empirically (summarized in table 1) based on whether the infection is community acquired or hospital acquired, suspected bacteria, and drug resistance profile in particular geographical area. Immunosuppression in host and presence of co-morbidities (e.g., diabetes mellitus) may necessitate aggressive (including intravenous antibiotics) treatment of longer duration.

**BOX 1 Approach to management of bacterial skin and soft tissue infections**

- The diagnosis is suspected by typical clinical presentation. The gold standard of the diagnosis is demonstration of bacteria by Gram stain, Ziehl–Neelsen stain, or other appropriate stain, and culture
- The sample is collected from focus of infection (pus, discharge, and/or tissue) collected from
- In toxin mediated diseases, sample needs to be collected from distant focus of infection, not from skin lesions. For example, skin lesions in Ritter's disease is usually sterile. *Staphylococcus aureus* can only be identified in material collected from primary focus on infection (usually pharangitis or distant skin infection)
- Similarly, skin lesions due to bacteremia are often diagnosed by blood culture, rather than culture from skin lesion
- After collection of sample, empirical antibiotic therapy is started, based on suspected infecting bacteria and may be continued or changed when culture and sensitivity reports are available
- Antiseptic dressing and topical antibiotics (fusidic acid, mupirocin) are useful adjunct to systemic antibiotic therapy and may suffice in milder skin infections

## CLASSIFICATION OF BACTERIAL SKIN INFECTIONS

Bacterial skin diseases may be described into four major categories:

1. Primary skin infection (Table 2)
2. Secondary skin infection of preexisting dermatoses
3. Dissemination of bacteria from primary infection
4. Reactive skin reaction.

## CLINICAL PRESENTATIONS

The clinical spectrum of pyogenic bacterial skin infections has been summarized in table 3.

### Impetigo (Bullous and Nonbullous)

Impetigo (Latin word "*impetere*" which means to attack or assail) is an acute, highly contagious gram-positive bacterial infection (primary) of the superficial layers of the epidermis. Methicillin-resistant *S. aureus* (MRSA) and gentamicin-resistant *S. aureus* strains are becoming an increasingly common cause of impetigo. Bullous impetigo results from exfoliative toxins of *S. aureus* termed exfoliatins A, B, and D. These toxins target desmoglein 1, responsible for cell adhesion in upper epidermal layers (granular layer). These exotoxins cause blisters and skin sloughing.

Impetigo is common in warm, humid conditions of tropical countries where frequent cutaneous disruption via insect bites,

**TABLE 1: Empirical antibiotic treatment for bacterial skin and soft tissue infections**

| Suspected bacteria | Effective antibiotic |
|---|---|
| Gram-positive bacteria | Penicillins (ampicillin, amoxicillin) including penicillinase resistant penicillins (dicloxacillin, oxacillin), cephalosporins (1st and 2nd generation), macrolides, clindamycin, and tetracyclines |
| Methicillin-resistant *Staphylococcus aureus* | Vancomycin and linezolid |
| Gram-negative bacteria | Broadspectrum penicillins (Ticarcillin-clavulanate, piperacillin-tazobactam), cephalosporins (2nd, 3rd, and 4th generation), aminoglycosides, quinolones (ciprofloxacin), monobactams (aztreonam), and carbapenems (imipenem) |
| *Pseudomonas spp.* | Ciprofloxacin, aminoglycosides, cephalosporins (4th generation), broad-spectrum penicillins, and carbapenems |
| Anaerobic bacteria | Metronidazole, clindamycin, Broad-spectrum penicillins, quinolones (gatifloxacin, moxifloxacin), and carbapenems |
| *Legionella, Mycoplasma,* Chlamydiae | Macrolides, quinolones |
| *Rickettsia,* Chlamydiae | Tetracyclines |
| *Rickettsia,* Chlamydiae, *Mycoplasma* | Chloramphenicol |
| *Listeria* | Ampicillin |

crowded conditions, and poor hygiene contribute to bacterial infection of skin. The precipitating factors have been summarized in box 2.

### Clinical Features

Bullous impetigo is common in children with 90% cases occurring below 2 years.

The lesions in bullous impetigo (Fig. 1) is characterized by small or large, superficial, and fragile bullae. These quickly rupture to leave remnant collarettes of scales around an erythematous moist base. Thick crust, perilesional erythema, and regional adenopathy are typically absent. The commonly affected sites are intertriginous areas such as the neck, the axillary and crural folds, and the diaper area, but lesions may appear on the face or anywhere on the body.

The lesions of nonbullous impetigo (Fig. 2) start as erythematous macule that rapidly evolves into a vesicle or pustule and rupture. The released contents then dry, leaving "honey-colored" crust over the erosion. Rapid spread follows by contiguous extension or to distal areas through inoculation. Lesions are usually asymptomatic or mildly pruritic.

### Prognosis and Complications

Nephritogenic strains can cause acute post-streptococcal glomerulonephritis. Exfoliative toxins of bullous impetigo can cause staphylococcal scalded skin syndrome.

### Treatment

Topical mupirocin or fusidic acid. Severe cases may require systemic treatment with β-lactamase-resistant penicillin or macrolides or first-generation cephalosporins.

## Ecthyma

Ecthyma is a deep form of impetigo.

### Clinical Features

This is characterized by painful ulcer with overlying crust that is gray-yellow or hemorrhagic, thick, hard, and tightly adherent. When removed, it reveals a shallow, punched out ulcer with raised and indurated surrounding margin.

### Complications

Secondary lymphangitis, cellulitis and poststreptococcal glomerulonephritis.

### Treatment

Ecthyma is usually treated with β-lactamase-resistant penicillin (e.g., dicloxacillin) or first-generation cephalosporin.

## Botryomycosis

Botryomycosis is a rare, chronic, purulent, and granulomatous bacterial infection. Immunosuppression due to human immunodeficiency virus (HIV) infection, alcoholism, and diabetes is a common predisposing factor. *S. aureus* is the most commonly implicated agent followed by *Pseudomonas aeruginosa, Proteus* and *Escherichia coli.*

Trauma-prone parts of the body, most often the feet and hands develop a slowly progressive subcutaneous nodules (resembling bunch of grapes), large verrucous (wart-like) lesions, ulcers, and fistulae and there may be draining of pus containing small yellow "grains". Infection may progress by continuity, affecting subcutaneous tissue, muscles, joints, bones, and the internal viscera.

### Differential Diagnosis

Actinomycosis, actinomycetoma, and eumycetoma. The diagnosis is established by demonstrating and culturing the responsible bacteria and grains in pus or skin biopsy specimens.

### Treatment

Long-term antibiotic therapy and surgical debridement. The choice of antibiotics depends on the bacteria isolated from lesion.

## Folliculitis

Folliculitis refers to inflammation of hair follicular unit. The various causes of folliculitis have been summarized in box 3.

**TABLE 2: Bacterial skin and soft tissue infections**

| | Bacterial species | Cutaneous disease |
|---|---|---|
| Gram-positive | *Staphylococcus aureus* and *Streptococcus pyogenes* | • *Superficial*: Impetigo and ecthyma<br>• *Deep*: Erysipelas, cellulitis, and necrotizing fasciitis<br>• *Follicular infections*: Folliculitis, furunculosis, and carbuncle<br>• *Miscellaneous infections*: Acute paronychia, blistering distal dactylitis, botryomycosis, mastitis, and secondary bacterial infections complicating skin lesions<br>• *Toxin-mediated S. aureus and S. pyogenes syndromes (Systemic symptoms are mediated by superantigens)*: Staphylococcal scalded skin syndrome, Toxic shock syndrome, and scarlet fever |
| | *Corynebacterium* sp. | Malodorous axillae, trichomycosis axillaris, erythrasma, pitted keratolysis, and cutaneous diphtheria |
| | *Erysipelothrix rhusiopathiae* | Erysipeloid |
| | *Bacillus anthracis, Bacillus cereus* | Cutaneous anthrax |
| | *Clostridium Perfringens* | Gas gangrene, Anaerobic cellulitis |
| Gram-negative | *Pseudomonas aeruginosa* | Green nail syndrome, pseudomonal pyoderma and blastomycosis like pyoderma, otitis externa and malignant otitis externa, pseudomonas folliculitis (hot tub folliculitis), pseudomonas hot foot syndrome, ecthyma gangrenosum, swimming pool rash, gram-negative toe web infection, and gram-negative folliculitis |
| | *Helicobacter cinaedi* | Atypical cellulitis (in HIV) |
| | *Bartonella henselae* | Cat-scratch disease and bacillary angiomatosis |
| | *Bartonella quintana* | Trench fever and bacillary angiomatosis |
| | *Bartonella bacilliformis* | Verruga peruana and oroya fever |
| | *Klebsiella rhinoscleromatis* | Rhinoscleroma |
| | *Vibrio vulnificus* | Gangrene |
| | *Borrelia burgdorferi, Borrelia garinii, Borrelia afzelii* | Lyme disease |
| | *Brucella abortus, Brucella canis, Brucella melitensis, Brucella suis* | Brucellosis |
| | *Francisella tularensis* | Tularemia |
| | *Legionella pneumophila* | Legionnaire's disease |
| | *Leptospira* species | Leptospirosis |
| | *Neisseria gonorrhoeae* | Gonorrhea, ophthalmia neonatorum |
| | *Neisseria meningitidis* | Meningococcemia |
| | *Rickettsia rickettsii* | Rocky mountain spotted fever |

**TABLE 3: Clinical spectrum of primary pyogenic infections of skin**

| Superficial pyodermas | |
|---|---|
| Skin | Bullous impetigo, nonbullous impetigo (Impetigo contagiosa), ecthyma, botryomycosis |
| Hair follicle | Superficial folliculitis (Bockhart impetigo), deep folliculitis, furuncle (Boil), carbuncle |
| Digital infections | Acute paronychia, blistering distal dactylitis |
| Intertriginous area | Perianal dermatitis |
| **Invasive soft-tissue infections** | |
| | Erysipelas, cellulitis, streptococcal gangrene, necrotizing fasciitis |

## Superficial Folliculitis

This involves superficial part of hair unit presents with a small, fragile, dome-shaped pustule at the opening of a hair follicle surrounded by a zone of erythema often on the scalp of children and in the beard area, axillae, extremities, and buttocks of adults. Stye is a specific superficial folliculitis affecting the eyelids and is caused by staphylococci.

**BOX 2 Precipitating factors for pyoderma**

- Breach in skin barrier
- Poor hygiene
- Altered resident flora, altered composition of sebum, desquamation, and loss of acid mantle
- Preexisting skin disease
- Infective focus in the body
- Impaired host immunity

Dermatitis cruris pustulosa et atrophicans (also known as Nigerian shin disease or "chronic folliculitis of the legs" in India) is a distinctive type of chronic superficial folliculitis, seen primarily in tropical countries mostly over anterior shin. The etiopathogenesis is complex; *S. aureus*, vegetable oils (coconut oil and mustard oil), physical injury during outdoor work, constant wetting of the skin, and occupational exposure to irritants are supposed to play a crucial role. There are recurrent crops of

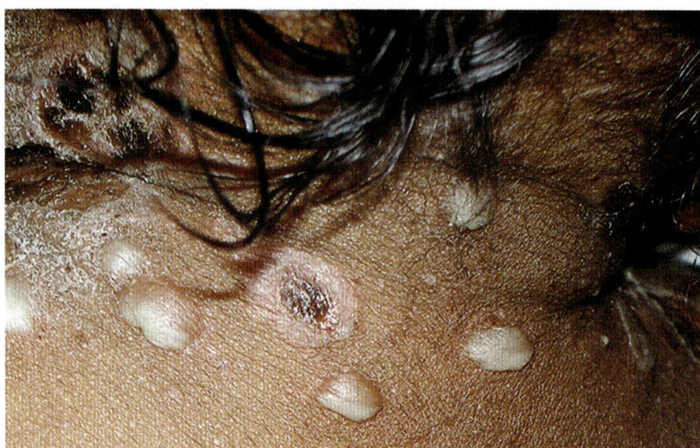

**FIG. 1:** Multiple bullae with purulent fluid and erosions with rim of pus around it—bullous impetigo.

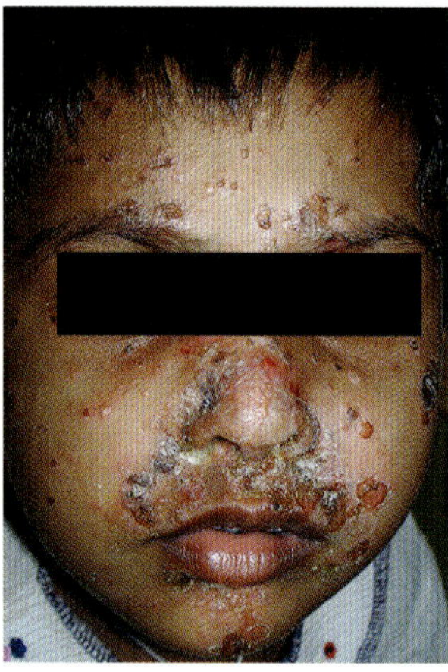

**FIG. 2:** Superficial erosions covered with honey-colored crusts—impetigo contagiosa.

| BOX 3 | Agents responsible for folliculitis |
|---|---|

- Infectious etiology
  - *Bacteria*—Staphylococcal folliculitis, Gram-negative folliculitis (organisms include *Enterobacter*, *Proteus*, and *Klebsiella*), Pseudomonas folliculitis ("hot-tub" folliculitis), and syphilitic folliculitis (*Treponema pallidum*)
  - *Fungi*—Pityrosporum folliculitis (*Malassezia furfur*), candidia folliculitis (*Candida aibicans*), dermatophytic folliculitis (Tinea barbae due to *Trichophyton mentagrophytes* or *Trichophyton verrucosum*; Majocchi's granuloma due to *T. mentagrophytes* or *Trichophyton rubrum*)
  - *Virus*—Molluscum contagiosum folliculitis (molluscum contagiosum virus), herpetic folliculitis (herpes simplex virus, varicella-zoster virus), and HIV infection
  - *Others*—Demodex folliculitis (*Demodex folliculorum*, Demodicidosis)
- Noninfectious etiology
  - Eosinophilic folliculitis/eosinophilic pustular folliculitis
  - Irritant folliculitis (topical tar, mustard oil, and friction
  - Drug-induced folliculitis (Topical/systemic corticosteroids, androgenic hormones, isotretinoin, epidermal growth factor receptor inhibitors, iodides, bromides, lithium, isoniazid, and anticonvulsants)
  - Actinic folliculitis (Seasonal; following initial summer sun exposure)
  - Disseminated recurrent infundibulofolliculitis (Hitch and Lund disease)
  - Pseudofolliculitis barbae (caused by intrafollicular and transfollicular penetration of tightly curled hair post shaving in beard area)
- Miscellaneous
  - Poor hygiene, obesity, perspiration, hyperhidrosis, occlusion, humidity, physical injury, etc

itchy follicular pustules, which resolve either spontaneously or with treatment, with eventual loss of hair and atrophy over the affected skin. The disease shows a marked seasonal variation, with exacerbations in the summer and monsoon months.

## Deep Folliculitis

It affects complete hair unit and presents with large, tender, and erythematous papules or nodules often with a central pustule. Sycosis barbae (also known as Sycosis vulgaris and Barber's itch) (Fig. 3) is an example of deep folliculitis affecting beard area. Sometimes, back of the neck too is affected (sycosis nuchae). Untreated disease may evolve into a condition called lupoid sycosis which presents as a circinate lesion—a central cicatrix surrounded by pustules and papules.

## Furuncle (Boil)

It is involvement of perifollicular tissue in addition to folliculitis (Fig. 4). This may be solitary or multiple and start as tender, red folliculocentric nodule that enlarges and becomes painful and fluctuant after several days and eventually ruptures discharging pus. Furunculosis (multiple or recurrent furuncles) can be associated with chronic *S. aureus* carriage. Topical mupirocin in nasal vestibule for 5 days, rifampin 600 mg orally daily for 10 days, dicloxacillin for methicillin-susceptible *S. aureus*, and trimethoprim-sulfamethoxazole, ciprofloxacin, and minocycline (for MRSA) have been effective in eradicating nasal carriage of *S. aureus*.

## Carbuncles

These are clusters of furuncles connected subcutaneously. There are multiple draining sinus tracts, ulceration, and scarring (Fig. 5). They are mostly seen in areas with thicker skin (e.g., nape of neck, back, and thigh).

## Paronychia

Acute paronychia is bacterial infection of the folds of tissue surrounding the nail. It usually results following trauma. *S. aureus* (most common), *Streptococcus* species, *Pseudomonas* species, gram-negative bacteria, anaerobic bacteria, and mixed infections too may cause acute paronychia. Gram staining, and culture from the pus should be done to identify causative agent. Clinically, green coloration of the nail suggests *Pseudomonas* species infection.

Chronic paronychia (Fig. 6) is a multifactorial inflammatory reaction of the proximal nail fold due to fungal infection, irritants, and allergens.

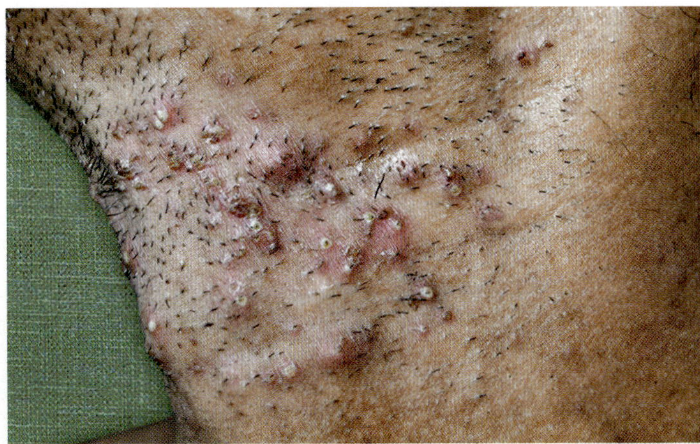

**FIG. 3:** Follicular pustules with erythema of surrounding skin—sycosis barbae.

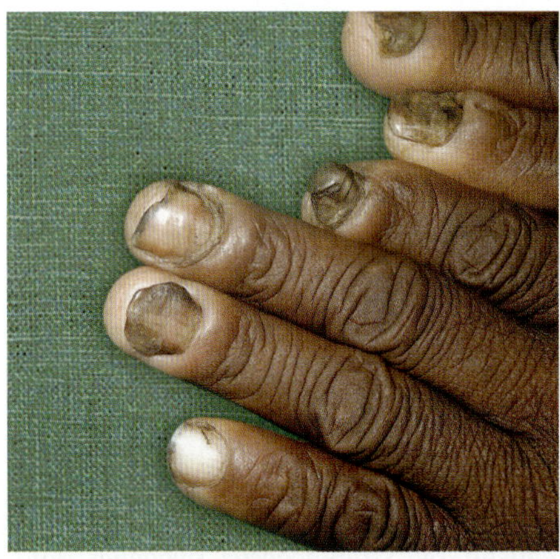

**FIG. 6:** Edematous nail folds with loss of cuticle—chronic paronychia.

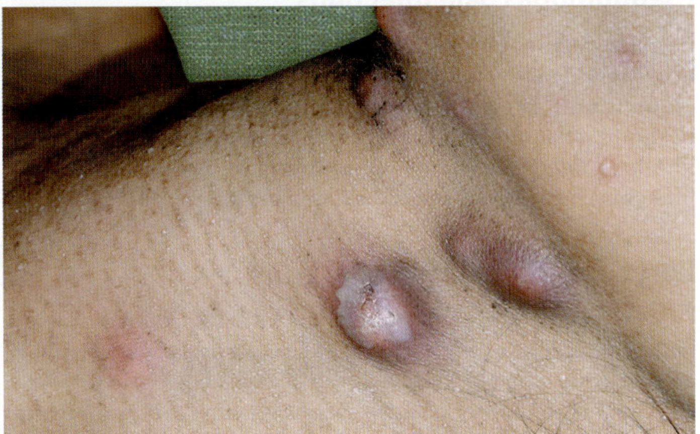

**FIG. 4:** Multiple erythematous nodules—furunculosis.

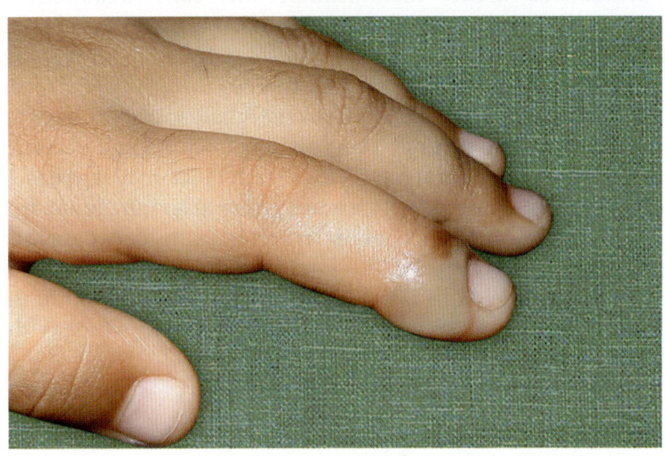

**FIG. 7:** Single blister on distal finger in a child—blistering distal dactylitis.

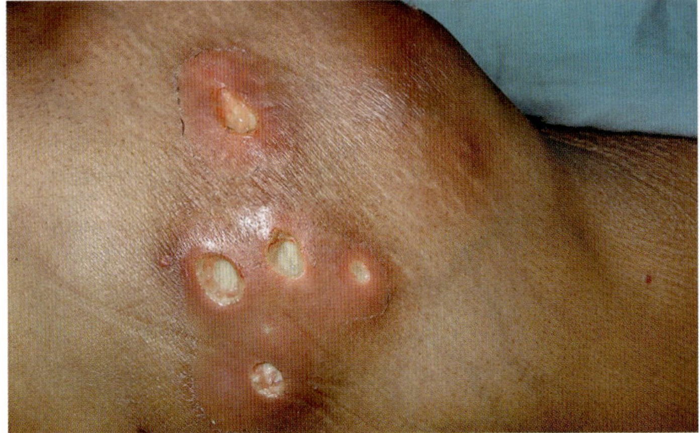

**FIG. 5:** Erythematous plaque with multiple ulcers on its surface—carbuncle.

## Blistering Distal Dactylitis

The disease usually seen in children aged between 2 years and 16 years is characterized by a single, purulent, and large bulla on tender erythematous base near the lateral nail folds (Fig. 7) and is most often caused by group A β-hemolytic streptococci (GABHS) and *S. aureus*. Untreated cases may result in onychomadesis, onycholysis, or permanent nail dystrophy.

## Intertriginous Streptococcal Infections

Streptococci may infect intertriginous areas like perineum or perianal region (Perianal dermatitis), vulva or vagina, axillae, inframammary region, groin, preputial sac, and web spaces of the feet. It is clinically characterized by painful fiery-red erythema, maceration, and a foul odor. There are no satellite lesions.

### Perianal Dermatitis

This is characterized by sharply demarcated perianal erythema, itching, rectal pain (may lead to fecal retention), anal fissures, and discharge of pus and/or blood from the rectum. It is seen in children between 6 months and 10 years of age and is caused by GABHS. It should be differentiated from diaper dermatitis, candidiasis, psoriasis, seborrheic dermatitis, sexual abuse, pinworm infestation, and local trauma from aggressive cleansing. A swab for bacterial culture will confirm the diagnosis.

## Soft-tissue Infections

Soft-tissue infections are acute, tender, progressive, edematous, and suppurative inflammation of the dermis, subcutaneous, or muscular tissues, often associated with systemic symptoms of malaise, fever, chills, and local pain. The usual causative agents are β-hemolytic streptococci (primarily group A), and *S. aureus*. Infections of deep fascia and muscle are usually caused by mixed anaerobic and facultative gram-positive and gram-negative organisms.

### Erysipelas and Cellulitis

Erysipelas and cellulitis are invasive soft-tissue infection, most frequently caused by *Streptococcus pyogenes,* and *S. aureus*. While erysipelas is the infection of upper demis with prominent lymphatic involvement, cellulitis affects deep dermis and subcutaneous tissue. Identification and early treatment is essential to prevent septicemia, skin necrosis, and permanent tissue damage.

In both erysipelas and cellulitis, there is abrupt onset of fever, chills, malaise, and nausea. The lesion is usually solitary and begins as erythematous patch that progressively enlarges and becomes edematous and indurated, vesicles and bulla may appear in severe cases and lesion may ulcerate, regional lymphadenopathy is usually present; and lesion resolves with desquamation and pigmentary changes. The clinical differentiation between erysipelas and cellulitis is made by observing the margin of the lesion. The margin in erysipelas is well-defined, whereas the cellulitis has ill-defined margins.

### Necrotizing Fasciitis

Necrotizing fasciitis (NF) is a very serious, potentially fatal bacterial infection involving the subcutaneous tissue and fascia, with relative sparing of the underlying muscle and is characterized by rapid destruction of tissue, systemic toxicity, gross morbidity, and sometimes mortality.

Microbiologically, NF has been classified as either type 1 (polymicrobial) or type 2 (monomicrobial). Polymicrobial infections are more common, and typically occur in the perineum and trunk in immunocompromised individuals such as patients with diabetes mellitus or chronic renal failure. The isolates reflect normal skin commensals found adjacent to the site of infection and consist of gram-positive organisms such as *S. aureus, S. pyogenes*, and enterococci; gram-negative aerobes such as *E. coli* and *Pseudomonas* species; and anaerobic organisms, such as *Bacteroides* or *Clostridium* species. Monomicrobial infections occur following trivial trauma and are caused by *S. pyogenes* and *S. aureus*. Occasionally, this might be associated with toxic shock syndrome.

## Pseudomonas Skin Infections

Primary cutaneous infection with *P. aeruginosa* can occur in otherwise healthy individuals in areas exposed to high level of moisture (maceration leading to breach in skin barrier). In immunosuppressed patients, it is associated with severe life-threatening infections. The common pseudomonal skin infections have been summarized in table 4.

## Corynebacterium Skin Infections

Corynebacteria are gram-positive rods that account for nearly half of normal skin flora especially in intertriginous areas (e.g., axillae, groin, and toe webs).

Cutaneous diphtheria (also known as ecthyma diphthericum) is now rare. *Corynebacterium diphtheriae* (Klebs-Loffler bacillus) is transmitted through respiratory secretions, infected skin lesions and fomites.

**TABLE 4: Common cutaneous infections by Pseudomonas**

| | Hot tub folliculitis (spa pool folliculitis) | Pseudomonas hot foot syndrome | Ecthyma gangrenosum |
|---|---|---|---|
| Risk factors | Inadequate pool care [Hot water, high pH (>7.8), and low chlorine level (< 0.5 mg/L)], depilation or vigorous rubbing with sponges, prolonged water exposure, and crowding | Hot tubs, swimming pools with less chlorine levels | Immunosuppression including patients with hematologic malignancies, immunodeficiency syndromes, severe burns, malnutrition, recent chemotherapy, immunosuppressive therapy, diabetes mellitus, and severe neutropenia |
| Clinical features | • Pruritic perifollicular erythematous papules and pustules arising 8–48 hours after exposure. The lesions are worse in intertriginous areas and under bathing suits<br>• Low-grade fever, malaise, otitis media and otitis externa, breast tenderness, or even frank mastitis, and painful lymphadenopathy | • Intense pain, marked swelling, redness, deep, exquisitely tender, red-to-purple, and 1–2 cm nodules on the weight-bearing surfaces<br>• Fever, malaise, and nausea, lymphangitis | • Painless erythematous/purpuric lesions that progressively form inflamed pustule, hemorrhagic bulla and necrotic ulcer with central black eschar surrounded by an erythematous halo<br>• Predominant in anogenital and axillary areas<br>• Accompanied by features of septicemia, i.e., fever, hypotension, and altered consciousness<br>• Always a sign of pseudomonas sepsis |
| Treatment | • Acetic acid 5% compresses for 20 minutes 2–4 times a day<br>• Gentamicin cream, oral ciprofloxacin<br>• Cleaning and disinfection of the pool | Cold compresses, analgesic agents, and elevation of the feet | Antipseudomonal penicillins, aminoglycosides, fluoroquinolones, third-generation cephalosporins, or aztreonam. An empirical treatment with piperacillin in conjunction with an aminoglycoside (gentamicin) should be started on clinical suspicion |

**TABLE 5: Common corynebacterial skin infections**

| | Erythrasma | Pitted keratolysis | Trichomycosis axillaris (pubis) |
|---|---|---|---|
| Etiology | *Corynebacterium minutissimum* | *Kytococcus sedentarius, Corynebacterium* sp. | *Corynebacterium* sp. |
| Risk factors | Friction, heat, obesity, humidity, poor hygiene, and diabetes mellitus | Hyperhidrosis, maceration, prolonged occlusion, increased skin surface pH, and hot humid weather | Sweating, heat, humidity, poor hygiene, and immunocompromised state |
| Site | Axilla, groin, submammary region, body folds | Weight bearing area of sole (and palms) | Axillary and/or pubic hair (most dense in central area) |
| Clinical features | Well defined, mildly scaly, and red-brown patches. The patch has a uniform appearance (Fig. 8) | Numerous noninflammatory small crateriform pits coalescing to form a large discrete defect (Fig. 10) | Asymptomatic tan/yellow/red/black dirty looking nodules or cylindrical sheaths (composed of bacterial colonies) on hair shafts (Fig. 11) |
| Wood's lamp examination | Coral-red fluorescence due to coproporphyrin III (Fig. 9) | No fluorescence | Pale yellow fluorescence |
| Gram staining | • Material—scales<br>• Finding—Gram-positive rods and filaments | • Material—Scrapping from bottom of crater<br>• Finding—Gram-positive small cocci and filamentous bacteria | • Material—Affected hair shaft<br>• Finding—Gram-positive rods |
| Treatment | • Topical—20% aluminum chloride, clindamycin, azole antifungals, Whitfield's ointment, and benzoyl peroxide face wash or gel<br>• Systemic—erythromycin, tetracycline, and clarithromycin (1 g single dose) | • Topical—20% aluminum chloride, 10% formalin, clindamycin, azole antifungals, Whitfield's ointment, benzoyl peroxide face wash or gel, fusidic acid<br>• Botulinum toxin (for hyperhidrosis) | • Shaving/clipping of hair, benzoyl peroxide's facewash, topical erythromycin, or clindamycin |

It presents with single or multiple ulcer with punched out margin, hard rolled edge, and variably grey pseudomembranous eschar. The bacteria may also complicate preexisting wounds or eczematous area. Post-diphtherial paralysis and potentially fatal cardiac complications due to exotoxin are known.

The management includes isolation of patient, intramuscular injection of diphtheria antitoxin (20,000–40,000 U) (rule out hypersensitivity through conjunctival or intradermal test) and broad-spectrum antibiotic like erythromycin or intravenous penicillin. The antibiotics have to be continued for sufficiently long period, and ulcer takes some 20–25 days to heal completely.

Nondiphtherial infections are common in tropical climate. One of most common manifestations is apocrine bromhidrosis. *Corynebacterium* species transform nonodoriferous precursors in sweat to more odoriferous volatile acids through the action of a specific zinc-dependent N-alpha-acyl-glutamine aminoacylase. Other common cutaneous infections by nondiphtherial corynebacteria have been summarized in table 5.

## Toxin-mediated Diseases

Many bacteria including *S. aureus, S. pyogenes* and *Listeria monocytogenes* secrete toxins which lead to clinical disease. The majority of these toxins produce their clinical effects in large part by functioning as superantigens (Box 4).

Toxin-mediated disease shares some common clinical features (Table 6). Frequently, focus of infection is throat, perianal area or cutaneous lesion. The blood culture usually does not grow any organism.

Treatment is directed at supportive and symptomatic management. Antibiotics, by inhibiting the toxin-producing bacteria, are often helpful in arresting the progress of the disease. However, their effects are not immediate, as they do not neutralize already secreted toxins.

**BOX 4 Superantigens**

Superantigens are unique group of proteins produced by bacteria and viruses, and have the ability to interact with T-cells in a relatively nonspecific fashion, resulting in activation of huge proportion of T-cells (5–30% of the entire T-cell population, in contrast to conventional antigens (0.01–0.1%). This large-scale activation of T-cells by superantigens leads to massive cytokine production, especially of tumor necrosis factor-a (TNF-a), interleukin (IL)-1, and IL-6, responsible for various clinical effects

## Miscellaneous Bacterial Infections

### Erysipeloid

Erysipeloid of Rosenbach is an acute infection of traumatized skin caused by *Erysipelothrix rhusiopathiae*, gram-positive, microaerophilic, nonmotile bacillus, and occurs most frequently in fishermen, butchers, kitchen workers, and others who handle raw fish, poultry, and meat products. The lesion is usually seen on a finger or the back of the hand, and often involves the web spaces but spares the terminal phalanges and does not progress beyond the wrist.

Clinically, the lesion is characterized by warm, tender, violaceous plaque expanding in centrifugal manner, and has well-defined, raised margins with an angular or polygonal border. Rarely, arthritis and sepsis, leading to endocarditis may occur.

*Treatment*: High-dose penicillin, ampicillin or third-generation cephalosporin, imipenem, or ciprofloxacin.

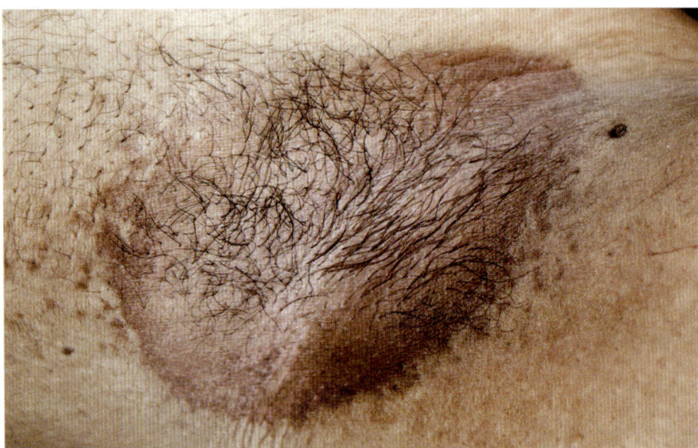

FIG. 8: Dry erythematous patch—erythrasma.

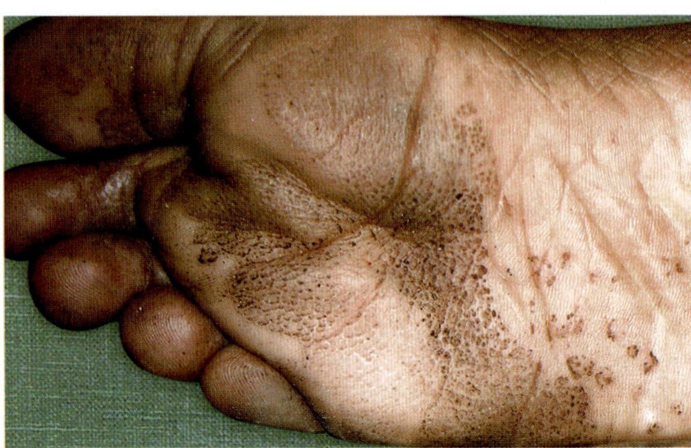

FIG. 10: Superficial noninflammatory pits of pitted keratolysis.

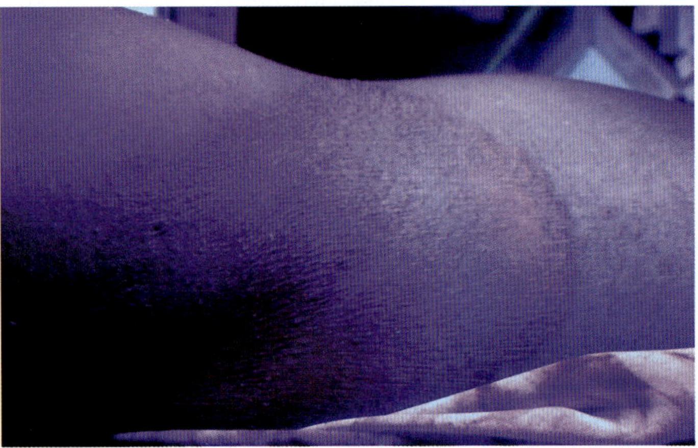

FIG. 9: Coral-red fluorescence in erythrasma on Wood's lamp examination.

*Courtesy*: Dr Rajesh Kumar Mandal, Associate professor, Department of Dermatology, North Bengal Medical College and Hospital, Siliguri, West Bengal.

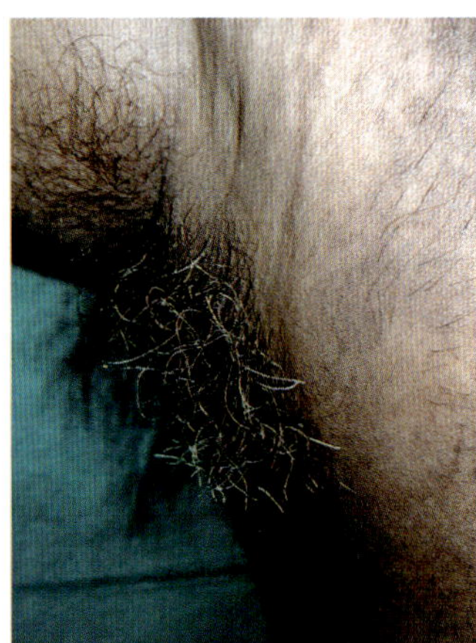

FIG. 11: Yellow-white material adherent to hair shafts—trichomycosis axillaris.

**TABLE 6: The salient features of toxin mediated skin diseases**

| | |
|---|---|
| Staphylococcal scalded skin syndrome | • *Synonyms*: Ritter's disease, Pemphigus neonatorum, and Dermatitis exfoliativa neonatorum<br>• Neonates and children less than 6 years of age (inadequate renal function leading to incomplete clearance of toxin). Adults, especially with renal compromise and immunosuppression<br>Phage group II strains (types 3A, 3C, 55, 71) of S. *aureus* releasing exfoliative toxins, e.g., A, B, D, staphylococcal enterotoxins and toxic shock syndrome toxin-1. These toxins cleave the desmogleins-1 leading to superficial vesicles and bullae.<br>• Source/focus of infection—pharyngitis, conjunctivitis, skin infections, otitis media, and septicemia<br>• Prodrome of malaise, fever, irritability, sore throat, and severe tenderness of the skin<br>• Sad man facies, perioral crusting, and radial fissuring with mild facial edema<br>• Erythema starts from head with generalization within 48 hours, flaccid bullae, leading to wrinkled appearance, sloughing, moist skin and areas of thin, varnish-like crust then scaling, and desquamation<br>• Flexural areas are the first to exfoliate. Palm/sole/mucosa are spared<br>• Nikolsky sign is positive<br>• Diagnosis—bullae are sterile. *S. aureus* may be cultured from the conjunctiva, nasopharynx, feces or pyogenic foci on the skin. Confirmation by examination of frozen sections of the lesions as well as double immunodiffusion or enzyme-linked immunosorbent assay tests that can identify the toxins<br>• Treatment is with a β-lactamase-resistant antibiotic (e.g., dicloxacillin, cloxacillin, cephalexin) for a minimum of 1 week. Extensive, generalized forms of staphylococcal scalded skin syndrome require hospitalization and parenteral antibiotics.<br>• Prognosis is good—mortality rate is 3% for children. Poor prognosis in adults. |

*Continued*

*Continued*

| | |
|---|---|
| Scarlet fever | • Characterized by exudative pharyngitis, fever, and bright-red exanthem<br>• Caused by exotoxin-producing group A beta-hemolytic streptococci<br>• Following streptococcal wound infections or burns, as well as upper respiratory tract infections<br>• Predominantly occurs in children aged 5–15 years. Rare in children younger than 2 years because of the presence of maternal anti-exotoxin antibodies<br>• Abrupt onset, usually heralded by sudden onset of fever associated with sore throat, headache, nausea, vomiting, abdominal pain, myalgias, and malaise<br>• Rash appears 12–48 hours after onset of fever, first on the neck and then extending to the trunk and extremities<br>• The rash first appears as erythematous patches below the ears and on the neck, and disseminates to involve trunk and extremities. The rash (erythematous patch) progresses to develop scarlet macules, seen overlying the generalized erythema ("boiled-lobster" appearance). The rash lasts for 4-5 days and heals with fine branny desquamation. Desquamation of palms and soles, and of skin around the fingertip is classical<br>• Increased capillary fragility results in linear arrays of petechiae and hyperpigmentation in the axillary, antecubital, and inguinal areas (Pastia lines, or the Pastia sign)<br>• Facial flushing with circumoral pallor<br>• Small vesicular lesions termed miliary sudamina may appear on the abdomen, hands, and feet<br>• Mucous membrane shows bright red, and scattered petechiae. On day 1 or 2, the tongue is heavily coated with a white membrane studded with edematous red hypertrophied papillae protrude (white strawberry tongue). By day 4 or 5, the white membrane sloughs off, revealing a shiny red tongue (red-strawberry tongue). Red, edematous, and exudative tonsillitis may be present<br>• Diagnosis—Cultures of suspected source area |
| Toxic shock syndrome (also see chapter on Dermatologic Emergency) | • Multisystem disease caused by an exotoxin produced by *S. aureus* and occasionally group A streptococci<br>• Staphylococcal toxic shock syndrome (TSS) is common in menstruating women using tampon, in patients who have undergone surgical procedures, pyodermas, postpartum infections, deep abscesses, and infections associated with nasal packing or insulin pump infusion sites. Signs of underlying soft tissue infection (e.g., localized swelling, tenderness, and erythema) is frequently present in streptococcal TSS<br>• The illness can be fatal with sudden onset of high fever with myalgias, vomiting, diarrhea, headache and pharyngitis, hypotension and shock<br>• Diffuse scarlatiniform exanthem that starts on the trunk and spreads in centripetal manner. Generalized nonpitting edema are also present. Desquamation of the hands and feet (seen in 20% cases) occurs 1–3 weeks after the onset of symptoms<br>• Generalized blanching macular erythema, edema of the palms and soles, erythema of the mucous membranes, a strawberry tongue, hyperemia of the conjunctivae |
| Recurrent toxin-mediated perineal erythema | • Caused by the action of toxins produced by both staphylococci and streptococci in young adults<br>• Diffuse erythema involving the perineum associated with perianal itching and swelling. Rapid resolution with desquamation is notable<br>• Erythema of the hands and feet and strawberry tongue are associated findings<br>• *Staphylococcus* and *Streptococcus* may be isolated from throat or perianal culture |
| Listeriosis | • Caused by *Listeria monocytogenes*, gram-positive bacillus with rounded ends<br>• Veterinary physician, pregnant patients, neonates, elderly individuals, alcoholics, and immunocompromised individuals are predisposed to listeriosis<br>• Usually acquired by contaminated food<br>• Common clinical manifestations are fever, nausea, vomiting, and diarrhea. Bacteremia, meningitis, encephalitis, and endocarditis are more serious manifestations seen in high-risk individuals. Petechiae may be noted in severe bacteremia.<br>• The lesion consists of tender erythematous papules and pustules on acral areas, associated with regional lymphadenopathy, and mild flu like symptoms<br>• *Treatment*: Sulphonamides |

## Tropical Ulcer

Tropical ulcers (tropical phagedenic ulcer or tropical phagedena, Aden ulcer, Malabar ulcer, and jungle rot) are necrotic painful ulcers caused by mixed bacterial (both anaerobic and aerobic bacteria together) infection. They are common in hot, humid, tropical or subtropical areas, and are usually seen on the lower legs or feet of children and young adults.

The lesion is usually solitary, mostly at the site of preexisting trauma; however, multiple ulcers (partly because of autoinoculation) may be seen. Ulcer has an undermined edge and a yellowish necrotic base, enlarges rapidly and involves muscle or even the periosteum.

It should be differentiated from ecthyma, cutaneous leishmaniasis, atypical mycobacteria, and ulcers due to arterial and venous diseases.

*Treatment*: Tetracycline, metronidazole, 0.01% potassium permanganate or 0.005% silver nitrate solution.

## Anthrax

Anthrax is a zoonotic infection caused by *Bacillus anthracis*, a large, spore-forming, gram-positive rod. The disease is rare except in cattlemen, woolsorters, tanners, butchers, and workers in the goat-hair industry. Most common presentation is cutaneous anthrax, acquired by exposure to the spores of *B. anthracis*. Pulmonary anthrax (Woolsorters' disease) is the next common presentation, resulting from inhaling anthrax spores and is usually fatal.

The cutaneous lesion begins as papule on exposed parts 1–7 days after exposure and progresses rapidly through vesicular, pustular, and escharotic phases. Well-developed lesion is characterized by painless hemorrhagic eschar or ulcer surrounded by vesicles and nonpitting edema ("malignant edema"). The lesion may spread as small satellite papules and vesicles, extending along lymphatics in a sporotrichoid manner. The progression is due to toxins and is unaffected by antibiotic therapy. Regional lymphadenopathy is common and may be painful. The eschar dries and separates in 1–2 weeks, leaving permanent scar. It may be fatal in up to 20% of untreated cases.

*Diagnosis:* Gram-stain of smears and cultures of the local material.

*Treatment:* Ciprofloxacin or doxycycline for 60 days. Individuals with inhalational anthrax should be treated by a multidrug regimen with either ciprofloxacin or doxycycline along with at least one more drug, including rifampin, tetracycline, vancomycin, imipenem, meropenem, chloramphenicol, clindamycin, or an aminoglycoside. Raxibacumab, a monoclonal antibody against antigen of *B. anthracis*, is available and is used along with appropriate antibiotics for treatment and prophylaxis of inhalational anthrax. Anthrax vaccine is available for use in high-risk situations, but its efficacy is questionable.

## Cat-scratch Disease

Cat-scratch disease is caused by *Bartonella henselae*. The papule appears at the inoculation site within 3–10 days of exposure, progresses through an edematous and crusted stage and lasts 1–3 weeks. The presence of inoculation papule along with adenopathy is a valuable sign in clinical diagnosis.

Dissemination causing endocarditis, hepatic and splenic granulomatosis, massive lymph node enlargement resembling lymphoma, ocular complications (neuroretinitis, focal retinochoroiditis, arterial and venous occlusion, and iridocyclitis) and neurologic complication (acute encephalopathy) is known. Erythema nodosum and rheumatoid factor-sero negative arthropathy of the larger joints are also seen.

*Diagnosis*: Histopathology, polymerase chain reaction (PCR) from affected lymph node, and also serology.

*Treatment*: Most cases are self-limiting. *B. henselae* is highly sensitive to macrolides, tetracycline derivatives, and second- and third-generation cephalosporins. For complicated cases with eye or central nervous system involvement, doxycycline 100 mg twice daily plus rifampicin 300 mg twice daily is recommended.

## Bacillary Angiomatosis

This is caused by *Bartonella henselae* and *B. Quintana* and is acquired from infected cats. Immunosuppressed persons have higher number of lesions, more systemic involvement and a progressive course.

The classical lesions are multiple, grouped, firm, tender, dusky-red, and violaceous papules and nodules that bleeds easily, resembling pyogenic granulomas. Subcutaneous nodules, and hyperpigmented indurated plaques are other known presenting lesions. Other organs like liver, spleen, and central nervous may be affected.

Bacillary angiomatosis needs to be differentiated from pyogenic granuloma, Kaposi sarcoma, and malignancies like amelanotic melanoma, squamous cell carcinoma, or basal cell carcinoma.

*Diagnosis:* Histopathology, blood culture and tissue culture.

*Treatment:* Erythromycin (500 mg four times a day) and doxycycline (100 mg twice a day) for 3 months is considered drug of choice.

**TABLE 7: The clinical spectrum of cutaneous tuberculosis**

| Exogenous | Endogenous | Tuberculids |
|---|---|---|
| Tubercular chancre | Scrofuloderma | Micropapular—Lichen scrofulosorum |
| Tuberculosis verrucosa cutis | Tubercular gumma | Papular—Papulonecrotic tuberculid |
| Bacille Calmette-Guérin vaccination-induced tuberculosis | Miliary tuberculosis | • Nodular<br>○ Erythema induratum of Bazin<br>○ Erythema nodosum |
| Lupus vulgaris* | Lupus vulgaris | – |
| – | Orificial tuberculosis | – |

*Exogenous lupus vulgaris at trauma prone sites is common in India.

## Cutaneous Tuberculosis

*Mycobacterium tuberculosis* is a slender, nonmotile, aerobic, non-spore-forming bacteria, filamentous acid and alcohol fast bacillus and is known to infect mankind since prehistoric times. Cutaneous tuberculosis may be caused by direct implantation of bacilli into skin (exogenous), dissemination of tubercular bacillus from viscera affected with tuberculosis (endogenous) or contiguous spread from underlying or nearby structure like lymph nodes, bones, or mucosa. The cutaneous tuberculosis and tuberculids have been summarized in table 7.

## Tuberculosis Verrucosa Cutis (Warty Tuberculosis)

Tuberculosis verrucosa cutis, also known as warty tuberculosis, is caused by exogenous reinfection (inoculation) in previously sensitized individuals with high immunity. The lesion is usually single and is frequently noted on trauma prone areas—extremities and buttock. The lesion begins as small verrucous papule, which enlarges in size with time. Regional lymphadenopathy is uncommon. The condition needs to be differentiated from wart, verrucous psoriasis, chromoblastomycosis, hyperkeratotic lupus vulgaris, and hypertrophic lichen planus.

## Lupus Vulgaris

Lupus vulgaris usually follows exogenous infection in previously sensitized individuals. However, it may develop secondarily from scrofuloderma or a Bacillus Calmette-Guérin (BCG) inoculation. The typical lesion is a red-brown plaque composed of papulonodules with an "apple-jelly" color on diascopy. The lesion characteristically shows tendency to heal at one end (with scarring) and to progress at another end. This may continue for

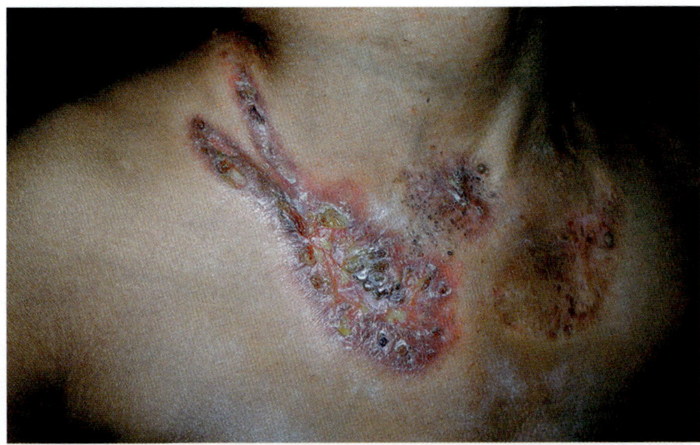

FIG. 12: Erythematous scaly plaque with scarring—lupus vulgaris.

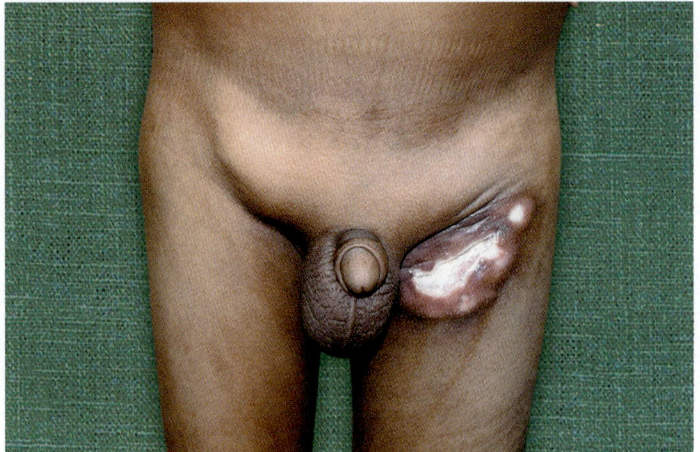

FIG. 13: Nontender erythematous nodule with overlying ulcers—scrofuloderma.

years, resulting in significant destruction and is often a helpful clinical clue for diagnosis (Fig. 12). Ulcerative or mutilating, hyperkeratotic type, tumor-like, and papulonodular are other known morphological variants.

## Scrofuloderma (Tuberculosis Colliquativa Cutis)

Scrofuloderma is subcutaneous tuberculosis resulting from contiguous involvement of the skin overlying another site of infection (lymph nodes, bones and joints, or epididymitis) and is commonly seen in children, adolescents, and the aged persons. The lesion begins as a firm, deep-seated, and subcutaneous nodule, best characterized as a "cold abscess". The suppuration follows and nodules become fluctuant and drains with secondary ulceration (Fig. 13) and sinus tract formation. The borders of the ulcers are often blue, the margins are undermined, and the base is covered with soft granulation tissue. After healing, keloids and retracted tethered scars may develop at the sites of infection.

## Tubercular Chancre (Primary Inoculation Tuberculosis)

Tubercular chancre develops 2–4 weeks after the inoculation of *Mycobacterium tuberculosis* into the skin. It starts as painless, firm, and reddish-brown papulonodule which eventually erodes to form a sharply demarcated ulcer. The ulcer is usually shallow with a granular or hemorrhagic base and ragged, undermined edges of a reddish-blue hue. Regional lymphadenopathy is common and develops 3–8 weeks after the infection. Gradually suppuration (cold abscess) develops and lymph nodes may drain to surface of skin, forming sinuses. The lesions may heal spontaneously within 3–12 months, leaving an atrophic scar and calcified regional lymph nodes.

## Bacillus Calmette–Guérin Vaccination-induced Tuberculosis

The usual course of BCG vaccination is characterized by development of an infiltrated papule approximately 2 weeks after vaccination. The papules enlarges and attains a size of approximately 10 mm after 6–12 weeks, ulcerates, and then slowly heals leaving a scar. Rarely, perforating regional adenitis, post vaccination lupus vulgaris and even, generalized BCG tuberculosis may develop.

## Tubercular Gumma

Tubercular gumma results from bacteremia with cutaneous seeding and extremities are commonly affected. The lesions start as firm subcutaneous nodule that slowly softens as an ill-defined fluctuant swelling. The skin overlying the swelling gradually erodes to form an undermined ulcer, often with sinus formation.

## Orificial Tuberculosis

Orificial tuberculosis is rare tuberculosis affecting mucosa and adjacent skin and occurs within or adjacent to a natural orifice that is draining an active internal tuberculous infection, primarily pulmonary, intestinal, or anogenital. The ulcer has a typical punched-out appearance, undermined edges, circular or irregular border, and the floor often exhibits multiple yellowish tubercles and bleeds easily. The ulcers are painful, recalcitrant to treatment, and do not tend to heal spontaneously. Orificial tuberculosis may have an exogenous origin too.

## Miliary Tuberculosis

The lesions in miliary tuberculosis are caused by bacteremia dissemination from the primary focus usually lungs and are characterized by pinhead-sized, bluish-red papules capped by minute vesicles. These vesicles develop a tiny central umbilication followed by the formation of crusts. When the papules heal, they leave a residual white scar with a brownish rim.

## Diagnosis and Management

The diagnosis of cutaneous tuberculosis is suspected clinically by their characteristic cutaneous lesions. Histopathology is often diagnostic and shows caseating or noncaseating epithelioid granuloma. These granuloma may demonstrate acid-fast bacilli by tissue staining, culture, and PCR. Other tests like tuberculin skin test (Mantoux), QuantiFERON-TB Gold blood test, and interferon-gamma release assays may be helpful in certain cases. Sputum culture, X-ray, and other imaging techniques may demonstrate visceral involvement. Under Revised National Tuberculosis Control Program, cutaneous tuberculosis is treated with four drugs (Isoniazid, rifampicin, pyrazinamide, and ethambutol) at

**TABLE 8: Tuberculids**

| | |
|---|---|
| Lichen scrofulosorum | • Also known as tuberculosis cutis lichenoides<br>• Usually seen in children with nodal or skeletal tuberculosis or following Bacille Calmette-Guerin(BCG) vaccination<br>• Asymptomatic, firm, grouped, follicular or perifollicular flat-topped skin-colored or reddish brown papules, and discoid plaques. It should be differentiated from keratosis pilaris, phrynoderma, lichen nitidus, and pityriasis rubra pilaris<br>• Positive Mantoux test and typical histopathology (tuberculoid granulomas in upper dermis, usually around hair follicles, and sweat ducts)<br>• Responds to antitubercular drugs |
| Papulonecrotic tuberculid | • Erythematous papules that become pustules and undergo central ulceration forming hemorrhagic crusted papules<br>• Symmetric, appear in crops, knees, elbows, and dorsum of the hands and the feet<br>• Lesions heal with pock like/varioliform scars<br>• *Differentials*: Insect bite reaction, pityriasis lichenoides et varioliformis acuta, and lymphomatoid papulosis<br>• On histopathology, granulomatous vasculitis with wedge-shaped dermal necrosis is characteristic. Mantoux test is usually positive<br>• Lesions respond well to antitubercular drugs |
| Erythema nodosum | Discussed in other chapter |
| Erythema induratum (EI) of Bazin | Discussed in other chapter |

**TABLE 9: Atypical mycobacteria**

| | | | |
|---|---|---|---|
| Group I | Photochromogens | Produces yellow pigment on photoexposure | *Mycobacterium marinum, M. kansasii, M. simiae* |
| Group II | Scotochromogens | Produces pigment without photoexposure | *M. scrofulaceum, M szulgai, M. gordonae* |
| Group III | Nonchromogens | Do not produce pigment | *M. malmoense, M. xenopi, M. avium intracellulare (MAC)* |
| Group IV | Rapid growers | Produce visible growth on standard agar within a week | *M. fortuitum, M. chelonae, M. abscessus* |

**TABLE 10: Cutaneous infections by atypical mycobacteria**

| | |
|---|---|
| *Mycobacterium marinum* | • Also known as fish tank granuloma, swimming pool granuloma, or aquarium granuloma<br>• Usually a single lump or pustule that breaks down to form a crusty sore or abscess. May develop nodules along lines of lymphatic drainage (sporotrichoid forms)<br>• Elbows, knees, feet, knuckles, or fingers<br>• Resistant to isoniazid, streptomycin, pyrazinamide, and para-aminosalicylic acid. Tetracyclines, fluoroquinolones, macrolides, and sulfonamides are effective |
| *M. ulcerans* | • Also known as Buruli ulcer, Bairnsdale ulcer and Searl ulcer<br>• *Pre-ulcerative stage:* Solitary, painless subcutaneous nodule develops about 7–14 days after infection. It ulcerates over 1–2 months<br>• Severe infections may destroy blood vessels, nerves, and invade bone<br>• Rifampin plus streptomycin for at least 4 weeks. Clarithromycin too is effective |
| *M. kansasii,*<br>*M. chelonae,*<br>*M. abscessus,*<br>*M. fortuitum,*<br>*M. haemophilum,*<br>*Mycobacterium avium complex* | • Usually seen in immunosuppressed people. *M. kansasii* is second most common nontuberculous mycobacterial infection associated with AIDS<br>• Presents as subcutaneous nodule, cellulitis-like lesion, pustule, abscess or non-healing wound, and even disseminated infection<br>• Rifampicin (Rifabutin in AIDS patients on highly active antiretroviral treatment), macrolides, tetracyclines, fluoroquinolones, aminoglycosides in combination |

thrice-weekly schedule for 2 months (Intensive phase), followed by 2 drugs (Isoniazid and rifampicin) at thrice-weekly schedule for 4 months (continuation phase). Surgical intervention may be necessary in case of visceral or bone involvement.

## Tuberculids

The tuberculids are a heterogeneous group of cutaneous disorders associated with tuberculous infections elsewhere in the body or in other parts of the skin and tend to be bilateral symmetrical as they result from hematogenous dissemination of bacilli. The lesions demonstrate mycobacterial DNA by PCR. The tuberculids have been summarized in table 8.

## Atypical Mycobacterial Infections

Various acid-fast mycobacteria which do not cause tuberculosis or Hansen's disease are grouped as atypical mycobacteria. These bacteria are often found naturally in environment and humans get infection by contact with contaminated soil, water, or animals. Runyon has classified atypical mycobacteria based on *in vitro* growth characteristics on agar plate. The classification has been summarized in table 9.

These atypical mycobacteria commonly cause infection of lung, lymph nodes, skin or soft tissue, and disseminated disease in acquired immunodeficiency syndrome. The skin and soft-tissue infections have been summarized in table 10.

The gold standard of diagnosis is by performing a tissue culture, preferably performed at multiple temperatures of 25°C, 37°C, and 42°C to ensure growth of all possible pathogens. Purified protein derivative test (Mantoux test) result is usually negative. PCR is a valuable aid in diagnosing these conditions.

### Management

Surgical excision, local heat (40°C), and hyperbaric oxygen are useful adjunct in severe lesions not responding adequately to medical treatment.

## SUGGESTED READINGS


1. Alqurashi AM. Anthrax threat: a review of clinical and diagnostic measures. J Egypt Soc Parasitol. 2013;43(1):147-66.
2. Bhambri S, Bhambri A, Del Rosso JQ. Atypical mycobacterial cutaneous infections. Dermatol Clin. 2009;27(1):63-73.
3. Blaise G, Nikkels AF, Hermanns-Lê T, et al. Corynebacterium-associated skin infections. Int J Dermatol. 2008;47(9):884-90.
4. Dias MF, Bernardes Filho F, Quaresma MV, et al. Update on cutaneous tuberculosis. An Bras Dermatol. 2014;89(6):925-38.
5. Gonzalez-Santiago TM, Drage LA. Nontuberculous Mycobacteria: Skin and Soft Tissue Infections. Dermatol Clin. 2015;33(3):563-77.
6. Santos JB, Figueiredo AR, Ferraz CE, et al. Cutaneous tuberculosis: epidemiologic, etiopathogenic and clinical aspects - part I. An Bras Dermatol. 2014;89(2):219-28.
7. Sethi A. Tuberculosis and infections with atypical mycobacteria. In: Goldsmith LA, Katz SI, Gilchrest BA, Paller AS, Leffell DJ, Wolff K (Eds). Fitzpatrick's Dermatology in General Medicine, 8th Edition. Philadelphia: The McGraw-Hill Companies Inc; 2012. pp. 2225-41.
8. Sharma S, Verma KK. Skin and soft tissue infection. Indian J Pediatr. 2001;68 Suppl 3:S46-50.
9. Wu DC, Chan WW, Metelitsa AI, et al. Pseudomonas skin infection: clinical features, epidemiology, and management. Am J Clin Dermatol. 2011;12(3):157-69.

# 59 CHAPTER Cutaneous Viral Infections

Rochelle C Monteiro, Ramesh Bhat M

## INTRODUCTION

Viruses are obligate intracellular parasites, which contain either RNA or DNA as nucleic acid, which is enclosed within a capsid. The peculiarity of viruses is the dependence on host ribosomes for translation and propagation.

## CLASSIFICATION

Viruses are classified (Table 1) based on their morphology, chemical composition, and mode of replication.

## PATHOGENESIS

This has been graphically represented in flowchart 1.

## VIRAL WARTS

Viral warts or verrucae are benign epidermal proliferations. They were described based on the appearance as "ficus" referring to genital warts, "thymion" (thyme plant) indicating the common wart and "*Myrmecia*"(anthill) which refers to the deep plantar wart by Celsus as early as the first century AD. Ciuffo first demonstrated transmission of warts in 1907 and Strauss is credited with isolation of the causative virus, called human papillomavirus (HPV) in 1949. Subsequently, the virus was identified as a double-stranded DNA virus belonging to the family Papovaviridae.

### Epidemiology

Warts are common in children and young adults. The estimated incidence is 10%. Common warts are 70%, plantar warts 24%, and plane warts 3.5%. The incidence of anogenital warts has increased in recent years, as also the incidence of HPV infections in patients with depressed cell-mediated immunity (CMI).

### Pathogenesis

Transmission of HPV usually occurs by close contact with an infected person. Autoinoculation results in spread to adjacent areas. Verruca takes 1–6 months to become apparent. The factors which determine the infectivity of HPV are:

- Number of viral particles
- Number of viral particles in the lesions
- Degree of exposure to the lesions
- Hosts defenses against the virus.

In case of genital warts, it was found that the longer they are present, the less infectious they become. Most genital warts contain HPV 6, 11, or 16, whereas common warts are due to HPV 1, 2, and 4.

### Clinical Features

Cutaneous warts include common warts (verruca vulgaris), filiform warts, flat warts (verruca plana), plantar warts (myrmecia and mosaic types), and anogenital warts.

Common warts can present over any cutaneous surface, more commonly over the dorsum of hands, fingers, or over the knees, as rough keratotic papules (Fig. 1A). They may be single or grouped. Periungual warts can cause nail dystrophy by involving the hyponychium and nail bed.

Flat warts are smooth, slightly elevated papules, generally less than 5 mm, gray or brown in color, and usually occur as multiple lesions on the face, hands, and legs.

Plantar warts are similar to common warts, occur over pressure points of the feet and cause pain on weight bearing. Mosaic warts are formed when multiple warts coalesce into a large plaque and myrmecia warts are deep endophytic lesions.

Anogenital warts can present as cauliflower-like lesions, hyperplastic, sessile papules, or keratotic papules (Fig. 1B).

### Differential Diagnosis

- Seborrheic keratosis
- Solar keratosis
- Acrochordons
- Epidermal nevi.

Flat warts have to be differentiated from lichen planus, epidermodyslasia verruciformis (EDV) and anogenital warts from epidermal nevi, benign keratosis, cysts and ectopic sebaceous glands.

**TABLE 1: Classification of viruses**

| DNA viruses | Family | Genera | Species |
|---|---|---|---|
| Double-stranded | Poxviridae | Orthopox | • Variola • Cowpox • Vaccinia • Monkeypox |
| | | Parapox | • Orf • Pseudocowpox |
| | | Molluscipox | Molluscum contagiosum |
| | | Yatapox | – |
| | Herpesviridae | Alpha herpes virus | (HHV 1 and 2) herpes simplex 1 and 2 |
| | | Varicella virus | (HHV-3) varicella |
| | | Gammaherpesvirus | (HHV-4) Epstein–Barr virus |
| | | Betaherpesvirus | (HHV-5) cytomegalovirus |
| | | Roseolavirus | • Human herpesvirus (HHV)-6 • HHV-7 • HHV-8 |
| | Adenoviridae | A-F strains | – |
| | Papovaviridae | Polyomavirus | • BK virus • JC virus |
| | Papillomaviridae | Human papillomavirus | – |
| | Hepadnaviridae | Hepatitis B | – |
| Single-stranded | Parvoviridae | Human parvovirus B19 | – |
| **RNA viruses** | | | |
| Single-stranded | Retroviridae | • Oncoviruses • Lentiviruses • HTLV-1, HTLV-2 • HIV-1, HIV-2, HIV-0 | – |
| | Coronaviridae | Coronavirus | – |
| | Togaviridae | • Rubella • Chikungunya • Alphaviruses • O'nyong-nyong • Ross river • Barmah forest • Sindbis • Equine encephalitis | – |
| | Caliciviridae | • Calicivirus • Hepatitis E | – |
| | Picornaviridae | Aphthovirus | Foot and mouth (cattle) |
| | | Enterovirus | • Polio • Coxsackie B • Coxsackie A-Hand-Foot-Mouth disease • Echovirus |
| | Rhabdoviridae | • Rabies • Vesicular stomatitis • Lyssa | – |
| | Filoviridae | • Marburg disease • Ebola virus | – |
| | Paramyxoviridae | • Measles • Parainfluenza • Mumps • Respiratory syncytial virus | – |
| | Orthomyxoviridae | Influenza A, B, C | – |
| | Arenaviridae | • Lymphocytic choriomeningitis • Lassa fever • Argentinian hemorrhagic fever • Bolivian hemorrhagic fever • Venezuelan hemorrhagic fever | – |
| | Bunyaviridae | • Crimean-Congo hemorrhagic fever • Rift valley fever | – |
| Double-stranded | Reoviridae | Rotavirus | – |

HTLV, human T-cell lymphotropic virus; HIV, human immunodeficiency virus; BK, ??; JC, ??; A-F, ??.

## Laboratory Diagnosis

This is mostly diagnosed clinically. Histopathologically, warts show acanthosis, hyperkeratosis, parakeratosis, and papillomatosis. Koilocytosis of upper keratinocytes is a characteristic feature. These vacuolated cells have a dark pyknotic nucleus with perinuclear halo. The dermis may show thrombosed capillary vessels. Application of 3–5% acetic acid and colposcopic visualization aids in the diagnosis of genital warts. Polymerase chain reaction (PCR) and HPV typing can be done.

## Treatment

- *Physical methods:* Surgery, electrosurgery, cryosurgery, laser
- *Chemical methods (topical):* Retinoic acid, salicylic acid, lactic acid, trichloroacetic acid, formic acid, cantharidin, formaldehyde, glutaraldehyde, chemotherapeutic agents (podophyllin, bleomycin, 5-fluorouracil)
- *Newer modalities:* Topical podophyllotoxin, interferon, and systemic retinoids. Retinoids may act through proliferation of keratinocytes, stimulation of both humoral and CMI and regulation of cell differentiation, blocking of viral replication, and preventing malignant transformation. Etretinate has been successfully tried in a dose of 1 mg/kg/day.

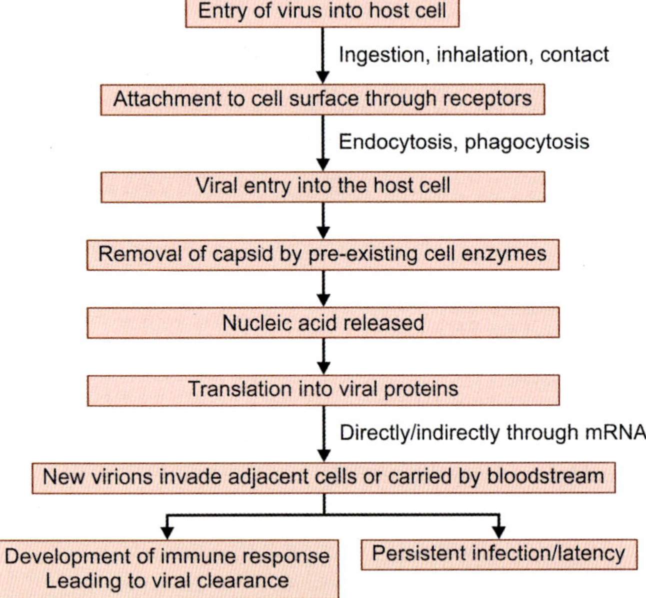


**FLOWCHART 1:** Pathogenesis of viral infections in human.

Podophyllotoxin is the purified active ingredient in podophyllin, which is a plant extract derived from *Podophyllum peltatum* or *Podophyllum emodi.* It can be applied as a 0.5% solution once or twice daily for 3 days a week for up to 6 weeks. Side effects are mild, transient and reversible, which includes local irritation, erythema, swelling, burning, and erosions.

Interferon-α is administered intralesionally in a low dose of $1 \times 10^6$ two or three times a week for 3–8 weeks. Side effects include fatigue, fever, chills, myalgias, headache, malaise, and transient leukopenia.

## Anogenital Warts

Anogenital warts can be classified morphologically into hyperplastic, cauliflower-like lesions, sessile papules, and keratotic verruca vulgaris-like lesions. The hyperplastic variety is soft, flesh colored and present over the urethral meatus, glans penis, inner surface of the prepuce, perianal area, anal mucosa, and labia. They can grow into exophytic lesions. Verruca over the penile shaft are usually sessile or keratotic. The sessile variety remains small in size. Condyloma can increase in size during pregnancy causing serious complications like obstructed labor, hemorrhage, or sepsis leading to birth. After birth, many cases of genital warts have been known to regress. Detection of these lesions can be aided by application of 5% acetic acid.

## Other Human Papilloma Virus-associated Disorders

Bowenoid papulosis, linked to HPV 16, is a disorder presenting in young adults over the anogenital region as multiple small, verrucous or velvety, pigmented papules. Histologically, it shows features of a carcinoma *in situ*. Lesions may undergo spontaneous regression, or may have to be surgically removed. Topically 5-fluorouracil has been found to be effective.

Vulvar papillomatosis is another HPV infection, which presents with lesions over the vulvar vestibule. These appear velvety, granular, or cobblestone-like. On colposcopic examination, they are described as having "Arizona cactus-like projections, "stony colonial pavement-like projections" or "camel hump-like projections".

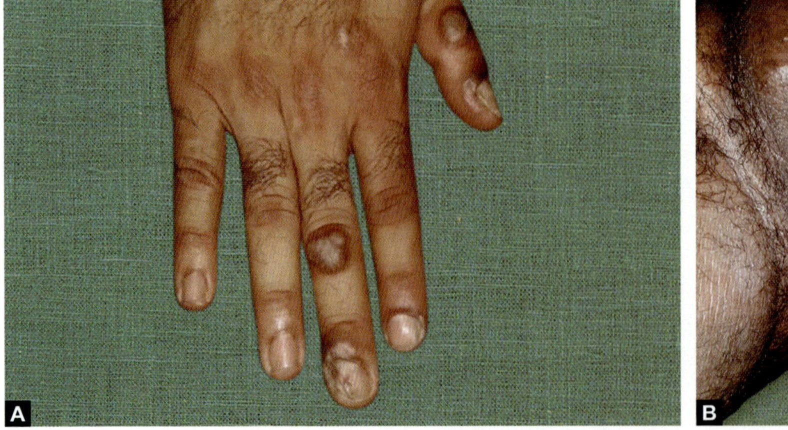


**FIG. 1:** **A,** Verrucae over the dorsum of the hands; **B,** Anogenital warts on the undersurface of the scrotum

## HERPES SIMPLEX

Herpes simplex virus (HSV) is a common viral infection affecting more than one-third of the world's population.

### Pathogenesis

Herpes simplex virus is a double-stranded DNA virus that enters the skin and mucosa through abrasions. Retrograde transport of the virus occurs to sensory ganglia and leading to lifelong latent infection. Triggers like immunodeficiency, trauma, fever, menstruation, and ultraviolet light cause reactivation of the virus. HSV exists as two types, i.e., HSV-1 and HSV-2. Generally, HSV-1 causes oral disease and HSV-2 causes genital disease (Fig. 2).

### Genital Herpes

Genital herpes is one of the most common genital sexually transmitted infection.

Risk factors include multiple sexual partners, increasing age, low socioeconomic status, and human immunodeficiency virus (HIV) infection.

#### Clinical Features

The incubation period is 2–12 days. It begins with a prodrome of itching, burning, and erythema. Multiple, painful, transient vesicles appear over the penis, perineum, vagina, vulva, and cervix. It may be associated with tender inguinal lymphadenopathy. The lesions heal with crusting by 2–3 weeks. There may be associated systemic features like malaise, headache, fever, myalgia, and abdominal pain. Similar to oral herpes, recurrence is common due to viral latency.

### Herpes Gingivostomatitis

Primary herpes gingivostomatitis presents as painful vesicles and ulcerative erosions on the tongue, gingiva, palate, buccal mucosa, and lips (Fig. 3). It usually affects young children under 5 years of age. Other features include edema, halitosis, drooling and tender submandibular, or cervical nodes. Systemic features like fever, malaise, and myalgia may be present.

Recurrent infections may occur two or three times a year. The episodes are shorter and less severe.

#### Laboratory Diagnosis

The diagnosis is most often clinical. Viral isolation by tissue culture is the gold standard in diagnosis. The limitation of culture being its sensitivity of 70–80% and it takes 4–5 days. Tzanck smears and antigen detection tests have a lower sensitivity rate (50–70%). Serologic testing for antibody is highly sensitive, but it cannot be done early in primary infection. PCR-enzyme-linked immunosorbent assay (ELISA) is the most sensitive (96%) and specific (99%), and it is not used to diagnose skin lesions, its limitation being its high cost. However, it is the diagnostic method of choice for herpes encephalitis.

#### Treatment

Table 2 highlights the treatment for herpes.

### Herpes Simplex Virus in Pregnancy

The prevalence of HSV in pregnant women varies worldwide, 7–8% in Europe, 22% in the United States. Most significant complication of genital herpes is transmission of infection to the fetus or neonate. This can cause spontaneous abortion, intrauterine growth retardation, preterm labor, and congenital and neonatal herpes infection and even fetal death.

Risk of acquiring neonatal infection is about 1% during early pregnancy, while later stages have a risk of 30–50%. About 85% of perinatal transmission occurs during the intrapartum period. Risk is higher for disseminated infection and HSV 2 infections.

The features of congenital infection are skin vesicles, scarring, eye involvement in the form of chorioretinitis, microphthalmia, cataract, neurologic manifestations like seizures, microcephaly, encephalomyelitis, intracranial calcifications, and others like psychomotor and growth retardation (see Chapter on Neonatal Dermatoses).

*Treatment of primary infection*: First trimester infections can be treated with acyclovir in case of severe maternal infection. Infections 4–6 weeks prior to delivery are an indication for cesarean section. If vaginal delivery is not possible, both the mother and child have to be treated with intravenous acyclovir.

*Recurrent infection*: In such cases, the mother has circulating immunoglobulin G (IgG) antibodies which pass through the placenta and reach the fetus; hence, risk of infection to the baby is minimal. If viral cultures at the time of delivery are positive, a

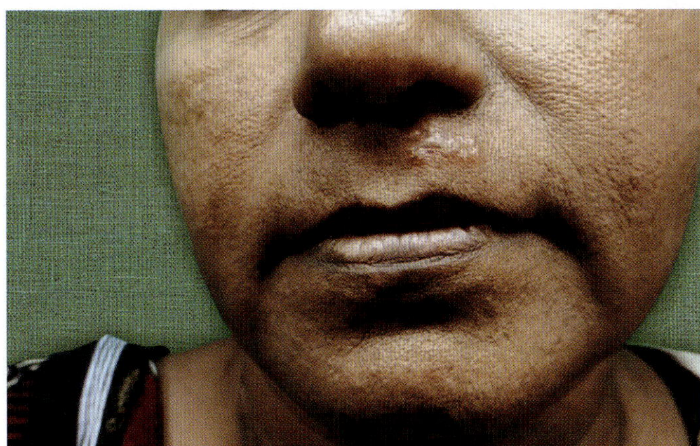

**FIG. 2:** Herpes simplex.

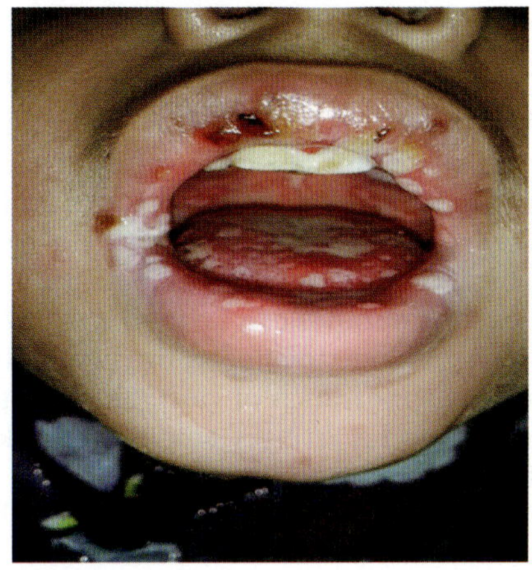

**FIG. 3:** Herpes gingivostomatitis.

**TABLE 2: Treatment of herpes**

| Genital herpes primary infection | Genital herpes recurrent episodes (chronic suppressive treatment) | Genital herpes episodic treatment | Orolabial herpes primary episode | Orolabial herpes recurrent episodes |
|---|---|---|---|---|
| • Acyclovir 200 mg five times daily for 10 days<br>• Famciclovir 250 mg three times daily for 10 days<br>• Valacyclovir 1 g twice daily for 10 days | • Acyclovir 400 mg twice daily<br>• Famciclovir 250 mg twice daily<br>• Valacyclovir 1g once daily | • Acyclovir 200 mg 5 times daily for 5 days or 800 mg twice daily for 5 days<br>• Famciclovir 125 mg twice daily for 5 days<br>• Valacyclovir 500 mg twice daily for 5 days | Acyclovir 200 mg five times daily for 5 days | • Acyclovir<br>• Famciclovir 250 mg three times daily |

cesarean section is indicated. Similarly, negative viral cultures are an indication for spontaneous delivery.

## VARICELLA-ZOSTER VIRUS

The varicella-zoster virus (VZV), which causes a primary infection varicella (chicken pox) and herpes zoster (shingles) due to reactivation, is a ubiquitous human alphaherpesvirus.

### Epidemiology

The VZV virus occurs in a wide geographical distribution, and is more common in temperate climates. Infection occurs in the first 5–10 years of life. Attacks are more common in late winter and spring. Second episodes of varicella are rare.

Herpes zoster occurs only in individuals who have had primary VZV infection. Hence, there is no seasonal pattern. In the United Kingdom, the incidence is 3.4 cases per 1,000 persons per year. The epidemiology is affected by host factors, i.e., advancing age, immunosuppression, and patients on long-term systemic steroid therapy.

### Pathogenesis

The incubation period is around 14 days. VZV is usually transmitted by the respiratory route.

The VZV from mucocutaneous sites is transported to the dorsal ganglia by an ascending route along neuronal axons or it may be transported by the mononuclear cells. During reactivation of the virus, the infectious particles are transported back to the skin in an area of a single sensory nerve.

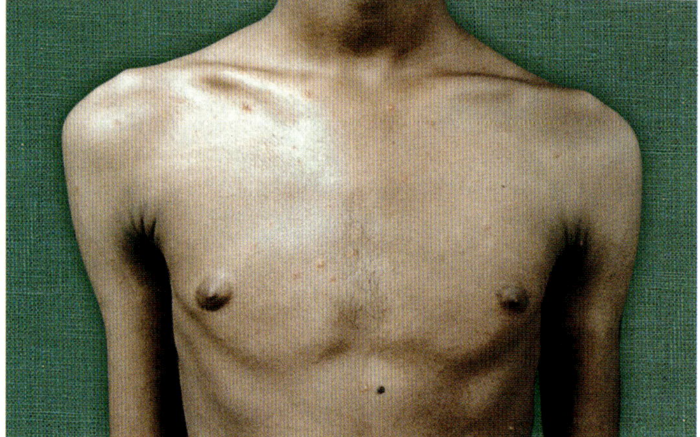

**FIG. 4** Vesicles of varicella over the trunk.

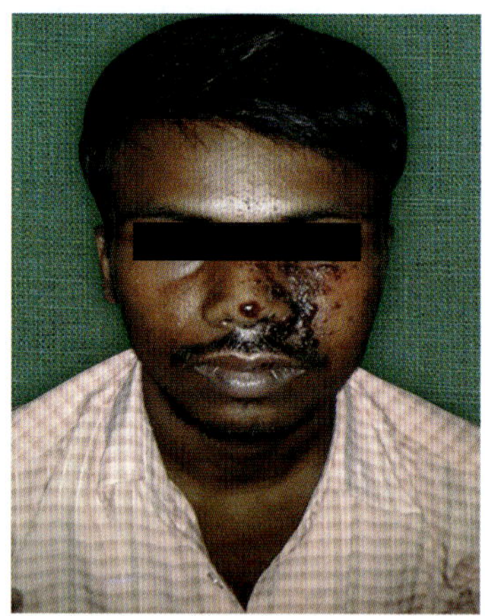

**FIG. 5:** Herpes zoster.

### Clinical Features

Varicella infection begins with a prodrome with varying symptoms like fever, malaise, headache, and abdominal pain. The initial cutaneous lesions involve the face, scalp and trunk and are erythematous, pruritic macules which evolve to form fluid-filled vesicles surrounded by an irregular zone of erythema giving it the "dew drops on a rose petal appearance" (Fig. 4). Mucous membranes can be involved. Several crops of new lesions may continue to appear. Crusting of lesions begin 24–48 hours after appearance of rash. The lesions heal with hypopigmentation and scarring. Complications like secondary bacterial infections, transient hepatitis, varicella pneumonia, meningoencephalitis, cerebellar ataxia, thrombocytopenia, nephritis, myocarditis, pericarditis, pancreatitis, and orchitis may be seen.

*Herpes zoster*: Reactivation of the VZV from its latent state causes the vesicular, localized, pruritic, dermatomal lesions which are usually unilateral in the distribution of one or more adjacent sensory nerves. The rash is often preceded by several days of localized neuropathic pain. The thoracic dermatomes are most commonly affected, followed by cranial, and lumbosacral (Fig. 5). The lesions typically resolve within 2 weeks. "Zoster sine herpete" is the occurrence of acute unilateral neuropathic pain without rash.

Postherpetic neuralgia (PHN) is the most common and debilitating complication of herpes zoster. The pain may last from weeks to years. The risk of PHN is higher in old age and in immunocompromised state. Other complications include encephalitis, facial palsy, ocular complications like conjunctivitis, dendritic keratitis, anterior uveitis, iridocyclitis, panophthalmitis when it involves the ophthalmic branch, loss of taste in seventh nerve involvement. Ramsay Hunt syndrome (herpes zoster oticus and facial palsy) occurs when reactivation of the virus takes place in the geniculate ganglion of the 7th and 8th cranial nerves. Lumbosacral zoster may result in bladder dysfunction or ileus. The motor deficits usually resolve over time.

### Laboratory Diagnosis

This is essentially a clinical diagnosis. Tzanck smears, cell culture, and serology can be done. Tzanck smear demonstrate the presence of multinucleated giant cells but it cannot differentiate VZV from other herpes viruses. Immunofluorescence or immunoperoxidase procedures with polyclonal or monoclonal antibodies to VZV are a means of rapid diagnosis. Hybridization and PCR methods are more sensitive for viral detection.

### Treatment

Aciclovir given in a dose of 800 mg five times daily for 5–7 days, Famciclovir (250–500 mg thrice daily for 5–7 days) or valacyclovir are used.

Sorivudine (BVaraU) is another nucleoside compound with high inhibitory activity against VZV. It is administered in a dose of 40 mg/day for 5 days. Foscarnet, cidofovir and interferon-α are indicated for acyclovir-resistant strains.

- *Prevention*: Varicella-zoster immunoglobulin is indicated for susceptible high-risk individuals, including immunocompromised children and pregnant women who have had close contact with an infected case. It has to be administered within 48–96 hours after exposure
- *Vaccine*: A live attenuated vaccine using the Oka strain is used. A single dose suffices for individuals in the 12 months to 13 years age group. For children more than 13 years and young adults, two doses are given, separated by a 4–8 week interval. The vaccine is contraindicated in immunodeficient states, pregnancy, exposure to varicella or herpes zoster within 21 days, administration of salicylates, immune globulins, or steroids.

## HUMAN HERPES VIRUS 8

Human herpesvirus (HHV)-8 is a gamma herpes virus, closely related to Epstein-Barr virus (EBV). It is associated mainly with Kaposi's sarcoma. Other associations are primary effusion lymphoma and multicentric Castleman's disease.

## HAND FOOT AND MOUTH DISEASE

### Epidemiology

Hand foot and mouth disease (HFMD) is a common, mild, self-limiting childhood infection. It is caused by the coxsackie A-16 virus and enterovirus 71. Transmission occurs from person to person through direct contact with respiratory droplets, vesicular fluid, saliva, and feces of an infected person. Infection is common in preschool children below 5 years of age and in summer or fall seasons. Sex incidence is equal. Symptoms appear 3–6 days after initial exposure to the virus. Infection usually occurs as epidemics. Infection in adults rarely occurs.

### Clinical Features

It begins with a brief prodromal fever, followed by pharyngitis, mouth ulcers, and vesicular rash over the hands and feet, perioral areas, knees, elbows, buttocks, and genitalia. In the oral cavity, the vesicles are common in the buccal mucosa, tongue, and hard palate. Complications are rare but pneumonia, encephalitis, and meningitis may occur (Fig. 6).

### Laboratory Diagnosis

No specific lab tests are indicated. Stool and throat cultures and PCR can be done for strain identification.

### Differential Diagnosis

Herpes gingivostomatitis, herpangina, varicella, aphthous stomatitis, drug eruption, and erythema multiforme have to be differentiated from HFMD.

**HFMD**

- Common, self-limiting childhood infection caused by coxsackie A16 and enterovirus 71
- Presents with painful vesicles over the mouth, hands, feet and buttocks

### Treatment

The disease runs a benign self-limited course and treatment is usually not necessary. Symptomatic treatment can be given.

## PARAPOXVIRUS INFECTIONS

### Molluscum Contagiosum

#### Epidemiology

Molluscum contagiosum (MC) is caused by a double-stranded DNA virus molluscipox, of the family Poxviridae. It was first described by Bateman in the beginning of the 19th century and the characteristic intracytoplasmic inclusions were later described by Henderson and Paterson. The virus is found worldwide, more commonly in the tropics. Children are more commonly affected. Predisposing factors include overcrowding, poor hygiene, and poverty. The virus has four strains, viz. MCV-I, MCV-II, MCV-III, and MCV-IV of which MCV-I is more prevalent.

#### Pathogenesis

The virus is transmitted by direct skin contact with an affected individual. Fomites might play a role in transmission. The incubation period is between 2 weeks and 7 weeks.

#### Clinical Features

The lesions are discrete, smooth, papular, dome shaped, skin colored, or opaque with central umbilication (Fig. 7). The average size is 2–6 mm in immunosuppressed individuals, size may exceed 1 cm. Sites of predilection are the face, trunk, and extremities. In adults, genitals are commonly involved and it may be a sexually transmitted disease.

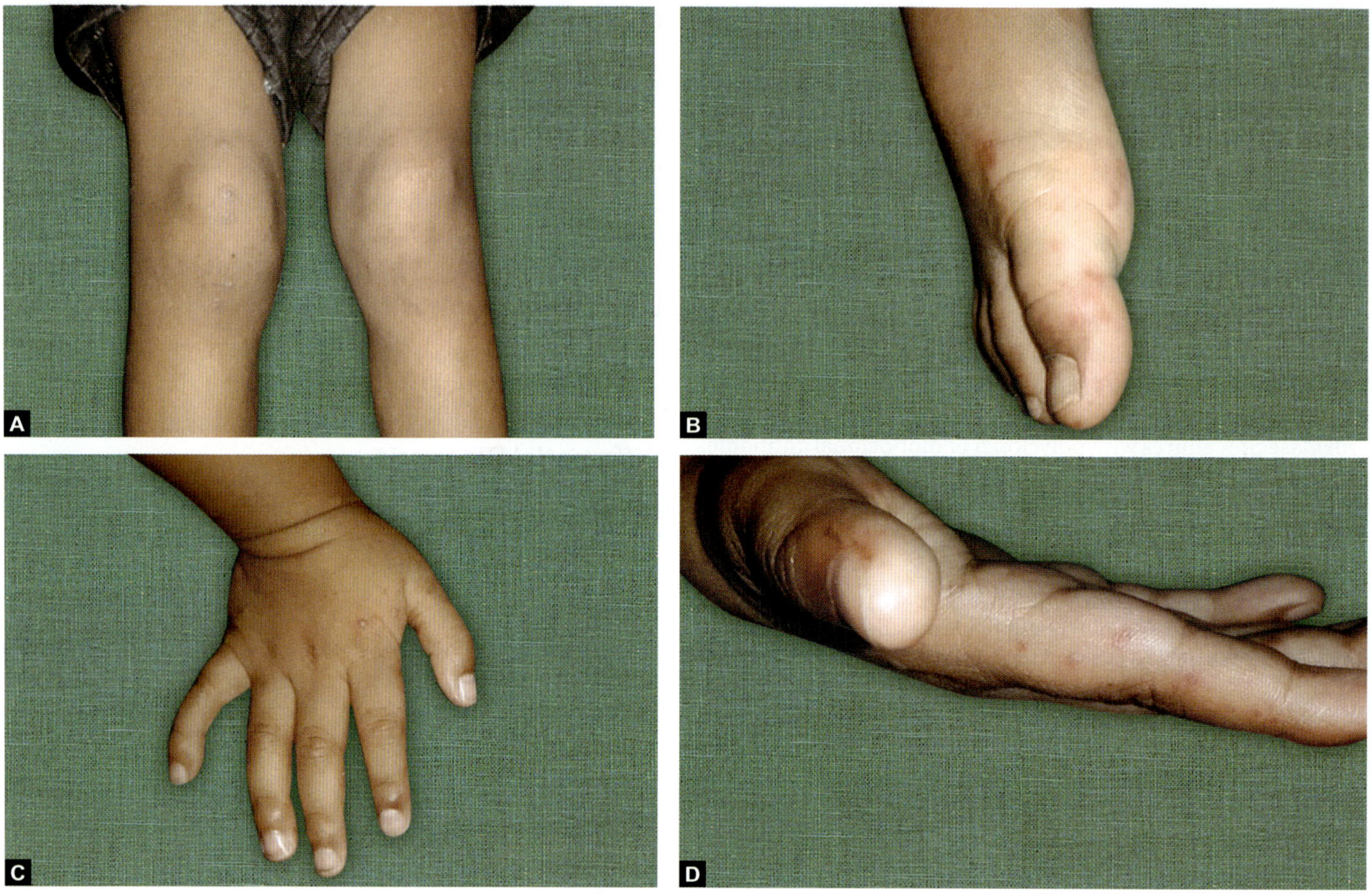

**FIG. 6: A,** Tender vesicles over the knees; **B,** Foot; **C,** Dorsum of the hands; **D,** Lateral border of the fingers.

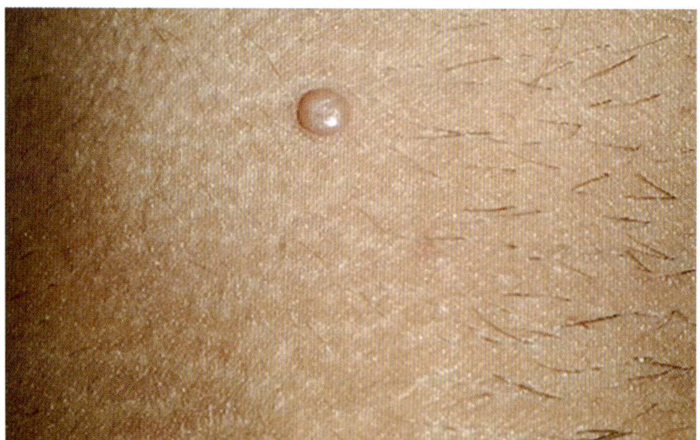

**FIG. 7:** Pearly, umbilicated papule of molluscum over the thigh.

> **Molluscum contagiosum**
>
> - Molluscum caused by the poxvirus, common in children, presents as smooth skin colored or pearly papules with central umbilication
> - Treatment is by physical or chemical removal.

## Laboratory Diagnosis

Histopathologically, the lesions show intraepidermal lobules with central viral and cellular debris. Enlarged basophilic nuclei and mitotic figures may be present in the basal layer. Other features include cytoplasmic vacuolization and eosinophilic globules at the granular cell layer, the nuclei become compressed and molluscum bodies lose their internal structure. The dermis can show an infiltrate which varies from lymphohistiocytic, neutrophilic, or granulomatous.

Polymerase chain reaction can detect MCV in skin lesions. The virus cannot be cultured in the laboratory. The central white core can be expressed and smeared on a slide and stained with Giemsa, Gram, Wright or papanicolaou stain which demonstrate the large brick-shaped inclusion bodies. Electron microscopy, PCR, and *in-situ* DNA hybridization can be done for research purpose.

## Differential Diagnosis

Verruca vulgaris, inclusion cysts, adnexal tumors, histoplasma infection, cryptococcosis.

## Treatment

Molluscum contagiosum can be self-limited. In atopic and immunocompromised individuals. It may have a protracted course. Commonly, it is treated with cryosurgery, evisceration, curettage, and electrocautery. Also used are topical imiquimod 5% cream, podophyllin and podophyllotoxin, cantharidin, iodine solution and salicylic acid plaster, tretinoin, potassium hydroxide, oral cimetidine, pulse dye laser, and topical cidofovir.

## ORF

### Epidemiology and Pathogenesis

Orf, also known as ecthyma contagiosum, scabby mouth, sore mouth, contagious pustular dermatosis, and infectious pustular dermatosis is a viral infection of sheep, goats, and humans. The distribution is worldwide. Transmission to humans is from infected animals or from fomites.

### Clinical Features

The disease starts as a maculopapular lesion over the hands, which progresses to form a target lesion, acute weeping nodule, regenerative dry stage and crusting, each stage lasting for around 6 days. Scarring does not occur. Secondary bacterial infection may rarely occur. In animals, a vesiculopapular eruption occurs over the gums, lips, nose, or groins.

### Laboratory Diagnosis

On histopathological examination, epidermis shows vacuolation and intracytoplasmic eosinophilic inclusions in early stages and multilocular vesicles in later stages. In the later stages, reticular degeneration of the epidermis, dilated hair follicles filled with debris and lymphohistiocytic dermal infiltrate are seen.

Electron microscopy shows "brick-shaped" viral particles 200–380 nm in length. Other methods of diagnosis are cell culture, complement fixation, and fluorescent antibody technique.

### Differential Diagnosis

Milker's nodule, herpetic whitlow, primary inoculation tuberculosis, anthrax, tularemia, atypical mycobacterial infection, syphilitic chancre, sporotrichosis, and pyogenic granuloma.

### Treatment

There is no specific treatment. Antibiotics can be given in case of secondary infection. A live vaccine is available for animals. Infection confers lifelong immunity in humans.

## MILKER'S NODULE

### Epidemiology

Milker's nodule, also called Paravaccinia or Pseudocowpox is a self-limiting viral infection which occurs in people working in close proximity with infected sheep and cattle. It is caused by a parapoxvirus which belongs to the poxvirus group. The disease is transmitted to human beings from infected animals or from contaminated objects. The organism may persist in the surroundings for some time, as it is resistant to heat, cold, and drying. Men are more commonly affected.

### Clinical Features

The incubation period is 4–7 days. It may begin with a prodrome of low-grade fever. Lesions usually occur on the hands, rarely on the face, as reddish macules, which evolve into papules, papulovesicles and then take on a target like appearance, i.e., a reddish center surrounded by a white ring and an outer red halo. The lesions then turn into violaceous, painful nodules which ulcerate and result in crusting. The lesions may last for 4–8 weeks (Fig. 8).

### Laboratory Diagnosis

Skin biopsy, electron microscopic examination of the blister fluid, DNA hybridization methods, and PCR are the diagnostic options available.

### Differential Diagnosis

Cowpox, herpetic whitlow, syphilitic chancre, pyogenic granuloma, sporotrichosis, anthrax.

### Treatment

The disease is self-limiting. If needed, large lesions can be surgically curetted.

## CYTOMEGALOVIRUS

Cytomegalovirus (CMV) is a DNA virus that belongs to the herpesvirus family. Once infected, latent infection is generally established in the host resulting in periodic reactivation. The virus has been isolated from body fluids like saliva, urine, feces, semen, genital secretions, and breast milk. The characteristic finding in infected tissue is the presence of cytomegalic cells with large intranuclear inclusions surrounded by a clear halo.

### Cytomegalovirus in Pregnancy

In utero transmission of CMV can occur as a result of reactivation of virus. Infection may be asymptomatic or may manifest as a mononucleosis like syndrome with a transient rubelliform rash (For congenital infection, see Neonatal Dermatoses chapter).

A mononucleosis like syndrome has been reported with CMV infection, similar to the EBV mononucleosis but less severe in nature. Disseminated CMV infections can occur in the immunocompromised and transplant patients. They are characterized by ulcerated lesions, indurated hyperpigmented nodules and plaques, and exanthematous rashes.

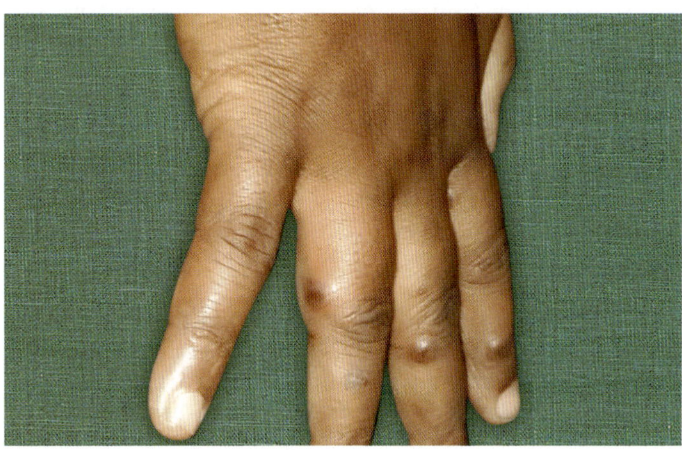

**FIG. 8:** Tender nodules of cowpox on the fingers.

## GIANOTTI–CROSTI SYNDROME

### Epidemiology

Gianotti-Crosti syndrome is a relatively common dermatosis of worldwide in distribution. It primarily affects children between 1 year and 6 years of age. The disease has no racial or sexual predilections.

### Etiology

Hepatitis B virus and EBV most commonly linked to it. Other associated viruses are the CMV, HHV-6, coxsackie virus A16, B4 and B5, rotavirus, parvovirus, MC, respiratory syncytial virus, mumps virus, and parainfluenza virus type 1 and 2. Rarely, bacteria like *Bartonella henselae*, *Mycoplasma pneumoniae*, and β-hemolytic streptococci are capable of triggering the disease. Immunization is also known to trigger the onset. Atopic dermatitis and immunosuppressive conditions may predispose.

### Pathogenesis

The pathogenesis is still unclear.

### Clinical Features

Following a prodrome of pharyngitis, upper airway infection or diarrhea, monomorphous, multiple, pruritic, pink to red-brown papules or papulovesicles, which can become confluent starts abruptly. They are symmetrically distributed over the cheeks, extensor aspects of the extremities, and buttocks. The trunk, knees, elbows, palms, and soles are usually spared. Less commonly, hemorrhage and scaling may be present. Systemic findings include malaise, low-grade fever, diarrhea, lymphadenopathy (usually cervical, axillary, or inguinal). Hepatosplenomegaly is rare.

### Laboratory Diagnosis

Peripheral blood can show lymphopenia or lymphocytosis. Monocytes may be elevated if associated with EBV. Histopathology is not diagnostic and shows features include acanthosis, spongiosis, exocytosis of lymphocytes in the epidermis with presence of Langerhans cells. The dermis shows an intense lymphocytic perivascular infiltrate consisting of T-cells and dendritic cells.

### Differential Diagnosis

Lichen planus, lichenoid drug eruptions, erythema multiforme, scabies, and popular urticaria.

### Treatment

Usually heal spontaneously without scarring over 10–60 days. The lymphadenopathy may persist for several months. Oral antihistaminics and topical anti-pruritics can be prescribed. In severe cases, systemic corticosteroid pulse therapy has been used.

## KAPOSI'S VARICELLIFORM ERUPTION

Kaposi's varicelliform eruption is a potentially life-threatening viral infection that arises in preexisting skin conditions.

### Etiology

A majority of cases are caused by the (HSV 1 and 2), when it is known as eczema herpeticum. Other etiological conditions are cocksackievirus A16 and vaccinia virus. Viral infection may result from autoinoculation from an infected contact or from latent infection in the host. The most important risk factor for infection is disruption of the epidermal skin barrier. The pre-existing skin disorders are atopic dermatitis, most commonly, pemphigus foliaceus, Darier's disease, pemphigus vulgaris, pityriasis rubra pilaris, Hailey-Hailey disease, irritant contact dermatitis,, cutaneous T-cell lymphoma, seborrheic dermatitis, psoriasis, Wiskott-Aldrich syndrome, congenital ichthyosiform erythroderma, and Sézary syndrome. The condition can occur at any age, but is more common in children. The incidence is unknown.

### Clinical Features

Typically, it presents with clusters of umbilicated vesicles and pustules over the skin. Systemic features include fever, chills, and malaise. The skin lesions progress to form painful, hemorrhagic, crusted, punched out erosions and ulcers. The eroded areas coalesce to form large areas of denuded skin which are further prone to develop secondary bacterial infection. The head and neck are commonly affected sites; also, the upper body can be involved. Ophthalmic involvement can occur and can be severe leading to keratitis.

### Laboratory Diagnosis

Diagnosis is mainly clinical, laboratory tests can be used for confirmation. A Tzanck smear for multinucleated giant cells can confirm herpes virus infection. Direct fluorescent antibody staining is a rapid and accurate diagnostic modality. Viral culture is the most sensitive and specific method but it takes at least 48 hours.

### Differential Diagnosis

Primary varicella infection, impetigo, and eczema vaccinatum.

### Treatment

Early diagnosis and therapy can be potentially lifesaving. Intravenous antibiotics, acyclovir or valacyclovir should be started immediately. Prophylactic silver sulfadiazine creams can be given for prevention of bacterial infection.

## PAPULAR-PURPURIC GLOVES AND SOCKS SYNDROME

Papular-purpuric gloves and socks syndrome (PPGSS) refers to an acute self-limited eruption which occurs in young adults, primarily during spring and summer. The incubation period is about 10 days.

### Etiology

Most cases are linked to parvovirus B19. Other etiological agents are measles virus, EBV, CMV, HHV6, coxsackie B6 and hepatitis B. However, among the above, parvovirus B19 is the only agent found to be present in skin biopsies and peripheral blood.

### Clinical Features

Patients appears nontoxic with a rash which begins as symmetric erythema and edema of the hands and feet, which progress to petechial and purpuric macules, papules, and patches which later desquamate. It is characterized by a sharp demarcation at the wrists and ankles. Pain or pruritus may be seen occasionally. Rarely, the rash may extend to nonacral sites such as the face, buttocks, trunk, groin, and extremities. Patients may have a polymorphous enanthem which includes diffuse hyperemia, aphthae, petechiae, erosions over the palate, pharynx, tongue, and inner lips. The rash is followed in 2–4 days by fatigue, arthralgia, myalgia, anorexia and lymphadenopathy.

### Laboratory Diagnosis

Lymphopenia or thrombocytopenia may be seen. Histopathological samples show a lymphocytic perivascular infiltrate in the papillary dermis with extravasation of red blood cells. Immunofluorescence shows parvovirus B19 in the dermal vessel endothelial cells, sweat glands, and epidermal ducts.

### Treatment

The treatment is symptomatic. Antihistamines and emollients may be prescribed if needed. PPGSS resolves in 1–2 weeks spontaneously without any known late sequelae.

## UNILATERAL LATERAL THORACIC EXANTHEMA (ASYMMETRIC PERIFLEXURAL EXANTHEMA OF CHILDHOOD)

The eruption was first described in 1962 as lichen miliaris. It mainly affects young children. The origin of this infection is unknown; however, an infectious etiology is suspected due to the presence of prodromal symptoms and a seasonal pattern.

The rash is unilateral, macules, or papules, which may be eczematous, scarlatiniform, or morbilliform. The primary lesion is a micropapule with a pale halo, begins unilaterally in the axilla or groin, spreads centrifugally, and resolves by 4 weeks. Although both sides of the body may be involved progressively, it continues to show unilateral predominance. Low-grade fever and lymphadenopathy are seen. The palms, sole, and mucous membranes are typically spared.

Serologic testing usually yields no results. Histology of the lesions shows a dermal lymphocytic infiltrate predominantly around sweat glands and to a lesser extent around hair follicles and blood vessels.

The treatment is symptomatic. Topical steroids are ineffective.

## PITYRIASIS ROSEA

Pityriasis rosea is an acute, self-healing exanthema characterized by erythemato-squamous oval macules affecting the trunk, limbs, and sparing the face, scalp, palms, and soles. It can occur at any age; however, individuals between 10 years and 35 years of age are more commonly affected. HHV 6 and 7 have been linked to the causation in recent times.

### Clinical Features

Constitutional symptoms like malaise, nausea, loss of appetite, headache, irritability, difficulty in concentration, joint pain, fever, and sore throat are reported. Cutaneous lesions begin with a "herald patch" or "mother patch" which is oval, erythematous, with finely scaled, slightly elevated borders, and pale depressed center. It is followed by the generalized eruption around 2 weeks later with lesions similar to the initial one, the exception being smaller size and symmetrical Christmas tree distribution. Pruritus is variable in intensity and frequency. Atypical presentations like vesicular, purpuric, urticarial, hemorrhagic forms have been reported. In the inverse form, the face and distal extremities are affected; oral mucosal lesions can rarely occur. Pityriasis circinata et marginata of Vidal is a distinctive form which has a course spanning months. The course varies from 2 weeks to 45 days.

### Diagnosis

The histopathological features are nonspecific and include focal parakeratosis, lymphocytic exocytosis, spongiosis, and mild acanthosis in the epidermis. The dermis shows a perivascular lymphocytic and eosinophilic infiltrate, with red blood cell extravasation. In addition, giant cells and Langerhans cells may be present.

### Differential Diagnosis

Secondary syphilis, seborrheic dermatitis, nummular eczema, pityriasis lichenoides chronica have to be differentiated from rosea.

### Treatment

The disease is self-limiting. Various therapeutic modalities like emollients, topical antihistamines and corticosteroids, systemic antihistamines, antiviral agents and artificial ultraviolet therapy have been tried. Oral erythromycin has been shown to decrease pruritus and shorten the course of the disease. Also, antivirals like acyclovir have proven efficacious in some patients.

## EPIDERMODYSPLASIA VERRUCIFORMIS

Epidermodysplasia verruciformis (EDV) is a rare, autosomal recessive genetic disorder. It is characterized by an increased susceptibility to cutaneous HPV in early life. Lewandowsky and Lutz first described the condition.

### Pathogenesis

Epidermodysplasia verruciformis is characterized by mutations in *EVER1* or *EVER2* genes on the chromosome 17q25. This leads to a defect in CMI, resulting in susceptibility to specific HPV genotypes known as EDV HPV, mainly HPV 5 and 8. Rarely HPV 14, 17, 20, and 47 can be involved which have oncogenic potential.

### Clinical Features

Pityriasis versicolor like hypopigmented macules and plane wart-like papules develop in childhood on the face and other areas. Other types of lesions including lesions mimicking seborrheic keratosis may also be seen.

Malignant transformation occurs after 40–50 years of age with Bowen's disease being the most frequent tumor, followed by invasive squamous cell carcinoma. Sun exposure potentiates the malignant risk.

### Treatment

Topical retinoids, interferon, immunotherapy, cryotherapy and electrodessication are used. Results are not very satisfactory. Surgical excision with reconstruction of the defects with split-thickness or full-thickness skin grafts or local skin flaps is a more satisfactory treatment.

## KIKUCHI'S DISEASE

### Etiopathogenesis and Epidemiology

Kikuchi-Fujimoto disease (KFD) or histiocytic necrotizing lymphadenitis is an idiopathic, uncommon, self-limited disease. It has been reported worldwide but it has a higher prevalence among the Japanese and Asians. It is more common in females and in individuals within the age of 30 years.

#### Etiology and Pathogenesis

The exact etiology is unknown and the pathogenesis is poorly understood. A viral or post viral etiology has been postulated. EBV, HIV, HSV, dengue virus, human T-cell lymphotropic virus (HTLV)-1 and *parvovirus B19* have been suggested as possible etiological agents. Few bacterial agents like *Toxoplasma, Yersinia, Bartonella, Brucella* have also been implicated. It has also been linked to systemic lupus erythematosus and hence an autoimmune hypothesis has been proposed. It has been postulated that the primary event is the activation of T lymphocytes and histiocytes. The proliferating T-cells undergo apoptosis and form necrotic areas in lymph nodes, which are later cleared by histiocytes.

### Clinical Features

This presents with tender cervical lymphadenopathy, accompanied by fever, upper respiratory tract symptoms, arthralgia, skin rashes, weakness, and night sweats. Other presenting features are weight loss, anorexia, diarrhea, nausea, vomiting, chills, chest and abdominal pain.

### Laboratory Diagnosis

Leucopenia, elevated erythrocyte sedimentation rate and C-reactive protein may be seen. A few patients have atypical peripheral blood lymphocytes. Histopathology of regional lymph node is diagnostic and shows irregular paracortical areas of coagulative necrosis with histiocytes at the margin and abundant karyorrhectic debris, which may distort the nodular architecture, are seen. The histiocytes are positive for lysozyme, myeloperoxidase and CD68.

### Differential Diagnosis

Systemic lupus erythematosus, lymphoma.

### Treatment

Management is supportive. Nonsteroidal anti-inflammatory drugs may be prescribed. Corticosteroids are reserved for severe disease. Intravenous immunoglobulin has been tried in some cases. The course is generally benign and the disease is self-limited, resolving in few weeks or months. A recurrence rate of 3–4% has been noted.

## INFECTIOUS MONONUCLEOSIS

Infectious mononucleosis or glandular fever is caused by the EBV or HHV-4. Transmission of the virus occurs through contact with saliva from an infected individual. The incubation period is around 1–2 months.

### Clinical Features

Patients present with fever, lymph node enlargement, and sore throat. Other features include splenomegaly, arthritis, hepatitis, interstitial pneumonia, pericarditis, glomerulonephritis, keratitis, uveitis, conjunctivitis, retinitis, autoimmune hemolytic anemia, neutropenia and thrombocytopenia, neurological manifestations like Bell's palsy, transverse myelitis, meningoencephalitis, and Guillain–Barré syndrome.

Skin involvement is seen in about 10% of patients and includes maculopapular rashes, which first appear on the trunk and upper arms and spread to face and forearms later. Other uncommon skin associations are Gianotti–Crosti syndrome, erythema multiforme, erythema nodosum, urticarial, urticarial vasculitis, annular erythema, acrocyanosis and chronic bullous disease of childhood.

### Diagnosis

Diagnosis is done using the monospot test. Atypical lymphocytes are characteristically seen.

### Treatment

The treatment is mainly symptomatic.

## HUMAN T-CELL LYMPHOTROPIC VIRUS

Skin lesions are common in infection with the HTLV-1 infection. Among all, the most severe diseases related to HTLV-1 are adult T-cell leukemia or lymphoma (ATLL), which is an aggressive condition that fails to respond to chemotherapy and infective dermatitis associated with HTLV-1 (IDH) which is a severe and recurrent form of childhood eczema. IDH may progress to HTLV-1 associated myelopathy or tropical spastic paresis (HAM/TSP) and to ATLL. Other dermatological associations of the virus are xerosis, acquired ichthyosis, seborrheic dermatitis, and infectious and parasitic dermatosis.

**TABLE 3: Classification of viral hemorrhagic fevers**

| Family | Genus | Virus | Disease | Vector |
|---|---|---|---|---|
| Flaviviridae | Flavivirus | Yellow fever | Yellow fever | Mosquito |
| | | Dengue | Dengue hemorrhagic fever | Mosquito |
| | | Kyasanur Forest disease | Kyasanur Forest disease | Tick |
| Arenaviridae | Arenavirus | Lassa | Lassa fever | Rodent |
| | | Machupo | Bolivian hemorrhagic fever | Rodent |
| | | Junin | Argentine hemorrhagic fever | Rodent |
| | | Sabia | Brazilian hemorrhagic fever | Rodent |
| | | Guanarito | Venezuelan hemorrhagic fever | Rodent |
| Bunyaviridae | Hantavirus | Hantaan | Hemorrhagic fever with renal syndrome (HFRS) | Rodent |
| | | Puumala | HFRS | Rodent |
| | | Sin nombre and Andes | Hantavirus | Rodent |
| | Phlebovirus | Rift valley fever | Rift valley fever | Mosquito |
| | Nairovirus | Crimean-Congo hemorrhagic fever | Crimean-Congo hemorrhagic fever | Tick |
| | | Omsk hemorrhagic fever (HF) | Omsk HF | Tick |
| Filoviridae | Ebola virus | Ebola | Ebola HF | Bat |
| | Marburg virus | Marburg | Marburg HF | Bat |

## VIRAL HEMORRHAGIC FEVERS

Viral hemorrhagic fevers (VHFs) are acute febrile infections characterized by multisystem involvement, with features of microvascular leak or hemorrhage. They are zoonoses, with humans being the accidental or dead-end host.

### Etiology and Pathogenesis

Humans are infected by the bite of an infected arthropod or by contact with animal excreta or rarely by airborne contact. The geographic distribution of the VHF corresponds to the location of the vector and other epidemiological factors. Rarely imported cases can be seen in different locations due to air travel.

### Classification

Table 3 enlists classification of viral hemorrhagic fevers.

### Clinical Features

As the name suggests, VHF are febrile illnesses with evidence of vascular damage or increased vascular permeability. The average incubation period is 1–2 weeks. They manifest with insidious onset of fever, and varied symptoms like abdominal pain and nausea.

The hemorrhagic manifestations could vary from skin and mucosal petechiae, hemorrhage, hematochezia, epistaxis, hemoptysis.

### Laboratory Diagnosis

Currently, there are no commercially available diagnostic tests available for VHFs. Confirmatory testing is done only at specialized centers. The diagnostic methods available are ELISA for either IgG or IgM or viral antigens; reverse transcription-PCR for viral RNA detection. In endemic areas, molecular methods can be used for field detection.

### Differential Diagnosis

Typhoid, shigellosis, pneumonia, malaria, rickettsial disease, leptospirosis, gram-negative sepsis, toxic shock syndrome.

Idiopathic thrombocytopenic purpura, leukemia, and thrombotic thrombocytopenic purpura may also mimic VHFs.

### Treatment

Antiviral therapy can be instituted in early stages and supportive care in later stages. Ribavirin is effective in Lassa fever, Crimean-Congo hemorrhagic fever and hemorrhagic fever with renal syndrome. Immune plasma transfusion is the mainstay of treatment for argentine hemorrhagic fever. For severely ill patients, mechanical ventilation, hemodialysis and other supportive measures need to be instituted. In patients with hantavirus disease extracorporeal membrane oxygenation has been found useful. Other agents useful in VHFs are steroids, and recombinant activated protein C.

## SUGGESTED READINGS


1. Aronson J. Viral hemorrhagic fevers. In: Fraire AE, Woda BA, Welsh RM, Kradin RL (Eds). Viruses and the Lung. Berlin: Springer-Verlag Berlin Heidelberg; 2014. pp. 123-32.
2. Arvin AM. Varicella-zoster virus. Clin Microbiol Rev. 1996;9(3):361-81.
3. Brandt O, Abeck D, Gianotti R, et al. Gianotti –Crosti syndrome. J Am Acad Dermatol. 2006;54:136-45.
4. Cobb MW. Human papillomavirus infection. J Am Acad Dermatol. 1990;22(4): 547-66.
5. Drago F, Broccolo F, Rebora A. Pityriasisrosea: An update with critical appraisal of its possible herpesviral etiology. J Am Acad Dermatol. 2009:303-15.
6. Emsen MI, Kabalar ME. Epidermodysplasia verruciformis: An early and unusual presentation. Can J Plast Surg. 2010;18(1):21-4.
7. Epps RE, Pittelkow MR, Su WP. TORCH syndrome. Semin Dermatol. 1995;14(2): 179-86.
8. Frisch S, MSIV, Sigfries EC. The clinical spectrum and therapeutic challenge of eczema herpeticum. Paediatric Dermatol. 2011;28(1):46-52.

9. Gelderblom HR. Structure and Classification of Viruses. In: Baron S (Ed.). Medical Microbiology, 4th Edition. Galveston, TX: University of Texas Medical Branch; 1996.
10. Groves RW, Jones W, MacDonald DM. Human orf and milker's nodule: A clinicopathological study. J Am Acad Dermatol. 1991;25:706-11.
11. Hanson D, Diven DG. Molluscum contagiosum. Dermatol Online J. 2003;9(2).
12. Kochhar AM, Reddy BSN. Cutaneous manifestations of hepatitis B and C virus infections: A study of 100 cases. Indian J Dermatol. 2003;48(2):73-7.
13. Lesher JL Jr. Cytomegalovirus infections and the skin. J Am Acad Dermatol. 1998;1333-8.
14. Martins C, Goncalo M, Mariano A, et al. Papular-purpuric gloves and socks syndrome. J Eur Acad Dermatol Venereol. 1996;6:173-8.
15. Scott LA, Stone MS. Viral exanthems. Dermatol Online J. 2003;9:4.
16. Sterling JC. Virus infections. In: Burns T, Breathnach S, Cox N, Griffiths C (Eds). Rook's Textbook of Dermatology. Oxford: Wiley-Blackwell; 2010. p. 33.1.
17. Straface G, Alessia Selmin A, Vincenzo Zanardo V, et al. Herpes simplex virus infection in pregnancy. Infect Dis Obstet Gynecol. 2012;2012:536037.
18. Tschachler E, Bergstresser PR, Stingl G. HIV-related skin diseases. Lancet. 1996; 348:659-63.

# Superficial Fungal Infections

*Uma S Agarwal, Puneet Agarwal, Vinita Garg*

## INTRODUCTION

Fungi, once believed to be a part of plant kingdom, actually represent a distinct kingdom different from bacteria and plants. Superficial fungal infections of skin are common in both temperate and tropical climates. They are often caused by overgrowth of transient or resident flora associated with a change in the microenvironment of the skin. Invasion by these fungi is restricted to skin, hair, nails and mucous membranes. In skin, they are usually found in the stratum corneum. Common superficial fungal infections and their causative agents are given in table 1.

Besides these, some moulds are also capable of producing disease in humans. *Scytalidium dimidiatum* and *Scytalidium hyalinum* may involve palms, soles, toe webs, and nails. These infections mimic tinea manuum and tinea pedis. Other nondermatophyte moulds, e.g., *Scopulariopsis brevicaulis, Acremonium, Fusarium* and *Aspergillus* can cause onychomycosis.

## DERMATOPHYTOSIS

Dermatophytosis is an infection of skin caused by specialized group of fungi, the dermatophytes, which are able to invade and colonize stratum corneum of skin and keratinized tissue, such as hair and nails. Tinea is a term used commonly for this condition. Severity of infection depends upon the dermatophyte species involved and the immunological response of the host. Clinical appearance of lesion varies according to the site of infection and the causative organism.

**TABLE 1: Common superficial fungal infections**

| Superficial fungal infections | Causative agents | Common species |
|---|---|---|
| Dermatophytosis (39 species) | *Microsporum* | *M. canis, M. ferrugineum, M. gypseum* |
| | *Trichophyton* | *T. mentagrophytes, T. rubrum, T. tonsurans, T. verrucosum, T. violaceum* |
| | *Epidermophyton* | *E. floccosum* |
| Pityriasis versicolor | *Malassezia* | *M. furfur, M. globosa, M. sympodialis, M. restricta* |
| Piedra | *Trichosporon beigelii* (white)<br>*Piedraia hortae* (black) | – |
| Tinea nigra | *Hortaea werneckii* | |
| Candidiasis | *Candida* | *C. albicans,C. tropicalis* |

### Etiopathogenesis

Dermatophytes are not a part of the normal skin flora and can be divided into three groups based on their natural habitat (Table 2).

Intact skin is a barrier to dermatophytes. Trauma and maceration due to sweat are predisposing factors for tinea cruris, tinea pedis and tinea corporis. Once they get a suitable environment, spores germinate and penetrate the stratum corneum either through horn cells or preferably making their way between horn cells. Keratinases and other proteolytic enzymes produced by dermatophytes may cause digestion of keratin.

### Transmission and Source of Infection

Transmission is indirect, e.g., infected scales, hair shed from hosts, spores (arthoconidia), clothings, towels, floor of showers and changing rooms, and contaminated combs and hair brushes cause scalp infections.

### Clinical Features

Skin infections caused by dermatophytes are known as tinea infections. Depending upon the site involved, they are called by different names like tinea capitis (scalp), tinea corporis (body), tinea faciei (face), tinea barbae (beard and moustache area), tinea cruris (folds), tinea pedis (feet), and tinea manuum (hands).

**TABLE 2: Classification of dermatophytes**

| Dermatophytes | Transmission/ habitat | Clinical feature |
|---|---|---|
| Anthropohilic | Only human | Chronic, mild to non-inflammatory |
| Zoophilic | Both animals and human | Acute, intense inflammation |
| Geophilic | Soil. Transmitted to human through contact | Moderate inflammation |

## Tinea Capitis

Tinea capitis accounts for more than 80% of fungal infections in children under 15 years of age. It is more common in boys than girls probably because of shorter hair, allowing easy access for fungal spores.

This is caused by *Trichophyton* and *Microsporum*. Tinea capitis may be of inflammatory and noninflammatory variants. Patchy loss of hair and inflammatory changes (erythema, scaling, pustulation) are the cardinal signs for diagnosis of tinea capitis. The scaling is a result of increased epidermal replacement following inflammation. Various clinical presentations are seen depending on the type of fungus and the degree of host immunological response (Table 3).

Tinea capitis may also be associated with tinea infections in other body sites in about one-fourth of the patients. (Fig. 9). Repeated itching and poor hygiene may result in secondary scalp infection, lymphadenopathy and subsequent cicatricial alopecia. Tinea capitis is much more common in children than adults.

Tinea capitis always requires systemic treatment because topical antifungal agents do not penetrate the hair follicle. Topical treatment is only used as adjuvant therapy to systemic antifungals. Not all drugs have ideal formulations (like syrup) to be used for children.

## Tinea Faciei

It is the dermatophytic infection of non-beard area of the face. *Trichophyton mentagrophytes* and *Trichophyton rubrum* are the common species causing it. Lesions begin as erythematous, scaly macules which extend peripherally and form an annular lesion with raised border (Fig. 10).

## Tinea Barbae

It is caused by *Trichophyton verrucosum* and *T. mentagrophytes* var. mentagrophytes. Inflammatory papules, pustules, exudation and crusting are seen in a beard and mustache area.

## Tinea Corporis

It is caused by *T. rubrum, T. mentagrophytes, Epidermophyton floccosum*, and *Microsporum canis*. The typical lesion of tinea corporis is an erythematous, annular or polycyclic plaque with vesicular or scaly border. Lesions show central clearing and sometimes show hyperpigmentation (Fig. 11).

## Tinea Incognito (Steroid Modified Tinea)

It is the infection in which usual signs of tinea are masked by application of potent topical steroids. Classical features of tinea like well-defined margins, erythema and scaling may be absent. Pustular lesions, nodules, and hyperpigmentation are commonly seen.

## Tinea Imbricata

It is a variant of tinea corporis, in which lesions are seen as multiple scaly concentric rings. It is caused by *Trichophyton concentricum* and is found only in Western Pacific area and Southeast Asia.

## Tinea Cruris

Tinea cruris is infrequent before puberty and seen more commonly in adolescent males. Humid climate, obesity and tight-fitting clothes are the predisposing factors. It may spread to thighs, perianal region and buttocks. Lesions are seen in groin as annular, scaly plaques with central clearing (Fig. 12). *T. rubrum, T. mentagrophytes*, or *E. floccosum* are the causative organisms.

## Tinea Pedis

Infection of the sole can have four different presentations. Tinea pedis may be associated with tinea manuum concurrently.

- *Bullous*: Disease may present with acute inflammatory reaction with vesicular eruptions involving the thin skin of the plantar arch, digits, sides of the feet, and heel. This may be associated with burning, itching and great discomfort. This is mostly caused by *T. mentagrophytes*
- *Moccasin type*: This is characterized by a dull erythema and pronounced silvery scaling that may involve the entire sole and sides of the foot, giving a moccasin or sandal appearance. This is often unilateral. Sometimes *T. rubrum* may involve both feet and one hand
- *Hyperkeratotic type*: Sometimes, it may also present as hyperkeratotic variant along the sides of the sole. It becomes important to differentiate with psoriasis, lichen planus, and

**TABLE 3: Clinical patterns of tinea capitis**

| Clinical type | Clinical features | Species |
|---|---|---|
| Gray patch/ seborrheic type (non-inflammatory type) | Erythematous papules, scaly plaques with partial or complete hair loss, dull gray and lusterless hair because of numerous arthrospores on surface of the hair (ectothrix). This appears as gray patches (Fig. 1), diffuse scaling with minimal hair loss, can be easily confused with seborrhea capitis (Fig. 5). Ear sign, if present, can be very helpful (Box 1) | • *Microsporum audouinii,*<br>• *M. canis,*<br>• *M. ferrugineum,*<br>• *Trichophyton tonsurans* |
| Black dot (non-inflammatory type) | Patches of hair loss and mild scaling with black dots. There is invasion within the hair shaft (endothrix) by the fungus. Black dots appear due to breakage of the hair at the level of scalp with minimum inflammation (Fig. 2) | *T. violaceum, T. tonsurans* |
| Favus (inflammatory type) | Yellow, confluent crusts that are dried up and appear as cup-shaped lesions (called scutula) at the follicular openings with characteristic mousy odor. Cicatricial alopecia may be seen later at the site of lesions (Fig. 3). It is endemic in some families in Kashmir | *T. schoenleinii* |
| Kerion (inflammatory type) | Caused by zoophilic or geophilic species, inflammed, indurated and boggy swelling, abscess, interconnecting tunnels studded with broken and intact hairs and pustules. Thick crusting and matting of hair is common. Lymphadenopathy and secondary infection are more common. Lesions heal with scarring (Fig. 4) | *T. verrucosum, T. mentagrophytes, M. canis, or M. gypseum* |

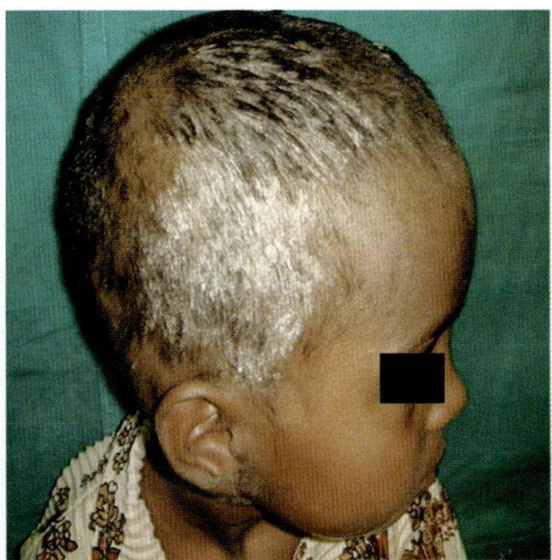

**FIG. 1:** Gray patch variety of tinea capitis.

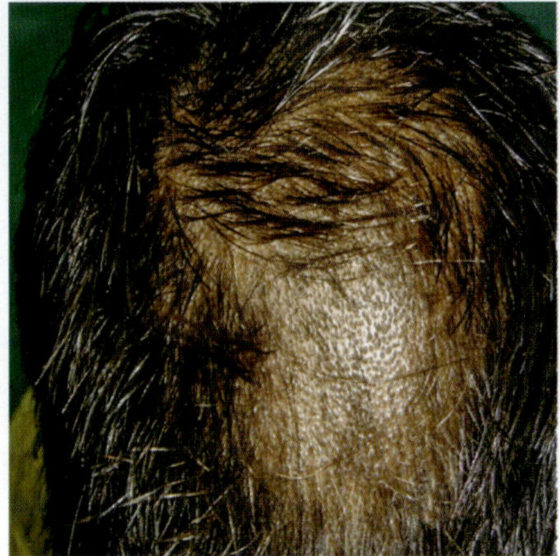

**FIG. 2:** Black dot variety of tinea capitis.

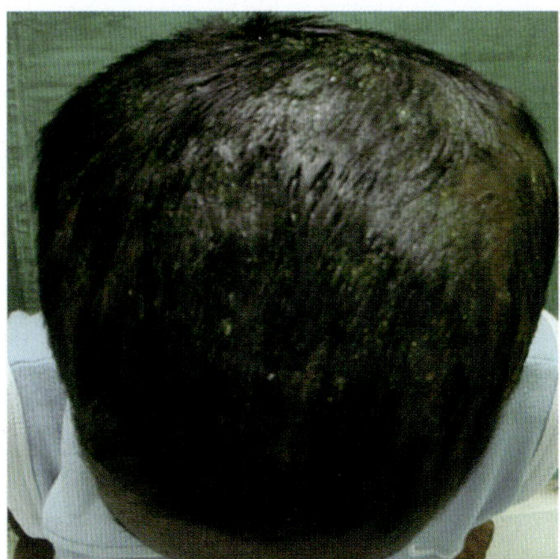

**FIG. 3:** Favus.

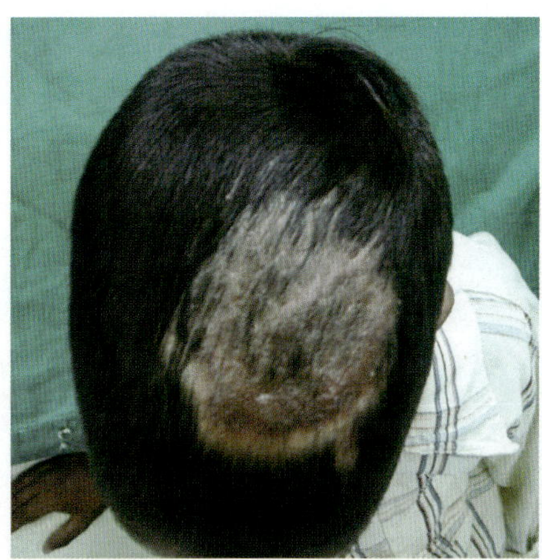

**FIG. 4:** Kerion.

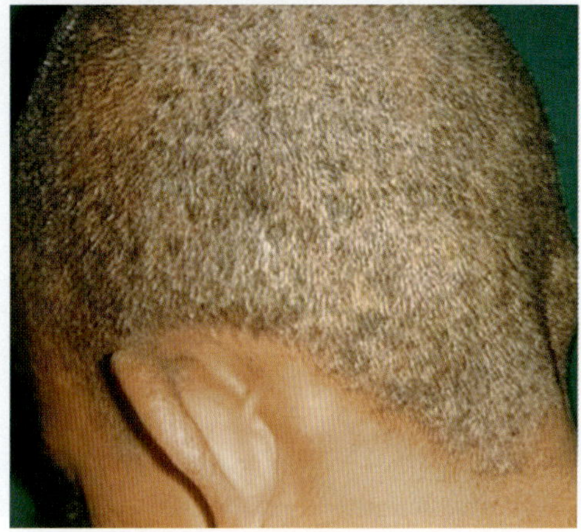

**FIG. 5:** Seborrheic type of tinea capitis.

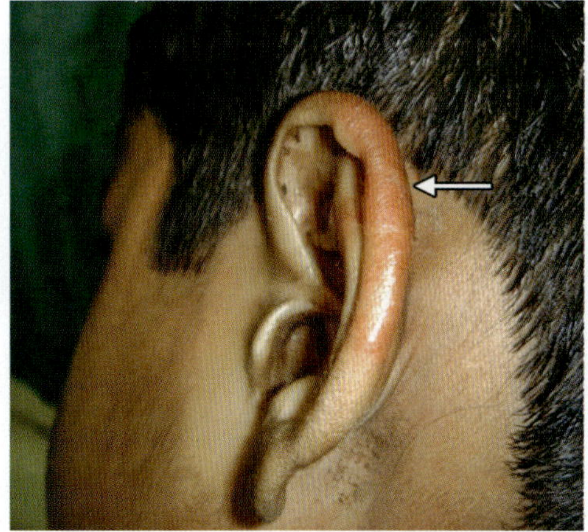

**FIG. 6:** Ear sign—showing scaly plaque over helix of external ear in tinea capitis.

**BOX 1 Ear sign**

It is a sign to easily diffrentiate tinea capitis from seborrheic capitis. In noninflammatory tinea capitis, at ; the curvature of helix, antihelix, the back of ear pina or near the tragus there may be present scaly plaques (Fig. 6) or papules (Fig. 7) along with lesions in scalp. In seborrheic capitis, the retroauricular fold is affected by erythema, scaling and fissuring (Fig. 8) (Fig. 6) or papules (Fig. 7). In seborrheic capitis, the retroauricular fold is affected by erythema, scaling and fissuring (Fig. 8).

hyperkeratotic dermatitis. Scraping may help in diagnosing the disease

- *Interdigitale type*: It is caused by anthropophilic *T. mentagrophytes*. It presents with erythema and desquamation between the toes with a white frilling border and may be associated with onychomycosis.

It may have to be distinguished from simple maceration, candidiasis and gram-negative toe web infection.

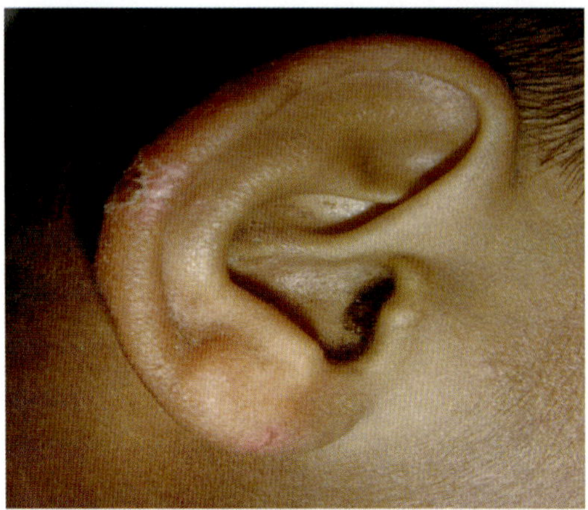

**FIG. 7:** Ear sign—papule presents over helix of external ear.

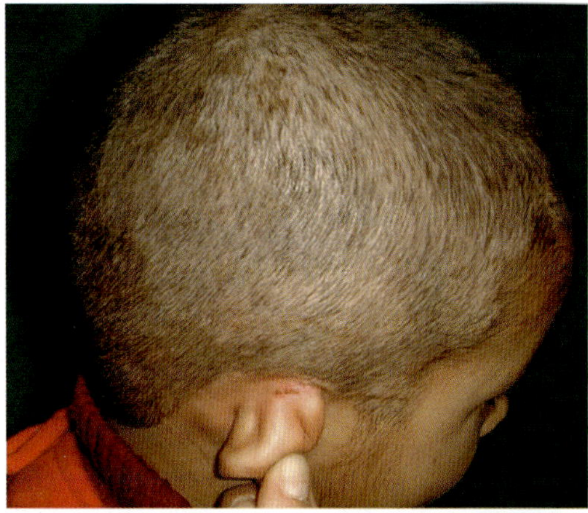

**FIG. 8:** Ear sign—seborrheic capitis with fissuring in retroauricular area.

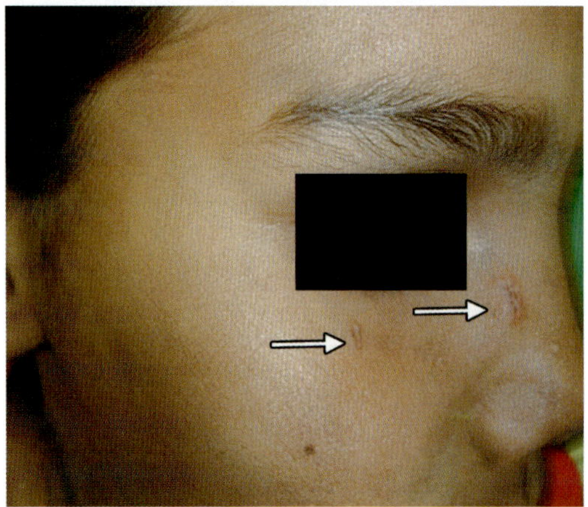

**FIG. 9:** Lesion of tinea presents over face along with tinea capitis.

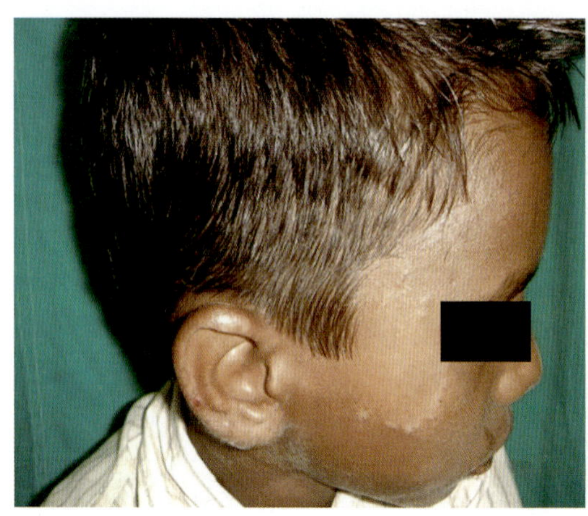

**FIG. 10:** Tinea faciei—showing the annular margin of lesion with ear involvement.

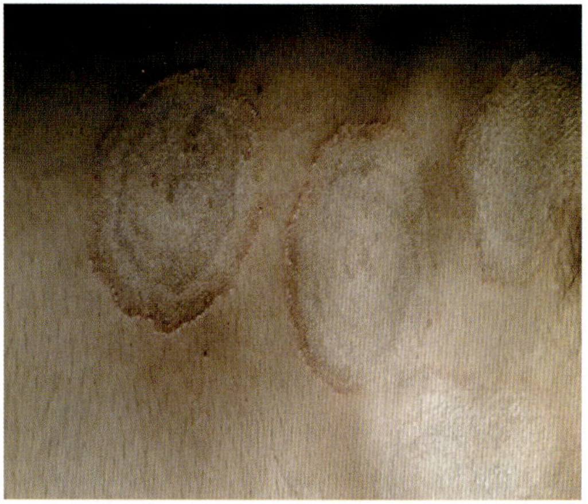

**FIG. 11:** Tinea corporis.

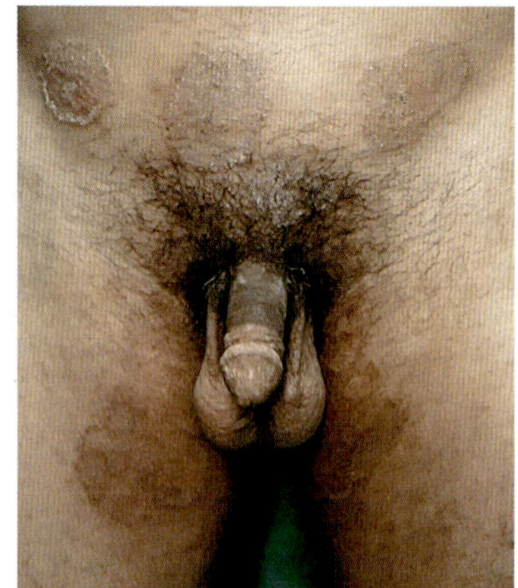

**FIG. 12:** Tinea cruris.

## Tinea Manuum

This presents as diffuse hyperkeratosis and scaling. Onychomycosis may be associated (Fig. 13). Similar to tinea pedis, tinea manuum is also often unilateral. The causative organism is *T. rubrum,* and *T. mentagrophytes.*

## Tinea Unguium

Dermatophytic infection of nails is known as onychomycosis. The causative organism is *T. rubrum* and *T. mentagrophytes. Tinea unguium* usually affects few nails only and is asymmetrical. It can however occur in association with tinea manuum or tinea

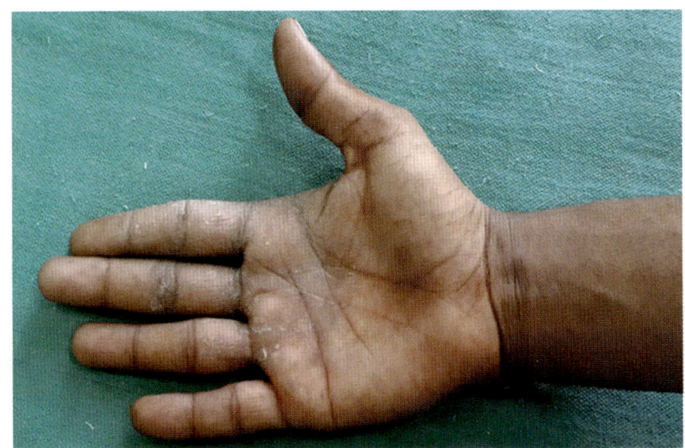

FIG. 13: Tinea manuum.

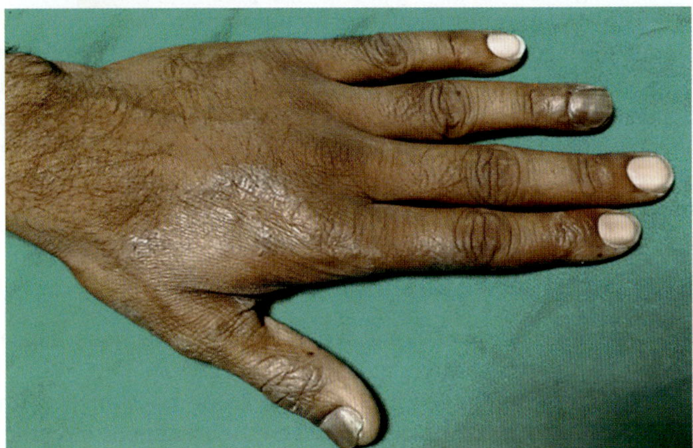

FIG. 14: Tinea manuum with onychomycosis.

pedis. Nail plate involvement starts from free edge and results in thickened yellow nail dystrophy, subungual hyperkeratosis and onycholysis (Fig.14). Following four clinical patterns of *Tinea unguium* have been reported:

- Distal and lateral subungual onychomycosis
- White superficial onychomycosis (SO)
- Proximal subungual onychomycosis (PSO)
- Total nail dystrophy.

Recently, a revised classification has been proposed in which it has been classified into following subtypes:

- Distal and lateral subungual onychomycosis (DLSO)
- Superficial onychomycosis
- Endonyx onychomycosis (EO)
- Proximal subungual onychomycosis
- *Mixed pattern onychomycosis (MPO)*: Combination of following patterns on same nail—DLSO plus SO, SO plus DLSO, SO plus PSO, DLSO plus PSO
- Totally dystrophic onychomycosis (TDO).

Distal and lateral subungual onychomycosis is commonly caused by *T. rubrum, T. mentagrophytes, E. floccosum, Candida albicans, Fusarium* species, *Scytalidium* species, and *Scopulariopsis brevicaulis*. Common etiologies of SO are *T. mentagrophytes, T rubrum, Fusarium* sp., *Acremonium,* and *Scytalidium*. Endonyx is generally caused by *Trichophyton soudanense* and *Trichophyton violaceum*, and PSO by *Tinea rubrum* and *Fusarium*.

Paronychia is an important associated condition with onychomycosis. This is caused by fungus like *Candida, Scytalidium dimidiatum, Scytalidium hyalinum, Fusarium* species, and bacteria. Frequently, there is significant inflammation that require anti-inflammatory treatment. Involvement of nail is often secondary to paronychia but can also be primary. Secondly, diseases of nail folds from other diseases like contact dermatitis may also lead to damage of nail and subsequent infection by the fungi.

## Majocchi Granuloma

Sometimes, tinea infection can lead to granulomatous eruptions; there may be perifollicular pustules.

## Diagnosis

Clinical diagnosis of dermatophytoses can be further confirmed by:

- *Wood's lamp examination*: It is helpful in screening the patients of tinea capitis. Examination is done in a darkroom. Certain dermatophytes produce a characteristic fluorescence when exposed to ultraviolet rays (365–400 nm) filtered by Wood's filter. *M. canis* and *Microsporum audouinii* produce brilliant green fluorescence, while *Trichophyton schoenleinii* produces paler green fluorescence
- *KOH mount*: Specimen from a skin lesion, hair or nail clippings are placed in a drop of 10–30% potassium hydroxide (KOH) on a slide and examined under light microscope. It shows branching hyphae with chains of arthroconidia (Fig. 15). Size and arrangement of spores in infected hair in tinea capitis helps in identification of species involved
  Fluorescent microscopy using either acridine orange or calcofluor white may aid in diagnosis
- *Culture*: Sabouraud dextrose agar is the most common medium used. Fungus grows within 2–4 weeks
- *Histopathological examination*: It is useful in confirmation of onychomycosis; rarely required for diagnosis of other dermatophytosis. The fungus-specific stain such as periodic acid–Schiff (PAS) can be used to assist in diagnosis.

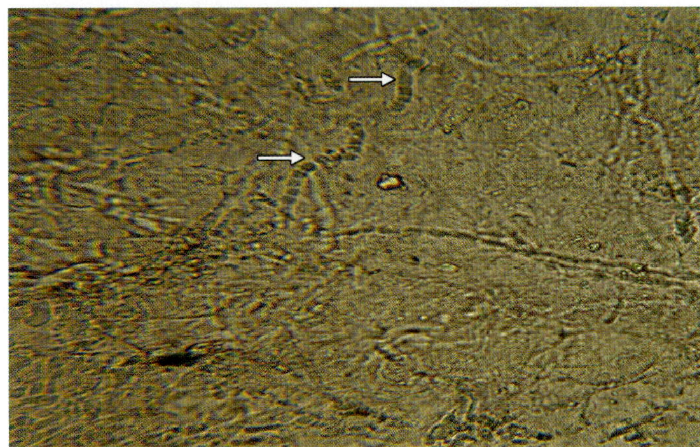

FIG. 15: Potassium hydroxide (KOH) mount—showing branched septate hyphae with chain of arthroconidia.

**TABLE 4: Differential diagnosis of dermatophytic infections**

| Dermatophytosis | Differential diagnosis |
|---|---|
| Tinea capitis | • If patchy hair loss<br>  ○ Alopecia areata<br>• If secondarily infected<br>  ○ Pyoderma capitis<br>  ○ Pediculosis capitis with secondary infection<br>• If noninflammatory<br>  ○ Seborrheic capitis<br>  ○ Psoriasis<br>  ○ Pityriasis amiantacea<br>• If cicatricial alopecia<br>  ○ pseudopelade |
| Tinea corporis | • Annular eczema<br>• Granuloma annulare<br>• Psoriasis |
| Tinea cruris | • Flexural psoriasis<br>• Seborrheic dermatitis<br>• Erythrasma<br>• Candidal intertrigo<br>• Napkin dermatitis in infants |
| Tinea pedis and tinea manuum | • Psoriasis<br>• Hyperkeratotic eczema<br>• *Candida* infection<br>• Pitted keratolysis |
| Tinea unguium | • Lichen planus<br>• Eczema<br>• Psoriasis<br>• *Candida* infection |

## Differential Diagnosis (Table 4)

Differential diagnosis of dermatophytic infections is given in table 4.

## Treatment

### Topical Therapy

Topical therapy is adequate to treat most of the localized tinea infections.

Topical antifungals include:

- *Imidazole derivatives*: Miconazole, clotrimazole, ketoconazole, oxiconazole, sertaconazole, bifonazole, tioconazole, and efinaconzole
- *Amines*: Allylamines (terbinafine), benzylamines (butenafine), and naftifine (amorolfine). Amorolfine is used as a lacquer in fungal infections of nail
- *Polyenes*: Nystatin ointment
- *Others*: Ciclopirox olamine and selenium sulfide
- *Newer topical antifungals*: Tavaborole.

### Systemic Therapy

Systemic therapy is required in extensive tinea infections, tinea unguium and tinea capitis. Drugs used in systemic therapy include:

- Griseofulvin
- *Azoles*: Ketoconazole, fluconazole, and itraconazole
- *Allylamines*: Terbinafine.

Griseofulvin, ketoconazole, fluconazole, and itraconazole are pregnancy category C drugs. Thus, they should be avoided during pregnancy. Terbinafine is pregnancy category B drug (animal studies has not shown any teratogenicity).

Ketoconazole has wider spectrum of activity against all three fungal species, such as dermatophytes, *Pityrosporum ovale*, and *Candida*. It is a hepatotoxic drug, so it should not be given in children below 5 years of age. Hepatitis due to ketoconazole is caused due to idiosyncratic reaction. Hepatitis and liver disorders are also reported after itraconazole use. However, this is much rare than ketoconazole.

Azoles like ketoconazole and itraconazole (but not fluconazole), are poorly absorbed when gastric pH is towards alkaline. Thus, concomitant administration with antacids, type-2 histamine antagonists can reduce their absorption. Fluconazole is one of the most commonly used drug for dermatophytosis.

All the azoles are metabolized in the liver by cytochrome P-450 enzymes. Thus, drugs that induce this enzyme (phenytoin, rifampicin, isoniazid, and carbamazepine) can decrease the efficacy of the azoles. Terbinafine is not metabolized through this enzyme. Dosages and adverse effects of commonly used antifungal drugs are mentioned in tables 5 and 6.

### Treatment of Tinea Capitis in Children

Griseofulvin is known to be active both in infections caused by *Trichophyton* species and *Microsporum* species. But its use is being gradually restricted with rising resistance to the drug. However, it is still considered as the treatment of choice, especially for cases caused by *Microsporum* species.

The reduction in the efficacy of griseofulvin over the years has been attributed to various factors like changes in patterns of epidemiology, fungal genetic mutations resulting in decreased susceptibility, long-term use of the drug, and poor compliance arising from the long duration of therapy.

Terbinafine, itraconazole, and fluconazole appear to have efficacy rates similar to those of griseofulvin in cases of tinea capitis caused by *Trichophyton* species in children. But the efficacy of griseofulvin is still superior to terbinafine in treating cases infected with *Microsporum* species. It is also considered as the cheaper effective alternative to the newer drugs.

Topical therapies like antifungal shampoos containing selenium sulphide, ketoconazole in shampoo or in lotion base may be helpful in eliminating the carriage of viable spores responsible for the disease transmission and reinfection. They may shorten the duration of treatment with oral antifungal. The topical fungicidal cream or lotion should be applied to the lesions once daily.

Clinical and mycologic examinations of the children should be conducted at regular intervals (2–4 weeks) till culture negative state.

### Treatment of Onychomycosis

Nail dystrophy may require surgical nail removal. Treatment of paronychia and tinea pedis, removal of associated predisposing conditions like contact dermatitis and treatment of diabetes are necessary.

**TABLE 5: Dosage of antifungal drugs**

| Type | Griseofulvin | Ketaconazole | Fluconazole | Terbinafine | Itraconazole |
|---|---|---|---|---|---|
| Tinea capitis (Tinea capitis caused by *Microsporum canis* may require higher dose/ longer duration than mentioned here) | • Micronized griseofulvin 20–25 mg/kg/day, for 6–12 weeks<br>• Ultramicronized griseofulvin- 10–15 mg/kg/day<br>• Ideally, treatment should continue 2 weeks after the clinical cure | 3–5 mg/kg for 4–6 weeks | 6–8 mg/kg for 8 weeks | • 62.5 mg/day (for body weight <20 kg)<br>• 125 mg/day (20–40 kg)<br>• 250 mg/day (>40 kg)<br>• It should continue for 4–6 weeks. | 5 mg/kg daily for 4–6 weeks or 5 mg/kg/day for first 7 days of every month for 2–4 months |
| Tinea corporis | 10 mg/kg for 4 weeks (ultramicronized) | 3–5 mg/kg for 2–4 weeks | 150–300 mg once weekly for 2–4 weeks | 250 mg/day for 4–6 weeks | 3–5 mg/kg daily for 2 weeks |
| Tinea unguium (onychomycosis) | 500–1000 mg/day until infection is cleared. This may require 3–6 months or more | 3–5 mg/kg for 3–6 months | 150–300 mg once weekly. *For fingernails*: 3–6 months. *Toenails*: 9–12 months | 250 mg/day for 6 weeks (finger nails) or 12 weeks (toe nails) | 200 mg/day continuously for 3 months<br>Or<br>400 mg/day for first 7 days of every month (28 days cycle) for 2 months (finger nails) or 3 months (toe nail) |

**TABLE 6: Adverse effects and contraindications of antifungal drugs**

| Drug | Adverse effects | Contraindications |
|---|---|---|
| Griseofulvin | Headache, gastrointestinal upset | Not active against *Candida* and *Malassezia* sp.<br>Pregnancy (category C) |
| Ketaconazole | Nausea, vomiting, headache, gynecomastia, loss of libido and hepatitis | Children below 5 years, hepatic diseases.<br>Pregnancy (category C) |
| Fluconazole | Headache, gastrointestinal upset | Ventricular dysfunctions, chronic or active liver disease, pregnancy (category D) |
| Terbinafine | Mild gastrointestinal upset, skin rash, elevation of liver enzymes, taste and visual disturbance | Chronic or active liver disease, pregnancy (category B) |
| Itraconazole | Dyspepsia, diarrhea, rash, headache, hepatic enzymes elevation | Ventricular dysfunctions, chronic or active liver disease, pregnancy (category C) |

Development of newer topical antifungal agents like efinaconazole and tavaborole mainly focuses on achieving broad-spectrum activity and formulation enhancement that facilitate enhanced penetration of the drug to achieve a better cure rate in onychomycosis, especially toenail onychomycosis. Efinaconazole (10%) is already approved by United States Food and Drug Administration (FDA) for toenail dermatophyte onychomycosis.

Efinaconazole has a broad spectrum of in vitro activity against dermatophytes, nondermatophytes, and yeasts. It is more potent against the most common pathogens, *T. rubrum*, *T. mentagrophytes* and *C. albicans* than currently marketed antifungal agents used to treat onychomycosis. In coming years, it can prove itself as a good adjuvant in treating onychomycosis along with the systemic agents.

Tavaborole represents a new class of protein synthesis inhibitors that exhibit antifungal properties. It interferes with protein synthesis in fungal cells by acting on cytoplasmic aminoacyl-transfer RNA (tRNA) synthetases. Tavaborole has been shown to effectively treat mild to moderate onychomycosis caused by dermatophytes without the need for debridement as it has better penetration of the nail plate. It is used as 5% solution.

## CANDIDIASIS

Candidiasis is an infection of the skin, mucous membranes, or nails caused by a dimorphic yeast known as *Candida*. *Candida* species are normal commensals in the mouth and gastrointestinal tract and infrequently on the skin also.

### Etiopathogenesis

*Candida albicans* is the major etiological agent for the superficial *Candida* infections being responsible for more than 70% cutaneous infections. Other *Candida* species in humans include *Candida tropicalis*, *Candida glabrata*, *Candida krusei*, and *Candida parapsilosis*. *C. tropicalis* is often implicated as the causative agent of fungemia in patients with leukemia. Epidemiological survey data from India showed that 67–90% of nosocomial candidemia cases were due to *Candida* non-albicans of which *C. tropicalis* was the most dominant.

- The most important source of *Candida* species in human disease is endogenous. Carriage rate of *Candida* in mouths of healthy subjects is up to 40%. Vaginal carriage rate of *Candida* species is less than 20%, which is more in pregnancy

- The change from a commensal status to pathogenic one is associated with underlying host factors like immunosuppressive therapy, immune deficiency disease, e.g., AIDS, pregnancy, endocrinal diseases like diabetes, local occlusion, maceration, and antibiotic therapy
- Neonates, especially premature infants are more susceptible to *Candida* infections, due to their immature immune mechanism. Occlusive effects of diapers and thumb sucking leading to maceration are important predisposing factors in infants.

## Clinical Features

### Oral Candidiasis

- *Oral thrush (Acute pseudomembranous candidiasis)*: It is seen as sharply defined curd-like or creamy white pseudomembrane on the buccal mucosa of cheeks, gums, palate and on lateral borders of the tongue (Fig. 16). Pseudomembrane consists of fungal hyphae, epithelial cells, fibrin, and leucocytes. When scrapped, it leaves erythematous base. Oral plaques may coalesce and become confluent. Lesions may extend to the throat causing dysphagia
- *Acute erythematous candidiasis (acute atrophic oral candidiasis)*: It is seen as atrophic lesions with erythematous base. It is associated with antibiotic therapy and inhaled steroids
- *Chronic erythematous candidiasis*: It is most common form of oral *candida* infection associated with oral prostheses used in orthodontics. It presents as edema and erythema of the area in contact with the dentures
- *Chronic plaque like candidiasis or candidal leukoplakia*: Lesions ranging from small white areas to large dense plaques are seen, which cannot be easily detached from the base. This is often associated with smoking. Median rhomboid glossitis is a variant of chronic plaque candidiasis
- Angular cheilitis (perleche) and chronic nodular candidiasis are the other manifestations.

### Other Manifestations of Candidial Infection

- *Napkin or diaper dermatitis:* This type of candidal rash is seen on the buttocks and perianal region of babies, associated with wearing diapers. Typical erythema, scaling and satellite pustular lesions may be seen in some cases

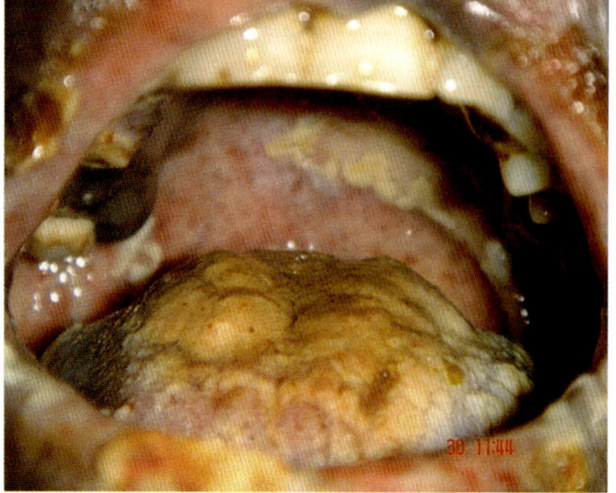

FIG. 16: Oral candidiasis.

- *Candidal vulvovaginitis*: It clinically presents as itching, burning in vulvar region or dysuria affecting mainly women of childbearing age. There is erythema and edema of vulva, white patches on vaginal mucosa and white curdy discharge
- *Candidal balanitis*: It is characterized by papules, pustules, fissuring with irritation over glans penis. Perianal and scrotal candidiasis may coexist with it
- *Paronychia*: It is an acute or chronic infections of the nail folds and nails. Nail fold becomes erythematous, swollen, and painful with pustular discharge. Nail plate invasion may occur which leads to discolored, ridged, and thickened nails. Finally, the nail becomes friable and detached from the nail bed
- *Congenital cutaneous candidiasis*: It is rare condition in newborn infant whose mother has had intrauterine *Candida* infection prior to delivery. It is characterized by generalized eruption of multiple pustules on an erythematous base
- *Neonatal candidiasis*: It occurs after the first week of life as oral thrush or diaper dermatitis. Infection is acquired during passage through birth canal or through nursery contacts
- *Chronic mucocutaneous candidiasis*: This is a rare syndrome that presents in infancy or childhood with recurrent oral, nail or cutaneous *Candida* infection which is resistant to treatment. It may be autosomal dominant type, autosomal recessive type or associated with autoimmune polyendocrinopathy
- *Candidal intertrigo*: Candidal intertrigo is candidal infections affecting skin folds like gluteal region or axilla. The lesions are moist, erythematous patches with fringed irregular edges. Papular or pustular satellite lesions may be seen
- *Candidal allergy*: Infection with *Candida* or gut carriage may be the cause of generalized pruritus or urticaria.

## Diagnosis

- Clinical picture is usually diagnostic, but microscopy and culture is confirmatory in all doubtful lesions
- Mucosal smear can be examined under microscope as unstained wet KOH mounts, heat fixed specimens may be Gram-stained or periodic acid-Schiff stained. Round or oval budding yeasts with long pseudohyphae are seen
- Fungal culture can be done on Sabouraud dextrose agar.

**TABLE 7: Differential diagnosis of candidal infections**

| Type | Differential diagnosis |
|---|---|
| Oral candidiasis | • Lichen planus<br>• Leukoplakia<br>• Herpes stomatitis<br>• Aphthous stomatitis<br>• Erythema multiforme |
| Napkin dermatitis | • Eczema<br>• Psoriasis |
| Paronychia | • Staphylococcal nail fold infections<br>• Dermatophytosis<br>• Psoriasis |
| Congenital cutaneous candidiasis | • Neonatal staphylococcal infection<br>• Transient neonatal pustulosis<br>• Congenital syphilis |

## Differential Diagnosis

Differential diagnosis of candidal infections is given in table 7.

## Treatment

Drugs used to treat dermatophytosis (except griseofulvin and terbinafine) are also effective for *Candida* infections. In addition, polyene antifungals like amphotericin B, nystatin, etc. are also effective.

### Topical Therapy

- *Imidazoles*: Clotrimazole, miconazole, ketoconazole, and econazole are highly effective
- Amphotericin B and nystatin are also effective
- For oral candidiasis oral solution of imidazoles or nystatin are used.

### Systemic Therapy

- Systemic therapy is indicated for chronic cases, reinfection, extensive lesions and in unresponsive cases
- Ketoconazole, fluconazole, and itraconazole may be used orally in the dosage as used for dermatophytosis; however, higher doses are required in patients with mucosal candidiasis.

### Newer Antifungal Drugs

- *Newer azoles*: Mainly used for systemic fungal infections, resistant candidal infection, e.g., voriconazole, ravuconazole, posaconazole
- *Other newer antifungal agents*:
  - *Echinocandins (caspofungin, micafungin)*: These are effective against resistant strains of *Candida* and dermatophytes and are fungicidal drugs available in parenteral form
  - *Pradimicins*: This antibiotic has shown therapeutic efficacy against lung candidiasis and aspergillosis, vaginal candidiasis, skin infection with *T. mentagrophytes* and 5-fluorocytosine- and azole-resistant *C. albicans* in mice with intravenous or topical treatment.

# PITYRIASIS VERSICOLOR

Asymptomatic, scaly, hypo- or hyperpigmented patches are seen, satellite lesions may be present. Few lesions may coalesce to form patches of various sizes and shapes (Fig. 17). The pigmentary changes may be due to production of substances like azelaic acid by enzyme activity of the yeast, which suppresses pigment synthesis. The disease occurs mainly on upper trunk and arms but face, and neck may also be involved.

It is caused by the yeast *Malassezia furfur* or *Pityrosporum ovale*, which is a part of the normal flora. It converts from yeast to mycelial phase in warm and humid climate, leading to pityriasis versicolor. Changes in the skin lipids during puberty could increase the fungal pathogenicity, which might be a possible explanation for its common occurrence in young adults.

KOH mount shows short, fragmented and wide mycelia, while the yeast is spherical, thick walled, known as spaghetti and meatball appearance. Wood's lamp examination of the lesions shows golden yellow fluorescence. Culture is not very useful as *Malassezia* is a part of human skin flora.

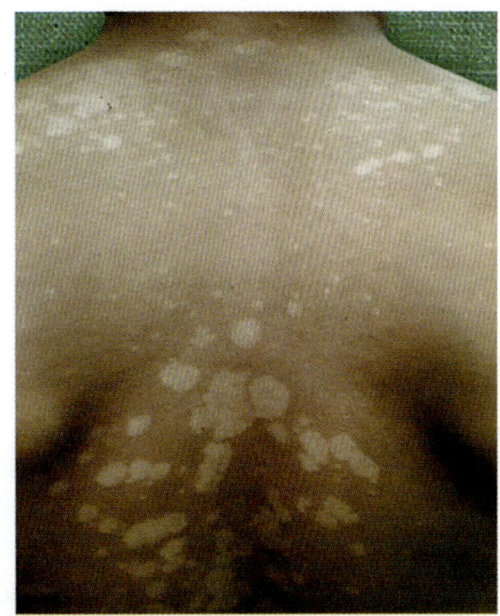

**FIG. 17:** Pityriasis versicolor.

Differential diagnosis includes vitiligo, seborrheic dermatitis, pityriasis rosea, secondary syphilis, tinea corporis, and erythrasma.

Oral azole antifungals like ketoconazole 3–5 mg/kg once daily for 15–20 days or single dose of fluconazole 3–6 mg/kg once a week for 4–6 weeks are given. Systemic antifungals should be combined with topical antifungals like clotrimazole or ketoconazole cream/lotion. In recalcitrant cases, itraconazole 200 mg/day for 5 days is given.

Hypopigmentation may persist for months after cure of fungus and may be treated with nighttime application of topical psoralens.

# TINEA NIGRA

It is an asymptomatic superficial fungal infection, caused by *Hortaea werneckii* or *Exophiala werneckii*. Lesions are brown or black colored, nonscaly, well-defined macules over palms, but may occur over soles, neck, and trunk also. The brown-black color represents silver nitrate stain. Pityriasis versicolor, syphilis, pigmented lesions of Addison's disease, nevi or melanoma, and exogenous pigments should be considered in differential diagnosis. Fungus can be demonstrated on KOH mount or culture and reveals abundant brown branched closely septate hyphae, and elongated budding cells. Topical azole creams like econazole and ketoconazole are effective. Topical application of benzoic acid and topical keratolytics may also give good result.

# PIEDRA

Piedra is a fungal infection of hair shafts. It is commonly caused by *Trichosporon beigelii* and *Piedraia hortae*. *Trichosporon inkin* and *Trichosporon mucoides* have been reported as an uncommon superficial agent for scalp white piedra. It leads to formation of superficial nodules on the hair shaft. There are two clinical types of piedra depending on the species affecting the hair shaft (Table 8).

White piedra may be sexually transmitted. The fungus grows both outside and inside the hair without affecting the skin. The hairs often break down due to weakening. Often the nodules may be misdiagnosed as the eggs of pediculi.

**TABLE 8: Differentiating features of piedra**

| Features | White piedra | Black piedra |
|---|---|---|
| Organism | *Trichosporon beigelii* | *Piedraia hortae* |
| **Nodules** | | |
| Color | White | Brown to black |
| Firmness | Soft | Hard |
| Adherence to hair shaft | Loose | Firm |
| Sites | Face, axillae, pubic area | Scalp > Face |
| KOH examination | Non-dematiaceous hyphae with blastoconidia and arthroconidia | Dematiaceous hyphae with asci and ascospores |
| Culture on Sabouraud dextrose agar | Moist cream-colored yeast like colonies | Slow-growing dark-green to dark-brown-black colored colonies |
| Treatment | • Cut affected hairs<br>• Antifungal shampoo<br>• Topical antifungals like azoles and allylamines may be helpful | • Cut affected hairs<br>• Antifungal shampoo<br>• Topical antifungals like azoles and allylamines may be helpful |

## SUGGESTED READINGS


1. Agarwal US, Mathur D, Mathur D, et al. Ear Sign. IDOJ. 2014;5:105-6.
2. Agarwal US, Saran J, Agarwal P. Clinico-mycological study of dermatophyte in a tertiary care centre in northwest India. IJDVL. 2014;80:194.
3. Agarwal US, Shukla SR. Fungal infections. In: Agarwal US, Shukla SR (Eds). Illustrated Textbook of Clinical Pediatric Dermatology, 1st Edition. New Delhi: PEEPEE; 2011. pp. 37-8.
4. Agarwal US, Sitaraman S, Panse G, et al. Useful sign to diagnose Tineacapitis—'ear sign'. Indian J Pediatr. 2012;79:679-80.
5. Alley MRK, Baker SJ, Beutner Kr, et al. Recent progress in the topical therapy of onychomycosis. Expert Opin Investig Drugs. 2007;16(2):157-67.
6. Amrinder JK, Dipankar De. Superficial fungal infections. In: Valia RG, Valia AR (Eds). IADVL Textbook of Dermatology, 2nd Edition. Mumbai: Bhalani Publishing House; 2008. p. 252.
7. Bao YQ, wan Z, Li RY. Invitro antifungal activity of micafungin&caspofungin against dermatophytes isolated from China. Mycopathologia. 2013;175:141-5.
8. Bhatt V, Sarpotdar P, Pillai R, et al. Development of an optimal formulation for efinaconazole a novel antifungal agent for the treatment of onychomycosis by topical application. Poster presented at 71st Annual Meeting. Miami Beach, FL: American Academy of Dermatology; 2013.
9. Elewski BE, Ca´ ceres HW, DeLeon L, et al. Terbinafinehydrochloride oral granules versus griseofulvin suspensionin children with tineacapitis: results of two randomized, investigator-blinded, multicenter,international, controlled trials. J Am Acad Dermatol. 2008;59:41-54.
10. Fischman O, Bezerra FC, Francisco EC, et al. Trichosporoninkin: an uncommon agent of scalp white piedra. Report of four cases in Brazilian children. Mycopathologia. 2014;178(1-2):85-9.
11. Grover C, Arora P, Manchanda V. Tineacapitis in the pediatric population: A study fromnorth India. IJDVL. 2010;76:527-32.
12. Huang DB, Zuchner L, Wu JJ, et al. Therapy of common superficial fungal infections. Dermatol Ther. 2004;17(6):517-22.
13. Jo Siu WJ, Tatsumi Y, Senda H, et al. Comparison of in vitro antifungal activities of efinaconazole and currently available antifungal agents against a variety of pathogenic fungi associated withonychomycosis. Antimicrob Agents Chemother. 2013;57(4):1610-6.
14. Kannan P, Janaki C, Selvi GS. Prevalence of dermatophytes and other fungal agents. Indian J Med Microbiol. 2006;24:212-5.
15. Kothari A, Sagar V. Epidemiology of Candida bloodstream infections in a tertiary care institute in India. Indian. J. Med. Microbiol. 2009;27:171-2.
16. Makimura K, Tamura Y, Mochizuki T, et al. Phylogenetic classification and species identification of dermatophyte strains based on DNA sequences of Nuclear Ribosomal Internal Transcribed Spacer 1 regions. J Clin Microbiol. 1999;37:920-4.
17. Oki T, Tenmyo O, Hirano M, et al. Pradimicins A, B and C: new antifungal antibiotics. II. In vitro and in vivo biological activities. J Antibiot. 1990;43:763-70.
18. Pai VV, Hanumanthayya K, Tophakhane R. Clinical study of Tineacapitis in Nothern Karnataka: A three year experience at a single institute. IDOJ. 2013;4:22-6.
19. Sharma M, Sharma R. Profile of dermatophytic and other fungal infections in Jaipur. Indian J Microbiol. 2012;52:270-4.
20. Sohnle PG. Dermatophytosis. In: Cox RA (Ed.) Immunology of Fungal Diseases. Florida: CRC Press; 1989. pp. 1-27.
21. Srinivasan B, Suyambu R, Thiyagarajan T, et al. Epidemiology of dermatophytosis in and around Tiruchirapalli, Tamil Nadu, India. Asian Pac J Trop Dis. 2012;2:286-9.
22. Tendolkar U, Shinde A, Baveja S, et al. Trichosporoninkin and Trichosporonmucoides as unusual causes of white piedra of scalp hair. Indian J Dermatol Venereol Leprol. 2014;80(4):324-7.
23. Trovato MJ, Schwartz AR, Janninger CK. Tineacapitis: current concepts in clinical practice. Cutis. 2006;77:93-9.

# 61 CHAPTER Subcutaneous and Secondary Cutaneous Fungal Infections

*Sarah A Ahmed, Wendy WJ van de Sande, Alexandro Bonifaz, Sybren de Hoog*

## INTRODUCTION

Invasive fungal infections involving the skin present a wide spectrum of clinical conditions ranging from subcutaneous to disseminated diseases, the latter often presenting with secondary cutaneous lesions. Subcutaneous infections frequently develop after traumatic inoculation of contaminated material from the environment. The most common subcutaneous mycoses are mycetoma, chromoblastomycosis, sporotrichosis, and lobomycosis, defined by different groups of etiologic agents. In contrast, disseminated infections generally are inhalation mycoses which are deep seated and finally affect multiple internal organs. Commonly involved are the lungs, abdominal viscera, bones and the central nervous system (CNS), while dissemination usually leads to manifestations in skin and subcutaneous tissues. Disseminated mycoses can be divided into three entities:

- Infections initially controlled by the cellular immunity of healthy hosts, mostly leading to recovery or dormancy. Endogenous reactivation and dissemination may occur. These mainly concern the dimorphic environmental pathogens. Examples—histoplasmosis, blastomycosis, coccidioidomycosis, paracoccidioidomycosis, talaromycosis, and adiaspiromycosis
- Infection emerging after impairment of innate immunity; these infections concern environmental saprobes which show opportunistic behavior in hosts with impaired immunity, such as leukemic patients or transplant recipients with gradual, chronic expansion of the infective biomass. Examples of this category are candidiasis and aspergillosis
- As yet insufficiently understood, third category is formed by the fungi that infect immunocompetent hosts but show chronic expansion rather than dormancy. Hosts may have hidden immune impairments, such as mutations in the *CARD9* gene which plays a role in the dectin signaling pathway. Examples of this category are particularly found among mucocutaneous candidiasis and black yeast-like organisms.

## SUBCUTANEOUS INFECTIONS

### Mycetoma

Mycetoma is a chronic progressive disease of the skin and subcutaneous tissues or even muscles and bones. It is clinically characterized by a painless subcutaneous mass, sinuses at the skin surface, and a discharge that contains grains (Figs 1 and 2). The disease is present worldwide but is mainly found in tropical and subtropical regions, with a particularly high prevalence in semiarid climate zones of Africa, Asia, and South America.

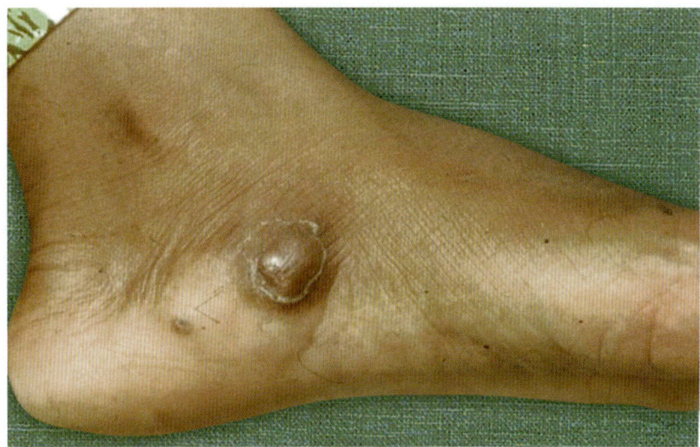

**FIG. 1:** Small mycetoma lesion.
*Courtesy*: Prof. Ahmed Fahal, Mycetoma Research Center, Khartoum, Sudan.

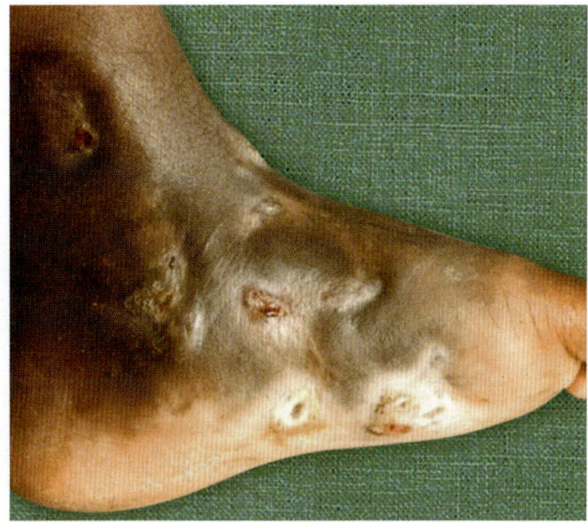

**FIG. 2:** Mycetoma lesion with discharging sinuses.
*Courtesy*: Prof. Ahmed Fahal, Mycetoma Research Center, Khartoum, Sudan.

## Pathogenesis and Clinical Presentation

Mycetoma starts after the organism is traumatically inoculated with a sharp object, such as from a thorn prick. A small, firm, progressive painless tumor appears with subsequent sinus formation, pus, blood, and grains exuded. The sinuses may close spontaneously (Figs 2 to 4) and new sinuses may open.

Grains are small granules, which consist of compacted material of the causative agent and host matrix materials.

Actinomycetoma, progresses faster than eumycetoma, is more inflammatory and destructive with an ill-defined margin, whereas lesions of eumycetoma are encapsulated (Figs 3 and 4). In general, these lesions are usually painless even when enlarged except in late stage. Fibrosis and hyperproliferation of the dermis may occur. Advanced disease may develop deformity and disability of the affected limbs. The foot is the most common site of infection but other body parts may also be affected. (Figs 1, 2, 5, and 6).

## Etiology

Agents of mycetoma are either bacteria or fungi, and therefore the disease is classified to eumycetoma (fungal mycetoma) or actinomycetoma (bacterial mycetoma) (Table 1). The most prevalent etiologic agent worldwide is *Madurella mycetomatis*.

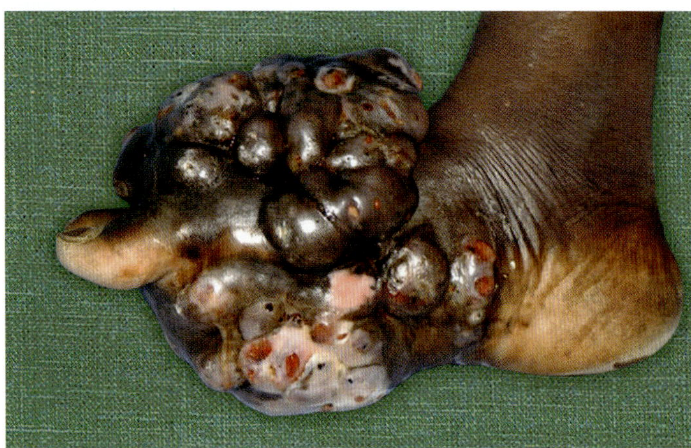

**FIG. 3:** Massive eumycetoma lesion of the foot.
*Courtesy*: Prof. Ahmed Fahal, Mycetoma Research Center, Khartoum, Sudan.

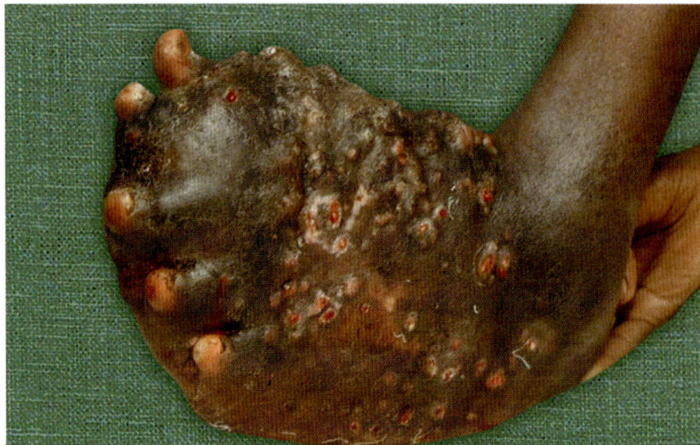

**FIG. 4:** Massive actinomycetoma lesion of the foot.
*Courtesy*: Prof. Ahmed Fahal, Mycetoma Research Center, Khartoum, Sudan.

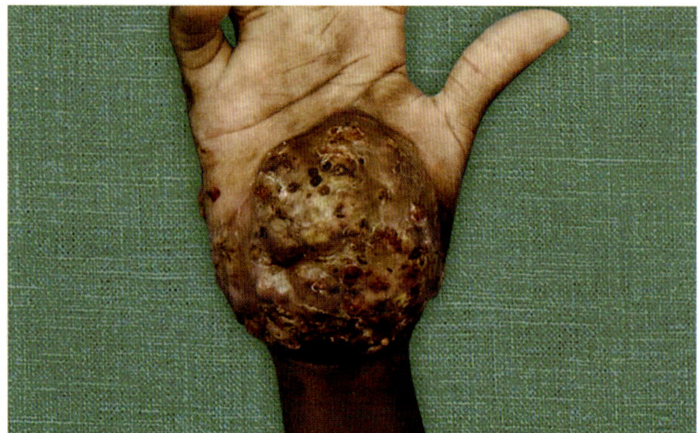

**FIG. 5:** Massive eumycetoma lesion of the hand.
*Courtesy*: Prof. Ahmed Fahal, Mycetoma Research Center, Khartoum, Sudan.

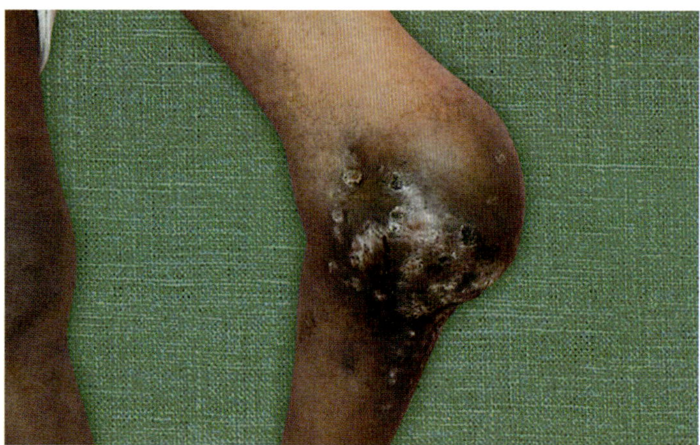

**FIG. 6:** Massive mycetoma lesion of the knee.
*Courtesy*: Prof. Ahmed Fahal, Mycetoma Research Center, Khartoum, Sudan.

**TABLE 1: Selected etiologic agents of eumycetoma and actinomycetoma**

| Eumycetoma | Color of grains |
|---|---|
| *Madurella mycetomatis* | Black |
| *Trematosphaeria grisea* | Black |
| *Falciformispora senegalensis* | Black |
| *Falciformispora tompkinsii* | Black |
| *Exophiala jeanselmei* | Black |
| *Medicopsis romeroi* | Black |
| *Biatriospora mackinnonii* | Black |
| *Scedosporium boydii* | White |
| *Aspergillus nidulans* | White |
| *Pleurostomophora ochracea* | Yellow |
| **Actinomycetoma** | **Color of grains** |
| *Actinomadura madurae* | White/yellow |
| *Streptomyces somaliensis* | Yellow/Brown |
| *Actinomadura pelletieri* | Red/Pink |
| *Nocardia brasiliensis* | White |
| *Nocardia asteroides* | White |

## Diagnosis

A fully developed mycetoma with discharging sinuses and grains is easily recognized clinically. Early disease (Fig. 1) may be confused with soft-tissue tumors (Kaposi's sarcoma, malignant melanoma, fibroma, foreign body granulomas) or other infections (chromoblastomycosis, sporotrichosis, actinomycetoma, atypical mycobacterial infection).

Diagnostic tools include cultural, cytological, histopathological, serological, and radiological techniques.

Eumycetoma grains differ in their histopathological appearance and color (Figs 7 to 9). However, many of the causative agents lack sporulation and characteristic morphological features. Sequencing of the ribosomal deoxyribonucleic acid (rDNA) spacer region is confirmatory. Recently, isothermal techniques have been introduced for rapid identification; these include loop-mediated isothermal amplification (LAMP), rolling circle amplification (RCA) and recombinase polymerase amplification.

## Management

Management is dependent on the type of the infection (eumycetoma or actinomycetoma), the causative pathogen, and the extent of the infection. Currently, actinomycetoma is treated with combination of amikacin sulfate (15 mg/kg/day) given intramuscularly in a divided dose every 12 hours for 3 weeks, and trimethoprim-sulfamethoxazole (8/40 mg/kg/day) given orally for 5 weeks. Several cycles of this combination can be administered (each cycle consisted of 3 weeks amikacin and 5 weeks trimethoprim-sulfamethoxazole) depending on the severity of the condition. Regular monitoring of renal and auditory functions is essential during these cycles. Other alternatives that can be used as second line in cases of resistance or development of side effect to the first-line therapy including, amoxicillin-clavulanic acid, rifampicin, moxifloxacin, and dapsone.

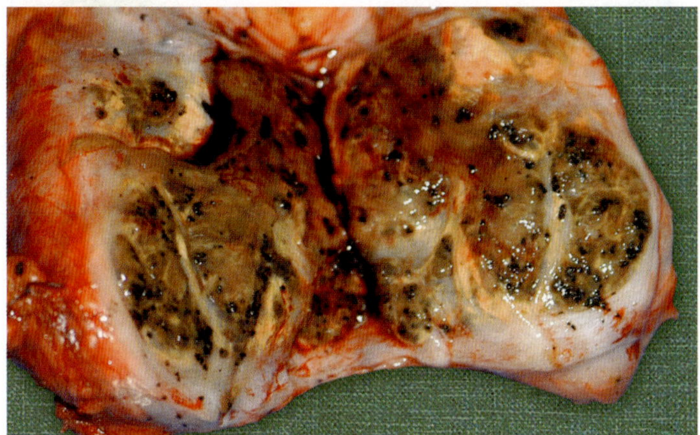

**FIG. 7:** Mycetoma with black grain in abscess.
*Courtesy*: Prof. Ahmed Fahal, Mycetoma Research Center, Khartoum, Sudan.

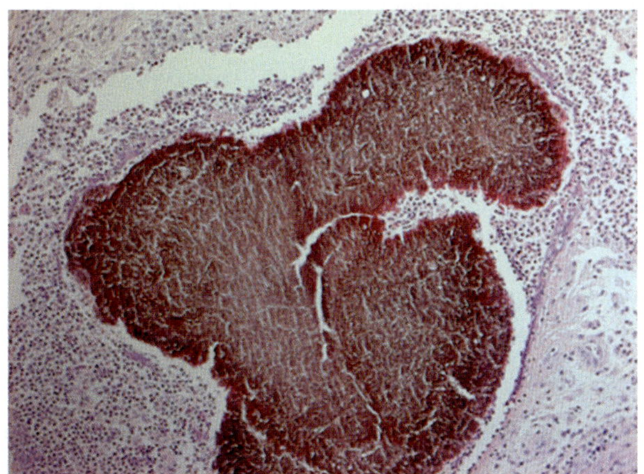

**FIG. 8:** Histology showing eumycetoma grains (*Madurella mycetomatis*).

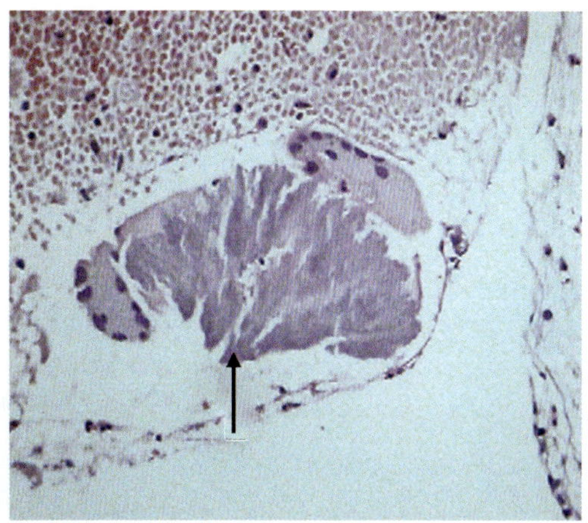

**FIG. 9:** Histology showing actinomycetoma grains (*Streptomyces somaliensis*).

The standard and first-line treatment for eumycetoma is complete surgical excision of the lesion combined with antifungal therapy, prior to and after surgery. Surgical options range from extended debulking to amputation in advance cases. Itraconazole (200–400 mg/day) is preferred antifungal drug. Due to nephrotoxic potential, the use of systemic ketoconazole is now limited. Terbinafine, posaconazole, and voriconazole have been used in few patients with variable success. The duration of antifungal therapy also depends on the extent of the infection, but in most cases, a minimum of 9–12 months is needed. Medical treatment must be continued until complete cure is achieved.

# Chromoblastomycosis

Chromoblastomycosis is a chronic infection of cutaneous and subcutaneous tissues caused by darkly pigmented fungi which form dark muriform cells (sclerotic bodies) in tissue. The disease is characterized by hyperproliferation of skin tissue. This has a worldwide distribution, particularly in hot areas, which may be semiarid or humid depending on the etiologic agent.

## Pathogenesis and Clinical Presentation

The infection is mostly post-traumatic and progresses slowly.

Clinically, it represents a polymorphous disease which can be recognized as verrucose, dry, scaly warty to cauliflower-like tumors, scaly plaques (psoriasis-like), as well as atrophic patches, and ulcerative lesions (Figs 10 and 11) (Table 2). The nodular, tumorous, and verrucous types are the most common forms. Lower limbs are the most common site but other parts of the body can be infected as well. Malignant transformation may occur.

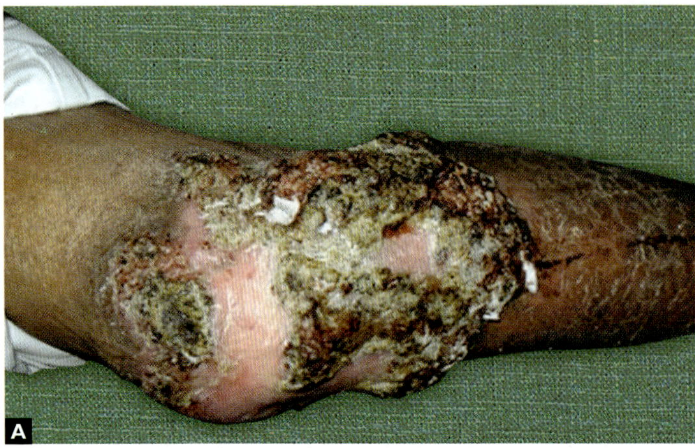


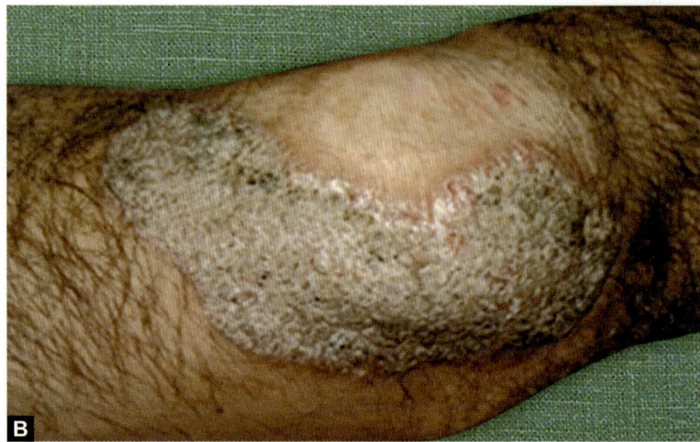


FIG. 10: Chromoblastomycosis—clinical appearance. **A,** Nodular; **B,** Verrucous.

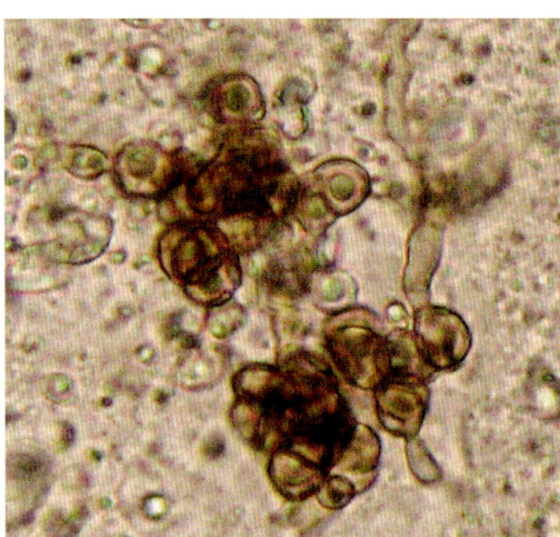

FIG. 11: Muriform cells in direct examination of patient's skin (10% KOH).

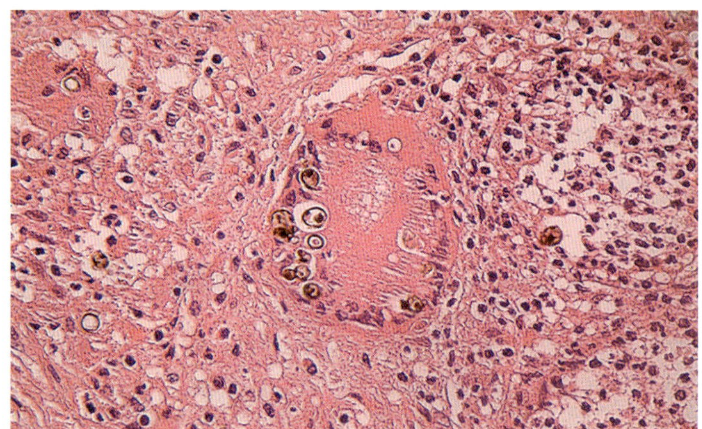

FIG. 12: Histology showing muriform cells.

**TABLE 2: Main clinical forms of chromoblastomycosis[a]**

| | |
|---|---|
| Nodular | Elevated, with smooth, verrucous or scaly surfaces, may gradually become tumorous |
| Tumorous | Tumor-like, papillomatous, and "cauliflower-like" covered with epidermal debris and crusts |
| Verrucous | Strongly hyperkeratotic |
| Cicatricial | Atrophic center (healed) with peripheral extension |
| Scaly plaque (or superficial) | Flat or slightly elevated and scaly lesions (psoriasis-like) |
| Sporotrichoid | Series of plaque-like patches |
| Lymphostatic | Extended verrucous with regional lymphostasis |

[a] Several clinical forms can coexist in the same patient.

## Etiology

All agents belong to the group of black yeasts. The most common species are *F. pedrosoi, Fonsecaea monophora,* and *Cladophialophora carrionii,* which prevalently occur in tropical rain forests and in semi-arid regions, respectively. Other prevalent species include *Phialophora verrucosa* and *Rhinocladiella aquaspersa.*

## Diagnosis

Chromoblastomycosis lesions are clinically polymorphic and differential diagnosis includes many fungal, bacterial, and other diseases, such as blastomycosis, paracoccidioidomycosis, lobomycosis, sporotrichosis, protothecosis, verrucose tuberculosis, leprosy, syphilis, leishmaniasis, squamous cell carcinoma, keratoacanthoma, lupus erythematosus, cutaneous sarcoidosis, and cutaneous granuloma. The hallmark for diagnosis is the muriform cells under direct examination of skin scrapings or histopathological specimens. Histologically, muriform cells are surrounded by a tissue reaction displaying hyperkeratosis, granulomatous response (mostly suppurative), neutrophil abscesses, and pseudoepitheliomatous hyperplasia (Fig. 12). Identification of the fungal pathogen requires culturing. The genera are distinguished morphologically, but for species identification, molecular data are required. Rapid molecular techniques have been introduced, e.g., LAMP, RCA, and multiplex ligation-dependent probe amplification (MLPA).

## Management

Recurrence rate is high. Therapeutic success depends on the etiologic agent, clinical form, and severity of the disease. Several treatment options have been used (Box 1). Treatment should be continued for several months until complete clinical resolution is ascertain.

**BOX 1 Chromoblastomycosis treatment options**

- Physical
  - Surgery
  - Local heat therapy
  - Local cold therapy (cryosurgery)
- Chemotherapy
  - Itraconazole (200–400 mg/day)
  - Posaconazole (800 mg/day)
  - Terbinafine (250–500 mg/day)
  - *Less common drugs include*: Amphotericin B and ketoconazole
- Combination therapy
  - Itraconazole + dry heat or cryosurgery
  - Terbinafine + dry heat or cryosurgery
  - Itraconazole + terbinafine
  - Itraconazole + 5-flucytosine
  - Amphotericin B + itraconazole
- Immunotherapy
  - Imiquimod

## Sporotrichosis

Sporotrichosis is a (sub)cutaneous infection that starts as a nodule which later breaks through the skin and is locally disseminated through the lymphatic system during the first 1–3 months. Lesions usually appear in a line following the regional lymphatics (Fig. 13). The disease is caused by species of the genus *Sporothrix*. The classical species *Sporothrix schenckii* has a worldwide distribution; Brazil and Eastern China are hyperendemic areas for *Sporothrix brasiliensis,* and *Sporothrix globosa*, respectively.

### Pathogenesis and Clinical Presentation

Sporotrichosis commonly affects people who work with soil and plants, such as farmers, gardeners, and agricultural workers, but also contact with cats and occasionally other animals is known to provide a transmission route for the disease. The primary lesion develops at the site of trauma, approximately 2–3 weeks after, and the clinical presentations vary according to the host immunity, the inoculum, and the virulence of the fungus. The disease is mostly localized to the skin and subcutaneous tissues and can be classified clinically into several forms (Table 3). The skin lesions are mostly ulcerative but may also be papular, nodular, or erythematous. Dissemination is commonly associated with alcohol abuse, uncontrolled diabetes or immunosuppression, especially AIDS and steroids use.

### Etiology

The main agents are the closely interrelated species *S. schenckii, S. globosa,* and *S. brasiliensis. S. schenckii* is mostly transmitted via plant material, causing isolated infections or small outbreaks. *Sporothrix globosa* causes sapronoses mainly in Eastern China. *S. brasiliensis* causes cat-borne zoonoses in Brazil. *Sporothrix luriei* is very rare and other *Sporothrix* species cause infections only exceptionally.

### Diagnosis

In the fixed form, cutaneous leishmaniasis is the main entity to be compared. Other conditions to be considered include non-tuberculous mycobacterial infections, nocardiosis, syphilis, chromoblastomycosis, blastomycosis, cryptococcosis, sarcoidosis, lymphomas, and skin cancer (Box 2). The fungus forms tear-shaped yeast cells in tissue (Fig. 14). Histological examination of biopsies may be difficult because the number of cells is often scant. Granulomatous inflammatory reactions may lead to characteristic asteroid bodies (Fig. 15). Nested polymerase chain reaction (PCR) from clinical specimen was described, but for species identification, after isolation, sequencing of the partial calmodulin is optimal. The rDNA internal transcribed space (ITS) is also useful marker.

### Management

Itraconazole (200 mg/day) is the most common applied antifungal for (lympho) cutaneous and osteoarticular cases of sporotrichosis. Treatment duration is 2–4 weeks and can be extended up to 3–6 months until complete clinical and mycological cure is achieved. Terbinafine, fluconazole, saturated solutions potassium iodide, and local hyperthermia (42–45°C, 107.6–113°F) can also be used (Table 4). Disseminated cases may require amphotericin B either alone or in combination with itraconazole as step-down therapy.

## Lobomycosis (Lacaziosis or Jorge Lobo's Disease)

Lobomycosis, also called lacaziosis, is a rare, chronic, granulomatous fungal infection of the skin and subcutaneous tissue characterized by skin nodules with a keloid-like appearance (Figs 16 and 17). The disease has been reported in humans and

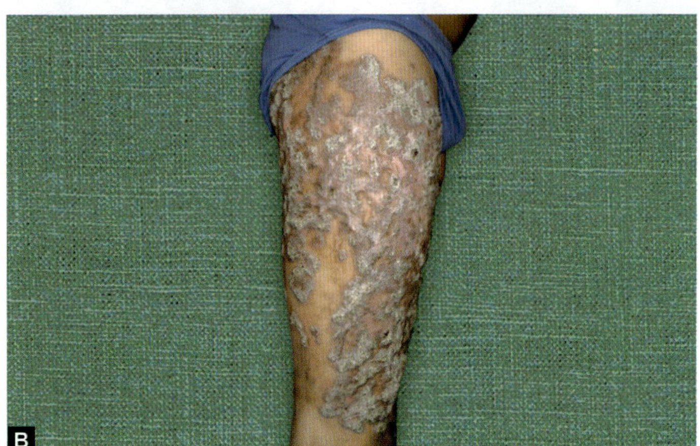

**FIG. 13:** Clinical aspect of sporotrichosis. **A,** Lymphocutaneous; **B,** Disseminated.

**TABLE 3: Clinical forms of sporotrichosis**

| | |
|---|---|
| Lymphocutaneous | Most common presentation. Series of painless nodules (rarely ulcers) develop along the lymphatic vessels, starting from the primary lesion. Regional lymph nodes are not involved and there are no systemic symptoms |
| Fixed cutaneous | Ulcers, verrucous or infiltrated plaques; small satellite lesions may be present that are confined to the inoculation site; no lymphatic involvement |
| Cutaneous disseminated | Usually starts as lymphocutaneous form, ulcerated nodules affect all the body. Associated with immunosuppression or underlying diseases |
| Pulmonary | Rare, caused by inhalation of conidia. Symptoms include common pneumonia-like symptoms with unproductive cough and fever |
| Osteoarticular | Infection of joints and bones and occurs by direct inoculation or hematogenous spread. Consists of cutaneous lesions near affected joints |
| Other forms | Ocular, meningeal, fungemia |

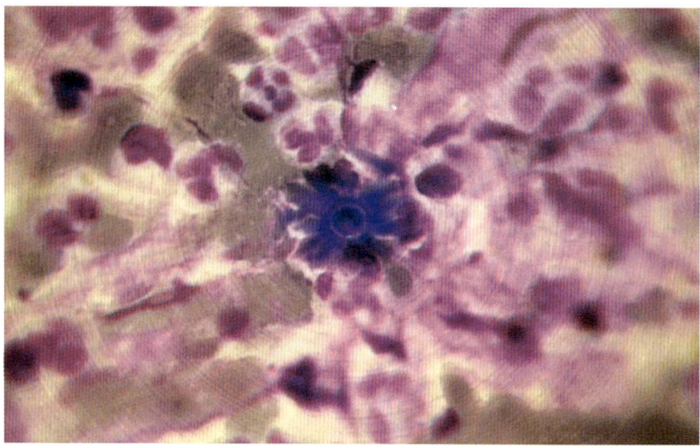

**FIG. 15:** Histology showing asteroid bodies.

**BOX 2 Conditions with sporotrichoid lymphocutaneous spreading presentation**

- Sporotrichosis
- Leishmaniasis
- Atypical *Mycobacterium* infection (*Mycobacterium marinum*)
- Metastatic squamous cell carcinoma
- Hyphomycosis
- Trichosporonosis
- Nocardiosis

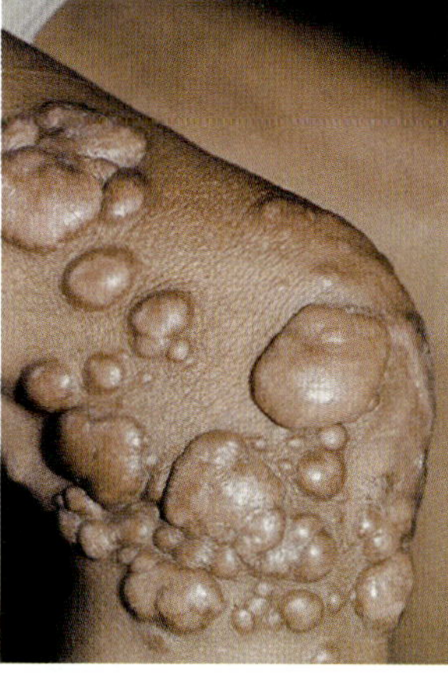

**FIG. 16:** Lobomycosis, clinical picture.

*Courtesy*: Professor Sinesio Talhari, Brazil with permission from Dr Flavio Queiroz-Telles

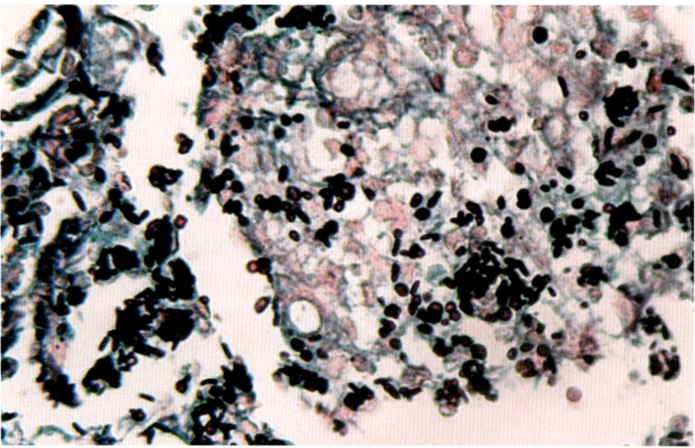

**FIG. 14:** Histology showing cigar-shaped yeast cells.

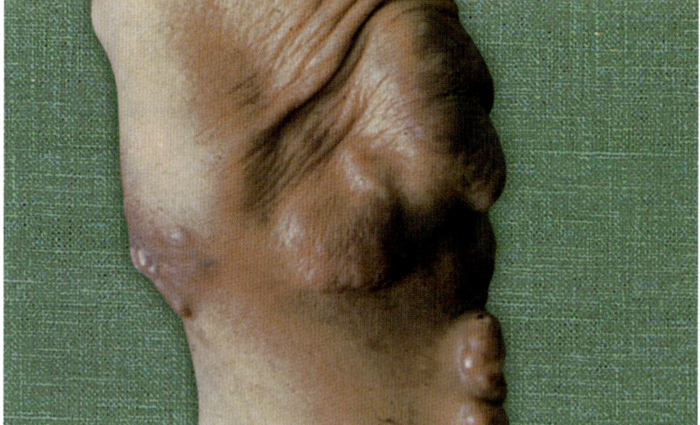

**FIG. 17:** Lobomycosis, skin nodules.

dolphins and is restricted to the South American Amazon rain forest.

## Pathogenesis and Clinical Presentation

The disease is acquired after a trauma or insect bite and begins as small, hard nodules that continue to develop over a period of many years. Lesions are pleomorphic, smooth and shiny, keloidal, verrucoid, or nodular, or present as crusty plaques and tumors. Pruritus occasionally reported and older lesions can become ulcerative. They are painless and usually found on arms, legs, face, or ears.

## Etiology

The disease is caused by a single species of a monotypic genus, *Lacazia (Loboa) loboi*, which as yet has proved unable to grow in culture.

**TABLE 4: Guidelines for the management of sporotrichosis.[a]**

| Clinical form | Preferred | Alternative |
|---|---|---|
| Lymphocutaneous and cutaneous | Itraconazole (200 mg twice/day) | Terbinafine (500 mg twice/day), fluconazole (400–800 mg/day), saturated solution potassium iodide, local hyperthermia |
| Pulmonary | Lipid amphotericin B (3–5 mg/kg/day) followed by itraconazole (200 mg twice/day) | Amphotericin B deoxycholate (0.7–1 mg/kg/day) followed by itraconazole (200 mg twice/day), surgical removal |
| Osteoarticular | Itraconazole (200 mg twice/day) | Lipid amphotericin B (3–5 mg/kg/day), amphotericin B deoxycholate (0.7–1 mg/kg/day) |
| Meningeal or disseminated | Lipid amphotericin B (5 mg/kg/day) followed by Itraconazole (200 mg twice/day) | Amphotericin B deoxycholate (0.7–1 mg/kg/day) followed by itraconazole (200 mg twice/day) |

[a]For doses in cases of children and pregnancy, please see the detailed guideline.

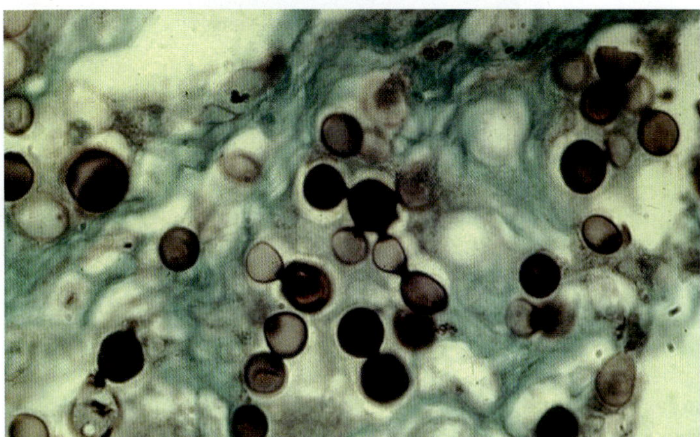

**FIG. 18:** Yeast cells of *Lacazia loboi* in direct examination of skin.
*Courtesy*: Professor Sinesio Talhari, Brazil with permission from Dr Flavio Queiroz-Telles.

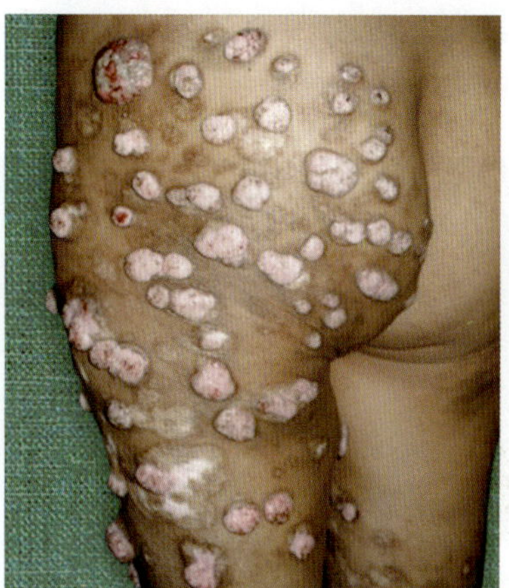

**FIG. 19:** Nodular disseminated phaeohyphomycosis.

## Diagnosis

Differential diagnosis of lobomycosis includes leishmaniasis, lepromatous leprosy, chromoblastomycosis, paracoccidioidomycosis, sporotrichosis, keloids, and malignant tumors. Clinical features and geographic location combined with laboratory findings are important. In tissue, the fungus has a characteristic, darkly pigmented, spheroidal to lemon-shape yeast-like morphology (Fig. 18) with cells that are often arranged in chains which may be branched.

## Management

Management of lobomycosis is difficult and relapses are common. The most successful treatment consists of surgical excision of the lesion, or cryosurgery. Antifungal agents appear to be less effective; however, posaconazole (400 mg, 2 times/day), itraconazole (100 mg/day) combined with clofazimine (100-200 mg/day) have been used, with some success.

## Phaeohyphomycosis

Fungal infections caused by darkly pigmented, melanized fungi producing hyphal elements or yeast-like cells in tissue are united under the umbrella term phaeohyphomycoses. Clinical presentations can be superficial (colonization), cutaneous or subcutaneous after traumatic implantation and the lesions may remain localized or slowly spread to the adjacent tissue and can show a nodule or a cystic form (Fig. 19). Epidermal hyperplasia and acanthosis may occur in initial phase of the cutaneous form which then develop to suppurative or sarcoid-like granulomas.

This is seen in both immunocompromised as well as in apparently healthy individuals. Disseminated infections are less frequent and mostly occur in severely compromised patients and present as dry secondary lesions, which often are nodular in appearance. Small number of fungal species belonging to the order *Chaetothyriales* (genera *Rhinocladiella, Exophiala, Cladophialophora,* and *Veronaea*) have been associated with the disseminated form of the disease. Members of *Pleosporales* (*Curvularia, Alternaria, Exserohilum, Bipolaris*) are associated with sub (cutaneous) or rarely disseminated forms in hosts with impaired innate immunity.

Diagnosis is by detection of fungal material (dark pigmented hyphae or yeast-like cells) in aspirate or biopsy from the infected site and by culturing (Fig. 20). Localized subcutaneous nodules are treated with surgery or other alternatives like cryotherapy, laser, heat, and photodynamic therapy. Multiple subcutaneous nodules are treatment with itraconazole (400 mg/day) or voriconazole (400 mg/day) is recommended.

## Hyalohyphomycosis

This term stands for a wide spectrum of fungal infections characterized by presence of hyaline hyphae in the infected tissue. Infection can be superficial or sub(cutaneous), but also disseminated infections with secondary cutaneous lesions occur (Fig. 21). Skin lesions are painful and usually indurated erythematous macula or papula with central area of necrosis.

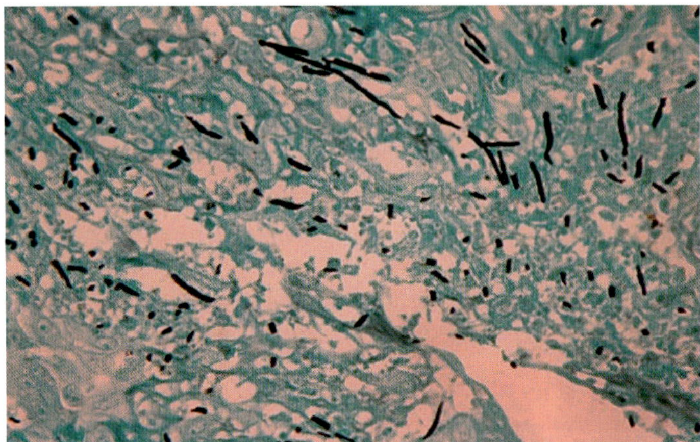

FIG. 20: Histology showing fungal elements in tissue.

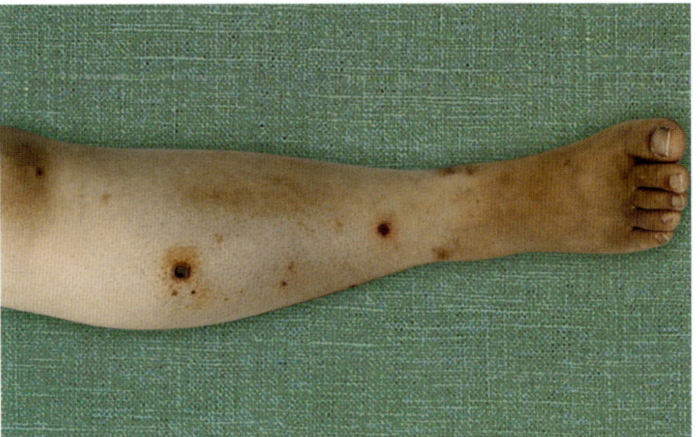

FIG. 21: Skin manifestation of disseminated *Fusarium* infection.

Patients with prolonged neutropenia, corticosteroid therapy, and human immunodeficiency virus (HIV) are at risk. The routes of entry are either through the skin following trauma or by inhalation. Causative agents belong to highly diverse groups of saprobes in genera, such as *Fusarium*, *Scedosporium*, *Scopulariopsis*, and *Acremonium*.

Diagnostic investigations include imaging (pulmonary) and isolation of the causative pathogen from the infected site (skin, sinuses, lungs, blood, and other parts). Identification of the clinical isolates is important and this can be achieved by molecular methods like multilocus sequence analysis or with the recently developed protein analysis matrix-assisted laser desorption ionization time-of-flight mass spectrometry. Species of *Fusarium* and *Scedosporium* are known to be resistant toward numerous antifungal agents. First-line treatment for systemic hyalohyphomycosis is voriconazole (200 mg twice a day); other treatment options can be used according to the clinical presentations and causative pathogen.

## SECONDARY CUTANEOUS INFECTIONS

### Blastomycosis

Blastomycosis is endemic in the Great Lake regions of North America and primarily affects the lungs. With hematogenous, spread infection can disseminate to other body sites, such as skin (Fig. 22), bones, genitourinary, and CNS.

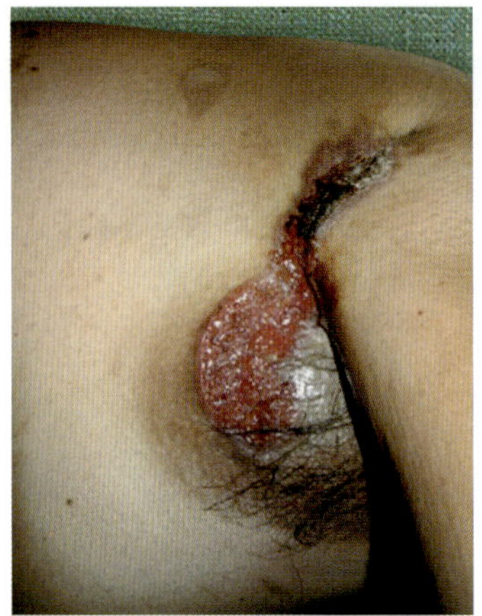

FIG. 22: Blastomycosis skin manifestation.

#### Pathogenesis and Clinical Presentation

Infection is mostly acquired by inhalation. Virulence ranges from subclinical to fatal disseminated infection. Most cases are asymptomatic while some may present with flu-like illness with reproductive cough, fever, myalgia, and chest pain. Skin lesions, commonly present over face, neck, and extremities present as papules, pustules, verrucous or ulcerative lesions, and subcutaneous nodules. Also, indolent abscesses and erythematous areas of induration have been reported. Other manifestations include osseous, CNS, and genitourinary involvement.

#### Etiology

The disease is caused by the dimorphic fungus *Blastomyces dermatitidis*. Dogs may be carriers of the disease.

#### Diagnosis

Clinically, the disease can be confused with a wide range of fungal, bacterial, or neoplastic diseases. Differential diagnosis of cutaneous manifestations are infections by dimorphic fungi, leishmaniasis, nocardiosis, cutaneous tuberculosis, syphilis, giant keratoacanthoma, lymphoma, basal and squamous cell carcinoma. Specific diagnosis is based on detection of the yeast form of *B. dermatitidis* in tissue, presenting large yeast cells with unipolar budding at a broad base (Fig. 23). Direct detection of *B. dermatitidis* from clinical sample can be achieved by real-time PCR assay. Identification after culture should be confirmed by sequencing of the rDNA-ITS region, as sporulation may be poor and uncharacteristic. Antigen detection is widely used.

#### Management

Mild-to-moderate forms of the disease can be managed with itraconazole, while severe, disseminated and CNS infections require amphotericin B (Table 5).

### Paracoccidioidomycosis

Paracoccidioidomycosis is a systemic fungal infection caused by the two currently recognized species of the thermally dimorphic genus *Paracoccidioides*. Paracoccidioidomycosis is geographically confined to South and Central America.

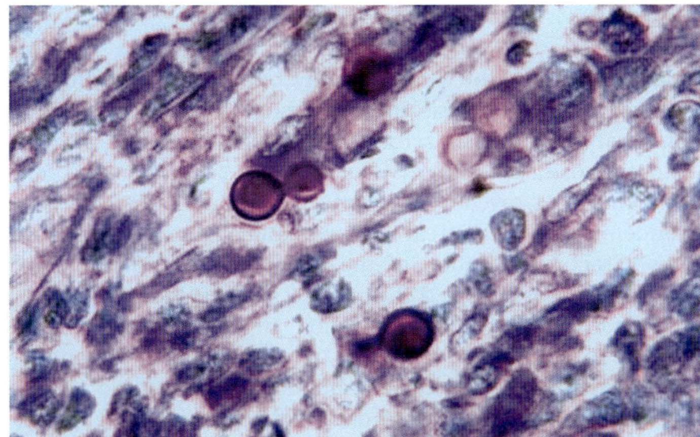

**FIG. 23:** Histology showing unipolar budding yeast of *Blastomyces dermatitidis*.

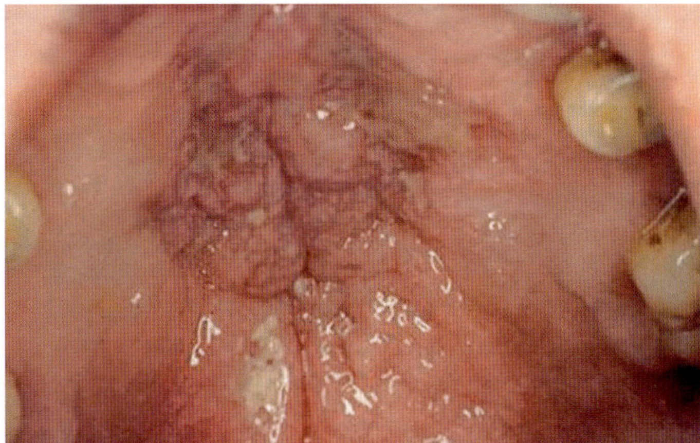

**FIG. 24:** Paracoccidioidomycosis involving oral mucosa.
*Courtesy:* Dr Antonio Guzmán-Fawcett, Bolivia.

**TABLE 5: Guidelines for the management of blastomycosis[a]**

| Clinical form | Preferred |
|---|---|
| Mild-to-moderate pulmonary or disseminated | Itraconazole (200 mg once or twice/day) for 6–12 months |
| Moderately severe-to-severe pulmonary or disseminated | Amphotericin B lipid complex (3–5 mg/kg/day), or amphotericin B deoxycholate (0.7–1 mg/kg/day) for 1–2 weeks, followed by itraconazole (200 mg/twice/day) for 6–12 months |
| Central nervous system | Amphotericin B lipid (5 mg/kg/day) for 4–6 weeks, then oral azole for at least 1 year |

[a]For doses in children and pregnant women, please see the guideline.

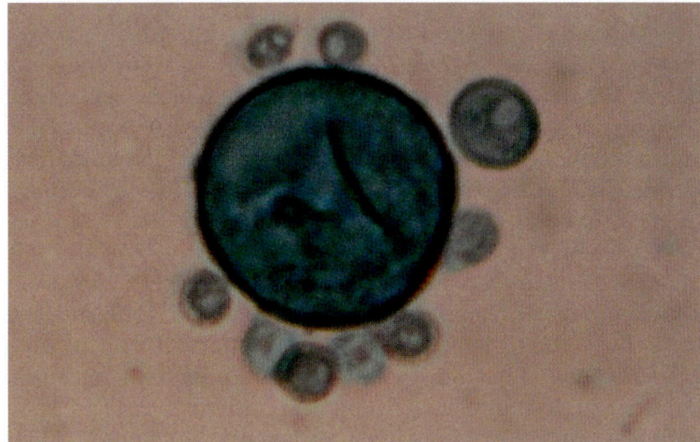

**FIG. 25:** Steering wheel appearance of *Paracoccidioides* in direct microscopic examination.
*Courtesy:* Dr Fernando Gomez-Daza, Venezuela.

## Pathogenesis and Clinical Presentation

Infection is acquired through inhalation of *Paracoccidioides* propagules, usually from soil dust in disturbed environments. Pulmonary infections are usually subclinical. This can resolve spontaneously, remain latent in the lung or give rise to symptomatic infection after many years.

The disease starts as an asymptomatic pulmonary infection which can disseminate to the oral and nasal mucosa, lymphatics, skin, and other organs (Fig. 24). Clinical manifestations are acute, subacute, or chronic. The acute form is rapidly progressive and is mostly seen in patients under the age of 30 years of poor socioeconomic status and involves lymph nodes, liver, spleen, bone marrow, and skin. The chronic form usually occurs in adults during the fourth decade of age and is characterized by involvement of oral and respiratory mucosa. Cutaneous lesions present as crusted papules, ulcers, nodules or plaque-like lesions and are particularly found on the face. Mucosal lesions are painful and can become ulcerative.

## Etiology

Two dimorphic species have been reported, *Paracoccidioides brasiliensis* and *Paracoccidioides lutzii*.

## Diagnosis

Differential diagnosis of the disease is aided by anamnesis and by clinical and radiologic findings and includes mucocutaneous leishmaniasis, coccidioidomycosis, histoplasmosis, blastomycosis, tuberculosis, syphilis, squamous cell carcinoma, and lymphoma. Diagnosis is confirmed by direct observation of characteristic "steering wheels", which are thick-walled yeast cells with multiple, narrow-based budding cells (Fig. 25). Histopathology is extremely useful and serological tools have been used but differ between the species. Final identification is made by isolation of the pathogen and sequencing the rDNA spacer region.

## Management

Itraconazole (200 mg/day) has proven to be most effective in mild and moderate forms of the disease. For severe forms of paracoccidioidomycosis, amphotericin B (0.5–1.0 mg/kg/day or in alternate days) is recommended. Sulfamethoxazole combined with trimethoprim have been used as alternatives.

# Coccidioidomycosis (Valley Fever)

Coccidioidomycosis generally causes mild lung infection and is self-limiting, but may progress to chronic pulmonary and disseminated disease involving skin and subcutaneous tissue, bone, meninges and visceral organs (Fig. 26). Endemic areas are Southwestern United States, Northwestern Mexico, and arid climate zones of Central and South America.

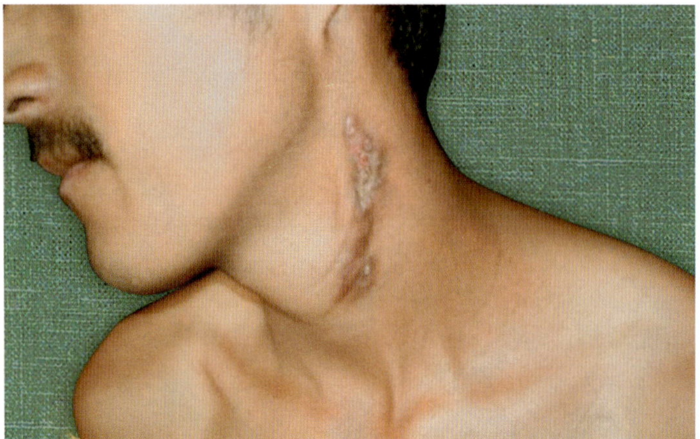

FIG. 26: Coccidioidomycosis skin manifestation.

## Pathogenesis and Clinical Presentation

Infection after inhalation of fungal particles from the environment, mostly in the form of soil dust derived from endemic, desert-like areas leads to formation of swollen fungal cells which become compartmented and ultimately release endospores which enhance hematogenous or lymphatic dissemination. Disease is mostly asymptomatic or with flu-like symptoms. After resolution, the fungus goes into dormancy and may be endogenously reactivated and disseminate to multiple organs. Disseminated and fulminant disease is seen in certain ethnic groups, pregnant women, and immunocompromised individuals. Skin manifestations are polymorphic and include granulomatous, ulcerative lesions, nodules, papules, pustules, or verrucous lesions usually found near the lymph node areas. In patients with acute pulmonary infection, erythematous macular rash-like erythema nodosum, erythema multiforme or swollen lymph nodes may appear. Primary cutaneous infection due to direct skin inoculation is rare and presents as an ulcerated nodule which can evolve into verrucous lesions and can spread to regional lymph nodes.

## Etiology

Two dimorphic environmental pathogens have been described: *Coccidioides immitis*, which is limited to Southwestern United States (California), and *Coccidioides posadasii*, which is found in semi-arid climate zones of the United States and the remainder of the American continent.

## Diagnosis

Cutaneous lesions of coccidioidomycosis are nonspecific and the differential diagnosis includes many conditions, such as pulmonary tuberculosis, scrofuloderma, paracoccidioidomycosis histoplasmosis, blastomycosis, squamous cell carcinoma, and nontuberculous mycobacterial infections. Anamnesis with visits to endemic desert-like areas is often helpful. Laboratory diagnosis is by direct visualization of the characteristic spherules with endospores in tissue (Fig. 27). For direct and specific identification of *Coccidioides*, *in-situ* hybridization and PCR-based methods have been employed. Culture is characteristically expanding, white, cottony, and produces abundant enteroarthric conidia (Fig. 28). Antibody and antigen detection are helpful for diagnosis. Species identification can routinely be achieved by rDNA-ITS sequencing, although PCR amplification may be difficult.

## Management

The management varies according to the extent of the disease and the patient condition.

Patients with primary infection normally do not require antifungal therapy. For patients with chronic or disseminated forms, the antifungal agents amphotericin B (doses are according to the formulation), itraconazole (200 mg/twice a day), fluconazole (400–800 mg/day), posaconazole (400 mg/day), and voriconazole (200–600 mg/day) have been used.

# Histoplasmosis

Histoplasmosis is a systemic infection caused by the dimorphic fungus *Histoplasma capsulatum*. It is a worldwide disease, but is mostly found in local pockets in the Americas, Africa, Asia, and Australia. Hyperendemicity in the United States is noted in the state of Ohio and in the Mississippi River valley.

## Pathogenesis and Clinical Feature

The infection starts by inhalation of fungal spores from soil contaminated with bat or bird droppings. Mostly, disturbance of sheltered environments are concerned, such as unused attics frequented by birds, or caves with bat guano. In most of the patients, infection is asymptomatic or mild but it can develop into an acute, chronic pneumonia, or may disseminate (Table 6). Skin manifestations, such as erythema nodosum and multiforme

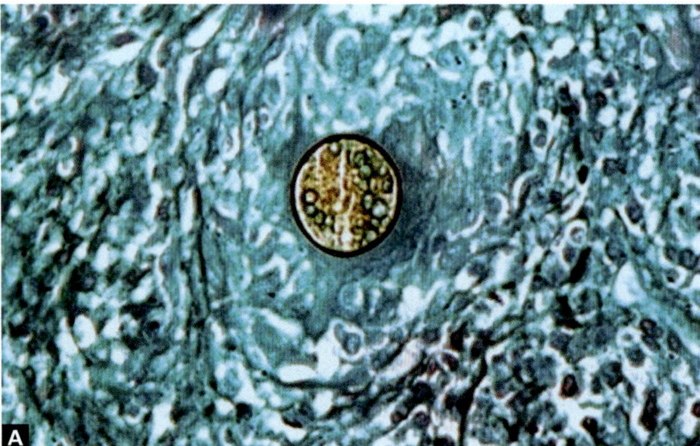


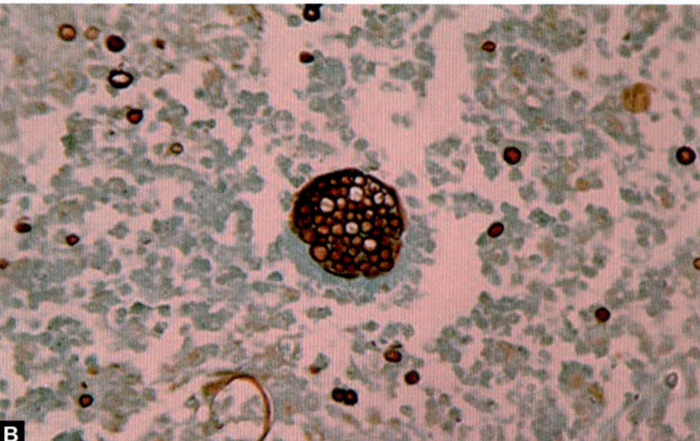


FIG. 27: **A,** Single spherule (grocott, 40x); **B,** Spherules with multiple endospores (grocott, 40x).

may occur as a result of the immune response to the pathogen in the acute phase of the disease while pustules, nodules, or plaques are associated with dissemination of the disease (Fig. 29). Most of cutaneous cases are associated with HIV infection and acquired immune deficiency syndrome and habitually affect the face and chest. In cases of dissemination, lesions may develop in the oral cavity involving the tongue, palate, buccal mucosa, and the pharynx. Primary cutaneous infection is rare.

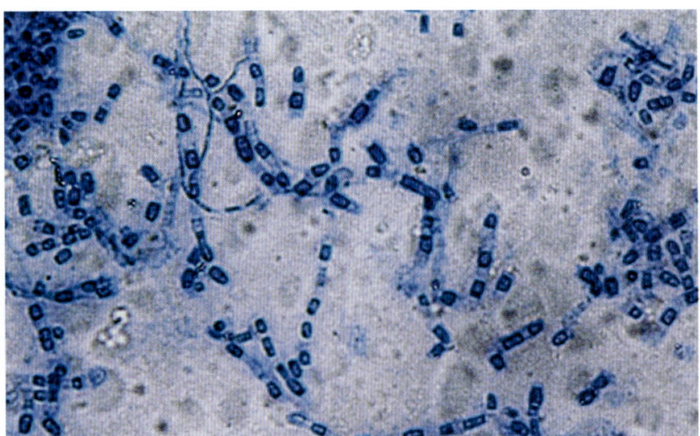

**FIG. 28:** *Coccidioides* arthroconidia.

**TABLE 6: Clinical manifestations of histoplasmosis**

| | |
|---|---|
| Acute and subacute pulmonary histoplasmosis | Self-limited; symptoms are dry cough, fever, chest pain, and fatigue; erythema nodosum and erythema multiforme |
| Chronic cavitary pulmonary histoplasmosis | Productive cough, night sweats, anorexia, weight loss, and fatigue (lung cavitation) |
| Progressive disseminated histoplasmosis | Extrapulmonary dissemination to central nervous system, skin, liver, and spleen. Symptoms are fever, weight loss, lymphadenopathy, hepatosplenomegaly, skin and mucosal lesions, and meningitis |
| Mediastinitis | Mediastinal granuloma can progress to fibrosing mediastinitis |

## Etiology

The thermodimorphic pathogen *Histoplasma capsulatum* is filamentous in culture with small, hyaline conidia in addition to large, brown, tuberculate conidia, while at 37°C, a yeast-like form is produced. This is the invasive form which develops inside the host's macrophages. An African variety *H. capsulatum* var. *duboisii* is known which produces large, broad-based budding cells.

## Diagnosis

Clinically, there are no specific symptoms for histoplasmosis and differential diagnosis includes a wide spectrum of conditions depending on the extent of the disease, including tuberculosis, paracoccidioidomycosis, coccidioidomycosis, blastomycosis, cryptococcosis, syphilis, squamous cell carcinoma, nontuberculous mycobacterial infections, and talaromycosis. Histopathology provides tentative diagnosis by demonstration of intracellular yeast cells inside macrophages (Fig. 30). The *Histoplasma capsulatum var. duboisii* has broad-based budding cells. Culture provides identification by characteristic morphology of the fungus. Rapid tools including serology, antigen detection and PCR-based techniques are in current use.

## Management

Individuals with mild forms of the disease generally do not require antifungal treatment, but in cases of severe, chronic, and disseminated forms, antifungal agents are needed. The most commonly used drugs are amphotericin B and itraconazole (Table 7).

# Talaromycosis (formerly Penicilliosis)

Talaromycosis is disseminated infection caused by the thermodimorphic fungus *Talaromyces (Penicillium) marneffei*. The disease is endemic in Southeast Asia and mostly affects patients with impaired cellular immunity; the infection is considered to be an AIDS-defining illness (Fig. 31). In endemic areas in Southern China, infection in immunocompetent individuals has been reported.

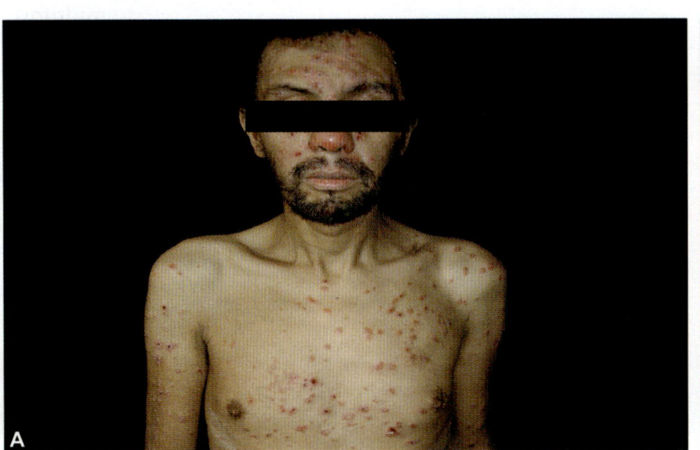

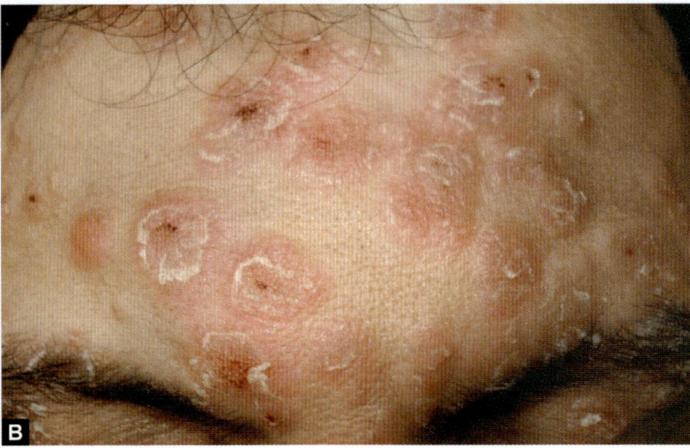

**FIG. 29:** **A,** Extensive papular lesions in patients with AIDS; **B,** Close-up of papular lesions.

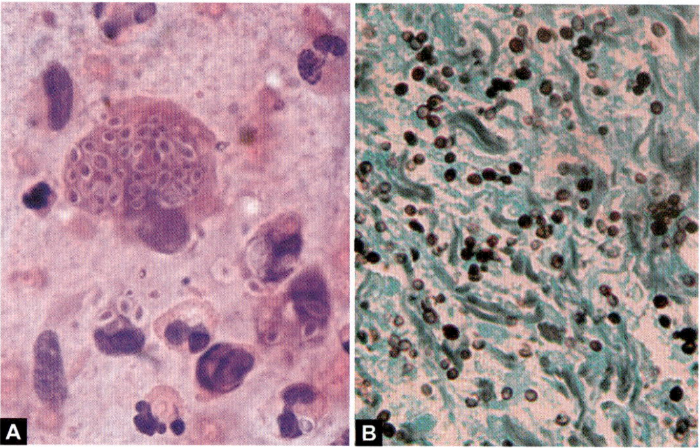


**FIG. 30: A,** Intracellular yeast of Polymorphonuclear (H&E, 100x); **B,** Multiple yeasts (grocott, 100x).

**TABLE 7: Guidelines for the management of histoplasmosis[a]**

| | |
|---|---|
| Acute pulmonary histoplasmosis | • Amphotericin B lipid (3.0–5.0 mg/kg daily) or amphotericin B deoxycholate (0.7–1.0 mg/kg daily) for 1–2 weeks, followed by itraconazole (200 mg twice daily for 12 weeks)<br>• Methylprednisolone (0.5–1.0 mg/kg daily intravenously for 1–2 weeks) |
| Chronic cavitary pulmonary histoplasmosis | Itraconazole (200 mg once or twice daily for 12 months) |
| Progressive disseminated histoplasmosis | Liposomal amphotericin B (3.0 mg/kg daily) or amphotericin B lipid (5.0 mg/kg daily) 1–2 weeks, followed by itraconazole (200 mg twice daily for at least 12 months) |

[a]In cases of mild-to-moderate pulmonary histoplasmosis, if symptoms <4 weeks, no treatment required, if the symptoms persist, itraconazole is recommended (200 mg once or twice daily for 6–12 weeks)

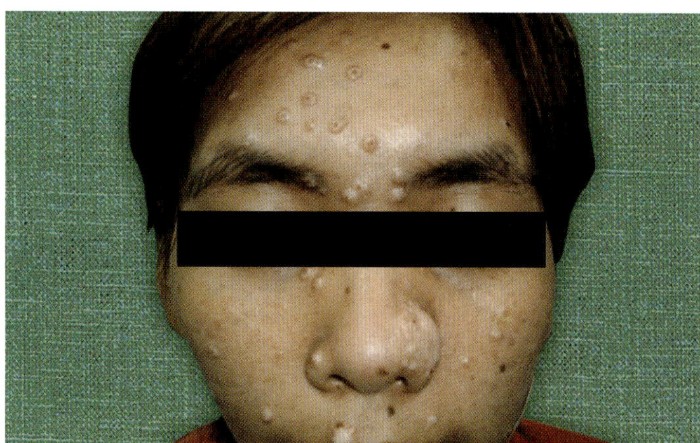

**FIG. 31:** HIV patient with disseminated talaromycosis.
*Courtesy*: Dr Rataporn Ungpakorn, Thailand.

## Pathogenesis and Clinical Presentation

*Talaromyces marneffei* is acquired by inhalation of fungal propagules. The disease presents as a subacute febrile illness with skin manifestations. The natural habitat of the fungus is in association with bamboo rats, which often have fungal cells in their pulmonary tissue but remain otherwise asymptomatic. The fungus may be dormant in the human host, but in case of impairment of the cellular immune system, such as with HIV coinfection, dissemination occurs. Clinical features of disseminated talaromycosis include fever, weight loss, lymphadenopathy, hepatomegaly, and skin lesions. The secondary cutaneous lesions are commonly seen on face, trunk and extremities presenting as papules, pustules, acneiform ulcers, subcutaneous abscesses, or molluscum contagiosum-like nodules (Fig. 32).

## Etiology

The single fungus *T. marneffei*, formerly classified in *Penicillium*.

## Diagnosis

Presence of oval to elongated yeast-like cells (arthroconidia) inside macrophages are characteristic for *T. marneffei* (Figs 33 and 34). The thermophilic form grows slowly with hyphae which fall apart into separate cells; *in vitro* this can be seen as a clear central septum in some of the "yeast cells" and is a characteristic feature of *T. marneffei*. Definitive diagnosis is made by culture, which provides a green and later yellow, powdery colony with penicillium-like morphology and exuding a brick-red pigment into the agar. Colonies of relatives of this species may show similar

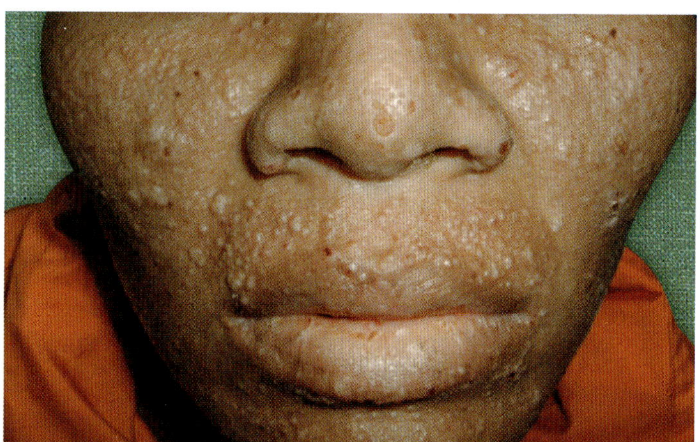

**FIG. 32:** Patient with disseminated talaromycosis.
*Courtesy*: Dr Rataporn Ungpakorn, Thailand.

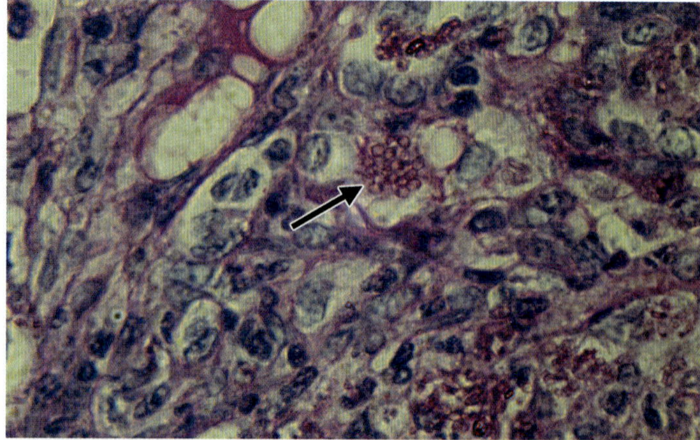

**FIG. 33:** Yeast-like cells of *Talaromyces marneffei*.
*Courtesy*: Professor Xi Liyan, China, with permission from Dr Peiying Feng.

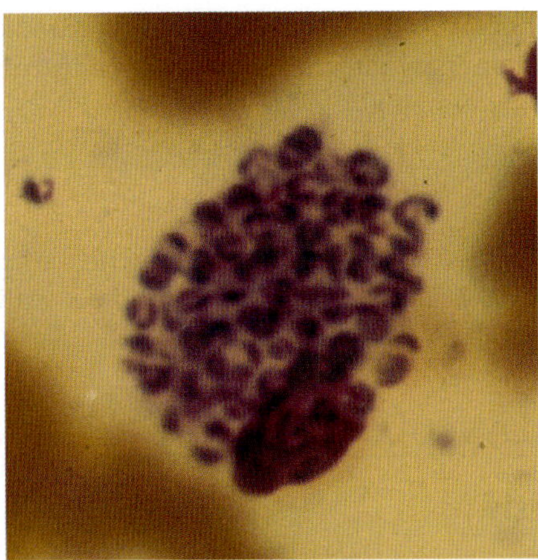

FIG. 34: Yeast-like cells of *Talaromyces marneffei* inside the macrophages.
*Courtesy*: Dr Rataporn Ungpakorn, Thailand.

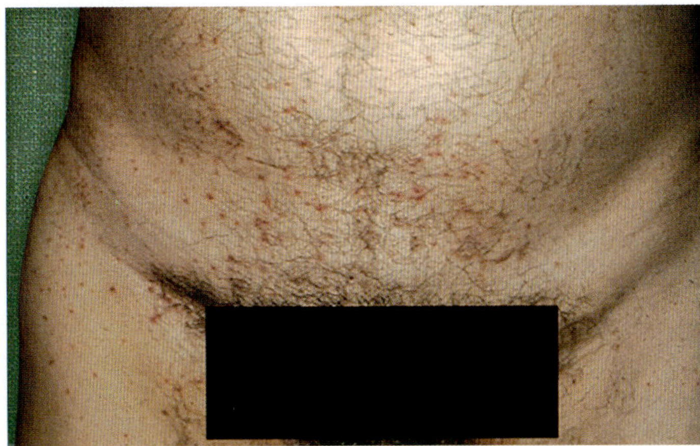

FIG. 35: Skin manifestation of disseminated candidiasis.

**TABLE 8. Antifungals used for treatment of *Talaromyces marneffei* infection**

| | |
|---|---|
| Mild infection | Itraconazole (200–400 mg/day), or voriconazole 400 mg twice a day on day 1 then reduce the dose to 200 mg twice daily for 12 weeks |
| Severe | Amphotericin B liposomal, 3–5 mg/kg/day intravenously for 2 weeks, followed by oral itraconazole, 200–400 mg/day for a subsequent duration of 6–10 weeks. Or intravenous voriconazole, 6 mg/kg every 12 hours on day 1 and then 4 mg/kg every 12 hours for a minimum of 3 days, followed by oral voriconazole, 200 mg twice daily for 12 weeks |

pigmentation but are unable to produce an arthroconidial form at 37°C. Molecular methods based on PCR for direct amplification of specific target gene have been described.

## Management

Itraconazole, amphotericin B, and voriconazole are the most commonly used antifungals for treatment of talaromycosis (Table 8). For prophylaxis, itraconazole and fluconazole has been used in some endemic areas.

# Disseminated and Systemic Candidiasis

Candidiasis is an opportunistic fungal infection caused by members of the genus *Candida. Candida* species are present as commensals on skin, intestinal tract, and female genitalia. Infection occurs as a result of break of cutaneous barriers or as a result of immunosuppression, debilitating diseases, drugs, or genetic disorders. The infection is either superficial or systemic invasive. Superficial candidiases comprise oropharyngeal, vulvovaginal, cutaneous infection, or paronychia and onychomycosis. *Candida* is able to colonize and invade internal organs; intra-abdominal colonization is common in high-risk patients. Dissemination through bloodstream leads to candidemia (blood stream infection) and is a common catheter-related disease. Secondary cutaneous manifestations as a result of systemic candidiasis have been reported in immunocompromised patient and present as macules, papules, or nodules (Fig. 35). Specific immunological and genetic disorders were recently identified as predisposing for or increasing susceptibility to candidiasis. These include mutation and abnormalities in signal transducer and activator of transcription (*STAT1*) and (*STAT3*), caspase recruitment domain-containing protein *CARD9*, myeloid differentiation factor (*MyD88*), mannose-binding lectin, and dectin-1 abnormalities. Patients with such immunological abnormalities or endocrinological disorders may develop recurrent or persistent form of the disease known as chronic mucocutaneous candidiasis (CMC). Infants with CMC often present with diaper dermatitis, oral thrush, and extensive skin and nail lesion.

## Etiology

Candida species concerned are particularly *Candida albicans, Candida tropicalis, Candida glabrata, Candida guilliermondii, Candida krusei,* and other ascomycetous yeasts currently classified in *Candida.*

## Diagnosis

Clinical data combined with direct observation, isolation, and identification of the pathogen from clinical specimen are main diagnostic. Molecular techniques (routinely with rDNA-ITS) and antigen detection for rapid diagnosis were reported.

## Management

Treatment depends on the clinical presentation. Antifungals include azoles; fluconazole 400–800 mg or voriconazole 6/3 mg/kg/day, echinocandins; anidulafungin 200/100 mg or caspofungin 70/50 mg or micafungin 100 mg; amphotericin B liposomal 3 mg/kg. For more details on doses and alternatives, please see the guideline (suggested reading 16, 55).

# Cryptococcosis

Cryptococcosis is a global opportunistic fungal infection caused by the encapsulated yeast *Cryptococcus.* Systemic disease of the CNS is common in patients with impaired cell-mediated immunity and considered as life-threatening infection in AIDS patients. Meninges are the most common sites of infection for *Cryptococcus neoformans*, while *Cryptococcus gattii* is predominantly found in the brain of immunocompetent individuals. Infection acquired via inhalation and starts as pulmonary symptoms with cough, fever, and chest pain. Afterward, dissemination can occur to the CNS leading to meningitis. Cutaneous cryptococcosis can occur as a result of dissemination in immunocompromised patients or in rare cases as primary infection in immunocompetent individuals. Skin lesions are polymorphic resembling molluscum contagious and can present as papules, pustules, plaques, ulcers, subcutaneous masses, cellulitis, or acneiform (Fig. 36).

### Etiology

Serotypes and varieties of *C. neoformans* and *C. gattii* are the prevalent agents of two forms of cryptococcosis described above. Other rare species were reported.

### Diagnosis

Diagnosis is by detection and isolation of the etiologic agent from tissue biopsies or body fluids. In direct microscopy of cerebrospinal fluid (stained by India ink) or histopathology, demonstration of yeast cells surrounded by a wide gelatinous capsule is suggestive for cryptococcosis by *C. neoformans* or *C. gattii* (Fig. 37). The two species differ by physiological parameters.

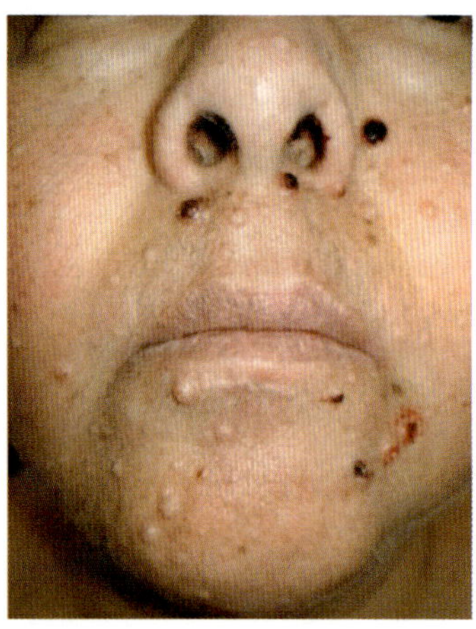

**FIG. 36:** Disseminated cryptococcosis with secondary cutaneous lesions.

Other investigations for disseminated cryptococcosis include radiology and antigen detection. Agents of cutaneous lesions are identified by sequencing.

### Management

Treatment of disseminated cases is with amphotericin B deoxycholate (0.7–1.0 mg/kg/day) combined with flucytosine (100 mg/kg/day) as first-line therapy.

## MISCELLANEOUS INFECTIONS

### Aspergillosis

Aspergillosis covers a wide range of diseases caused by species of the genus *Aspergillus*. Pulmonary aspergillosis is the most common clinical form and occurs in patients with severe immunodeficiency commonly in patient with hematologic malignancy or hematopoietic stem cell transplant. Cutaneous aspergillosis is a rare condition and occurs as a manifestation of disseminated infection or as a primary infection after a trauma, affected patients regularly have severe neutropenia. Lesions may present as erythematous papules, ulcerative nodules, macules, plaques, or hemorrhagic bullae with progressive central necrosis (Fig. 38). Skin biopsy for microbiology and histopathology is required for diagnosis and detection of hyaline, dichotomously branched septate hyphae which is suggestive for *Aspergillus* (Fig. 39) or another hyaline fungus, to be identified by culture and sequencing. *Aspergillus fumigatus* and *Aspergillus flavus* are the most common reported species. The recommended treatment of invasive aspergillosis is voriconazole (6 mg/kg/12h intravenously for 1 day, reduced to 4 mg/kg) or oral dosage (200 mg every 12 h). For primary cutaneous aspergillosis, itraconazole can be used as alternative and if required, surgical debridement or wide margin surgical resection.

### Mucormycosis (Zygomycosis)

Mucormycoses are infections caused by a group of fast-growing fungi belonging to the order Mucorales, which were previously classified under the zygomycetes. In patients with severe malignant hematological disorders or uncontrolled diabetes mellitus, especially diabetic ketoacidosis, the disease

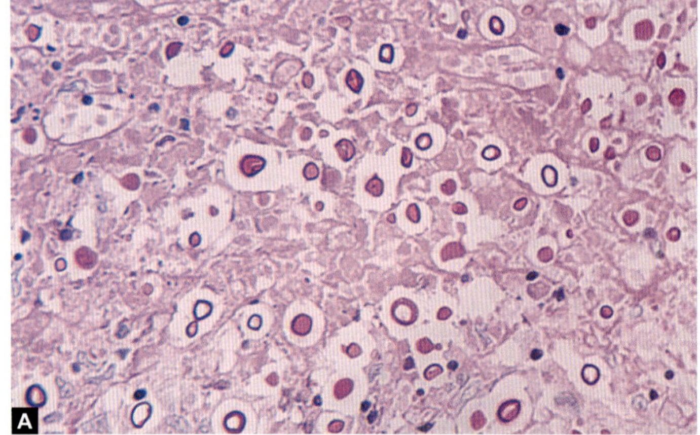


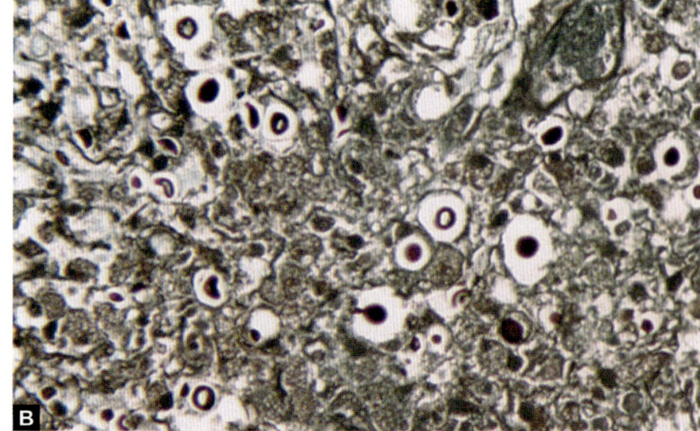


**FIG. 37:** **A,** Multiple yeasts with capsule halo (PAS, 100x); **B,** Multiple yeast with capsule (grocott, 100x).

is acute and mostly fatal, with rhinocerebral, pulmonary, or gastrointestinal presentations. Infections with Mucorales are associated with angioinvasion, thrombosis, and necrosis. Cutaneous mucormycosis can start in two ways—primary and secondary cutaneous form. Primary cutaneous form occurs after severe trauma or contamination of large open wounds or burns. Necrotic lesions with erythema and induration are typical for mucormycosis (Fig. 40A). Secondary cutaneous form constitutes the rhinocerebral form spreading to the skin, showing palpebral fistulae and developing necrotic lesions (Fig. 40B). The causative species present as broad branched aseptate hyphal elements in the infected tissue (Fig. 41). When the causative species belonged to the order *Entomophthorales*, the infection is called entomophthoramycosis. Two clinical forms of entomophthoramycosis can be recognized and mostly seen in tropical areas; conidiobolomycosis is an infection of mostly mucocutaneous sites caused by *Conidiobolus* species also called (rhinoentomophthoromycoses), basidiobolomycosis is cutaneous or subcutaneous infections caused by *Basidiobolus* species. Unlike Mucorales, Entomophthorales infects primarily immunocompetent individuals and rarely associates with angioinvasion.

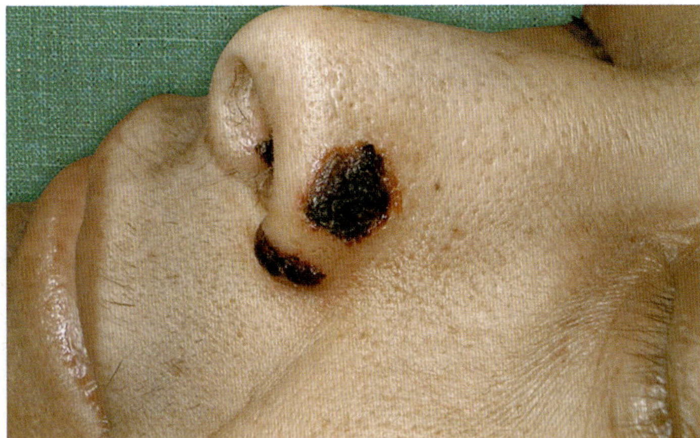

**FIG. 38:** Cutaneous aspergillosis associated to leukemia.

## Management

For management of mucormycosis and to increase the survival rate, surgery supported by antifungals (amphotericin B, posaconazole, caspofungin) is recommended.

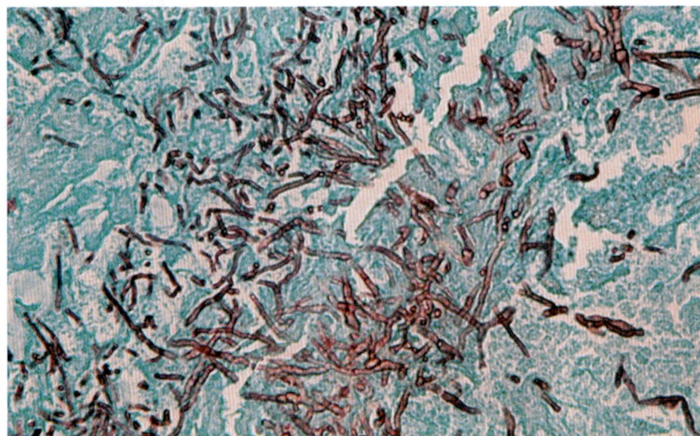

**FIG. 39:** Histology showing dichotomous branching hyphae of *Aspergillus*.

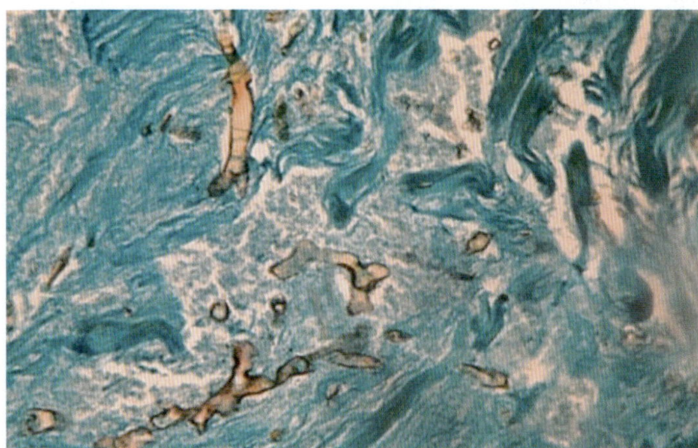

**FIG. 41:** Histopathology showing broad aseptate hyphae of Mucorales.

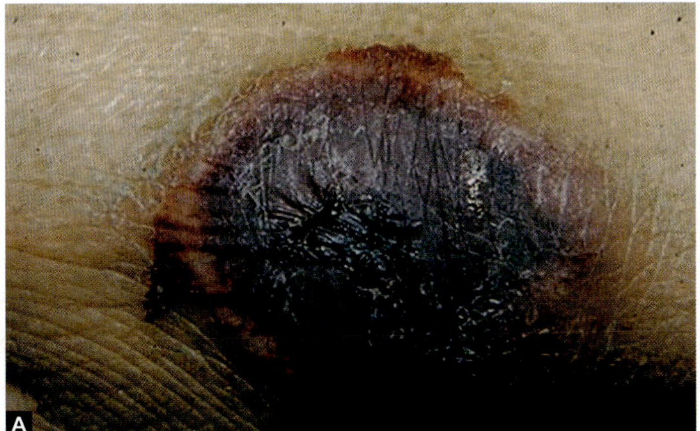


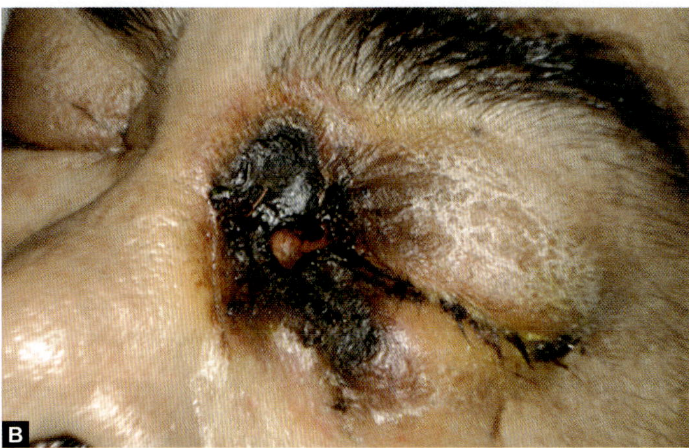


**FIG. 40:** Clinical presentation of cutaneous mucormycosis. **A,** Primary; **B,** Secondary.

## SUGGESTED READINGS


1. Ahmed SA, van de Sande WWJ, Desnos-Ollivier M, et al. Application of isothermal amplification techniques for identification of Madurella mycetomatis, the prevalent agent of human mycetoma. J Clin Microbiol. 2015;53:3280-5.
2. Ampel NM. The diagnosis of coccidioidomycosis. F1000 Med Rep. 2010;2:2.
3. Barros MB, de Almeida Paes R, Schubach AO. Sporothrix schenckii and sporotrichosis. Clin Microbiol Rev. 2011;24:633-54.
4. Bialek R, González GM, Begerow D, Zelck UE. Coccidioidomycosis and blastomycosis: advances in molecular diagnosis. FEMS Immunol Med Microbiol. 2005;45:355-60.
5. Bocca AL, Amaral AC, Teixeira MM, et al. Paracoccidioidomycosis: eco-epidemiology, taxonomy and clinical and therapeutic issues. Future Microbiol. 2013;8:1177-91.
6. Bonifaz A, Vázquez-González D, Perusquía-Ortiz AM. Endemic systemic mycoses: coccidioidomycosis, histoplasmosis, paracoccidioidomycosis and blastomycosis. J Dtsch Dermatol Ges. 2011;9:705-14.
7. Bonifaz A, Vázquez-González D, Tirado-Sánchez A, et al. Cutaneous zygomycosis. Clin Dermatol. 2012;30(4):413-9.
8. Bonifaz A, Vázquez-González D. Sporotrichosis: an update. G Ital Dermatol Venereol. 2010;145:659-73.
9. Bradsher RW, Chapman SW, Pappas PG. Blastomycosis. Infect Dis Clin North Am 2003;17:21-40.
10. Brandt ME, Warnock DW. Epidemiology, clinical manifestations, and therapy of infections caused by dematiaceous fungi. J Chemother. 2003;15:36-47.
11. Bustamante B, Seas C, Salomon M, et al. Lobomycosis successfully treated with posaconazole. Am J Trop Med Hyg. 2013;88(6):1207-8.
12. Cardone JS, Vinson R, Anderson LL. Coccidioidomycosis: the other great imitator. Cutis. 1995;56:33-6.
13. Chapman SW, Dismukes WE, Proia LA, et al. Infectious Diseases Society of America. Clinical practice guidelines for the management of blastomycosis: 2008 update by the Infectious Diseases Society of America. Clin Infect Dis. 2008;46:1801-12.
14. Chowdhary A, Meis JF, Guarro J, et al. ESCMID and ECMM joint clinical guidelines for the diagnosis and management of systemic phaeohyphomycosis: diseases caused by black fungi. Clin Microbiol Infect. 2014;20:47-75.
15. Cornely OA, Arikan-Akdagli S, Dannaoui E, et al. ESCMID and ECMM joint clinical guidelines for the diagnosis and management of mucormycosis 2013. Clin Microbiol Infect. 2014;20 Suppl 3:5-26.
16. Cornely OA, Bassetti M, Calandra T, et al. ESCMID* guideline for the diagnosis and management of Candida diseases 2012: non-neutropenic adult patients. Clin Microbiol Infect. 2012 (18 Suppl 7):19-37.
17. Das S, Saha R, Bhattacharya SN, et al. Hyalohyphomycosis: An unusual presentation and review of literature. IJMS. 2010;1:123-9
18. Deng S, de Hoog GS, Pan W, et al. Three isothermal amplification techniques for rapid identification of Cladophialophora carrionii, an agent of human chromoblastomycosis. J Clin Microbiol. 2014;52:3531-5.
19. Deorukhkar SC, Saini S. Laboratory approach for diagnosis of candidiasis through ages. Int J Curr Microbiol Appl Sci. 2014;3:206-18.
20. de Sousa MD, Belda W, Spina R, et al. Topical application of imiquimod as a treatment for chromoblastomycosis. Clin Infect Dis 2014;58:1734-7.
21. DiCaudo DJ. Coccidioidomycosis: a review and update. J Am Acad Dermatol. 2006;55:929-42.
22. Duong TA. Infection due to Penicillium marneffei, an emerging pathogen: Review of 155 reported cases. Clin Infect Dis. 1996;23:125-30.
23. Esterre P, Queiroz-Telles F. Management of chromoblastomycosis: novel perspectives. Curr Opin Infect Dis. 2006;19:148-52.
24. Fahal AH. Mycetoma. Clinicopathological Monograph. Khartoum: Khartoum University Press; 2006.
25. Fahal AH. Review: Management of mycetoma. Expert Rev Dermatol. 2010;5:87-93.
26. Galgiani JN, Ampel NM, Blair JE, et al. Coccidioidomycosis. Clin Infect Dis 2005;41:1217-23.
27. Guimarães AJ, Nosanchuk JD, Zancopé-Oliveira RM. Diagnosis of histoplasmosis. Braz J Microbiol. 2006;37:1-13.
28. Hector RF, Laniado-Laborin R. Coccidioidomycosis—A fungal disease of the Americas. PLoS Med. 2005;2:e2.
29. Joosten SA, Hannan L, Heroit G, et al. Penicillium marneffei presenting as an obstructing endobronchial lesion in an immunocompetent host. Eur Respir J. 2012;39:1540-3.
30. Kauffman CA, Bustamante B, Chapman SW, et al. Infectious Diseases Society of America. Clinical practice guidelines for the management of sporotrichosis: 2007 update by the Infectious Diseases Society of America. Clin Infect Dis. 2007;45:1255-65.
31. Kauffman CA. Histoplasmosis: a clinical and laboratory update. Clin Microbiol Rev. 2007;20:115-32.
32. Krzy ciak PM, Pindycka-Piaszczy ska M, Piaszczy ski M. Chromoblastomycosis. Postepy Dermatol Alergol. 2014;31:310-21.
33. Lionakis MS. Genetic Susceptibility to fungal infections in humans. Curr Fungal Infect Rep. 2012;6:11-22.
34. Lopez Martinez R, Mendez Tovar LJ. Chromoblastomycosis. Clin Dermatol. 2007;25:188-94.
35. Marques SA. Paracoccidioidomycosis: epidemiological, clinical, diagnostic and treatment up-dating. An Bras Dermatol. 2013;88:700-11.
36. Mason AR, Cortes GY, Cook J, et al. Thiers BH. Cutaneous blastomycosis: a diagnostic challenge. Int J Dermatol 2008;47:824-30.
37. Oliveira MM, Almeida-Paes R, Gutierrez-Galhardo MC, et al. Zancope-Oliveira RM Molecular identification of the Sporothrix schenckii complex. Rev Iberoam Micol. 2014;31:2-6.
38. Paniz-Mondolfi A, Talhari C, Sander Hoffmann L, et al. Lobomycosis: an emerging disease in humans and delphinidae. Mycoses. 2012;55:298-309.
39. Perfect JR, Dismukes WE, Dromer F, et al. Clinical practice guidelines for the management of cryptococcal disease: 2010 update by the infectious diseases society of America. Clin Infect Dis. 2010;50:291-322.
40. Perusquía-Ortiz AM, Vázquez-González D, Bonifaz A. Opportunistic filamentous mycoses: aspergillosis, mucormycosis, phaeohyphomycosis and hyalohyphomycosis. J Dtsch Dermatol Ges. 2012;10(9):611-21.
41. Petrikkos G, Skiada A, Lortholary O, et al. Epidemiology and clinical manifestations of mucormycosis. Clin Infect Dis. 2012;54(Suppl 1):S23-34.
42. Queiroz-Telles F, Esterre P, Perez-Blanco M, et al. Chromoblastomycosis: an overview of clinical manifestations, diagnosis and treatment. Med Mycol. 2009;47:3-15.
43. Ramos-E-Silva M, Aguiar-Santos-Vilela F, Cardoso-de-Brito A, et al. Lobomycosis. Literature review and future perspectives. Actas Dermosifiliogr. 2009;100 Suppl 1:92-100.
44. Revankar SG, Sutton DA. Melanized fungi in human disease. Clin Microbiol Rev. 2010;23:884-928.
45. Ribes JA, Vanover-Sams CL, Baker DJ. Zygomycetes in human disease. Clin Microbiol Rev. 2000;13(2):236-301.
46. Richardson MD, Jones BL, Shaw F. Therapeutic Guidelines in Systemic Fungal Infections. London: Current Medical Literature Ltd.; 2003.
47. Rowen JL. Mucocutaneous candidiasis. Semin Perinatol. 2003;27:406-13.
48. Saccente M, Woods GL. Clinical and laboratory update on blastomycosis. Clin Microbiol Rev. 2010; 23:367-81.
49. Sidrim JJ, Costa AK, Cordeiro RA, et al. Molecular methods for the diagnosis and characterization of Cryptococcus: a review. Can J Microbiol. 2010;56:445-58.
50. Skiada A, Petrikkos G. Cutaneous zygomycosis. Clin Microbiol Infect. 2009;15 (Suppl 5):41-54.
51. Subramanian S, Mathai D. Clinical manifestations and management of cryptococcal infection. J Postgrad Med. 2005;(51 Suppl 1):S21-6.
52. Talhari S, Talhari C. Lobomycosis. Clin Dermatol. 2012;30:420-4.
53. Teles FR, Martins ML. Laboratorial diagnosis of paracoccidioidomycosis and new insights for the future of fungal diagnosis. Talanta. 2011;85:2254-64.
54. Tortorano AM, Richardson M, Roilides E, et al. ESCMID and ECMM joint guidelines on diagnosis and management of hyalohyphomycosis: Fusarium spp., Scedosporium spp. and others. Clin Microbiol Infect. 2014;20 Suppl 3:27-46.
55. Ullmann AJ, Cornely OA, Donnelly JP, et al. ESCMID* guideline for the diagnosis and management of Candida diseases 2012: developing European guidelines in clinical microbiology and infectious diseases. Clin Microbiol Infect. 2012;(18 Suppl 7):53-67.
56. van de Sande WWJ, Fahal AH, Goodfellow M, et al. Merits and pitfalls of currently used diagnostic tools in mycetoma. PLoS Negl Trop Dis. 2014;8:e2918.
57. van de Sande WWJ. Global burden of human mycetoma: a systematic review and meta-analysis. PLoS Negl Trop Dis. 2013;7:e2550.
58. Walsh TJ, Anaissie EJ, Denning DW, et al. Treatment of aspergillosis: clinical practice guidelines of the Infectious Diseases Society of America. Clin Infect Dis. 2008;46(3):327-60.
59. Welsh O, Al-Abdely HM, Salinas-Carmona MC, Fahal AH. Mycetoma medical therapy. PLoS Negl Trop Dis. 2014;8:e3218.
60. Welsh O, Vera-Cabrera L, Rendon A, et al. Coccidiodomycosis. Clin Dermatol. 2012;30:573-91.
61. Wheat J. Histoplasmosis: recognition and treatment. Clin Infect Dis. 1994;19 Suppl 1:S19-27.
62. Wheat LJ, Freifeld AG, Kleiman MB, et al.. Clinical practice guidelines for the management of patients with histoplasmosis: 2007 update by the Infectious Diseases Society of America. Clin Infect Dis. 2007;45:807-25.
63. Wong SYN, Wong KF. Penicillium marneffei infection in AIDS. Patholog Res Int. 2011;(764293):1-10.
64. Yapar N. Epidemiology and risk factors for invasive candidiasis. Ther Clin Risk Manag. 2014;10:95-105.

# 62 CHAPTER Skin Disease Caused by Protozoa and Nematodes

Monica Chahar, Sanjay K Rathi, Paschal V D'Souza

## INTRODUCTION

Protozoa are single celled organisms divided into classes according to their morphology and means of locomotion. Here we discuss few of protozoan infection with cutaneous findings.

## LEISHMANIASIS

More than 90% of leishmaniasis cases occur in Afghanistan, Algeria, Brazil, Iraq, Iran, Peru, Saudi Arabia, and Syria.

The disease can manifest in the following patterns—cutaneous leishmaniasis (CL), which can be localized or disseminated [diffuse cutaneous leishmaniasis (DCL)]; mucocutaneous leishmaniasis (MCL), which affects the skin and mucosal surfaces; and visceral leishmaniasis (VL), which affects organs of the reticuloendothelial system. The various species causing disease according to different locations have been summarized here:

- Old world cutaneous leishmaniasis (Oriental sore)
  - *Leishmania tropica (L. tropica)* complex (Asia, Africa, Mediterranean Europe)
    - *L. tropica* minor—dry or urban cutaneous leishmaniasis
    - *L. tropica* major—wet or rural cutaneous leishmaniasis
    - *Leishmania aethiopica*—cutaneous leishmaniasis (Ethiopia and Kenya).
- New world cutaneous and mucocutaneous leishmaniasis (American cutaneous leishmaniasis) (South and Central America)
  - *Leishmania mexicana* complex (*L. mexicana, L. amazonensis, and L. venezuelensis*)—cutaneous leishmaniasis
  - *Leishmania braziliensis* complex (subgenus *Viannia*): *L. (V.) braziliensis, L. (V.) guyanensis, L. (V.) panamensis, and L. (V.) peruviana*—mucocutaneous or cutaneous leishmaniasis
- Visceral leishmaniasis
  - *L. donovani* (Asia, Africa, and Southeast Asia)
  - *L. infantum* (Mediterranean basin; Middle East and Central Asia to Pakistan; China; Central and South America)
  - *L. chagasi* (South and Central America).

### Transmission

Arthropods (sandflies) from the genus *Phlebotomus* (Old World) or *Lutzomyia* (America) are the vectors for the protozoan. *Leishmania* species exists in two forms—one is the motile, flagellated promastigotes seen in the culture and in the gut, pharynx, and proboscis of sandflies; second is the intracellular amastigote form. During feeding by female sandflies, the parasites are transmitted to mammalian tissues either by regurgitation or after being rubbed in when the sandfly is crushed by the host. These transform to amastigote forms within macrophages (Leishman-Donovan Bodies) wherein they multiply by binary fission and infect other macrophages. The incubation time till the first clinical manifestation can vary from 2 months (ulcers of CL) to more than 2 years (MCL lesions).

In the Amazon Rain Forest, the most important reservoirs are wild animals, such as tree-living anteaters (*Tamandua tetradactyla*), opossums (*Didelphis albiventris*), and wild rats. In cases of Old World CL, the rock hyrax (*Procavia capensis*) is a reservoir for *L. tropica*, the fat desert rat (*Psammomys obesus*) is a reservoir for *L. major*, and dogs and foxes are reservoirs for *L. infantum*.

Apart from the bite of an infected sandfly, transmission may also occur through the accidental inoculation of laboratory cultured parasites, blood transfusion or through the congenital or sexual route.

### Clinical Features

Old world cutaneous leishmaniasis (oriental sore/bouton d'Orient/Delhi boil/Aleppo boil) (Figs 1 and 2).

It has two forms—(1) anthroponotic cutaneous leishmaniasis (ACL), primarily caused by *L. tropica*, and (2) zoonotic cutaneous leishmaniasis (ZCL) caused by *L. major. L. tropica* usually presents with a solitary lesion whereas *L. major* causes multiple lesions. It presents as an erythematous papule or nodule or "oriental button" at the site of insect bite, usually on exposed parts such as the face, neck, and arms. It can lead to an ulcer formation with a violaceous border. Satellite lesions may be seen. The lesion heals spontaneously after several weeks to months leaving a scar. ACL lesions may develop into recidivans leishmaniasis. Various morphological variants of this form have been described such as verrucous, keloidal, psoriasiform, and eczematous. Other forms of Old World CL include the self-healing *L. infantum* infections, which are most often seen in Europe and frequently involve children, and *L. aethiopica* infection, which may cause diffuse and localized CL in Africa.

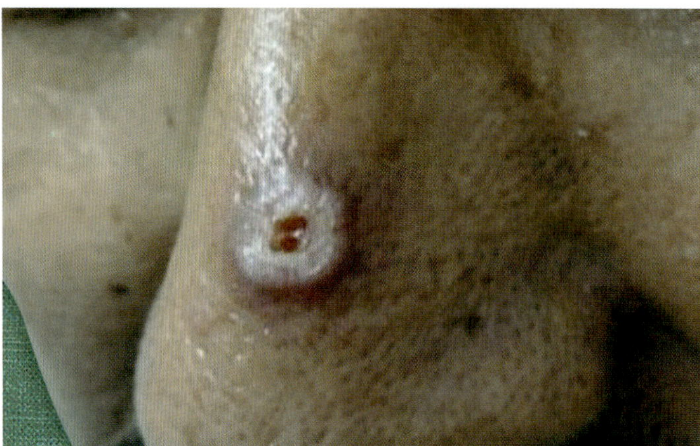

FIG. 1: Cutaneous leishmaniasis nose.

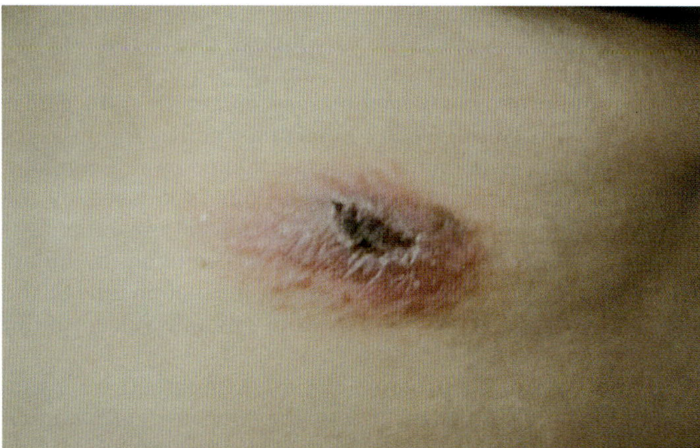

FIG. 2: Oriental sore.

### New World Cutaneous Leishmaniasis

It usually presents as a pruritic nodule or a papule which ulcerates over a period of few weeks. The ulcer has a prominent raised edge. In Mexico and Central America, the ulcers characteristically involve the pinna of the ears (chiclero ulcers), while in Brazil the lower limbs are more commonly affected (Bauru ulcers). The lesions heal giving rise to a thin scar over the ulcer site surrounded by a hyperpigmented halo.

*L. braziliensis* infection can disseminate hematogenously causing mucosal lesions. Within 1–2 years of the presentation of the initial lesion, the patient may present with clinical lesions of MCL (Espundia). Nasal involvement is the most common leading to nodular infiltration and crusting of the inferior turbinate and the septum. The result could be the complete destruction of the septum, a massive infiltration of the face, and the development of "tapir face". Mucosal lesions are characterized by ulcerations and infiltrated lesions of the nose, lips, mouth, and pharynx.

### Diffuse Cutaneous Leishmaniasis (Anergic/Lepromatous or Pseudolepromatous Leishmaniasis)

It is characterized by diffuse distribution of skin-colored papules, nodules, and tuberous lesions that affect the face and the limbs, sparing the trunk. The face can show a massive infiltration similar to the "lion face" or leonine facies of lepromatous leprosy.

### Borderline Disseminated Cutaneous Leishmaniasis

It is an intermediate form of leishmaniasis, between localized CL and anergic DCL. It is usually caused by *L. amazonensis*. After 2 years of the appearance of the primary skin lesion, an erythematous and infiltrated plaque develops usually on the face and upper or lower limbs. There is lymphatic spread of the infection with lymph node enlargement. The delayed hypersensitivity skin test is usually negative.

### Visceral Leishmaniasis

It is also known as kala-azar or black fever and is characterized by the spread of the parasite to the bone marrow, spleen, and liver. The incubation period varies from 1 month to 36 months. The symptoms include high grade fever, anorexia, diarrhea, pallor, abdominal pain, cough, and epistaxis. The skin of the face, hands, feet, and abdomen may become hyperpigmented. Other signs include hepatosplenomegaly, generalized lymphadenopathy and oral, nasal, and intestinal hemorrhage. VL occurs both in the Old World (China, Russia, India, Pakistan, and Africa) and in South America (Brazil). The skin lesions present as papules, nodules, or ulcers at the inoculation site.

Nonspecific findings including yellowish discoloration of fine brittle hair, purpura, and xeroderma may occur.

## Diagnosis

The most important diagnostic method is the detection of the amastigotes in a tissue smear from a lesion. Smears are stained using Giemsa or Leishman stain which reveals the intramacrophagic Leishmania donovani (LD) bodies. Giemsa stains the cytoplasm of the LD bodies blue while the nucleus and the kinetoplast stain reddish-purple. Parasites can also be found in skin biopsies or cultured from biopsy samples in a biphasic medium, such as Novy-MacNeal-Nicolle (NMN).

Montenegro skin test (Leishmanin test, a delayed hypersensitivity reaction)—phenol-killed promastigotes are injected into the dermis and read after 72 hours. A papule more than 5 mm is characteristic of a positive Montenegro test. The test can be negative in cases of both VL and DCL, and also in cases of CL and MCL with 3 months of evolution. Its positivity indicates contact with Leishmania organisms but is not diagnostic for disease.

Enzyme-linked immunosorbent assay (ELISA) and Western blot are only useful in evaluating the response to treatment.

More recently, flow cytometry antielive promastigote antibody (FC-ALPA) was described. Combined FC-ALPA IgG1/FC-ALPA IgG2 analysis can be used to distinguish between those infections, when necessary. Polymerase chain reaction (PCR) is highly sensitive and specific. Further analysis with single-strand conformational polymorphism or restriction fragment length polymorphism has been shown to be effective for species typing.

## Treatment

*Local treatment*: Topical paromomycin, cryotherapy, localized controlled heat, carbon dioxide laser therapy and intralesional meglumine antimoniate. Paromomycin, or aminosidine ointment, is a parenteral aminoglycoside antibacterial agent that also has considerable activity against protozoa.

*Systemic*: Pentavalent antimony or pentamidine salts is standard treatment for leishmaniasis.

Amphotericin B is a second-line therapy and also used in CL. Liposomal amphotericin B is very effective even in leishmaniasis associated with HIV disease.

Other systemic treatments include interferon, allopurinol, rifampicin, dapsone, azole antifungals, and immunotherapy.

Among the pentavalent antimonies, sodium stibogluconate, and meglumine antimonies now considered standard therapy for CL. Cure rates after 14-day treatment regimens with intramuscular antimony have varied from 41% to 77%. Intralesional injections of pentavalent antimonies have variable cure rates ranging from 55.6% to 92% in Old World CL.

Imiquimod induces tumor necrosis factor-alpha (TNF-α), interferon-gamma (IFN-γ), and interleukin-12 (IL-12), leading to the inhibition of interleukin-5 (IL-5). In a randomized, double-blind clinical trial in Peru, combined antimony plus imiquimod treatment was well tolerated, led to the accelerated healing of lesions, and improved scar quality.

Pentamidine isethionate is a widely available treatment option. Permanent hyperglycemia may result from long-term administration.

Miltefosine is the first oral agent with demonstrable efficacy against both visceral and cutaneous forms of leishmaniasis. Miltefosine is a lecithin analog that inhibits phosphatidylcholine biosynthesis in the causative parasites. Diarrhea and vomiting are common side effects along with reproductive toxicity in animals.

## Post-kala-azar Dermal Leishmaniasis

Post-kala-azar dermal leishmaniasis (PKDL) is a sequel of untreated VL, commonly seen in Sudan and Indian subcontinents. PKDL was first described in 1922 as distinct clinical entity, manifest usually 6 months to 5 years following an attack of VL and affect around 5–10% of patients. Most common clinical presentations are hypopigmented macules, papules, nodules and butterfly erythema. In India, commonly mixed pattern (Fig. 3) is seen of macules, infiltrated papules, and nodules; but sometimes hypopigmentation may be only presentation (Fig. 4). The central part of face is most commonly affected (Fig. 5) and then spread to rest part of body including mucous membrane involvement in some.

Diagnosis of PKDL is mostly by history and clinical presentation. An accurate diagnosis is a challenge due to few parasites, the *Leishmania donovani* bodies (LD bodies) in lesions and blood; if found they are a gold standard.

Antibody based tests, such as rK39 rapid dipstick test, and direct agglutination tests (DAT) are both sensitive and specific for VL and PKDL, but sometimes differentiating them is not possible. The rK39 rapid diagnostic tests in skin slit smears is promising and can be used as an initial diagnostic screening for PKDL in tertiary centers.

### Treatment

Post-kala-azar dermal leishmaniasis is known for its refractoriness to various modalities tried. They are sodium antimony gluconate (SAG), miltefosine, rifampin, ketoconazole, nystatin, terbinafine, itraconazole, amphotericin-B, and immunotherapy.

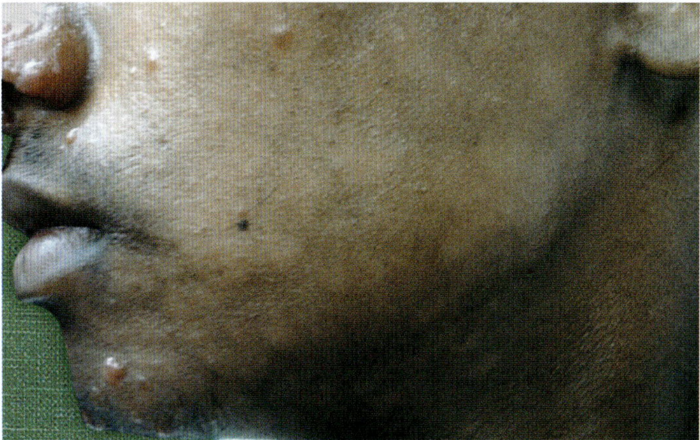

**FIG. 3:** Mixed (infiltrated nodule and hypopigmented macules) pattern post-kala-azar dermal leishmaniasis.

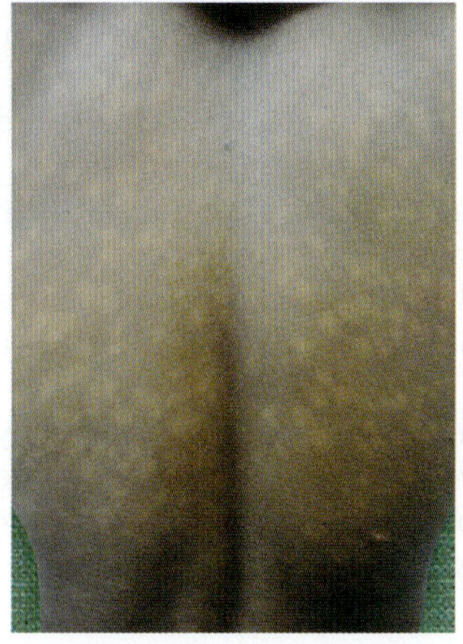

**FIG. 4:** Hypopigmented macules of post-kala-azar dermal leishmaniasis on back.

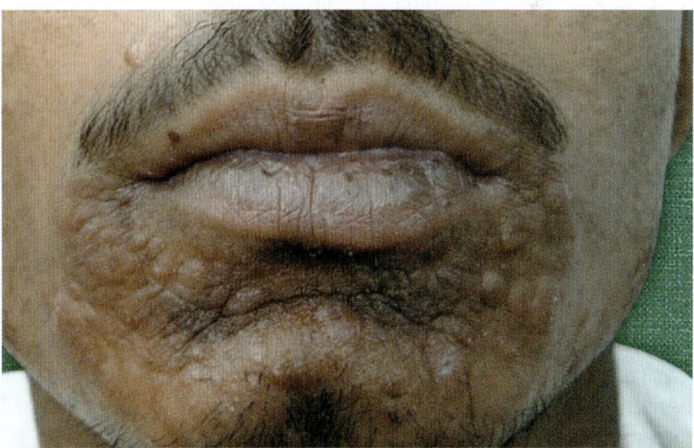

**FIG. 5:** Infiltrated nodules on central part of face in post-kala-azar dermal leishmaniasis.

# AMEBIASIS

## Entamoeba Histolytica

Cyst is the infective form of the parasite and is transmitted in contaminated water or food, especially salads, or by hands or flies, or by male homosexual intercourse. The most common sites affected in cutaneous amebiasis are the perianal region, perineum, genitalia, and groin.

Clinically the lesion is a well demarcated deep seated ulcer with indurated and undermined margins which may become irregular to serpiginous in shape.

Treatment of invasive amebiasis is with oral or intravenous metronidazole. Intestinal cysts may be eliminated using diloxanide furoate or diiodohydroxyquin.

## TRYPANOSOMIASIS

### African Trypanosomiasis (Sleeping Sickness)

It is caused by the parasite *Trypanosoma brucei* (*T. brucei gambiense, T. brucei rhodesiense*). *Glossina palpalis, G. tachinoides*, and *G. fuscipes* are the three species of tsetse flies involved in the transmission of Gambian sleeping sickness.

The initial lesion is the trypanosomal chancre which is an indurated red or violaceous nodule, 2–5 cm in diameter, often accompanied by regional lymphadenopathy. Hemolymphatic stage begins 3–10 days after the chancre develops causing general malaise, anemia, headache, pyrexia, weight loss, and weakness. Late stage consists of neurologic, neuroendocrine, and psychiatric symptoms, is referred to as the meningoencephalitic stage and coincides with invasion of the central nervous system (CNS) by the parasites. Somnolence is the classic symptom of the disease.

Suramin is the drug of choice for the early hemolymphatic stage before CNS invasion occurs. Pentamidine is an alternative drug. Melarsoprol, nitrofurazone, and difluoromethylornithine are for the cases with CNS involvement.

### American Trypanosomiasis (Chagas Disease)

It is caused by the flagellated trypanosome *T. cruzi*, which is transmitted to humans via reduviid or kissing bugs.

Cutaneous lesions seen during the acute stage of disease are seen at the site of inoculation—chagoma which are furuncle-like violaceous lesions. If feces are accidentally rubbed by the individual into the eyes, an eyelid swelling, known as the Romana sign may form. If it is associated with local lymphadenopathy (preauricular), it is known as oculoglandular complex or Parinaud's syndrome. Chronic Chagas disease causes Chagasic heart disease and gastrointestinal manifestations such as achalasia, chronic constipation, megasyndromes, including megaesophagus or megacolon.

Treatment for the acute stage includes nifurtimox or benznidazole. Allopurinol has been tried for the treatment of chronic infection.

## TOXOPLASMOSIS

The disease is caused by *Toxoplasma gondii*. Cats are definitive hosts; rodents and birds are the intermediate hosts. Larger mammals including humans are infected incidentally, by eating raw, infected meat or by ingesting oocysts in contaminated food or water. Toxoplasmosis causes four types of disease in humans:

1. An acute febrile lymphadenopathy
2. Fetal infection, causing brain damage
3. Ocular disease, usually due to reactivation of fetal infection
4. Disseminated disease in immunocompromised patients, including those with HIV infection, causing fulminating encephalitis.

Congenital infection usually manifests as hemorrhagic or necrotic papules found commonly on the trunk. The most effective treatment is sulfadiazine in combination with pyrimethamine.

## INFECTION WITH NEMATODES

### Tissue Nematodes

This group includes the filarial worms, the guinea worm (*Dracunculus medinensis*) and *Trichinella spiralis*.

### Filarial Worms

Filariasis refers to parasitic infection caused by filarial parasites that require an arthropod vector for their transmission. The worms inhabit either the lymphatic system or the subcutaneous tissues of man. The female worm gives rise to a young worm called microfilaria. The microfilariae, when taken by the arthropod intermediate host during biting, develop into filariform larvae, which are the infective stages. Humans get infected when bitten by the infected arthropod intermediate host.

#### Epidemiology

It has been estimated that approximately 1 billion people in tropical and subtropical countries are exposed to the risk of filarial infections and at least 200 million are infected with filariasis. The species, vector, geographical location, and diseases caused are given in table 1.

#### Pathogenesis

Filariasis is spread from host-to-host via the bites of certain flies and mosquitoes that act as vectors for the parasites. The nematode is usually in its third larval stage in the vector when it enters the host. These mature into adults settling in lymphatics, body cavities or subcutaneous tissue of skin where they mate and produce microfilariae. These are taken up by the vector during a bite and the cycle is completed.

Cutaneous and other manifestations are due to:

- Adult worms causing lymphatic blockage and immune response to the dead and dying worms in the lymphatic system as seen in bancroftian and malayan filariasis
- Death of microfilariae in subcutaneous and ocular tissue as in onchocerciasis
- Host's response to the worm or its metabolic products as in Loasis
- Embolism and localized inflammation of pulmonary vessels in dirofilariasis
- Presence of a type of *Rickettsia* (*Wolbachia* spp.) which has a symbiotic relationship with filarial nematodes. The bacteria initiate the filarial disease process with a severe adverse inflammatory reaction.
- Humans may be infected as accidental hosts. The larva wanders through the human body and finally forms a nodule as in dirofilariasis.

**TABLE 1: Epidemiology of filariasis**

| Filarial parasite | Vector | Geographical location | Filarial disease |
|---|---|---|---|
| *Onchocerca volvulus* | Blackfly (*Simulium* species) | Africa, Latin America Yemen (Arabian Peninsula) | Onchocerciasis |
| *Wuchereria bancrofti* | Culicidae (mosquitoes) | Africa, India, and the Far East | Bancroftian filariasis (lymphatic filariasis) |
| *Brugia malayi* and *Brugia timori* | Culicidae (mosquitoes) | Southeast Asia | Malayan filariasis (lymphatic filariasis) |
| *Loa loa* | *Chrysops* species | West and Central Africa | Loiasis |
| *Mansonella* species | *Culicoides* (biting midges) | Africa, and South America | Mansonelliasis |
| • *Dirofilaria* species<br>• *D. immitis* and *D. repens* | Culicidae (mosquito) | Americas, Asia, Australia, and Mediterranean region of Europe | Dirofilariasis |

**TABLE 2: Patterns of skin dermatoses due to onchocerciasis**

| Classification | Skin features |
|---|---|
| Acute papular onchodermatitis | Widespread itchy papules, vesicles and pustules over face, trunk, and extremities |
| Chronic papular onchodermatitis | Severely itchy scattered flat-topped papules and areas pigmentation over shoulders, buttocks, and extremities is most common pattern |
| Lichenified onchodermatitis | Thickened, scaly, hyperpigmented plaque over lower extremities with lymphadenopathy |
| Onchocercal atrophy | Presents as thin dry inelastic skin over buttocks and lower back |
| Onchocercal depigmentation | Also called "leopard skin" seen over lower extremity having areas of perifollicular normopigmentation within large areas of depigmented skin |
| Palpable onchocercal nodules (onchocercoma) | Subcutaneous nodules of size few millimeters to several centimeters are found over bony prominences, which contain the adult worms |

## Clinical Manifestation

The cutaneous and systemic signs and symptoms vary depending on the type of filarial infection.

## Onchocerciasis (River Blindness)

### Cutaneous

Most common sign/symptom of onchocerciasis and six different patterns of skin dermatoses due to onchocerciasis are described in table 2.

Other skin findings include ichthyotic changes, the "lizard skin" and "hanging groin" where folds of inelastic atrophic skin are present in the groin.

The dead microfilariae can produce inflammation and bleeding in the eye. Symptoms range from itching, redness, pain, and photophobia (light sensitivity) to blurring of vision, night blindness, glaucoma, visual field loss (restricted area of vision), and eventually blindness.

## Bancroftian and Malayan Filariasis (Lymphatic Filariasis)

Many patients are asymptomatic. There may be fever, lymphangitis, and lymphadenitis involving lower extremities, genital, and breast. Edema may resolve or gradually result in thickening and verrucous changes in the skin known as elephantiasis (Fig. 6). The genital manifestation may be in form of hydrocele or scrotal lymphedema. Obstruction of renal lymphatics may lead to rupture into the urinary tract producing chyluria. In *B. malayi*, unlike *Wuchereria bancrofti*, genital involvement, hydrocele, and chyluria are rare.

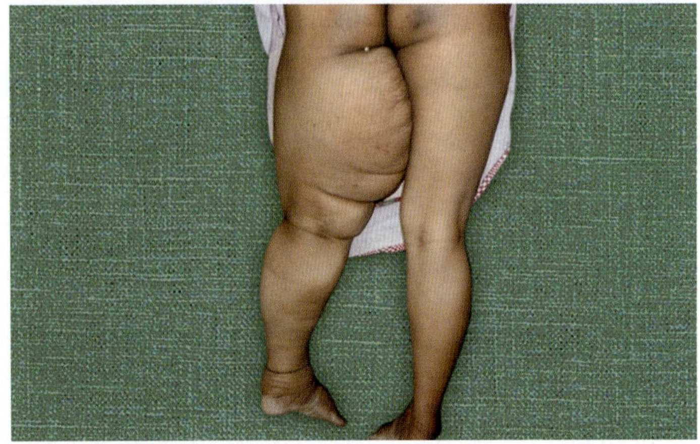

**FIG. 6:** Lymphatic filariasis.
*Courtesy*: Dr Akhilesh Shukla, MD

## Loiasis

The initial bite causes redness, swelling, and itching. Patients later are either asymptomatic or develop Calabar swellings, which are localized subcutaneous edema commonly in the extremities lasting 1–3 days, usually accompanied by localized pain, urticaria. Sometimes adult worm can be seen crossing the eye. There may be fever, pain, pruritus, urticaria, allergic reactions, retinopathy, glomerulonephritis, and meningoencephalitis.

## Mansonelliasis

Most patients infected with *M. perstans* do not experience any symptoms. Newcomers to an endemic area who become infected appear to experience more symptoms than local inhabitants. Symptoms include swelling of the arms, shoulders, and face, abdominal pain, itchiness, fatigue, and joint pain. The most common symptom of a patient infected with *M. streptocerca* is chronic itching dermatitis that is often confined to one part of the torso. Constant scratching may thicken the skin.

## Dirofilariasis

Humans are poor hosts for this filarial parasite as the worm usually dies before reaching sexual maturity. However in recent years there has been a reported increase in the number of human dirofilariasis cases. The head, neck, breasts, arms, legs, and scrotum are most commonly affected where tender subcutaneous nodule develops. This can be painful and cause burning and itching. Human pulmonary dirofilariasis is characterized by the formation of pulmonary nodules which may be frequently misdiagnosed as a malignant lesion. Symptoms are nonspecific and include coughing with pleural or nonpleural thoracic pain, hemoptysis, and dyspnea in the minority of cases, fever, and other nonspecific signs such as malaise and myalgia. Dirofilaria repens-related infections can occur in ocular regions. Some of these cases have serious consequences, with damaged vision, floaters, or loss of sight due to complications such as retinal detachment, glaucoma, and opacity of the vitreous humor.

### Diagnosis

- *Detection of microfilariae: collection of specimens*: The specimen collection times should be selected in accordance with the patient's clinical symptoms, travel history, and known feeding pattern of the vector. Blood film examination can be done after staining by Giemsa or Leishman stain to detect microfilaria. When skin specimen is taken it is allowed to stand for 30 minutes in saline before it is examined microscopically for microfilariae. Site with time of collection and morphological features of microfilariae of different species are given in table 3
- *Biopsy*: Superficial biopsy (skin snip) taken from the skin in cases of onchocerciasis and mansonelliasis and biopsy from subcutaneous and ocular tissue in dirofilariasis may also pick up microfilariae or adult worm
- *Urine examination*: If lymphatic filariasis is suspected, urine should be examined macroscopically for chyluria and then concentrated to examine for microfilariae
- *Hematological and serological tests*: Eosinophilia, high IgE level and high antifilarial antibody titers are seen in most of these disorders. PCR, immunohistochemical staining and ELISA may also be helpful
- *Imaging studies*: Diffuse pulmonary infiltrates is seen in tropical pulmonary eosinophilia. Ultrasonography may pick up lymphatic obstruction of the inguinal and scrotal lymphatics, deep onchocercomas, and vitreous changes in the eye. It can also demonstrate the presence of viable worms (filarial dance sign). Lymphoscintigraphy can assess extent of limb involvement in lymphatic filariasis
- *Mazzotti test*: An intense pruritus within hours after a single small dose of DEC (50–100 mg) denotes a positive test. Steroids may be necessary to control this inflammatory reaction. It should be performed with caution in individuals suspected to be heavily infected, as a severe systemic reaction may occur
- *Other investigations*: Microfilariae may be directly observed during slit lamp examination of the eye in onchocerciasis.

### Treatment

Broad outlines of treatment for various filarial worms including oral or injectable antihelminthic therapy, antibiotic therapy against *Wolbachia* bacteria, surgical excision, and needle aspiration/injection depending on the infecting parasite are given in table 4.

### Prevention

Following measures are to be adopted for control of filariasis:
- Vector control
- Individual and mass treatment
- Use of repellents such as DEET
- Protective clothing like wearing long-sleeved shirts and pants
- Long-term or intermittent treatment with antihelminthic therapy.

## Dracunculiasis

*Dracunculus medinensis* is a nonfilarial parasite causing infection known as dracunculiasis or guinea worm disease. Infection is acquired by drinking unclean and unboiled water that contains *Cyclops* species. The larvae released in the stomach reach the subcutaneous tissue where they mature to adults. The fertilized

**TABLE 3: Helpful Features for laboratory diagnosis of various microfilariae**

| Species | Microfilaria (present in) | Time of collection (Blood/skin samples ) | Size of microfilariae | Morphology of microfilariae |
|---|---|---|---|---|
| *W. bancrofti* | Blood | 10 PM to 2 AM | 210–320 µm | Sheathed, tail pointed, and clear |
| *B. malayi* | Blood | 10 PM to 2 AM | 170–260 µm | Sheathed, tail pointed with 2 nuclei |
| *Loa loa* | Blood | 10 PM to 2 PM | 230–300 µm | Sheathed, tail blunt with nuclei |
| *Mansonella perstans* | Blood | Any time | 200 µm | Unsheathed, tail blunt with nuclei |
| *Mansonella Streptocerca* | Skin, occasional in blood and urine | Skin snipping anytime | 180–240 µm | No sheath, curled tail with nuclei |
| *Onchocerca volvulus* | Skin, occasional in blood and urine | Skin snipping anytime | 280–330 µm | No sheath, pointed tail, and clear |
| *Dirofilaria* species: *D. immitis* and *D. repens* | Skin, eye, and lungs | Excision of skin nodule, eye lesion any time | 290–330 µm | Straight tail and a spindle-shaped cephalic extremity |

**TABLE 4: Therapeutic options for various filarial diseases**

| Filarial disease | Drug | Surgical Treatment | Comments |
|---|---|---|---|
| Onchocerciasis | • Ivermectin drug of choice single dose of 150–200 µg/kg body weight every 3–12 months<br>• Doxycycline given to treat *Wolbachia* | Nodulectomy | Corticosteroids in eye involvement to prevent ocular damage |
| Lymphatic filariasis | • Diethylcarbamazine (DEC) 2 mg/kg 3 × daily for 2 weeks<br>• Ivermectin and DEC appears to be effective combination as they act synergistically<br>• Doxycycline to kill *Wolbachia* bacteria | Surgical decompression of the lymphatic system | Combination of lower limb exercise and regular cleansing helps in decreasing the morbidity |
| Loiasis | DEC drug of choice 9 mg/kg of body weight for 21days | Adult worms can be extracted as they traverse the eye | Ivermectin contraindicated (cause retinal hemorrhage and severe or fatal encephalopathy) |
| • Mansonelliasis<br>• Ivermectin appears to be effective treatment against M streptocerca infections | • Combination treatment with DEC (8–10 mg/kg body weight) for 21 days and mebendazole 100 mg per day for 30 days appears to be the ideal treatment for *M. perstans* infections<br>• Ivermectin appears to be effective treatment against *M. streptocerca* infections | – | Doxycycline is used to eradicate *Wolbachia*, an endosymbiont found in most filarial species |
| Dirofilariasis | – | Surgical removal of the lesion or extraction of the worm only method of treatment | – |

female worms travel through the subcutaneous tissue reaching the lower limbs and provoke the formation of a burning blister which bursts on contact with water forming an ulcer. The best treatment for removing the adult worm is a slow process of daily gently rolling the worm round a small stick and slowly pulling it out of the skin.

## CUTANEOUS LARVA MIGRANS

*Synonyms*: Sandworms, creeping verminous dermatitis, creeping eruption, plumber's itch, and duck hunter's itch.

### Etiology

Causes of creeping eruption include *Ancylostoma brasiliense, A. caninum, A. ceylonicum, Uncinaria stenocephala,* and *Bunostomum phlebotomum*. The threadworms *Strongyloides papillosus, S. westeri, S. stercoralis, S. procyonis,* and *S. myopotami* can cause a very similar clinical syndrome. Other parasites such as *Gnathostoma spinigerum* and *Dirofilaria repens* can travel through the skin and cause dermatitis or swelling. Some authors consider these syndromes to be cutaneous larva migrans.

### Transmission

Transmission usually occurs by walking barefoot on sand or soil contaminated with animal feces. Larvae penetrate the skin and usually stay there (if *Ancylostoma* spp.) as it is believed they lack collagenase necessary to break through the basement membrane.

### Clinical Features

The most common sites of entry are the interdigital spaces of toes, dorsa of feet, and medial aspect of sole. Other sites like buttocks, backs, and thighs, which may have rested on contaminated sand, are susceptible (Fig. 7). The incubation period ranges from 1 to 6 days. The primary lesion is a pruritic, erythematous serpiginous burrow. The larvae travel at a speed of 3 cm per day. It is a self-limited disease, although it can be complicated by bacterial superinfection. *A. caninum* larvae can migrate to the small intestine and can cause eosinophilic enteritis. Transient eosinophilia is also described.

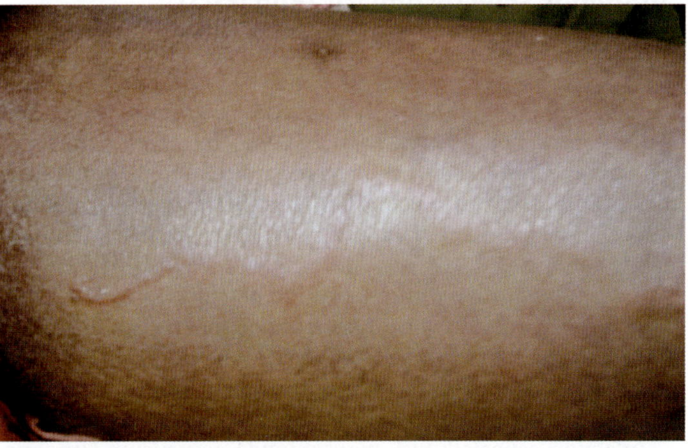

**FIG. 7:** Cutaneous larva migrans.

### Diagnosis

Biopsy is of no value as the larvae advance ahead of the clinical tract. Epiluminescence microscopy is an effective noninvasive method to detect larva and confirm the diagnosis.

### Treatment

The most effective agents in treating CLM are topical or oral antihelminthics, including albendazole, thiabendazole, and ivermectin. The more common regimens include topical thiabendazole 10–15% cream twice to three times daily for 5–10 days; oral albendazole 400 mg daily for 3–5 days; and one dose of 12 mg (150–200 µg/kg) oral ivermectin.

Oral thiabendazole is less well-tolerated than either oral albendazole or ivermectin and also has lower cure rates.

### Visceral Larva Migrans: Toxocariasis

*Toxocara canis* and *T. cati*, the common roundworms of dogs and cats respectively, which can cause visceral larva migrans (VLM) and ocular larva migrans (OLM). Common skin manifestations are chronic pruritus or prurigo, different forms of eczema and chronic urticaria.

## TRICHINOSIS

Trichinosis is caused by eating raw or undercooked meat from pork or wild game animals infected with *Trichinella spiralis*. In early stages of infection there may be a transient maculopapular rash of the extremities and splinter hemorrhages beneath the nails.

## INFECTION WITH TREMATODES

### Cutaneous Schistosomiasis (Bilharzia)

#### Etiology

Humans are the definitive host for five *schistosome* species: *Schistosoma haematobium, S. japonicum, S. mansoni, S. mekongi,* and *S intercalatum*. Schistosomes have a trematode vertebrate-invertebrate lifecycle (infecting both vertebrate and invertebrate), with humans being the definitive host. There are five cutaneous manifestations:

1. *Schistosomal dermatitis*: A pruritic maculopapular eruption may occur at the site of penetration of the epidermis by cercariae. This rash is self-healing within hours or days
2. *Katayama fever*: Acute schistosomiasis (Katayama's fever/ urticarial fever) may occur weeks (2–8 weeks) after the initial infection, especially by *S. mansoni* and *S. japonicum*. Urticaria, fever, lethargy, malaise, and myalgia are the most common symptoms of Katayama syndrome. Other manifestations include abdominal pain, cough, diarrhea, eosinophilia, fever, fatigue, and hepatosplenomegaly. Symptoms usually resolve without treatment over several weeks, but occasionally can be fatal
3. Late nonspecific allergic dermatitis
4. *Perigenital infiltrative granulomata*: Perigenital lesions in the form of verrucous or granulomatous can occur due to the direct spread of adult flukes to adjacent vasculature
5. *Extragenital infiltrative lesions*: Ectopic cutaneous deposition may occur when the ova get deposited on the skin and other ectopic sites, such as conjunctiva, lungs, and CNS. It occurs after embolism of ova from adults and presents as skin-colored or erythematous papules which may coalesce to form slightly raised plaques with irregular contours.

#### Diagnosis

Ova may be found in stools or urine. Rectal biopsy is an alternative method. Serological methods such as immunofluorescence and ELISA are useful for screening. Ectopic cutaneous schistosomiasis is diagnosed by biopsy which shows characteristic epithelioid cell granulomas around the eggs.

#### Treatment

Praziquantel 20 mg/kg taken over a single day; *S. japonicum* and *S. mekongi* require the higher dosing. Treatment for swimmer's itch is mostly symptomatic.

### Cercarial Dermatitis (Swimmer's Itch, Clam Digger's Itch, Sedge Pool Itch, Kogan Byo, and Sawah Itch)

There are three main types of cercarial dermatitis: Fresh-water avian cercarial dermatitis (genera *Trichobilharzia, Gigantobilharzia,* and *Ornithobilharzia*); Sea-water avian cercarial dermatitis, and fresh-water mammalian cercarial dermatitis. It occurs on the exposed skin and is associated with a tingling sensation and erythema at the site of penetration.

### Paragonimiasis (Endemic Hemoptysis, Oriental Lung Fluke Infection, Pulmonary Distomiasis)

*Paragonimus westermani* is regarded as the most common and widely distributed human pathogen in Asia. *P. heterotremus* infection is common particularly in South and Southeast Asia. Humans usually acquire infection by ingestion of uncooked or undercooked crustaceans containing metacercariae. The typical skin lesion is a migratory subcutaneous nodule, which usually appear on the anterior chest wall. Praziquantel is the drug of choice for both pulmonary and extrapulmonary paragonimiasis.

## INFECTION WITH CESTODES

### Echinococcosis/Hydatid Disease

*Echinococcus granulosus* and *E. multilocularis* can infect humans, their larval stage causes echinococcosis. Humans acquire hydatid cysts when they ingest eggs passed by dogs and other canids. The common sites for hydatid cysts are the liver and the lungs but the CNS, the spleen and other organs may be involved. Subcutaneous cysts may occasionally develop as firm, painless swellings which may be fluctuant. If they rupture, anaphylaxis, and the formation of metastatic cysts may occur. The treatment is surgical removal. If inoperable, the use of albendazole is recommended.

### Cysticercosis

*Taenia solium*, the pork tapeworm causes human intestinal infection and its larval stage (Cysticercus cellulosae) causes cysticercosis. It can occur through heteroinfection—by eating food contaminated with infected human feces containing the eggs; external autoinfection—when eggs are ingested from the patient's own contaminated fingers, or internal autoinfection—when eggs which are regurgitated up in a proglottid from a worm in the patient's intestine are reswallowed from the stomach. Cysticercosis cellulosae cutis is the term given to the formation of subcutaneous nodules by the cysticerci and their surgical excision can be done.

## SUGGESTED READINGS


1. Bryceson AD, Hay RJ. Parasitic Worms and Protozoa. In: Champion RH, Burton L, Ebling FJ (Eds). Text book of Dermatology, 5th edition. Oxford: Blackwell; 1992. pp. 1217-64.
2. Desjeux P, Ghosh RS, Dhalaria P, et al. Reports of the Post kala-azar dermal leishmaniasis (PKDL) consortium meeting, New Delhi, India 27-29 June 2012. Parasit Vectors. 2013;6:196-217.
3. Haddad V Jr, Lupi O, Lonza JP, et al. Tropical dermatology: marine and aquatic dermatology. J Am Acad Dermatol. 2009;61(5):733-50.
4. Jacobson CC, Abel EA. Parasitic infestations. J Am Acad Dermatol. 2007;56(6): 1026-43.
5. John DT, Petri WA. Markell and Voge's Medical Parasitology, 9th edition. Missouri, USA: Elsevier; 2006. pp. 274-321.
6. Klion A, Nutman TB. Loiasis and Mansonella Infections. In: Guerrant R, Walker DH, Weller PF (Eds). Tropical Infectious Diseases: Principles, Pathogens and Practice. Philadelphia: Churchill Livingstone; 2011. pp.735.
7. Lupi O, Bartlett BL, Haugen RN, et al. Tropical dermatology: tropical diseases caused by protozoa. J Am Acad Dermatol. 2009;60(6):897-925.
8. Nutman TB, Kazura J. Lymphatic Filariasis. In: Guerrant R, Walker DH, Weller PF (Eds). Tropical Infectious Diseases: Principles, Pathogens, and Practice, 2nd edition. Philadelphia: Churchill Livingstone; 2011. pp.729.
9. O'Quinn JC, Dushin R. Cutaneous larva migrans. Case report with current recommendations for treatment. J Am Pediatr Med Assoc. 2005;95:291-4.
10. Peters W, Gilles HM. Tropical medicine and parasitology, 4th edition. London: Mosby-Wolfe; 1997. pp. 42-7.
11. Rathi SK, Pandhi RK, Khanna N, et al. Mucosal and peri-orificial involvement in Post-Kala-Azar dermal leishmaniasis. Indian J Dermatol Venereol Leprol. 2004;70:280-2.
12. Semenovitch I, Lupi O. Trypanosomiasis. In: Tyring SK, Lupi O, Hengge UR (Eds). Tropical dermatology. New York: Elsevier Inc.; 2006. pp. 29-39.
13. Sra KK, Sracic J, Tyring SK. Treatment of protozoan infections. Dermatol Ther. 2004;17:513-6.
14. Vega-López F, Hay RJ. Parasitic worms and Protozoa. In: Burns T, Breathnach S, Cox N, Griffiths C (Eds). Rook's Textbook of Dermatology, 8th edition. UK: Wiley-Blackwell Publications Ltd.; 2010. pp. 37.1-44.
15. WHO expert committee on filariasis. Lymphatic filariasis: diagnosis and pathogenesis. Bull World Health Organ. 1993;71:135.

# 63 CHAPTER Skin Diseases Caused by Arthropods, Bites, and Stings

*Monica Chahar, Paschal V D'Souza, Sanjay K Rathi*

## INTRODUCTION

Arthropods are one of the most widely distributed animal species. Their bites and stings can cause a variety of clinical reactions which can be broadly divided into immunological (allergic) and nonimmunological reactions (toxin or trauma mediated). Arthropods consists of the following main classes—Insecta, Arachnida, Diplopoda, and Chilopoda.

## ARTHROPOD BITE REACTION

Arthropods produce their effects on the skin through the following main mechanisms:
- Mechanical trauma
- Injection of irritant, cytotoxic or pharmacologically active substances
- Injection of potential allergens
- Contact reactions
- Reactions to retained mouthparts
- Transmission of disease.

### Clinical Features

The most commonly seen response is papular urticaria which consists of small, 3–10 mm diameter, pruritic, urticarial papules present on exposed areas which may show a central hemorrhagic punctum (Fig. 1). Bullous reactions and secondary infection are not uncommon. Bite reactions may persist for months.

### Histopathology of Arthropod Bites and Stings

Papular urticaria shows prominent papillary dermal edema and a perivascular chronic inflammatory infiltrate having eosinophils. There may be spongiosis with exocytosis and vesicle formation. Presence of T lymphocytes (CD45RO, CD3) and macrophages (CD68) were detected but B lymphocytes (CD20) and dendritic antigen-presenting cells (S100) were not found.

Chronic reactions show a dense dermal inflammatory infiltrate consisting of lymphocytes, histiocytes, eosinophils, plasma cells, atypical mononuclear cells having hyperchromatic nuclei and sometimes a foreign body type granulomatous (if mouthparts are present).

### Treatment

The ideal treatment is the identification and removal of its cause. Mild topical steroids, systemic antihistamines, and oral antibiotics may be given.

## CLASS INSECTA

This comprises around 60% of the arthropod species in the world.

### Orders

1. Lepidoptera
2. Hymenoptera
3. Coleoptera
4. Diptera
5. Hemiptera
6. Dictyoptera
7. Siphonaptera
8. Thrips (Thysanoptera)
9. Locusts (Orthoptera)
10. Phthiraptera.

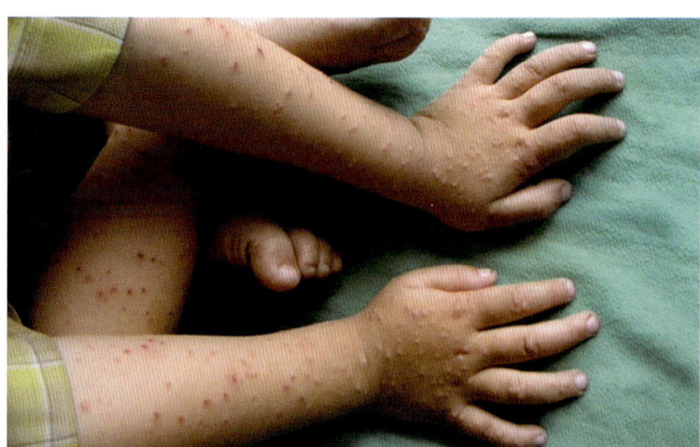

**FIG. 1:** Papular urticarial.
*Courtesy*: Dr TK Dhali, ESIPGIMSR, Basaidarapur, New Delhi.

## Lepidoptera (Butterflies, Caterpillars, and Moths)

Injuries caused by lepidopterans are called erucism (larval form) and lepidopterism (adult form).

### Pathogenesis

Epithelial penetration by the "hairs" (setae) can cause foreign body reaction. The venom present may cause toxin-mediated reactions due to histamine, kinins, plasminogen activators, and other proteinaceous toxins.

### Clinical Features

Local edema and erythema (within few hours) and occasionally, conjunctivitis, keratitis, ophthalmia nodosa, and iritis can be observed. Contact with *Lonomia* caterpillars can cause a potentially fatal hemorrhagic syndrome. Pararama, caused by contact with *Premolis* larvae, can cause periarticular fibrosis and ankylosis.

### Management

Local application of cold compresses, baths, and corticosteroid creams along with systemic antihistamines is recommended. Setae can be removed from the skin by "stripping" with adhesive tape. The therapy of choice for envenomation by caterpillars is local blockade with 2% lidocaine.

## Hymenoptera (Ants, Bees, Hornets, and Wasps)

Medically important species of this group are shown in the table 1.

There are three subfamilies within the family Formicidae which are of medical importance—Ponerinae (genus *Paraponera—Poneratoxin* and *Dinoponera*), Dorylinae (genus *Eciton*), and Myrmicinae (*Solenopsis* genus—fire ants).

### Pathogenesis

Hymenoptera venom contains vasoactive amines, small polypeptides, and larger protein molecules. Bee venom contains histamine, melittin, hyaluronidase, a high molecular weight substance with acid phosphatase activity, and phospholipase A. The three major allergens in vespid venoms are phospholipases, hyaluronidase, and antigen. Ants of the *Solenopsis* genus have venom containing oily alkaloids. Its major fraction is solenopsin A, which has a cytotoxic effect that can degranulate mast cells.

### Clinical Features

Stings produce immediate burning and pain, followed by an intense, local, erythematous wheal. Anaphylactoid reactions may also occur (Figs 2 and 3).

### Management

Cold compresses and topical corticosteroids with systemic antihistamines may help in pruritus. Massive envenomation may require oral corticosteroids. Treatment for anaphylaxis includes subcutaneous epinephrine hydrochloride. In cases of bee stings, early extraction with clamps decreases the amount of the venom injected and improves the prognosis.

**TABLE 1: Clinically important hymenoptera**

| | |
|---|---|
| Superfamily Apoidea (bees) | Honeybees (*Apis mellifera*); Humblebees; Bumblebees (*Bombus spp.*) |
| Superfamily Vespoidea | Family Vespidae (social wasps)-Vespa, *Vespula*, and *Polistes* |
| Superfamily Bethyloidea | *Scleroderma domesticum, Epyris californicus* and *Cephalonomia gallicola* |
| Superfamily Scolioidea | Family Formicidae (ants) |

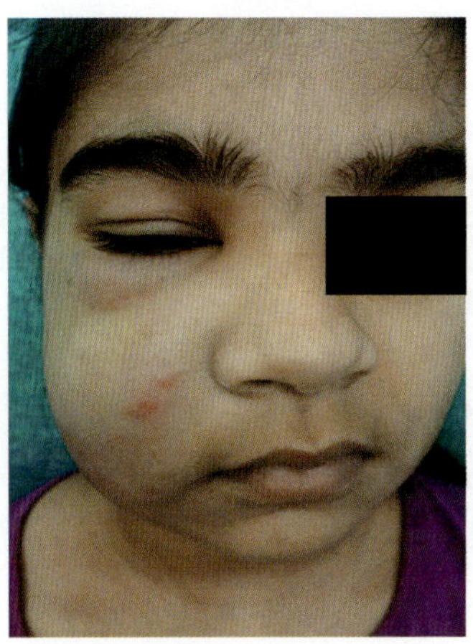

**FIG. 2:** Angioedema caused by wasp sting.
*Courtesy*: Dr Saurabh Singh, ESIC Medical College, Faridabad, Haryana.

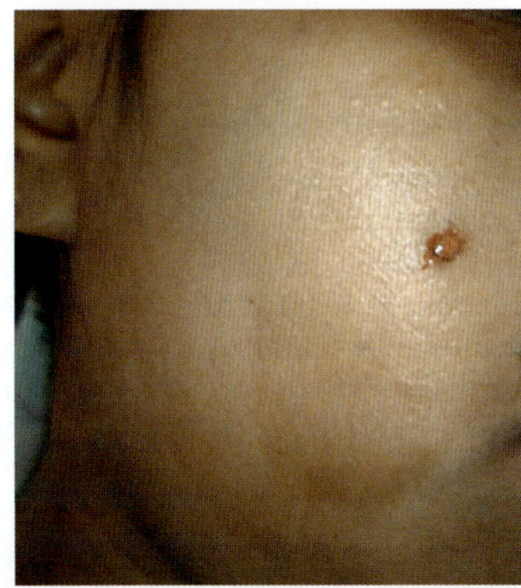

**FIG. 3:** Bee sting.
*Courtesy*: Dr Rajkumar Kothiwala, JLN Medical College, Ajmer Rajasthan.

## Coleoptera (Beetles)

Blister beetle dermatitis occurs after contact with several groups of beetle. Medically important members of this order are shown in table 2.

### Pathogenesis

Meloidae and Oedemeridae families (genus *Lytta* and *Epicauta*) release a vesicating agent, cantharidin. Cantharidin acts by activating neutral serine proteases, leading to the

**TABLE 2: Classification of order Coleoptera**

| | |
|---|---|
| Family Meloidae (oil beetles, blister beetles) | Genus *Lytta (L. vesicatoria); Epicauta; Mylabris; Psalydolytta; Cylindrotheca melanocephala* |
| Family Staphylinidae (rove beetles) | Genus *Paederus* |
| Family Oedemeridae | Genus *Oxycopis; Sessinia; Thelyphassa* |
| Family Paussinae | *Cerapterus concolor* |
| Family Tenebrionidae (darkling beetles) | *Tribolium castaneum* (rust-red flour beetle) |

degeneration of desmosomes. Members of the family Staphylinidae (genus *Paederus*) contain the vesicant *pederin* which can block mitosis by acting on cellular DNA. The beetles release their blistering fluid if they are brushed against, pressed, or crushed on the skin.

## Clinical Features

Elongated or linear lesions comprising of erythema, pruritus, and burning and vesicles are seen. "Kissing lesions" are observed when the blister beetle's excretion is deposited in the flexures of the elbows or other folds (Figs 4 and 5).

## Management

Immediate cleaning with water and potassium permanganate compresses. Corticosteroid creams are often needed.

# Diptera (Flies and Mosquitoes)

The different families of flies are discussed here.

Black flies of the family Simuliidae are vectors for onchocerciasis (African river blindness) and tularemia. Cutaneous myiasis may be caused by the deposition of fly larvae into open wounds. Other important flies worldwide are the sand fly (*Phlebotomus*), which is a vector for leishmanial parasites, and the tsetse fly, which is a vector for trypanosomes that cause sleeping sickness. Culicidae (mosquitoes) are vectors of many important diseases, such as filariasis, malaria, dengue, and yellow fever.

## Pathogenesis

Bite reactions due to insects of order Diptera are mostly due to allergens in saliva of insect and not due to toxin. Salivary gland surface proteins of mosquitoes are major immunogenic components.

## Clinical Features

Sandfly bites are responsible for the syndrome known as harara (urticarial multiformis endemic). The sites of the bites of Simuliidae are often marked by a small blood crust with surrounding ecchymosis. Nodules and discoid eczematous areas persist at the sites of the bites for several months. Urticaria papules, ulcers, or bullae often persist for weeks.

Myiasis is the general term given for infestation of maggots feeding on the host's necrotic or living tissue. Cutaneous myiasis usually presents as slowly growing nodules, furuncles or as ulcers. This can also be nasal, aural, or ophthalmic (Fig. 6).

Mellanby has described five stages of reaction to repeated mosquito bites.

Stage 1: No observable reaction, induction of hypersensitivity
Stage 2: Pruritic papules
Stage 3: Additional immediate wheal
Stage 4: Only immediate wheal without delayed papule
Stage 5: Complete tolerance with no reaction.

A disease has been described in which there is a triad of hypersensitivity to mosquito bites, chronic Epstein–Barr virus infection, and natural killer cell leukemia or lymphoma. Skeeter syndrome is a mosquito saliva-induced large local inflammatory reaction clinically resembling cellulites.

## Management

Thorough cleaning with soap and water, topical steroids, and systemic antihistamines. Treatment of myiasis includes the use of forceps, excision, occlusion or suffocation approaches (e.g., tape,

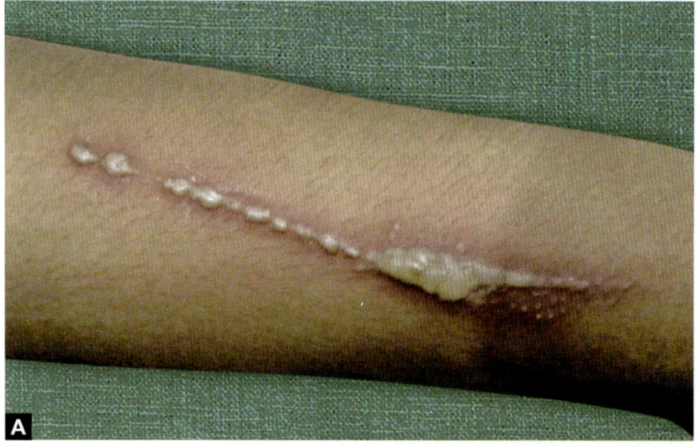


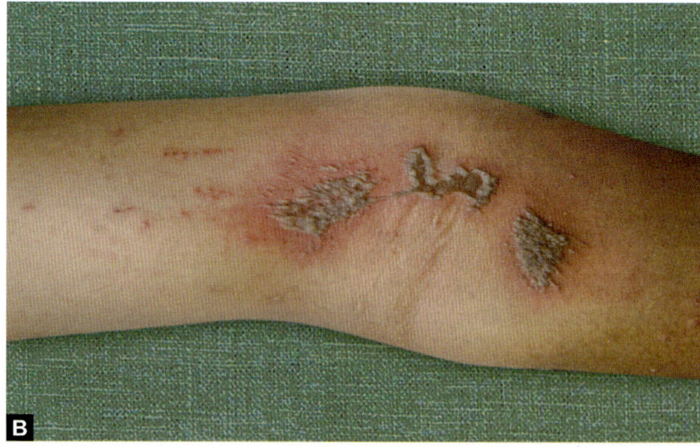


**FIG 4:** Paederus dermatitis showing **A,** Streaked vesiculo-pustular lesions with background erythem; ***B,** Irregularly linear inflammatory lesion showing central cauterization and surrounding vesiculopustules, erythema, and edema

**Courtesy*: Dr Mayank Kaushik, ESIPGIMSR, Basaidarpur, New Delhi.

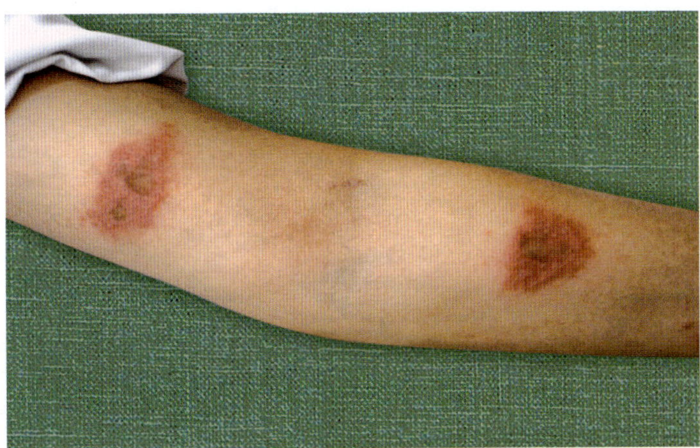

**FIG. 5:** Kissing lesions.
*Courtesy*: Dr Mayank Kaushik, ESIPGIMSR, Basaidarapur, New Delhi

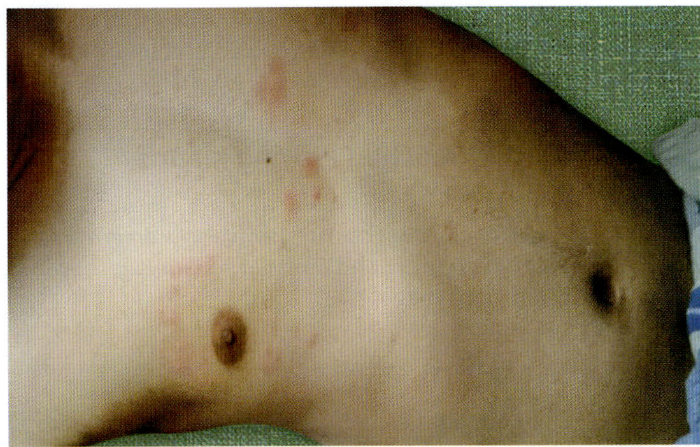

**FIG. 7:** Bed bug bites.

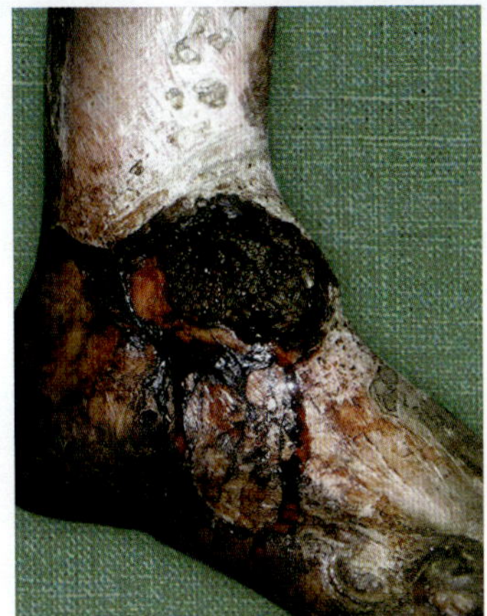

**FIG. 6:** Myiasis.
*Courtesy*: Dr Rajkumar Kothiwala, JLN Medical College, Ajmer Rajasthan.

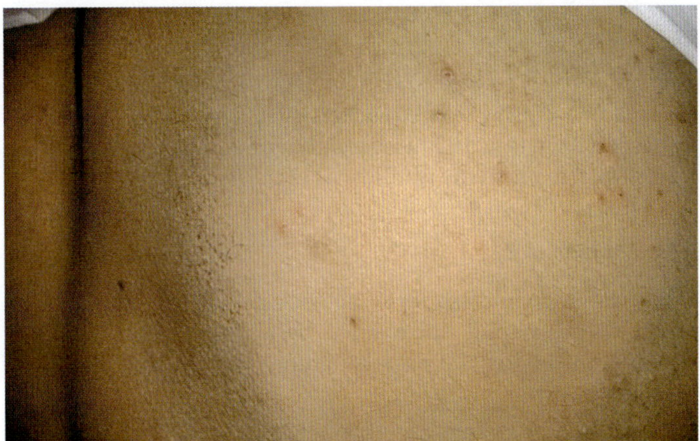

**FIG. 8:** Bed bug bites.
*Courtesy*: Dr Rajkumar Kothiwala, JLN Medical College, Ajmer Rajasthan.

**TABLE 3: Classification of Hemiptera**

| | |
|---|---|
| Family Cimicidae | • Genus *Cimex- Cimex lectularius* (common bed bugs), *Cimex pipistrelli* (batbug), *Cimex hemipterus* (tropical batbug)<br>• Genus *Leptocimex- L. boueti*<br>• Genus *Oeciacus* (martin bug, swallow bug)-*Oeciacus hirundinis; O. vicarius*<br>• Genus *Haematosiphon* (Mexican chicken bedbug)-*H. inodorus* |
| Family Anthrocoridae | *Lyctocoris campestris*, *Anthocoris kingi*, and *Anthocoris nemorum* |
| Family Pantatomidae | Palomena prasina (green shield bug) |
| Family Reduviidae | Triatoma sanguisuga |

nail polish, glue, or petroleum jelly) or use of an irritant (chewing tobacco, snuff, or camphor oil).

## Hemiptera (Bugs)

Medically important families belonging to this order are listed in the table 3.

### Pathogenesis

Triatomine reduviid bugs (kissing bugs, assassin bugs, conenose bugs) feed on the exposed areas of people while they sleep. Triatomine bugs infest cracks and crevices, and infestation is associated with poor housing conditions. Arilus cristatus, the wheal bug, is widely distributed.

### Clinical Features

Multiple bites arranged in an irregular, linear fashion are seen. Bites that occur in a row of three are sometimes referred to as "breakfast, lunch, and dinner". Local response consists of wheals and papules with a small hemorrhagic punctum at the center (Figs 7 and 8). Bullous reactions can occur. The bite of the reduviid bugs is typically painless with swelling and itching occurring within hours of the bite. Romana's sign is the unilateral eye swelling caused by a triatomine bug. This sign may occur after a bite in absence of *Trypanosoma cruzi* transmission.

### Management

Cracks and crevices should be eliminated, and the area treated with an insecticide such as dichlorvos or permethrin. Removal of infested furniture can also help. Treatment with antihistamines and topical steroids may be given. Topical antibiotics may be needed in cases of secondary infections.

## Dictyoptera (Cockroaches, Praying Mantis, and Termites)

Main pest species of cockroaches are *Periplaneta americana, P. australasiae, Blatta orientalis*, and *Blattella germanica*. They may cause urticaria and dermatitis.

## Siphonaptera (Fleas)

The order Siphonaptera contains three families of medical importance (Table 4).

The rat fleas (Xenopsylla cheopis and X. braziliensis) transmit bubonic plague and typhus. Tunga penetrans (smallest flea) causes Tungiasis.

### Pathogenesis

Fleas are exclusive blood suckers and their saliva is highly antigenic. Tungiasis is caused by penetration of the skin by the adult flea, usually in the web spaces of the feet.

### Clinical Features

Tungiasis is characterized by a black dot at the center of an erythematous papule surrounded by a white halo. Secondary bacterial infections and even gangrene with autoamputation of toes may occur.

### Diagnosis

Confirmation of flea infestation can be done by microscopical examination of debris from the animal's bedding material in case of suspected flea infestation from pet animals.

### Management

Treatment involves extraction, cryotherapy, or occlusion/suffocation of the flea. In tungiasis, topical ivermectin, metrifonate, and thiabendazole have been used. Oral thiabendazole (25 mg/kg/day) has been used in heavily infested patients.

**TABLE 4: Classification of order Siphonaptera**

| | |
|---|---|
| Tungidae | *Tunga penetrans* (sand flea, jigger or chigoe) |
| Pulicidae | *Pulex irritans* (human flea); *Ctenocephalides canis* (dog flea); Ctenocephalides felis (cat flea); *Xenopsylla cheopis* (tropical rat flea) |
| Ceratophyllidae | Bird fleas |

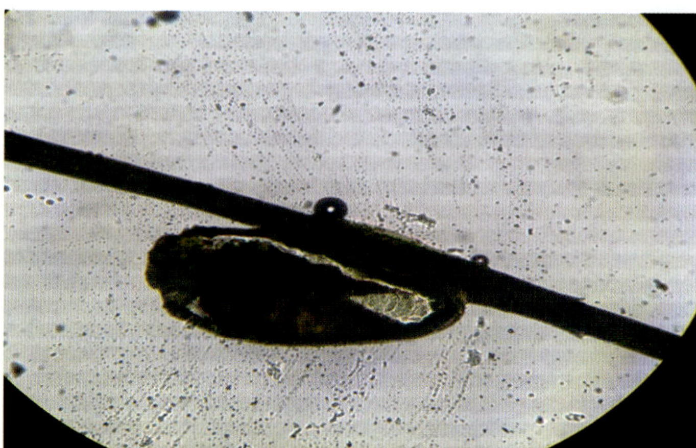

**FIG. 9:** Live nit of head lice as seen under microscope (10x.)
*Courtesy*: Dr Akhilesh Shukla, MD.

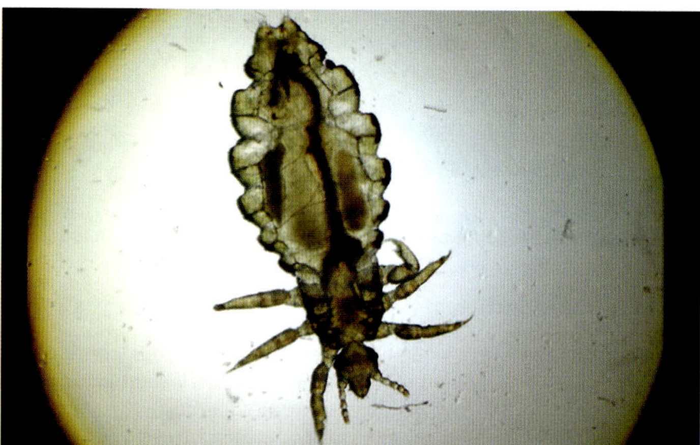

**FIG. 10:** Head lice as seen under microscope (10x).
Courtesy: Dr Akhilesh Shukla, MD.

## Thrips (Thysanoptera)

Thrip bites, which occur on exposed skin, produce tiny puncta and small, pink macules, or papules.

## Locusts (Orthoptera)

Reactions occur due to an allergen present in the gut of locusts which manifests as asthma, allergic rhinitis, and contact urticaria.

## Lice (Phthiraptera)

Lice are blood-sucking, strictly obligatory, species-specific insects that have no free-living stage in their life cycle. Pediculosis can primarily involve head (*Pediculus humanus var. capitis*), the body (*P. humanus var. corporis*), or the pubic region (Pthirus pubis). Body lice are the only disease vector of the complex, capable of transmitting bacterial diseases including trench fever, epidemic typhus, and louse-borne relapsing fever. Pubic lice infestations are not a reportable condition in many countries, but are considered a sexually transmitted disease.

### Lice Characteristic

Head lice are the most common lice. They are hematophagous that survive by sucking the blood, several times a day (every 2–3 hours). The female (3–4 mm in size) head lice lives 30 days after fertilization and lays 8–10 eggs close to the base of the scalp per day for a total of 50–300 eggs during its lifetime of 30 days (Figs 9 and 10). Young lice hatch within 1 week and go through nymphal instar stages, maturing to adults over a period of 7 days. Most spread of infection is related to the third instar forms and adults.

Head lice can survive for up to 3 days off the host. Body lice live on the body surface and lay their eggs on clothing. Pubic lice is 1–3 mm long, is sedentary, found usually in pubic region, groin, and on eyelashes.

## Pathogenesis

Head lice are the most common infestation. The transmission may be direct contact, or indirect, through clothing, hair brushes, blankets, and wardrobes. A genetically close "cousin", *P. humanus var. corporis*, is responsible for body lice and is more commonly associated with poverty, overcrowding, poor hygiene, and disaster. Pubic lice are transmitted by intimate and/or sexual contact.

A louse feeds by sucking blood and simultaneously injects saliva with vasodilatory and anticoagulation properties into the host. Deposition of saliva fecal matter on the scalp elicits an inflammatory response leading to scratching and secondary impetiginization.

## Clinical Features

Pruritus, exudation, and crusting are present. Nits can be seen (Fig. 11).

The hair can become tangled with exudates, predisposing the area to fungal infection. This results in a malodorous mass called plica polonica (plica neuropathica). Countless lice and nits can be found under the entangled hair mass. Secondary cellulitis may develop. In longstanding infestation, the skin may become lichenified, hyperpigmented with scars and excoriations particularly on the trunk, so called vagabond's skin. Pubic lice may uncommonly infest eyebrows and eyelashes. Physical findings include visible opalescent nits or live lice and blue macules (maculae ceruleae), a characteristic finding at feeding sites (Fig. 12).

## Diagnosis

All lice infestations are diagnosed by identification of live adult lice, and viable eggs (nits) on the hair shafts in the specific body regions giving them their names. Empty egg cases attached to hair shafts are not diagnostic of an active infection.

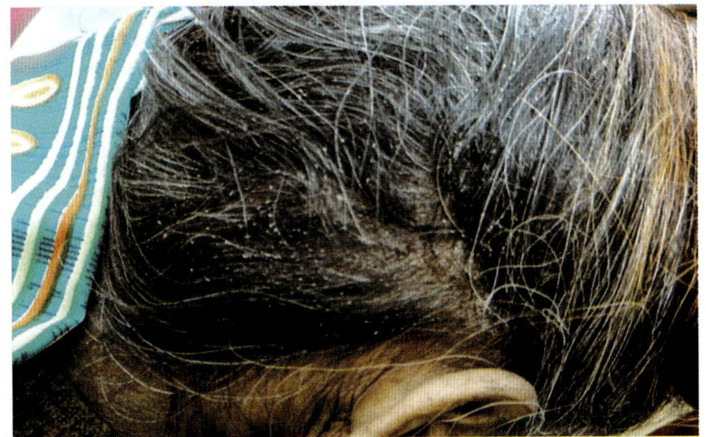

**FIG. 11:** Pediculosis capitis.

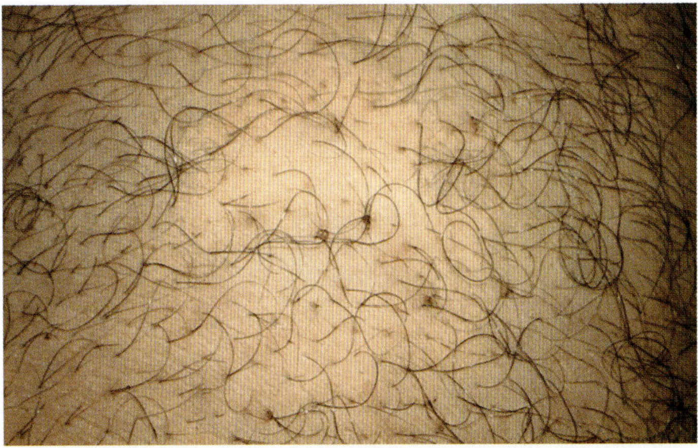

**FIG. 12:** Pubic lice.
*Courtesy*: Dr Saurabh Singh, ESIC Medical College, Faridabad, Haryana.

### *Differential Diagnosis*

Pediculosis capitis needs to be differentiated from inner root sheath remnants (hair casts), black piedra, white piedra, trichodystrophies (monilethrix and trichorrhexis nodosa), psoriasis, hair spray debris, seborrheic dermatitis, and psocids (book lice).

Pediculosis corporis may be confused with other causes of prurigo simplex by the uninitiated.

## Treatment

Treatment of lice infection in general is based on topical or oral drugs, physical agents, and wet combing.

- *Pediculosis capitis—nonpharmacological treatment*: Wet combing after prior priming of nit infested hair with vinegar (4% acetic acid) for 3 minutes. This is not recommended internationally
- *Pediculosis capitis—pharmacological treatment*: Pediculicide treatment is summarized in tables 5 and 6. Any suspected bacterial infection should be treated with anti-staphylococcal antibiotic. Topical steroid may help in symptomatic relief for eczematization

Treatment failures are often due to noncompliance, improper application of pediculicides, or reinfestation, and rarely, resistance to pediculicides.

Some patients may require a second application of topical therapy after 3–7 days. Infestation of the eyelashes should be treated by application of an occlusive ointment, such as petroleum jelly, twice daily for 10 days.

## Resistance to Pediculocidal Drugs

Pyrethroid resistance in human lice which is now been extensively reported is due to three knockdown resistance (kdr)-type point mutations (M815I, T917I, and L920) in the voltage-sensitive sodium channel *alpha-subunit* gene.

## Prevention and Control

Community-based treatment with oral ivermectin has given promising results. Proper education of the public and health professionals and clear treatment plans are essential.

**TABLE 5: Recommended local pediculicide treatments for pediculosis**

| Therapy | Use | Mechanism of action | Safety profile | Comments |
|---|---|---|---|---|
| 1% permethrin cream rinse | Applied after shampoo, left on for 10 min and then rinsed off | Neurotoxin | – | First-line treatment for head lice. Residual activity lasting for over 2 weeks. It is both pediculicidal and ovicidal |
| Malathion (0.5%) | Applied to the hair, left to air dry, and washed off after 8–12 hours | Causing respiratory paralysis in the arthropod | Flammable, organophosphate poisoning risks | 95% ovicidal in susceptible strains, rapid killing, good residual activity |
| Lindane (1%) | Be left on for no more than 10 min | – | Potential central nervous system (CNS) toxicity from organochlorine poisoning | 95% ovicidal, no residual activity |
| Ivermectin 0.8 % shampoo | Apply to hair, wash off after 5 min. | – | Excellent | Excellent |
| Spinosad 0.9% cream | Left on the scalp and hair for 10 min and then rinsed | It causes involuntary muscle contractions and excitation of the arthropod CNS system, eventually resulting in spastic and then later flaccid paralysis | 4 years and older | – |

**TABLE 6: Oral drugs used for pediculosis**

| Therapy | Use | Mechanism of action | Safety profile | Comments |
|---|---|---|---|---|
| Ivermectin | 200 µg/kg of body weight. Two oral doses of 12 mg once a day at 7–10 days apart | It results in hyperpolarization, leading to flaccid paralysis culminating in the death of the parasite | – | Not recommended below 5 years of age, children who weigh <15 kg pregnancy and lactation |
| Cotrimoxazole | – | Gut flora of pediculosis is killed, and thereby depriving the lice of essential vitamins | – | Not approved by US-FDA for treatment of head lice |

**TABLE 7: Classification of Order Arachnida**

| Family Theridiidae (widow spiders) | Genus Latrodectus |
|---|---|
| Family Hexathelidae (funnel-web spiders) | Genus *Atrax/Hadronyche* and *Macrothele* |
| Family Sicariidae ("fiddleback", "violin", "brown recluse" spiders) | Genus *Loxosceles: L. reclusa, laeta, deserta, arizonica and rufescens* |
| Family Lycosidae (wolf spiders) | Genus *Lycosa* |

## ARACHNIDA

Unlike insects, where the body is divided into three segments (head, thorax, and abdomen), arachnids have only two, the cephalothorax, from which the legs arise, and the abdomen. The Arachnida are classified in seven orders, only three of which are of medical importance:

1. Araneae (spiders)
2. Scorpiones (scorpions)
3. Acari (ticks and mites).

### Araneae (Spiders)

Clinical syndrome following the bite of a spider is known as arachnidism. They are classified in table 7.

#### Pathogenesis

Potent toxin venom induces skin necrosis.

#### Clinical Features

The bite of *Latrodectus* species is initially painless, but soon local erythema, edema, and severe pain develops and becomes generalized. Cramp-like or colicky abdominal pain is particularly common. There is frequently profuse sweating, and neuromuscular involvement causes paraesthesia, incoordination, and paralysis. The symptoms usually resolve within 2–3 days.

The bite of funnel-web spiders is painful and can be accompanied by nausea, vomiting, abdominal pain, profuse sweating, piloerection, muscle fasciculation, lacrimation, excess salivation, dyspnea, and pulmonary edema.

There are two distinct clinical forms of loxoscelism: necrotic cutaneous loxoscelism, and the much less frequent viscerocutaneous loxoscelism. There are local erythema, edema, and central bulla (Fig. 13). In cases of necrotic cutaneous loxoscelism, a "target" lesion surrounded by an ischaemic halo and an outer ring of erythema (the "red, white and blue" sign)-*marble plaque* sign are found (Fig. 14). In viscerocutaneous loxoscelism, systemic symptoms are fever, malaise, restlessness, and headache. Presence of ecchymoses, jaundice, hematuria, and hemoglobinuria indicate massive intravascular hemolysis, which may result in death.

#### Management

The compression bandage-splinting method helps in delaying onset of envenomation. Species-specific antivenoms are available for *Latrodectus* bites. Rest, ice compresses, and elevation (RICE therapy) help to reduce inflammation and pain in loxoscelism. Dapsone can be used (controversial). The

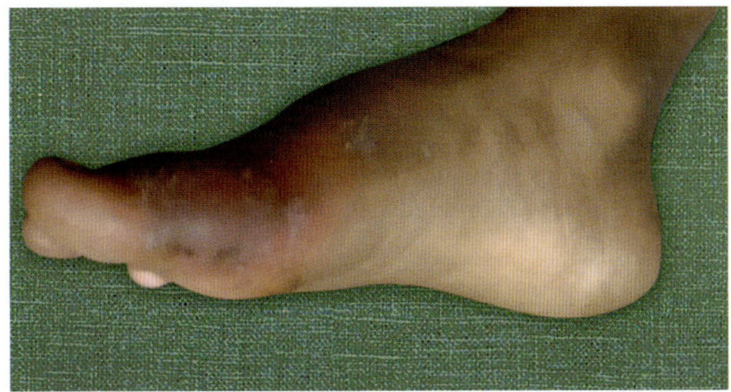

**FIG. 13:** Bullae at the site of spider bite.
*Courtesy*: Dr MA Haroon, Integral Institute of Medical Sciences & Research, Lucknow.

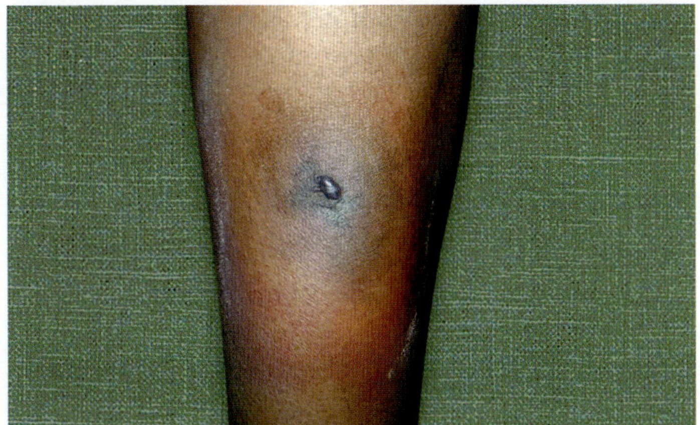

**FIG. 14:** Spider bite.
*Courtesy*: Dr Rajkumar Kothiwala, JLN Medical College, Ajmer, Rajasthan.

lesions of tarantulas can be treated with topical corticosteroids and oral antihistamines.

## Scorpiones (Scorpions)

There are six families of scorpions, but almost all scorpions dangerous to humans are in the Buthidae family. The venom of Tityus serrulatus (T. serrulatus), from Tityinae subfamily of Buthidae, is the most potent.

### Pathogenesis

The principal components of their venom are neurotoxins. The venom of T. serrulatus contains tityustoxin which binds to sodium and potassium ion channels causing sialorrhea, lacrimation, and rhinorrhea. The toxin from Hemiscorpius lepturus is hemicalcin, which is active on ryanodine-sensitive calcium channels and causes neurotoxic symptoms.

### Clinical Features

Local effects are severe burning pain and hyperaesthesia. Systemic effects include restlessness, profuse sweating, muscle spasms, marked increase in salivary and lacrimal secretion, nausea, vomiting, convulsions, hypertension, cardiac arrhythmias, myocarditis, and pulmonary edema. Death is usually due to respiratory or cardiac failure.

### Management

Ice packs and the injection of local anesthetic around the sting site help to reduce the pain. Specific antivenoms are available. In 2011, the Food and Drug Administration (FDA)-approved the first treatment specifically for scorpion stings—Centruroides (Scorpion) Immune F(ab)2 injection.

## Acari (Ticks)

There are two major families: the Ixodidae (hard ticks) and the Argasidae (soft ticks). Medically important species in Ixodidae family are: *Ixodes scapularis* (deer tick), *Dermacentor andersoni* (American wood tick), and *D. variabilis* (American dog tick).

### Pathogenesis

Most ticks are parasites of wild animals, and humans are incidental hosts. Tick bites are not painful, as an anesthetic and anticoagulant substance is introduced. Tick bites may induce foreign body and hypersensitivity reactions. Granulomatous foreign body reactions occur when mouthparts are retained in the patient's skin after vigorous attempts at removal of the tick.

Among diseases transmitted by ticks are Lyme disease, ehrlichiosis, and babesiosis (*Ixodes scapularis*); rocky mountain spotted fever (*Dermacentor variabilis* and *D. andersoni*); Colorado tick fever, Q-fever, and tularemia (D. andersoni); and other rickettsial diseases. Ticks are also responsible for transmitting arboviruses that are responsible for encephalitis and hemorrhagic fevers.

### Clinical Features

Tick bite may cause papular urticaria. Classic sign of tick's (or mite's) or their nymph's bites is the "comet" sign, where many bites spread from initial points in the distal areas of the ankles and legs, with a cone distribution (Fig. 15).

*Lyme disease* is caused by the spirochete *Borrelia burgdorferi.* The hallmark cutaneous disease is erythema migrans. Hematologic spread of the spirochetes may trigger systemic flu-like symptoms along with urticarial and lichenoid exanthemas. Multiple organs may be involved eventually.

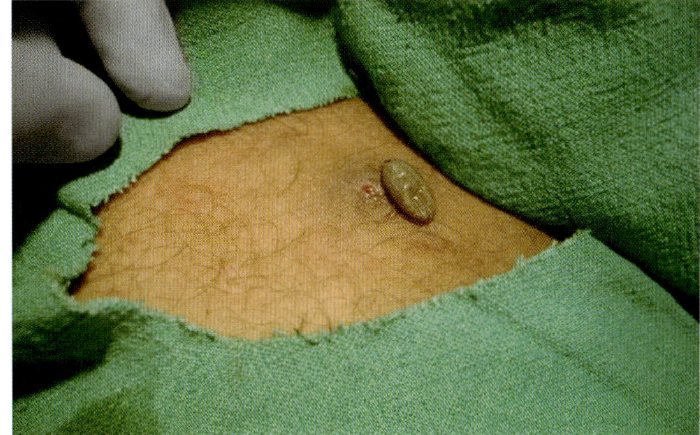

**FIG. 15:** Tick bite.
*Courtesy*: Dr Mayank Kaushik, ESIPGIMSR, New Delhi.

*Tick paralysis*: Hard ticks can inject certain toxins that can cause tick paralysis. It starts usually after a week the tick begins feeding, paralyzing the legs, and affecting speech, swallowing, and breathing. Rickettsiae diseases spread by Ixodes include Q-fever (*Coxiella burneti*) and arboviruses that cause serious encephalitis.

### Treatment

Ticks should not be removed by a sudden force. Use of forceps and gentle traction usually succeeds when other methods have failed.

Prevention of bites is the most important measure. Permethrin, when applied directly to clothing, may be the most effective tick repellent, give nits long duration of action, and actual ability to kill ticks. DEET can be applied to exposed skin surfaces.

## Mites

### Scabies

Scabies is a contagious skin infestation caused by the obligate human parasitic mite *Sarcoptes scabiei var. hominis* (Fig. 16).

#### *Epidemiology*

The disease is widespread though it tends to mainly affect the children living in poor, overcrowded tropical areas mainly in developing countries. Racial differences are probably attributable to socioeconomic and behavioral factors. Hygiene appears to have limited role in spread of scabies.

#### *Transmission*

The primary source of transmission is prolonged skin-to-skin contact with an infected individual. Fomites may bear potential source of transmission. The developmental cycle from egg through three active intermediate stages or instars to adult is about 2 weeks. In classical scabies only about 10–12 mites are present on the entire body.

#### *Pathogenesis*

The protective immune response in ordinary scabies is dominated by a Th1-type cytokine profile associated with CD4+ T-lymphocytes, whereas the severe form of crusted scabies is dominated by a nonprotective Th2 cytokine profile with the predominant effector cells being CD8+ lymphocytes. An aspartic protease of the scabies mite facilitates digestion of host skin and serum while the scabies mite serine protease inhibitors mediate overall inhibition of the complement system protecting scabies mites from complement-mediated gut damage.

#### *Clinical Features*

Human scabies is characterized clinically by pruritus with nocturnal exacerbation. The clinical types are:

- *Classical scabies*: Itchy, excoriated, papular lesions appear predominantly over the hands between the fingers, wrists, elbows, shoulders, genital area, including the penis, lower legs, particularly the ankles, the scrotum in males, and the breasts in women (Figs 17 to 19). Small raised or flattened burrows may be seen which represent curved linear lesions that often end in a tiny papule or pustule, and are diagnostic. Usually, the head is not affected, although it may be involved in infants and babies. Pustular or vesicular lesions may be seen on palms and soles in infants. Secondary infections are common
- Nodular scabies (NS): Larger, very itchy, papules or small nodules, are seen on the genitalia, axilla or groin though it may occur elsewhere in children. They result from developing immune reaction to mite antigens. NS often shows pseudolymphoma-like histopathology with predominant T lymphocytes

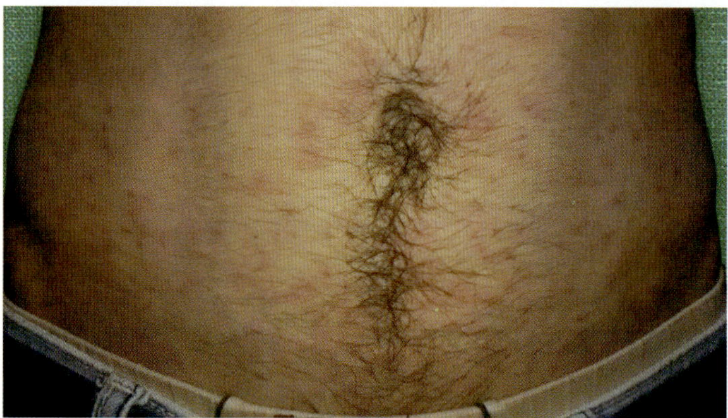

**FIG. 17:** Scabies.
*Courtesy*: Dr MA Haroon, Integral Institute of Medical Sciences & Research, Lucknow.

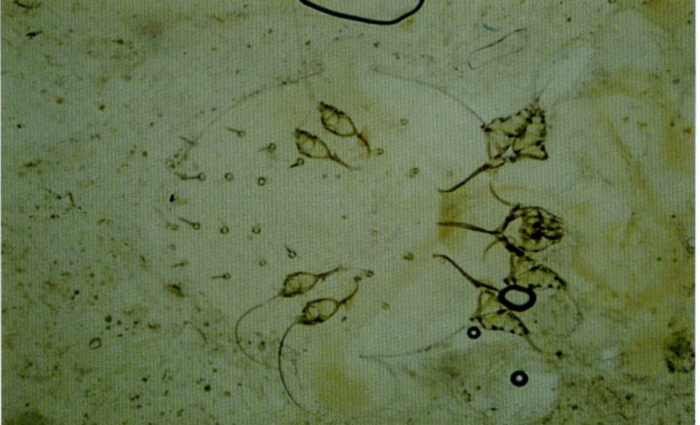

**FIG. 16:** Scabies mite.
*Courtesy*: Dr Saurabh Singh, ESIC Medical College, Faridabad, Haryana.

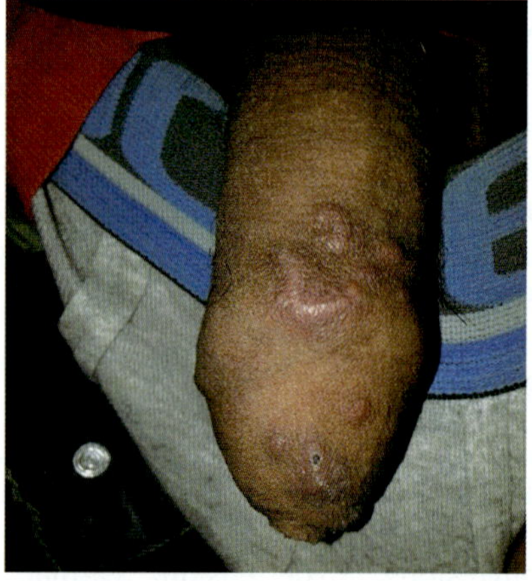

**FIG. 18:** Scabies.
*Courtesy*: Dr Devraj Dogra, Government Medical College, Jammu.

- *Crusted scabies*: Also known as Norwegian scabies, which is seen in the severely ill or immunocompromised or in disorders like Down syndrome. The clinical features manifests as rash without itch. It may mimick psoriasis. There may be dry scales and crusts that are most marked over prominences such as the dorsum of the fingers, wrists, and ears. The face may be involved, and one or more nails show hyperkeratosis and thickening. These crusted infections are caused by a superinfection with thousands of mites, and such patients are very contagious
- *Scabies of the cleanly (Braun-Falco's)*: Seen in the super hygienic people wherein there is severe pruritus without obvious skin lesions except for occasional scattered papules. Secondary infection by group A streptococci and the development of glomerulonephritis has been reported.

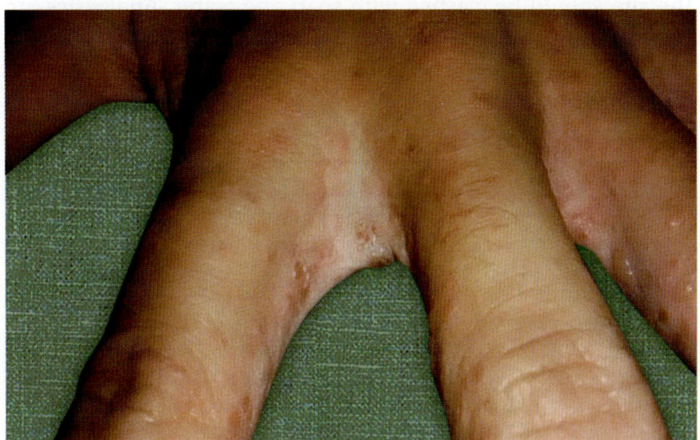

**FIG. 19:** Scabies (burrow).
*Courtesy*: Dr MA Haroon, Integral Institute of Medical Sciences & Research, Lucknow.

### *Diagnosis*

Diagnosis usually rests on clinical features such as the presence of itching that is worse at night, the anatomical distribution of lesions, presence of burrows in the skin, and coupled with itching in other members of the family.

Confirmation of the diagnosis by direct tests which demonstrate adult or immature scabies mites, ova, or even feces in scrapings taken from a skin burrow, requires both skill and perseverance. The burrow ink test is a simple, rapid, noninvasive test that can be used to screen a large number of patients. Hand held dermatoscopy which identifies triangular structures is an accurate test. Polymerase chain reaction or serodiagnosis has not been assessed in a tropical environment.

### *Treatment and Control Measures*

It is important to treat all cases and household contacts including recent sexual partners with antiscabetic treatment. An ideal antiscabetic is one which is effective against adult and egg, easily applicable, nonsensitizing, nonirritating, nontoxic, and economical. Secondary bacterial infection should also be treated simultaneously. The rash and itch may take up to 2 weeks or more to clear after a successful treatment. Oral antihistamines and topical soothing lotions and even brief application of topical corticosteroids can help with itching. Specific treatment can be topical or oral.

### *Topical Antiscabetic Agents*

A number of topical agents are highly effective. They should be applied to the entire skin surface below chin for the period specified, and then completely washed off. Children and the

**TABLE 8: Topical antiscabetic drugs**

| Topical agent | Instructions | Remarks |
|---|---|---|
| Permethrin 5% | Apply overnight (8–14 hours) | • Expensive<br>• Widely used agent<br>• Few side effects<br>• There is increasing concern about potential resistance of the scabies mite to permethrin<br>• Safe for younger children, pregnancy and lactation<br>• In the USA, approved for infants aged >2 months |
| Benzyl benzoate 10–25% | Leave on skin for 24 hours. Apply daily for 3 days | • Availability and cost vary<br>• Widely used agent in developing countries<br>• Transient skin irritation and burning, immediately after application<br>• Neurological complications possible<br>• May be diluted to 12.5% for children and to 6.25% for infants |
| Crotamiton 10% | Apply for 24 hours, and then wash and reapply. Repeat applications for 3–5 days | • Less effective but safe alternative for infants<br>• Multiple treatments needed<br>• Safe in pregnancy and lactation |
| Gamma benzene hexachloride (lindane) 1% | Apply for 8 hours then wash | • Second-line treatment in developed countries<br>• Widely used in tropical and developing countries<br>• Cheap and effective<br>• Aplastic anemia, convulsions, potential complications.<br>• Resistance and treatment failures reported<br>• Not advised for infants, pregnant women, and lactating women |
| Malathion 0.5% | Apply for 24 hours | Infrequently used |
| Sulfur ointment 6% (2–10%) | • Apply for 24 hour, and then wash and reapply<br>• Repeat applications for 3 days | • Effective in outbreaks in regions without available alternatives<br>• Poor acceptance, being messy, malodorous, and cause skin irritation |

A Cochrane review concluded that permethrin was the most effective agent for the treatment of scabies.

elderly, who more commonly have lesions in the scalp, require application to the head. Important ones are listed in table 8.

### *Oral Agents*

Ivermectin is the agent mainly used for treatment, of crusted scabies, in institutional outbreaks, and for mass administration in highly endemic communities. A dose of 200 mcg/kg orally stat can be repeated after 1-2 weeks due to its poor ovicidal activity. Ivermectin is a substrate for the cytochrome P450 3A4 pathway, and so caution should be exercised in people taking medications that induce or inhibit this pathway. Ivermectin is not recommended for use in children of less than 15 kg and pregnant women. Crusted scabies is difficult to treat and may require multiple doses of oral ivermectin with repeated topical permethrin and keratolytic therapy.

Nodular scabies is usually treated with topical steroids or with intralesional steroids. Topical tacrolimus has also been used with encouraging results.

Each treatment with scabicide should be followed the next morning by hot-wash laundering or dry cleaning of sheets and pillow cases and any clothes worn against the skin over the last week. Nonwashable items should be sealed in a plastic bag and stored above 20°C for 1 week.

Treatment failure may be due to incorrect diagnosis, dermatitis secondary to the mite or topical agent, incorrect application of the topical agent, poor penetration of thickened skin, or nails, or re-infestation. Drug resistance to ivermectin and permethrin is reported.

Treatment of close contacts, including recent sexual partners, is recommended.

### Animal Scabies

Transmission of animal scabies to humans can occur with *Sarcoptes scabiei* var. *canis* and *Notoedres cati*.

### Mites of Stored Products

Mites of the family Acaridae, Carpoglyphidae, and Glycyphagidae are found in various food products such as flour, grain, dried meat, cheese, and dried fruit and can cause "copra itch" or "grocer's itch".

### House Dust Mites

*Dermatophagoides pteronyssinus* is the most common species. The major house dust mites' allergens (Der p1 and Der f1) are present in the fecal pellets. Their role in atopic eczema remains controversial.

### Follicle Mites (Demodicidae)

*Demodex folliculorum* has been implicated in the pathogenesis of pityriasis folliculorum, rosacea, and blepharitis.

## DIPLOPODA AND CHILOPODA

Centipedes and millipedes belong to the classes Chilopoda and Diplopoda, respectively.

### Pathogenesis

The venom of the chilopedes contains several enzymes (metalloproteases) which have myotoxic, cardiotoxic, and neurotoxic activities. Millipedes have lateral glands that produce cyanide and quinones to repel predators.

### Clinical Features

Centipede bites causes local pain, erythema, and edema. Systemic symptoms include nausea, dizziness, and pyrexia. Contact of millipede secretions with the skin produces a local burning sensation and a yellowish-brown pigmentation due to oxidation of the quinones in the secretions. The lesions usually heal and desquamate in 10-14 days.

### Management

The site should be washed with soap and water. Analgesics are essential for pain control. The immediate use of alcohol or ether on the site could dissolve toxins.

## SUGGESTED READINGS

1. Bush SE, Rock AN, Jones SL, et al. Efficacy of the Louse Buster, a new medical device for treating head lice (Anoplura:Pediculidae). J Med Entomol. 2011;48:
2. Dodd CS. Interventions for treating headlice. Cochrane Database Syst Rev. 2001(3):CD001165.
3. Golant AK, GolantAK, Levitt JO. Scabies: a review of diagnosis and management based on mite biology. Pediatr Rev. 2012;33(1):e1-e12.
4. Haddad V Jr, Cardoso JL, Lupi O, et al. Tropical dermatology: Venomous arthropods and human skin: Part I. Insecta. J Am Acad Dermatol. 2012;67(3):331.e1-14.
5. Haddad V Jr, Cardoso JL, Lupi O, et al. Tropical dermatology: Venomous arthropods and human skin: Part II. Diplopoda, Chilopoda, and Arachnida. J Am Acad Dermatol. 2012;67(3):347.e1-9.
6. Hay RJ, Steer AC, Engelman D, et al. Scabies in the developing world—its prevalence, complications, and management. Clin Microbiol Infect. 2012;18:313-23.
7. Hicks MI, Elston DM. Scabies. Dermatol Ther. 2009;22:279-292.
8. Jayaraj R, Hales B, Viberg L, et al. A diagnostic test for scabies: IgE specificity for a recombinant allergen of Sarcoptes scabiei. Diagn Microbiol Infect Dis. 2011;71:403-7.
9. Karthikeyan K. Treatment of scabies: newer perspectives. Postgrad Med J. 2005;81(951):7-11.
10. Leung V, Miller M. Detection of Scabies: A Systematic Review of Diagnostic Methods. Can J Infect Dis Med Microbiol. 2011;22(4):143-6.
11. Madke B, Khopkar U. Pediculosis capitis: An update. Indian J Dermatol Venereol Leprol. 2012;78:429-38.
12. Mahmood W, Viberg LT, Fischer K, et al. An Aspartic Protease of the Scabies Mite Sarcoptes scabiei is Involved in the Digestion of Host Skin and Blood Macromolecules. PLoS Negl Trop Dis. 2013;7(11):e2525.
13. Mika A, Reynolds SL, Mohlin FC, et al. Novel Scabies Mite Serpins Inhibit the Three Pathways of the Human Complement System. PLoS ONE. 2012;7(7):e40489.
14. Mumcuoglu KY, Barker SC, Burgess IE, et al. International guidelines for effective control of head louse infestations. J Drugs Dermatol. 2007;6(4):409-14.
15. Pilger D, Heukelbach J, Khakban A, et al. Household-wide ivermectin treatment for head lice in an impoverished community: Randomized observer blinded controlled trial. Bull World Health Organ. 2010;88:90-6.
16. Roberts LJ, Huffam SE, Walton SF, et al. Crusted scabies: clinical and immunological findings in seventy-eight patients and a review of the literature. J Infect. 2005;50:375-81.
17. Rufi T. Diseases caused by Arthropods. In: Burgdorf WHC, Plewig G, Wolff HH, et al. (Eds). Braun-Falco's Dermatology, 3rd edition. Springer: Berlin Heidelberg; 2009. pp. 323-42.
18. Steen CJ, Carbonaro PA, Schwartz RA. Arthropods in dermatology. J Am Acad Dermatol. 2004;50(6):819-42.
19. Strong M, Johnstone P. Interventions for treating scabies. Cochrane Database Syst Rev. 2007;CD000320.
20. Usha V, Nair TVG. A comparative study of oral ivermectin and topical permethrin cream in the treatment of scabies. J Am Acad Dermatol. 2000;42:236-40.
21. Walton SF, Currie BJ. Problems in diagnosing scabies, a global disease in human and animal populations. Clin Microbiol Rev. 2007;20:268-79.
22. Woodley D, Saurat JH. The burrow ink test and the scabies mite. J Am Acad Dermatol. 1981;4:715-22.

# 64 CHAPTER Sexually Transmitted Infections

*Yogesh S Marfatia*

## INTRODUCTION

Unprotected sexual contact is responsible for transmission of many infections, horizontally or vertically. The term venereal disease was previously used to describe sexually transmitted disease (STD). Currently the term "sexually transmitted infection" (STI) is preferred which aptly includes the spectrum of both symptomatic and asymptomatic infections, which covers more than 30 pathogens. Bacterial STDs of previous decades are being replaced by persistent and recurrent viral infections resulting not only in morbidity but also mortality [human immunodeficiency virus (HIV)] and malignancy [human papillomavirus (HPV)]. Viral infections like herpes simplex virus (HSV) and HPV are dominating the STIs scenario.

Sexually transmitted infections can cause not only local symptoms but its dissemination further leads to sequelae and consequences like pelvic inflammatory disease (PID), infertility, and abortion.

Both ulcerative and nonulcerative STIs increase the potential of HIV transmission by manyfolds. HIV and STDs are the perfect example of epidemiologic synergy and they are cotransmitters of each other. As per demographic profile of India, a large proportion of population belongs to the sexually active age group and migrants, thus increasing potential of dissemination of STIs.

Comprehensive details of etiology, incubation period, clinical features, and complications are included in table 1.

## SEXUALLY TRANSMITTED DISEASES CHARACTERIZED BY ANOGENITAL ULCERS

These include genital herpes, syphilis, chancroid, lymphogranuloma venereum (LGV), donovanosis. The clinical features are discussed here. Diagnosis and treatment of each disease is included in tables 2 and 3, respectively.

**TABLE 1: Commonly occurring sexually transmitted infections and diseases**

| Etiology | Incubation period | Clinical manifestations | Sequelae/complications |
|---|---|---|---|
| **Bacterial** | | | |
| *Neisseria gonorrhoeae* | 1–14 days (average 2–7 days) | • Acute gonococcal urethritis in male<br>• Cervicitis in female—may be asymptomatic<br>• Local dissemination to urogenital tract | Infertility, ectopic pregnancy, pelvic inflammatory disease (PID), disseminated gonococcal infection (DGI) |
| *Chlamydia trachomatis (D-K)* | 7–21 days | • Nongonococcal urethritis in male<br>• Cervicitis in female | Same as in *N. gonorrhoeae*, except DGI, Reiter's syndrome |
| *Chlamydia trachomatis (L1, L2, L3)* | 3–30 days | • Lymphogranuloma venereum<br>• Acute transient genital ulcers and suppurative inguinal lymphadenitis (bubo) | Esthiomene, anorectogenital syndrome, proctocolitis |
| *Treponema pallidum* | 9–90 days | • Syphilis<br>• Primary—painless genital ulcer and lymphadenopathy<br>• Secondary:<br>○ Generalized lymphadenopathy<br>○ Generalized skin rash<br>○ Condyloma lata | Adverse outcomes of pregnancy, congenital syphilis |
| *Haemophilus ducreyi* | 3–10 days | Chancroid—multiple painful ulcers over genitalia and suppurative inguinal lymphadenitis (bubo) | Phimosis, paraphimosis, balanitis |
| *Calymmatobacterium granulomatis* | 9–50 days | • Donovanosis–ulcerogranulomatous<br>• Lesions over genitalia | Squamous cell carcinoma, pseudoelephantiasis |

*Continued*

*Continued*

| Etiology | Incubation period | Clinical manifestations | Sequelae/complications |
|---|---|---|---|
| *Gardnerella vaginalis** | – | Bacterial vaginosis—malodorous, white homogeneous vaginal discharge, pruritus, pain during coitus | Vaginal cuff cellulitis, PID, miscarriage/ preterm delivery |
| *Mycoplasma genitalium* | – | • Acute gonococcal urethritis in male<br>• Cervicitis in female | Pelvic inflammatory disease |
| **Viral** | | | |
| Herpes simplex virus-2 | 5–7 days | Primary/recurrent genital herpes—multiple genital erosions on erythematous base | Neurological complications, miscarriage, potential chances of transmission during labor and neonatal herpes |
| Human papillomavirus | 3 weeks to 2 years | Condyloma accuminata—warty growth over genitalia, perianal region | Laryngeal papilloma in infants, squamous epithelial neoplasia of cervix, anus, vagina, vulva and penis |
| Hepatitis B virus | 2–4 weeks | Hepatitis B (acute/chronic/fulminant) | Cirrhosis, hepatocellular carcinoma |
| Molluscum contagiosum virus | 2 weeks to 6 months | Genital molluscum contagiosum: umbilicated pearly white papules | Secondary infection |
| Human immunodeficiency virus | 2–15 years | AIDS and related conditions | Opportunistic infections, death |
| **Fungal** | | | |
| *Candida albicans** | – | Vulvovaginitis, balanitis, balanoposthitis | – |
| **Parasite** | | | |
| *Trichomonas vaginalis* | 4–21 days | Vaginitis, urethritis, prostatitis | PID, preterm delivery and low birth weight baby |
| **Ectoparasite** | | | |
| *Pthirus pubis* | 1–2 weeks | Pubic lice infestation | – |
| *Sarcoptes scabiei* | 3–4 weeks | Genital scabies | Secondary bacterial infection, glomerulonephritis, post-scabietic pruritus |

*It is a primarily an endogenous reproductive tract infection with potential for sexual transmission.

**TABLE 2: Laboratory diagnosis**

| Condition | *Smear* | *Culture* | *Serology* | *Other* |
|---|---|---|---|---|
| Chancroid | • Gram's, Giemsa stain or Wright's stain—gram-negative coccobacilli<br>• School of fish appearance or railroad track pattern | • Gold standard for diagnosis. 80% sensitive<br>• Mueller-Hilton's agar with 5% chocolatized horse blood | – | • Polymerase chain reaction (PCR)<br>• Indirect immunofluorescence<br>• Enzyme immunoassays |
| Donovanosis | Giemsa or Leishman stain: the Donovan bodies intracellular pinkish bodies with a "closed safety pin" appearance due to bipolar condensation of chromatin | – | Complement fixation tests | • PCR<br>• Colorimetric detection system |
| Gonococcal urethritis | Gram staining—intracellular gram-negative kidney-shaped diplococci in polymorphonuclear leukocytes | • Modified Thayer–Martin media<br>• Martin Lewis media<br>• Chacko–Nayar medium<br>• New York city medium | Complement fixation, latex agglutination, fluorescent antibody tests, coagglutination test, radioimmunoassay,ELISA | • Rapid carbohydrate utilization test<br>• Positive oxidase and glucose fermentation tests (negative maltose fermentation)<br>• Multiplex PCR |



*Continued*

*Continued*

| Condition | *Smear* | *Culture* | *Serology* | *Other* |
|---|---|---|---|---|
| Lymphogranuloma venereum | Giemsa–Romanowsky staining—inclusion bodies | HeLa229, baby Hamster kidney cells and McCoy cells have been widely used for culture | • Complement fixation test, microimmune fluorescence test (most accurate), radio-isotope precipitation test to detect type specific anti-bodies to L1, L2, L3 in serum<br>• Enzyme immunoassays and rapid assays—for antigen detection<br>• NAAT | • Frei's intradermal test—delayed type hypersensitivity<br>• PCR |
| Syphilis | Dark-field microscopy—corkscrew movement | – | • DFA-TP, TPHA<br>• VDRL/RPR (nontreponemal serological tests) | • PCR-using DNA polymerase gene polA sequence<br>• NAATs |
| Bacterial vaginosis | Wet mount and Gram's stain—clue cells | – | – | • pH and Whiff test;<br>• detection of proline iminopeptidase |
| Genital warts (condyloma acuminata) | – | – | – | • Biopsy for confirmation if needed<br>• *PCR*: most sensitive for latent infection<br>• *Southern blot hybridization*: gold standard due to high sensitivity and specificity |
| Hepatitis B | – | – | HBsAg (first serological marker), HBeAg, HBV-DNA, anti-HBc antibodies (IgM and IgG) | – |
| Genital herpes<br>(the classical presentation helps in the diagnosis) | Tzanck smear—shows multinucleated giant cells. Less sensitive, cannot differentiate between HSV-1 and HSV-2 | Viral culture gold standard | Type specific antibodies IgG and IgM—useful in differentiation between HSV-1 and 2 infection, enzyme immunoassay, Western blot, CFT | Immunofluorescence, PCR |
| Genital molluscum contagiosum<br>(the clinical diagnosis is obvious) | – | – | – | • ELISA—detection of antibodies. Hybridization or PCR techniques—molecular analysis of DNA<br>• HP—lobular proliferation of surface epithelium showing an aggregation of enlarged keratinocytes engorged with viral inclusions (molluscum bodies) usually at center of lesion |
| Candidal vulvo-vaginitis, balanitis, balanoposthitis | 10% KOH or Gram staining—yeast cells with pseudohyphae | Sabouraud's agar | – | – |
| Trichomoniasis | Wet mount; stain with Giemsa, acridine orange | Gold standard diamond, modified diamond, Kupferberg, Lash, NIH, Feinberg-Whittington. | – | – |
| Genital scabies<br>(typical history of pruritus with nocturnal exacerbations, and the distribution of the eruption of inflamma-tory papules, should suggest the diagnosis) | – | – | – | • Microscopical examination and discovery of burrows<br>• Dermatoscopy—useful for detecting burrows<br>• the mite in burrow resemble a "jet-with-contrail" |
| Pubic lice infestation (phthiriasis) | – | – | – | Demonstration of louse or nits |

ELISA, enzyme-linked immunosorbent assay; NAAT, nucleic acid amplification tests; DFA-TP, direct fluorescent antibody-T.pallidum; TPHA, treponema pallidum hemagglutination assay; VDRL, venereal disease research laboratory; RPR, rapid plasma reagin; HBV-DNA, Hepatitis B virus-deoxyribonucleic acid; IgM, immunoglobulin M; IgG, immunoglobulin G; HSV-1, herpes simplex virus type 1; HSV-2, herpes simplex virus type 2; CFT, complement fixation test.

**TABLE 3: Treatment**

| WHO recommendations | NACO recommendations |
|---|---|
| **Genital herpes** | |
| **First clinical episode**<br>*Acyclovir 200 mg orally, five times daily for 7 days<br>Or<br>Acyclovir 400 mg orally, three times daily for 7 days<br>Or<br>Famciclovir 250 mg orally, three times daily for 7 days<br>Or<br>Valacyclovir 1 g twice daily for 7 days | **First clinical episode**<br>Acyclovir 200 mg orally, five times daily for 7 days<br>Or<br>Acyclovir 400 mg orally, three times daily for 7 days<br>**Episodic treatment in recurrent infections**<br>Acyclovir 200 mg orally, five times daily for 7 days<br>Or<br>Acyclovir 400 mg orally, three times daily for 7 days<br>Or<br>Acyclovir 800 mg orally, twice daily for 7 days |
| **Suppressive therapy in persons with frequent recurrences** | **Suppressive therapy** |
| Aciclovir 400 mg orally twice daily<br>Or<br>Famciclovir 250 mg orally twice daily<br>Or<br>Valacyclovir 500 mg orally once daily<br>Or<br>Valacyclovir 1,000 mg orally once daily | Acyclovir 400 mg orally, twice daily continuously for at least 1 year recurrence rate should than be re-assessed after the stoppage of acyclovir |
| *Note*: Acyclovir resistance which occurs mostly in immunocompromised patients is caused due to mutations in either the thymidine kinase/DNA polymerase genes. Management of acyclovir-resistant HSV infections includes the use of the foscarnet and cidofovir. | |
| **Early acquired syphilis** | |
| Benzathine benzylpenicillin 2.4 million IU IM at a single session<br>Or<br>Procaine benzylpenicillin 1.2 million IU IM daily for 10 consecutive days<br>Or<br>Doxycycline 100 mg PO 12 hourly for 14 days<br>Or<br>Tetracycline 500 mg PO 6 hourly for 14 days<br>Or<br>Azithromycin 2 g PO single dose*<br>Or<br>Erythromycin 500 mg PO 6 hourly is given for 14 days | Benzathine benzylpenicillin 2.4 million IU deep IM in a single session<br>Or<br>Procaine benzylpenicillin 1.2 million IU IM once daily for 10 days<br>Or<br>Doxycycline 100 mg BD for 15 days#<br>Or<br>Minocycline 100 mg BD for 15 days<br>Or<br>Erythromycin base/stearate 500 mg QID for 15 days*<br>Or<br>Tetracycline 500 mg QID for 15 days |

*Continued*

*Continued*

| WHO recommendations | NACO recommendations |
|---|---|
| **Late-acquired syphilis** | |
| Benzathine benzylpenicillin 2.4 million IU IM once weekly for 3 weeks<br>Or<br>Procaine benzylpenicillin 1.2 million IU IM daily for 20 consecutive days<br>Or<br>Doxycycline 100 mg PO orally for 30 days#<br>Or<br>Tetracycline 500 mg PO 6 hourly for 30 days<br>Or<br>Erythromycin 500 mg PO 6 hourly for 30 days* | Benzathine benzylpenicillin 2.4 million IU deep IM weekly for 3 consecutive weeks<br>Or<br>Procaine benzylpenicillin 1.2 million IU once daily for 20 consecutive days<br>Doxycycline 100 mg orally twice daily for 30 days#<br>Or<br>Tetracycline 500 mg orally four times daily for 30 days<br>Or<br>Erythromycin base/stearate 500 mg orally four times a day for 30 days* |
| **Chancroid** | |
| Ciprofloxacin 500 mg orally, twice daily for 3 days<br>Or<br>Erythromycin 500 mg orally, four times a day, for 7 days<br>Or<br>Azithromycin 1 g orally as a single oral dose.<br>Or<br>Ceftriaxone 250 mg IM as a single dose | Erythromycin stearate/ erythromycin base 500 mg QID for 7 days<br>Or<br>Erythromycin ethylsuccinate 800 mg QID for 7 days<br>Or<br>Ciprofloxacin 500 mg 3–5 days<br>Or<br>Ceftriaxone 250 mg IM single dose<br>Or<br>Azithromycin 1 g single dose<br>Or<br>Doxycycline 100 mg twice daily for 7 days<br>Or<br>Trimethoprim (80 mg) + Sulfamethoxazole (400 mg) 2 tabs BD for 14 days<br>Hot fomentation |
| **Lymphogranuloma venereum (tropical bubo, climatic bubo, poradinitis inguinale)** | |
| Doxycycline 100 mg, orally BD for 2 weeks<br>Or<br>Erythromycin 500 mg orally, QID for 2 weeks<br>Or<br>Tetracycline 500 mg QID for 2 weeks | Doxycycline 100 mg BD for 21 days<br>Or<br>Tetracycline 500 mg QID for 21 days<br>Or<br>Trimethoprim (80 mg) + Sulfamethoxazole (400 mg) 2 tabs BD for 21 days<br>Or<br>Erythromycin stearate or base 500 mg orally QID for 2 weeks* |

*Continued*

*Continued*

| Donovanosis (granuloma venereum/granuloma inguinale) | |
|---|---|
| Azithromycin 1 g orally on the first day, then 500 mg orally once a day<br>Or<br>Doxycycline 100 mg orally twice daily.<br>Or<br>Erythromycin 500 mg orally four times daily<br>Or<br>Tetracycline 500 mg orally four times daily<br>Or<br>Trimethoprim 80 mg/ Sulfamethoxazole 400 mg two tabs orally twice daily, minimum of 14 days | Doxycycline 100 mg BD orally for 14 days<br>Or<br>Tetracycline 500 mg orally QID for 14 days<br>Or<br>Erythromycin base/stearate 500 mg orally QID for 14 days<br>Or<br>Co-trimoxazole double-strength (160/800) |

| Gonococcal urethritis | |
|---|---|
| Ceftriaxone 250 mg by (IM)<br>Or<br>Cefixime 400 mg PO<br>Or<br>Spectinomycin 2 g IM<br>Or<br>Ciprofloxacin 500 mg PO | Ceftriaxone 250 mg IM single dose |

| Nongonococcal urethritis | |
|---|---|
| Doxycycline 100 mg BD for 7 days<br>Or<br>Azithromycin 1 g single dose<br>Or<br>Amoxycillin 500 mg orally TDS for 7 days<br>Or<br>Ofloxacin 300 mg BD for 7 days<br>Or<br>Tetracycline 500 mg QID for 7 days<br>Or<br>Erythromycin 500 mg QID for 7 days* | Azithromycin 2 g single dose<br>Or<br>Amoxycillin 500 mg orally three times a day for 7 days on empty stomach<br>Or<br>Erythromycin base/stearate 500 mg orally four times a day for 7 days* |

| Bacterial vaginosis | |
|---|---|
| Metronidazole 400 mg or 500 mg orally, twice daily for 7 days<br>Or<br>Metronidazole 2 g orally as a single dose | Metronidazole 400 mg orally twice daily for 7 days<br>Or<br>Metronidazole 2 g orally as a single dose<br>Or<br>Tinidazole 2 g orally as a single dose<br>*Pregnancy*: Metronidazole is contraindicated during the first trimester of pregnancy. Metronidazole 0.75% gel, 5 g intra-vaginally twice daily for 5 days can be used |

*Continued*

*Continued*

| Vulvovaginal candidiasis | |
|---|---|
| Miconazole or clotrimazole 200 mg intravaginally daily for 3 days<br>Or<br>Clotrimazole 500 mg intravaginally, as a single dose<br>Or<br>Fluconazole 150 mg orally as a single dose<br>Or<br>Nystatin 100,000 IU intravaginally, daily for 14 days | Miconazole or clotrimazole 100 mg intravaginally daily for 6 days<br>Or<br>Clotrimazole 500 mg intravaginally, as a single dose<br>Or<br>Fluconazole 150 mg orally as a single dose |

| Trichomoniasis | |
|---|---|
| Metronidazole 2 g orally in a single dose<br>Or<br>Tinidazole 2 g orally in a single dose<br>Or<br>Metronidazole 400 mg or 500 mg orally, BD × 7 days<br>Or<br>Tinidazole 500 mg orally, BD × 5 days | Metronidazole 2 g orally in a single dose<br>Or<br>Metronidazole 400 mg orally, BD × 7 days<br>Or<br>Tinidazole 2 g orally in a single dose |

| Genital warts (condyloma acuminata) | |
|---|---|
| Patient applied:<br>Podofilox 0.5%, solution or gel, twice daily for 3 days followed by 4 days of no treatment, up to four times.<br>Or<br>Imiquimod 5% cream applied at bedtime three times a week for up to16 weeks.<br>*Provider administration*:<br>Podophyllin 10 to 15%<br>Or<br>Trichloroacetic acid (TCA) 80–90 % at weekly interval<br>*Alternative regimen*:<br>Cryotherapy with liquid nitrogen, solid carbon dioxide or a cryoprobe every 1–2 weeks<br>Or<br>Electrosurgery<br>Or<br>Surgical removal | |

*Treatment for pregnant female.
#For penicillin allergic nonpregnant patients.

## Genital Herpes

Herpes simplex virus-2 is endemic throughout the world. It is one of the most common STIs afflicting both men and women having diverse symptomatology and varied clinical presentations. It is a chronic infection of sensory ganglion. HSV genome is maintained in host cell nucleus for the entire lifetime. Due to its persistent and recurring nature, it is often troublesome to patients. More than 70% transmission of HSV-2 is associated with asymptomatic and subclinical reactivation and viral shedding. Recurrent nonhealing herpetic ulcer is an acquired immunodeficiency syndrome (AIDS) defining illness.

## Etiology

DNA virus, herpesvirus hominis type 2; HSV-1 is seen in one-third of the cases.

## Clinical Features

- *First episode*:
    - *True primary*: It occurs in seronegative individuals. Lesions start as grouped vesicles on erythematous base but rapidly become pustular and ulcerate often with polycyclic margins (Fig. 1). Systemic symptoms like fever, myalgia, and malaise are prominent and prolonged. New lesions continue to form in the first 8–10 days and complete re-epithelialization may take as long as 3 weeks or more. Scarring is uncommon.

      Urethral and vaginal discharge and local lymphadenopathy are common but suppurative lymphadenopathy does not occur
    - *Nonprimary*: First episode in a previously infected individual.
- *Recurrent herpes*: It generally follows first episode of infection, but in many cases the first episode may be asymptomatic or so mild that it may remain unrecognized. Recurrent episodes are milder, lasting only 5–7 days
- *Genital herpes and pregnancy*: In most cases, herpes is acquired early during pregnancy and hence seroconversion occurs before onset of labor, which does not pose any danger to fetus. However, in certain cases where HSV is acquired late in pregnancy, risk of vertical transmission increases up to 40% as seroconversion is not completed by the time of labor
- *Atypical presentations of HSV in patients with AIDS* (Fig. 2):
    - With increase in immunosuppression in an HIV-infected person, HSV lesion tends to become subacute or chronic, indolent and atypical responding less promptly to oral antivirals

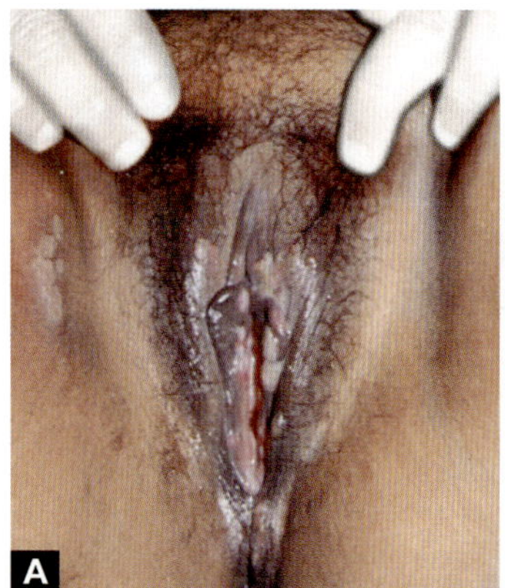
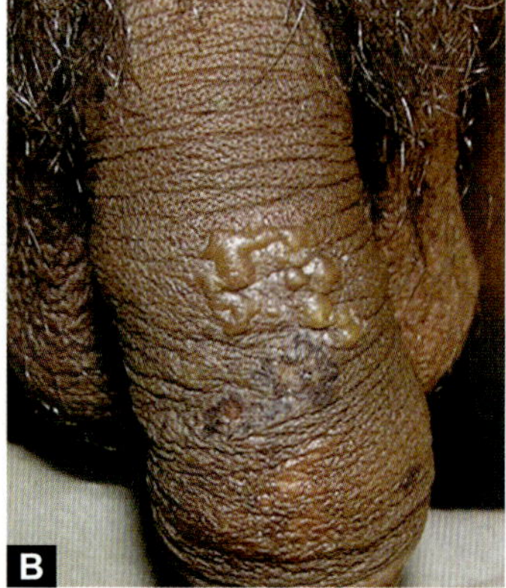

**FIG. 1:** Genital herpes.

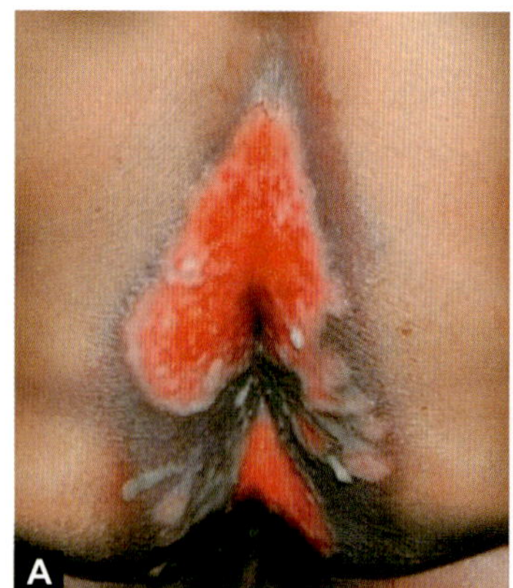
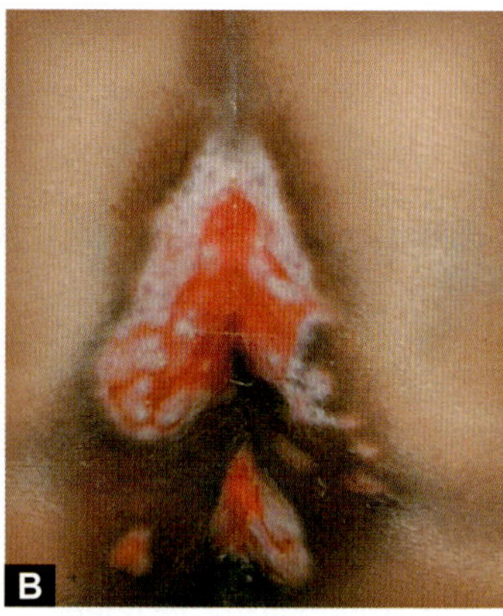

**FIG. 2:** Herpetic ulcer in an AIDS case. **A,** Pretreatment; **B,** Post-treatment.

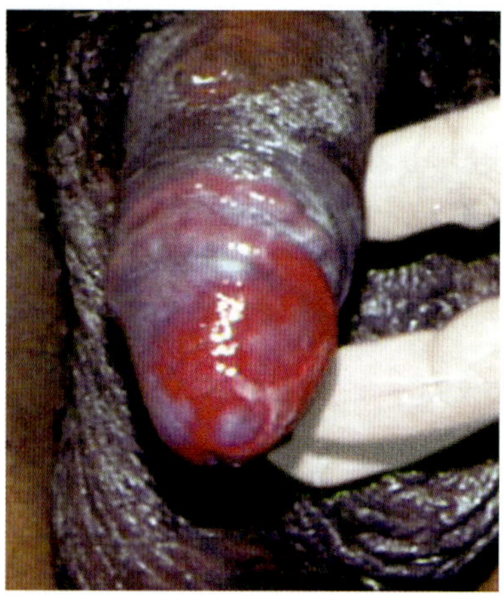

**FIG. 3:** Herpetic balanitis.

    - Deep progressive hemorrhagic ulceration or hyperkeratotic verrucous lesions resembling condyloma lata and other complications like esophagitis, hepatitis, pneumonitis, aseptic meningitis or life-threatening disseminated infections may occur in these patients.
- Varied presentations of herpes (herpes en masquerade) include vaginal discharge (unrelated to candidiasis), genitourinary pain, nonspecific vulvar erythema, prostatitis, lower back pain, itching, burning, soreness and pain over genitalia, unexplained systemic symptoms, vulvar, penile and perianal fissures, folliculitis and balanitis (Fig. 3)
- Cryptic herpes includes herpetic cervicitis (seen in >80% cases of primary infection and less common in recurrent diseases), herpetic esophagitis (common in HIV-positive cases), and herpetic urethritis.

For diagnosis and treatment refer to tables 2 and 3, respectively.

## Syphilis

Syphilis is defined as a chronic infectious disease due to *Treponema pallidum* which is systemic from the outset; capable of involving practically every structure of the body in its course.

**Key Points**

- It may present to dermatologist as a sexually acquired, contagious disease or as a congenitally acquired infection
- Distinguished by florid manifestations on the one hand and years of completely asymptomatic latency on the other
- Known as "the greatest imitator". It mimics many cutaneous and medical conditions

## Etiology

*Treponema pallidum*, a closed coiled, slender, spiral organism.
Acquired syphilis is divided into:

- Early syphilis (infectious phase)
  - Primary syphilis
  - Secondary syphilis
  - Early latent syphilis (detection within 2 years of infection)*
- Late syphilis (noninfectious phase).
  - Late latent syphilis (detection after 2 years of infection)*
  - Tertiary syphilis
    - Benign tertiary
    - Cardiovascular syphilis
    - Neurosyphilis.

*The dividing line of 2 years between early and late latent syphilis indicates substantially diminished infectivity potential after 2 years of infection.

## Clinical Features

- *Primary syphilis*: Primary chancre or hard sore occurs at the site of entry of *T. pallidum* which is characterized by a single well-defined painless, nontender, indurated ulcer, round to oval in shape with rolled borders and clean looking floor which do not bleed on touch (Fig. 4). Lymph nodes are multiple, small, discrete, shotty, nontender, firm and rubbery. Females come more frequently with secondary lesions as asymptomatic primary lesions on the hidden parts may be missed
- *Secondary syphilis*: If not treated, primary lesion resolves spontaneously and after 2–8 weeks patient presents with secondary lesions (Figs 5 to 11). The most common tissue involved is skin, mucous membrane and lymph node with or without constitutional symptoms. It may also involve bones, eyes, nervous system, and abdominal organs

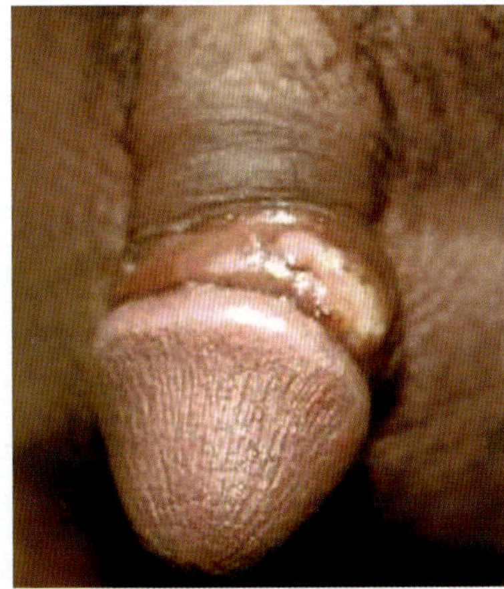

FIG. 4: Primary chancre.

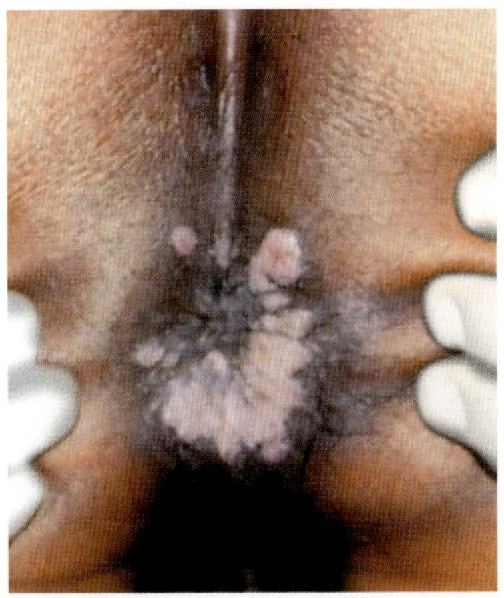

FIG. 5: Secondary syphilis.

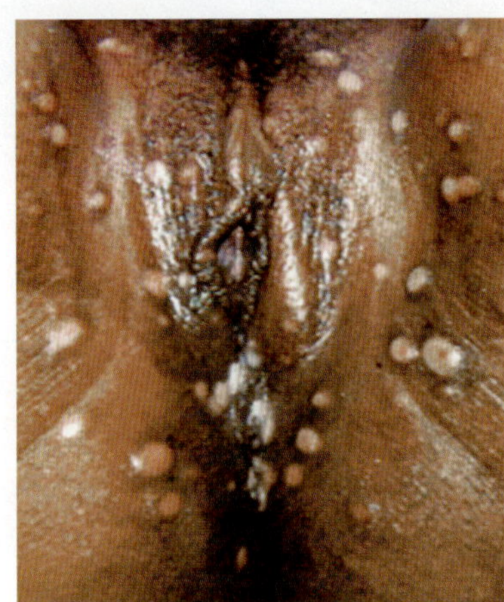

FIG. 6: Secondary syphilis—condylomata lata.

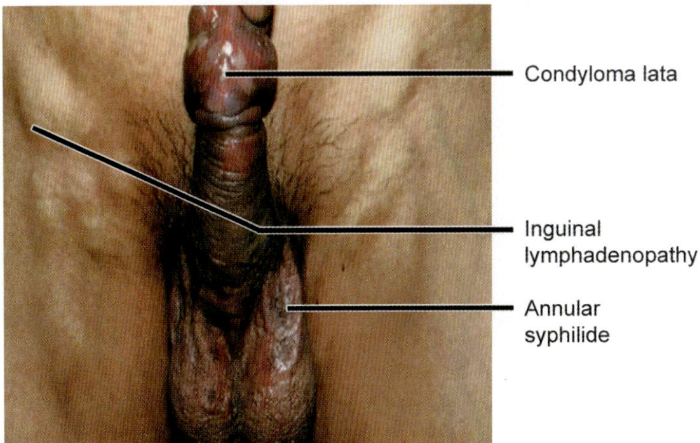


FIG. 7: Secondary syphilis—condylomata lata, inguinal lymphadenopathy and annular syphilide.

- *Tertiary syphilis*: It occurs many years after the primary and secondary lesions. It includes cardiovascular and neurosyphilis.

For diagnosis and treatment refer to tables 2 and 3, respectively.

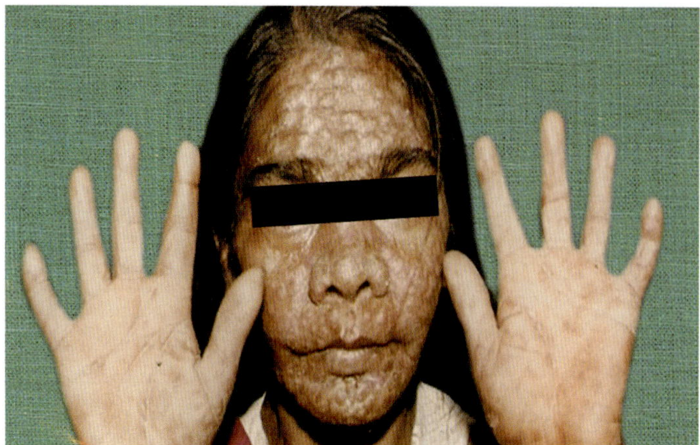

FIG. 8: Secondary syphilis—facial and palmar lesions.

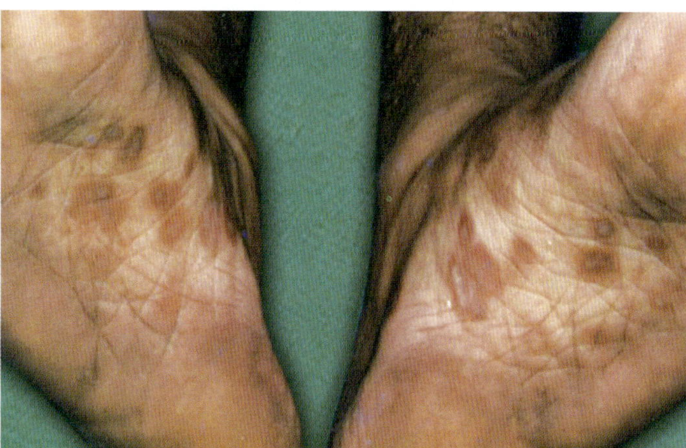

FIG. 9: Secondary syphilis—plantar lesions.

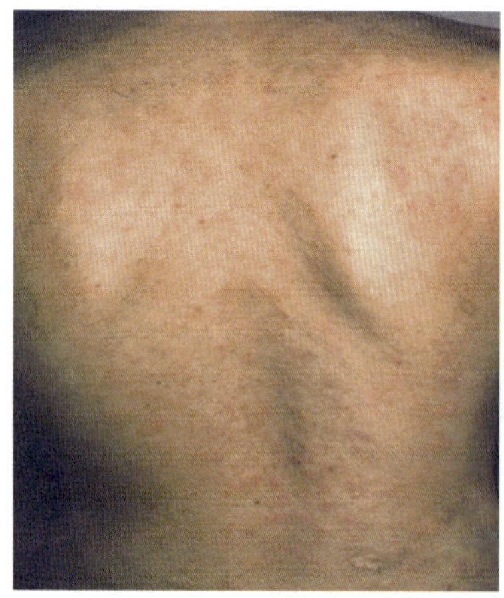

FIG. 10: Secondary syphilis (roseolar syphilide).

### Smear

Dark-field microscopy.

### Motility

- For locomotion—rotation and propulsion
- For change in shape—angulation, buckling, undulation, coil compression and expansion and looping. Angulation where the organism bends on itself at an acute or obtuse angle is most typical. It is seen in fresh specimens.

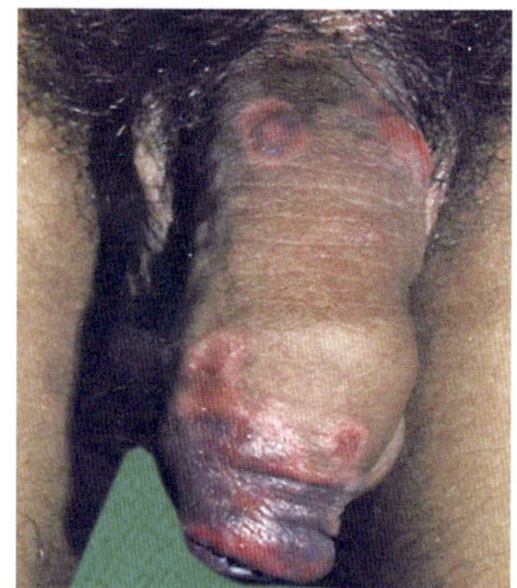

FIG. 11: Secondary syphilis with annular lesion.

### Serology

- Nontreponemal tests—detect nonspecific treponemal antibodies—venereal disease research laboratory (VDRL)/rapid plasma reagin (RPR)
- Treponemal tests—detect specific treponemal antibodies—*T. pallidum* hemagglutination assay (TPHA), fluorescent treponemal antibody absorption and treponemal enzyme immunoassay
- Others—nucleic acid amplification tests (NAATs).

### Testing Strategy

An important principle is to detect treponemal antibody by a highly sensitive screening test (VDRL/RPR) coupled with a specific confirmatory test (TPHA). TPHA remains positive lifelong so quantitative VDRL is used to assess prognosis as it becomes negative with treatment.

## Chancroid (Soft Sore, Soft Chancre, Ulcus Molle)

- It is an acute, localized, autoinoculable infection of the genitals seen mainly in uncircumcised men and tropical regions
- Other variants include giant chancroid, phagedenic chancroid (superinfection with fusospirochetes) (Figs 12 to 15), transient chancroid, follicular chancroid, papular chancroid, and dwarf chancroid

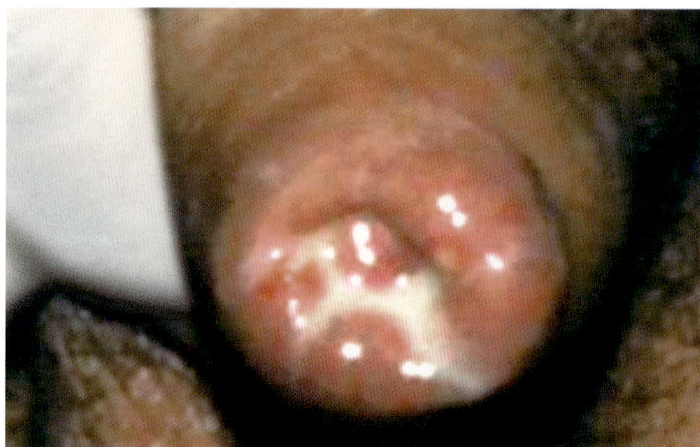

FIG. 12: Phagedenic chancroid with phimosis.

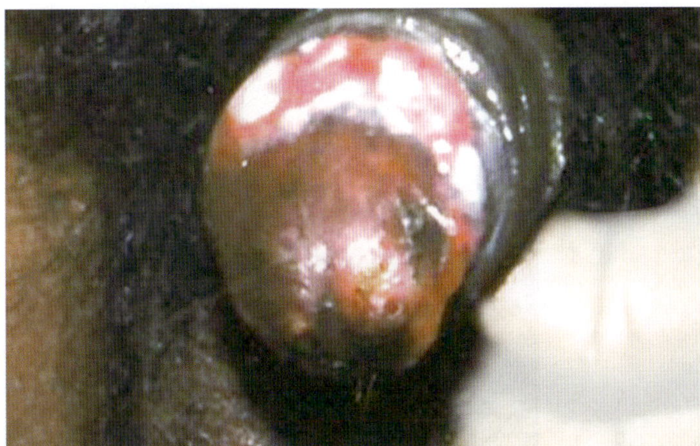

FIG. 13: Phagedenic chancroid.

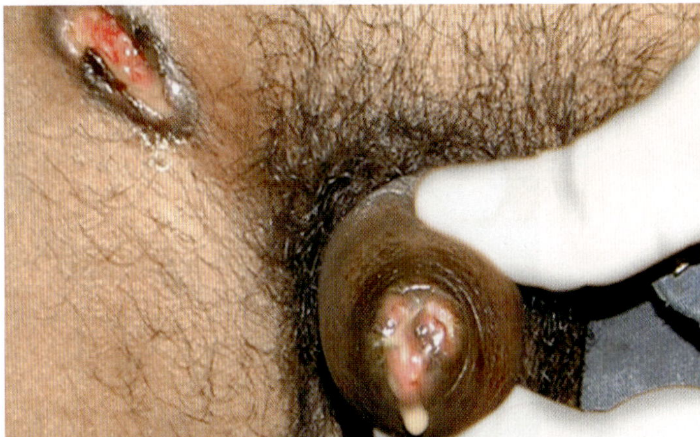

FIG. 14: Mixed infection. Chancroid (ruptured bubo) with gonorrhea.

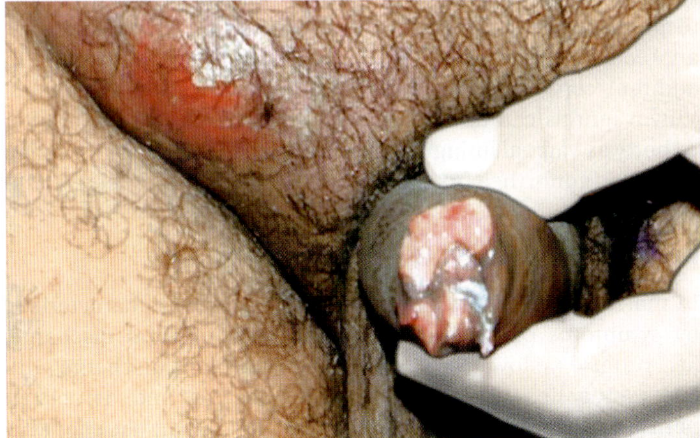

FIG. 15: Mixed infection. Chancroid with inguinal bubo.

## Etiology

*Hemophilus ducreyi*, a gram-negative facultative anaerobic bacillus.

## Clinical Features

Multiple small sharply demarcated painful ulcers with ragged undermined margins and yellow necrotic purulent base are present. The base of the ulcer is nonindurated.

This is commonly seen over prepuce, frenulum, coronal sulcus and occasionally external urinary meatus in males. It is more common in uncircumcised males. In females, it commonly involves fourchette, vestibule, labia, clitoris, vagina and the perianal area. Presenting symptoms in females are pain on urination or defecation, vaginal discharge and dyspareunia. Unilateral, painful, tender, and suppurative inguinal lymphadenitis (unilocular bubo) can be seen in 30–60% cases which, if not treated, can burst and form a giant chancroid.

For diagnosis and treatment refer to tables 2 and 3, respectively.

# Lymphogranuloma Venereum (Tropical Bubo, Climatic Bubo, Poradenitis Inguinale)

The disease is usually present as a transient, primary genital lesion followed by suppurative regional adenitis.

## Etiology

Gram-negative bacteria, *Chlamydia trachomatis* biovars—L1, L2, L3.

## Clinical Features

- *Early manifestations*: The primary genital lesion presents as an asymptomatic transient small painless papules, pustules, vesicles, herpetiform, or nodular ulcerations. Inguinal adenitis or inguinal syndrome is characterized by enlarged tender regional lymphadenopathy or "bubo (multilocular)", above the Poupart's (inguinal) ligament and below it of femoral lymph nodes resulting into characteristic "groove sign of Greenblatt" (Fig. 16)
- *Late manifestations*: Genital elephantiasis or esthiomene and anorectal syndrome.

For diagnosis and treatment refer to tables 2 and 3, respectively.

# Donovanosis (Granuloma Venereum/Granuloma Inguinale)

It is a slowly progressive, mildly contagious and chronically destructive STI that usually involves genital region.

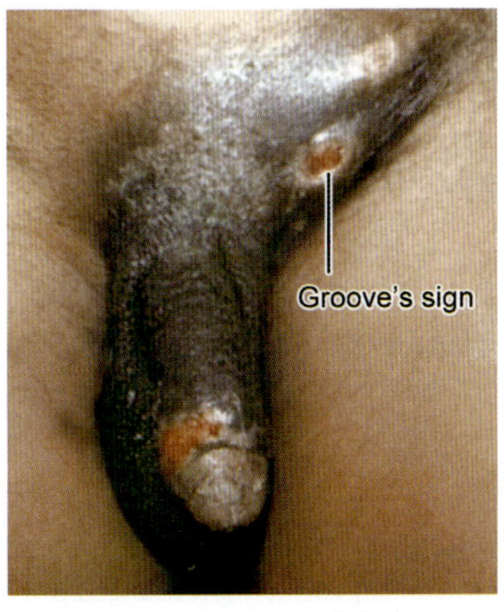


FIG. 16: Lymphogranuloma venereum with bubo.

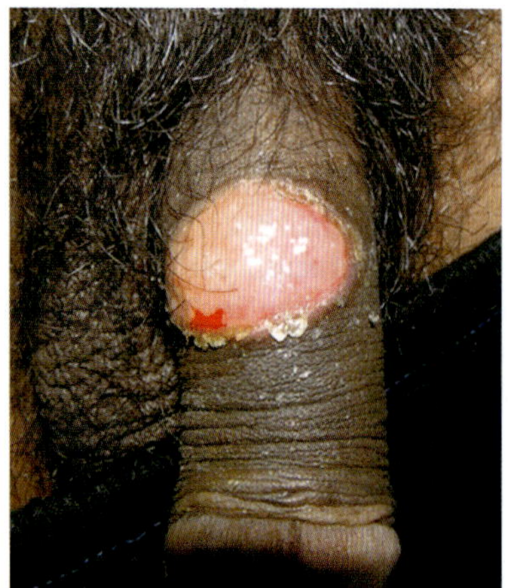

FIG. 17: Granuloma inguinale (donovanosis).

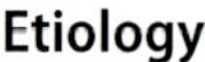

## Etiology

Gram-negative intracellular pleomorphic bacterium, *Calymmatobacterium granulomatis* or *Klebsiella granulomatis.*

## Clinical Features

It is characterized by single or multiple granulomatous ulcers affecting genital area. There develops a painless papule or nodule at the site of entry which ulcerates and develops into a beefy red ulcerogranulomatous mass that bleeds on touch (Fig. 17). Lymph node involvement is unusual. Spread of infection in groin by direct contiguity along the dermis may present as "pseudobubo". Four classical types have been described here.

1. Ulcerogranulomatous
2. Hypertrophic or verrucous type
3. Destructive necrotic
4. Sclerotic or cicatricial.

For diagnosis and treatment refer to tables 2 and 3, respectively.

# DISEASES CHARACTERIZED BY URETHRITIS

Urethritis is a clinical syndrome, characterized by urethral inflammation with or without urethral discharge.

Sexually transmitted urethritis is classified into two types:

1. Gonococcal urethritis
2. Nongonococcal urethritis.

## Gonococcal Urethritis

Second most common prevalent bacterial STD globally and a major public health concern worldwide.

### Etiology

*Neisseria gonorrhoeae* is a gram-negative, aerobic, capnophilic, nonflagellated and nonsporulating reniform diplococcus.

### Pathogenesis

*Gonococcus* has a predilection for columnar epithelium which it attacks and penetrates, producing a marked polymorphonuclear response in the submucosa. The common sites include urethra, anorectum, conjunctivae, and oropharynx in both sexes and in addition cervix uteri as well as Bartholin's glands in females. Vulvovaginitis can occur in prepubertal girls but not seen after puberty as vaginal lining becomes stratified. The risk of a woman acquiring gonorrhea from an infected male is much greater.

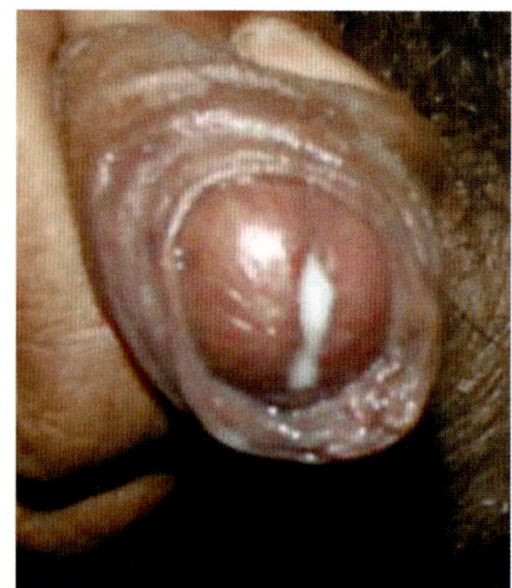

FIG. 18: Acute gonococcal urethritis.

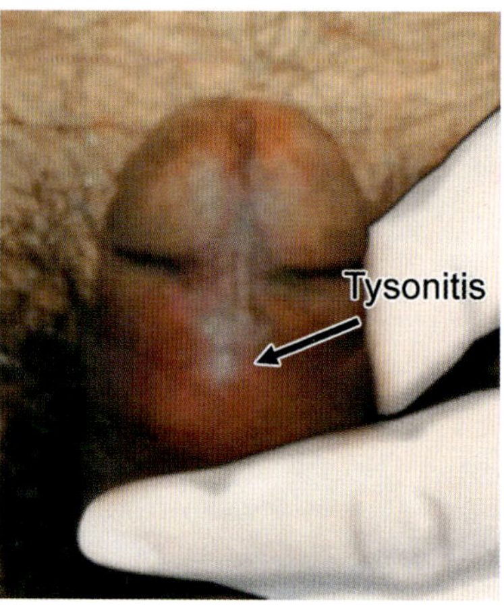


FIG. 19: Gonococcal tysonitis.

### Clinical Features (Table 1)

In males, it mainly presents as anterior urethritis characterized by symptoms of dysuria and voluminous urethral discharge, i.e., profuse yellow to yellowish green purulent discharge with edematous lips of external urethral meatus and associated perimeatal erythema with tender inguinal lymphadenopathy (Figs 18 and 19). The female urethra often escapes infections, because it is very short and lined by stratified squamous epithelium. Gonococcal cervicitis can occur, but it is usually asymptomatic.

For diagnosis and treatment refer to tables 2 and 3, respectively.

### Drug Resistance

*Neisseria gonorrhoeae* has developed resistance to almost all antimicrobials introduced for the treatment of gonorrhea. Resistance to antimicrobials occurs as high-level plasmid mediated resistance in case of penicillins [penicillinase-producing *N. gonococci* (PPNG)] and tetracyclines and as chromosomally mediated resistance in other groups. This resistance is mainly acquired by intrastrain mutations and/or interstrain transfer of DNA.

Penicillinase-producing *N. gonococci* possess a plasmid containing a gene responsible for β-lactamase production, possibly acquired from ampicillin-resistant *Haemophilus influenzae* or *Enterobacteriaceae*. Treatment of choice for PPNG is third-generation cephalosporins like ceftriaxone and cefotaxime.

### Multiplex Polymerase Chain Reaction

Recently molecular amplification assays like polymerase chain reaction (PCR) and ligase chain reaction (LCR) have been found to be highly sensitive and specific methods for detection of *N. gonorrhoeae* and *C. trachomatis* not only in urethral and cervical specimens but also in urine especially in asymptomatic cases.

## Nongonococcal Urethritis

### Etiology

The most common organism implicated is *C. trachomatis* which may coexist with gonorrhea. Other organisms include *Mycoplasma genitalium, Ureaplasma urealyticum, Trichomonas vaginalis*, herpes simplex, adenovirus and *Candida* species.

### Clinical Features

Patients may be asymptomatic or may present with clear, creamy white, yellow, or green urethral discharge with or without dysuria.

### Laboratory Diagnosis

- *Smear (preferably first morning sample/after 2 hours of passing urine)*: Gram stain of urethral secretions—more than or equal to 5 white blood cells (WBCs) per oil immersion field
- *Microscopic examination of first void urine*: Positive leukocyte esterase test, more than or equal to 10 WBC per high-power field
- *Recommendation for pregnant females*: Repeat testing to document chlamydial eradication (preferably by NAAT) 3 weeks after completion of therapy is recommended for all pregnant women to ensure therapeutic cure, taking into consideration the severe sequelae that might occur in mothers and neonates if the infection persists.

For treatment refer table 3.

### Vaginal Discharge

It may be physiological or pathological. Scanty, odorless asymptomatic discharge is usually physiological while copious, malodorous, frothy discharge associated with symptoms like vulval pruritus and dysuria may be due to vaginitis or cervicitis. Common causes of vaginitis include candidiasis, trichomoniasis, and bacterial vaginosis. Candidiasis and bacterial vaginosis are primarily endogenous reproductive tract infections. Cervicitis is usually caused by gonococci or *chlamydia*. Endocervical smear can be taken for the diagnosis of cervicitis.

# OTHER SEXUALLY TRANSMITTED INFECTIONS

## Genital Warts (Condyloma Acuminata)

### Definition

Most common manifestations of sexually transmissible HPV infection and prevalence peaks during the 2nd and 3rd decades of life.

Viruses causing genital warts and common skin warts are antigenically and biologically different.

### Etiology

DNA virus with cytopathic effects on epithelium—HPV strains 6, 11 (most common); other strains 1–5, 10, 16, 18, 30, 31, 33, 35, 39–45, 51–59, 70, 83. It establishes persistent and multifocal infection.

### Clinical Features

Grouped, pedunculated, filiform lesions (hyperplastic warts) on any part of male or female genitalia but more common on moist surfaces (Figs 20 and 21).

In males, they are usually seen over the subpreputial sac, terminal urethra, perianal region and walls of anal canal. Lesions may fuse into a cauliflower-like mass appearing as a Buschke-Löwenstein tumor or giant condyloma acuminatum have been described on the penis are mostly histologically benign.

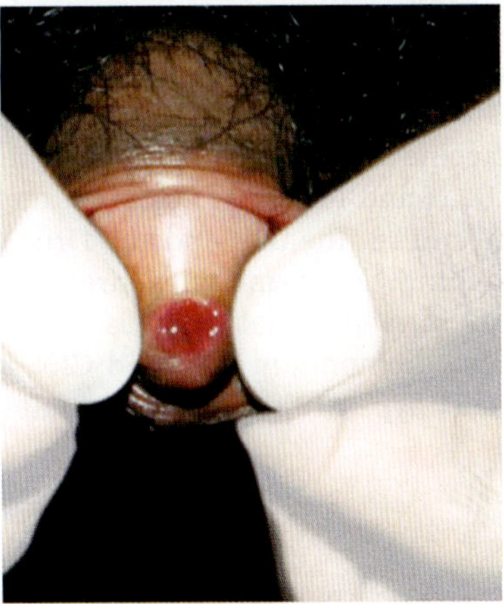

**FIG. 20:** Intrameatal wart.

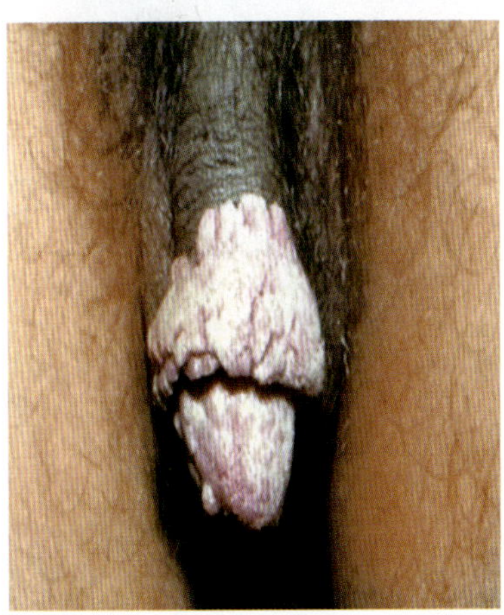

**FIG. 21:** Condyloma Accuminata.

In females, they are seen commonly on the vulva, particularly posterior part of introitus, vaginal wall and vaginal portion of cervix.

The HPV-related lesions can be distinguished from other lesions by application of 5% acetic acid for 5 minutes. Warts and intraepithelial neoplasia become white called acetowhite showing asymptomatic colonization of the virus.

## Human Papillomavirus and Human Immunodeficiency Virus

Human immunodeficiency virus-induced immunosuppression increases the risk for benign and malignant manifestations of HPV infections. HPV-16 and HPV-18 cause various grades of squamous intraepithelial lesion and invasive carcinoma. Invasive cervical carcinoma is an AIDS defining illness. HIV-positive women should be screened with Pap smear twice (every 6 months) within the first year after initial HIV diagnosis and, if both tests are normal, annual screening is recommended thereafter.

### Human Papillomavirus and Malignancy

Human papillomavirus types 16, 18, 31, 33, 35, 39, 45, 51, 52, 54, 56, 66, and 68 are frequently associated with several types of cancers like cervical, vulvar, vaginal, penile, anal, and oropharyngeal.

### Human Papillomavirus Vaccine

Currently, there are two prophylactic vaccines. Both use virus-like particles of the recombinant major capsid (L1) protein of HPV to stimulate a protective immune response. Gardasil® is a quadrivalent vaccine and induces a protective response against HPV types 16, 18, 6, and 11 while Cervarix® is a bivalent vaccine against types 16 and 18. The US Food and Drug Administration (FDA)-approved indication includes prevention of cervical cancer, cervical intraepithelial neoplasia (CIN) grade 2 or worse and adenocarcinoma in situ, and CIN grade 1, caused by oncogenic HPV types 16 and 18, in females after 25 years of age.

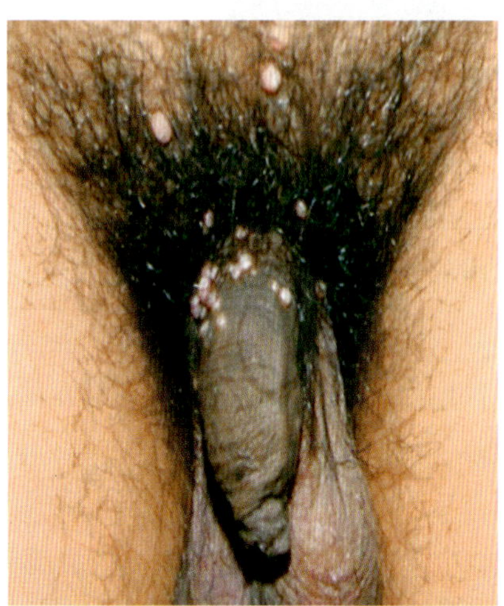

FIG. 22: Genital molluscum contagiosum.

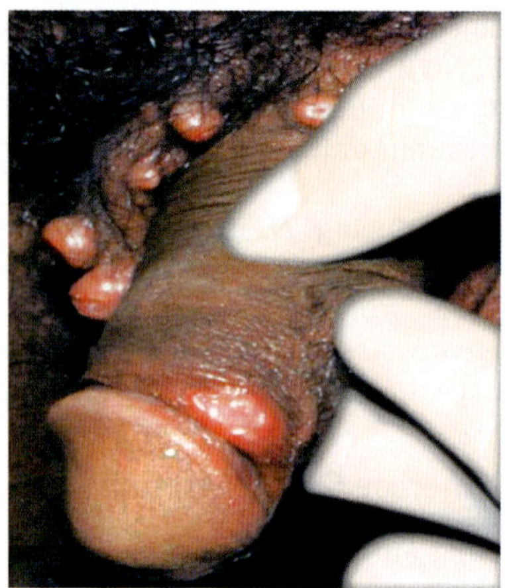

FIG. 23: Genital molluscum in HIV.

**TABLE 4: Common syndromes***

| Genital ulcer disease | Vaginal discharge | Urethral discharge (mainly in males) |
|---|---|---|
| Genital herpes | Trichomoniasis (vaginitis) | Gonorrhea |
| Syphilis | Bacterial vaginosis (vaginitis) | *Chlamydia* |
| Chancroid | Candidiasis (vaginitis) | |
| | Gonorrhea (cervicitis) | |
| | *Chlamydia* (cervicitis) | |

*As per the National AIDS Control Organisation guidelines.

### Diagnosis

It is mainly clinical. For laboratory diagnosis and treatment refer to tables 2 and 3, respectively.

For brief description of other STIs like genital molluscum contagiosum (Figs 22 and 23), genital scabies and pubic lice infestation (phthiriasis) refer to tables 1 and 2.

## SYNDROMIC APPROACH

Ideal approach to manage STDs is etiologic which is laboratory based. Laboratory diagnosis of STI needs facilities, increases the cost and delays initiation of treatment.

Syndromic approach is to diagnose and treat cases on the basis of easily identifiable clinical syndromes (Table 4).

*Syndrome*: Constellation of symptoms reported by patient and signs identified by clinicians.

Syndromic approach is promoted as a public health approach so as to treat a STD case at first point of contact (primary care level). It increases compliance and decreases chances of transmission of STIs including HIV. The major limitation of syndromic approach is that the patient may be overtreated and there is potential for drug resistance. Validation of syndromic approach by laboratory tests at a tertiary care center is recommended (enhanced syndromic case management).

As per the National AIDS Control Organisation (NACO) guidelines, there are nine syndromes. An attempt is made to highlight the most common among them, i.e., urethral discharge (Flowchart 1), genital ulcer (Flowchart 2), and vaginal discharge (Flowchart 3).

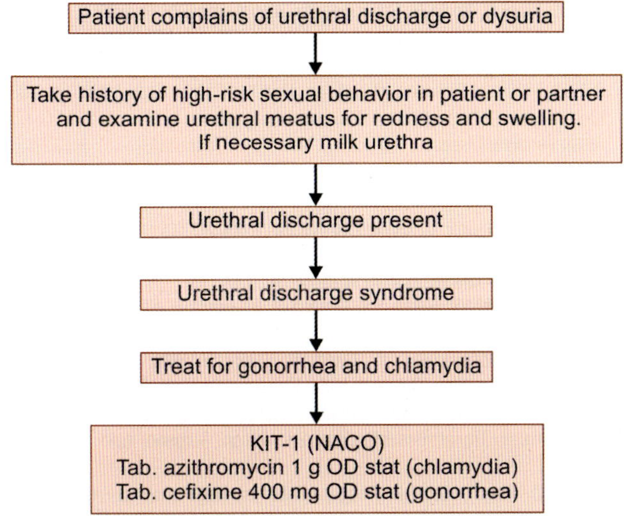


NACO, National AIDS Control Organisation.

**FLOWCHART1:** Management of urethral discharge/burning micturition in males.

## PREVENTION

Early diagnosis and treatment of STI is important to interrupt the chain of transmission. This should be coupled with partner management. Patients and partners should be educated and counseled regarding risk reduction, safe sex, and behavior modification. Males should be educated about correct and consistent use of good quality latex condoms. Condom is less protective against HPV and HSV but maximum effectiveness is seen in gonorrhea, *chlamydia*, HIV, and hepatitis B. Though male condom is a useful primary prevention option, it is male-driven and less acceptable. Promotion of female-driven protective measures like female condom and vaginal microbicides is the need of the hour. Among microbicides tenofovir gel could potentially fill an important HIV prevention gap, especially for women unable to successfully negotiate mutual monogamy or condom use. Limited evidence suggests that vaginal tenofovir microbicides may reduce the risk of acquisition of HIV and HSV-2 infections in women.

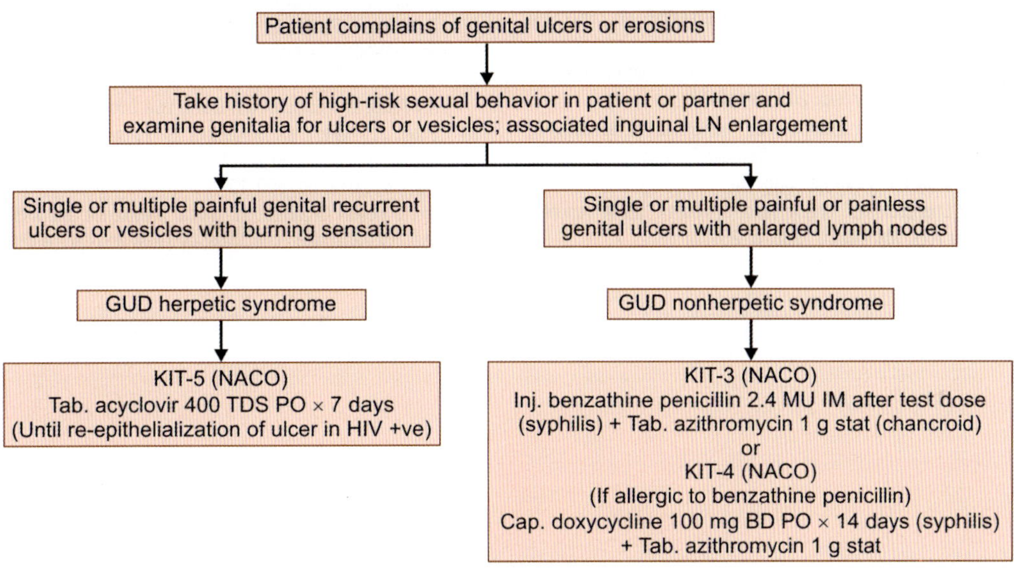


NACO, National AIDS Control Organisation.

**FLOWCHART 2:** Management of genital ulcer diseases.

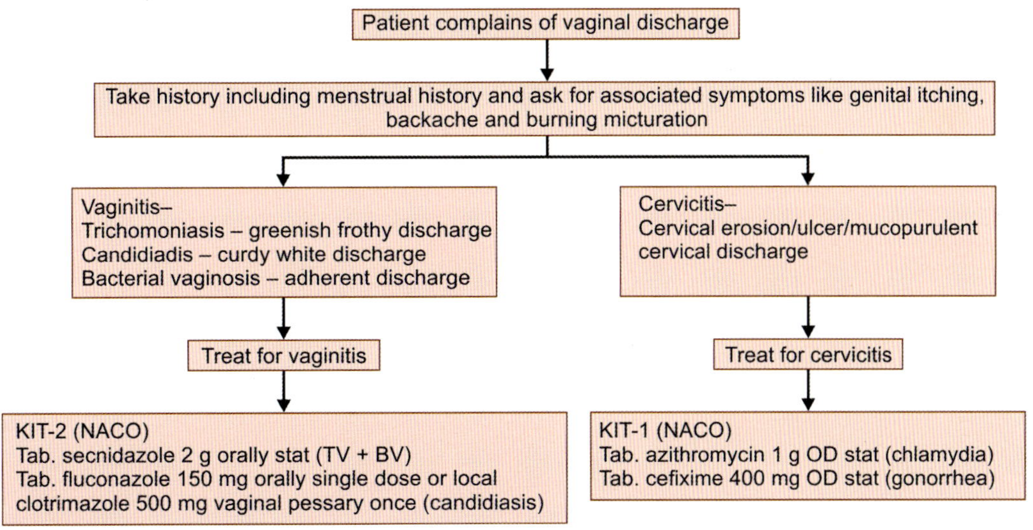


NACO, National AIDS Control Organisation.

**FLOWCHART 3:** Management of vaginal discharge in females.

Circumcision in men lowers the risk of chancroid and syphilis. There is strong evidence that medical male circumcision reduces the acquisition of HIV by heterosexual men.

Except HPV no vaccine is available currently against STI. Taking into account epidemiologic synergy between STI and HIV, STI prevention is crucial for HIV prevention.

## ACKNOWLEDGMENTS

Dr Dimpal Patel and Dr Ipsa Pandya, M.D. (SKIN-VD), Department of Skin-VD, Medical College Baroda, Gujarat, India.

## SUGGESTED READINGS

1. Aggarwal K, Sharma VK. Comparative (WHO/CDC/NACO) treatment of sexually transmitted diseases. Sexually Transmitted Diseases and HIV/AIDS, 2nd edition. New Delhi: Viva Books Pvt Ltd; 2012. pp. 852-8.
2. Balachandran C, Pai S, Chancroid. In: Sharma VK (Ed). Sexually Transmitted Diseases and HIV/AIDS, 2nd edition. New Delhi. Viva Books Pvt Ltd; 2012. p. 341.
3. Carter JS, Bowden FJ, Bastian I, et al. Phylogenetic evidence for reclassification of Calymmatobacterium granulomatis as Klebsiella granulomatis comb. nov. Int J Syst Bacteriol. 1999;49(4):1695-700.
4. Centers for Disease Control and Prevention. Sexually transmitted diseases treatment guidelines. Morb Mortal Wkly Rep. 2010;59:40-55.
5. Galloway DA. Biology of genital human papilloma virus. In: Holmes KK, Sparling PF, Mardh PA, Lemon SM, Stamm WE, Piot P (Eds). Sexually Transmitted Diseases, 3rd edition. New York: McGraw-Hill; 1999. pp. 335-46.
6. King A, Nicol C, Rodin P. Chancroid. In: King A, Nicol C, Rodin P (Eds). Venereal Diseases, 4th edition. New York: Macmillan; 1980. p. 251.
7. King A, Nicol C, Rodin P. Gonorrhea. In: King A, Nicol C, Rodin P (Eds). Venereal Diseases, 4th edition. New York: Macmillan; 1980. pp. 173-99.
8. King A, Nicol C, Rodin P. Lymphogranuloma venereum. In: King A, Nicol C, Rodin P (Eds). Venereal Diseases, 4th edition. New York: Macmillan; 1980. pp. 258-67.
9. King A, Nicol C, Rodin P. Other lesions of the genitalia. In: King A, Nicol C, Rodin P (Eds). Venereal Diseases, 4th edition. New York: Macmillan; 1980. p. 362.
10. King A, Nicol C, Rodin P. Syphilis. In: King A, Nicol C, Rodin P (Eds). Venereal Diseases, 4th edition. New York: Macmillan; 1980. p. 6.
11. Latif AS, Mutandwa C. Guidelines for the management of sexually transmitted infections. In: Gupta S, Kumar B (Eds). Sexually Transmitted Infections, 2nd edition. Gurgaon, India: Elsevier; 2012. pp. 1301-9.
12. Nanda S, Reddy VB, Reddy BS. Chancroid. In: Gupta S, Kumar B (Eds). Sexually Transmitted Infections, 2nd edition. Gurgaon, India: Elsevier; 2012. pp. 522-32.
13. O'Farrell N. Donovanosis. In: Gupta S, Kumar B (Eds). Sexually Transmitted Infections, 2nd edition. Gurgaon, India: Elsevier; 2012. pp. 534-41.
14. Reddy BS, Khandpur S, Sethi S, et al. Gonococcal infections. In: Gupta S, Kumar B (Eds). Sexually Transmitted Infections, 2nd edition. Gurgaon, India: Elsevier; 2012. p. 488.
15. Rowen D, Fox P, Goon P. Anogenital human papillomavirus infection: natural history, epidemiology, and vaccination. In: Gupta S, Kumar B (Eds). Sexually Transmitted Infections, 2nd edition. Gurgaon, India: Elsevier; 2012. p. 363.
16. Sharma VK. Syphilis: clinical features and natural course. In: Sharma VK (Ed). Sexually Transmitted Diseases and HIV/AIDS, 2nd edition. New Delhi:Viva Books Pvt Ltd; 2012. p. 262.
17. Sundharam JA, Herpes genitalis. In: Sharma VK (Ed). Sexually Transmitted Diseases and HIV/AIDS, 2nd edition. New Delhi: Viva Books Pvt Ltd; 2012. pp. 410-4.
18. Usman N. Anogenital warts. In: Sharma VK (Ed). Sexually Transmitted Diseases and HIV/AIDS, 2nd edition. New Delhi: Viva Books Pvt Ltd; 2012. pp. 439-40.
19. Vries JC, Reddy BS, Khandpur S. Lymphogranuloma venereum. In: Gupta S, Kumar B (Eds). Sexually Transmitted Infections, 2nd edition. Gurgaon, India: Elsevier; 2012. pp. 509-13.
20. World Health Organization. Global prevalence and incidence of selected curable sexually transmitted infections: overview and estimate. Geneva: WHO; 2001.

# 65 CHAPTER Skin Manifestations of HIV/AIDS

Vinay Kulkarni

## INTRODUCTION

Almost every person (child or adult) living with human immunodeficiency virus (PLHIV) suffers from one or the other skin problem during the course of the disease. So, the prevalence is 100%. With the advent of highly effective antiretroviral treatment (ART), PLHIV are surviving for decades and so the nature of presentation has drastically changed. When the disease is diagnosed on time and treated appropriately, the immunological status of the person remains optimal for many years; also for those with advanced immunodeficiency, there is remarkable reversal of the immune status. In general, the manifestations, such as opportunistic infections are on decline; while on the other hand, those with long-term exposure to treatment and survival, such as malignancies, are on the rise.

As the pathogenesis, presentation and management of majority of these diseases remain the same with or without human immunodeficiency virus (HIV) and has been described in details elsewhere in this book, the same will not be repeated. Also, only the clinical photographs of unusual and rare presentations are presented.

The cutaneous manifestations associated with HIV can be classified as infections and noninfectious inflammatory disorders and malignancies. Infections could be due to either known pathogens or with the hitherto unknown or rare organisms. The possibility of infections with opportunistic microbes, as well as the severity and chronicity of lesions increases with the degree of immunodeficiency.

The plethora of noninfectious inflammatory disorders seen are associated with the immune dysregulation related to HIV infection. Various malignancies are also associated with such prolonged immune dysregulation or with certain viruses [e.g., human papillomavirus (HPV), hepatitis B virus (HBV), etc.]. Certain cutaneous complications occur early in the disease and may be associated with HIV itself.

## CUTANEOUS MANIFESTATIONS (TABLE 1)

- Infectious
- Noninfectious.

## INFECTIOUS

These could be:

- Viral infections
- Bacterial infections
- Fungal infections
- Bacillary angiomatosis
- Mycobacterial infections
- Arthropod infestations.

### Viral Infections

#### Acute HIV Exanthema

In approximately 40% persons recently infected with HIV, several signs and symptoms may occur. This is called acute retroviral disease or also seroconversion illness. Symptoms of “seroconversion” illness include—fever, rigors, myalgia, sore throat, headache, neck stiffness, etc. Skin lesions may appear during this early phase. They are coppery red, macular or papulosquamous lesions, mainly on the upper trunk, palms and soles. Oral lesions may also occur. They are similar to viral exanthema. As the presentation is similar to any acute viral illness, only a high index of suspicion may alert the clinician to diagnosis.

#### Herpes Zoster

This probably could be the most common cutaneous manifestation encountered in HIV disease, occurring in 15–30% of HIV patients. It is seen throughout the course of the disease. May erupt early in the disease and could be the presenting feature of HIV or may appear when the immune status declines or could be seen as a consequence of immune reconstitution.

Clinically, the manifestations vary from mild to extremely severe eruption. Severity is indicative of the immune status. Multidermatomal lesions and hemorrhagic vesicles that leave behind necrotic ulceration and scars or systemic dissemination suggest advanced immunodeficiency (Figs 1 to 4). It may run a very chronic course.

Recurrences are common.

**TABLE 1: Differential diagnosis of skin lesions occurring in HIV disease**

| Type | Diagnosis |
|---|---|
| Papules, Nodules | Staphylococcal abscess, furunculosis, verrucae, bacillary angiomatosis, molluscum contagiosum, Kaposi's sarcoma, cryptococcosis, squamous/basal cell carcinoma |
| Crusted papule, nodule | Impetigo, ecthyma, herpes simplex ulcer, Kaposi's sarcoma |
| Vesicles, bullae, pustules | Bullous impetigo, drug reactions, herpes simplex, herpes zoster, pustular psoriasis, erythema multiforme |
| Acneiform | Acne vulgaris, drug rash (INH), rosacea, papular eruption of AIDS |
| Folliculitis | *Staph. aureus*, pityrosporum ovale, eosinophilic folliculitis, pustular eruption of AIDS, demodex folliculitis |
| Psoriasiform | Psoriasis, seborrheic, dermatitis, drug rash, secondary syphilis, pityriasis versicolor, dermatophytosis, scabies |
| Eczematous lesions | Seborrheic dermatitis, atopic dermatitis, scabies |
| Urticarial lesions | Drug reaction |
| Morbilliform eruption | Acute seroconversion illness, drug rash, CMV, histoplasmosis, etc. and other exanthems |
| Purpuric | Thrombocytopenic purpura, vasculitis, drug rash |
| Erosions/ulcers | HSV, herpes zoster, CMV, ecthyma, fixed-drug eruption, malignant syphilide, lupus vulgaris |
| Generalized pruritus | Scabies, drug rash, atopic dermatitis, HIV associated pruritus, seroconversion illness |

INH, isonicotinylhydrazide; AIDS, acquired immune deficiency syndrome; CMV, cytomegalovirus; HSV, herpes simplex virus; HIV, human immunodeficiency virus.

*Source*: Reproduced with permission from Vinay Kulkarni. HIV/AIDS: Diagnosis and Management—A Physician's Handbook. Pune: Prayas; 1999.

Any herpes zoster at any age, of any severity should raise a suspicion and the person should be screened for HIV. The cost of a missed diagnosis of HIV, both for the individual as well as the society, is tremendous.

*Complications*: Atrophic or hypertrophic scars, chronic verrucous hyperkeratotic nodules or granulomatous lesions at the site, meningitis or encephalitis, severe postherpetic neuralgia.

## Herpes Simplex Virus (HSV-1 and HSV-2)

Vesicles and ulcers may be superficial as seen commonly in immunocompetent persons or may be chronic and painful. Apart from genital lesions, perianal, mucosal as well as cutaneous lesions are commonly seen. Perianal lesions are more frequent in men having sex with men but should also raise a suspicion of anal sex among heterosexuals. With advanced immunodeficiency, recurrences become more frequent and lesions may become chronic. Lesions may become confluent, resulting in deep ulcers with necrotic margins (Figs 4 to 6).

Any chronic painful nonhealing ulcer in an HIV-infected individual should be treated as due to HSV unless otherwise proved.

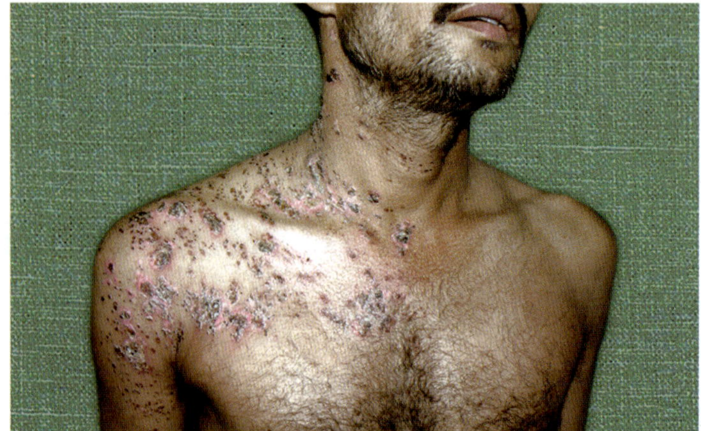

**FIG. 1:** Multidermatomal herpes zoster.

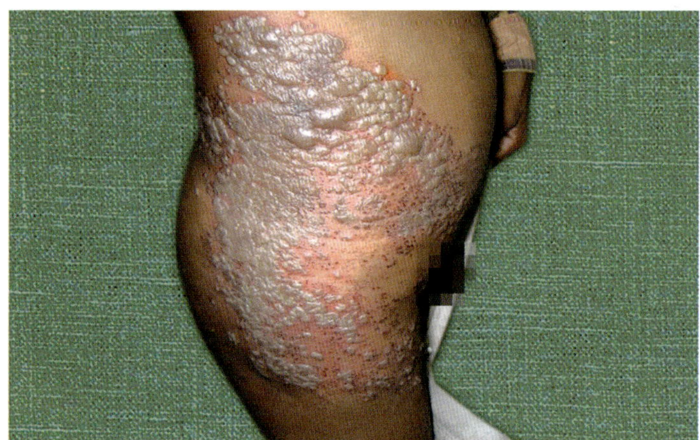

**FIG. 2:** Severe herpes zoster.

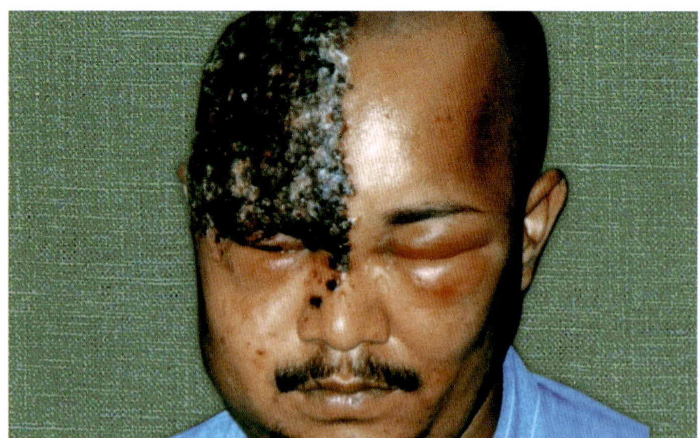

**FIG. 3:** Hepres zoster ophthalmicus.

## Molluscum Contagiosum

Mollusca are extremely common with incidence increasing by 18-fold in PLHIV. Lesions tend to be larger and widespread. Face and genitals are frequently involved (Fig. 7). Several large mollusca can become confluent to give a "cluster of grapes" appearance (Fig. 8). Perigenital or perianal molluscum contagiosum should be suspected to be sexually transmitted and investigated appropriately. Recurrences after treatment are extremely common.

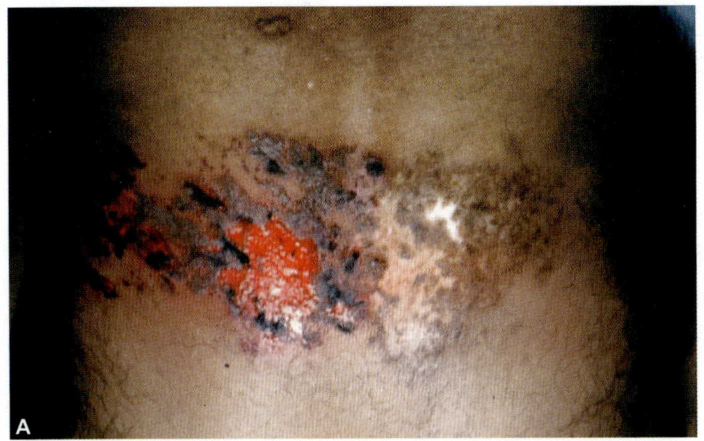

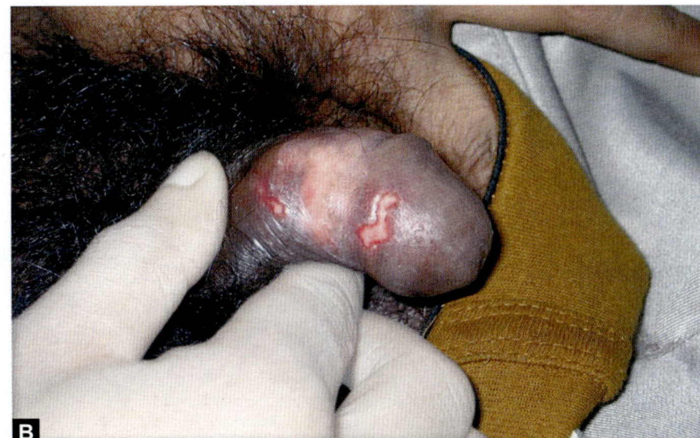

FIG. 4: **A,** Bilateral herpes zoster; **B,** Herpes simplex.

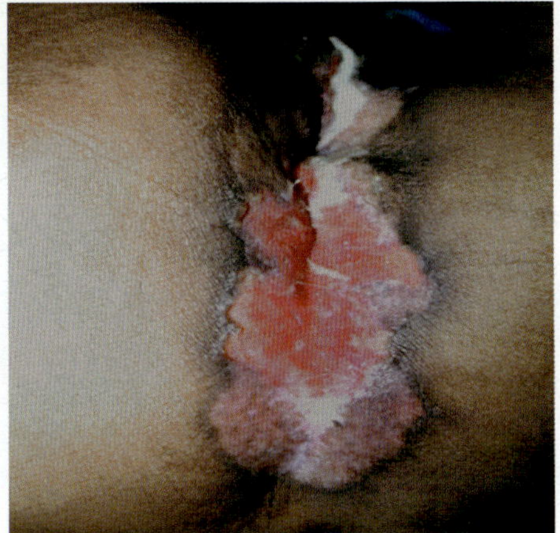

FIG. 5: Herpes simplex.

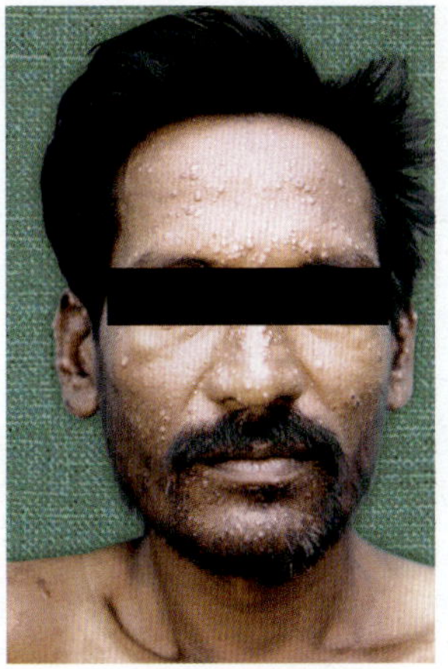

FIG. 7: Extensive molluscum contagiosum.

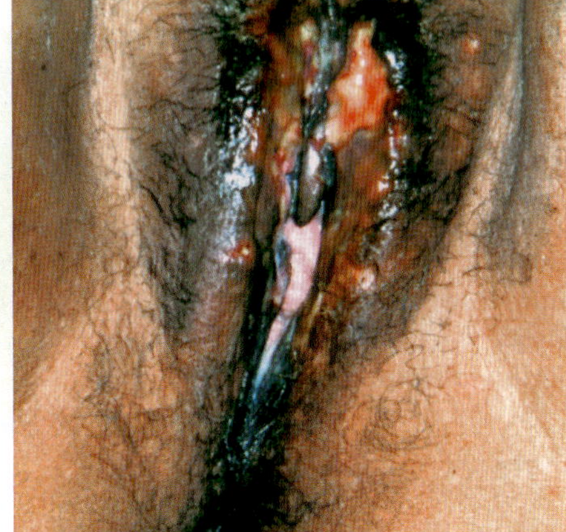

FIG. 6: Herpes simplex.

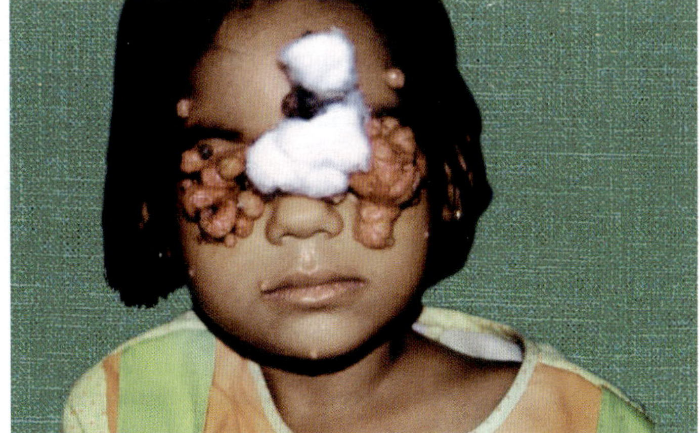

FIG. 8: Giant molluscum contagiosum.

## Human Papillomavirus (Viral Warts)

Human papillomavirus infection leading to warts is very common in PLHIV. Disseminated verruca vulgaris can occur in immunodeficient persons. Warts tend to be larger in size and refractory to treatments as immunodeficiency advances (Fig. 9). When the transmission is sexual, there could be condylomatous lesions (perigenital, perianal or oropharyngeal). Malignant changes with intraepithelial carcinoma and frank invasive squamous cell carcinoma can also occur.

## Oral Hairy Leukoplakia

Oral hairy leukoplakia (OHL) is due to infection of the oral epithelium by the Epstein–Barr virus (EBV). It presents as white-colored verrucous or corrugated plaques on the lateral aspect of

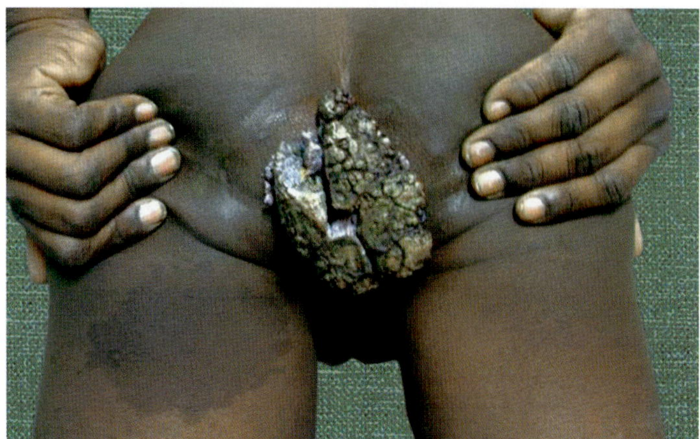

FIG. 9: Giant perianal warts.

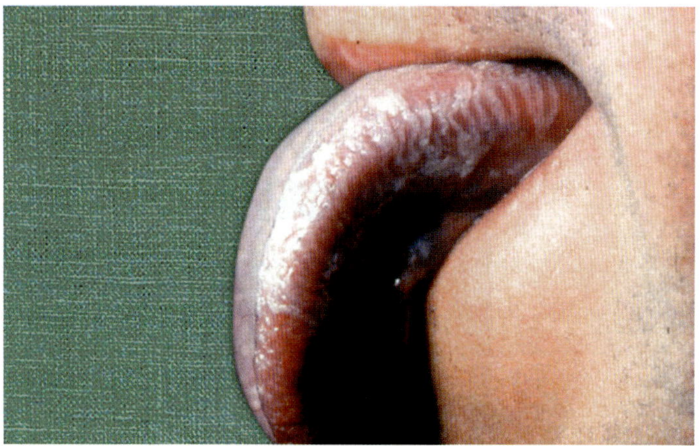

FIG. 10: Oral hairy leukoplakia.

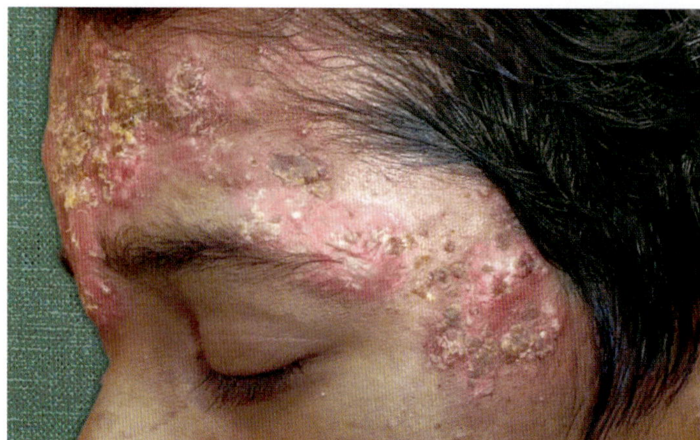

FIG. 11: Recurrent bacterial infections.

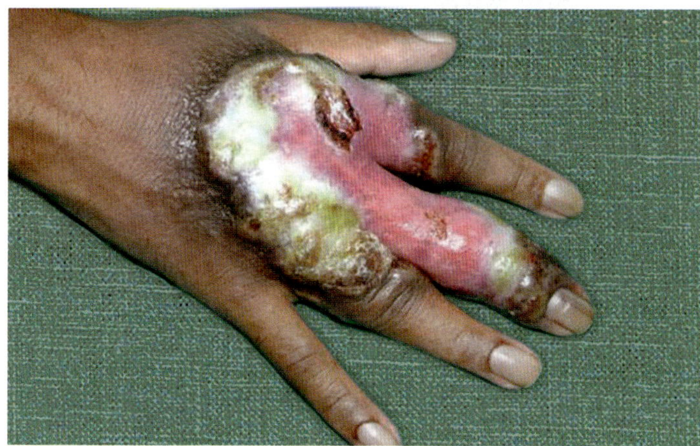

FIG. 12: Brucellosis.

the tongue (Fig. 10). It is asymptomatic. Initially thought to be pathognomonic of HIV infection, OHL has now been shown to occur also in other immunocompromised patients. A biopsy will show epithelial hyperplasia with "hairs." Electron microscopy will demonstrate the presence of EBV. No treatment is required, as it is asymptomatic.

## Bacterial Infections

Common pyogenic bacteria, such as *Staphylococcus aureus* commonly cause skin and soft tissue infections in HIV disease. Multiple recurrent furunculosis (boils) is common (Fig. 11). *Streptococcus pyogenes* can cause ecthyma, impetigo, and folliculitis. Ecthyma lesions may be unusually deep and necrotic. Other dermatoses, such as scabies, eczema, seborrheic dermatitis, pruritic eruption of HIV, and HSV ulceration may get secondarily infected. Unusual infections, such as brucellosis may also occur (Fig. 12). Diagnosis is done by bacterial cultures and treatment as per antibiotic sensitivity.

### Syphilis

Syphilis is on the rise in many parts of the world recently. Primary syphilis is an important cause of genital, perianal as well as perioral ulcerations. Syphilis may rapidly progress to secondary as well as tertiary stage in immunocompromised persons. It is described in detail elsewhere in the book. High index of suspicion and proper clinical examination aided by appropriate laboratory investigations will help in diagnosis and management (Figs 13 and 14).

## Fungal Infections

The superficial fungal infections seen in HIV disease comprise of:
- Dermatophytoses
- Candidiasis
- Pityrosporum infections.

### Dermatophytoses

Almost 30–40% of PLHIV patients have superficial infections with dermatophytoses. The lesions may be extensive, may be conspicuous by absence of any inflammation (presenting as just powdery flaking of extensive areas) (Fig. 15). Nail involvement is quite common and usually involves all nails. The "proximal onychomycosis" of toenails is quite characteristic.

### Candidiasis

Oral and oropharyngeal candidiasis is almost pathognomonic of HIV disease. Other sites affected are the genitalia and other intertriginous areas. Oral mucosal lesions may be whitish curds

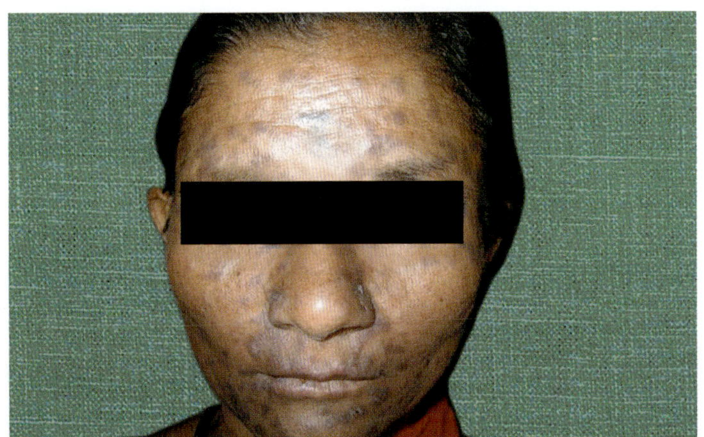

FIG. 13: Secondary syphilis.

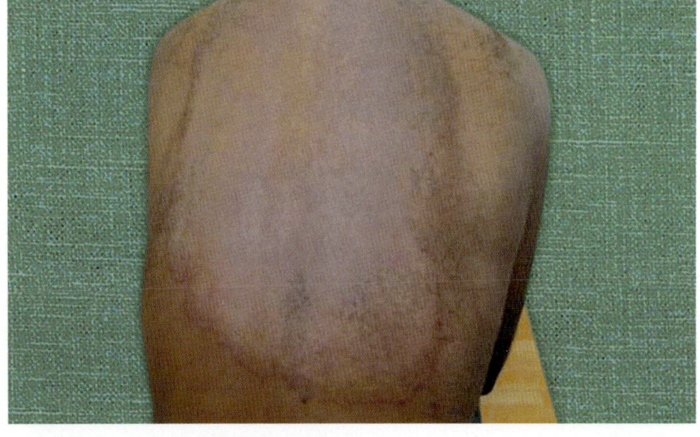

FIG. 15: Extensive dermatophytosis.

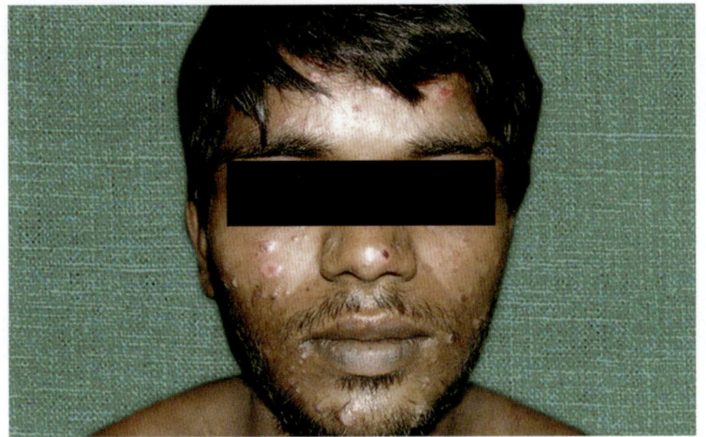

FIG. 14: Secondary syphilis.

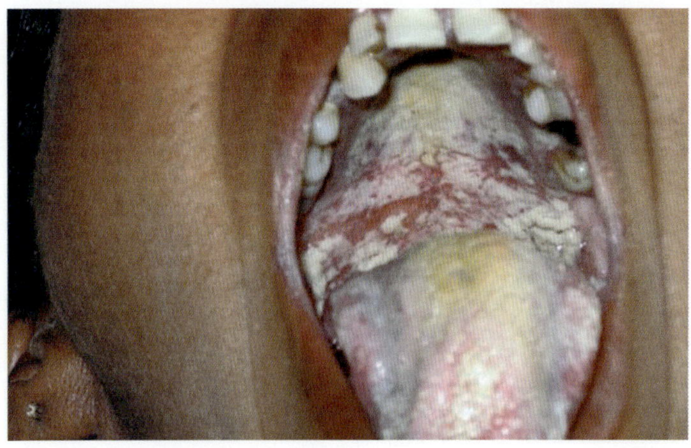

FIG. 16: Oral candidiasis.

like plaques, erythematous membranous, erosive or hypertrophic lesions or as chronic angular stomatitis (Fig. 16). In advanced disease, esophageal involvement may present as dysphagia, odynophagia, and retrosternal pain. Candidal paronychia is also common.

Dysphagia or odynophagia in PLHIV should empirically be treated as candidal infection while seeking definitive diagnosis.

## Pityrosporum Infections

Pityriasis versicolor, usually presenting as florid hypopigmented or hyperpigmented scaly macular eruption may be recalcitrant to routine treatment. Pityrosporum folliculitis may present as wide spread itchy follicular pustular lesions over back and arms. Pityrosporum species may be an important etiological factor in seborrheic dermatitis commonly seen in PLHIV.

## Deep (Systemic) Fungal Infections

In patients with immunodeficiency cryptococcosis (Fig. 17), histoplasmosis (Fig. 18), aspergillosis (Fig. 19), sporotrichosis, candidiasis, coccidioidomycosis, actinomycosis, pheohyphomycosis, mucormycosis (Fig. 20), penicilliosis (caused by *Penicillium marneffei*), etc. have been reported. Cutaneous

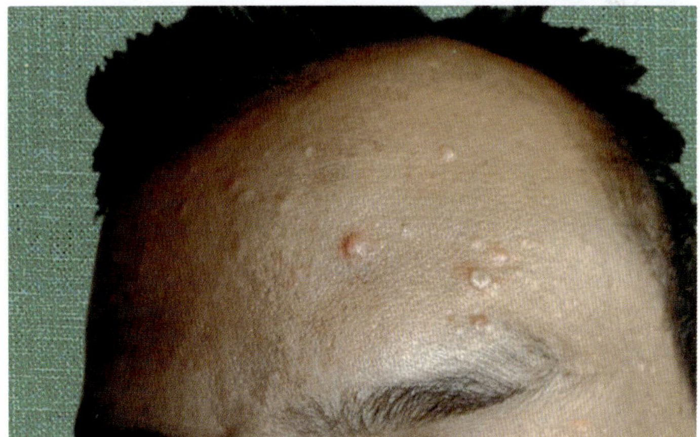

FIG. 17: Molluscum-like lesions of cutaneous cryptococcosis.

cryptococcal lesions are commonly seen on the head and neck as pearly 2–5 mm translucent papules resembling mollusca but may be widespread. They are usually associated with other systemic manifestations. Cutaneous histoplasmosis lesions vary in presentation. There may be nonspecific erythematous macules, papules, or eczematous lesions. These are also usually a part of systemic infection and the presentation is almost

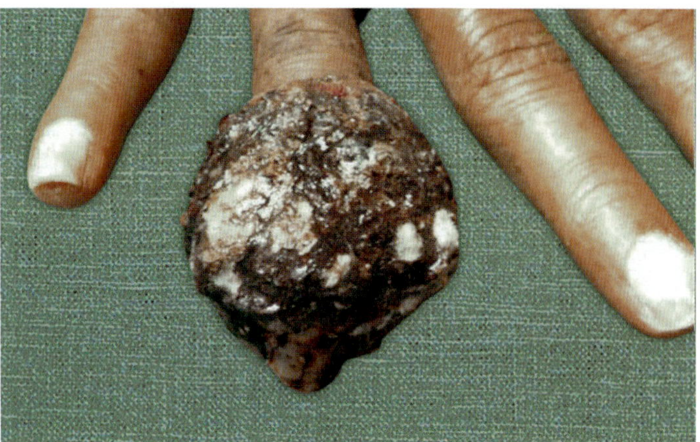

FIG. 18: Cutaneous histoplasmosis.

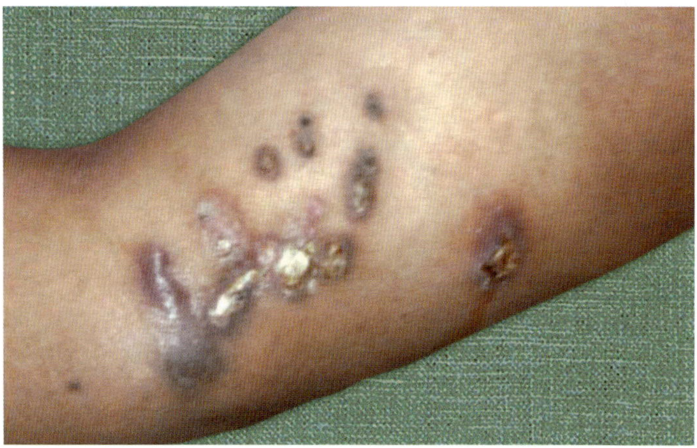

FIG. 19: Cutaneous aspergillosis.

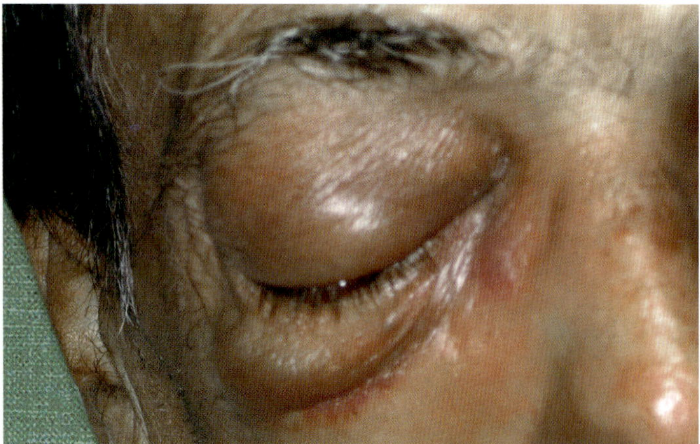

FIG. 20: Mucormycosis.

indistinguishable from disseminated tuberculosis. Diagnosis is by looking at the histopathology or by cultures.

## Mycobacterial Infections

*Mycobacterium tuberculosis* infection is probably the most common coinfection in PLHIV. In persons with advanced immunodeficiency (CD4 counts below 50 cells/mm$^3$) *Mycobacterium avium* intracellulare complex (MAC) disease is also common and has myriad presentations. These infections may be disseminated, unusual, and severe. Cutaneous lesions caused by these organisms are unusual. Common clinical presentation is in the form of chronic sinuses over involved lymph nodes (scrofuloderma) or chronic ulcerations. If suspected histopathology specimens should be also stained for acid-fast bacilli. Treatment with appropriate antimycobacterial agents is needed and it must be ensured that the same is completed without default. *Mycobacterium kansasii* can rarely cause cutaneous infections which on histopathology look like a spindle cell proliferation resembling Kaposi's sarcoma (KS).

Bacillus Calmette-Guérin immunization may cause disseminated *Mycobacterium bovis* infection and so has to be avoided in clinically sick infants born to HIV-infected mothers and other PLHIV.

## Arthropod Infestations

- Scabies
- Demodex folliculorum.

### Scabies

What has been described as the Norwegian scabies, a disseminated form with thousands of mites on the body, may present with an intensely pruritic lesions with extensive erythema scaling and exfoliative dermatitis in persons with advanced immunodeficiency. Otherwise, scabies might just present as intense pruritus without any rash.

### Demodex Folliculorum

This infestation may present with an itchy follicular, papular eruption distributed over the back, head, and neck.

# NONINFECTIOUS DISORDERS

There are several noninfectious disorders associated with HIV disease. The exact pathogenetic role of HIV is not clearly defined. The understanding of HIV disease not just a disease of immune deficiency but also of immune dysregulation and of chronic inflammation has paved the way for studying the underlying mechanisms leading to these disorders. Following is the list of disorders commonly associated with HIV.

- Xerosis and ichthyosis
- Psoriasis
- Seborrheic dermatitis
- Papular pruritic eruptions
- Eosinophilic pustular folliculitis
- Nail and hair changes
- Cutaneous drug reactions
- Malignancies.

## Xerosis and Ichthyosis

Dry, scaly, hyperpigmented lesions on extremities and trunk are commonly seen. They worsen in winter and in dry weather conditions. The worsening in advanced HIV disease may be associated with malnutrition. Persons with atopic diathesis may be severely affected. Frequent bathing and excessive use of soap also worsen the condition. Treatment is with liberal applications of emollients on moist or hydrated skin and appropriate use of mild topical steroids.

## Psoriasis

There is a strong association between psoriasis and HIV infection. However, whether HIV increases the incidence of HIV (except for the flexural type of psoriasis) is not established. Psoriatic erythroderma is also common. Severe pruritus is often a feature and secondary infection following scratching may be a serious complication. Treatment of psoriasis in HIV-infected persons is not different; however, response seems to be poorer as compared to a noninfected person. Though not commonly reported from India, tar therapy and psoralen plus ultraviolet A (PUVA) have been suspected to increase chances of development of KS, and low-dose methotrexate has been associated with worsening of the immunodeficiency. There are several reports that psoriatic lesions resolve after starting ART.

## Seborrheic Dermatitis

This is the most common cutaneous manifestation associated with HIV. Severity of seborrheic dermatitis has been associated with extent of immune deficiency and therefore can be good marker of the progression of HIV disease. It involves all hairy regions. There is intense erythema and greasy adherent scaling (Fig. 21). The disease shows remissions and exacerbations. It is linked with growth of *Pityrosporum ovale (Malassezia furfur)* due to immunosuppression. Lesions may heal with vitiligo like depigmentation. Treatment may be frustrating and is with topical steroids, topical imidazole derivatives and coal tar creams. But, lesions may be recalcitrant to treatment and may require use of systemic antifungal agents such as ketoconazole or itraconazole.

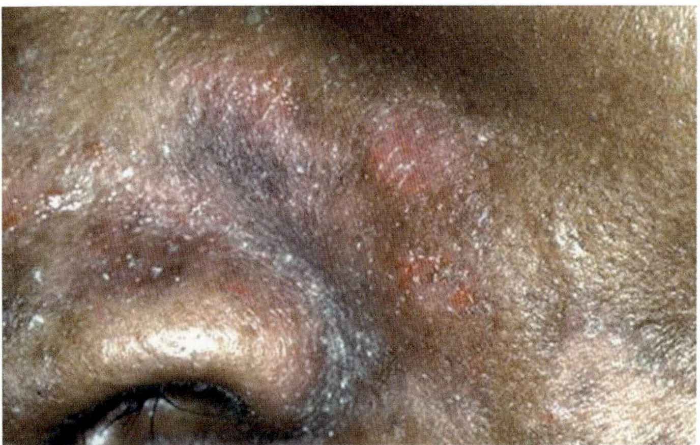

**FIG. 21:** Seborrheic dermatitis.

## Papular Pruritic Eruptions

These are extremely common in PLHIV and are seen as tiny, flesh-colored, itchy papules on neck and trunk (Figs 22 and 23). The etiology is unclear. Empiric treatment for infective focus (staphylococcal) antihistaminics to control the pruritus and topical steroids may help. PUVA therapy has been recommended but needs to be given with caution.

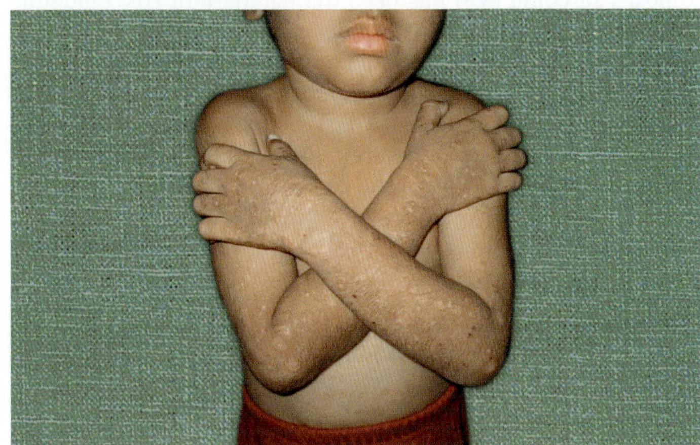

**FIG. 22:** Papulopruritiic eruption.

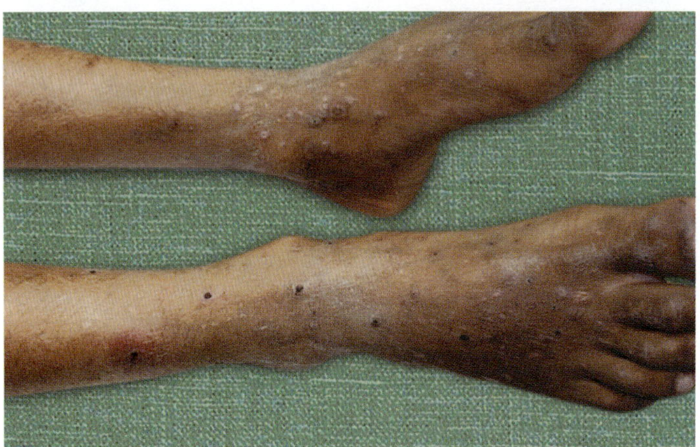

**FIG. 23:** Pruritic papular eruption.

## Eosinophilic Pustular Folliculitis

This is a form of chronic, pruritic, and pustular eruption. This is not associated with infection and on histopathological examination shows eosinophils. Treatment with antibiotics is futile. Narrowband ultraviolet B treatment, antihistamines, and a course of itraconazole may be tried.

## Nails and Hair Changes

- *Nails*: A yellowish discoloration of nails associated with pneumocystis infection has been observed. Nails may show pallor, fragility, and bluish pigmentation (associated with use of zidovudine)
- *Hairs*: Thinning of scalp hairs with alopecia is common. Hypertrichosis with elongation of eyelashes has also been observed in some cases.

## Cutaneous Drug Reactions

The incidence of adverse cutaneous drug reactions is very high in HIV disease. Helper T-cells, which are the target of HIV infection and which are depleted, should actually reduce the chances of hypersensitivity, so the pathogenesis remains unclear. PLHIV are on multiple drugs for HIV (ART), opportunistic infections (tuberculosis being the most common) and prophylaxis of opportunistic infections (e.g., trimethoprim or sulfamethoxazole). Generalized or localized rash, urticarial reactions, exfoliative erythroderma, fixed drug eruption, erythema multiforme, and toxic epidermal necrolysis (Fig. 24) have all been reported.

Another important aspect of long-term treatment with antiretroviral medicines, that is rapidly emerging is the disfigurement caused by several drugs, commonly described as the lipodystrophy. This could be in the form of lipoatrophy (sunken cheeks, thinning of extremities) (Fig. 25) or lipohypertrophy (Fig. 26) ("buffalo hump"-like accumulation of fat on the nape of the neck, gynecomastia, and protruding abdomen).

## Malignancies

### Kaposi's Sarcoma

Kaposi's sarcoma (KS) has been the hallmark of HIV epidemic since beginning; however, it is quite uncommon in Indian PLHIV. The reasons for this remain unknown. KS is linked to human herpesvirus 8 (HHV-8). It is a neoplasm of vascular endothelium and presents as with blue-red or dark-brown plaques and nodules especially on the lower extremities (Fig. 27). Lesions may occur in lymph nodes and other visceral organs. Advent of ART has had a declining impact on KS. Surgery, radiotherapy, chemotherapy with vincristine, vinblastine, and bleomycin are the available treatment options.

### Immune Reconstitution Inflammatory Syndrome

Initiation of ART will reduce the viral load and will lead to increase in the CD4 counts. While this is a welcome effect, there could at times be a dysregulated immune recovery leading to the phenomenon described as immune reconstitution inflammatory syndrome (IRIS). The manifestations are of two types—paradoxical worsening of existing opportunistic infection with exacerbation of inflammatory lesions, worsening of existing infectious lesions or the other type called unmasking IRIS in which latent opportunistic infections may manifest. Lower the nadir CD4 at the initiation of ART, higher the viral load, increased are the chances of IRIS. Isolated cutaneous IRIS is rare but cryptococcosis, histoplasmosis, tuberculosis, and leprosy have been reported. IRIS does not warrant discontinuation of ART. Appropriate treatment of any infection along with oral steroids for reducing the inflammation may be needed. Central nervous system or respiratory IRIS, however, may lead to increased morbidity and mortality. It is possible that if ART is started at high CD4 counts, as per evolving guidelines, the incidence of IRIS may go down.

## OROPHARYNGEAL LESIONS OF IMPORTANCE

Since ancient times, the mouth has been regarded as a mirror reflecting the health of the rest of the body. This remains true even in case of HIV infection. Oral lesions can lead to the initial diagnosis, inform about the progression, and indicate the prognosis.

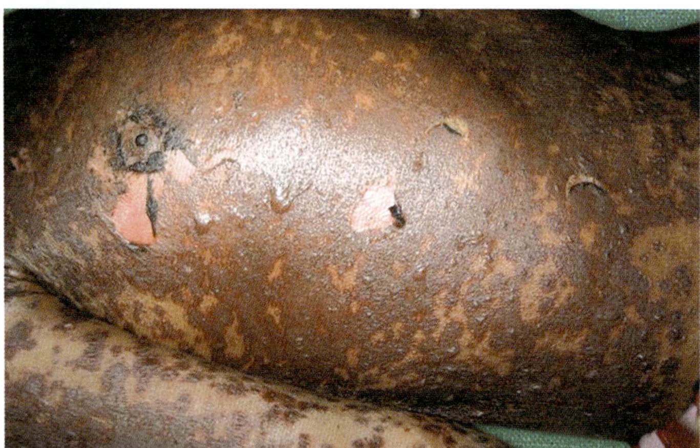

**FIG. 24:** Toxic epidermal necrolysis.

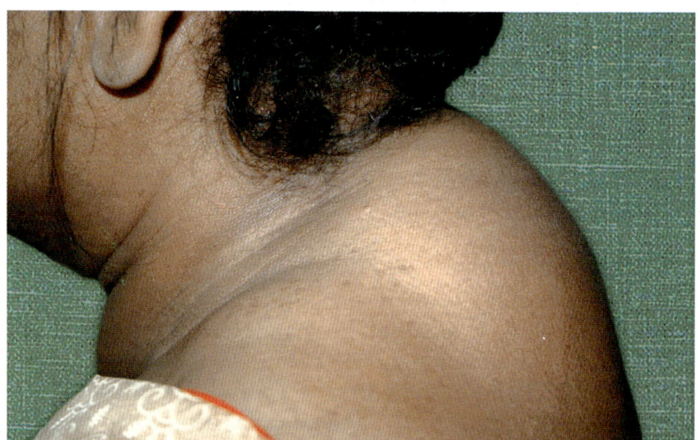

**FIG. 26:** Lipohypertrophy.

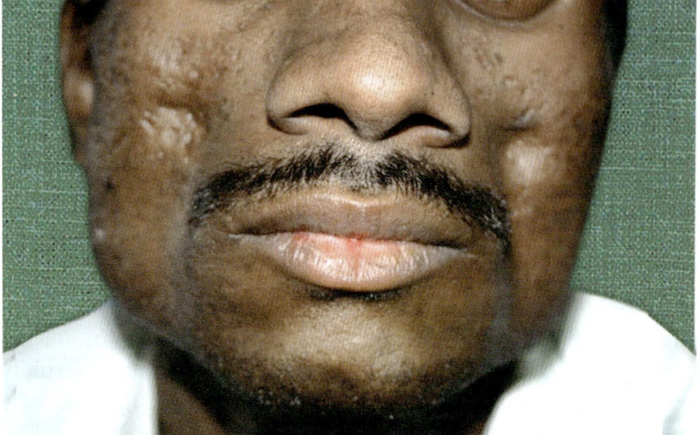

**FIG. 25:** Lipoatrophy.

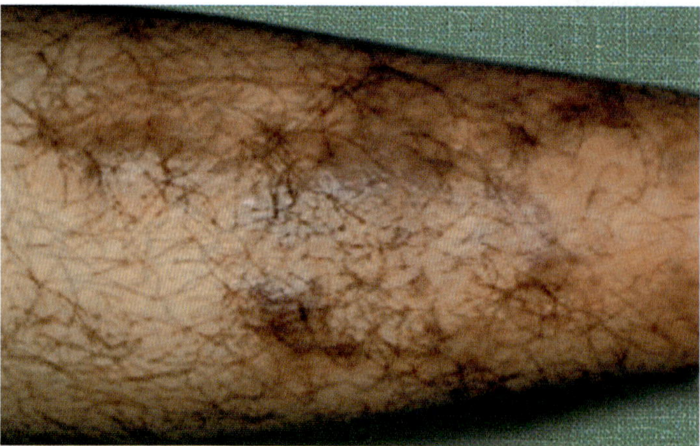

**FIG. 27:** Kaposi's sarcoma.

Common manifestations are:

- Candidiasis
- Oral hairy leukoplakia
- Kaposi's sarcoma
- Non-Hodgkin's lymphoma
- Periodontal disease
- Necrotizing (ulcerative) stomatitis
- Viral infections (herpes simplex, human papillomavirus (warts), varicella zoster virus)
- Drug reactions (ulcerative, erythema multiforme, toxic epidermolysis, lichenoid)
- Recurrent aphthous stomatitis.

Those not described before and are common—discussed here.

### Recurrent Aphthous Stomatitis

The etiology of this disorder is unknown. Typically, the ulcers are preceded by a prodromal irritation followed by crops of ulcers (1–10 mm diameter). The ulcers are shallow with a yellow sloughing base. They can last from a week to a month. At times, the ulcers may be greater than 1 cm in diameter especially on the soft palate. They are extremely painful and may take up to 3 months to heal. The diagnosis is clinical. There may be an underlying nutritional deficiency. There may also be neutropenia. It is crucial to maintain good oral hygiene. Chlorhexidine (0.2%) mouthwashes are invaluable. Topical steroids preferably in Orabase, a mouthwash prepared from tetracycline 250 mg capsule 4 times a day, mouth rinse with local anesthetics and in very severe cases oral prednisolone, starting at 40 mg/day tapered over next month is recommended.

### Necrotizing Ulcerative Periodontitis and Gingivitis

This condition is thought to be due to anaerobic fusiform bacteria and spirochetes. There is ulceration at the tips the interdental papillae leading to their loss. There is gingival bleeding, soreness and fetor (Fig. 28). Diagnosis is clinical. Topical antiseptics like povidone iodine, chlorhexidine in the form of rinses, antibiotics (amoxicillin, clindamycin, and metronidazole (400 mg tid) can be used.

## OVERVIEW OF MANAGEMENT OF HIV

Management of HIV has evolved tremendously in last couple of decades. Treatment of HIV disease is not ART alone, it also involves prevention, diagnosis, and treatment of opportunistic infections, nutrition and mental health issues as well as dealing with social rehabilitation. However, initiation of ART at the right time and adherence to treatment are the keys to successful management of HIV disease for prolonged periods of time; and remains the backbone of management. Currently, more than 20 different antiretroviral drugs are available, belonging to 5 different classes (entry inhibitors, fusion inhibitors, nucleoside, and non-nucleoside reverse transcriptase inhibitors, integrase inhibitors and protease inhibitors). Many new drugs are in the pipeline and some new targets for suppression of the virus are under investigation. Many new different strategies that could lead to "cure" are being experimented upon. Treatment of HIV is a rapidly evolving field. Guidelines are being modified and changed almost on annual basis. Safer and durable combinations are now being recommended. One needs to keep abreast with these developments by referring to contemporary recommendations. It is beyond the scope of this chapter to discuss management of HIV disease in its fullest details.

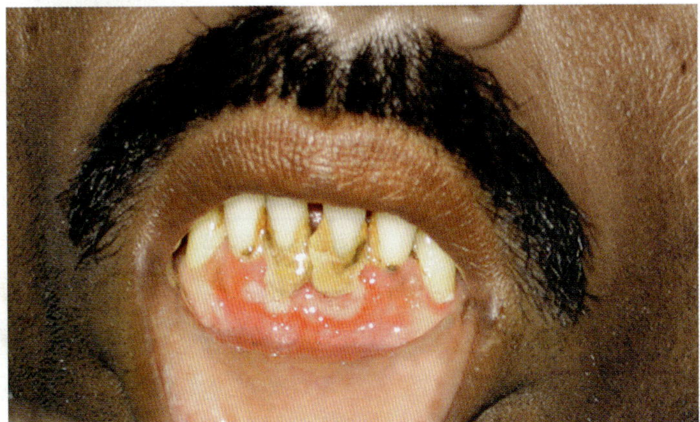

**FIG. 28:** Acute necrotizing gingivitis.

## GOALS OF ANTIRETROVIRAL TREATMENT

### Clinical Goals

- Extend life expectancy and quality of life in HIV infected individuals
- Prevent disease progression
- Reduce risk of opportunistic infections.

### Virological Goals

Reduce viral load to the lowest level possible and maintain as such (<25 or 400 HIV RNA copies/mL) depending upon the assay used.

Limit development of antiretroviral resistance.

### Immunological Goal

Restore and preserve immunologic function by maintaining CD4 cell counts.

### Epidemiological Goal

Reduce transmission of HIV to others.

### Challenges in Achieving these Goals

- Maximizing drug adherence
- Avoiding adverse drug reactions
- Avoiding drugs to which resistance has been demonstrated and also preserving future options for ART, in case drug resistance develops.

## SUGGESTED READINGS


1. Kreuter A, Schugt I, Hartmann M, et al. Dermatological diseases and signs of HIV infection. Eur J Med Res. 2002;7:57-62.
2. Paul S, Evans R, Maurer T, et al. Treatment of Dermatological Conditions Associated with HIV/AIDS: The Scarcity of Guidance on a Global Scale. AIDS Res Treat. 2016;2016:3272483.
3. Schneider JW, Dittmer DP. Diagnosis and treatment of Kaposi sarcoma. Am J Clin Dermatol. 2017;18(4):529-39.
4. Sharma G, Oberoi SS, Vohra P, et al. Oral manifestations of HIV/AIDS in Asia: Systematic review and future research guidelines. J Clin Exp Dent. 2015;7:e419-27.

# 66 CHAPTER Leprosy

*Vivek V Pai, Vanaja P Shetty, Nilendu Sarma, Sayantani Chakraborty*

## INTRODUCTION

Leprosy, one of the major diseases of mankind, has been declared eliminated in many endemic countries. As per World Health Organization (WHO) documents, since the introduction of multidrug therapy (MDT) in 1981, an estimated 16 million patients have been cured globally and disabilities have been prevented in some 4 million individuals. The seemingly great success of MDT had therefore prompted the World Health Assembly in 1991 to call for elimination of leprosy as a public health problem by the year 2000 which was further revised and strategized by WHO to achieve one or less than one, grade 2 disability among new cases/one million population and zero grade 2 disability in newly detected child cases.

However, in a recent review, PSS Rao observed that the incidence rates have continued to remain high in several countries. Owing to stigma and other factors, many patients especially of multibacillary (MB) type, delay treatment resulting in irreversible disabilities and continued transmission of the disease. Inadequate surveillance, poor research and lack of dissemination of accurate information have added to the problems of not developing more effective strategies to eradicate leprosy.

## EPIDEMIOLOGY

### Leprosy Case Detection Trends in the World and in India

Elimination of leprosy as a public health problem is currently monitored through measurement of prevalence and through annual new case detection which serves as an indicator for incidence.

The rate of new cases with grade two disabilities per 100,000 population is the current indicator for a global target given it is less influenced by operational factors, focuses attention on impairments and stimulates improvements in case detection. There has been no appreciable reduction in new case detection.

The data reveal highest numbers and rates in the southeast Asia region. In India, as a whole, the reduction in prevalence is 95.6%, and the mean reduction in case detection is 81.2% as of 2005. The comparative figures of new cases detected in India and in the rest of the World vis a vis the total new cases detected in the World indicates that 60% of the new cases detected are from India (Fig. 1).

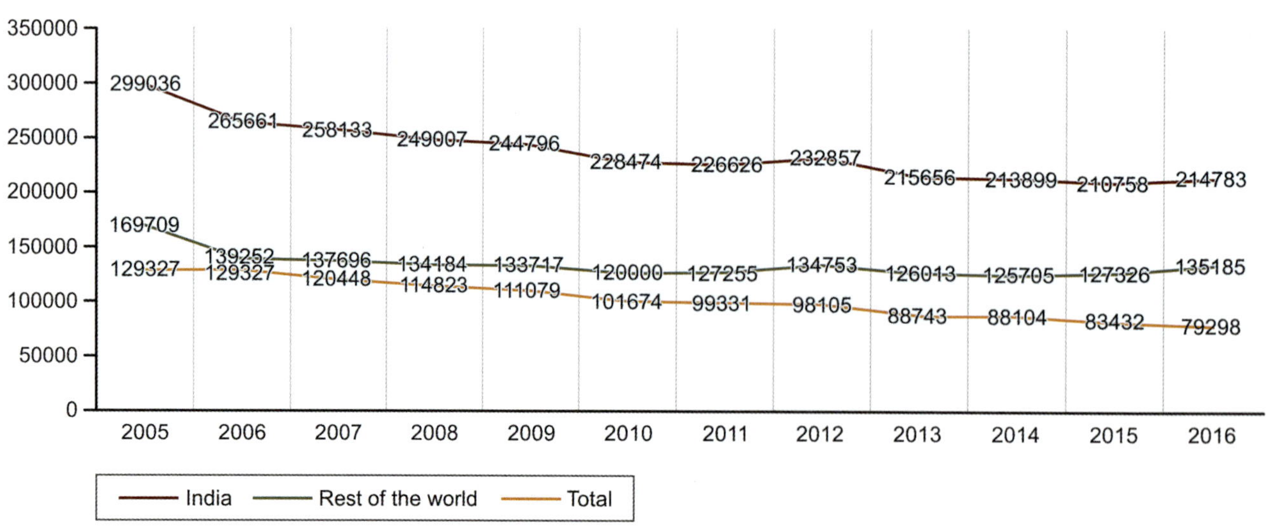


**FIG. 1:** The comparative figures of new cases detected in India and in the rest of the World.

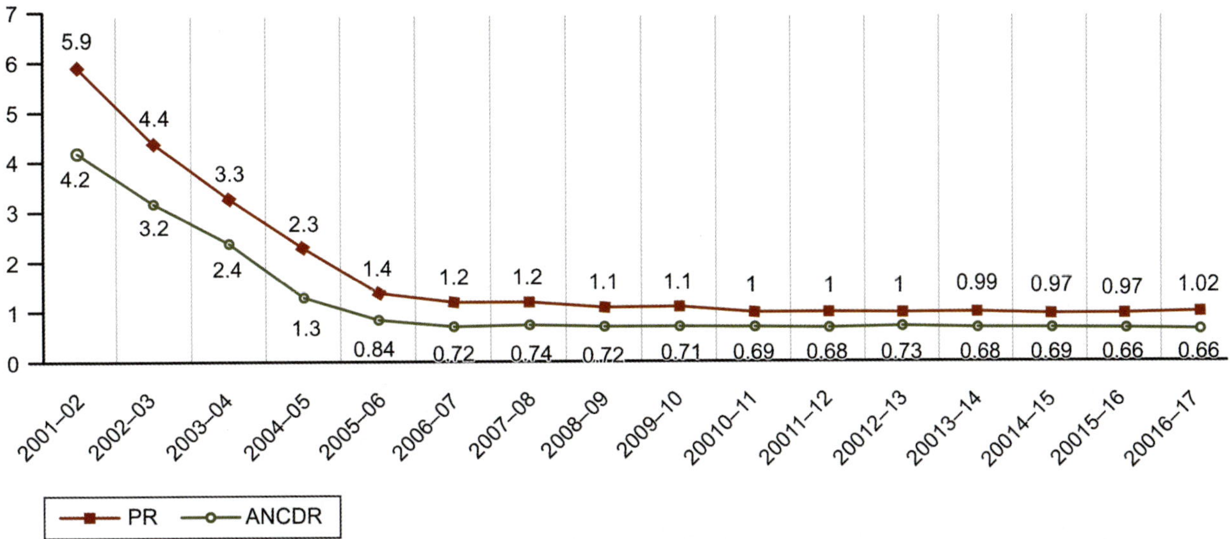


**Note:** The increase in new cases and prevalance during 2012–13 was attributable to the NLEP strategy to carry out extensive house to house survey for new case detection. Further increase in ANCDR during 2016–17 is attributable to leprosy case detection campaign.

**FIG. 2:** Trends of leprosy prevalence (PR) and annual new case detection (ANCDR) in India.

## Trends of Prevalence Rate and Annual New Case Detection Rate in India

A total of 0.86 lakh cases were on record as on 1st April 2014 giving a prevalence rate (PR) of 0.68/10,000 population. A total of 1.27 lakh new cases were detected during the year 2013–14 giving an Annual New Case Detection Rate of 9.98/100,000 population. Graph showing the trend of prevalence rate and new case detection rate from 2001-02 to 2016-17 (Fig. 2). The number of new cases with grade 2 disability increased from 4,069 during 2009–10 to 5,256 during 2013–14.

## PATHOGEN

Leprosy is an obligate intracellular infection caused by a pathogen, *Mycobacterium leprae* in man. This was first demonstrated by the Norwegian physician G.H.A Hansen in 1873 followed by Danielssen who came across globi, solid and beaded rods, coccoid forms, etc. both within and outside cells in leprosy lesions. In 1960, Shepherd, demonstrated a limited but reproducible growth of *M. leprae* in the footpad of mouse. This landmark discovery proved to be a major contribution as it made possible the screening of drugs, assessment of their efficacy, and detection of drug-resistant strains. Further Rees RJW showed enhanced growth of *M. leprae* in the footpads of thymectomized, irradiated mice in the year 1966 and later in nude mice. In 1971, Kirchheimer and Stores demonstrated unlimited multiplication of *M. leprae* in nine-banded armadillo (a South American rodent). Meanwhile, several attempts at cultivating the organism *in vitro* turned futile.

The genome sequencing of *M. leprae* was completed in 2000 by Stewart Cole. *M. leprae* barely maintains its existence with a minimal gene set.

*Mycobacterium leprae* has several traits that together make it a unique pathogen in human disease (Box 1).

**BOX 1 Important features and facts of *Mycobacterium leprae***

- Specific affinity for Schwann cells of the peripheral nerves where it multiplies freely and seems to escape immune detection
- Very slow multiplication rate (generation time of 13–15 days)
- Ability to go into a dormant stage where it can survive for years
- It is extremely nontoxic. Some polar lepromatous leprosy patients in spite of high load of bacilli barely show any clinical signs of disease
- Most of the bacilli in a leprosy patient are beaded, probably dead, thus leaving the host with a vast amount of bacillary waste
- It has not yet been grown successfully on an artificial medium thus hampering all kinds of research considerably

## PATHOGENESIS

Tuberculoid disease is the result of high-cell mediated immunity (CMI) with a largely Th1 type immune response. Lepromatous leprosy, on the other hand, is characterized by low CMI with high humoral (Th2) response. The borderline part of the spectrum is immunologically dynamic, and shift between the two polar forms occur.

Highly conserved toll-like receptors (TLRs) on the surface of monocytes and macrophages recognize mycobacterial lipoproteins and leads to monocyte differentiation into macrophages and dendritic cells. In tuberculoid cases, interferon-γ and interleukin-2 (IL-2) are secreted in lesions and result in intense phagocytic activity. T-cells in tuberculoid granulomas produce the antimicrobial protein granulysin.

Lepromatous disease is characterized by poor granuloma formation. IL-4 has been shown to downregulate TLR2 on monocytes, and IL-10 will suppress production of IL-12. This is associated with a preponderance of CD8+ lymphocytes in lepromatous lesions.

There is evidence to show that *M. leprae* was able to reduce and evade immune activity that is dependent on vitamin D. This vitamin D dependent immune pathway is suppressed through some particular micro-RNA that acts through MIR-21.

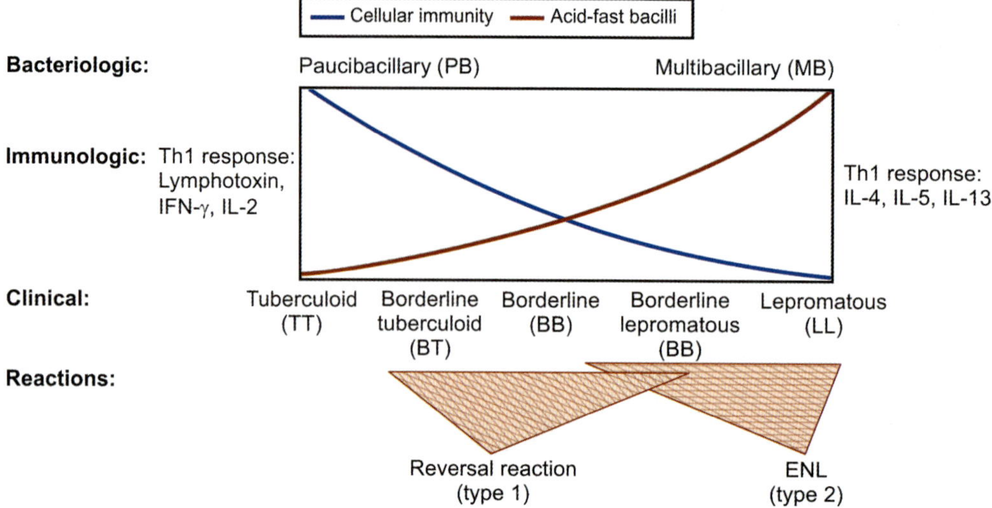


**FIG. 3:** Bacteriologic, immunologic, and clinical spectrum of leprosy.

Schematic representation of the clinical and immunological spectrum of leprosy is presented in fig. 3.

### Portal of Entry and Host Response

Mucous membranes of the respiratory tract and penetrance through the skin are the primary route of entry into human.

### Genetic Susceptibility to Leprosy

A large number of host genes have been implicated in conferring susceptibility to leprosy, e.g., TLR1 and TLR2 clusters, LTA genes, HLA genes, IFN-γ, vitamin D receptors, PARK2/PARKG regions, HLA-DR2, and MICA/MICB.

## CLASSIFICATION

Ridley–Jopling classification, proposed in 1966, classified leprosy patients into five groups viz. polar tuberculoid (TT), borderline tuberculoid (BT), borderline (BB), borderline lepromatous (BL) and lepromatous (LL) based on the clinical symptoms was amongst the earliest systems with remarkable scientific validity.

Subsequently, another subtype, called indeterminate leprosy was added to this list. Another special variant called "pure neuritic leprosy" was seen among Indians. In 1982, WHO proposed the "operational classification" into MB and paucibacillary (PB) leprosy. The PB category of patients comprise of patients with indeterminate, TT, and BT cases. Similarly, the MB group consists of BT, BB, BL, and LL cases. Thus, there is some scope for ambiguity and misclassification.

The WHO operational classification was further simplified to consider the number of skin lesions, i.e., patients with less than five lesions are grouped as PB and more than five lesions as MB. This operational classification finds its apt use in hyperendemic resource-poor settings where it is imperative to classify the patients into respective treatment groups.

Likewise, histopathological classification is important from the epidemiological and research point of view where there is a need for stratification and in-depth analysis. Both these classifications need to be used by a harmonizing approach rather than as exclusive.

## CLINICAL FEATURES OF LEPROSY

Leprosy primarily involves skin, nerves, eyes, and certain organs like testicles. Systemic organ involvement is found in long-standing disseminated disease. Disease severity and thus extent of involvement actually correlates with the disease severity and host immunity. Clinical manifestation depends on extent of skin and systemic involvement, reactions, and complications (Tables 1 and 2).

## LEPROSY REACTIONS

Leprosy reactions are immunological phenomena that may occur in leprosy. This may be spontaneous, related to treatment or there may be some precipitating factors (Box 2).
There are two types of leprosy reactions:

### Type 1 or Reversal Reaction

This happens in patients with unstable CMI. This is commonly an upgrading reaction (increase in CMI) but may be a downgrading reaction. Borderline leprosy cases (especially BT) are prone to develop type 1 reaction. This is a type 4 hypersensitivity reaction.

Significant inflammation leads to clinical signs of inflammation on the existing skin lesions. They may ulcerate. There may be edema of the hands, feet, and the face. Some previously unnoticed or nonvisible patches may become visible but actually, there are no new lesions (Fig. 4).

Inflammation in the affected nerves and its surrounding areas may lead to sudden swelling and entrapment. This can lead to sudden paralysis (wrist drop, foot drop) necessitating urgent management. Paralysis of trigeminal nerve and the facial nerve may lead to corneal anesthesia and lagophthalmos.

Histopathology of the lesions shows edema and infiltration by increased number of lymphocytes.

**TABLE 1: Clinical features of each subtype of leprosy**

| Leprosy type | Clinical features | Histopathology and other investigations |
|---|---|---|
| Indeterminate leprosy | • Very early form of disease<br>• Ill-defined, variable-sized, hypopigmented patch. There may be mild or no loss of sensation, slight dryness, and wrinkled appearance | Lepromin reaction varies from strong to weak. In histopathological examination, there may be presence of perineural and periappendageal lymphohistiocytic infiltration and even acid–fast bacillus (AFB) in the nerve sheath, arrectores pilorum muscle, or subepidermally |
| Tuberculoid leprosy (TT) | • Erythematous or coppery colored plaque with well-defined borders, single to few in number. Size is usually small<br>• Margin may show inward slope<br>• Surface is dry, sweating is lost, atrophy may be prominent, and sensory loss is marked<br>• A thickened feeding nerve twig may be present close to the lesion<br>• There may be enlargement of smaller feeding nerve of one to few peripheral nerves. This is usually stable without any signs of downgrading or reaction. A subpolar form of TT is known to exist that may rarely downgrade to BT | • Lepromin test is strongly positive<br>• AFB on slit-skin smear is not found<br>• Presence of epithelioid granuloma in close approximation with the epidermis, even reaching epidermis is characteristic. Scanty Langhans giant cells are present |
| Borderline tuberculoid (BT) | • Hypopigmented hyposthetic or anesthetic patch or plaque<br>• Margin is well defined, may show inward slope with areas of break (loss of definition) at some places (Fig. 5)<br>• Size and number of lesions may vary. Size may be very big Loss of sensation, and dryness are prominent (may be less conspicuous than in TT) (Fig. 6)<br>• Smaller satellite lesions are typically present surrounding the lesion in many cases<br>• There may be enlargement of several nerve trunks but in asymmetrical fashion<br>• Type 1 reaction is common as its complications like nerve paralysis, muscle atrophy and deformity (Fig. 7) | • Epithelioid granuloma is often admixed with macrophages, loosely distributed and has a tendency to spread. Fair number of lymphocytes and a good number of giant cells are found. A clear subepidermal zone is found<br>• Few fragmented AFBs may be found |
| Borderline-borderline leprosy (BB) | • Most unstable form and quickly downgrade toward lepromatous pole<br>• Multiple skin lesion with tendency to symmetry<br>• Characteristic clinical presentation is punched out annular lesions and large geographical lesion. There may be nodular lesions also. These lesions have well-defined inner edge and ill-defined outer edge<br>• Nerve damage may be variable | • Here there is admixture of almost equal number of macrophages and epithelioid cells. Lesser and scattered lymphocytes are usually present. Giant cells are scanty<br>• AFB are present in fair number |
| Borderline lepromatous leprosy (BL) | • Skin lesions are numerous in number<br>• They may range from macules, papules, plaques and nodules. Margins of BL lesions are usually vague<br>• Peripheral nerve involvement may be more in number, approaching toward symmetry<br>• Type 1 and 2 reactions (more common) are common<br>• It may downgrade to LL overtime | Predominantly macrophage granuloma with isolated clump of epithelioid cells is found. Foamy nature of macrophages is characteristic. Lymphocytes are sparse and scattered. Plenty of AFBs are found |
| Lepromatous leprosy (LL) | • Innumerable number of smaller sized lesions distributed symmetrically<br>• Lesions are composed of macules, papules, and nodules. Margin is ill-defined and surface is typically shiny. There may be diffuse infiltration of the skin with innumerable indistinct macules and patches. Nodules when present are often plenty and may appear as discrete or grouped (Figs 8 to 10)<br>• Along with broadening of the nasal, infiltrated eyebrows, and face acquires leonine appearance. Nodules and plaques on ear are classical (Fig. 11). Multiple peripheral nerves are grossly thickened symmetrically. This leads to symmetric loss of acral sensation (glove and sticking area). Silent loss of sensation is typical and may lead to trophic ulcers, deformity, digital resorption, swollen digits, lagophthalmos, corneal opacity, uveitis, and blindness<br>• Autonomic dysfunction may lead to swelling of feet<br>• Dense bacilli in nasal and oral mucosa may cause epistaxis, ulcer, resorption and perforation of cartilage<br>• Amyloidosis of vital organs like kidney is a long-term complication | • Granuloma rich in macrophage is characteristic. Often in advanced stage, the entire dermis is loaded with foamy macrophages loaded with bacilli. The epidermis is usually thinned due to pressure from the granuloma. A compressed strip of subepidermal zone is present (grenz zone). Lymphocytes are few in number. Innumerable number of bacilli are present<br>• Lepromin test is negative |

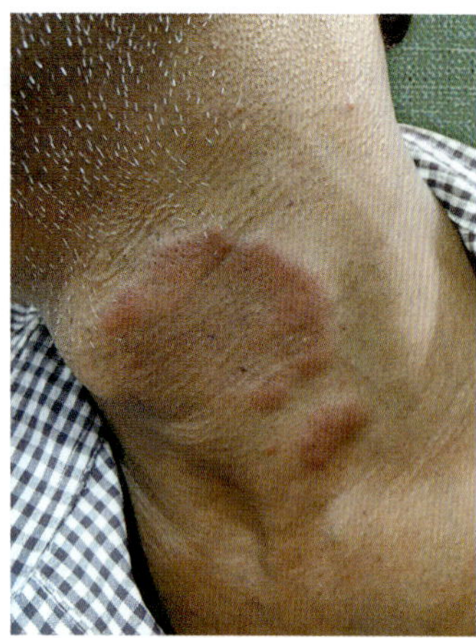

**FIG. 4:** Inflammed lesion of borderline tuberculoid leprosy with a satellite lesion during type 1 reaction.

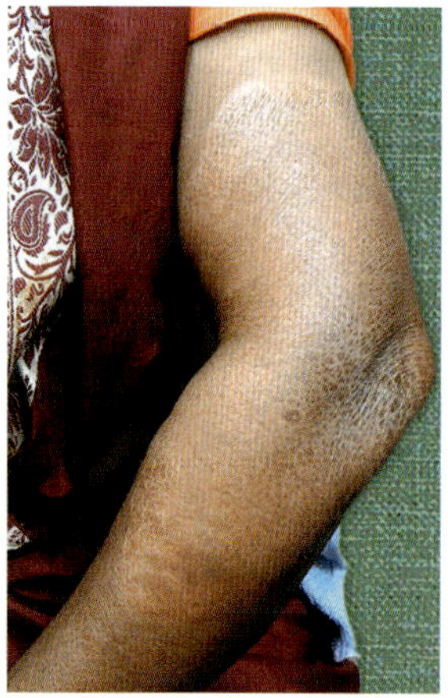

**FIG. 5:** Large well-defined patch of borderline tuberculoid leprosy with surface dryness and anesthesia.

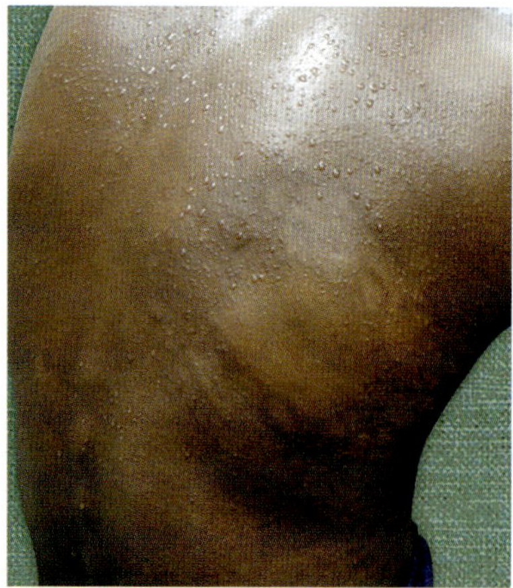

**FIG. 6:** Borderline tuberculoid leprosy showing significant loss of sweating due to autonomic loss.

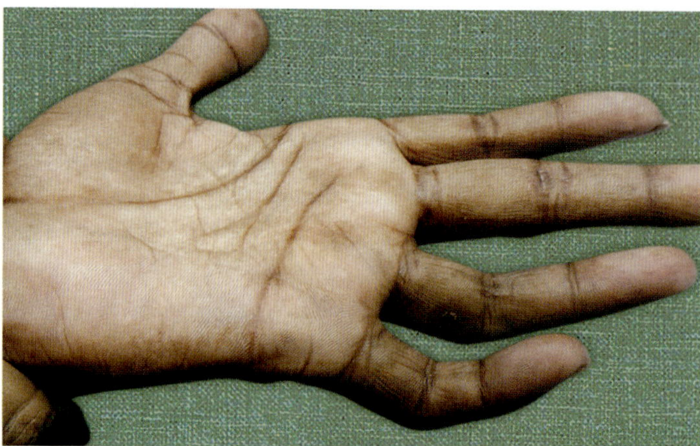

**FIG. 7:** Ulnar nerve palsy after type 1 reaction leading to ulnar clawing and muscle atrophy.

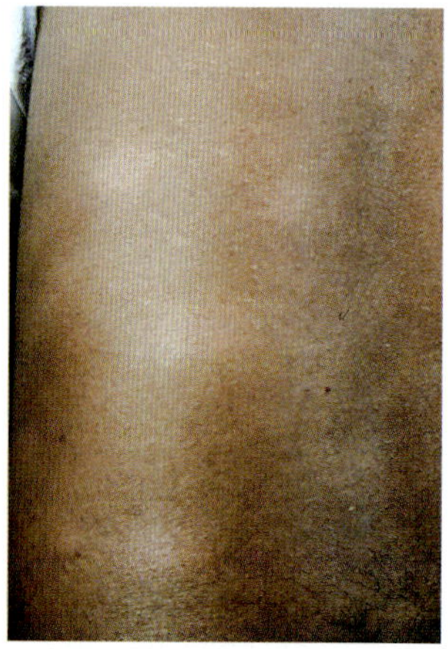

**FIG. 8:** Indistinct macules on the trunk in BL.

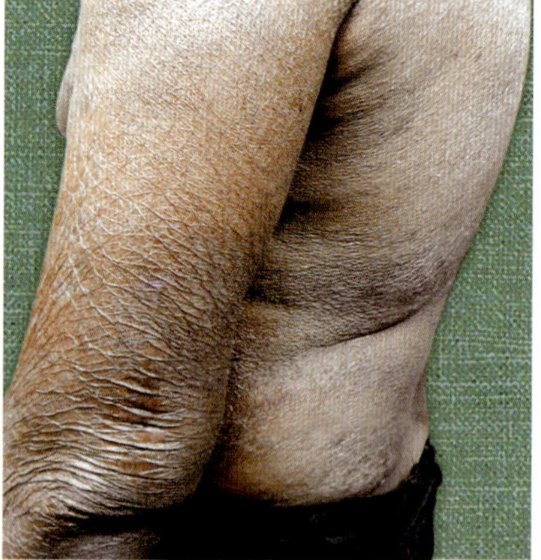

**FIG. 9:** Diffuse involvement of skin in lepromatous leprosy with indistinct patches.

There is inflammation induced destruction of the Schwann cells.

## Type 2 Reaction

This is a form of type 3 hypersensitivity reaction. Skin lesion in this reaction is typical. Such lesions are called erythema nodosum leprosum (ENL). This occurs in MB smear positive patients having a heavy load of bacilli (BL and LL). It may occur in the early stages of treatment and also long after completion of the treatment with MDT. This is because body takes a long time to clear the dead bacilli. ENL may become chronic or recurrent.

Immune complex are deposited in skin, eyes, joints, lymph nodes, kidneys, liver, spleen, bone marrow, endothelium, and testes. Thus, this may involve multiple organs causing generalized symptoms.

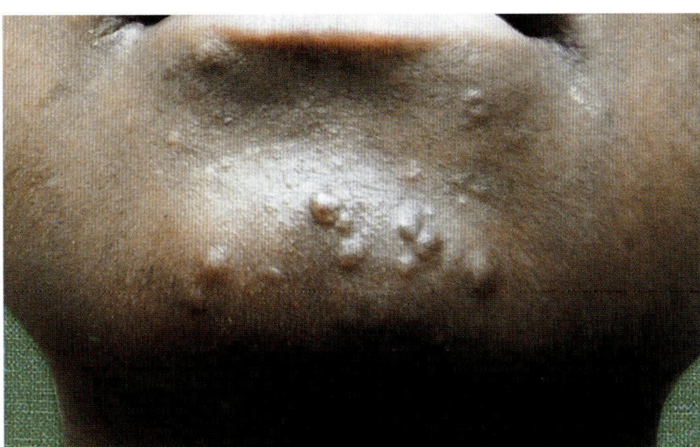

FIG. 10: Papulonodular lesions in lepromatous leprosy.

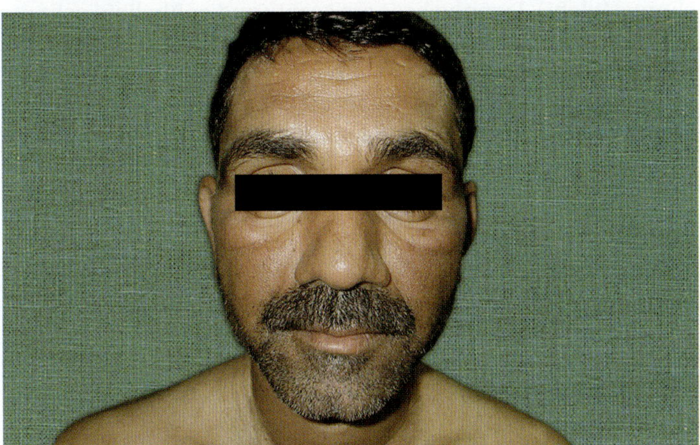

FIG. 11: Diffuse infiltration in early lepromatous leprosy.
*Courtesy*: Bombay Leprosy Project.

**TABLE 2: Special variants of leprosy**

| | |
|---|---|
| Histoid leprosy | • Smooth, shiny, dome-shaped, button-like, firm papules, and nodules. The intervening skin is normal (Fig. 12)<br>• The lesions may be located on face, back, buttocks, extensor areas of limbs, and joints. Histopathology is characteristic and shows granuloma formed of spindled cells arranged in whorled pattern. The bacilli are arranged in parallel stacks like "sheaves of wheat" |
| Pure neuritic leprosy | This type is characterized by involvement of one or more peripheral nerve trunk in absence of skin lesions. This is more common in India and Nepal. Wide spectrum of disease (pauci to multibacillary) may present with this form. Histology reveals features characteristic of the particular spectrum of disease |
| Lucio leprosy | Common in Mexico, this form of leprosy is a diffuse disease which is slowly progressive. This involves skin of face and body without any discrete lesions. The skin looks waxy with shiny appearance; there is diffuse infiltration of the earlobes and forehead. There occurs loss of eyebrows and eyelashes |
| Lazarine leprosy | This is characterized by borderline tuberculoid lesions undergoing spontaneous ulceration due to exaggerated hypersensitivity in type 1 reactions |

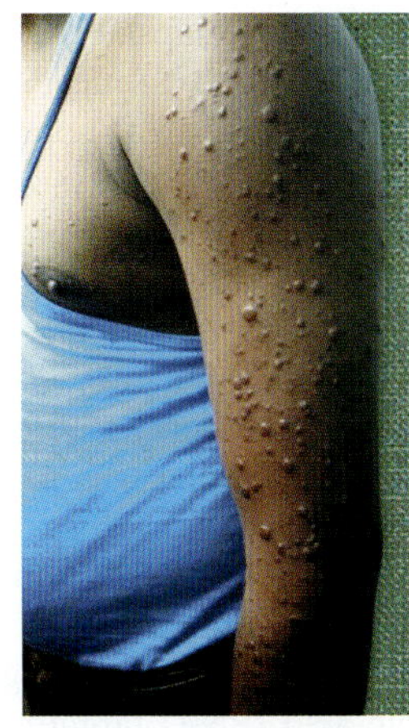

FIG. 12: Histoid leprosy.
*Courtesy*: Dr Pradip Bhakat, Consultant Dermatologist, Purulia, West Bengal.

**BOX 2 Proposed precipitating factors for leprosy reactions**

- Infections and infestations
- Vaccination
- Hormonal changes
- Puberty
- Pregnancy
- Childbirth
- Psychological stress

It manifests with fever, headache and bodyache, periosteal pain (especially tibiae), muscle pain (myositis), pain and swelling of the tendons and joints, rhinitis, epistaxis, painful dactylitis, swollen tender lymph nodes especially femoral, acute epididymo-orchitis, hepatosplenomegaly with hepatitis and endocarditis, and typical skin lesions.

Characteristic skin lesions are crops of new red, firm, painful, tender cutaneous and subcutaneous nodules (about 1–2 cm across), and variable-sized plaques. Nodules blanch on pressure. Usually multiple, they tend to be distributed bilaterally and symmetrically. Rarely they can break down and suppurate or necrose (called erythema necroticans/ulcerative ENL). When nodules fade, these leave bluish/brownish pigmentation. Nerves may also get affected in type 2 reactions.

Involvement of the eyes may lead to the development of iritis or iridocyclitis (inflammation of the iris and ciliary body) and impairment of vision. Eye becomes red, watery, and painful; pupil becomes constricted and nonreactive.

There is dense infiltrate of neutrophil within the granuloma and formation of microabscess. There may be vasculitis. Lymphocytes predominate at later stage.

### Lucio Phenomenon

This is analogous to type 2 reaction which occurs in untreated case of lucio leprosy. It presents as well-defined angular ulcerations often massive spreading in ascending fashion over the extremities and healing with atrophic scarring.

Histopathologically, there is necrosis of the epidermis and the dermis with histiocytic and neutrophilic infiltrate in and around the nerve fibers, blood vessels and the adnexa.

## RELAPSE AND PERSISTENT INFECTION

Relapse after MDT is most likely to be due to persisters and only could be due to resistance.

Several risk factors for relapses in leprosy have been suggested, including persisters, reinfection, drug resistance, inadequate/irregular therapy, use of monotherapy, high initial bacterial indices (BI), number and even size of skin lesions, and lepromin negativity. The risk of relapse in patients coinfected with HIV is a possibility and needs further investigation.

Currently, diagnosis of relapse is based mainly on clinical features, such as appearance of a new lesion and BI positivity after remaining smear negative. Some studies have demonstrated the utility of histopathological changes and simple serological tests in confirming the diagnosis of relapse. There is a possibility of developing molecular tests based on polymerase chain reaction (PCR) for early identification of relapses. There are several PCR methods to amplify different gene stretches of *M. leprae*. The ribonucleic acid (RNA) targeting probes are 10–100 fold more sensitive than deoxyribonucleic acid (DNA) targeting probes and can be used to monitor responses to therapy and also for identifying true relapses while differentiating them from reactions.

In patients who relapsed after WHO-MDT, retreatment with the same regimen showed a good response indicating persisters or drug-sensitive bacilli to be the cause of relapse. In our experience, relapses are observed in practically every regimen.

Recently published WHO operational guidelines recommend that it may be advisable to treat an MB patient with high BI for more than 12 months, taking careful consideration of the clinical and bacteriological evidence. A number of studies have reported that retreatment of relapses following dapsone monotherapy or MDT with another course of standard MDT regimens is highly successful. Long-term observations to assess relapse after fixed duration therapy (FDT) for 12 months is required.

## DIAGNOSIS

The WHO global strategy for further reducing the leprosy burden and sustaining leprosy control activities recommends the presence of any one of the following three cardinal signs to be used as the diagnostic criteria for leprosy worldwide; (WHO 2005).

1. Definite loss of sensation in a pale (hypopigmented) or erythematous skin patch
2. A thickened or enlarged peripheral nerve with loss of sensation and/or weakness of the muscle supplied by that nerve
3. Presence of AFB in a slit-skin smear.

### Laboratory Diagnosis of Leprosy

#### Cytology

Slit skin smear examination has been the major tool used in the laboratory diagnosis and classification and follow-up of patients with leprosy. Although highly specific, sensitivity is low, and 70% of all leprosy patients are smear negative.

#### Histopathology

Histopathological evaluation of affected skin is a vital step in confirmation and in classification of the disease spectrum. Histopathology of the tissue reflects the on-going immunological mechanisms.

In TT, the pole with highest immunity, macrophages are activated forming many epithelioid cells that form well-formed granuloma around the dermal neurovascular bundles. Lymphocytes are plenty and are present surrounding the granulomas. Dermal nerves are destroyed early and Langhans cells giant cells are not found.

In borderline leprosy (BT, BB and BL), histological features represent the gradual shift in immunological status in the body. Epithelioid cells and lymphocytes are prominent towards BT. Well-formed granulomas tend to develop in BT and are not seen in BL. Granulomas are distributed along superficial neurovascular bundles in dermis (Fig. 13). Number of lymphocytes gradually decreases from BT towards BL. Foam cells may be present in BL although much less commonly than in LL. Small sized Langhans giant cells may be seen in BT. Infiltrations and granuloma in all borderline cases are separated from epidermis (grenz zone).

In LL, there is diffuse non-granulomatous infiltration of the dermis with macrophage that shows abundant eosinophilic cytoplasm and many solid and fragmented bacilli. Wide-Fite stain can detect lepra bacilli that are often present in large clumps (globi). Lymphocytes are scanty and epithelioid cells are not seen. With treatment, and with time, even without treatment, macrophages are seen to contain tiny vacuoles that are formed from degenerated bacilli. These vacuolated cells are typical of late LL. Vacuolated macrophages are known as 'lepra cells' or 'Virchow cells' (Figs 14 and 15).

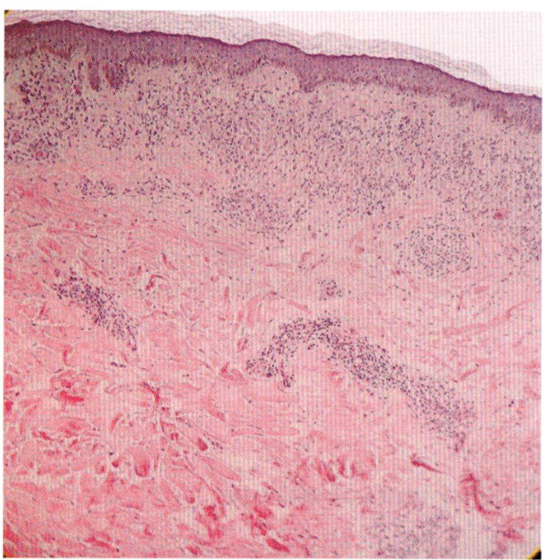

**FIG. 13:** Borderline tuberculoid leprosy. Lymphohistiocytic infiltration and formation of granuloma in superficial dermis and around neurovascular bundles

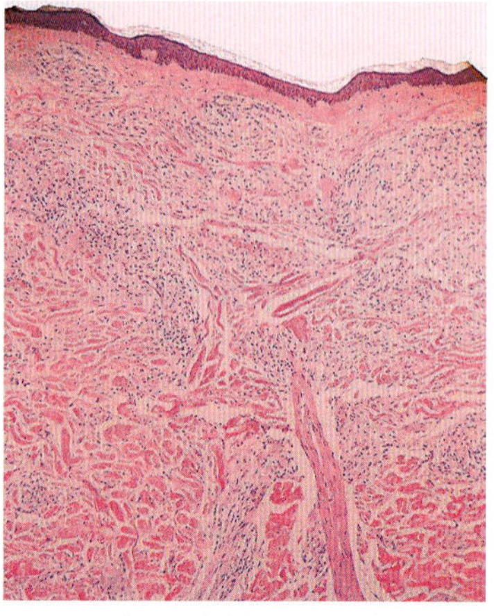

**FIG. 14:** Lepromatous leprosy. Diffuse macrophage infiltration in the dermis, flattened epidermis and prominent grenz zone.

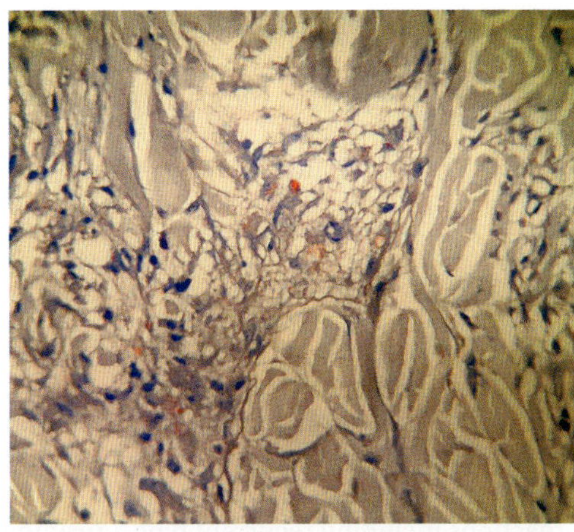

**FIG. 15:** Wide-Fite stain in lepromatous leprosy. Extensive foamy macrophages and numerous acid fast bacilli (red colored).

### Histopathology of Leprosy Reactions

- *Type 1 reaction*: There is distinct edema in and around the granuloma. Fibrinoid necrosis may be seen, epithelioid cells increase and Langhans giant cells are becomes bigger in size. Granuloma may encroach upon the epidermis in upgrading reaction. In downgrading reaction, necrosis is less frequent. Differentiation between upgrading and down grading is difficult. Tissue may have both features of initial stage along with upgraded/ downgraded newer stage.
- *Type 2 reaction*: Histological section is often dominated by numerous neutrophils. However, this feature may not be present in all cases.

### Molecular Markers for *M. leprae*

*M. leprae* specific genetic markers, such as 16S rRNA, RLEP and TTC repetitive sequences.

### Detection of *M. leprae* in the Environmental Sources

In addition to human cases, number of recent studies has detected the presence of viable *M. leprae* in soil and water samples in areas with high prevalence of leprosy. The presence of 16S rRNA in both patient samples and environmental samples may be assessed for its risk potential.

### Serological Markers

Serological markers like phenolic glycolipid I (PGL-I), 45 kD antigen, ESAT-6, and CPF-10 have been tested in India and a combination of all these antigens reported to detect *M. leprae* in 73% of PB cases as well. PGL-I has been widely studied but its diagnostic potential as a single marker in India may be limited due to cross reactivity with *Leishmania donovani*. Nonspecific markers, such as cytokines, levels of nitric oxide, and oxidative radicals have been tested, however, their value in prognosis of leprosy remains limited.

## TREATMENT

Chemotherapy of leprosy has undergone a sea change over the last several years (Table 3).

**TABLE 3: Changing regimens in leprosy**

| Regimen | Duration |
|---|---|
| DDS monotherapy | MB for lifelong and PB for 10 years |
| WHO-MDT (21 days intensive therapy) | MB therapy for 24 months or till skin smear negativity |
| WHO-MDT (modified) | MB therapy for 24 months or till skin smear negativity |
| WHO-MDT (FDT-24) | MB therapy for 24 months |
| WHO-MDT (FDT-12) | MB therapy for 12 months |
| WHO-MDT (FDT-6) | PB therapy for 6 months |
| ROM-12 | MB therapy for 12 months (monthly) |
| ROM-6 | PB therapy for 6 months (monthly) |
| RO | PB/MB therapy for 28 days (daily) |
| ROM-1 | Single dose |
| PMMx-1 | Single dose MB |
| MxRM-12 | Monthly MB |
| MxRM-6 | Monthly PB |

**Note:** No. 1–4: Not in vogue; No. 5 and 6: universally recommended by WHO; No. 7, 8, 9, 11, 12, 13: Trials in progress; No. 10: In vogue for some time now given up.

DDS, domiciliary dapsone; WHO, World Health Organization; MDT, multidrug therapy; FDT, fixed duration therapy; MB, multibacillary; PB, paucibacillary; R, rifampicin; O, ofloxacin; M, minocycline; P, rifapentine; Mx, moxifloxacin.

## Fixed Duration Therapy

Presently, recommended MDT regimen for MB leprosy is 12 months and for PB leprosy, is 6 months FDT.

The Government of India (National Leprosy Eradication Programme) made the following recommendations for the treatment of leprosy for control or eradication purposes to be adopted uniformly throughout the country:

- *FDT for MB leprosy*: All MB leprosy patients (patients with more than five lesions, irrespective of skin smear positivity) may be put on 12 months of standard WHO-MB MDT. These patients after release from treatment (RFT) will be kept on general surveillance for 5 years. All MB leprosy patients who have received 12 months or more of MDT should be released from treatment
- *FDT for PB leprosy*: All PB leprosy cases, including single skin lesion (SSL-PB) cases will be treated with 6 months of standard WHO-PB MDT and thereafter released from treatment. They should be kept under surveillance for 2 years.

## Newer Chemotherapeutic Agents in Leprosy

The recommended duration of treatment, particularly for MB leprosy currently in vogue, is still too long. Dapsone and clofazimine are weakly bactericidal against *M. leprae*. Hence, further shortening the duration of treatment by this regimen might result in higher relapse rate. Administration of the daily components dapsone and clofazimine cannot be supervised. Patients who cannot tolerate any of the drugs in standard WHO-MDT-MB need safer and effective alternative drugs. Thus, to further improve the efficacy of treatment and shorten the duration of treatment, several newer drugs are being studied in combination with rifampicin to achieve a better cure in PB and MB leprosy.

The following are the various group of drugs:

- *Fluoroquinolones*: Ofloxacin, pefloxacin, sparfloxacin, temafloxacin, moxifloxacin, and sitafloxacin
- *Tetracyclines*: Minocycline—bacteriostatic
- *Macrolides*: Clarithromycin—bactericidal
- *Ansamycins*: Rifabutin, rifapentine, and R-76-1—bactericidal
- *Dihydrofolate reductase inhibitors*: Brodimoprim and K-130 bacteriostatic
- *Fusidic acid*: Bacteriostatic
- *Beta-lactam antibiotics*: Cephaloridine, cefuroxime and amoxycillin plus clavulanic acid bactericidal
- *Diarylquinoline R20791068*: Bactericidal.

### Moxifloxacin-based Regimens

The flouroquinolone moxifloxacin has been shown to be the most powerful bactericidal agent against *M. leprae*. Some preliminary reports suggest use of a combination of moxifloxacin with rifapentine and minocycline. Clinical trials for the first time conducted by Bombay Leprosy Project have shown excellent clinical results and efficacy in moxifloxacin based regimens both in multibacillary and paucibacillary leprosy.

### Other Regimens for Special Situations

*Multibacillary adult patients who cannot tolerate rifampicin*: Daily administration of 50 mg clofazimine together with 400 mg of ofloxacin, and 100 mg of minocycline or 500 mg of clarithromycin for 6 months followed by daily administration of 50 mg of clofazimine together with 100 mg of minocycline or 400 mg of ofloxacin for at least an additional 18 months.

Rifampicin-resistant *M. leprae* are very often also resistant to dapsone and their treatment depends almost entirely on clofazimine. Daily treatment with the combination of ofloxacin plus minocycline shows promising bactericidal activity.

For patients who do not accept clofazimine, the 1993 Study Group recommended using ofloxacin 400 mg daily, or minocycline 100 mg daily as substitutes for clofazimine. The committee suggested that they could also be treated by monthly administration of rifampicin, ofloxacin, and minocycline (ROM) for 24 months.

*Dapsone toxicity*: Dapsone is stopped. No other modification is required for patients with MB leprosy. However, clofazimine may be substituted for dapsone for a period of 6 months in the dose employed in WHO-MDT regimen for PB leprosy.

## MANAGEMENT

### Type 1 Reaction

Corticosteroids are effective in the treatment of leprosy reaction and in acute nerve function impairment (NFI) in leprosy. A standardized steroid schedule recommended by WHO is presented below:

| | | | |
|---|---|---|---|
| Tablet prednisolone | 40 mg/day | × | 2 weeks |
| | 30 mg/day | × | 2 weeks |
| | 20 mg/day | × | 2 weeks |
| | 15 mg/day | × | 2 weeks |
| | 10 mg/day | × | 2 weeks |
| | 5 mg/day | × | 2 weeks |

A study was undertaken in Bombay Leprosy Project concluded that low dose regimen (40 mg) was associated with a higher incidence of recurrence (48.3%) as compared to high dose (60 mg) regimen (16%).

Newer alternative drugs, such as cyclosporine, azathioprine, and others are under investigation.

### Type 2 Reaction

Steroids are drug of choice in type 2 reactions but as ENL reaction is episodic in nature with chances of recurrence and chronicity in some individuals. Long-term administration or maintenance therapy with steroids is avoided as this may lead to steroid dependency and steroid adverse effects.

Type 2 reactions including recurrent type 2 reactions, steroid dependent cases, those with steroid adverse effects, severe, and chronic ulcerative ENL reactions could be controlled well with long-term administration of thalidomide as a maintenance therapy; however, recurrence to the extent of 20% is observed and among the patients with recurrence some patients despite being smear negative continue to have recurrent ENL reactions, which means there could be other factors responsible for recurrence apart from bacterial positivity as a possible precipitating factor. A suitable standardized dosage schedule as per the study is given below:

Capsule thalidomide 300–400 mg/day in divided doses × 2 weeks
200 mg/day in divided doses × 2 weeks
100 mg/day × 4 weeks
50 mg/day × 3–6 months
100 mg twice weekly × 3–6 months.

Clofazimine is also useful in type 2 reactions when given in anti-inflammatory dosage and particularly useful in recurrent and chronic type 2 reactions. Clofazimine when given in high doses (300 mg) will not only help to control type 2 reactions but will also help to wean off patients from long-term steroid administration and adverse effects and those dependent on steroids.

### Disability in Leprosy

Risk factors for disability in leprosy are mentioned in box 3.

### Nerve Damage in Leprosy

Identification of thickened or tender nerves is an important parameter to prioritize patients needing frequent follow-up to prevent NFI.

### Quiet Nerve Paralysis (Silent Neuritis)

It is generally believed that corticosteroid treatment is effective in cases with neural impairment of "recent" (an arbitrary time limit of 6 months) onset. The sensory impairment responded to prednisolone satisfactorily with a recovery rate of 73.8%, 76.5%, and 81% in ulnar, median, and posterior tibial nerves, respectively. However, field observations in South India did not suggest any role for steroids in preventing or correcting quite nerve paralysis.

### Nerve Function Assessment

In general practice, pain sensation is tested using the tip of the ballpoint pen and weakness of the skeletal muscles is examined

| BOX 3 | Risk for developing disability |
|---|---|
| • Registration delay | • Number of nerves involved |
| • High bacterial index | • Acute and silent neuritis |
| • More than five skin lesions | |

either by simple function involving groups of muscles or individual muscles. In addition, other tests, such as tendon, reflexes, vibration sense, position sense, and coordination should be performed routinely in control programs.

### Sensory Function

While testing with the tip of a ballpoint pen is widely practiced, sensory testing using graded nylon monofilaments is much more reliable and reproducible. Loss of hot and cold sensation discrimination in the suspected lesion is often the earliest sign.

### Motor Function

Voluntary muscle testing (VMT), as described by the Medical Research Council (MRC), is an accurate method of assessing muscle function, but is difficult to practice in the field. For practical purpose, the 0–5 scale recommended by MRC has been modified as 3–1 (paralysis, weak, and normal) and one synergic action of a muscle supplied by individual nerves commonly affected in leprosy is tested. A simple and inexpensive pinch meter to detect subclinical muscle weakness among leprosy patients by testing the pinch pressure has been developed. This finger dynamometer is an accurate and reproducible method of testing the muscle strength of the hands. VMT of the intrinsic muscles, innervated by the posterior tibial nerve, is difficult to grade. While using a 9-point or even higher VMT scale, caution should be exercised while interpreting the results, because of possible intertester variability.

## NEUROPATHIC PAIN IN LEPROSY

Neuropathic pain was associated with nerve enlargement and tenderness, painful skin lesions, and with psychological morbidity. The Douleur Neuropathique four questionnaire had a sensitivity of 100% and specificity of 92% in diagnosing neuropathic pain. The Douleur Neuropathique four is a simple tool for the screening of neuropathic patients. Using 12-item General Health Questionnaire to identify neuropathic pain and psychological morbidity was detected in 15% of the patients.

## PHYSICAL APPROACH TO PREVENT WORSENING OF DISABILITIES IN LEPROSY

The following are some of the simple field techniques that can be applied to treat disabilities in leprosy:

- Prefabricated splints for the prevention and correction of hand deformities
- Grip aid to patients with grossly mutilated hand deformities
- Application of "mini-plaster cast" for the treatment of plantar ulcers
- Special microcellular rubber (MCR) footwear
- Use of an "ulcer care" kit for offering foot care
- Eye care.

## CONCLUSION

"Elimination" of leprosy using chemotherapy based on WHO regimens has been achieved at the national level in a majority of countries. However, in the authors' experience, the occurrence of lepromatous cases with a high transmission potential is a matter of great and continued concern.

Hence, the dire need to identify early multibacillary smear positive individuals with diffuse infiltration of face, ears, trunk, back, and extremities which has to be emphasized during training of health staff and community volunteers and also to shift the training focus from the conventional patch oriented to look for individuals with early lepromatous leprosy eventually will do a lot of good to the program.

While MDT can cure patients under treatment, its impact on transmission within the community will depend upon treatment of all or nearly all patients in the community.

Achieving the elimination target with regard to the disease burden and social issues associated with leprosy demand an integrated comprehensive health services program with active community participation. A substantial hidden caseload exists in the community and numerous cases are being treated by private practitioners who are still not reporting their cases. The absence of effective field strategies for disability prevention and care would make the concept of elimination less meaningful.

## ACKNOWLEDGMENTS

The authors gratefully acknowledge the assistance provided by Mr R Gupta and Mr S Kulkarni and all other clinical and secretarial staff of Bombay Leprosy Project. The authors are also grateful to the patients for their cooperation and to the donors for their support in the various studies undertaken and helping to understand several aspects of the disease.

## SUGGESTED READINGS

1. Algood HM, Lin PL, Flynn JL. Tumor necrosis factor and chemokine interactions in the formation and maintenance of granulomas in tuberculosis. Clin Infect Dis. 2005;41(Supp.3):189-93.
2. Antia NH. The significance of nerve involvement in leprosy. Plast Reconstr Surgery. 1974;54:55-62.
3. Cole ST, Eiglmeier K, Parkhill J, et al. Massive gene decay in the leprosy bacillus. Nature. 2001;409:1007-11.
4. Colston MJ, Hilson GRF. Growth of M. leprae and M. marinum in congenitally athymic (nude) mice. Nature. 1976;262:399-401.
5. Demangel C, Britton WJ. Interaction of dendritic cells with mycobacteria; where the action starts. Immunol Cell Biol. 2000;78:318-24.
6. Estrella Lasry-Levy, Hietaharju A, Pai V, et al. Neuropathic pain and psychological morbidity in patients with treated leprosy; a cross sectional prevalence study in Mumbai. PLOS Neglected Tropical Diseases. 2011;5(3):e981.
7. Fitness J, Floyd S, Warndroff DK, et al. large-scale candidate gene study of leprosy susceptibility in the Karonga district of northern Malawi. Am J Trop Med Hyg. 2004;71:330-40.
8. Frytche TJ. The prevalence of disabling ocular complications of leprosy: a global study. Indian J Lepr. 1998;70:49-59.
9. Gupte MD, Srinivasan H, Paul SK, et al. Quiet nerve paralysis assessment with respect to MDT and corticosteroid therapy. Abstracts of 14th International Leprosy Congress. Orlando, Florida: International Leprosy Congress; 1993.
10. Ganapati R, Pai VV, Khanolkar SA et al. Clinical trials with moxifloxacin based regimens in leprosy - A Preliminary communication. Revista de Leprologia. 2009; XXVii(1).

11. Iyer CGS. Predilection of M. leprae for nerves neuropathologic observations. Int J Lepr. 1965;33:634-45.
12. Katoch VM, Lavania M, Chauhan DS, et al. Recent advances in molecular biology of leprosy. Indian J Lep. 2007;79(2&3):115-66.
13. Krieg RE, Mayers WH, Wolcott JH. Mycobacterial infections of the skin. Arch Dermatol. 1979;110:783-8.
14. Levy L, Shepherd CC, Faisal P. Death of M. leprosy bacilli following treatment of leprosy patients with 1500 mg Rifampicin in a single dose. Int J Lep. 1973;41:489-90.
15. Levy L. Studies of the mouse footpad technique for cultivation of Mycobacterium leprae – doubling time during logarithmic multiplication. Lepr Rev. 1976;47:103-6.
16. Little D, Khanolkar-Young S, Coultharta, et al. Immunohistological analysis of cellular infiltrate and gamma interferon, interleukin-12, and inducible nitric oxide synthetase expression in leprosy type 1 (reversal) reactions before and during prednisolone treatment. Infect Immun. 2001;69:3413-7.
17. Mira MT, Alcais A, Thuc NV, et al. Susceptibility to leprosy is associated with PARK2 and PACRG. Nature. 2004;427:636-40.
18. Pai VV, Pai RR, Nagpur NG, et al. Role of thalidomide in maintenance therapy in leprosy. Abstracts. Hyderabad: International Leprosy Congress; 2008.
19. Pai VV, Taysetye PU, Ganapati R. A study of standardized regimens of steroid treatment in reactions in leprosy at a referral centre. Indian J Lepr. 2012;84:9-15.
20. Pattyan SR, Deckx P, Rollier MT, et al. M. leprae persisters after treatment with dapsone and rifampicin. Int J Lep. 1976;44:154-8.
21. Pai VV, Gawali R, Khanolkar SA, et al. Moxifloxacin based regimens in Leprosy - Clinical Observations on occurrence of Reaction and bacterial decline. Abstracts, 19th International Leprosy Congress, Beijing, China, 2016.
22. Rees RJW, Meade TW. Comparison of the modes of spread and the incidence of tuberculosis and leprosy. Lancet. 1974;1:47.
23. Rees RJW, Weddell AG. Transmission of human leprosy to the mouse and its clinical implications. Trans Roy Soc Trop Med Hyg. 1970;64:31.
24. Sarno EN, Grau GE, Viera LM, et al. Serum levels of tumor necrosis factor-alpha and interleukin-1 beta during leprosy reactional states. Clin Exp Immunol. 1991;84:103-8.
25. Spellberg B, Edwards JE Jr. Type 1/Type 2 immunity in infectious diseases. Clin Infect Dis. 2001;32:76-102.
26. Van Brakel, Nicholls P. The INFIR cohort study: assessment of sensory and motor neuropathy at baseline. Lep Rev. 2005;76:277-9.
27. Van Brakel WH, Khawas IB. Nerve damage in leprosy: an epidemiological and clinical study of 396 patients in west Nepal- part 1. Definitions, methods and frequencies. Lepr Rev. 1994;65:204-21.
28. WHO Expert Committee on Leprosy. TRS 768. Geneva: WHO; 1988.

# 18 SECTION Disorders of Mucosa, Genitalia, and Skin Appendages

# 67 CHAPTER Disorders of Lip and Oral Mucosae

*Vijay Zawar, Tarang Goyal*

## INTRODUCTION

Oral cavity is a unique anatomical location with structures such as teeth, mucosa, and junction of stratified epithelium at vermillion of lips. Certain cutaneous and systemic diseases often manifest onto oral cavity and thus, the knowledge of diseases of oral cavity is extremely important in diagnosis and management of several disorders.

## WHITE SPONGE NEVUS

White sponge is inherited in an autosomal dominant, extremely rare condition.

### Etiology

Mutation in keratin K4 or K13 results in keratin instability and abnormal keratin aggregation. Spontaneous mutations have been reported.

### Clinical Features

Patients usually within first two decades of life develop poorly demarcated, diffuse, and painless white plaques on the oral mucosa and tongue. It affects both oral and genital mucosa, usually in a symmetric distribution.

### Diagnosis

Biopsy or exfoliative cytology shows perinuclear eosinophilic condensations (showing abnormal keratin aggregation) and distinguishes it from other mucosal disorders.

### Management

No treatment is needed. Some patients reported response to tetracycline.

## HEREDITARY BENIGN INTRAEPITHELIAL DYSKERATOSIS (WITKOP-VON SALLMANN SYNDROME)

This is a rare autosomal dominant benign condition.

### Etiology

It is associated with chromosome four anomalies. It is mainly seen in some groups of mixed ethnic origin, predominantly in North Carolina, the United States of America.

### Clinical Features

Presents as oral milky white, smooth, and translucent plaques that appear in childhood and become obvious in adolescence. It predominantly affects the buccal mucosa, lips, and ventrum of the tongue.

Ocular lesions include conjunctivitis with gelatinous conjunctival plaques and become evident in infancy. Photophobia and corneal involvement may be seen.

### Diagnosis

Histopathology shows epithelial acanthosis, vacuolization in the stratum spinosum, and eosinophilic cells engulfed by normal squamous cells (tobacco cells).

### Treatment

No treatment is required.

## PACHYONYCHIA CONGENITA (JADASSOHN–LEWANDOWSKY SYNDROME)

It is a benign disorder associated with mutations in keratin 16. About 60% of patients have oral keratosis, 16% have natal or neonatal teeth, and 10% have angular stomatitis. Some develop chronic intraoral candidiasis. Keratosis requires no treatment. Dental advice should be given regarding natal or neonatal teeth (Fig. 1).

## MORSICATIO MUCOSAE ORIS (PATHOMINIA MUCOSAE ORIS, CHRONIC BITE INJURY)

This is a more intense local factitial injury of the oral mucosa, caused by a chewing habit, leading to reactive keratosis and benign epithelial hyperplasia.

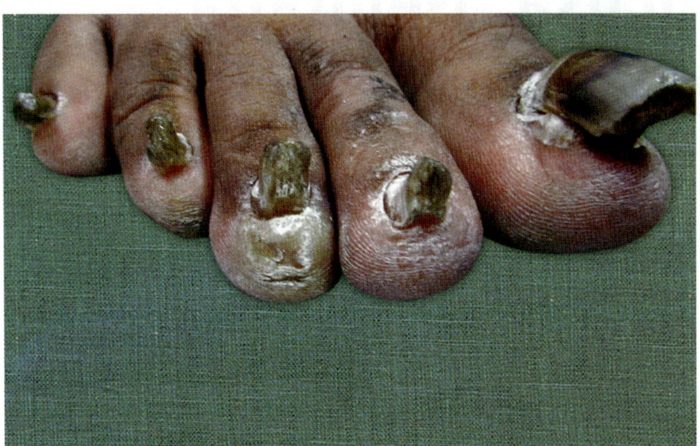

**FIG. 1:** Pachyonychia congenita.

## Clinical Features

It presents as white papules and plaques on either side of *linea alba* on the buccal mucosa, lower labial mucosa, or the lateral tongue usually caused by raking of teeth over the mucosa.

Lesions presents as shaggy, rough surface, poorly demarcated, and occasionally show evidence of erythema and ulceration. It should be differentiated from candidiasis, lichen planus, leukoplakia and erythroleukoplakias.

## Diagnosis

Biopsy shows varying degrees of parakeratosis with impetiginization and benign epithelial hyperplasia.

## Treatment

Protection from injury.

# LEUKOEDEMA

It is likely to be a reactive lesion. It occurs in 20–70% with chewing habits or smoking.

## Clinical Features

Painless, fine grayish white, ill demarcated, diffuse, and opalescent reticulations are present bilaterally on the buccal mucosa or ventral tongue. Stretching the mucosa completely eliminates these fine lines since this is not a keratotic lesion, rather caused by intracellular edema of damaged superficial keratinocytes. It should be differentiated from reticular lichen planus.

## Diagnosis

Histopathology shows typical findings of keratinocyte edema or hydropic degeneration.

## Treatment

No treatment is necessary.

# APHTHOUS ULCER

Aphthous stomatitis or canker sores are common, recurrent, and painful mucosal erosions that appear on the inner cheeks, lips, gums, tongue, palate, and pharynx (nonkeratinized tissues). Adults and females are more commonly affected.

## Etiology

Trauma is most important factor. Pleomorphic α-hemolytic *Streptococcus sanguis* are sometimes found in aphthous. Nicotine may have a beneficial effect. Aphthous ulcers may develop in systemic diseases like Crohn's disease and cyclical neutropenia (Box 1).

## Pathogenesis

The presence of antimucosal antibodies indicates an immunologic reaction to damaged epithelial tissue. There is depressed or reversed CD4:CD8 ratio, increased T-cell receptor γ-delta T-cells and an increase in tumor necrosis factor-α (TNF-α) levels. Human leukocyte antigen types A2 and B12 are common in patients with recurrent aphthae.

## Clinical Findings

Single or multiple, small (1–10 mm diameter), shallow erosions with clearly defined borders covered by a gray membrane and surrounded by an intense erythematous halo. There is often pain, tingling, or burning sensation (Fig. 2).

## Stages

- *Premonitory stage*: Last for up to 24 hours and is characterized by tingling, burning, painful, or hyperesthetic sensations in absence of any clinical changes
- *Preulcerative stage*: Flat or raised indurated areas surrounded by a red halo, lasts for 18 hours to 3 days with variable but often moderately severe pain
- *Ulcerative stage*: Lasts for 1–16 days and lesions are severely painful
- *Healing stage*: May last for few to many days.

**BOX 1** **Etiological or precipitating factors**

- Trauma
- Physical and mental stress
- Premenstrual period (often remits during the third trimester of pregnancy)
- Drug and food
- Hematinic deficiency (iron, folate, vitamin B12)
- Behçet syndrome
- Infections, *Helicobacter pylori* and Epstein–Barr virus, human immunodeficiency virus, herpes (Fig. 3), cytomegalovirus
- Autoinflammatory syndromes
- Malignancy

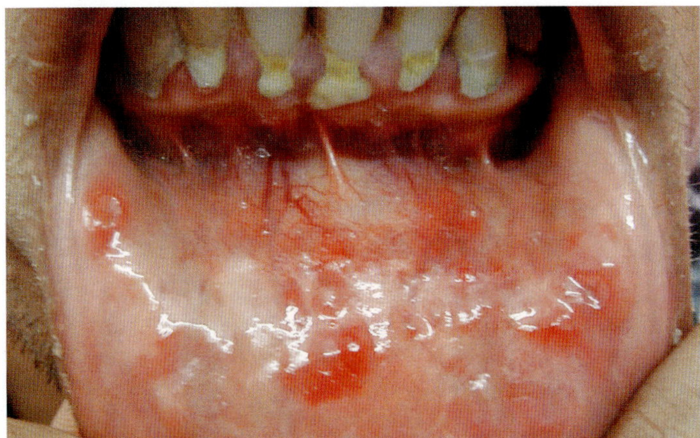

**FIG. 2:** Aphthous stomatitis.

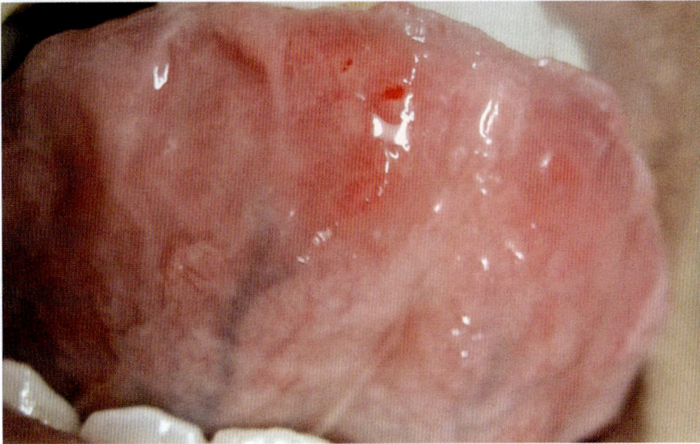

**FIG. 3:** Herpetic glossitis.

## Types of Aphthae

- *Minor aphthae*: This is the most common form, accounting for 80% of the cases. They measure between 1 and 5 mm and last for 7–14 days. Pain is minimal to moderate and there is no scarring
- *Herpetiform aphthae*: More numerous and grouped lesions
- *Major aphthae or Sutton's disease*: These are larger, fewer, and very painful and heal slowly (2–4 weeks). They frequently involve the soft palate and oropharynx. Scarring may develop.

## Differential Diagnosis

- Acute herpes simplex gingivostomatitis
- Candidiasis
- Vincent's angina
- Traumatic ulcers
- Aphthae seen in diseases like Behcet's syndrome, Crohn's disease.

## Management

Topical anesthetics (dicyclomine hydrochloride solution), topical steroids, topical 5% aminosalicylic acid (5-ASA) are commonly used.

Suppression of oral streptococci by topical antibiotics is a logical approach.

Systemic corticosteroids may be effective if used during prodromal stage.

Tetracycline capsules (250–1,000 mg) dissolved in 30 mL of water or elixir of Benadryl and apply for 10–20 minutes four to six times/day for 5–7 days.

Cephalexin monohydrate (250 mg) capsule dissolved in 30 mL of water and apply for 10–20 minutes four to six times a day.

Also helpful are colchicine, dapsone and pentoxifylline, low dose interferon-α, cyclosporin topical solution, granulocyte-macrophage colony-stimulating factor, and carbon dioxide laser ablation has been used.

# ORAL ULCERATIVE LESIONS ASSOCIATED WITH GASTROINTESTINAL DISEASE

Oral ulcers are a very common problem and are sometimes a marker of gastrointestinal disease like Crohn's disease, ulcerative colitis, malabsorption syndromes affecting hematopoiesis.

## Crohn's Disease

Oral lesions are seen in up to 20% of patients with Crohn's disease. Ulcers are persistent, linear, and deep ulcer. Other oral manifestations are cobblestoning of oral mucosa, diffuse swelling of lips, indurated polypoid tag like lesions in the vestibule erythema and inflammation of mucosa sometimes associated with *Staphylococcus aureus* infection.

## Ulcerative Colitis

Pyostomatitis vegetans (oral analog of pyoderma gangrenosum) presents as scattered, clumped, or linear pustules with ulcers on an erythematous base giving it an appearance of snail-track.

## Management

Antiseptic mouth rinse, local anesthetics, and oral and topical corticosteroids in severe cases and in absence of gastrointestinal findings are generally used. This may respond to dapsone.

# CHEMOTHERAPY-ASSOCIATED ULCERATIVE MUCOSITIS

Mucositis are common and occur due to apoptosis of dividing epithelial cells mediated through cytokines. Chemotherapy agents often causing this are fluorouracil, cytarabine, methotrexate, and cisplatin especially when combined with radiation.

Common chemotherapeutic agents causing mucositis include:
- Methotrexate
- Cyclophosphamide
- Hydroxyurea
- Doxorubicin and analogs
- Vinca alkaloids
- Taxanes.

## Clinical Findings

Lesions are seen on unkeratinized movable mucosa, with frequent involvement of keratinized hard palate, dorsal surface of the tongue, or gingiva. These ulcerative lesions begin 3–4 days after the initiation of chemotherapy. Lesions are extremely painful and large.

## Treatment

Lesions are self-limiting. Treatment is directed toward pain control and prevention of infection. Oral hygiene and topical analgesics or anesthetics are generally all that are required.

- Cryotherapy
- Cytokines—Treated with granulocyte colony-stimulating factor to reduce period of neutropenia
- Amifostine—topical application
- Dinoprostone
- Antimicrobials/antifungals/antiviral agents
- Chamomile.

# CANDIDIASIS

*Candida* reside in oral cavity as a commensal in approximately 50% of population as carriers. Fungal infections are extremely common in oral cavity and most common being the *Candida albicans.* In immunocompromised hosts, other species such as *Candida tropicalis, Candida krusei, Candida glabrata, Candida guilliermondii, Candida parapsilosis,* and *Candida dubliniensis.* Risk factors of oral candidiasis include:

- Cancers
- Antibiotic therapy
- *Nutritional*: Iron deficiency
- Diabetes
- *Immunosuppression*: Diabetes, HIV
- Dentures, drugs (Corticoids, steroid-sparing agents, and cancer chemotherapy)
- Infants and old age
- Anemia
- Steroid treatment, salivary secretion abnormality (Hyposalivation)
- Immunosuppressive therapy
- Smoking
- *Pneumonic*: Candidiasis.

Saliva has anticandidal properties. Flow of saliva dilutes and moves *Candida* from mucosal surfaces. Saliva contains defensins, lactoferrin, lysozyme, and anticandidal antibodies that inhibits growth of organisms. Denture wearers are prone to oral candidiasis because of poorly fitted dentures leading to minor mucosal injuries and poor oral hygiene.

## Clinical Findings

Oral candidiasis may manifest with burning mouth, altered taste, burning to spicy food, and change in sense of smell. Dysphagia and odynophagia may occur, if involvement extends to oropharynx. Various forms of candidiasis are mentioned below:

### Acute Pseudomembranous Candidiasis (Oral Thrush)

It is the most common type and is characterized by discrete white patches over buccal mucosa, tongue, palate, and gingivae covered by pseudomembrane. This pseudomembrane resembles cottage cheese or milk curds and consists of desquamated epithelial cells, fungal elements, inflammatory cells, fibrin, and food debris. On removal, the membrane reveals erythematous base. The disease can extend to the esophagus or pharynx and may cause ulceration. AIDS and other hospitalized, debilitated, and elderly patients are common sufferers.

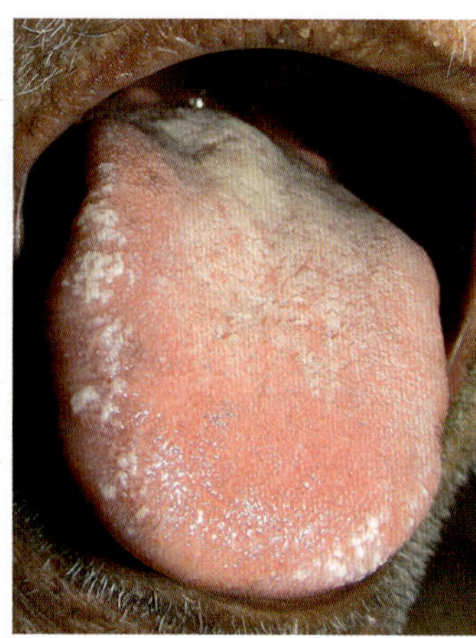

**FIG. 4:** Oral candidiasis.

### Chronic Pseudomembranous Candldiasis

The lesions are similar to acute type but are more persistent. Such a manifestation is seen in immunocompromised patients (Fig. 4).

### Acute Atrophic Candidiasis (Erythematous Candidiasis)

It occurs after sloughing of the thrush pseudomembrane with presence of a denuded, atrophic, and inflamed membrane commonly over the dorsum of the tongue. This is generally seen following the use of broad-spectrum antibiotic or systemic glucocorticoid therapy and HIV infection.

### Chronic Hyperplastic Candidiasis (Candidal Leukoplakia)

It presents as a very persistent, firm, and irregular white plaque present over the cheeks or tongue surrounded by an erythematous margin. Other areas like lips and floor of mouth may be involved. The plaque, unlike oral thrush, cannot be easily removed. Smokers are more prone to develop this type. A malignant change may develop. It may clear with prolonged anticandidal therapy.

### Median Rhomboid Glossitis

It is an acquired condition where dorsum of tongue shows a diamond shaped area with loss of papillae. It can be a true invasion by *Candida albicans* or a developmental abnormality invaded secondarily by *Candida albicans.*

### Chronic Atrophic Candidiasis (Denture Stomatitis or Denture Sore Mouth)

It is common among denture wearers and more commonly occurs in women. This is often confined to the upper denture bearing areas, i.e., the palate and gums. It is characterized by dusky-red, sharply defined shiny and atrophic patches at the denture margin.

### Angular Cheilitis (Candidal Cheilosis or Perleche)

It is characterized by erythema, fissuring, maceration, and soreness at the angles of the mouth. This is common in habitual lip lickers and in elderly patients, loss of dentition, poorly fitting dentures, malocclusion, and riboflavin deficiency.

### Diagnosis

Culture is not particularly useful since many individuals are carriers except when speciation or sensitivity is required or to identify carriers. A potassium hydroxide preparation using scrapings from oral lesions is a good way to identify infection. Biopsies show typical candidal organisms.

### Treatment

Topical antifungals are the first line of treatment for uncomplicated oral candidiasis. These include:

- Nystatin suspension (4–6 lakh U qid) held in the mouth for 5 minutes and swallowed
- Nystatin oral tablets (1 lakh U qid) dissolved slowly in the mouth
- Clotrimazole troches 10 mg one tablet dissolved in mouth 5 times/day
- Gentian violet 1–2%, chlorhexidine rinses, ketoconazole 2% cream, and amphotericin gel are also used.

For reinfection, or unresponsive and chronic cases, systemic therapy with the following is indicated:

- Ketoconazole 200 mg/day for 1–2 weeks, fluconazole 50–100 mg/day for 1 week, or itraconazole 100 mg/day for 3 weeks.

## HAIRY LEUKOPLAKIA

This benign and self-limiting condition presents as asymptomatic, white plaques on the margins of tongue, usually with a corrugated surface. This is caused by Epstein–Barr virus. Oral hairy leukoplakia is reported to occur in patients on immunosuppressive therapy and occasionally in immunocompetent individuals. This does not involve other mucosal or extramucosal sites.

Treatment options include topical podophyllin, topical retinoids, topical gentian violet, cryotherapy, surgical excision, oral acyclovir, famciclovir, and valaciclovir, but it responds to highly active antiretroviral therapy.

## MIGRATORY GLOSSITIS OR STOMATITIS (GEOGRAPHIC TONGUE)

It affects about 1–3% of the population and can occur at any age, sex, and race but seen more commonly in females and in psoriasis.

### Clinical Features

Sharply demarcated, geographic, or circinate areas of erythematous atrophic patches appear on the dorsum of the tongue. Rarely, lesion may arise elsewhere in the floor of the mouth or buccal mucosa and palatal mucosa (Fig. 5).

This is asymptomatic but burning or irritation while taking hot, spicy, or acidic foods is often reported. Acute flares are associated with emotional and physical stress (menstruation, pregnancy).

Histological alterations are similar to psoriasis.

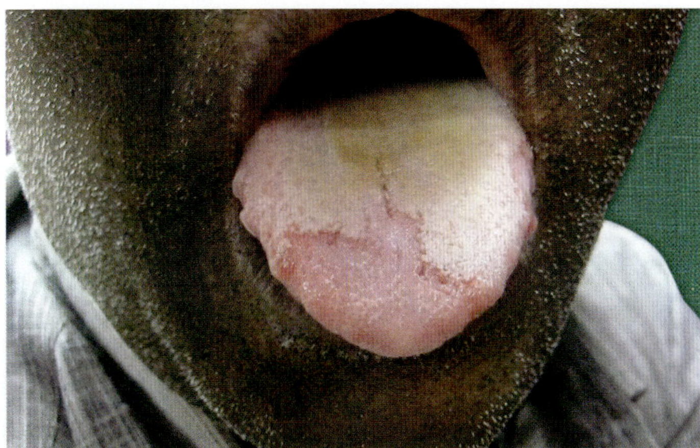

**FIG. 5:** Migratory glossitis or geographic tongue.

### Treatment

Reassurance is necessary. Antiseptic and anesthetic agents may be given.

## SMOKELESS TOBACCO KERATOSIS

It develops due to direct contact with toxicity of the smokeless tobacco on the mucosa (early lesions) and from effects of carcinogens within the snuff, namely tobacco-associated nitrosamines (late lesions that represent true leukoplakias).

### Clinical Findings

Lesions are found where snuff is placed, usually the mandibular sulcus or vestibule, between the teeth and the buccal mucosa. The area looks grayish white, opalescent, and wrinkled, often with fissures.

Lesions are generally painless and poorly demarcated.

### Diagnosis

Biopsy reveals thin parakeratosis, intracellular edema and devitalization of superficial keratinocytes.

### Treatment

Most early lesions are caused by contact injury and are reversible if the habit is discontinued.

However, the development of a dense white plaque or erythema may signal transformation to malignancy and these areas should be biopsied.

## SUBMUCOUS FIBROSIS

Submucous fibrosis is a chronic disease of the oral mucous that appears to be caused by exposure to constituents of areca nut, which is almost exclusively used in Indian subcontinent.

### Clinical Findings

It develops insidiously, often initially presents as oral dysesthesia and nonspecific vesicular stomatitis. Later develops symmetrical fibrosis of cheeks, lips, or palate which may be symptomless and

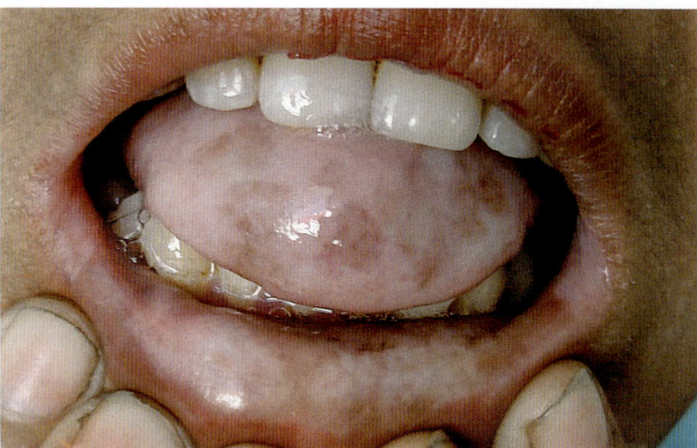

FIG. 6: Submucous fibrosis.

noted as band running through mucosa. Severe form presents as white and firm with severely restricted opening of the mouth. It appears to be restricted to mouth (Fig. 6).

## Diagnosis

Submucous fibrosis is confirmed by biopsy, which shows subepithelial chronic inflammatory reaction with fibrosis extending to submucosa and muscle. Epithelial changes range from atrophy to keratosis and there may be dysplasia.

## Treatment

Management is somewhat difficult. Intralesional corticosteroids and jaw exercises may be helpful in early stages but surgery may be needed to relieve the fibrosis. Pentoxifylline and lycopene have been used in some cases.

# HAIRY TONGUE (BLACK HAIRY TONGUE, COATED TONGUE)

Hairy tongue is an extremely common condition that causes much confusion.

## Etiology

Hairy tongue is caused by retention of keratinaceous debris on the tongue dorsum resulting from dehydration, poor oral intake, and/or overgrowth of chromogenic bacteria. These bacteria reside in the tongue produce metabolic by-products that sometimes stain the tongue, as do food dyes.

## Clinical Findings

Tongue dorsum appears dark brown to black, rough with foul smell. This needs to be differentiated from candidiasis and black tongue caused by exogenous pigment due to ingestion of bismuth subsalicylate.

Culture for *Candida* is positive in 20–30% of patients and likely indicate carrier status.

## Treatment

Vigorous hydration, normal diet with fresh fruits and vegetables, brushing and maintenance of oral hygiene is all that are necessary.

# CHEILITIS GRANULOMATOSA (OROFACIAL GRANULOMATOSIS/MIESCHER'S CHEILITIS)

This is a chronic swelling of the lip due to inflammation of unknown cause. Melkersson, in 1928, described labial edema in association with recurrent facial palsy. Role of genetic factors and scrotal tongue to the syndrome was added by Rosenthal in 1930. This is thus called as Melkersson–Rosenthal syndrome.

## Etiology

Cause is unknown, but there may be genetic predisposition and familial cases, even presenting with partial manifestations (like scrotal tongue) are reported. Sarcoidosis or ectopic Crohn's disease is suspected to be the etiology. Allergy to cobalt or to food additives such as cinnamic aldehyde is also suspected.

## Clinical Features

Both the sexes equally affected. The earliest manifestations usually develop in childhood or adolescence but may be delayed until middle or old age. There is sudden development of diffuse or nodular swellings or cobblestoning involving the upper lip, lower lip, and/or both cheeks in decreasing order of frequency. The swelling is originally relapsing-recurring and then becomes persistent, often with fissuring of the lips. There may be history of facial swelling (periorbital or zygomatic) and sometimes VII nerve palsy. Linear ulcers in the maxillary and mandibular vestibule/sulcus, more typical of Crohn's disease, may be seen.

## Differential Diagnosis

Early Crohn's disease, sarcoidosis, cellulitis, and lymphoma. Isotretinoin therapy can occasionally lead to swollen lips (Fig. 7).

## Diagnosis

Biopsy reveals the presence of nonnecrotizing granulomas without foreign material or identifiable infectious agent.

## Treatment and Prognosis

Topical and intralesional steroid injections are the mainstay. Oral prednisone (1 mg/kg), thalidomide, minocycline, and more

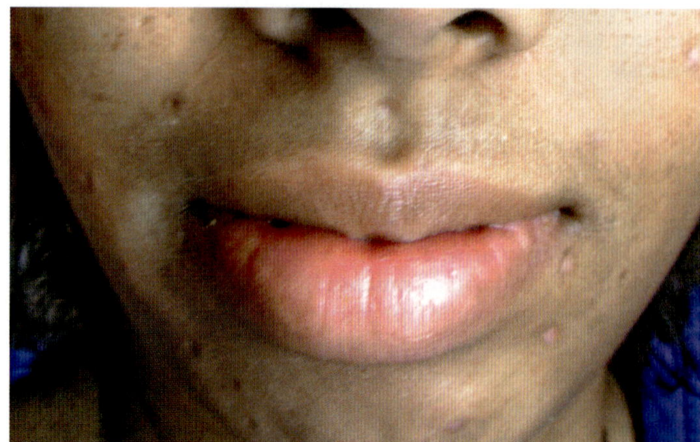

FIG. 7: Macrocheilia due to isotretinoin therapy.

recently, monoclonal antibodies against TNF-α can be used. Surgical reconstruction may be done in fibrotic lips.

## ANGULAR CHEILITIS/ANGULAR STOMATITIS

Angular cheilitis is an acute or chronic inflammation of the skin and contiguous labial mucous membrane at the angles of the mouth. This is more common in denture wearers. It may be painful and usually bilateral. It presents with maceration of the corners of the mouth with ulceration, crusting, cracking, and in severe cases, fissuring. Lesions may heal and recur within days or weeks (Fig. 8).

### Etiology

Most cases in adults are due to mechanical and/or infective causes, but in children nutritional or immune defects are prominent causes. Infection with *Candida*, streptococci or staphylococci, nutritional deficiency, immune deficiency, diabetes, and HIV infection, may present with this condition.

### Management and Prognosis

Usual anticandidal regimens, antibiotics, hematinic repletion and management of other causes.

## EXFOLIATIVE CHEILITIS (FACTITIOUS CHEILITIS/LE TIC DES LÈVRES)

It is a chronic superficial inflammatory disorder of the vermillion borders of the lips characterized by persistent scaling.

### Etiology

Repeated lip sucking, chewing, or other manipulation of the lips.

### Management

Some cases resolve spontaneously or with improved oral hygiene. Reassurance and topical corticosteroids or tacrolimus may be helpful in some cases. Some cases require psychotherapy, antidepressants or tranquilizers.

## PIGMENTED DISORDERS OF THE ORAL MUCOSA

### Drug-induced Hyperpigmentation

The pathogenesis of drug-induced hyperpigmentation varies, depending on the drug causing it. It may be due to deposition of melanin, deposit of the drug or its metabolites. Minocycline and tetracycline causes pigmentation of the alveolar bone and hard palate which can be seen through thin overlying mucosa. Chloroquine and other quinine derivatives cause direct stimulatory effect on the melanocytes and are restricted to the palatal mucosa. Pegylated interferon used with ribavirin may stimulate melanin production (Fig. 9).

#### Laboratory Tests

Biopsy reveals pigment granules that stain for both iron and melanin.

#### Treatment

Discontinuation of the drug may lead to resolution of the lesion.

### Melanoacanthosis

Melanoacanthoma is a rare, inflammatory, benign, and pigmented lesion that presents most commonly on the buccal mucosa.

#### Clinical Findings

It is seen exclusively in blacks with female predilection, occurs in second to fourth decade of life. Buccal mucosa is the most frequent site of involvement. Palate and gingival may also be affected. Lesions are brown, black, or blue macule, which spreads rapidly. This needs to be differentiated from dysplastic nevi and melanoma.

#### Treatment

No treatment is required; it regresses over time.

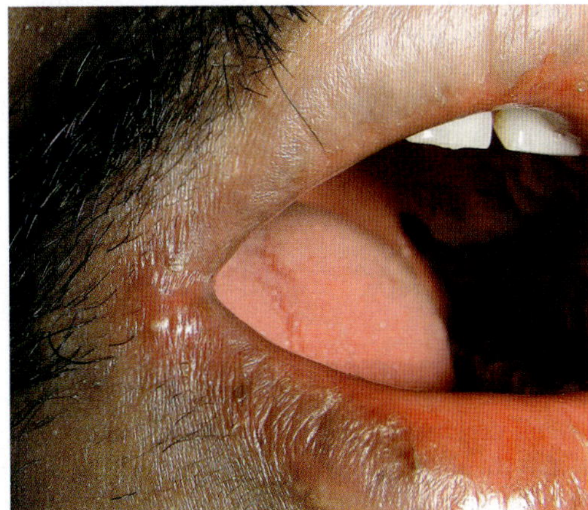

**FIG. 8:** Angular cheilitis.

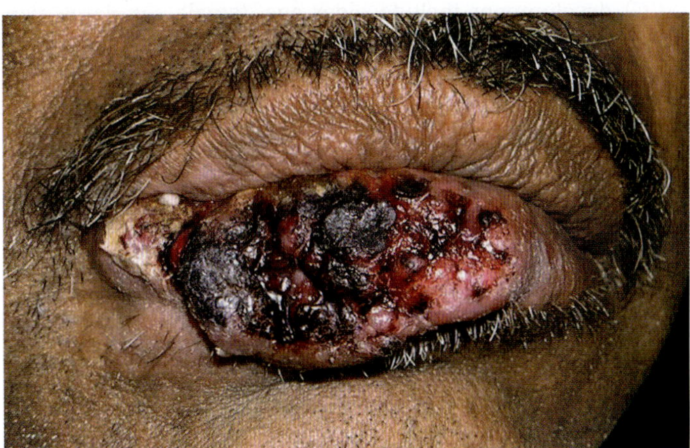

**FIG. 9:** Squamous cell carcinoma lower lip.

## NEVOMELANOCYTIC NEVI

Nevomelanocytic nevi is the most common intramucosal nevus which accounts for two-thirds of cases, followed by the compound nevus and blue nevus (17%) each, junctional nevus constitute only 3%.

### Clinical Findings

The most common sites are the palate and gingival but also may be encountered in the lips and buccal mucosa. Lesions are brown and may be macular or nodular, sharply defined. It is less than 0.5 cm in size.

### Histopathology

Nevomelanocytic cells in nests in the lamina propria and epithelial-connective interface.

### Treatment

Excisional or shaved biopsy.

## MALIGNANT AND PREMALIGNANT CONDITIONS

### Leukoplakia and Erythroplakia

Oral leukoplakia (OL) is a clinical term that refers to predominantly white lesion of the oral mucosa that cannot be rubbed off or characterized by any other definable lesion or known disease. Leukoplakia is the most common precancerous lesion of the oral mucosa.

The term erythroplakia is applied to leukoplakia that has not lost the thick keratin layer. This is present on the floor of the mouth, soft palate, or buccal mucosa, or under the tongue.

### Etiology

Tobacco, smokeless tobacco, *areca*, or betel nut chewing, reverse smoking, alcohol, poorly fitting dentures, sharp and chipped lips, and oral cavity may progress to leukoplakia.

Predictors of a higher risk of squamous cell carcinoma (SCC) development include older age, female sex, large size, nonsmokers, presence on the lateral or ventral tongue, floor of mouth, erythroleukoplakia, and a nonhomogenous morphology.

### Clinical Features

Oral leukoplakia is subdivided into homogenous and nonhomogenous. Homogenous OL appears as white, flat, and uniform lesion that may have shallow cracks and a smooth, wrinkled, or corrugated surface. Nonhomogenous OL has a risk of malignant transformation that is four to five times higher than that of homogenous OL.

### Histopathology

Biopsy of these lesions may reveal orthokeratosis or parakeratosis with minimal inflammation, or these may be evidence of varying degrees of dysplasia. The degree of epithelial atypia may be considered in staging the risk of developing malignancy. Atypical cells are present in only about 10–20% of leukoplakia whereas carcinoma *in situ* or invasive carcinoma is found in 90% of lesions of erythroplakia.

### Treatment

Tobacco chewing should be stopped and proper dental care obtained. Fulguration, simple excision, cryotherapy, and $CO_2$ ablation are effective methods of treatment. Medical therapies that have been the subject of randomized clinical trials may lead to temporary resolution of the lesions, but relapses and adverse effects are common and there is no evidence that they prevent the transformation to malignancy. Complete surgical removal may be required in many cases.

## ACTINIC CHEILITIS

This is a dysplastic premalignant keratosis of lip caused by exposure to solar irradiation.

### Etiology

- Prolonged sun exposure
- Fair-skinned people (Skin types I and II).

### Clinical Features

This presents as single or multiple crusted or scabbing, slightly scaly lesions and plaques on the vermillion of the lower lip, most commonly seen on lower lip. It occurs on a whitish, keratotic background. Fissuring and erosions of the vermillion may be present. The vermillion of lower lip receives a high dose of ultraviolet irradiation because it is almost at right angles to the rays of the midday sun and is poorly protected by keratin and melanocytes.

### Histopathology

Histopathology is diagnostic and shows a flattened or atrophic epithelium, beneath which is a band of inflammatory infiltrate in which plasma cells may predominate.

### Treatment

- *Topical agents*: 5% fluorouracil three times daily for 10 days is suitable. Topical tretinoin, trichloroacetic acid or diclofenac gel may also be effective
- Vermilionectomy (lip shave)
- Laser ablation
- Photodynamic therapy.

## ORAL SQUAMOUS CELL CARCINOMA

Squamous cell carcinoma accounts for 90% of all oral cancers. The oral SCC is the most common malignant tumor of the lip, oral cavity and oropharynx (90% of the cases) while the remaining 10% of the cases are mainly melanomas, sarcomas, minor salivary gland carcinomas, and metastatic cancers.

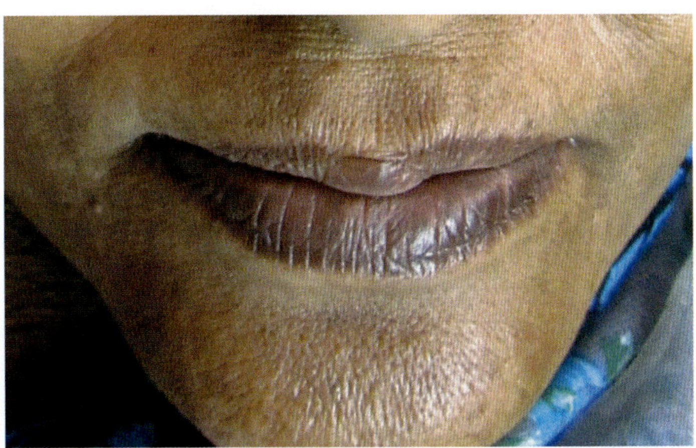

**FIG. 10:** Pigmentation lips due to vitamin $B_{12}$ deficiency.

## Risk Factors

Trauma from sharp teeth, tobacco, betel quid, heavy drinking, diet low in fresh fruits and vegetables, and chronic sun exposure are well-known risk factors. Oral erosive lichen planus leukoplakia, erythroplakia, and actinic chronic cheilitis are known precancerous condition.

## Clinical Presentation

The lip is the most common location. The paramedial area of the inferior lip is the region most often affected by lip cancer. Early lesion generally presents with loss of superficial tissue, erosion, and ulcers. Developed cases may appear as keratotic, exophytic, verrucous or vegetant. Lip is everted (lip on balcony). A significant atrophy of the vermillion area with scales that do not tend to shed and therefore accumulate to form keratosis can often be observed (Fig. 10).

Tongue carcinoma represents 30–40% of oral cancers, and is the most commonly observed oral cancer into the oral cavity. The lateral tongue being the most frequent situation (80%), followed by ventral and dorsum. Lymph nodes are usually enlarged. Tumors located in the anterior half of the tongue usually lead to lymphadenopathy in the suprahyoid region while those located in the posterior half lead to submaxillary, carotid and retropharyngeal nodes.

## Treatment

Surgery is the preferred first-line treatment of small, accessible oral SCCs. However, advanced-stage oral SCC is usually treated by a combined treatment program of surgery, chemotherapy, and radiotherapy. In cases of recurrent oral SCC, epidermal growth factor receptor inhibitor, coupled with chemoradiotherapy, is the first line of treatment.

Squamous cell carcinoma is managed by surgery, radiation, and chemotherapy singularly or in amalgamation. The 5-year survival rate is impecunious at about 50%.

# ORAL DISEASE IN CHRONIC GRAFT-VERSUS-HOST DISEASE

Chronic graft-versus-host reaction is the leading long-term complication of allogenic stem cell transplantation. The oral lesions in chronic graft-versus-host disease (GVHD) are consistent with skin lesions. Oral lesions in chronic GVHD are estimated to occur in 45–83% of patients.

Oral manifestations of chronic GVHD may be of different types namely, lichenoid plaques or striae, xerostomia, restriction of mouth opening due to sclerosis, mucosal atrophy, erythema and pain, pseudo membranes and ulcers, mucocele, mucositis, and salivary gland dysfunction. Often, the condition mimicks several autoimmune conditions. There may be depressed salivary IgA levels in minor salivary gland saliva. There may also be increased risk of developing oral SCC in patients with chronic GVHD. Biopsy is useful to confirm the clinical diagnosis.

# SUGGESTED READINGS


1. Axell T, Pindborg JJ, Smith CJ, et al. Oral white lesions with special reference to precancerous and tobacco- related lesions: conclusions of an international symposium held in Uppsala, Sweden, May 18-21 1994. International Collaborative Group on Oral White Lesions. J Oral Pathol Med. 1996;25(2):49-54.
2. Bork K. Diseases of the Lips and Mouth. In: Burgdorf WHC, Plewig G, Wolff HH (Eds). Braun-Falco's Dermatology. Landthaler M: Springer; 2009. pp. 1081-107.
3. Burket LW, Greenberg MS, Glick M. Burket's Book of Oral Medicine, 10th Edition. Hamilton (Canada): BC Decker; 2008. pp. 42-8.
4. Davenport S, Chen SY, Miller AS. Pemphigus vulgaris: clinicopathologic review of 33 cases in the oral cavity. Int J Periodontics Restorative Dent. 2001;21(1): 85-90.
5. Eisen D. The clinical features, malignant potential, and systemic associations of oral lichen planus: a study of 723 patients. J Am Acad Dermatol. 2002;46:207-14.
6. Francis V Howell. Oral mucous membrane lesions: Pathologic features. California medicine.1964;100:186-91.
7. Goncalves LM, Bezerra JR, Cruz MC. Clinical evaluation of oral lesions associated with dermatologic diseases. An Bras Dermatol. 2010;85:150-6.
8. Gupta S. (2017). Mucosal Candidiasis Clinical Presentation. [online] Available from http://emedicine.medscape.com/article/1075227-clinical#b5. [Accessed May 2018].
9. Jahanbani J, Sandvik L, Lyberg T, et al. Evaluation of oral mucosal lesions in 598 referred Iranian patients. Open Dent J.2009;3:42–7.
10. Kramer IR, Pindborg JJ, Bezroukov V, et al. Guide to epidemiology and diagnosis of oral mucosal diseases and conditions. World Health Organization. Community Dent Oral Epidemiol. 1980;8(1):1-26.
11. Patton LL, Bonito AJ, Shugars DA. A systematic review of the effectiveness of antifungal drugs for the prevention and treatment of oropharyngeal candidiasis in HIV-positive patients. Oral Surg Oral Med Oral Pathol Oral Radiol Endod. 2001;92:170-9.
12. Ramírez-Amador VA, Esquivel-Pedraza L, Orozco-Topete R. Frequency of oral conditions in a dermatology clinic. Int J Dermatol. 2000;39:501-5.
13. Ranganathan K, Umadevi M, Saraswathi TR, et al. Oral lesions and conditions associated with human immunodeficiency virus infection in 1000 South Indian patients. Ann Acad Med Singapore. 2004;33:37-42.
14. Smith KJ, Skelton HG, Yeager J, et al. Cutaneous findings in HIV-1-positive patients: A 42-month prospective study. Military medical Consortium for the advancement of retroviral research (MMCARR). J Am Acad Dermatol. 1994;31:746-54.
15. Spruance SL, Jones TM, Blatter MM, et al. High-dose, short-duration, early valacyclovir therapy for episodic treatment of cold sores: results of two randomized, placebo-controlled, multicenter studies. Antimicrob Agents Chemother. 2003;47: 1072-80.
16. Suliman NM, Astrøm AN, Ali RW, et al. Oral mucosal lesions in skin diseased patients attending a dermatologic clinic: A cross-sectional study in Sudan. BMC Oral Health. 2011;11:24.
17. Thoppay JR. (2018). Aphthous Ulcers. [online] Available from http://emedicine.medscape.com/article/867080-clinical. [Accessed May 2018].
18. Weedon D, Strutton G, Rubin AI, et al. The vesiculobullous reaction pattern. In: Weedon D (Ed.) Weedon's Skin Pathology, 3rd Edition. Edinburgh: Churchill Livingstone/Elsevier; 2010. pp.151-2.

# 68 CHAPTER Nonvenereal Genital Dermatoses

*Somesh Gupta, Vishal Gupta, Riti Bhatia*

## INTRODUCTION

External genitalia is a psychologically sensitive site, as many patients suffer from anxiety when a dermatosis, no matter how trivial, affects the genitals. This behavior stems from the belief prevalent not only among the patients but also their doctors, that any genital disease maybe sexually transmitted and the social stigma thereof. Sometimes, just the reassurance regarding the noninfectious nature of the disease may be therapeutic for the patient's psyche. Thus, it becomes important for the dermatologist to recognize many nonsexually transmitted diseases affecting this particular anatomic site. In this chapter, we discuss some of the common nonvenereal genital dermatoses briefly.

## PEARLY PENILE PAPULES

Pearly penile papules (PPP, synonyms—hirsutoid papillomas, corona capilliti, and Tyson glands) is a common entity seen predominantly in pubertal boys and young men, more common among negroes and uncircumcised men. Its prevalence varies from 14.3–48% depending on the study setting.

The PPPs are smooth monomorphic acuminate or dome-shaped papules of size 1–4 mm, arranged around the coronal sulcus in a single or double row (Fig. 1).

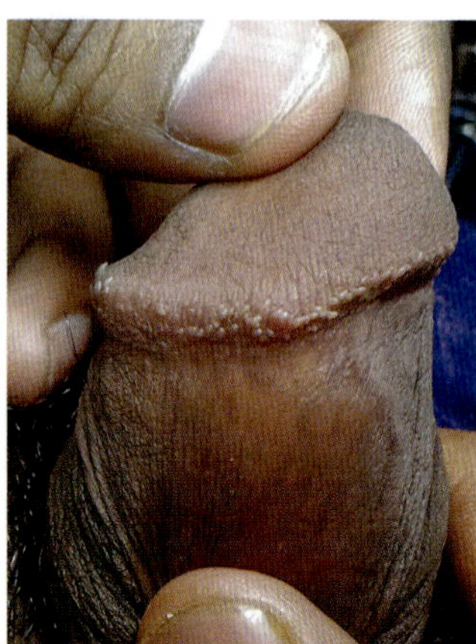

**FIG. 1:** Pearly penile papules: Fleshy filiform papules arranged circumferentially on the coronal sulcus.

*Courtesy*: Dr Nilendu Sarma, Associate Professor and Head, Department of Dermatology, Dr BC Roy Post Graduate Institute of Pediatric Sciences, West Bengal.

Structurally, PPPs are related to acral angiofibromas. They histology resembles those of adenoma sebaceum, subungual and periungual fibromas, fibrous papule of the nose, and oral fibroma. The histological features include dermal fibrosis, increased number of plump stellate fibroblasts and dilated capillaries in the papillary dermis.

Though not a pathological entity, at times PPP may be confused with condyloma acuminata, lichen nitidus, and ectopic sebaceous gland.

Reassuring the patient about its benign nature is usually sufficient; hence, PPPs do not require any specific treatment. Cryotherapy, electrodesiccation, podophyllin, curettage, and carbon dioxide laser ablation have been tried.

## LICHEN SCLEROSUS

Lichen sclerosus (LS, synonyms—lichen sclerosus et atrophicus, balanitis xerotica obliterans, and kraurosis vulvae) is a chronic inflammatory disease which preferentially affects the anogenital region. Rarely, only the extragenital sites may be involved. It is reportedly more common in females. Though it may occur at any age, prepubertal children, postmenopausal women, and middle-aged men are more commonly affected. Factors such as autoimmunity, genetic factors, infections like borreliosis, trauma and chronic irritation have been proposed to play a role in its pathogenesis.

The lesions of LS appear as ivory-white sclerosed and atrophic plaques (Fig. 2). It can be asymptomatic, or the patient may complain of itching, burning, painful erections, or a poor urinary stream. Glans penis and foreskin are most commonly affected in males, other sites which may be affected include the frenulum and urethral meatus. Secondary changes like hemorrhagic bullae, fissures, and erosions are not uncommon. As the disease advances, the sclerotic lesions can lead to phimosis or paraphimosis, and even difficulty in urination. The common sites affected in females are the labia minora, labia majora, and clitoris. Unlike in men, the perineum and perianal area are also quite commonly involved giving rise to the characteristic "figure-of-eight" shape. The most common symptom in women is itching, and chronic scratching may lead to erosions, subepithelial hemorrhage, and lichenification of the plaques. Other symptoms may include burning, dysuria, and dyspareunia. Squamous cell carcinoma may complicate genital LS in about 3–5% women,

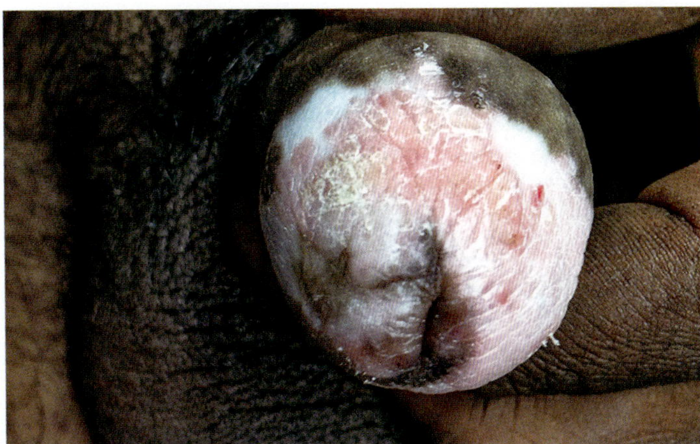

FIG. 2: Lichen sclerosus: Depigmented sclerosed plaque on the glans penis, with overlying erythema, atrophy, and scaling.

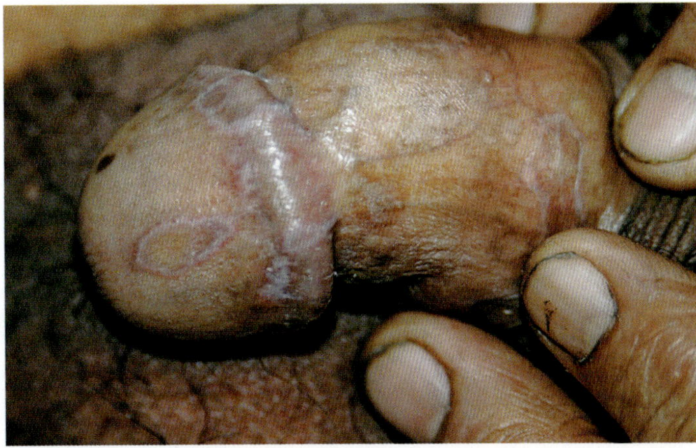

FIG. 3: Lichen planus: Annular violaceous plaques on the glans penis and prepuce.

especially if there is vulvar involvement. However, malignant change is relatively uncommon in men.

Vitiligo and lichen planus (LP) can be confused with LS. The histology is characterized by epidermal atrophy, interface dermatitis, papillary dermal sclerosis, and a lichenoid infiltrate.

Treatment options include emollients, topical corticosteroids (potent or ultrapotent) and topical calcineurin inhibitors. Photochemotherapy and photodynamic therapy have also been tried. Circumcision may be required in patients who have not responded to medical therapy or have an advanced disease.

## LICHEN PLANUS

Lichen planus is characterized by violaceous plane-topped polygonal pruritic papules. Isolated mucosal involvement either genital or oral is seen in upto 15% cases. Male genital involvement has been seen in upto 25% cases, with glans penis being the most commonly affected site.

Genital LP manifest as violaceous papules similar to the lesions present on the skin. Frequently, the lesions assume an annular morphology due to either arcuate arrangement of the papules or central clearing of the lesions along with their peripheral extension (Fig. 3). Fine white streaks in a reticulate network may also be seen. While glans penis and prepuce are the common sites in males; vulval skin, labia majora and minora are frequently involved in females. Sometimes, papules may become eroded and may lose their distinct characteristic morphology. The vulvovaginal-gingival syndrome is a variant of mucosal LP characterized by erosive lesions affecting the vulva, vagina, and gingivae.

Usually, the genital lesions are a part of the generalized cutaneous eruption. The presence of typical lesions of LP elsewhere including the oral mucosa should always be searched for which helps the dermatologist in reaching the correct diagnosis. However, a biopsy may be required in case of exclusive genital involvement to make a conclusive diagnosis.

Mid-potent topical corticosteroids or topical calcineurin inhibitors (tacrolimus, pimecrolimus) are effective treatment for genital LP.

## PSORIASIS

Psoriasis is a common papulosquamous disorder which presents on the skin as well-defined erythematous or salmon-colored plaques with silvery scales. Though it may occur solely on the genitals, more commonly it is a part of a more generalized disease with upto 40% psoriasis patients having genital lesions as well. It is the most common inflammatory dermatosis to affect the male genitalia.

In circumcised individuals, the morphology of the genital lesions is similar to their cutaneous counterparts. The lesions appear as erythematous scaly plaques usually on the glans penis and coronal sulcus. However, the clinical picture differs in uncircumcised men where the psoriatic plaques are non-scaly (or less scaly), probably due to the increased moisture content due to the local factors. Genital psoriasis in females is less common than in males, and can affect vulva and labia majora (Fig. 4). Frequently, genital lesions of psoriasis are accompanied by non-scaly plaques in the inguinoscrotal region and the intergluteal cleft (also called inverse psoriasis). More common sites like scalp, elbows, and knees may also be affected by the typical scaly plaques concomitantly.

The presence of typical psoriatic plaques at other sites usually helps in confirming the diagnosis. A biopsy may be required in the occasional doubtful case.

Topical mid-potent corticosteroids constitute the primary modality of treatment. Topical calcineurin inhibitors and vitamin D3 analogues have also been tried with good results.

## ZOON'S BALANITIS

Zoon's balanitis (synonyms—plasma cell balanitis, balanitis circumscripta plasma cellularis) first described by Zoon in 1952, is a benign chronic balanitis affecting the middle-aged or elderly uncircumcised men. Though exact cause is not known, constant exposure to urine and smegma in the preputial sac leading to chronic irritation may play a role in its pathogenesis. A somewhat similar condition has been described to affect the vulva and oral cavity.

The typical clinical picture is that of a moist, shiny, glistening, and well-defined red-brown plaque with a glazed appearance affecting the glans penis and prepuce (Fig. 5). Multiple minute red specks—the so-called cayenne pepper stippling, may be visible on the surface. Uncommonly, it may assume erosive or vegetative morphology. Though usually solitary, multiple lesions have also been reported. Usually, it is asymptomatic, indolent and may persist for months to years.

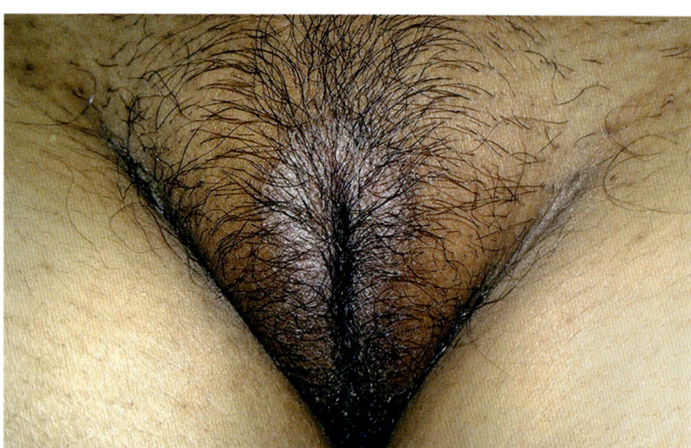

**FIG. 4:** Psoriasis: Well-defined erythematous scaly plaque present on the vulva.

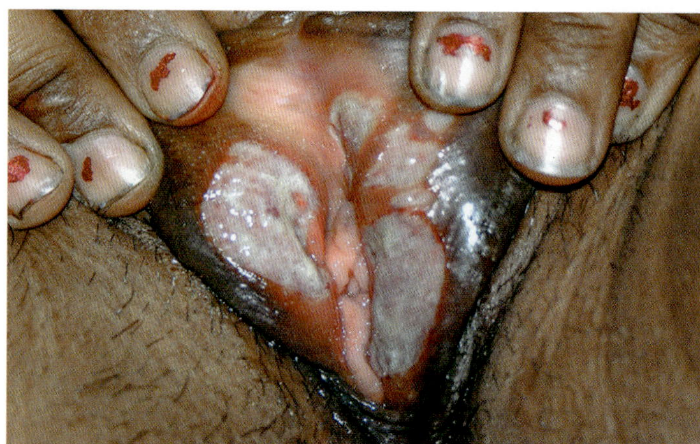

**FIG. 6:** Aphthous ulcers: Well-defined round to oval ulcers with white fibrinous material on the floor, on the vulva.

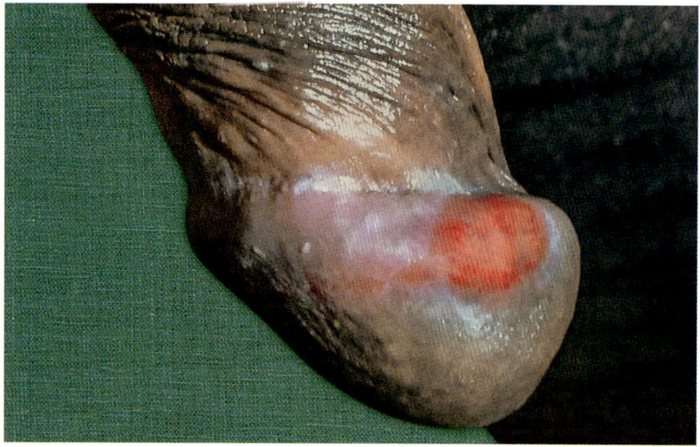

**FIG. 5:** Typical lesion of Zoons' balanitis.

*Courtesy:* Dr Nilendu Sarma, Associate Professor and Head, Department of Dermatology, Dr BC Roy Post Graduate Institute of Pediatric Sciences, West Bengal

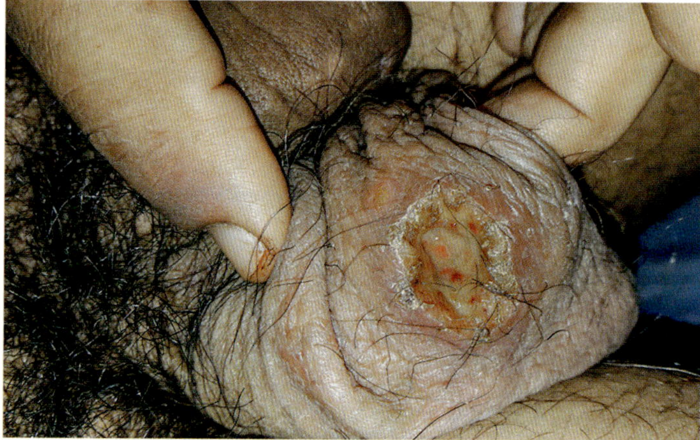

**FIG. 7:** Aphthous ulcer: Single oval ulcer with yellowish necrotic slough on the floor, on the scrotum of a young man with Behcet's disease.

The principal differential diagnosis is erythroplasia of Queyrat (carcinoma *in-situ*) which manifests as a red velvety plaque. Erosive LP, Kaposi sarcoma and fixed drug eruption may lead to a diagnostic confusion.

The histopathology is characterized by epidermal attenuation (with absence of horny and granular layers), diamond or lozenge-shaped keratinocytes with mild spongiosis and occasional dyskeratosis. There is a dense band-like infiltrate in the upper dermis comprising of plasma cells of varying density admixed with lymphocytes. Erythrocyte extravasation and hemosiderin deposition is responsible for "cayenne pepper speckling".

Mild topical corticosteroids and calcineurin inhibitors provide temporary relief with recurrence of the lesion following discontinuation of therapy. Circumcision is the definitive treatment. Carbon dioxide and erbium-YAG laser ablation have been tried for recalcitrant cases.

## APHTHOUS ULCERS

Aphthous ulcers (synonym—canker sores) are a common entity, characterized by painful ulcers affecting the oral and/or genital mucosa. These are known to recur commonly. Though patients with genital aphthae almost always have oral lesions as well, aphthous ulcers at both sites may not occur concomitantly.

The typical morphology of an aphthous ulcer is a round-oval ulcer, its floor covered with a white fibrinous material, and surrounded by an erythematous halo (Fig. 6). However, in comparison to their oral counterparts, genital aphthous ulcers are usually larger and more irregular. The ulcers are usually shallow and quite painful. Deeper ulcers are also known to occur, and may heal with scarring. The usual sites affected are the vulva (in females) and scrotum and penis (in men) (Fig. 7). Lipschutz ulcers, considered by many to be a variant of vulvar aphthosis, present as acute-onset painful vulvar ulcers in young women, frequently accompanied by fever and other constitutional symptoms.

Complex aphthosis is defined as recurrent oral and genital aphthae (bipolar aphthosis) or the near constant presence of multiple (>3) oral aphthae in the absence of a systemic illness. Diseases such as Behcet's disease, cyclic neutropenia, HIV infection, inflammatory bowel disease, and reactive arthritis should be ruled out in such a setting.

Genital aphthae are often mistaken for sexually-transmitted genital ulcers, most commonly genital herpes, chancroid, and sometimes donovanosis.

Mild cases may respond to topical steroids. For patients having severe involvement, interfering in routine activities, a short course of oral steroids may be warranted. Dapsone, colchicine and thalidomide have been used successfully for recurrent cases.

## CIRCINATE BALANITIS

Circinate balanitis is usually described as one of the mucocutaneous manifestations of Reiter's disease reported in 12–70%, upto 50% of patients. Rarely, it may occur in the absence of other features of Reiter's disease.

Clinically, it presents as erythematous moist plaques with well-defined raised margins studded with pustules affecting the glans penis. The plaques are often, but not always, annular or circinate with geographical margins (Fig. 8). The lesions are more dry and scaly, and may resemble psoriasis in circumcised individuals.

The presence of associated psoriasiform plaques on the skin, keratoderma blenorrhagicum and inflammatory arthritis point toward the diagnosis. Biopsy is indistinguishable from that of pustular psoriasis.

Treatment modalities include mild to mid-potent topical corticosteroids, calcineurin inhibitors and vitamin D3 analogs. Dapsone has been successfully tried in a few cases resistant to topical therapy.

## FIXED DRUG ERUPTION

Fixed drug eruption (FDE) is a cutaneous adverse drug reaction characterized by recurrence of the lesions at the site of previous reaction everytime the drug is given to the patient. Though lesions may appear anywhere, mucocutaneous junction-like glans penis is a favored site for FDEs. Several drugs have been implicated for FDEs, common ones include sulfonamides, nonsteroidal anti-inflammatory drugs, β-lactam antibiotics, and tetracyclines.

Clinically, the lesions present as sharply defined round-oval erythematous edematous plaques. Usually, a central zone of dusky erythema due to epidermal necrosis is present. Sometimes, a central bulla may be present. The lesions generally subside in a few days leaving behind brown-black pigmentation, once the implicated agent has been stopped. The lesions first appear within a few days after administration of the causative drug, but it takes usually only a few hours for the lesions to recur following a repeat drug exposure. Drug rechallenge may result in lesions not only at the sites of previous drug reaction, but may affect additional sites as well.

It may be confused with erosive LP, immunobullous diseases, and sexually transmitted genital ulcer diseases. Well circumscribed morphology of the lesion, a strong temporal correlation with drug intake and recurrent episodes of inflammatory changes on a hyperpigmented macule point towards a diagnosis of FDE.

Topical corticosteroids can be given during the early stages of FDE to attenuate the inflammatory response, however the postinflammatory pigmentation tends to persist for long.

## ANGIOKERATOMA OF FORDYCE

The term "angiokeratoma" is derived from three Greek words meaning vessels, horn and tumor, respectively. It is a vascular malformation and not a tumor in true sense. Angiokeratomas affecting the scrotum were first described by Fordyce in 1896. Though the exact prevalence is not known, it is estimated to be 0.6% between 16 and 20 years, to 16.6% in the 70s. Varicocele, by virtue of increased venous pressure may contribute in its pathogenesis.

The lesions are described as small (1–6 mm), discrete erythematous keratotic papules which may be present either in isolation or in clusters. As the lesion grows old, it becomes firm, keratotic, and non-compressible. It may be asymptomatic, or may be pruritic and associated with occasional bleeding. The common sites include scrotum and penile shaft, glans penis, and the adjoining groins and thighs may also be involved. Some patients may have angiokeratomas in their oral cavity as well.

It may occasionally be confused with anogenital warts. A biopsy may be required in doubtful cases. Dilated capillaries in the papillary dermis are the characteristic histological feature, with overlying basket-weave hyperkeratosis and acanthotic epidermis.

Treatment options include radiofrequency ablation, carbon dioxide laser ablation, and pulsed-dye laser.

## PSEUDOEPITHELIOMATOUS, KERATOTIC, AND MICACEOUS BALANITIS

Pseudoepitheliomatous, keratotic, and micaceous balanitis (PEKMB) is a rare genital dermatosis affecting elderly men (usually age >50 years). Phimosis and circumcision in adult life may be a predisposing factor. It was first described by Lortat-Jacob and Civatte in 1966.

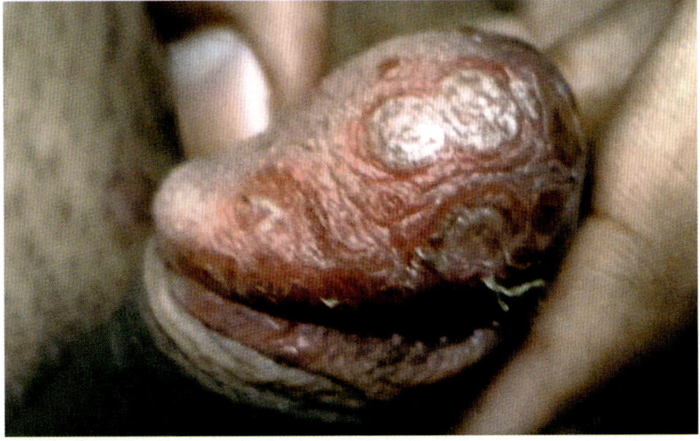

**FIG. 8:** Circinate balanitis: Erythematous serpiginous plaques with central heaped-up yellowish scales, present on the glans penis of a patient with Reiter's disease.

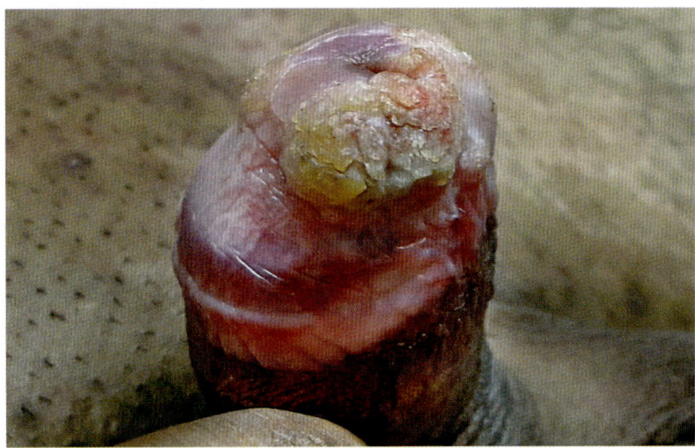

**FIG. 9:** Pseudoepitheliomatous keratotic and micaceous balanitis: Yellowish keratotic scaly plaques on the glans penis.

The PEKMB is characterized by verrucous excrescences on the glans penis with overlying scaling (Fig. 9). The scale is typically described as micaceous which can be easily peeled off. Overlying ulcerations and fissuring may also be present. There is a risk of malignant transformation with reports of verrucous carcinoma and invasive squamous cell carcinoma developing overtime.

Clinical differential diagnoses include penile horn, giant condyloma, verrucous carcinoma (Buschke-Löwenstein tumor), and squamous cell carcinoma. Histologically, PEKMB is characterized by pseudoepitheliomatous hyperplasia alongwith marked hyperkeratosis and parakeratosis. The acanthotic epidermis may assume a crateriform morphology.

The treatment is usually surgical excision. Topical 5-fluorouracil has also been used successfully. Long-term follow-up is advised due to its potential for malignant change.

## CONCLUSION

Nonvenereal genital dermatoses may behave differently from their extragenital counterparts because of the different anatomic features and local environment. Some of these diseases may manifest exclusively on the genitalia posing a diagnostic challenge. The readers of this chapter are likely to develop a better understanding of some of the commonly seen nonvenereal genital dermatoses including their differential diagnosis and management.

## SUGGESTED READINGS


1. Ackerman AB, Kronberg R. Pearly penile papules. Acral angiofibromas. Arch Dermatol. 1973;108(5):673-5.
2. Agrawal SK, Bhattacharya SN, Singh N. Pearly penile papules: a review. Int J Dermatol. 2004;43(3):199-201.
3. Bakkour W, Chularojanamontri L, Motta L, et al. Successful use of dapsone for the management of circinate balanitis. Clin Exp Dermatol. 2014;39(3):333-5.
4. Buechner SA. Common skin disorders of the penis. BJU Int. 2002;90(5):498-506.
5. Bunker CB. Topics in penile dermatology. Clin Exp Dermatol. 2001;26(6):469-79.
6. Das S, Ghoshal L. Pseudoepitheliomatous keratotic and micaceous balanitis of Civatte. Indian Dermatol Online J. 2014;5(2):148-50.
7. Farber EM, Nall L. Genital psoriasis. Cutis. 1992;50(4):263-6.
8. Fistarol SK, Itin PH. Diagnosis and treatment of lichen sclerosus: an update. Am J Clin Dermatol. 2013;14(1):27-47.
9. Gaffoor PM, George WM. Fixed drug eruptions occurring on the male genitals. Cutis. 1990;45(4):242-4.
10. Goldman BD. Common dermatoses of the male genitalia. Recognition of differences in genital rashes and lesions is essential and attainable. Postgrad Med. 2000;108(4):89-91, 95-6.
11. Huppert JS. Lipschutz ulcers: evaluation and management of acute genital ulcers in women. Dermatol Ther. 2010;23(5):533-40.
12. Imperial R, Helwig EB. Angiokeratoma. A clinicopathological study. Arch Dermatol. 1967;95(2):166-75.
13. Ive FA. The umbilical, perianal and genital regions. In: Champion RH, Burton JL, Burns DA, Breathnach SM (Eds). Rook/Wilkinson/Ebling Textbook of Dermatology, 6th edition. Oxford: Blackwell Science; 1998. pp. 3163-238.
14. Kanerva L, Kousa M, Niemi KM, et al. Ultrahistopathology of balanitis circinata. Br J Vener. Dis. 1982;58(3):188-95.
15. Khaitan BK. Non-venereal diseases of genitalia. In: Sharma VK. Sexually transmitted diseases and HIV/AIDS, 2nd edition. New Delhi: Viva Books; 2009. pp. 677-91.
16. Kumar B, Sharma R, Rajagopalan M, et al. Plasma cell balanitis: clinical and histopathological features--response to circumcision. Genitourin Med. 1995;71(1):32-4.
17. Lassus A, Tiilikainen A, Stubb S, et al. Circinate erosive balanitis and HL-A 27. Acta Derm Venereol. 1975;55(3):199-201.
18. Letsinger JA, McCarty MA, Jorizzo JL. Complex aphthosis: a large case series with evaluation algorithm and therapeutic ladder from topicals to thalidomide. J Am Acad Dermatol. 2005;52(3 Pt 1):500-8.
19. Majumdar S, Saha SS. Angiokeratoma of scrotum (fordyce). Indian J Dermatol Venereol Leprol. 1996;62(1):52-4.
20. Neinstein LS, Goldenring J. Pink pearly papules: an epidemiologic study. J. Pediatr. 1984;105(4):594-5.
21. Perry D, Lynch PJ, Fazel N. Pseudoepitheliomatous, keratotic, and micaceous balanitis: case report and review of the literature. Dermatol Nurs Dermatol Nurses Assoc. 2008;20(2):117-20.
22. Rappaport I, Shiffman MA. Multiple phlebectasia involving jejunum, oral cavity, and scrotum. JAMA. 1963;185:437-40.
23. Robinson SS, Tasker S. Angiomas of the scrotum (angiokeratoma, Fordyce); compilation of cases and discussion of nomenclature. Arch Dermatol Syphilol. 1946;54(6):667-74.
24. Sehgal VH, Gangwani OP. Genital fixed drug eruptions. Genitourin Med. 1986;62(1):56-8.
25. Sonnex TS, Dawber RP, Ryan TJ, et al. Zoon's (plasma-cell) balanitis: treatment by circumcision. Br J Dermatol. 1982;106(5):585-8.
26. Souteyrand P, Wong E, MacDonald DM. Zoon's balanitis (balanitis circumscripta plasmacellularis). Br J Dermatol. 1981;105(2):195-9.
27. Teichman JM, Sea J, Thompson IM, et al. Noninfectious penile lesions. Am Fam Physician. 2010;81(2):167-74.
28. Torgerson RR, Edwards L. Genital dermatoses. In: Holmes KK, Sparling PF, Stamm WE (Eds). Sexually transmitted diseases. 4th edition. New York: McGraw Hill; 2008. pp. 1209-26.
29. Yoganathan S, Bohl TG, Mason G. Plasma cell balanitis and vulvitis (of Zoon). A study of 10 cases. J Reprod Med. 1994;39(12):939-44.
30. Yoshida M, Maeyama Y, Yasumoto S, et al. Vulvo-vaginal-gingival syndrome of lichen planus. Int J Dermatol. 2006;45(10):1252-4.

# 69 CHAPTER Disorders of Eccrine and Apocrine Glands

Eswari Loganathan, Shashi Kumar BM, Raghunatha Reddy R

## INTRODUCTION

Eccrine, apocrine and sebaceous glands are the three glandular appendages of the skin. Sebaceous glands and their disorders are dealt elsewhere.

## ECCRINE SWEAT GLANDS

Eccrine sweat glands are distributed over the whole skin surface, including the glans penis and foreskin, but not on the lips, external ear canal, clitoris, or labia minora. Highest density is found on palms and soles. The total number on the body surface is between 2 and 5 million. Up to 10 L/day of sweat is produced by acclimatized individuals. Embryologically, sweat glands are derived from a specialized downgrowth of the epidermis at about the 3$^{rd}$ month of intrauterine and they resemble adult glands by 8 months. No new eccrine glands develop afterbirth. They are composed of coiled secretory glands, a coiled duct, a straight duct, an intraepidermal coil, and an eccrine pore. The three eccrine cell types are: (1) clear (secretory), (2) dark (mucoid), and (3) myoepithelial (contractile).The eccrine sweat glands and the vasculature of the skin help in thermoregulation. Hypothalamic temperature is the strongest stimulus for sweating. Both adrenergic and cholinergic fibers innervate the glands. Acetylcholine is the major stimulus secreted by sympathetic nerves. Various techniques for studying the function of eccrine sweat glands have been explained in box 1.

## APOCRINE GLANDS

Apocrine glands are adnexal glands that are distributed in the scalp, the axillae, the anogenital region and the eyelids (Moll's glands). The external auditory meatus (ceruminous glands), and the mammary glands are modified apocrine glands. Embryologically, apocrine glands develop from the upper bulge of the hair follicle late in the 4$^{th}$ month of gestation, with continued development as long as hair follicles develop. Apocrine glands are composed of three components: (1) the intraepithelial duct, (2) the intradermal duct, and (3) a coiled gland in the deep dermis or at the junction of the dermis and subcutaneous fat, which contains the secretory portion. The predominant mode of apocrine secretion is decapitation, a process where the apical portion of the secretory cell cytoplasm pinches off and enters the lumen of the gland. Apocrine sweat consists mainly of sialomucin. The exact function of apocrine glands is unclear, although they are thought to represent scent glands. Their primary sympathetic stimulation is adrenergic, epinephrine being the stimulant.

## DISORDERS OF ECCRINE GLANDS

### Hyperhidrosis

Hyperhidrosis is the excessive production of sweat which significantly impairs the quality of life and has a worldwide prevalence rate of 2.8%. Hyperhidrosis can be primary or secondary in nature and may have general, regional, or focal manifestations. Primary hyperhidrosis is most often focal and generally causes idiopathic, symmetrically bilateral excessive sweating of the axillae, palms, soles, or craniofacial region. Secondary hyperhidrosis manifests most often as generalized excessive sweating that is related to an underlying medical condition or use of medication. The criteria of diagnosing primary and secondary hyperhidrosis are given in table 1.

#### Primary Hyperhidrosis

This is the most common type of hyperhidrosis with typical distribution involving the axillae, palms, soles, and craniofacial sites. Onset is between 14 and 25 years, with prepubertal onset

**BOX 1 Techniques for studying the function of the eccrine sweat glands**

- Collection of sweat in pads at rest and after cholinergic stimulation (Gravimetry)
- Visualization of the individual sweat droplets by direct microscopy, by *in vivo* staining, by forming plastic impressions or by indicators, such as the starch/iodine technique, bromophenol blue, and quinizarin
- Microcannulation of the duct or coil
- Cutaneous microdialysis–microperfusion of the skin with perfusate containing various pharmacological agonists and antagonists allows for the study of continuous stimulation of sweat glands
- Measurement of electrical potential and resistance of skin.

**TABLE 1: Criteria for diagnosis**

| | |
|---|---|
| Primary hyperhidrosis | • Focal, visible, and excessive sweating of at least 6-month duration without apparent cause<br>• At least two of the following:<br>○ Bilateral and relatively symmetric<br>○ Impairs daily activities<br>○ At least one episode per week<br>○ Age of onset <25 years<br>○ Family history of hyperhidrosis<br>○ Cessation of focal sweating during sleep<br>• Exclusion of secondary causes of excessive sweating |
| Secondary generalized hyperhidrosis | Generalized excessive sweating attributable to a definitive underlying medical cause; most commonly drugs, substance abuse, cardiovascular disorders, respiratory failure, infections, malignancies, endocrine/metabolic disorders, or neurologic disease |
| Secondary regional hyperhidrosis | • Localized anhidrosis with compensatory excessive sweating in other areas<br>• Identification of a definitive underlying cause; most commonly stroke, peripheral nerve damage, spinal cord lesion, neuropathy, or Ross syndrome |
| Secondary focal hyperhidrosis | • Excessive sweating in typical anatomic sites (palms, soles, axillae, and craniofacial) or in a well-defined anatomic distribution (trunk, inguinal folds, buttocks, legs, submammary folds, neck, or wrist)<br>• Identification of a definitive underlying cause; most commonly Frey syndrome, eccrine nevus, social anxiety disorder, neurologic disorder, or tumor |

*Source*: Adapted from Moraites E, Vaughn OA, Hill S. Incidence and prevalence of hyperhidrosis. Dermatol Clin. 2014;32(4):457-65.

**TABLE 2: Management of hyperhidrosis**

| Type | Treatment route of administration and dosage | |
|---|---|---|
| Craniofacial, gustatory | *Glycopyrrolate*: 1 mg BID; increase up to 2 mg three to four times daily.<br>*Clonidine*: 0.6–1.2 mg/day in two or three divided doses | – |
| Axillary, palmar-plantar, craniofacial | 20% aluminum chloride in anhydrous ethyl alcohol | – |
| Palmar–plantar | *Iontophoresis unit (Fig. 1)*: 15–30 mA using tap water; glycopyrrolate can be added, making a 0.1% solution | Immerse hands, feet for 30 min once or twice daily, or 20 min at each site every 2–3 days, or 10 min at each site three to five times weekly; anode site is most effective so switch sides after one-half of each treatment; direct current more effective |
| Palmar–plantar, axillary, gustatory, recalcitrant | Botulinum toxin A injection | Given via high intradermal injections to ~1 $cm^2$ anesthetized skin areas; for botulinum toxin A, total of 12–20 injections (50 units total) given per axilla, 50–75 injections in the palm/each foot; benefit lasts 2–8 months; reinjection is effective |
| Axillary | Liposuction and curettage of sweat glands in dermis | – |
| Palmar, axillary; resistant to other treatment modalities | Sympathetic surgery | – |

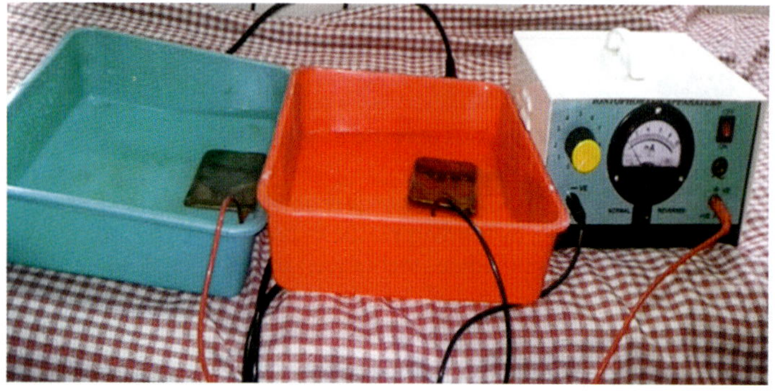

**FIG. 1:** Iontophoresis unit.

*Courtesy*: Bowring and Lady Curzon Hospital, Bengaluru.

associated with palmoplantar disease and postpubertal onset associated with axillary disease. Men may have higher incidence. It is autosomal dominant with greater than 35% of patients having positive family history.

*Management*: Treatment for various types of hyperhidrosis has been summarized in table 2.

## Anhidrosis/Hypohidrosis

This is a condition with scant or absent sweating. The skin is dry and coarse. Scaling and mild itching occurs, and fever may be produced by exercise because of lack of perspiration. The various causes of anhidrosis are given in table 3.

**TABLE 3: Causes of anhidrosis**

| | |
|---|---|
| Congenital absence of sweat gland function | Hypohidrotic ectodermal dysplasia |
| Metabolic disorders | Hypothyroidism, dehydration, thermic fever, Fabry's disease |
| Neurological disorder | Disorder of the hypothalamus and spinal cord, alcoholic neuritis, leprosy, diabetic neuropathy |
| Plugging of the eccrine pores | Ichthyosis, seborrheic dermatitis, atopic dermatitis, erythroderma, psoriasis |
| Atrophy or damage of sweat glands | Scleroderma, systemic sclerosis, Sjögren syndrome, systemic lupus erythematosus, solar elastosis |

**TABLE 4: Types of miliaria**

| Type | Location of obstruction | Age group | Clinical features |
|---|---|---|---|
| Miliaria crystallina (Fig. 2) | Stratum corneum | Neonates <2 weeks, Adults and children in hot climate | Clear, fragile, nonpruritic, 1 mm vesicles on face and trunk with brawny desquamation |
| Miliaria rubra (Fig. 3) | Mid epidermis | Infants, adults, and children in hot climate | Pruritic, erythematous 1–3 mm vesicles, papules or pustules on neck and upper trunk |
| Miliaria profunda | Dermo-epidermal junction | Adults in hot climates | Nonpruritic, white 1–3 mm papule on trunk, and proximal extremities |

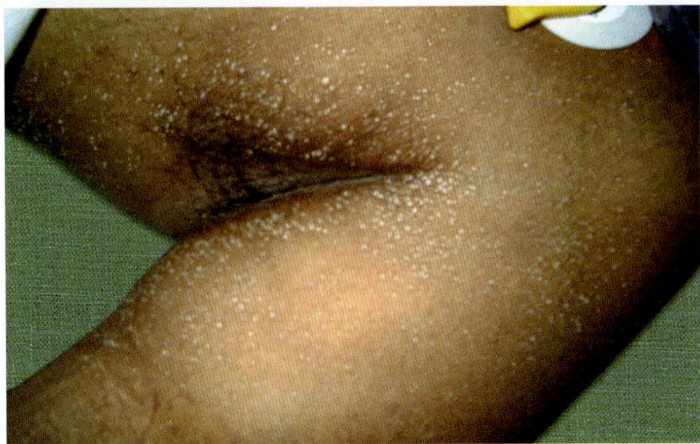

**FIG. 2:** Miliaria crystalline.
*Courtesy*: Bowring and Lady Curzon Hospital, Bengaluru.

## Management

Patients should maintain cool body temperature by being in a cool environment where air conditioning is there. They should carry water bottles to keep themselves from dehydration. They should chill their neck and axilla often with cold water.

Intravenous pulse therapy with systemic corticosteroids have been tried in various isolated cases. No proper randomized studies regarding the management of anhidrosis are available. They have also used antihistamines based on evidence that histamine inhibits the acetylcholine-induced sweating function of eccrine glands. Use of immunosuppressants, such as cyclosporine, acetylcholine receptor agonists (e.g., pilocarpine hydrochloride and cevimeline hydrochloride hydrate), and Chinese herbal medicines has also been an option, but the clinical effects appear inconsistent. Intravenous immunoglobulin has also been tried to prevent recurrences.

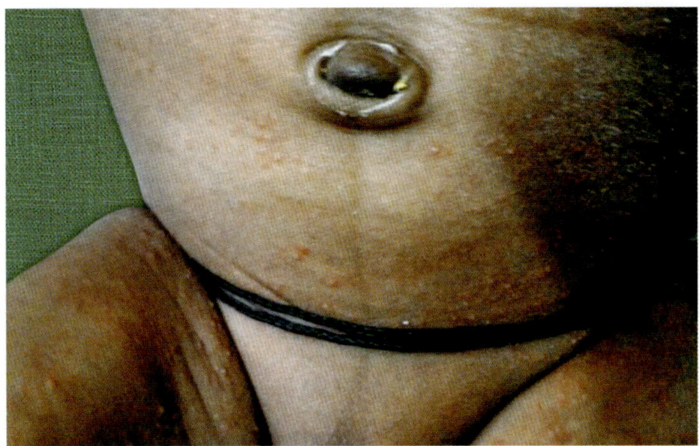

**FIG. 3:** Miliaria rubra.
*Courtesy*: Bowring and Lady Curzon Hospital, Bengaluru.

## Miliaria

It is commonly called heat rash which is caused by obstruction to the eccrine sweat ducts. Three forms of miliaria occur depending on the level of obstruction: miliaria crystallina (sudamina), miliaria rubra (prickly heat) and miliaria profunda. The types and clinical features are summarized in table 4.

The most important complications of miliaria are secondary infection and disturbance of heat regulation. Periporitis staphylogenes is the name given to multiple staphylococcal abscesses superimposed on miliaria rubra in young infants.

## Management

Moving away from tropical climates may be essential. Avoidance of excessive sweating, clothing, friction from clothing, excessive use of soap, and contact of the skin with irritants will reduce the incidence. The large number of treatments are advocated but with disappointing results. Calamine lotion is effective but because of its drying effect, a bland emollient may be required subsequently to prevent further epidermal damage.

# DISORDERS OF APOCRINE GLANDS

## Bromhidrosis

Also known as fetid sweat, osmidrosis, and malodorous sweating, bromhidrosis is chiefly encountered in the axillae. Individuals have increased levels of 5α-reductase in their apocrine glands. Bacterial decomposition of apocrine sweat, producing fatty acids with distinctive offensive odors, is considered to be the cause. The best characterized short chain fatty acid causing odor is trans-3-methyl-2-hexenoic acid. True bromhidrosis is usually not recognized by the patient.

Fish odor syndrome should be considered in patients presenting with complaints of offensive odor. It is caused by excretion of trimethylamine (which smells like rotten fish) in the eccrine sweat, urine, saliva, and other secretions. This chemical is produced from carnitine and choline in the diet and is normally metabolized in the liver.

### Management

Antibacterial soaps and deodorants are quite effective in controlling axillary malodor. Frequent bathing, changing of underclothes, shaving of the axillae, and topical application of aluminum chloride are all helpful measures. Surgical removal of the glands either by excision or tumescent liposuction is possible, as in axillary hyperhidrosis, but this is rarely indicated. Botulinum toxin A injections in the axilla have controlled body odor in this site as well in the pubic area.

## Chromhidrosis

Chromhidrosis, or colored sweat, is an exceedingly rare functional disorder of the apocrine sweat glands, frequently localized to the face or axilla. It has been less often noted on the abdomen, chest, breasts, thighs, groin, genitalia, and lower eyelids. The colored sweat may be yellow (most common), blue, green, or black. The colored secretion appears in response to adrenergic stimuli, which cause myoepithelial contractions. Colored apocrine sweat fluoresces and is caused by lipofuscin which can be appreciated clinically using Woods lamp. Different types have been mentioned in table 5.

Eccrine chromhidrosis is caused by the coloring of the clear eccrine sweat by dyes, pigments, or metals on the skin surface.

Treatment with botulinum toxin A or topical capsaicin has been reported to be effective.

**TABLE 5: Types of chromhidrosis**

| Color of sweat | Condition |
|---|---|
| Red sweat | Flight attendants from the red dye in the labels in life-vests |
| Blue–green sweat | Copper workers |
| Brownish sweat | Ochronosis |
| Bile stained sweat | Liver failure |

## Fox–Fordyce Disease

Fox–Fordyce disease is rare, occurring mostly in women during adolescence or soon afterward. It may occasionally be familial in nature.

### Clinical Features

It is characterized by conical, flesh-colored or grayish, intensely pruritic, and discrete follicular papules in areas where apocrine glands occur. The axillae and areolae are the primary sites of involvement, but the umbilicus, pubes, labia majora, and perineum may be affected (Fig. 4). Pregnancy invariably leads to improvement.

### Histopathology

There is obstruction of the follicular ostia by orthokeratotic cells. An inflammatory infiltrate of lymphocytes surrounds the upper third of the hair follicles and upper dermal vessels. There is an associated spongiosis of the infundibulum at the site of entrance of the apocrine duct into the hair follicle. Foam cells are the histologic markers.

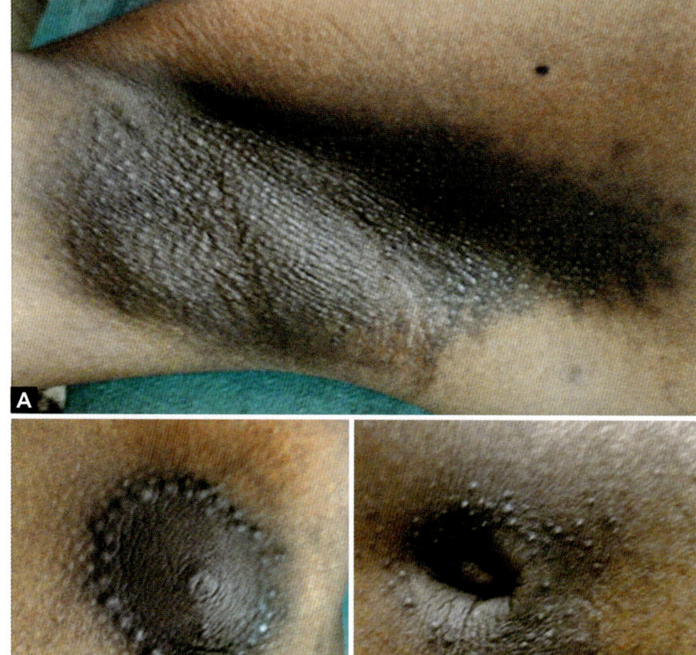


**FIG. 4:** Fox–Fordyce Disease. **A,** Papules seen in axilla; **B,** Papules seen around nipple; **C,** Papules seen around umbilicus.
*Courtesy*: Bowring and Lady Curzon Hospital, Bengaluru.

### Management

There is no effective treatment. Oral contraceptive pills, topical tretinoin or adapalene, topical pimecrolimus or weak corticosteroid creams, intralesional steroids, topical clindamycin solution, benzoyl peroxide, isotretinoin, and UV phototherapy have all been effective in small numbers of patients. Excision or liposuction-assisted curettage may be successful in axillary sites.

## SUGGESTED READINGS

1. Arseculeratne G1, Wong AK, Goudie DR, et al. Trimethylaminuria (fish odor syndrome). Arch Dermatol. 2007;143:81.
2. Collins KJ. Measurement of sweating and sweat gland function. In: Greaves MW, Shuster S (Eds). The Pharmacology of the Skin. Berlin: Springer; 1989.
3. Eisenach JH, Atkinson JL, Fealey RD. Hyperhidrosis: Evolving therapies for a well-established phenomenon. Mayo Clin Proc. 2005;80(5):657-66.
4. Heckman M, Teichmann B, Pause BM, et al. Amelioration of body odor after intracutaneous axillary injection of botulinum toxin A. Arch Dermatol. 2003;139:57.
5. Kamada A, Saga K, Jimbow K. Apoeccrine sweat duct obstruction as a cause for Fox–Fordyce disease. J Am Acad Dermatol. 2003;48:453-5.

6. Lowe N, Campanati A, Bodokh I, et al. The place of botulinum toxin type A in the treatment of focal hyperhidrosis. Br J Dermatol. 2004;151:1115-22.
7. Lubowe II, Perlman HH. Periporitis staphylogenes and other complications of miliaria in infants and children. Arch Dermatol Syphil. 1954;69:543-53.
8. Masuda T, Obayashi K, Ueda M, et al. Therapeutic effects and prevention of recurrence of acquired idiopathic generalized anhidrosis via IV immunoglobulin treatment. J Dermatol. 2016;43:336-7.
9. Matarasso SL. Treatment of facial chromhidrosis with botulinum toxin type A. J Am Acad Dermatol. 2005;52:89.
10. Matsui S, Murota H, Takahashi A, et al. Dynamic analysis of histamine-mediated attenuation of acetylcholine-induced sweating via GSK3beta activation. J Invest Dermatol. 2014;134:326-34.
11. Moraites E, Vaughn OA, Hill S. Incidence and prevalence of hyperhidrosis. Dermatol Clin. 2014;32(4):457-65.
12. Ohshima Y, Yanagishita T, Ito K, et al. Treatment of patients with acquired idiopathic generalized anhidrosis. Br J Dermatol. 2013;168:430-2.
13. Polat M, Dikilitaş M, Gözübüyükoğullari A, et al. Apocrine chromhidrosis. Clin Exp Dermatol. 2009;39:e373.
14. Seo SH, Jang BS, Oh CK, et al. Tumescent superficial liposuction with curettage for treatment of axillary bromhidrosis. J Eur Acad Dermatol Venereol. 2008;22:30.
15. Shelley WB, Horvath PN, Pillsbury DM. Anhidrosis. Medicine. 1950;29:194-224.
16. Strutton DR, Kowalski JW, Glaser DA, et al. US prevalence of hyperhidrosis and impact on individuals with axillary hyperhidrosis: results from a national survey. J Am Acad Dermatol. 2004;51:241-8.
17. Szabo G. The regional anatomy of the human integument with special reference to the distribution of hair follicles, sweat glands and melanocytes. Philos Trans R Soc Lond Biol. 1967;252:447-85.

# 70 CHAPTER Hair Disorders

*Savitha AS, Shashi Kumar BM*

## INTRODUCTION

Hair has no vital function in the human body, but lack of it or excess has an immense psychological impact. Hair abnormalities may be inherited or acquired. Androgenetic alopecia (AGA) is the most common type of hair loss seen in men. A detailed history, physical examination, and special investigations like hair microscopy, dermatoscopy, and histopathology may be required to diagnose hair disorders.

## HAIR BIOLOGY

On the scalp, and some other regions of the skin, hair follicles are arranged in groups of three or more follicles known as follicular units. The follicular unit is defined as a group of one to three hairs that grow naturally together, includes one to two fine vellus hairs, glands, muscle, nerves, and blood vessels (Fig. 1).

There are different types of hair on human body. Any particular follicle can produce different types of hair under the influence of hormones or advancing age. Table 1 summarizes the different types of hair (Fig. 2).

## EMBRYOLOGY

During embryonic development, human hair follicles appear at about 9 weeks. Initially it emerges in the regions of the chin, eyebrows, and upper lip, and by 4th month covers the entire body. Hair is an ectodermal derivative.

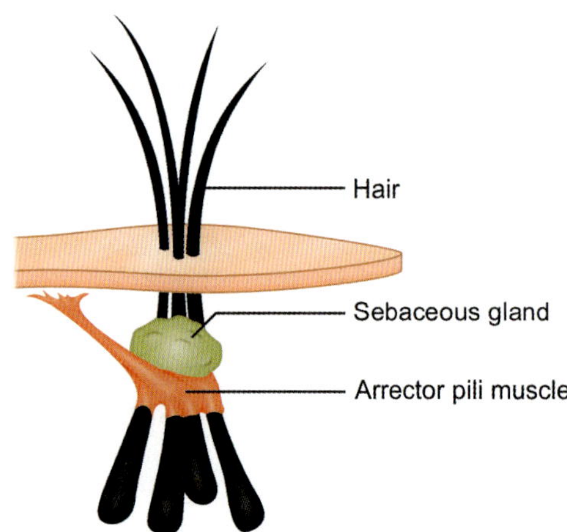


**FIG. 1:** Follicular unit.

## ANATOMY OF THE HAIR

The structure of hair is divided into two components: (1) the hair shaft and (2) hair root. Hair shaft is the portion of hair which emerges from the scalp. The hair root is divided anatomically into four parts from below upward (Fig. 3).

1. The bulb consisting of the matrix and dermal papilla
2. The suprabulbar area extends from the matrix to the insertion of the arrector pili muscle
3. The isthmus extends from the insertion of the arrector pili muscle to the sebaceous gland
4. The infundibulum extends from the sebaceous gland to the follicular orifice.

- *Dermal papilla*: The dermal papilla is a flask-shaped structure that invaginates the base of the hair follicle. In large follicles, it contains a loop of capillary blood vessels. This is the primary target of androgen action in the hair follicle. The volume of the dermal papilla probably determines the size of the hair follicle
- *Hair color*: It is determined by the melanocytes found in the matrix area of the follicle at the base of the cortex directly above the follicular papilla. Eumelanin is the dominant global pigment and confers black or brown hair. Pheomelanin, a mutation of eumelanin, is the predominant pigment found in blond hair. The proportions of eumelanin and pheomelanin and the total amount of melanin determine the hair color. Graying of hair is a normal manifestation of aging and illustrates progressive reduction in melanocyte function
- *Rate of hair growth*: Human hair generally grows at a rate of 1 cm/month or 0.35 mm/day
- *Follicle density*: There are approximately 100,000 hair follicles on the scalp. It varies with the age, sex, race, and area of the body. The forehead and cheeks have the highest hair follicle density, which is approximately 800/cm$^2$ and in women on cheeks it is 400–450/cm$^2$. Chest and back show lower hair density of 50–100/cm$^2$.

## HAIR CYCLE (FIG. 4)

Hair follows a specific growth cycle with three distinct and concurrent phases: (1) anagen, (2) catagen, and (3) telogen

**TABLE 1: Different types of hair**

| Type of hair | | Description | Clinical significance |
|---|---|---|---|
| Prenatal hair—lanugo | | Fine, soft, unmedullated and usually unpigmented hair, covers the entire body in humans in *utero* and is normally shed in the $8^{th}$–$9^{th}$ months of gestation | • In adults with anorexia nervosa and bulimia<br>• Congenital hypertrichosis lanuginosa<br>• Hypertrichosis lanuginosa acquisita |
| Postnatal hair | Vellus | Soft, unmedullated, occasionally pigmented, seldom grows more than 2 cm long and present over much of the body area | Eruptive vellus hair cyst |
| | Terminal | Pigmented, longer, coarser hair and consistently possesses a medulla. After puberty, they replace vellus hairs in areas like beard, axilla, and pubic area | • Hypertrichosis<br>• Hirsutism |
| | Intermediate | Have characteristics of both vellus hairs and terminal hairs. Intermediate hairs have a medulla and contain a moderate amount of pigment, less than that found in the terminal hair type | Androgenetic alopecia |

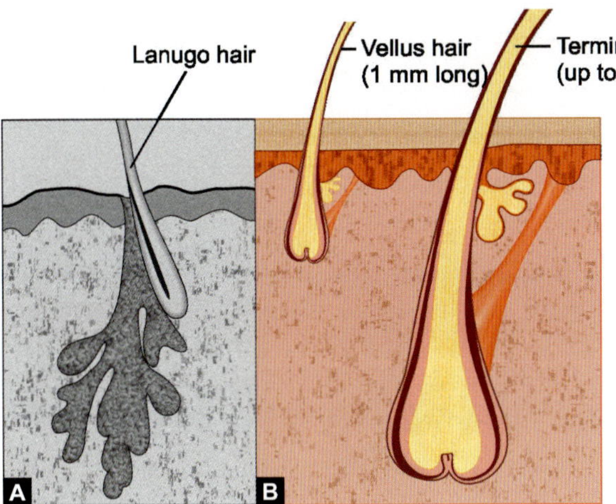


**FIG. 2:** Different types of hair.

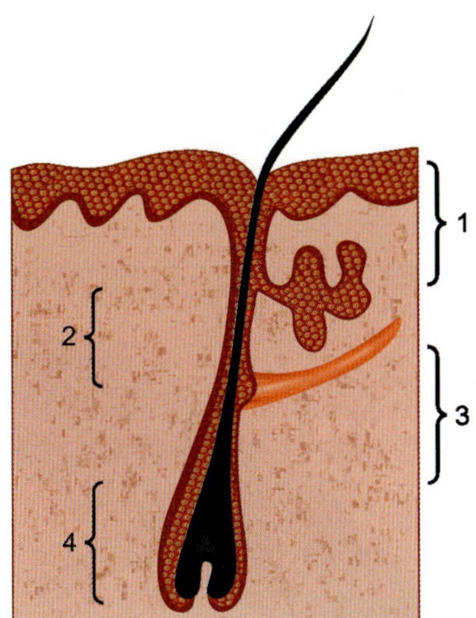


**FIG. 3:** Different parts of the hair bulb: 1. infundibulum; 2. isthmus; 3. suprabulbar region; 4. bulb.

phases. Each phase has specific characteristics that determine the length of the hair. All three phases occur simultaneously; one strand of hair may be in the anagen phase, while another is in the telogen phase.

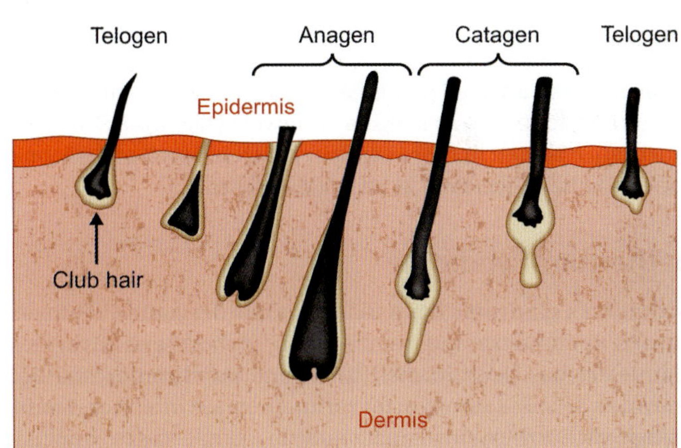


**FIG. 4:** Hair cycle.

## Anagen Phase

It is the period of active hair growth. The final length of hair is determined by anagen phase. At any one time, normally 80–90% of hair follicles on the human scalp are in anagen phase. Anagen phase lasts for about 2–6 years.

## Catagen Phase

Catagen phase is an involutionary phase in which the mitotic activity declines and ceases, usually lasts for about 3 weeks. During this phase, the proximal end of the hair shaft keratinizes to form a club-shaped structure and the lower part of the follicle involutes by apoptosis and thickens to form the "glassy membrane".

## Telogen Phase

The period between the completion of follicular regression and the onset of the next anagen phase is termed telogen, which lasts for about 3 months. The club hair is eventually shed through an active process termed exogen.

Fifty to one-hundred club hairs are shed daily from a normal scalp. In human scalp, hair follicles may remain in a state of latency, also known as kenogen, for a prolonged period after the club hair is shed.

## HAIR STRUCTURE DISORDERS

The function of scalp hair is mainly cosmetic; though in other regions of the body, it has a variety of functions. Hair shaft defects may give the hair an unusual appearance, make it fragile or act as a marker for a syndrome. These disorders may be congenital or acquired.

### Monilethrix

This term indicates the resemblance of the hair to a string of beads or a necklace. It is an autosomal dominant (AD) disorder. Abnormalities are attributed to mutations in human keratin type II genes *hHb1* and *hHb6* on chromosome 12q31. The hair shaft is beaded and breaks easily. Keratosis pilaris is almost invariably associated with monilethrix. Sites of predilection are the scalp, nape of the neck, and extensor surfaces of the upper arm and thigh (Fig. 5).

### Pili Torti

In pili torti, the affected hair is flattened and twisted through 180° along their long axis at irregular intervals (Fig. 6). AD mode of inheritance is seen in those cases in which pili torti of early onset appears to have occurred as an isolated defect.

### Netherton's Syndrome

Netherton's syndrome has a triad of atopic dermatitis, ichthyosis linearis circumflexa and bamboo hair/trichorrhexis invaginata. The defect has been located to a gene on chromosome 5q32 known as *SPINK 5* acronym for serum protease inhibitor. Finding a single trichorrhexis invaginata node in a single hair is conclusive of Netherton's syndrome. Characteristic "bamboo" shape under light microscopic examination is due to invagination of the distal part of the hair shaft to its proximal part (Fig. 7). The proximal remnant of the invaginate node may resemble a golf tee and can allow diagnosis where a classic node is absent.

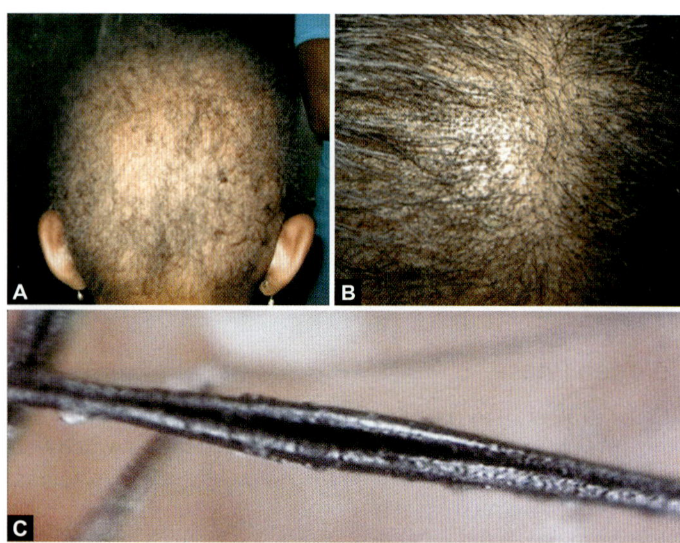

**FIG. 5: A,** Sparse, fragile hair in monilethrix; **B,** follicular prominence on scalp; **C,** microscopic appearance of hair shaft showing fusiform nodes.

### Trichorrhexis Nodosa

One of the most common hair shaft defects a dermatologist encounters is trichorrhexis nodosa (TN). TN is a distinctive response of hair shaft to injury. The cuticular cells become disrupted allowing the cortical cells to splay out to form nodes. The cumulative effect of shampooing, brushing, sea bathing, and sunlight has led to seasonal recurrences. A primary congenital form of TN is inherited as an AD trait in some families.

The frayed cortical fibers project out giving the appearance of two paint brushes thrust into one another (Fig. 8).

### Trichoptilosis

Trichoptilosis is the most common macroscopic response of the hair shaft to trauma. Thermal, mechanical, and chemical stress can cause split ends. The distal end of the shaft is split

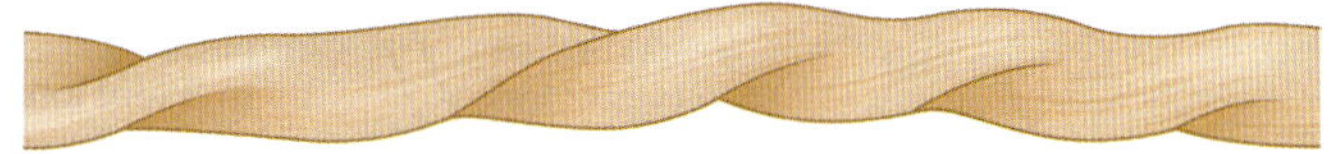

**FIG. 6:** Schematic representation of pili torti.

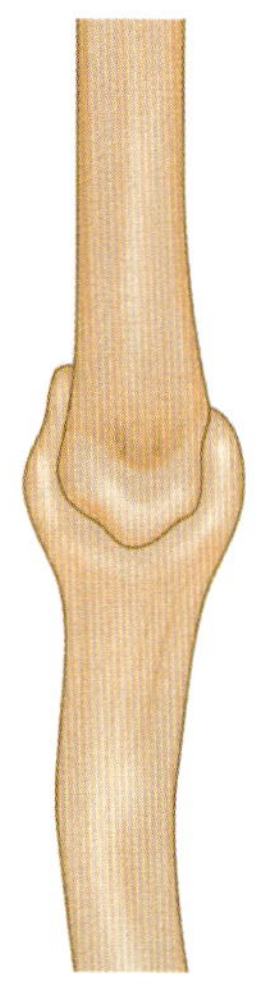

**FIG. 7:** Schematic representation of trichorrhexis invaginata.

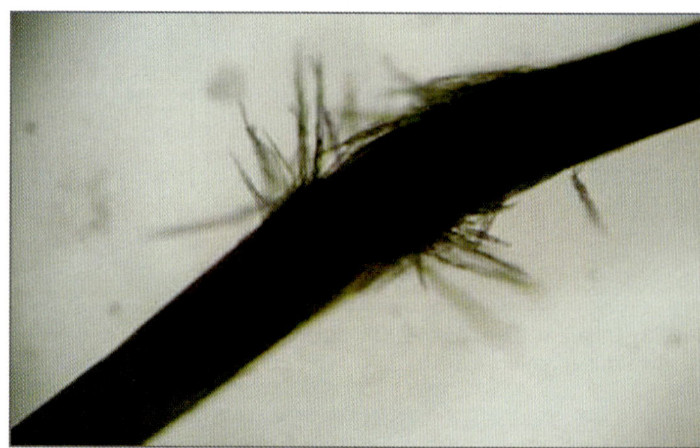

**FIG. 8:** Trichorrhexis nodosa under light microscope.

*Source*: Savitha A, Sacchidanand S, Revathy T. Bubble hair and other acquired hair shaft anomalies due to hot ironing on wet hair. Int J Trichology. 2011;3:118-20.

longitudinally into two or several divisions. Other microscopic evidence of hair damage may be present. The split commences from the distal tip thus distinguishing the problem from pili bifurcati or multigemini. TN and trichoptilosis are often present in the same patient (Fig. 9).

### Treatment

Careful explanation to the patient is necessary to avoid further hair trauma, otherwise the condition will definitely recur. Short hair and frequent trimming solves the problem.

## Trichonodosis

Incidental clinical finding of trauma-induced knotting of the naturally curly/wavy hair shaft is seen frequently over lower occipital regions. Microscopic examination may be needed to differentiate from piedra and the pediculosis capitis ova.

## Hair Casts (Pseudonits)

Hair casts often occur in great numbers and may mimic nits in scalp. They are 2–5 mm, firm, and tubular movable structures around the hair shafts (Fig. 10). They are found frequently in association with parakeratotic scalp disorders like psoriasis, lichen planus, seborrheic dermatitis or trichotillomania, and hair styles requiring traction. While nits are firmly cemented to hair shaft, hair casts slide freely along shaft (Table 2).

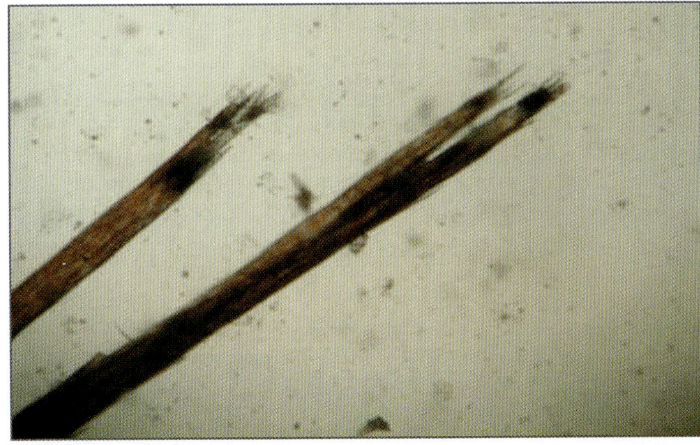

**FIG. 9:** Light microscopy of distal trichoptilosis.
*Source*: Savitha A, Sacchidanand S, Revathy T. Bubble hair and other acquired hair shaft anomalies due to hot ironing on wet hair. Int J Trichology. 2011;3:118-20.

# ALOPECIA

Loss of hair is termed alopecia. It can be broadly divided into two types: (1) scarring and (2) nonscarring (Flowchart 1).

## Alopecia Areata

Alopecia areata (AA) is a common nonscarring alopecia that occurs in 0.1–0.2% of the general population and accounts for 0.7–3% of all cases seen in dermatology practice. The disease is an inflammatory disease that manifests in the hair follicles and can occur in the nails up to 66% patients. Prevalence rates peak between the ages of 20–40 years of life; however up to 60% of patients with AA will present with their first patch before the age of 20 years.

### Etiology

Alopecia areata is most likely an organ-specific autoimmune disease.

- *Genetics*: Studies in AA found 28% of patients have at least one affected family member
- Autoimmunity is believed to play a central role in the development of AA. Patients with AA have been found to have an increased frequency of hair follicle-specific autoantibodies. The inferior portion of the normal hair follicle is an "immune privileged" site which is protected from surveillance by T-cells.

**TABLE 2: Differences between nits and pseudonits**

| True nits | Pseudonits |
|---|---|
| Tiny yellow, brown, or tan dots attached to the hair shaft near the scalp | Firm, shiny, white, and freely movable tubular accretions that encircle the hair shafts of the scalp |
| Caused by pediculus humanus capitis, female lays eggs at the base of the follicle | Etiology unknown |
| Common in childhood | Seen in all age groups |
| Contagious | Noncontagious |
| Causes an itchy scalp | Usually asymptomatic |

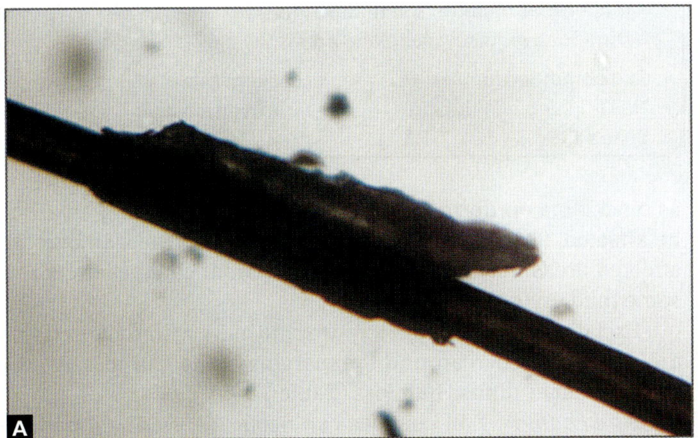

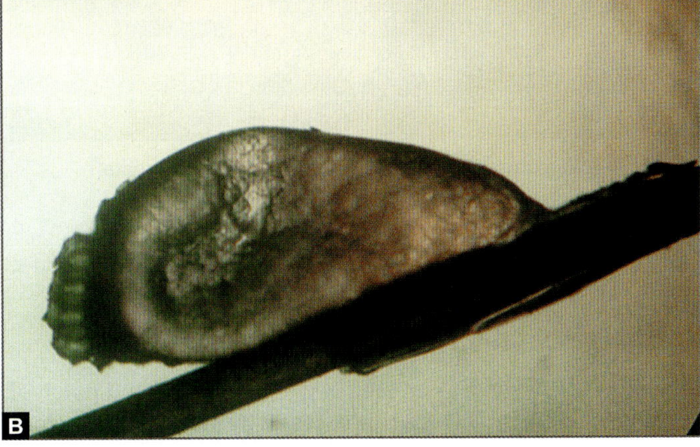

**FIG. 10: A,** Hair cast; **B,** nits.

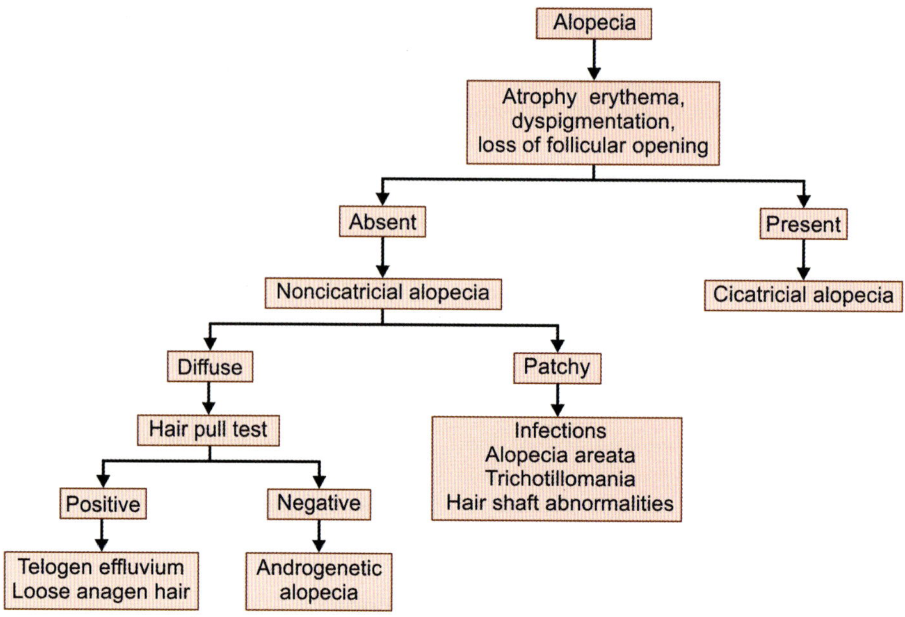


**FLOWCHART 1:** Classification of alopecia.

**TABLE 3: Ikeda's classification of alopecia areata**

| | |
|---|---|
| Type I | Common type. The onset is in older children or adults between 20–40 years of age. The isolated alopecic patches dating for less than 3 years. The separate lesions show aptitude for spontaneous recovery within 6 months |
| Type II | Atopic type—frequent early onset in childhood, prolonged course of more than 10 years |
| Type III | Prehypertensive type. Young adults, with personal or family history of hypertension, manifests rapid often fluctuating course |
| Type IV | Combined type—adult onset around 40 years. Frequently associated with autoimmune and endocrine diseases |

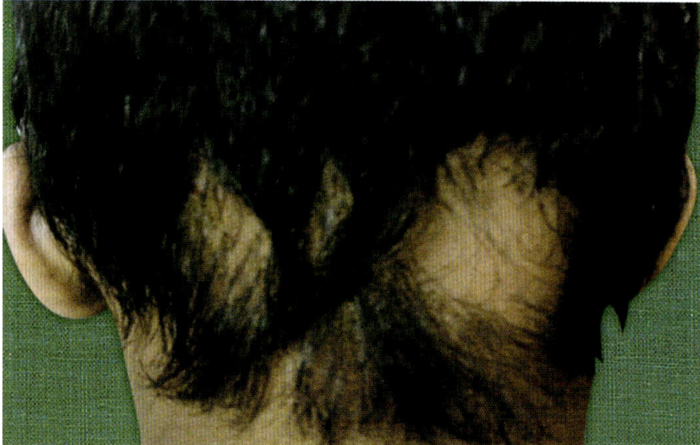

**FIG. 11:** Well-circumscribed patchy hair loss in alopecia areata.

## Ikeda's Classification

Ikeda's classification of alopecia areata has been shown in table 3.

## Clinical Presentation

Clinically, AA presents as an area of well-circumscribed patch of sudden hair loss (Fig. 11). The initial loss is by hair breakage, close to or just below the surface of the skin. Hair remnants are visible as black dots on dermoscopy. While any hair-bearing area may be affected, 90% of lesions occur on the scalp. The skin over the affected areas may have no overt epidermal changes except for some mild erythema and atrophy.

Exclamation mark hairs, dystrophic hairs with fractured tips, are commonly seen around the margins of the hair loss. AA can also present as diffuse hair loss (Table 4).

- *Nail changes*: Nail changes can occur in 10–66% of patients with AA (Box 1).

**TABLE 4: Morphological classification of alopecia areata**

| Type | Description |
|---|---|
| Patchy AA | This is the most common presentation of AA. Hair loss is localized and patchy |
| AA totalis | Total hair loss on the scalp |
| AA universalis | Complete hair loss of all hair-bearing areas |
| Acute diffuse and total alopecia (ADTA) | ADTA may present as a short clinical course ranging from acute hair loss to total baldness. The prognosis is favorable and there is rapid resolution of the condition—at times without treatment |
| Diffuse AA | Diffuse hair loss which can mimic telogen effluvium |
| Ophiasis | Hair loss is localized to the sides of the scalp and the nape |
| Sisaipho | Hair loss spares the sides of the scalp and the nape. This presentation is rare |
| Reticular patches | Several patches of AA may coalesce to form a reticular pattern |

**BOX 1 Nail changes in alopecia areata**

- "Scotch plaid" effect or "ripples"
  - Superficial, uniform, and minute pits
  - Arranged regularly along and across the nail
- Red or mottled lunulae
- Nail thinning and ridging
- Beau's lines
- Leukonychia
- Trachyonychia

## Differential Diagnosis

Tinea capitis and trichotillomania both produce hair breakage and patchy hair loss. In tinea capitis, the scalp skin may be scaly. In trichotillomania the border of the alopecia is angular rather than circular. Secondary syphilis will present with moth-eaten alopecia.

## Investigations

Diagnosis of AA is usually made on clinical examination and routine tests are not indicated. If there is uncertainty regarding the diagnosis, a scalp biopsy may be performed. Fungal culture, lupus serology and syphilis serology can also be taken to exclude other differentials.

## Histopathology

The histopathological features vary depending on the stage of the disease. In acute stages, terminal hairs are surrounded by bulbar lymphocytes, which can take the classical appearance of a "swarm of bees" (Fig. 12).

## Management

While spontaneous remission will occur in up to 50% of patients in 1 year, most people seek active treatment.

- *Intralesional corticosteroids*: Intralesional corticosteroids are the treatment of choice for patchy hair loss in AA. Triamcinolone acetonide (5–10 mg/mL) and hydrocortisone acetate (25 mg/mL) are the most commonly used intralesional corticosteroids. 0.1 mL of solution is injected into multiple sites 1 cm apart into deep dermis using a 30-gauge needle. This process is repeated every 4–6 weeks
- *Systemic corticosteroids*: Systemic corticosteroids are highly effective in the treatment of AA. Short-term use up to 3 months is generally well tolerated. Prednisolone may be given at a starting dosage of 0.5 mg/kg/day. Pulse corticosteroid therapy has been tried in an attempt to minimize the risk of steroid-related side effects and there have been reports of successful therapy with 250 mg intravenous (IV) methylprednisolone for 3 days in patchy AA

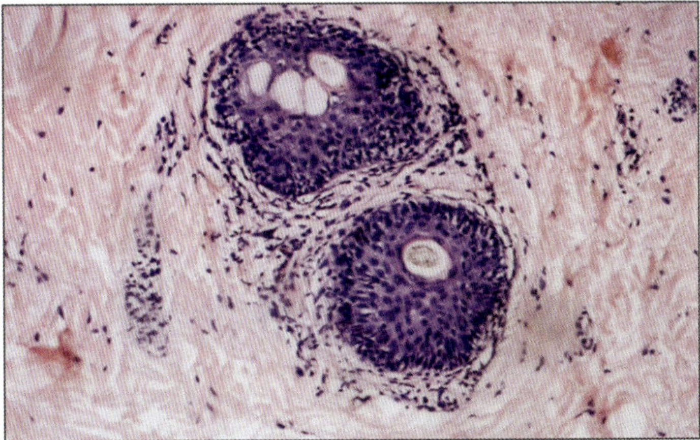

FIG. 12: "Swarm of bees" appearance on hematoxylin and eosin (H&E) staining.

- *Topical corticosteroids*: Topical corticosteroids are commonly used to treat AA. Treatment with topical corticosteroids needs to be continued for at least 3 months before regrowth is seen
- *Psoralen and ultraviolet A (PUVA)*: Psoralen and ultraviolet A light deplete inflammatory cell infiltrate and can produce satisfactory regrowth in patients with AA totalis and AA universalis with relatively low relapse rates
- *Minoxidil*: It is an effective topical preparation that stimulates proliferation at the base of the bulb and differentiation above the dermal papilla. A concentration of 2–5% minoxidil is used twice daily as a topical application to the affected area with good results in patient with mild to moderate AA
- *Topical immunotherapy*: Topical immunotherapy is useful for severe and refractory cases of AA. It is hypothesized that the allergic reaction created by the topical immunotherapy generates suppressor T-cells that inhibits an autoimmune reaction against the hair follicle. Diphenylcyclopropenone and squaric acid dibutylester are commonly used topical immunotherapy in the treatment of AA
- *Miscellaneous treatment*: 0.5–1% anthralin, sulfasalazine, cyclosporine, calcineurin inhibitors, biologic drugs, mesotherapy, and excimer lasers.

Poor prognostic factors in alopecia areata have been shown in box 2.

# Androgenetic Alopecia

Androgenetic alopecia is the most common causes of hair loss. The male pattern hair loss describes the temporal, and vertex balding seen in men due to AGA. Female pattern hair loss (FPHL) describes the mid-frontal scalp hair thinning seen in women with AGA.

## Etiology

Androgentic alopecia is familial with a complex polygenic mode of inheritance. Polymorphism of the androgen receptor gene, the 5-α reductase gene and two others, as yet unidentified genes on chromosomes 3 and 21 have been associated with premature balding.

## Pathogenesis

Circulating and locally produced androgens bind to androgen receptors in the hair follicle bulb. These androgens mediate an alteration in the size of the dermal papilla during early anagen

**BOX 2 Poor prognostic factors in alopecia areata**

- Early age of onset
- Positive family history
- *Severe patterns*: Ophiasis/reticular/sisaipho/alopecia totalis/alopecia universalis
- Extensive scalp involvement
- Recurrent episodes
- Loss of eyebrow and eyelashes
- *Nail involvement*: Pitting, dystrophy, onycholysis, and anonychia
- Associated systemic and genetic disorders
- Patchy regrowth of terminal hairs within a patch

that reduces the size of the anagen follicle and of the emerging hair and also reduces the duration of the anagen phase of the hair cycle. In addition, the onset of anagen is delayed. Initially, miniaturization affects some but not all of the hairs within an individual follicular unit, so that on affected zones of the scalp each unit has a reduced number of hairs rather than a total absence of hairs. The sparing of one or two hairs within each follicular unit results in diffuse thinning and increased hair shedding that precedes the development of baldness. Eventually, when all the hairs within a follicular unit are lost, a bald scalp becomes apparent.

## Clinical Presentation

Hair loss typically follows a defined pattern. In males, bitemporal recession of the frontal hairline usually precedes diffuse thinning over the vertex of the scalp which eventually produces vertex baldness (Fig. 13).

Thinning over the mid-frontal scalp eventually joins the receding frontal hairline and vertex bald spot. This highly reproducible pattern of hair loss is illustrated by the Norwood-Hamilton scale. In FPHL, the anterior hair line is often maintained, or there may be mild bitemporal recession (Fig. 14).

The severe bitemporal recession seen in men with AGA is not common in women. The usual pattern of hair loss in women is a diffuse reduction in hair density over the crown. A "Christmas tree" (Fig. 15) pattern can be observed with widening of the central part line. This hair thinning may extend over the parietal scalp to the ears.

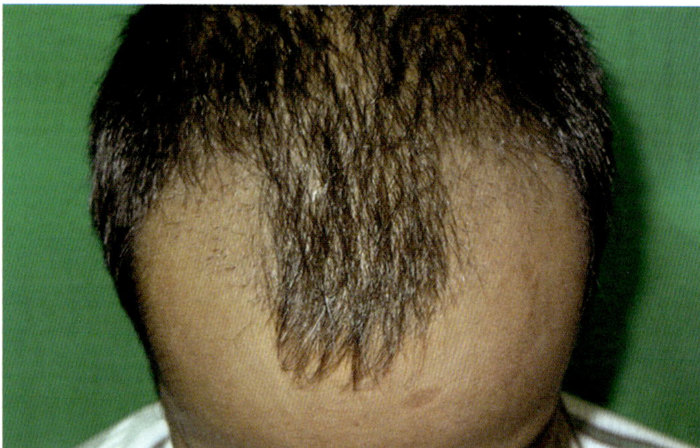

**FIG. 13:** Male pattern hair loss.

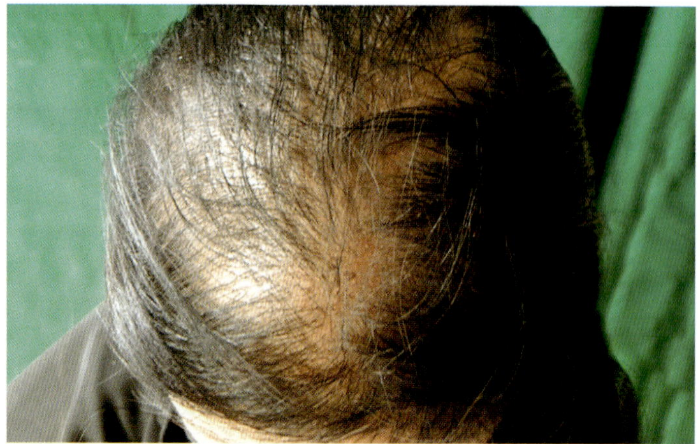

**FIG. 14:** Female pattern hair loss (FPHL). Hairline is spared.

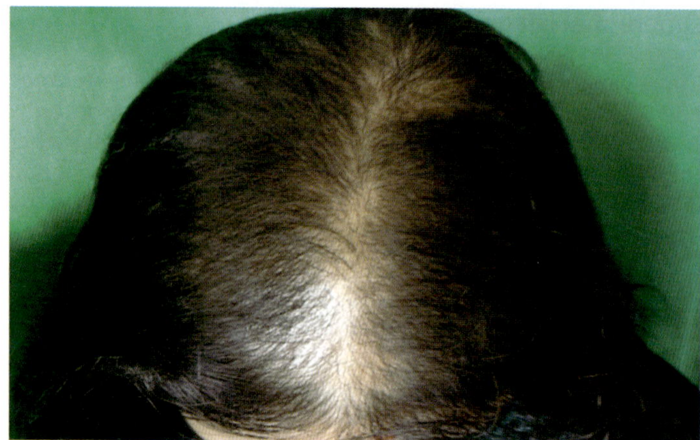

**FIG. 15:** Christmas tree pattern of hair loss in FPHL.

## Diagnosis

Diagnosis of AGA in males is straightforward; however, in females the diagnosis may not be so clear-cut. A careful history should be obtained from the patient. Information, including family history of AGA and drug history should be collected and a history of menstrual irregularities or hirsutism should be noted in females as this requires further investigation to exclude an underlying cause. Laboratory investigations are not usually indicated for patients with AGA and diagnosis is made on clinical grounds. However, in females who have features of hyperandrogenism, appropriate investigations include follicle-stimulating hormone (FSH), luteinizing hormone (LH), prolactin, serum androgen, and estrogen levels, fasting lipids and triglyceride levels. Scalp biopsies are not indicated in the diagnosis of AGA. Biopsies, however, are useful in distinguishing between chronic telogen effluvium and FPHL.

## Histopathology

Biopsies sectioned transversely at the opening of the sebaceous duct show differing hair shaft diameters reflecting the progressive miniaturization of hair follicles. The terminal to vellus ratio in AGA is usually less than 4:1. A fibrous tract or a follicular streamer leading to the miniaturize hair indicates the position of the original terminal follicle. Up to 40% of patients may show perifollicular fibrosis on microscopic examination.

## Management

### *Medical Treatment*

- *Minoxidil*: It is a potent arteriolar vasodilator. It has been shown to be effective in converting vellus hair to terminal hair in 30% of patients when applied in a 2% solution with a 10% propylene glycol water base. 1 mL of the solution is applied to the scalp twice daily. A temporary telogen effluvium may occur in the first 2–8 weeks. Treatment with a 5% solution yields superior hair growth compared to the 2% solution in both males and females
- *Oral finasteride*: Finasteride is a potent antagonist of 5-α-reductase type 2. It binds irreversibly to this enzyme to

inhibit the conversion of testosterone to dihydrotestosterone (DHT). This reduction of DHT production then limits the miniaturization of hair follicles. A dose of 1 mg orally is the optimal dose for treatment of male pattern baldness

- *Dutasteride*: Dutasteride inhibits both types 1 and 2 5-α-reductase isoenzymes. It is 100 times more potent in inhibiting the type 1 isoenzyme than finasteride. Off label indication for MPHL is 0.5 mg twice-weekly
- *Managing female pattern hair loss*: Topical minoxidil 2% is commonly used in women. Oral antiandrogen therapies that are thought to be beneficial in preventing progression of AGA in females include cyproterone acetate, spironolactone, and flutamide.

### *Surgery*

- Surgical treatment options for the treatment of AGA include hair transplant and scalp reduction procedures. Hair transplantation is ideal for patients who have high-density donor hair.
- *Camouflage products and hair pieces*: Products designed to camouflage hair loss are the simplest and cheapest way of treating androgenetic hair loss. Hair building fibers, topical shading, and scalp spray thickeners are among the most commonly used camouflaging products.

## Cicatricial Alopecia

Cicatricial or scarring alopecia is a group of disorders leading to permanent hair loss. The essential features of all cicatricial alopecia are visible loss of follicular ostia, clinically and destruction of the hair follicle, histopathologically.

### Classification

The North American Hair Research Society has proposed a working classification of cicatricial alopecia based on the histological findings. A modified combined classification based on both etiology and histopathology is shown in table 5. This classification is currently used as a guide for both diagnosis and treatment.

Salient clinic histological features of primary cicatricial alopecias are summarized in table 6.

**TABLE 5: Classification of cicatricial alopecia**

| Primary cicatricial alopecia | | | |
|---|---|---|---|
| Inflammatory | Lymphocytic | • Chronic cutaneous lupus erythematosus<br>• Lichen planopilaris (LPP)<br>• Graham-Little syndrome<br>• Frontal fibrosing alopecia | • Pseudopelade of Brocq<br>• Central centrifugal cicatricial alopecia<br>• Alopecia mucinosa<br>• Keratosis pilaris spinulosa decalvans |
| | Neutrophilic | • Folliculitis decalvans (including tufted folliculitis) | • Dissecting cellulitis/folliculitis |
| | Mixed | • Acne keloidalis<br>• Acne necrotica | • Nonspecific or end-stage cicatricial alopecia |
| **Secondary cicatricial alopecia** | | | |
| Traumatic | | • Radiodermatitis<br>• Mechanical trauma<br>• Postoperative (e.g., flap necrosis)<br>• Burns | • Accidental alopecia<br>• Dermatitis artefacta<br>• Traction alopecia<br>• Hot comb alopecia |
| Sclerosing disorders | | • Morphea<br>• Scleroderma<br>• Lichen sclerosus | • Sclerodermoid porphyria cutanea tarda<br>• Chronic graft-versus-host disease |
| Granulomatous | | • Sarcoidosis<br>• Necrobiosis lipoidica | • Infectious granulomas |
| Infectious | Bacterial | • Folliculitis | • Carbuncle/furuncle |
| | Fungal | • Kerion<br>• Favus | • Tinea capitis (rarely scarring) |
| | Viral | • Shingles<br>• Varicella | • HIV |
| | Protozoal | Leishmaniasis | |
| | Treponemal | Syphilis | |
| | Mycobacterial | Tuberculosis | |
| Neoplastic | Benign | • Cylindroma<br>• Other adnexal tumors | |
| | Malignant | • Basal cell carcinoma<br>• Squamous cell carcinoma | • Cutaneous T-cell lymphoma<br>• Metastases |
| Developmental defects and hereditary disorders | | • Aplasia cutis<br>• Facial hemiatrophy (Romberg's syndrome)<br>• Epidermal nevi<br>• Hair follicle hamartomas<br>• Incontinentia pigmenti<br>• Focal dermal hypoplasia of Goltz | • Porokeratosis of Mibelli<br>• Ichthyosis<br>• Epidermolysis bullosa<br>• Polyostotic fibrous dysplasia<br>• Conradi–Hünermann syndrome (chondrodysplasia punctata) |

**TABLE 6: Salient clinico–histological features of primary cicatricial alopecias**

| Disease | Clinical | Histopathology |
|---|---|---|
| Pseudopelade of Brocq | Often mistaken for alopecia areata; alopecic patches coalesce into irregular white patches resembling "footprints in the snow" (Fig. 16); localized only in the scalp; few solitary hairs within the patches of atrophy | Absence of marked inflammation, scarring, and follicular plugging; perpendicular columns of fibrous tissue (follicular ghosts); abnormally increased elastic tissue around the fibrous column (Fig. 17) |
| Lichen planopilaris | Pruritic, spinous, hyperkeratotic, follicular papules; perifollicular erythema and scaling; center of the bald patch is smooth and atrophic with active margins (Fig. 18) | Prototypical form of lymphocyte-mediated primary cicatricial alopecia; hypergranulosis within the affected infundibula; concentric lamellar fibrosis around follicles (Fig. 19) |
| Frontal fibrosing alopecia | Postmenopausal women; progressive frontoparietal recession; loss of eyebrows | Features similar to lichen planopilaris |
| Lupus erythematosus | Commonly affects the scalp, face, and ears; discoid, erythematous scaly plaques; telangiectasia, atrophy, dyspigmentation, and follicular plugging in the center of bald patch; "carpet tack sign" | Focal basal cell vacuolation; funnel-shaped keratotic plugs; patchy dermal infiltrate; thickening of the basement membrane zone; immunopathologically deposition of IgG, IgM, and C3 in a granular band like pattern at the dermal interface |
| Folliculitis decalvans | Crops of pustules with erythema and crusting around the rim of alopecic patches; center of the bald area shiny and atrophic | Prototypical of neutrophil-mediated primary cicatricial alopecia; intense infiltrate around the upper portion of the follicle; often, numerous foreign body giant cells around remnants of hair follicles; inflammatory cells in the follicular lumen |
| Dissecting cellulitis | Perifolliculitis; painful suppurative nodules; interconnecting sinus tracts, and extensive scarring; part of follicular occlusion tetrad | Mixed infiltrate; follicular perforation and abscess formation; granulomatous reaction; extensive fibrosis in dermis and subcutis |
| Central centrifugal cicatricial alopecia | Middle aged black women; focus of cicatricial alopecia over vertex spreading centrifugally | Premature desquamation of inner root sheath; perifollicular lymphocytic infiltrate; concentric lamellar fibroplasia |
| Acne keloidalis | Common in young black men; follicular papules/pustules, keloidal plaques over the occipital scalp and neck | Mixed infiltrate at the level of isthmus and lower infundibulum; granulomatous inflammation; lamellar fibroplasias |

IgG, immunoglobulin G; IgM, immunoglobulin M.

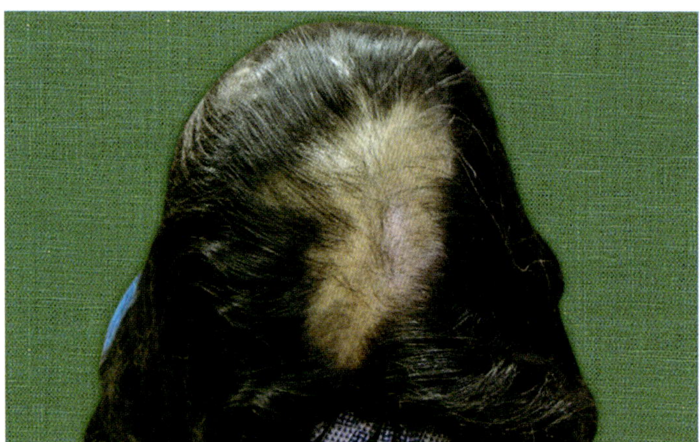

**FIG. 16:** Pseudopelade of Brocq—footprints in snow appearance.

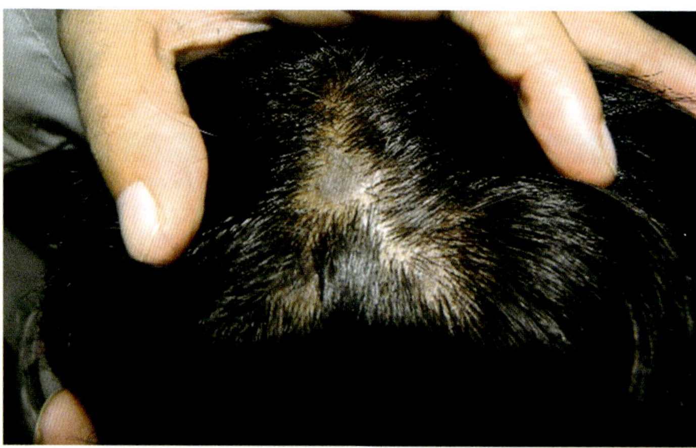

**FIG. 18:** Cicatricial alopecia due to lichen planopilaris.

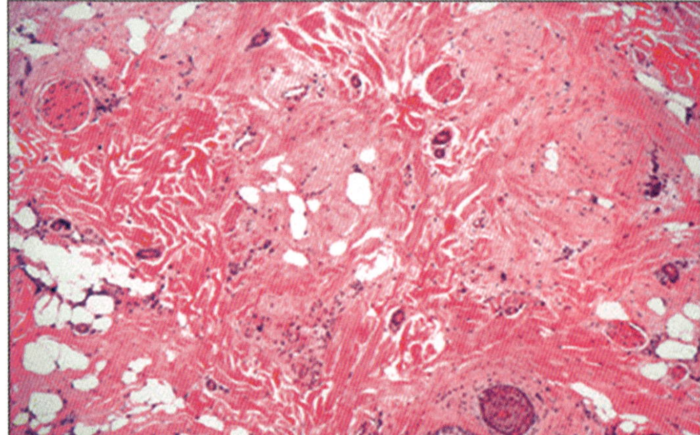

**FIG. 17:** Histopathology of pseudopelade of Brocq.

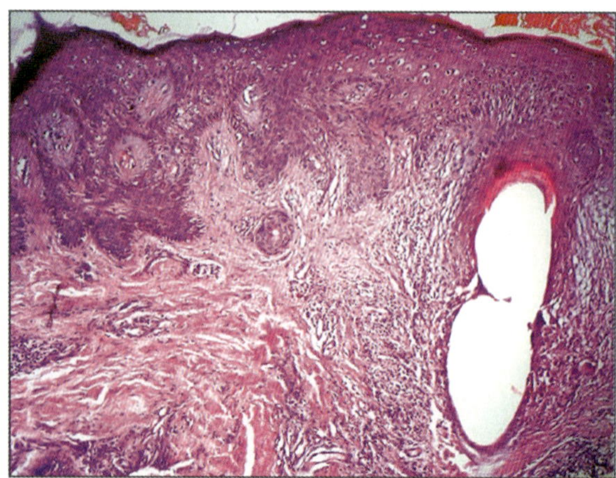

**FIG. 19:** Histopathology of lichen planopilaris.

## HIRSUTISM AND HYPERTRICHOSIS

The term "hirsutism" is of Latin origin which means excessive growth of stiff hair or hairiness, especially in women or children, with an adult male pattern of distribution.

Hypertrichosis is defined as excessive hair growth for a particular site of the body or age of a patient that is not hormone-dependent. Hypertrichosis and hirsutism need to be differentiated as the latter occurs in response to androgens and thus selectively affects the androgen-dependent hair (Table 7).

Approach to a patient with hirsutism is summarized in flowcharts 2 and 3.

**TABLE 7: Differences between hypertrichosis and hirsutism**

| Hypertrichosis | Hirsutism |
|---|---|
| Excessive hair growth on face and body | Excessive hair growth in androgen-dependent areas |
| Congenital/acquired | Due to androgen excess states |
| Both males and females affected | Females |
| Generalized or localized in distribution. Commonly seen over face and trunk | Seen over androgen-dependent areas |
| Type of hair involved can be lanugo, vellus or terminal | Vellus hairs transformed to terminal hair |
| Congenital forms show poor response to medical line of treatment | Good response when underlying cause is treated |
| Physical methods of management preferred | Can be managed medically |

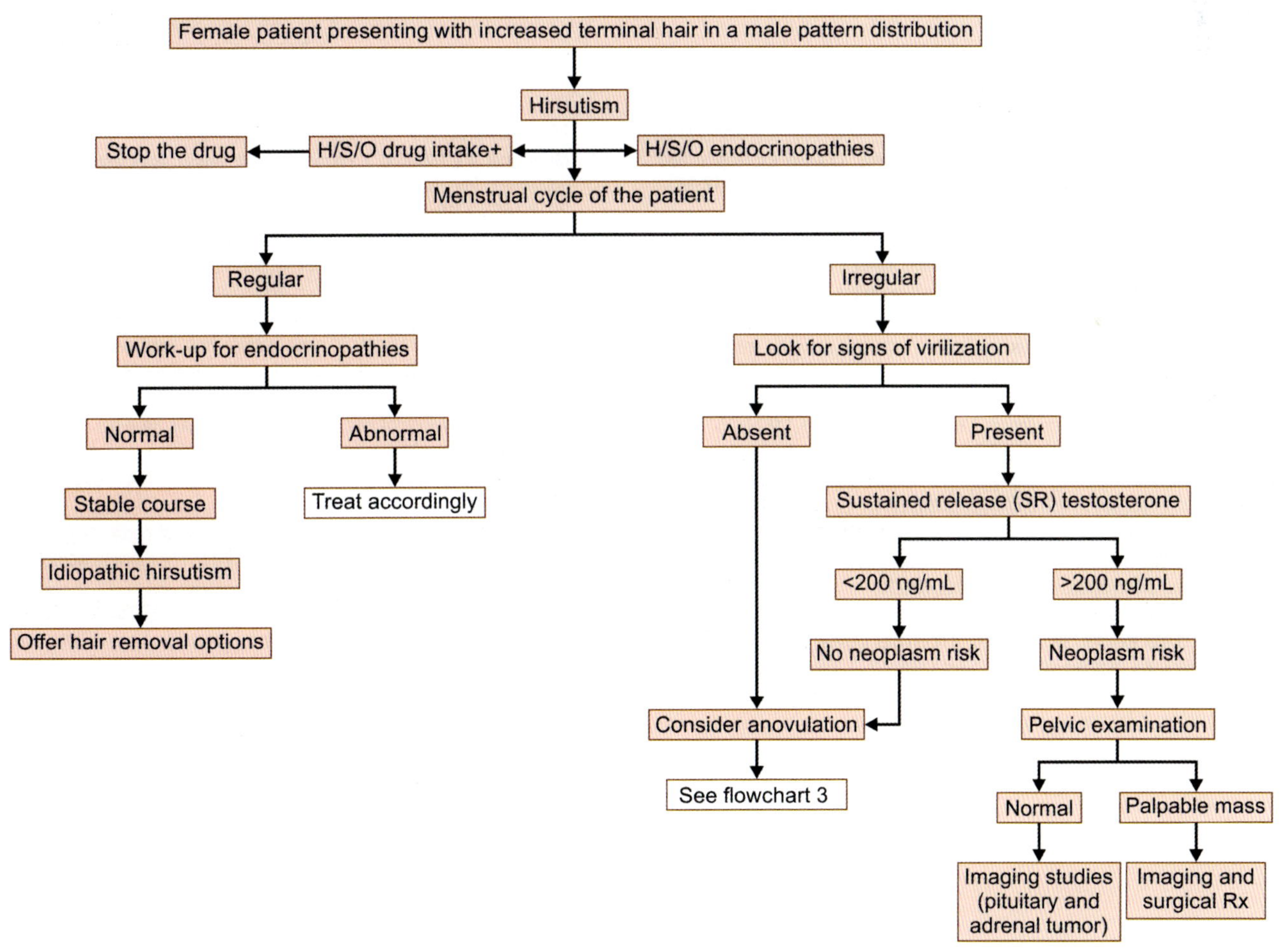


H/S/O, history suggestive of.

**FLOWCHART 2:** Approach to a patient with hirsutism.

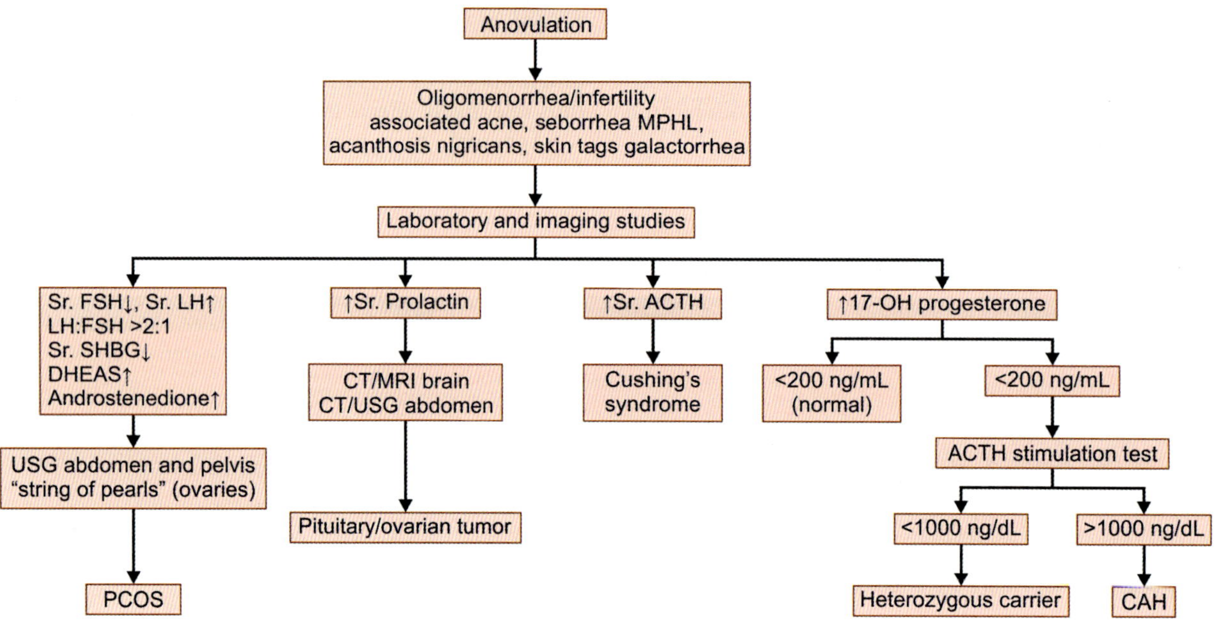


FSH, follicle-stimulating hormone; LH, luteinizing hormone; SHBG, sex hormone-binding globulin; DHEAS, dehydroepiandrosterone sulfate; Sr, serum; MPHL, male pattern hair loss; ACTH, adrenocortical-stimulating hormone; CAH, congenital adrenal hypoplasia; PCOS, polycystic ovarian syndrome.

**FLOWCHART 3:** Anovulation.

## SUGGESTED READINGS


1. Bitoun E, Chavanas S, Irvine AD. Netherton syndrome: disease expression and spectrum of SPINK5 mutations in 21 families. J Invest Dermatol. 2002;118:352-61.
2. Blume U, Ferracin J, Verschoore M, et al. Physiology of the vellus hair follicle: hair growth and sebum excretion. Br J Dermatol. 1991;124:21-8.
3. Cheng AS, Bayliss SJ. The genetics of hair shaft disorders. J Am Acad Dermatol. 2008;59:1-22.
4. Dhurat R, Saraogi P. Hair evaluation methods: merits and demerits. Int J Trichol. 2009;1(2):108-19.
5. Ellis JA, Stebbing M, Harrap SB. Polymorphism of the androgen receptor gene is associated with male pattern baldness. J Invest Dermatol. 2001;116(3):452-5
6. Fantauzzo KA, Kurban M, Levy B, et al. Trps1 and its target gene Sox9 regulate epithelial proliferation in the developing hair follicle and are associated with hypertrichosis. PLoS Genet. 2012;8(11):e1003002.
7. França K, Villa RT, Silva IR, et al. Hair casts or pseudonits. Int J Trichol. 2011;3:121-2.
8. Gilhar A, Paus R, Kalish RS. Lymphocytes, neuropeptides, and genes involved in alopecia areata. J Clin Invest. 2007;117(8):2019-27.
9. Hardy MH, Van Exan RJ, Sonstegard KS, et al. Basal lamina changes during tissue interactions in hair follicles: an in vitro study of normal dermal papillae and vitamin A-induced glandular morphogenesis. J Invest Dermatol. 1983;80(1):27-34.
10. Ibrahim L, Wright EA. A quantitative study of hair growth using mouse and rat vibrissal follicles. I. Dermal papilla volume determines hair volume. J Embryol Exp Morphol. 1982;72:209-24.
11. Majid I, Keen A. Management of alopecia areata: an update. Br J Med Pract. 2012;5(3):a530.
12. Messenger AG, McKillop J, Farrant P, et al. British Association of Dermatologists' guidelines for the management of alopecia areata 2012. Br J Dermatol. 2012;166(5):916-26.
13. Mohamed Z, Bhouri A, Jallouli A, et al. Alopecia areata treatment with a phototoxic dose of UVA and topical 8-methoxypsoralen. J Eur Acad Dermatol Venereol. 2005;19(5):552-5.
14. Olsen EA, Hordinsky M, Whiting D, et al. The importance of dual 5-alpha-reductase inhibition in the treatment of male pattern hair loss: results of a randomized placebo-controlled study of dutasteride versus finasteride. J Am Acad Dermatol. 2006;55(6):1014-23.
15. Pinkus H. Embryology of hair. In: Montagna W, Ellis RA (Eds). The Biology of Hair Growth. New York: Academic Press; 1958. pp. 1-32.
16. Rebora A, Kenogen GM. A new phase of the hair cycle? Dermatology. 2002;205(2):108-10.
17. Sinclair R, Jolley D, Mallari R, et al. The reliability of horizontally sectioned scalp biopsies in the diagnosis of chronic diffuse telogen hair loss in women. J Am Acad Dermatol. 2004;51(2):189-99.
18. Sinclair R. Male pattern androgenetic alopecia. BMJ. 1998;317(7162):865-9.
19. Trueb RM. Possibilities and limitations for reversal of age-related hair loss. In: Trueb RM, Tobin DJ (Eds). Aging Hair. Berlin: Springer-Verlag; 2010. pp. 193-206.
20. Yildiz BO, Bolour S, Woods K, et al. Visually scoring hirsutism. Hum Reprod Update. 2010;16(1):51-64.

71

CHAPTER

# Disorders of the Nails

*Bianca M Piraccini, Aurora Alessandrini*

## INTRODUCTION

Nails are cutaneous appendages which play important role in bearing mechanical functions, such as gripping, providing mechanical support to the digits. Nails may be affected in variety of dermatological and systemic diseases as well as disorders indigenous to the nail itself. Certain nail changes are specific to some diseases. They are frequently affected by nutritional status of the patient, systemic illness or some drug administration. There are several genetic disorders that present with some specific nail changes.

## NAIL ANATOMY AND PHYSIOLOGY

The "nail unit" is composed by four important elements. In particular, the nail plate production is due to the nail matrix, which is protected proximally and laterally by nail folds. Nail bed permits nail plate adhesion during growth and at the distal margin of the digit the hyponychium is present.

The nail plate emerges from the proximal nail fold to the distal one, well attached to the nail bed, up to detach toward the hyponychium.

The proximal nail fold is composed by two layers of epithelium: the dorsal one is the continuation of the skin of the dorsum of the digit, while the ventral one is continuous with the nail matrix. The nail plate is an epithelium that produces keratinocytes without the formation of a granular layer.

Because nail matrix keratinization occurs along an oblique axis, the proximal portion of the nail matrix produces the dorsal portion of the nail plate, while the distal matrix produces the ventral nail plate.

The distal part of the nail matrix is visible through the nail plate and is called lunula. The matrix encloses quiescent melanocytes that can be activated. The nail bed lies below the nail plate that strictly adheres to it during growth, its ventral part being produced by nail bed epithelium keratinization. Connective tissue separates nail bed dermis from the distal phalangeal bone.

The adherence between the nail plate and the nail bed is due to the nail isthmus, which is the site of primary damage in onycholysis.

The blood capillaries of the nail unit are oriented in different ways, depending on the location, and when they are damaged, a splinter hemorrhage can appears.

During embryonic life (around the $15^{th}$ week), nail plate production starts and go on until death (Table 1). Mean growth rate of fingernails is 3 mm/month, while for toenail this rate is lower (1 mm/month), as a result, complete regrowth of a fingernail in general require 4–6 months, and up to 1 year for a toenail.

## NAIL CHANGES: NOMENCLATURE

### Changes of the Nail Surface

#### Beau's Lines (Box 1)

A Beau's line appears as a transverse depression of the nail plate, resulting from a damage to the proximal nail matrix, like

**TABLE 1: Embryogenesis of the nail apparatus**

| Weeks of gestation | Milestones of nail development |
|---|---|
| 10 weeks | Primary nail fold can be seen with proximal, lateral, and distal grooves |
| 13 weeks | Invagination of the proximal nail fold on the matrix primordium that is moving proximally |
| 14 weeks | Emergence of the nail plate |
| 15 weeks | Formation of the hard keratin throughout the matrix and nail bed |
| 17 weeks | The nail plate covers most of the nail bed |
| 20 weeks | The nail plate extends to the distal ridge, now termed hyponychium |
| 25 weeks | Completion of nail unit differentiation |

**BOX 1 Causes of Beau's lines**

- Acute diseases (severe)—erythroderma, pustular psoriasis, Stevens–Johnson syndrome and toxic epidermal necrolysis
- High fever
- Viral illnesses
- Drugs
- Chronic paronychia
- Eczema
- Immunobullous diseases
- Excessive manicuring
- Raynaud's disease
- Trauma
- Zinc deficiency
- Acute hypocalcemia

mechanical trauma, as manicures, or diseases as chronic eczema, that affects the proximal nail fold. Beau's lines grow distally with the nail plate, and their depth corresponds to the level of the damage to the matrix, caused by the temporary decrease of the keratinocyte mitotic activity. The depth of the depression indicates the extent of the damage within the matrix, while their width along the longitudinal axis suggests the duration of the insult. Beau's lines grow distally with the nail plate. When Beau's lines are present in all nails at the same level a systemic disease should be suspected.

### Onychomadesis

Onychomadesis represents a more severe degree of Beau's lines, because the damage has involved the whole matrix, with complete temporary arrest of nail plate production. It appears as a sulcus that replaces the proximal nail plate.

The hand, foot, and mouth disease, caused by coxsackie virus is the most common cause of onychomadesis in children, while in adults is acute paronychia, which often involves only one fingernail (Fig. 1).

In toenails, the ingrowing of the new nail can be a consequence of an episode of onychomadesis.

### Pitting

Pitting appears as small depressions on the nail plate surface, typically on fingernails. Pits are due to foci of abnormal keratinization of the proximal nail matrix that result in parakeratotic cells in the dorsal nail plate.

They are distributed along one or more longitudinal lines and sometimes they may be arranged in crisscross patterns, in a random or regular way.

Depending on size and distribution, pitting may be diagnostic for a specific disease, like psoriasis and alopecia areata are characterized by diagnostic pitting: in particular, in the first case they are large, irregular in shape, and distribution, while in alopecia areata of the nails, pits are superficial, regular, and geometrically distributed in lines.

### Onychorrhexis

The term onychorrhexis describes nail plate brittleness in longitudinal direction. It can involve the whole or a part of the nail plate. Disease commonly responsible of this sign are lichen planus (LP), trauma, tumors, etc.

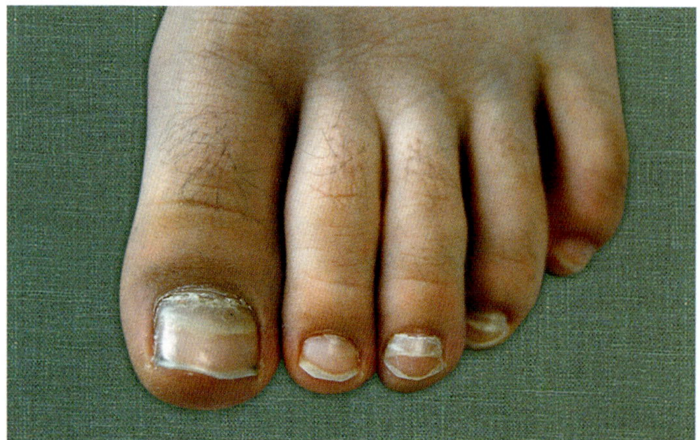

**FIG. 1:** Onychomadesis secondary to hand, foot, and mouth disease in a child.

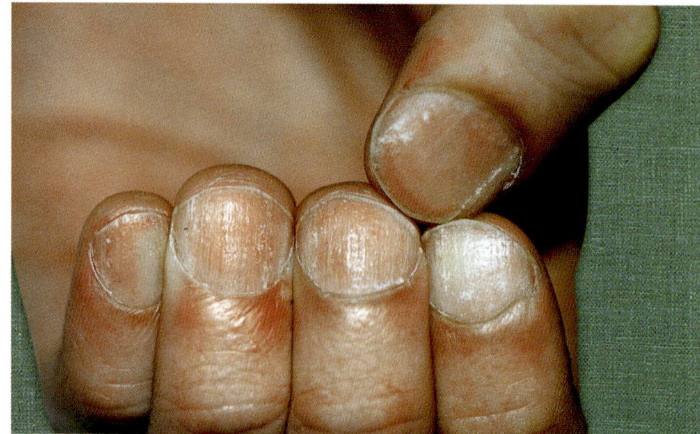

**FIG. 2:** Fine longitudinal striations covered by minute scales are typical of trachyonychia.

### Trachyonychia (Twenty Nail Dystrophy)

Trachyonychia is a sign of mild and diffuse damage to the proximal nail matrix caused by inflammatory disease like alopecia areata, nail psoriasis, LP, or eczema. It may also be idiopathic, congenital, and familial. A diffuse homogeneous roughness distinguishes this nail change (Fig. 2). The most common type presents with an opaque nail plate due to thin longitudinal striations covered by minute scales. Mild nail thinning can be present. The other variant is vertically striated sand paper dystrophy, which may be found in alopecia areata.

In some variants there may be spongiotic inflammation mediated by T-cell. Spongiotic trachyonychia seems to be associated with alopecia areata.

### Longitudinal Furrows

They are the result of a compression of the nail matrix by a tumor localized on the proximal nail fold, usually a mucous cyst or a fibroma/fibrokeratoma running through the plate length.

### Lamellar Nail Splitting (Onychoschizia Lamellina)

Household workers whose nails are constantly soaked in water or are subjected to repeated wear and tear, show splitting of the nails in lamellae along the distal border. This condition is more common in women and has also been reported in polycythemia vera and chondrodysplasia punctata and with intake of retinoids.

## Changes of the Nail Shape and Size

### Anonychia/Micronychia

One or several—all nails are very small or absent. It can be congenital or acquired (Table 2).

### Koilonychia (Spoon Nails)

The nail has an abnormal concavity, resembling a spoon. This nail change is common and transitory in the $2^{nd}$–$4^{th}$ toenails of children aging from 1 to 3-4 years, while in adults it is rare and

**TABLE 2: Causes of anonychia/micronychia**

| Congenital | Acquired |
|---|---|
| • Amniotic bands<br>• Teratogens (drugs, alcohol)<br>• Nail-patella syndrome<br>• Epidermolysis bullosa<br>• Ectodermal dysplasia<br>• DOOR syndrome<br>• Iso-Kikuchi syndrome | • Trauma<br>• Bullous diseases<br>• Idiopathic atrophy of the nails<br>• Psoriasiform acral dermatitis<br>• Ischemia |

DOOR, deafness, onychdystrophy, osteodystrophy, and mental retardation.

occurs in the fingernails because of a damage of the nail plate caused by irritant agents. It may be rarely a sign of severe iron deficiency anemia.

## Pincer Nails

The nails are transversally hypercurved, with their lateral edges traumatizing the lateral folds causing pain. This sign is rare in the fingernails, and it is related to exostosis or arthritis of the distal phalanx, while is common in the toenails of adults-elderly.

## Clubbing

The term clubbing describes a bulbous appearance of the digit, where the nail plate is enlarged and excessively curved. Its pathogenesis seems to be the accumulation of soft tissues around and underneath the nail plate, due to hypoxia caused by several respiratory and cardiac diseases. Causes of clubbing are listed in box 2.

## Pachyonychia/Onychogryphosis

In pachyonychia the nail plate is diffusely thickened, especially the distal portion of toenail, making difficult to cut it. Pachyonychia congenita is a very rare autosomal dominant skin disorder involving all nails and palms and soles.

Onychogryphosis describes a nail that resembles a claw or an oyster shell: the nail plate is thicker, yellow-brown in color, and distorted (Fig. 3). This condition is usually seen in the elderly with podiatric abnormalities or peripheral vascular deficiencies.

**BOX 2 Systemic condition associated with clubbing**

- Congenital\genetic
  - Congenital heart disease
  - Pulmonary arteriovenous malformations
  - Cystic fibrosis
  - Pachydermoperiostosis
- Acquired
  - Pulmonary/pleural neoplasm
  - Tuberculosis
  - Bronchiectasis
  - Sarcoidosis
  - Pulmonary fibrosis
  - Bacterial endocarditis
  - Congestive cardiac failure
  - Inflammatory bowel disease
  - Amebiasis, ascariasis
  - Liver disorders (hepatitis, cirrhosis)
  - HIV infection
  - Arterial graft sepsis
  - Thyroid disease (hyperthyroidism)
  - Secondary hyperparathyroidism

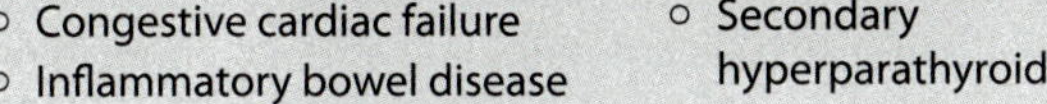

HIV, human immunodeficiency virus.

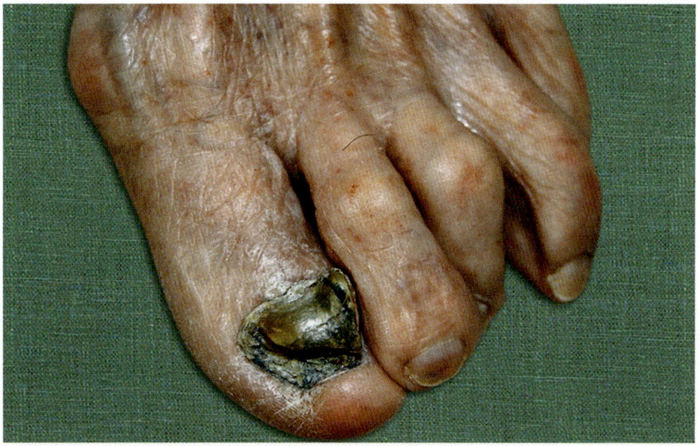

**FIG. 3:** Onychogryphosis—the nail plate is thick, yellow-brownish, and distorted.

# Changes of the Nail Color

## Leukonychia

This term describes a white discoloration of the nail and can be distinguished in three types, which are different in clinical appearance and pathogenesis.

- In true leukonychia, the nail plate is pigmented and the white color moves distally with nail growth. A defect of the keratinocytes of the distal nail matrix, with persistence of parakeratotic cells within the nail plate, causes the white discoloration, because these cells are light reflecting. Three types exist—punctate, striate, and diffuse
- In apparent leukonychia, the whitish discoloration disappears with pressure, as it is due to nail bed abnormalities. According to the clinical features, it can be distinguished in different types:
  - Terry's nails, commonly observed in patients with liver cirrhosis, where the whole nail is affected, except a 1–2 mm pink to brown distal b and, and the lunula may or may not be visible
  - Half and half nails (Lindsay's nails), observed in hemodialysis patients, where there is a definite border between the proximal area (opaque white) and the distal area (pink or reddish brown)
  - Muehrcke's lines, where multiple transverse whitish bands, parallel to the lunula are visible. This change is commonly seen after chemotherapy
- Pseudoleukonychia, where the nail discoloration has an exogenous origin, like in white superficial onychomycosis (WSO).

## Splinter Hemorrhages

They can be described as red-brown longitudinal lines in the distal portion of the nail, corresponding to hemorrhages of the blood capillaries of the nail bed. Splinter hemorrhages are usually due to trauma, psoriasis, and onychomycosis.

## Longitudinal Melanonychia

The term longitudinal melanonychia describes a longitudinal brown-gray or black band and is due to presence of melanin within the nail plate, due to nail matrix melanocytes activation.

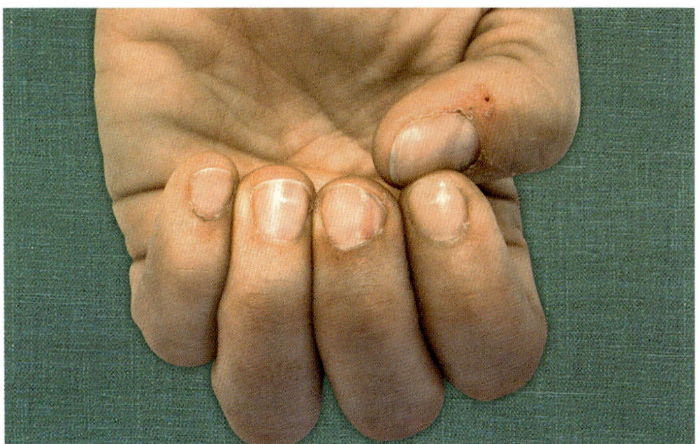
FIG. 4: Longitudinal erythronychia due to glomus tumor.

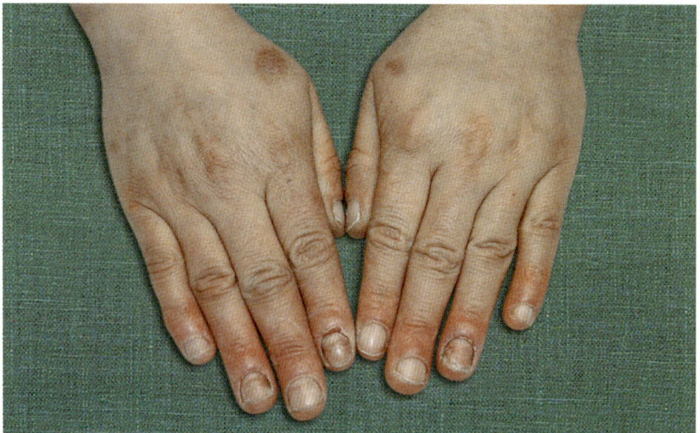
FIG. 5: Chronic paronychia.

The pigmentation may extend to the periungual soft tissues (Hutchinson's sign). We can therefore distinguish melanonychia due to melanocyte activation, and melanonychia due to benign (hyperplasia or nevus) or malignant (melanoma) proliferation. Diagnosis of the origin of melanonychia relies on clinical history, age and race of the patient, clinical examination and dermoscopy. A biopsy may be necessary for differential diagnosis.

### Longitudinal Erythronychia

This term describes a longitudinal red band, which originates at the lunula level up to the distal border. The red band is due to the presence of a subungual mass at the lunula level. An onychopapilloma or a subungual fibroma usually cause a single thin band with longitudinal nail plate fissure, while a glomus tumor typically produces a larger band (Fig. 4), as well as Bowen's disease. Multiple bands of erythronychia of several nails white bands and distal fissures are typical of Darier's disease.

## Changes of Nail Plate—Nail Bed Adhesion

### Onycholysis

The term describes detachment of the nail plate from the underlying nail bed. Pigmentation of the onycholytic area may occur as a consequence of microbial colonization or blood extravasation. Onycholysis is one of the most common nail signs and is usually not specific.

### Subungual Hyperkeratosis

The nail plate is detached and lifted up, with accumulation of scales under it, resulting in excessive proliferation of nail bed/ hyponychium keratinocytes. It is common in psoriasis, contact dermatitis, or in distal subungual onychomycosis (DSO).

## Changes of the Periungual Tissues

Changes of nail fold capillary patterns are typical of connective tissues diseases like systemic sclerosis, dermatomyositis, and systemic lupus erythematosus.

Capillary abnormalities include disorganization of the capillary architecture, dilated capillaries microhemorrhages, avascular areas, etc.

### Paronychia

Paronychia is an inflammation of the proximal and lateral nail folds, with erythema, swelling, pain, and pus production. The most common form is acute paronychia, which involves one fingernail as a result of a microtrauma or a bacterial infection, mainly in children.

Chronic paronychia is instead more frequent in adult females, which are in contact with irritants or water (Fig. 5) or often make manicure.

Other causes of acute paronychia of several digits, complicated by periungual pyogenic granulomas, are drugs, such as retinoids, antiretrovirals (indinavir), epidermal growth factor receptor (EGFR) inhibitors, etc.

Repetitive trauma of a nail spicule into the lateral soft tissues can determine ingrowing nail, characterized by paronychia and pyogenic granuloma.

# NAIL CHANGES IN DERMATOLOGICAL DISEASES

The most common inflammatory skin diseases that may involve the nail are psoriasis, LP, and other less common disorders, such as alopecia areata of the nails.

## Nail Psoriasis

Involvement of the nails occurs in up to 50% of patients with skin psoriasis, especially in adults and in case of severe disease. Interestingly, nail psoriasis is considered a risk factor for development of joint disease. Fingernail involvement is more common than toenail localization, where the pathology usually causes nonspecific signs like onycholysis and subungual hyperkeratosis. One or all nails may be affected, with various degrees of severity. Typical signs of nail psoriasis that allow diagnosis are: onycholysis with erythematous border (symptom of nail bed involvement); irregular pitting, which is typical of the fingernails and indicates nail matrix involvement, and salmon patches of the nail bed (oil drop sign), which appears as an irregular area of yellow-orange discoloration visible through the nail plate. These signs are often present together in the same patient and are typically well seen in the fingernails (Fig. 6). Other signs of nail psoriasis are nail plate surface abnormalities, subungual hyperkeratosis (common in toenails), splinter hemorrhages, and paronychia, but they are not diagnostic.

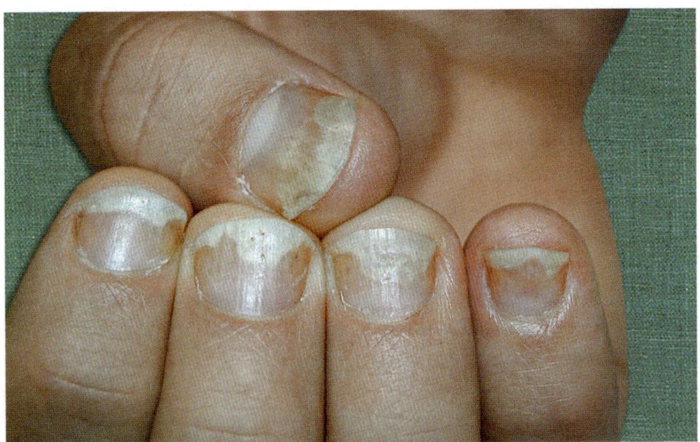

**FIG. 6:** Nail psoriasis presenting with onycholysis surrounded by an erythematous border.

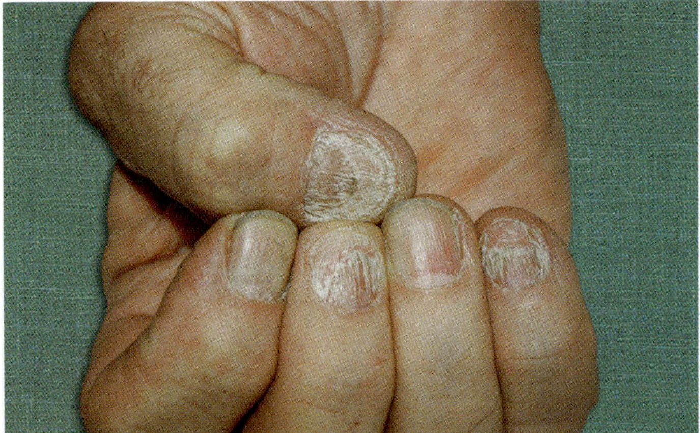

**FIG. 7:** Nail matrix lichen planus—longitudinal fissuring reaching the distal margin, nail plate thinning, and shortening.

### Differential Diagnosis

- Onychomycosis, as onycholysis and subungual hyperkeratosis are the clinical signs in toenails. Mycology is mandatory for diagnosis
- Idiopathic and traumatic onycholysis, where onycholysis is not surrounded by erythematous rim and subungual hyperkeratosis is not present
- Alopecia areata of the nails, in which pits are small and geometrically distributed.

Nail psoriasis has a chronic course and treatments are chosen in order to induce remission and maintain it, with the lower risk or side effects. The importance of trauma like manicure, nail biting, in triggering the disease should be explained to patients. Nails must be cut short.

Many topical therapies exist, like combination of betamethasone and calcipotriol, vitamin D3 analogs and tazarotene. Patients with involvement of a few nails may be treated with intralesional steroids like triamcinolone acetonide. In more severe cases, acitretin or methotrexate can be an option. When nail psoriasis is associated with involvement of other body sites, biologics can be considered. The use of these drugs for psoriasis limited to the nails is not approved.

### Pustular Psoriasis and Hallopeau's Acrodermatitis Continua

Pustular psoriasis may affect the nail, alone or in association with skin involvement. It is usually very painful and causes severe functional limitation and cosmetic discomfort. In the acute phase, the disease is characterized by periungual inflammation with formation of pustules and yellow crusts and onycholysis. In chronic phase, the nail shows subungual hyperkeratosis and periungual scaling. When one digit is involved (Hallopeau's acrodermatitis), differential diagnosis includes other causes of acute paronychia (bacterial/viral paronychia, eczema). Pustular psoriasis of several nails is associated with plantar or plantar skin involvement and is treated with systemic acitretin, at a dosage of 0.3–0.4 mg/kg/day, with good results. In Hallopeau's acrodermatitis continua, topical therapy with combination of steroids and vitamin D derivatives is the treatment of choice.

### Nail Lichen Planus

Nail abnormalities are present in about 10% of patients. Nail LP may however occur without skin or mucosal signs. Similarly to scalp LP, nail LP has an aggressive behavior that may lead to a scarring outcome.

Nail matrix LP is the most common type and is characterized by nail thinning with longitudinal ridging and fissuring (Fig. 7). Dorsal pterygium indicates irreversible destruction of a part of the nail matrix. In the toenails, clinical signs of LP are associated with marked nail thickening.

When suspecting nail LP, a longitudinal nail biopsy should be taken to confirm the diagnosis. Differential diagnosis includes systemic amyloidosis and graft versus host disease.

Treatment of nail LP is based on steroids: they can be locally injected if 1–3 nails are involved, or can be used systemically for 5–6 months (triamcinolone acetonide 0.5 mg/kg/month). Unfortunately, relapses after cure occur in about 60% of patients.

### Alopecia Areata of the Nails

Patients with alopecia areata often present with nail abnormalities including trachyonychia, geometric pitting, geometric leukonychia, mottled lunulae and onychomadesis, which are more common in children than in adults and in the most severe forms (alopecia areata totalis and universalis). Nail changes may involve one, several, or all nails. Evolution of nail signs does not parallel the course of alopecia.

## NAIL CHANGES IN SYSTEMIC DISEASES

### Yellow Nail Syndrome

The yellow nail syndrome (YNS) is a rare disorder, characterized by the triad: yellow nails, respiratory problems, and lymphedema. The three features are not always present together and the diagnosis can be done when two of them are present and even with nail changes alone. Pleuropulmonary symptoms and lymphedema usually precede the onset of nail signs of 3–5 years. The patient is typically an adult. A congenital abnormality of the lymphatic vessels is possibly involved in the pathogenesis of the syndrome.

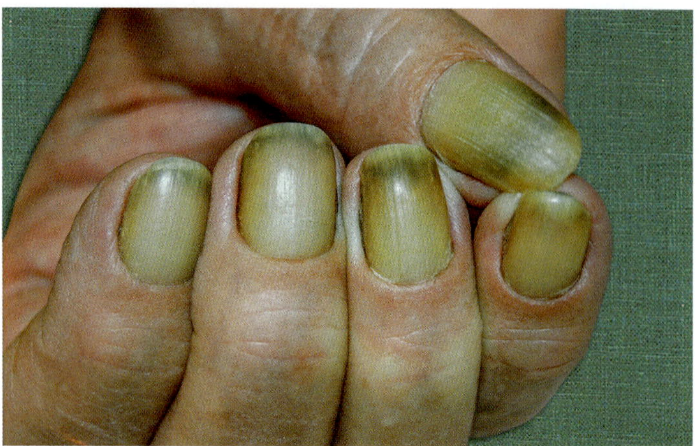

FIG. 8: Yellow nail syndrome—nail plate thickening and yellow-green discoloration is clearly evident.

Usually all 20 nails are involved. Diagnostic signs include: arrest or reduced nail growth, nail plate thickening, lack of cuticles, yellow-green discoloration, increased transverse curvature and onycholysis (Fig. 8). An ultrasound examination of lower limbs and chest X-ray are recommended. YNS may occasionally be paraneoplastic.

Treatment is based on oral vitamin E at doses of 1,200 IU/day for 8–12 months, that is effective in about 50% of the cases, or/in association of itraconazole in pulse regimen (400 mg/day for 1 week a month for 6–7 months).

### Autoimmune Connective Tissue Disorders

Abnormalities in the proximal nail fold capillaries are common in dermatomyositis, scleroderma, and lupus erythematosus. Pterygium inversum unguis is typical of scleroderma, together with parrot's beak nails.

### Peripheral Neuropathies

Depending on the severity of the nerve's injury, nail changes vary from Beau's lines, onychomadesis associated with pseudo-pyogenic granuloma, and necrosis.

### Clubbing

It can be isolated or part of the syndrome of hypertrophic osteoarthropathy, which includes periostosis of long bones, joint pain, and clubbing. Systemic conditions associated with clubbing are listed in box 1. Clubbing may be sometimes idiopathic and benign.

### Terry's Nails

Terry's nails, a variety of apparent leukonychia, are observed in patients with liver cirrhosis, congestive heart failure and adult-onset diabetes mellitus. They can also be observed in healthy individuals.

### Half and Half Nails

Half and half nails (Lindsay's nails) are frequent in patients with chronic renal disease, especially those in hemodialysis stage.

## NAIL CHANGES DUE TO DRUGS

Drug-induced nail abnormalities can present with a variety of clinical manifestations and they are often dose-related, disappearing after drug withdrawal. The drugs most commonly responsible are anticancer agents, including the classical drugs and the new ones, such as taxanes and tyrosine kinase inhibitors of the EGFR, retinoids and antiretrovirals.

Drug-induced nail changes usually involve several or all the 20 nails and appear in temporal correlation with the drug intake. The pathogenesis is not always readily explained, in most cases, nail alterations are the result of a toxic effect of the drug on the nail epithelia.

Clinical features of nail changes will depend on the extent of the damage and on the site of insult (Table 3). Antineoplastic agents may cause a reduction of growth rate, nail fragility, Mees lines and Beau's lines. Nail hyperpigmentation (total, transverse or longitudinal melanonychia) can occur with the use of cyclophosphamide, hydroxyurea, and fluoropyrimidines (e.g., 5-fluorouracil) and especially with the use of anthracyclines (e.g., doxorubicin, daunorubicin). Painful onycholysis and subungual abscesses are a common side effect of taxanes (e.g., docetaxel, paclitaxel) and anthracyclines (e.g., doxorubicin). Ingrown nails with paronychia and pyogenic granulomas are associated with the use of tyrosine kinase inhibitors of the EGFR (e.g., erlotinib, gefitinib).

Painful hemorrhagic onycholysis (Fig. 9) and subungual abscesses may be the result of the use of taxanes (docetaxel,

**TABLE 3: The most common nail changes caused by systemic drugs**

| Affected area | Symptoms |
|---|---|
| Matrix | • Beau's lines<br>• Onychomadesis<br>• Nail fragility<br>• Melanonychia |
| Nail bed | • Onycholysis<br>• Photo-onycholysis<br>• Hemorrhagic onycholysis<br>• Apparent leukonychia |
| Nail folds | • Paronychia<br>• Pyogenic granulomas |
| Vessels | • Subungual hemorrhages<br>• Ischemia |

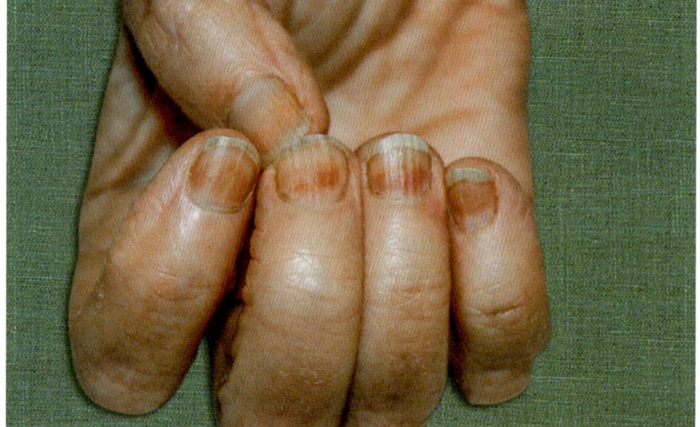

FIG. 9: Hemorrhagic onycholysis of the fingernail due to taxanes.

paclitaxel), anthracyclines (doxorubicin), and immunosuppressive drugs (sirolimus, rituximab, and methotrexate), which cause epidermolysis and loss of adhesion of the nail plate to the nail bed, with formation of a hemorrhagic blister.

Clipping away the onycholytic nail plate, the nail bed is exposed, avoiding bacterial infection thanks to antimicrobial solution for daily soaking, followed by application of creams with combination of steroids and antibiotics as local therapy. Acute paronychia with pyogenic granulomas is a possible side effect of several drugs (taxanes, capecitabine), is usually dose-related and intensely painful. Although uncommon, photo-onycholysis is a side effect of tetracyclines, taxanes, psoralens and photodynamic therapy. Topical drugs may induce nail changes, like dyschromia and irritant or allergic contact dermatitis.

## NAIL INFECTIVE DISEASES

### Onychomycosis

Onychomycosis is the most common nail infective disorder. It is frequent in the toenails of elderly, where it can reach a prevalence of 40%. Three main clinical varieties of onychomycosis are described, according to typical clinical features. Total onychomycosis is characterized by the involvement of the nail plate.

In most of the cases onychomycosis is caused by dermatophytes, *Trichophyton rubrum* or *Trichophyton interdigitale.* Nondermatophytes, like *Scopulariopsis brevicaulis, Fusarium solani or Fusarium oxysporum, Aspergillus* spp. and *Acremonium* spp., are responsible of 15% of cases; *Candida* nail infection is more rare and occurs only when predisposing factors are present, including immunosuppression and diabetes. Clinical diagnosis of onychomycosis always requires laboratory confirmation.

### Distal Subungual Onychomycosis

Fungi reach the nail through the hyponychium, invading the undersurface of the nail unit plate spreading proximally. In general, DSO involves one or both the great toenails and Tinea pedis plantaris (moccasin-type) is often associated. The nail plate appears with yellow-white, is detached due to onycholysis, with distal subungual hyperkeratosis (Fig. 10).

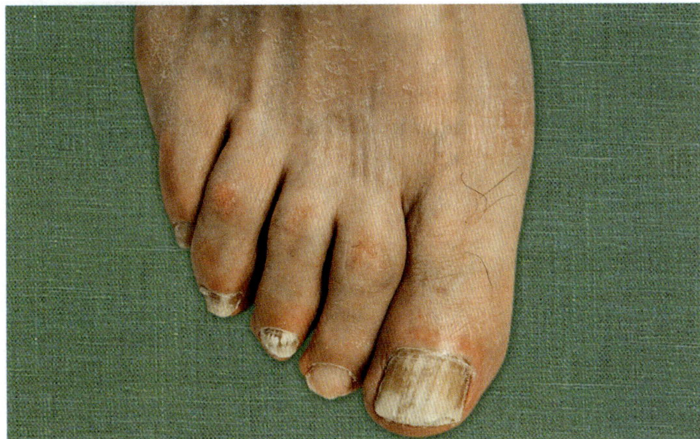

**FIG. 10:** Distal subungual onychomycosis.

A subungual accumulation of hyphae and scales, called dermatophytoma, is a possible presentation of distal subungual onychomycosis due to dermatophytes, and it is scarcely reached by antifungals. Distal subungual onychomycosis may be associated with black pigmentation of the nail, when the pathogen is the melanoides variant of *Trichophyton rubrum.* When a marked periungual inflammation is present, we should suspect onychomycosis due to non-dermatophytes. Differential diagnosis of DSO include traumatic onycholysis (usually symmetrical, and subungual hyperkeratosis is absent) and nail psoriasis (diffuse hyperkeratosis, several/all toenail involved).

### White Superficial Onychomycosis

Fungi invade the dorsal nail plate, forming white opaque formations, easily scraped away. It is exclusive of the toenails. The classical form is due to *Trichophyton interdigitale*, but also *Fusarium* spp. and other molds may cause a WSO causing a deeper nail invasion. Tinea pedis interdigitalis (Athlete's foot) due to *T. interdigitale* is commonly associated.

Differential diagnosis includes superficial nail fragility due to prolonged wearing of nail polish and transverse toenail leukonychia due to trauma.

### Proximal Subungual Onychomycosis

Fungi reach the ventral part of the proximal nail plate via proximal nail fold, so they are located under the proximal part of the nail. Proximal subungual onychomycosis (PSO) due to dermatophytes is very rare and is characterized by a white area under the proximal nail plate, in the lunula area. The form due to *Trichophyton rubrum* was considered as a sign of AIDS, but can be seen in immunocompetent individuals. *Aspergillus* spp. and *Fusarium* spp. which as mentioned are nondermatophyte mold infection, instead, can often cause a PSO. This form is associated with acute periungual inflammation with possible pus formation. Differential diagnosis includes acute bacterial paronychia.

### Total Onychomycosis

It results from all types of nail invasion, especially from long-standing DSO. The nail plate is diffusely thickened, friable, and yellowish.

### Treatment of Onychomycosis

It depends on clinical type, number of involved nails, and severity of the infection.

- *Topical treatment*: Nail lacquers are effective in monotherapy, for 6–12 months, in the treatment of WSO and of DSO located to the distal nail of few digits. Other possible options include amorolfine or ciclopirox in nonwater soluble lacquers and ciclopirox in water-soluble nail lacquer, applied once a day at bed time. Efinaconazole 10% nail solution is new promising treatment
- *Systemic treatment*: Systemic treatment is required for DSO extending to the proximal nail and PSO due to dermatophytes. Terbinafine (250 mg daily or as "pulse therapy" at the dosage of 500 mg daily for 1 week a month) or itraconazole (administered in pulse therapy at the dosage of 400 mg daily for 1 week a month) are very effective treatment, even

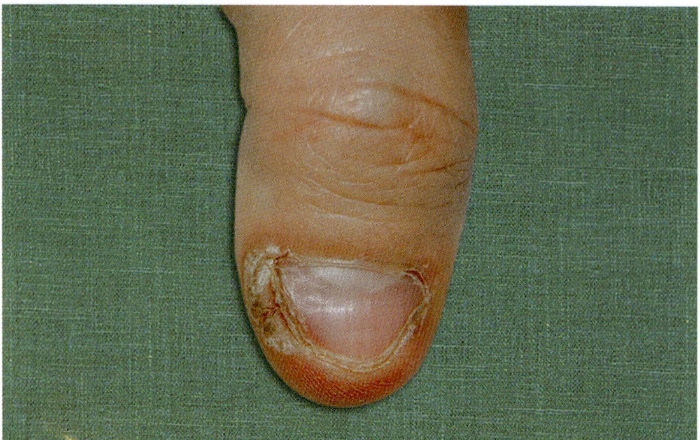

FIG. 11: Periungual viral wart.

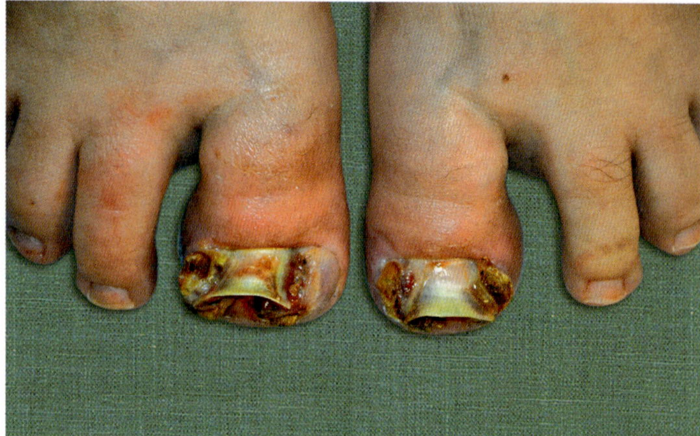

FIG. 12: Pyogenic granulomas due to ingrowing toenail.

associated with topical nail lacquers. Treatment duration is 6 weeks for fingernails and 3–4 months for toenails. Periodic removal of the affected nail plate, done by a podiatrist or by topical application of urea ointment may speed cure. Recurrences and reinfection are not uncommon, ranging up to 20% of cured patient.

## Viral Warts

Viral warts [human papillomavirus (HPV)-related] are periungual masses with rough surface, which induce onycholysis and subungual/periungual keratotic mass. Diagnosis is usually very easy and facilitates by dermoscopy, which shows a demarcated hyperkeratosis with small hemorrhages (Fig. 11). Long-standing lesions of the nail bed should be biopsied if they are nonresponding to therapy, as they may be Bowen's disease.

Treatment choice depends on number and location of the warts and on patient age. Single warts can be treated with keratolytic agents, like salicylic acid in concentrations ranging from 20–60%. Other therapies include cryotherapy, $CO_2$ laser, Er:YAG laser, pulsed dye laser, topical immunotherapy, or intralesional bleomycin.

### Herpes Simplex Infection (Herpetic Whitlow)

The classical clinical presentation is that of an acute recurring paronychia with pulsating pain, frequently misdiagnosed as a bacterial paronychia. In the typical case, one finger shows grouped vesicles appearing in 1–2 days. Clinical examination, Tzanck smear and cultures are important for diagnosis. Treatment should be started in the first 1–2 days: options include systemic antivirals and topical antibiotics, used to prevent superimposed bacterial infection.

# NAIL TUMORS

## Benign Tumors

### Pyogenic Granuloma (Botriomycoma)

Pyogenic granuloma is a common acquired benign vascular tumor that frequently involves the nail, including the periungual tissues and the nail bed. The tumor appears as a bleeding, friable, and soft red nodule. When localized in the nail bed, it appears as a red macule associated with oozing and onycholysis. Common causes of pyogenic granulomas include ingrowing toenails (Fig. 12), mechanical trauma, and drugs. Treatment is surgical. Topical application of high potency steroids (clobetasol propionate ointment) may reduce the lesions, decreasing inflammation and pain.

### Fibroma/Fibrokeratoma

It is a very common benign tumor usually arising from the proximal nail fold, subungual location being rare. Multiple fibrokeratomas (Koenen tumors) are a pathognomonic feature tuberous sclerosis disease, and usually appear after puberty in up to 50% of patients. A fibrokeratoma is characterized by a hyperkeratotic tip and may be surrounded by a collarette of raised skin. Periungual fibrokeratoma appears as pink filiform mass with hyperkeratotic tip originating from the proximal nail fold. Typically, compression of the underlying nail matrix produces a longitudinal groove in the nail plate. Sometimes, fibrokeratoma may grow underneath the nail plate producing a longitudinal erythronychia or onycholysis. Clinical features are usually diagnostic, but only histopathology can confirm the clinical suspicion.

### Myxoid Cyst (Mucoid Cyst)

It is the most common nail tumor, often occurring in adult-old women affected by osteoarthritis of the terminal joints. They appear as small soft nodules located in the proximal nail fold of fingernails, and a viscous transparent fluid from underneath the proximal nail fold can be present, due to cyst discharge (Fig. 13). Physical examination can be added of ultrasound and MRI, which is mandatory for myxoid cysts located under the nail plate. Recurrences after surgery are common, and other cyst may arise in different digits.

### Onychopapilloma

It is a frequent tumor that usually involves one fingernail, producing a thin (1–3 mm) longitudinal band of erythronychia starting from the lunula region and reaching the distal margin, where it can be associated with onycholysis or with a fissure (Fig. 14). Splinter hemorrhages are often present, especially in the distal part of the band. Histopathology is mandatory.

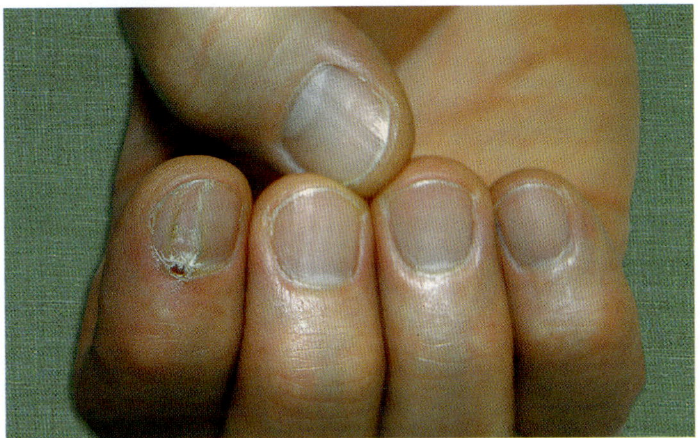

FIG. 13: Mucoid cyst.

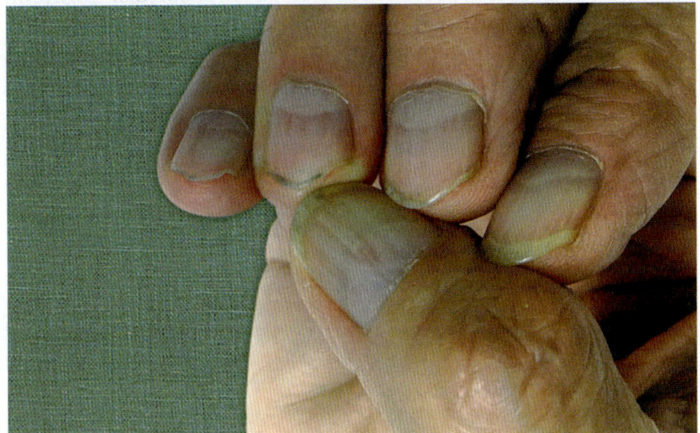

FIG. 14: Onychopapilloma appears as a thin longitudinal band of erythronychia starting from the lunula region, associated with a fissure.

Bands that produce only discoloration may be followed in time, while surgical removal is necessary when the tumor produce a distal fissure of the nail, which causes discomfort in manual activities.

## Subungual Exostosis

Subungual exostosis is a benign bone tumor of the distal phalanx beneath the nail and the most common nail tumor of young adults. The tumor appears as a pink-colored firm subungual mass under the free edge of the nail, which is detached and uplifted. It can also rise under the central part of the nail, increasing nail transverse curvature and producing pincer deformity (Fig. 15). X-ray is mandatory and surgical removal of the bone overgrowth is necessary. Recurrences are not rare, occurring in up to 20% of the cases.

## Glomus Tumor

It is an uncommon tumor of the neuromyoarterial glomus bodies located in the nail bed dermis.

The 1st and 2nd fingernails are the most common localizations. Subjective symptoms typically exceed clinical signs. The clinical triad of intense paroxysmal pain, localized tenderness and sensitivity to cold is a typical feature of the tumor. When visible, this tumor is a red-purple subungual mass, resembling a longitudinal. Bigger masses may be associated with onycholysis, nail plate thinning and fissuring. MRI permits detection of the subungual lesion, which can also be seen by ultrasound if bigger than 3 mm in diameter. Surgical removal is mandatory.

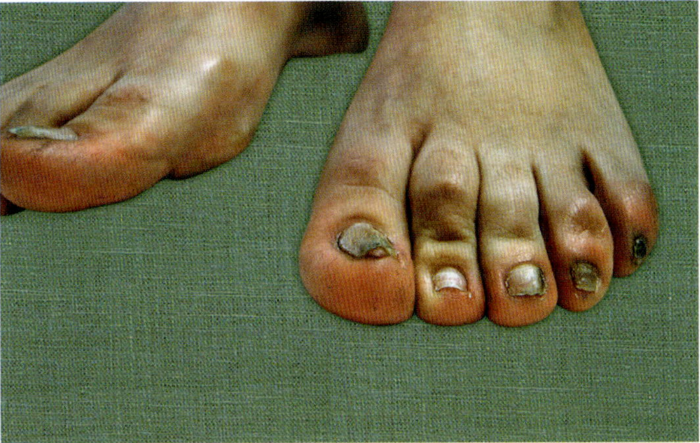

FIG. 15: Increasing nail transverse curvature and pincer deformity due to subungual exostosis.

## Onychomatricoma

It is a rare nail tumor arising from the epithelium and the connective tissue of the nail matrix, which produces localized or diffuse nail thickening and yellow discoloration with longitudinal lines involving the whole or part of the nail plate. Sometimes, splinter hemorrhages can be visible. At the distal margin of the nail, dermoscopy shows the honeycomb holes that correspond to the tunnels within the tumor.

## Nail Matrix Nevi

They produce total nail brown-black pigmentation or band of longitudinal melanonychia. The most important criterion for diagnosis of nail matrix nevi is the onset in childhood of a band of melanonychia. In Caucasian children, the ABCD should not be applied in evaluating a band of melanonychia.

The clinical and dermoscopic characteristics of nail matrix nevi are in fact not diagnostic, as these lesions are often irregular with tendency to modification in time, indicating increasing of the melanogenic activity of the melanocytes, and not malignant transformation.

Pigmentation of the periungual tissues, a well-known criterion suggestive for nail melanoma in adults (Hutchinson's sign), in often present in children, as nevi may be located both in the nail and in the periungual skin. Therefore, in children, this feature is a sign of nevus. Histopathology permits the definitive diagnosis of nail matrix nevus.

# Malignant Tumors

## Bowen's Disease and Squamous Cell Carcinoma

Squamous cell carcinoma (SCC) *in situ* variety (Bowen's disease) is the most common malignant tumor of the nail. Exposure to ionizing radiation, chronic trauma and HPV type 16 are predisposing factors. SCC usually involves one fingernail, especially the 2nd and 3rd of the dominant hand. Clinical features include a warty aspect of the exposed nail bed and lateral nail fold, with lateral onycholysis.

The presence of a band of melanonychia in the nail plate adjacent to a warty nail bed is diagnostic of Bowen's disease. Subungual erosion with mild serum oozing from under the nail is another way of presentation of the tumor.

Surgical removal is the rule for invasive SCC and it is the best approach for Bowen's disease, in particular, the Mohs micrographic. Other noninvasive techniques, including photodynamic therapy, 5% fluorouracil cream or 5% imiquimod cream after curettage are valid options but they are burdened by a high incidence of relapses.

Nail SCC tends to become an invasive tumor more quickly, bony involvement may occur but metastases are very rare.

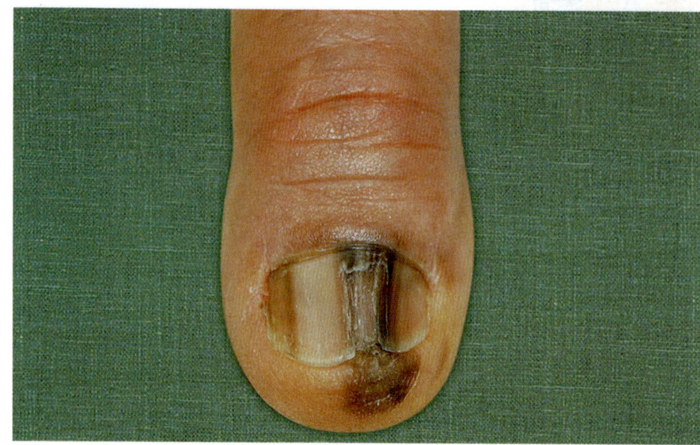

**FIG. 16:** Nail melanoma with Hutchinson's sign.

## Melanoma

Nail melanoma represents the 1–2% of melanomas in Caucasians, 10–23% in Asians and 25% in Afro-Americans. It is characterized by a bad prognosis and a delayed diagnosis.

Nail melanoma is typically located in the first digit of hand and feet, where it presents as a band of longitudinal melanonychia of a single digit. The ABCDEF rule proposed some parameters to helping early diagnosis of subungual melanoma: (A) Age—peak incidence $5^{th}$–$7^{th}$ decades with Africans, Asians, and Native Americans, in particular dark skinned races, representing up to one-third of all cases; (B) Black or brown band with a width of 3 mm or more; (C) Change in the nail or lack of improved change with treatment; (D) Digit most commonly involved (as mentioned, usually finger or thumb); (E) Extension of pigment into the proximal or lateral nail-fold, which is called Hutchinson's sign; and (F) Family or personal history of dysplastic nevus or melanoma. This last criterion is considerate not relevant for nail melanoma compared to the others.

A nail melanoma should be suspected when facing a band of a single digit with onset in adulthood without any cause that could explain its origin. The band of melanonychia is typically dark black in color and its width is broader than 3–4 mm.

Other clinical features include the destruction of the nail plate, and the Hutchinson's sign (Fig. 16), that is well visible with dermoscopy. A pigmentation of periungual tissue seen with dermatoscope but not with naked eye is called micro-Hutchinson's sign, and even in this case, dermoscopy helps the diagnosis. Clinical features, the history of the nail pigmentation and dermoscopy are all factors to consider together.

One-fourth of nail melanomas are amelanotic, characterized by the lack of melanin pigment, absence of the nail plate and nail bed hyperkeratosis or ulceration.

Excision is mandatory. Conservative surgery is indicated in melanoma *in situ*. The most important indicator of prognosis is the American Joint Committee on Cancer stage at diagnosis. In addition, thickness of the lesion (Breslow classification), depth of invasion (Clark level), presence of ulceration, absence of pigment, and histopathological data as infiltration by lymphocytes, and mitotic rate are also relevant. Melanoma metastasis affects typically regional lymph nodes. Invasive nail melanoma has a worse prognosis than cutaneous melanoma, mainly because the diagnosis is delayed. In addition, melanoma in acral sites has a very aggressive behavior. The prognosis is poor, with a 15 years survival rate of about 35%.

## SUGGESTED READINGS


1. de Berker D. Erythronychia. Dermatol. 2012;25(6):603-11.
2. Hasegawa M. Dermoscopy findings if nail fold capillaries in connective tissue disease. J Dermatol. 2011;38(1):66-70.
3. Herschthal J. McLeod MP, Zaiac M. Management of ungual warts. Dermatol Ther. 2012;25(6):545-50.
4. Lecerf P, Richert B, Theunis A, et al. A retrospective study of squamous cell carcinoma of the nail unit diagnosed in a Belgian general hospital over a 15-year period. J Am Acad Dermatol. 2013;69:253-61.
5. Piraccini BM, Alessandrini A, Bruni F, et al. Acute periungueal dermatitis induced by application of urea-containing cream under occlusion. J Dermatol Case Rep. 2012;6:18-20.
6. Piraccini BM, Alessandrini A. Drug-induced nail changes. Clin Dermatol. 2013;31:618-26.
7. Piraccini BM, Gianni C. Update on the management of onychomycosis. G Ital Dermatol Venereol. 2013;148(6):633-8.
8. Piraccini BM, Urciuoli B, Starace M, et al. Yellow nail syndrome: clinical experience in a series of 21 patients. J Dtsch Dermatol Ges. 2014;12(2):131-7.
9. Samaniego E, Crespo A, Sanz A. Key diagnostic features and treatment of subungual glomus tumor. Actas Dermosifiliogr. 2009;100:875-82.
10. Spicknall KE, Zirwas MJ, English JC 3rd. Clubbing: an update on diagnosis, differential diagnosis, pathophysiology, and clinical relevance. J Am Acad Dermatol. 2005;52:1020-8.
11. Tosti A, Baran R, Piraccini BM, et al. Nail matrix nevi: a clinical and histopathologic study of twenty-two patients. J Am Acad Dermatol. 1996;34:765-71.
12. Tosti A, Piraccini BM, de Farias DC. Dealing with melanonychia. Semin Cutan Med Surg. 2009;28:49-54.
13. Zaias N. The Nail in Health and Diseases, 2nd edition. Connecticut: Appleton & Lange; 1990.

# 19 SECTION Nevi, Neoplasia and Related Disorders

# 72 CHAPTER Nevi and Related Disorders

*Nilendu Sarma, Sayantani Chakraborty*

## INTRODUCTION

"Nevi" or birth marks are circumscribed, fixed, non-neoplastic cutaneous or mucosal lesions. Mostly, they arise early but can manifest later.

Cutaneous hamartoma is defined as increase or decrease of a given cellular structure and thus the lesions may comprise of abnormal mixture of a tissue's usual components.

Nevi originate due to genetic mosaicism and never show malignant neoplasia with the exception of melanocytic nevi. Nevi are not transmissible to offspring unless the mutation involves gonadal cells.

## CLASSIFICATION OF NEVI

Nevi can be of following types:

- Nevomelanocytic nevi
- Epidermal nevi
- Dermal and subcutaneous nevi
- Vascular nevi
- Nevus syndromes (syndromes with venous malformation, epidermal nevus syndromes).

## EPIDERMAL NEVI

Epidermal nevi are noncancerous hamartomatous patch of skin comprised of epithelium. They develop at birth or may develop later. Often, they are distributed along the lines of Blaschko.

### Classification

Epidermal nevi have been classified based on the predominant histological cell types of differentiation. Epidermal nevi showing involvement of only keratinocytes are called keratinocytic nevi or non organoid nevi. Other group showing prominent differentiation toward some adnexal structures, such as sebaceous glands, hair follicle, and apocrine or eccrine glands are called organoid nevi. Common organoid nevi are sebaceous nevi, eccrine nevi, apocrine nevi, and follicular nevi.

Pure keratinocytic nevus may have histological presence of epidermolysis and based on these findings, this has been divided into epidermolytic and nonepidermolytic variety.

### Pathogenesis

This has been subclassified based on their histopathological characteristics into two subtypes—(1) epidermolytic and (2) non-epidermolytic.

Epidermolytic hyperkeratosis literally means presence of perinuclear vacuolization of the keratinocytes as well as premature and excessive formation of the keratohyaline granules. This is seen in bullous ichthyosiform erythroderma (BIE) which is a generalized disease that develop due to mutation in *KRT1* and *KRT10* genes. It is important to note that although by rule nevi are always sporadic and not transmitted to the next generation, this may happen in some special situation. If same mutation also affects gonadal cells, this will be transmitted to the offspring who will develop BIE.

In contrast, nonepidermolytic verrucous epidermal nevi (VEN) may develop due to various mutations and many of these are yet not known. Epidermal nevi have been reported to harbor activating fibroblast growth factor receptor 3 (*FGFR3*) mutations, which is also present in some low-grade malignant bladder tumors and acquired benign conditions like seborrheic keratoses. Recently, activating mutations of the p110 subunit of phosphoinositide-3-kinase (*PIK3CA*) with substitution at E542K, E545K and H1047R oncogene that have been identified in a broad spectrum of malignant tumors has also been detected to be present in some epidermal nevi with a different spot of substitution (E545G). *HRAS* mutation is reported to cause epidermal nevi. *PTEN* is implicated in epidermal nevi associated with Proteus syndrome (PS).

Proposed mechanism of inflammatory linear verrucous epidermal nevus (ILVEN) is occurrence of "rescue" mosaicism for a dominant mutation that would be otherwise lethal. According to Happle, it may reflect the action of partly expressed and partly silenced "retrotransposons", a retroviral transposable element, infected at an early stage of development.

### Clinical Features

Epidermal nevi are usually present at birth and are persistent. Prevalence of these nevi in adults is between 0.1% and 0.5% with equal sex distribution.

Clinical manifestations vary widely. The lesion starts at birth with a white macerated appearance which later becomes pink velvety streaks and gradually as age progresses, it becomes darker and warty. In flexural areas the lesions may become macerated and foul smelling (Fig. 1).

Distribution may be limited or wide and extensive. Generally they are distributed along Blaschko's lines but may show different patterns like round or ovoid shapes (PENS syndrome) (Fig. 2).

They may be flat or raised, papular, verrucous, and may show signs of inflammation. ILVEN appears as pruritic, erythematous scaly (Fig. 3). Clinically, the lesions appear psoriasiform (clinically and histopathologically) and are eczematous. This appears within first 5 years of life, mostly by first 6 months. Commonly unilateral, but it may be bilateral and widespread.

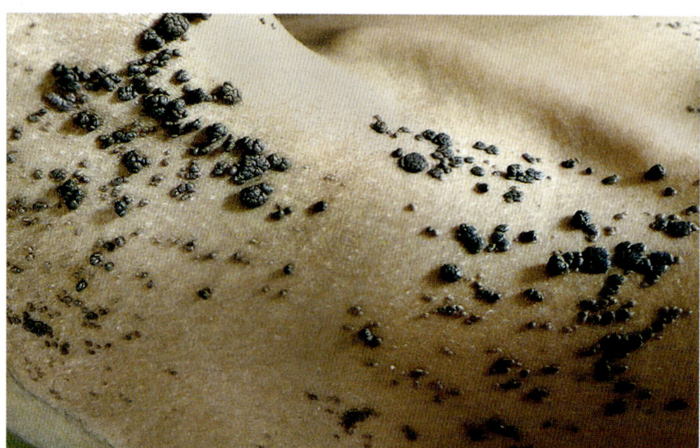

**FIG. 1:** Warty papular eruptions in verrucous epidermal nevi.

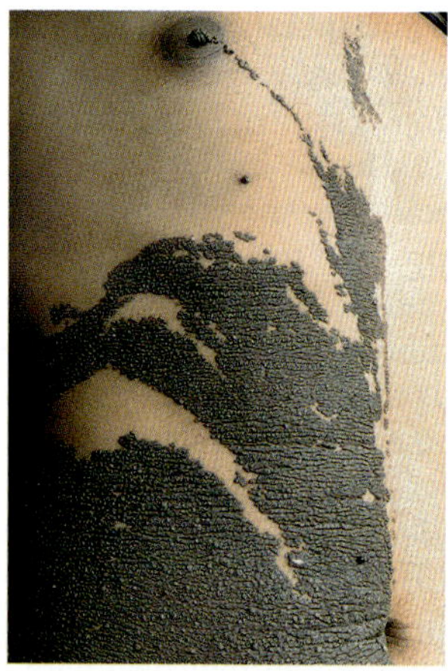

**FIG. 2:** Extensive epidermal nevi in Blaschkoid distribution.

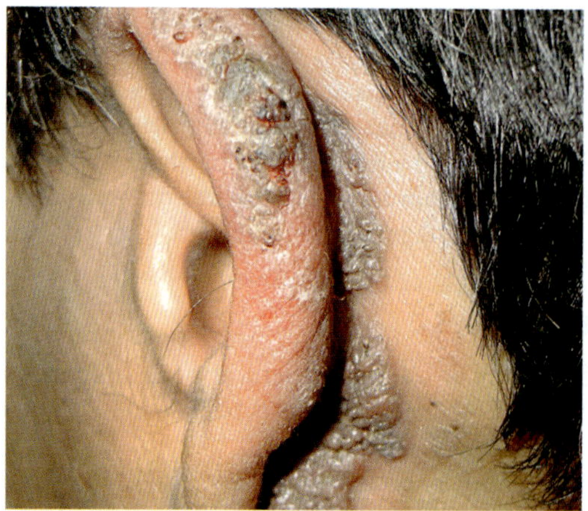

**FIG. 3:** Inflammatory linear verrucous epidermal nevus.
*Courtesy*: Dr Devesh Shukla.

They may be the sole manifestation without any systemic involvement or may be associated with different types of nevi and other systemic involvement (syndromic) as in Proteus syndrome and Congenital hemidysplasia with ichthyosiform erythroderma and limb defects (CHILD) syndrome. Few syndromic entities have been proposed in recent times. These are *PIK3CA*-related overgrowth syndrome, PENS syndrome, HRAS mosaicism (RASopathy), and *FGFR3* epidermal nevus syndrome.

## Histopathology

Nonepidemolytic epidermal nevi show hyperkeratosis, acanthosis, and papillomatosis with focal hypergranulosis. Epidermolytic variety shows presence of epidermolytic hyperkeratoses. ILVEN shows columns of hypergranulosis with orthokeratotic hyperkeratosis, columns of agranulosis with parakeratotic hyperkeratosis and occasional spongiosis.

## Management

Topical therapies may decrease the hyperkeratosis to certain degree; these are salicylic acid, lactic acid, or retinoic acid. Few cases treated with calcipotriol, 5-fluorouracil, and retinoic acid have responded well. Systemic therapy with acitretin or isotretinoin may alleviate the hyperkeratosis in epidermolytic type of lesions.

For successful surgical treatment the underlying dermis needs to be removed along with removal of the epidermal component. Cryotherapy may be used for smaller lesions. Multiple sessions with $CO_2$ laser (pulsed or continuous mode) have been used with success in selected cases. Newer Er-YAG lasers with high coagulative capacity and minimal tissue destruction may produce good clearance without major tissue destruction and scarring.

Overall, ILVEN is resistant to treatment. Calcipotriol may show prolonged clearance. Potent topical corticosteroid under occlusion may provide symptomatic relief. Other options are cryotherapy and flashlamp-pumped pulsed tunable dye laser. $CO_2$ laser resurfacing may also clear the lesion.

## CHILD Nevus and CHILD Syndrome

CHILD nevus is characterized by congenital hemidysplasia with ichthyosiform nevus and limb defects. The "CHILD syndrome" features association of CHILD nevus, and various other extracutaneous features.

### Clinical Features

CHILD nevus appears as asymptomatic, well-circumscribed areas of erythema, waxy scaling and often, verrucous surface distributed in a linear pattern along the Blaschko's lines, closely mimicking ILVEN but involving wider areas of one half of body with distinctive "lateralization". There might be a tendency toward flexural involvement. Bony defects and various other systemic defects are associated. Hypoplasia of metacarpals/phalanges to complete absence of the limbs, unilateral hypoplasia of the brain, cranial nerves or spinal cord, mental retardation, and sensory defects are seen.

### Pathogenesis

Defective cholesterol metabolism during early embryogenesis is the key mechanism. There is paroxysomal deficiency in the fibroblasts with elevated plasma 8-dehydrocholesterol and 8(9)-cholesterol. This is caused by mutation in the *NSDHL* gene (nicotinamide adenine dinucleotide phosphate steroid dehydrogenase like protein), required for cholesterol biosynthesis.

### Histopathology

Histopathologically, there is orthokeratosis along with areas of marked acanthosis and parakeratosis. There is focal collection of neutrophils and the dermis contains patchy lymphohistiocytic infiltrates. There may be lipid-laden histiocytes in the dermal papillae.

### Treatment

This condition is extremely resistant to treatment. However, retinoids can be tried.

## Nevus Sebaceous of Jadassohn

Nevus sebaceous was described by Jadassohn in 1895. This is an epidermal hamartoma composed predominantly of sebaceous glands but also consists of epidermal, follicular, and apocrine elements.

### Pathogenesis

Nevus sebaceous is a sporadic disorder reflecting lethal genes rescued by mosaicism; occasionally familial cases are found. Mutation in *HRAS* gene and *KRAS* gene is found. The same mutations are also found in Schimmelpenning syndrome. Development of secondary tumors is proposed to develop due to these particular mutations.

### Clinical Features

Nevus sebaceous involves 0.3% of all neonates with equal sex distribution. The most common sites of involvement are head and neck region involving the scalp, ears, forehead, and central part of the face in the descending order.

It has three stages of evolution. Initially, there is papillomatous epithelial hyperplasia and underdeveloped hairs. Clinically, this appears as a bald patch, or smooth surfaced circumscribed slightly raised pinkish/yellowish orange plaques.

This is followed by hyperplasia of the sebaceous glands along with epidermal verrucous hyperplasia and maturation of apocrine glands during the puberty. At this stage, it appease as verrucous, hyperpigmented nodule or plaque (Fig. 4).

In the third stage, benign and malignant epithelial neoplasm may develop in 5% of the cases. The most common malignancy arising from nevus sebaceous is basal cell carcinoma. Other malignant tumors are squamous cell carcinoma, sebaceous carcinoma, trichilemmal carcinoma, etc. Benign tumors like syringocystadenoma papilliferum and trichoblastoma may also develop from the lesion.

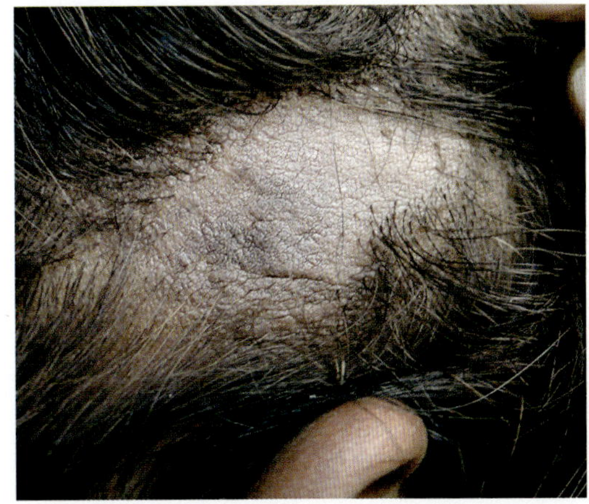

**FIG. 4:** Nevus sebaceous with verrucous surface.

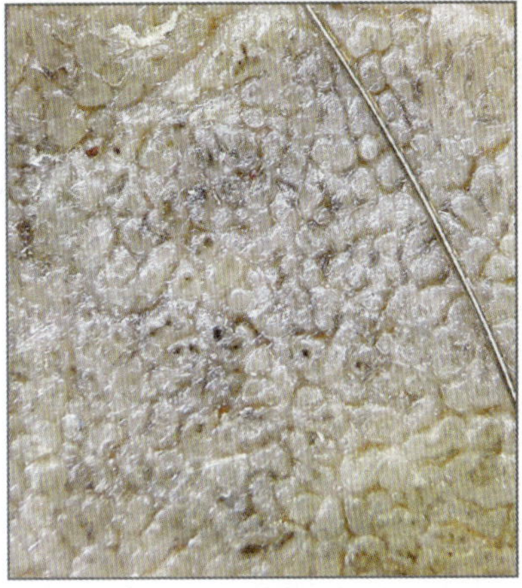

**FIG. 5:** Cerebriform appearance in dermatoscopy in nevus sebaceous.

### Dermatoscopy

Dermatoscopy in early childhood stages shows yellowish globular structures and cerebriform appearance in full developed adult stages (Fig. 5).

### Histopathology

Histopathologically, in the early and underdeveloped lesion, the sebaceous and apocrine glands are sparse and underdeveloped. Cords and buds of poorly differentiated epithelial cells representing primordial pilosebaceous follicles are the diagnostic features. In developed lesion, slight to prominent epidermal hyperplasia is noted. It may be simple, verrucous, seborrheic keratosis-like, and acrochordon type. Sebaceous glands may appear absolutely normal and as in normal follicle, these may be present, absent, immature, or hyperplastic. Basaloid epithelial proliferation of cells that are basically immature hair germs may be found. These often mimic basal cell carcinoma (Fig. 6).

### Treatment

Recurrence may occur following superficial dermabrasion, $CO_2$ laser, or electrosurgery. Excision of scalp lesion with primary closure gives an excellent cosmetic result.

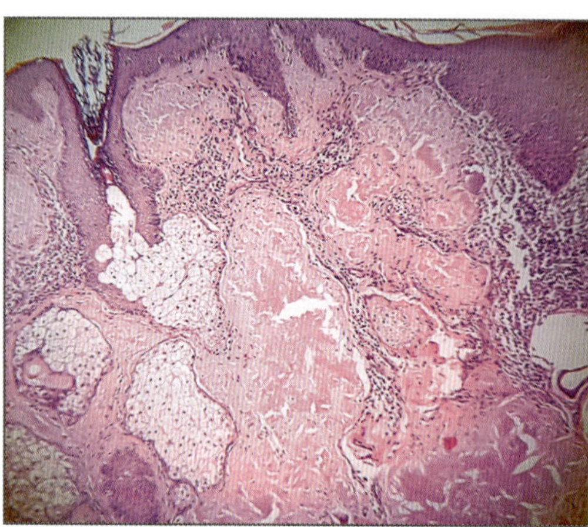

FIG. 6: Histopathology of nevus sebaceous showing proliferation of mature sebaceous cells, epidermal hyperplasia, and dilated infundibula with keratin plug but absence of mature hair follicular cells.

## Nevus Sebaceous Syndromes

Sebaceous nevi are associated with two syndromes: (1) Linear nevus sebaceous syndrome (LNSS) and (2) Muir–Torre syndrome (MTS).

Linear nevus sebaceous syndrome also known as Schimmelpenning syndrome and is considered as a type of epidermal nevus syndrome. It presents with triad of linear nevus sebaceous, seizures, and mental retardation. However now it is known to have many other features including wide range of neurologic, ophthalmic, skeletal, cardiovascular, and urological defects.

Muir–Torre syndrome is caused by mutations in DNA mismatch repair genes. The diagnosis of this syndrome requires concurrent or sequential diagnosis of multiple sebaceous neoplasms and keratoacanthomas, associated with internal malignancy. There should be a minimum of one internal malignancy or a family history of MTS.

## Nevus Comedonicus

Nevus comedonicus presents linear lesion of numerous keratin filled pits with acneiform pustules. Munro and Wilkie hypothesized that mosaicism for a dominant inherited disorder featuring severe acne might account for this disorder.

### Clinical Features

Commonly, this is present since birth or may appear during childhood and adolescence involving the face, neck, trunk, and upper arm as common sites. Palm, sole, and glans penis are also affected. It is characterized by "pits" with black keratinous plugs. Intervening epidermis may appear normal, slightly hyperkeratotic, or slightly hypo- and hyperpigmented. There may be other developmental anomalies may be associated like ipsilateral cataract, extensive nevus flammeus, and transverse myelitis.

### Histopathology

Epidermis shows epidermolytic hyperkeratosis and acanthosis without any signs of para or dyskeratosis. Grouped dilated follicular ostia devoid of any hair are found to have deep and wide invagination and are filed up with keratin material. Single rudimentary sebaceous gland is sometimes detected at the base of the invagination. Sometimes, small or even large cystic invaginations and cysts may be seen lined by keratinizing squamous epithelium.

Arrector pili muscles are absent. Interfollicular epidermis may be normal, acanthotic, and hyperkeratotic.

### Treatment

Treatment of choice is surgical excision. Topical therapies include retinoic acid and ammonium lactate (12%). Tacalcitol and tazarotene (0.05%) with calcipotriene (0.005%) are also effective.

## Eccrine Nevi

Three forms of eccrine nevus are found.

### Pure Eccrine Nevi

Pure eccrine nevi may present at any age but clinical appearance is variable. Histopathologically, numerous coils of both secretory and ductal elements can be found deep within the dermis.

### Eccrine Angiomatous Nevus

This is a rare, benign condition characterized by presence of solitary or multiple erythematous or sometimes violaceous/blue/yellow/brown/skin colored nodule or plaque having combined vascular and eccrine elements. The nevi appear as the lesions, which are distributed usually on the distal limbs, particularly over the palms and soles. It is present since birth or may appear later in childhood and usually enlarges with growth of the patient and this is often painful especially when pressed. Hyperhidrosis and hypertrichosis over the lesion are commonly observed distinctive features. Pain may necessitate surgical excision.

Histopathological, examination reveals numerous large but normal eccrine glands enmeshed within loose fibrous tissue which contains numerous thin walled blood vessels and lymphatics. Surgical excision is the definitive treatment.

### Porokeratotic Eccrine Ostial and Dermal Duct Nevus

This usually present asymptomatically since birth. It appears as localized area of plugged pores in a linear distribution usually on the palm and sole. The lesion may be anhidrotic or hyperhidrotic.

Histopathologically there are comedo-like epidermal invaginations filled with parakeratotic plug. Granular layer is absent at the base of this column.

Surgical excision is the treatment of choice.

## Apocrine Nevus

Apocrine nevus is rare and is commonly present as solitary or multiple nodules or plaques on the scalp, face, axilla, presternal skin and vulva in association with other forms of apocrine proliferations like apocrine carcinoma, extramammary Paget's disease, and syringocystadenoma papilliferum.

Histopathologically, true apocrine nevi comprises of large number of mature apocrine glands extending from the upper dermis to the subcutaneous fat.

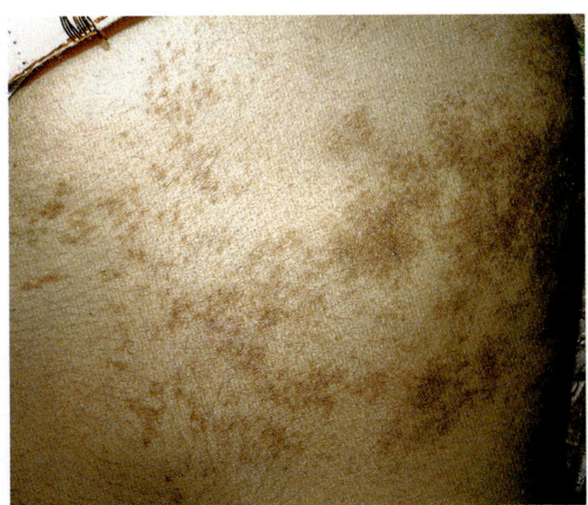

FIG. 7: Becker's nevus.

## Becker's Nevus

This is a common anomaly affecting predominantly males. It may present with two different morphological patterns, a single hyperpigmented lesion or multiple hyperpigmented macules in a checkerboard pattern. The lesion is characterized by the presence of a light or dark brown macule with a well-defined margin and irregular border (Fig. 7).

Most common sites of distribution are unilateral over the front of the chest or the scapular region but other sites may also be affected. The skin is thickened toward the center and increased terminal hairs may appear on and around the lesion. In few instances Becker's nevus may be associated with breast hypoplasia, supernumerary nipples, lipoatrophy, spina bifida and scoliosis, limb reduction, and maxillofacial dysplasia. There is frequent occurrence of acne within the nevi. There is report of coexistence of accessory scrotum.

### Pathogenesis

Becker's nevus is generally sporadic but familial cases have been reported. This has been explained by the genetic mechanism called paradominant inheritance and mutation results in mosaicism and is manifested in the checkerboard presentation. This concept is also applicable for Becker's nevus syndrome.

Higher sebum secretion resulting in frequent occurrence of acne, pityriasis versicolor over the nevus supports the androgenic influence. Presence of an increased number of androgen receptors, and androgen receptor messenger RNA, are strong evidence in support of the fact that this nevus is androgen dependent.

### Histopathology

Well-developed lesions show hyperkeratosis, acanthosis, papillomatosis, hyperplasia of hair follicles, and sebaceous glands. The basal and suprabasal keratinocytes are heavily pigmented with presence of few melanophages in the upper dermis. Dermis shows thickened smooth muscle bundles.

### Treatment

Treatment of Becker's nevus requires laser ablation, by either of the Q-switched ruby laser, Er:YAG laser, and Nd:YAG laser.

**BOX 1 Conditions included in epidermal nevus syndrome**

- Schimmelpenning syndrome
- Phacomatosis pigmentokeratotica
- Nevus comedonicus syndrome
- Becker nevus syndrome
- Proteus syndrome
- Angora hair nevus syndrome
- FGFR-3 epidermal nevus syndrome
- CHILD syndrome
- Type 2 segmental Cowden disease

# EPIDERMAL NEVUS SYNDROME

Epidermal nevus syndrome (ENS) is a heterogeneous group of mosaic conditions with variable clinical presentations characterized by concurrent occurrence of organoid or non-organoid epidermal nevi along with many other cutaneous and extracutaneous lesions.

At present there are nine conditions included under ENS. These are mentioned in box 1.

The first five are organoid nevus syndromes and the last four are keratinocytic nevus syndromes.

## Pathogenesis

It occurs due to mosaicism. Genetic defects associated with these syndromes are mosaic *FGFR2* mutations, mosaic *FGFR3* mutations and loss of heterozygosity for a *PTEN* mutation.

## Clinical Presentations

Common cutaneous manifestations are nevus sebaceous, verrucous epidermal nevus, syringocystadenoma papilliferum, wooly hair, and follicular hyperkeratosis. Less common cutaneous manifestations are infantile hemangioma, nevus flammeus, hypochromic nevi, congenital melanocytic nevi, spitz nevi, and dermatomegaly. Other manifestations are hypodontia, maxillary giant cell granuloma, and neurological manifestations like spasms, seizures, mental retardation, deafness, and cranial nerve palsies.

## Schimmelpenning Syndrome

Schimmelpenning syndrome features presence of nevus sebaceous and abnormalities in brain, eyes, or bone. Basal cell carcinoma may develop within sebaceous nevi. However, preventive excision of all sebaceous nevi is not advocated.

This is almost always sporadic and is caused by genetic mosaicism of a lethal autosomal dominant gene. Familial cases, reported only occasionally, might have been caused by paradominant inheritance. Genomic integration of human papillomavirus in diseased skin has also been suggested.

Systemic involvement is common (Table 1). Angiomatous growth can develop within the sebaceous nevi, bone, or lungs. It often releases some chemicals causing vitamin D resistant hypophosphatemic rickets. Surgical excision should be attempted it this happens.

## Phacomatosis Pigmentokeratotica

Cooccurrence of speckled-lentiginous nevus, epidermal nevus with sebaceous differentiation and skeletal and neurologic

**TABLE 1: Systemic involvement in Schimmelpenning syndrome**

| | |
|---|---|
| Skeletal defects | • Congenital dislocation of the hip, limb abnormalities like unilateral hypoplasia of any bony structure, benign cortical defect of the humerus, medial bowing of the distal ulna<br>• Craniofacial defects like frontal bossing<br>• Ameloblastoma of the mandible<br>• Lytic defects of ribs<br>• Hypoplastic iliac wings<br>• Kyphoscoliosis<br>• Hypophosphatemic rickets |
| Dental defect | Hypoplastic dentition |
| Neurological defect | • Hemimegalencephaly with resulting contralateral motor disease<br>• Mental and cognitive deficiency<br>• Seizures<br>• Cortical agyria, microgyria, or pachygyria<br>• Cerebral heterotopia<br>• Agenesis of corpus callosum<br>• Dysplasia of brain vessels<br>• Dandy–Walker malformation |
| Eye defect | • Ectropion<br>• Corneal vascularization<br>• Unilateral cataract<br>• Coloboma<br>• Epibulbar lipodermoid<br>• Ocular hemangiomas<br>• Defects of the optic nerve<br>• Cortical blindness |

defects is called phacomatosis pigmentokeratotica (PPK). The underlying mechanism is proposed as twin spotting (didymosis). Recent study however negated the twin spot theory. Postzygotic-activating *HRAS* mutation has been detected in both the sebaceous and a melanocytic nevus tissue (mosaicism).

Most of the systemic involvements present in Schemmelpenning syndrome and speckled lentiginous syndrome are also found in this condition.

There is slightly increased risk of malignancy within the pigmented lesions and the epidermal nevus in later life. The chance to develop basal cell carcinoma and vitamin-D resistant hypophosphatemic rickets are higher than in Schimmelpenning syndrome. Another interesting finding is occasional presence of brown papules or patch around the margin of the nevus sebaceous. This is non-organoid nevi and is called "nevus marginatus".

## Proteus Syndrome

This syndrome first described by Cohen and Hayden1 (1979) but the terminology "Proteus" was coined later by Wiedemann and coworkers after the Greek sea-god who was known for his ability to change his shape.

This is characterized by overgrowth of the various parts of the body in an asymmetric pattern. Overgrowth starts to manifest during infancy and progress with age. A typical cerebriform connective tissue nevus is highly characteristic feature of Proteus Syndrome. This frequently involves soles (Fig. 8).

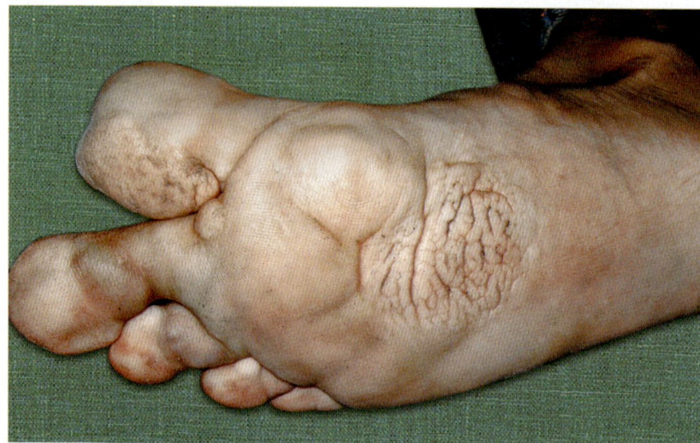

**FIG. 8:** Cerebriform plaque on the sole and overgrowth of toes in Proteus syndrome.

Patient may have a characteristic facies (long face, down-slanting palpebral fissures, and an open-mouth expression). There may be neurological abnormality, vascular malformations with high chance of deep vein thrombosis and pulmonary embolism.

Proteus syndrome is a constellation of various features. Thus it is often missed as well as overdiagnosed. To overcome this problem, diagnostic criteria have been developed by recommendations from National Institutes of Health. Other features are epidermal nevi, and lipoma. In contrast to hemihyperplasia multiple lipomatosis syndrome where lipomas generally develop at birth, lipoma develops at a later age in Proteus syndrome. Unilateral Proteus syndrome is also reported.

Mosaicism of an oncogenic *AKT1* gene is proposed to cause Proteus syndrome. Mutations in PTEN have also been suspected. This is often misdiagnosed for Klippel-Trenaunay syndrome, epidermal nevus syndromes, and Bannayan-Riley-Ruvalcaba syndromes which are important differential diagnoses.

No effective treatment is available. Surgery is discouraged because of high chances of recurrence and painful scarring that may make the situation worse.

## Becker's Nevus Syndrome

Becker's nevus can sometimes be associated unilateral breast hypoplasia and abnormalities of muscle, skin, and/or bone. Majority of the developmental anomalies are hypoplastic and are usually ipsilateral (Box 2).

**BOX 2 Conditions associated with Becker's nevus syndrome**

- Ipsilateral breast hypoplasia (most common associated anomaly in females)
- Musculoskeletal anomalies like scoliosis, limb asymmetry
- Aplasia of the pectoralis major muscle
- Patchy hypoplasia of the ipsilateral extramammary fatty tissue
- Supernumerary nipples
- Segmental odontomaxillary dysplasia
- Accessory scrotum
- Patchy hypoplasia of the ipsilateral temporal region
- Lipoatrophy

## SUGGESTED READINGS


1. Almaani N, Nagy N, Liu L, et al. Revertant mosaicism in recessive dystrophic epidermolysis bullosa. J Invest Dermatol. 2010;130(7):1937-40.
2. Aschinberg LC, Solomon LM, Zeis PM, et al. Vitamin D-resistant rickets associated with epidermal nevus syndrome: demonstration of a phosphaturic substance in the dermal lesions. J Pediatr 1977;91:56-60.
3. Biesecker LG, Happle R, Mulliken JB, et al. Proteus syndrome: diagnostic criteria, differential diagnosis, and patient evaluation. Am J Med Genet. 1999;84:389-95.
4. Biesecker LG, Peters KF, Darling TN, et al. Clinical differentiation between Proteus syndrome and hemihyperplasia: description of a distinct form of hemihyperplasia. Am J Med Genet. 1998;79:311-8.
5. Carlson JA, Cribier B, Nuovo G, et al. Epidermodysplasia verruciformis-associated and genital-mucosal high-risk human papillomavirus DNA are prevalent in nevus sebaceus of Jadassohn. J Am Acad Dermatol. 2008;59:279-94.
6. Cohen MM Jr, Hayden PW. A newly recognized hamartomatous syndrome. Birth Defects Orig Artic Ser. 1979;15:291-6.
7. Domingo J, Helwig EB. Malignant neoplasms associated with nevus sebaceus of Jadassohn. J Am Acad Dermatol 1979;1:545-56.
8. Downs AM, Mehta R, Lear JT, et al. Acne in a Becker's naevus: an androgen-mediated link? Clin Exp Dermatol 1998;23:191-2.
9. Eisen DB, Michael DJ. Sebaceous lesions and their associated syndromes: Part II. J Am Acad Dermatol. 2009;61:563-78.
10. Glinick SE, Alper JC, Bogaars H, et al. Becker's melanosis: associated abnormalities. J Am Acad Dermatol. 1983;9:509-14.
11. Gorlin RJ, Cohen MM Jr, Hennekam RC. Syndromes of the head and neck 4th edition. Oxford: Oxford University Press; 2001. pp. 480-8.
12. Groesser L, Herschberger E, Ruetten A, et al. Postzygotic HRAS and KRAS mutations cause nevus sebaceous and Schimmelpenning syndrome. Nat Genet. 2012;44(7):783-7.
13. Hafner C, Landthaler M, Happle R, et al. Nevus marginatus: a distinct type of epidermal nevus or merely a variant of nevus sebaceus? Dermatology. 2008;216:236-8.
14. Hafner C, Toll A, Gantner S, et al. Keratinocytic epidermal nevi are associated with mosaic RAS mutations. J Med Genet. 2012;49(4):249-53.
15. Haple R. Paradominant trait: a possible explanation for Becker's pigmented hairy nevus. Eur J Dermatol. 1992;2:39-40.
16. Happle R, Koopman RJ. Becker nevus syndrome. Am J Med Genet. 1997;68:357-61.
17. Happle R. Mosaicism in human skin: understanding the patterns and mechanisms. Arch Dermatol. 1993;129:1460-70.
18. Happle R. The group of epidermal nevus syndromes Part I. Well defined phenotypes. J Am Acad Dermatol. 2010;63:1-22.
19. Happle R. Transposable elements and the lines of Blaschko: a new perspective. Dermatology. 2002;204:4-7.
20. Kishida ES, Muniz Silva MA, da Costa Pereira F, et al. Epidermal nevus syndrome associated with adnexal tumors, Spitz nevus, and hypophosphatemic vitamin D-resistant rickets. Pediatr Dermatol. 2005;22:48-54.
21. Kwon O, Oh S, Kim S, et al. Eccrine angiomatous hamartoma. Int J Dermatol 1998;37:787-9.
22. Orloff MS, Eng C. Genetic and phenotypic heterogeneity in the PTEN hamartoma tumor syndrome. Oncogene. 2008;27:5387-97.
23. Pelle MT, Pride HB, Tyler WB. Eccrine angiomatous hamartoma. J Am Acad Dermatol. 2002;47:429-35.
24. Person JR, Longcope C. Becker's nevus: an androgen-mediated hyperplasia with increased androgen receptors. J Am Acad Dermatol. 1984;10:235-8.
25. Sarma N, Malakar S, Lahiri K. Unilateral proteus syndrome. Indian J Dermatol Venereol Leprol. 2005;71(2):122-4.
26. Sarma N. Pigmentary nevi on face have unique patterns and implications: the concept of Blaschko's lines for pigmentary nevi. Indian J Dermatol. 2012;57(1):30-4.
27. Schwartz RA, Torre DP. The Muir-Torre syndrome: a 25-year retrospect. J Am Acad Dermatol. 1995;33:90-104.
28. Tsubota A, Akiyama M, Sakai K, et al. Keratin 1 Gene mutation detected in epidermal nevus with epidermolytic hyperkeratosis. J Invest Dermatol. 2007;127:1371-4.
29. Turner JT, Cohen MM Jr, Biesecker LG. Reassessment of the Proteus syndrome literature: application of diagnostic criteria to published cases. Am J Med Genet A. 2004;130:111-22.
30. Uitto J, Bauer EA, Santa Cruz DJ, et al. Decreased collagenase production by regional fibroblasts cultured from skin of a patient with connective tissue nevi of the collagen type. J Invest Dermatol. 1982;78:136-40.
31. Wiedemann HR, Burgio GR, Aldenhoff P, et al. The Proteus syndrome: partial gigantism of the hands and/or feet, nevi, hemihypertrophy, subcutaneous tumors, macrocephaly or other skull anomalies and possible accelerated growth and visceral affections. Eur J Pediatr. 1983;140:5-12.
32. Zhang W, Simos PG, Ishibashi H, et al. Neuroimaging features of epidermal nevus syndrome. Am J Neuroradiol. 2003;24:1468-70.

# 73 CHAPTER Cutaneous Neoplasms: Benign and Malignant

Vijay Vanchinathan, Ann M John, W Clark Lambert, Robert A Schwartz

## INTRODUCTION

Cutaneous neoplasms encompass a wide array of entities both benign and malignant. Understanding their origin and learning to recognize their salient features are critical to successful management. Here, we summarize some of the most frequently encountered cutaneous neoplasms in clinical practice.

## SEBORRHEIC KERATOSIS

Seborrheic keratosis is a common benign cutaneous condition affecting middle-aged to older adults. The lesion presents as multiple papules or plaques that are light brown to black in color with an ovular shape. They have classically been described as having a "stuck-on" appearance and waxy texture (Figs 1 and 2). They are usually located on the chest and back, measure less than 3 cm in diameter, and are occasionally associated with itching and bleeding.

While the pathogenesis is unknown, age and sun exposure are purported risk factors. Moreover, mutations in *FGFR3* and *PI3K* genes may be involved. Of note, the sudden development of multiple seborrheic keratoses is known as the Leser–Trelat sign and has been thought to indicate the presence of an underlying gastrointestinal malignancy.

Histologically, seborrheic keratosis demonstrates hyperkeratosis, acanthosis, and horn cysts.

### Treatment

Treatment consists of destruction or removal, specifically if lesions are symptomatic or cosmetically unappealing. Laser or cryosurgical destuction, shave excision, and electrodessication and curettage are all methods of removal that have been employed.

## ACTINIC KERATOSIS

Actinic keratoses (AKs) are premalignant neoplasms of the skin characterized by partial thickness atypia of the epidermis. Risk factors for their development include older age, light skin, and chronic sun exposure. AKs initially present as erythematous macules or patches with overlying scale on sun-exposed areas of the body, including the head, neck, shoulders, and forearms (Fig. 3).

### Clinical Features

Clinically and histologically, there are five major actinic keratosis variants: hypertrophic, pigmented, lichenoid, atropic, and when on the lips, solar cheilosis (actinic cheilitis). Hypertrophic AKs are hyperkeratotic papules and plaques with prominent scaling over an erythematous base, from which a cutaneous horn may develop. Pigmented AKs lack the classical erythema and instead have a

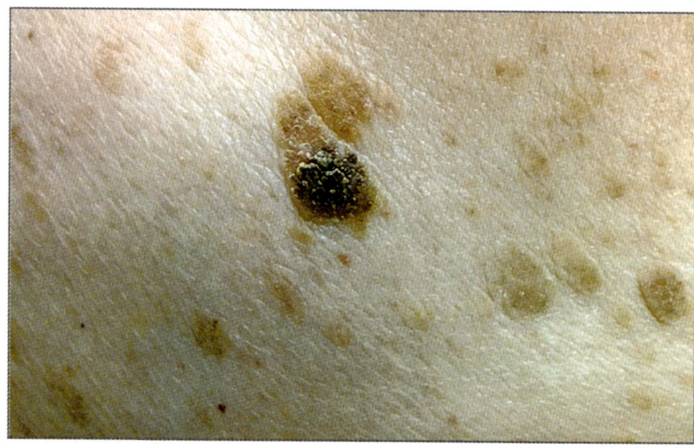

**FIG. 1:** Seborrheic keratosis demonstrating waxy, stuck-on appearance with variation in color.

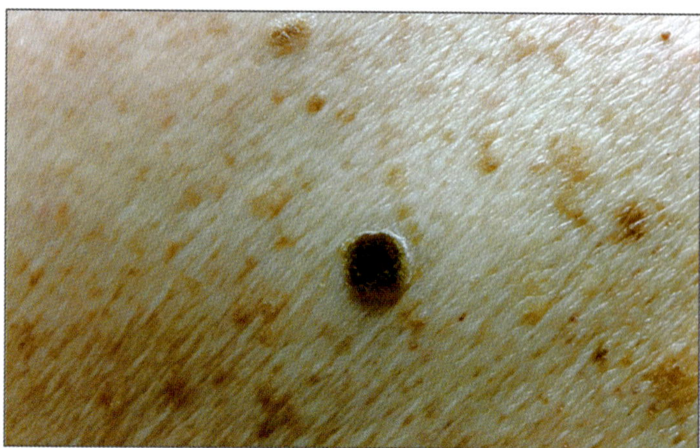

**FIG. 2:** Seborrheic keratosis on sun exposed, aged skin.

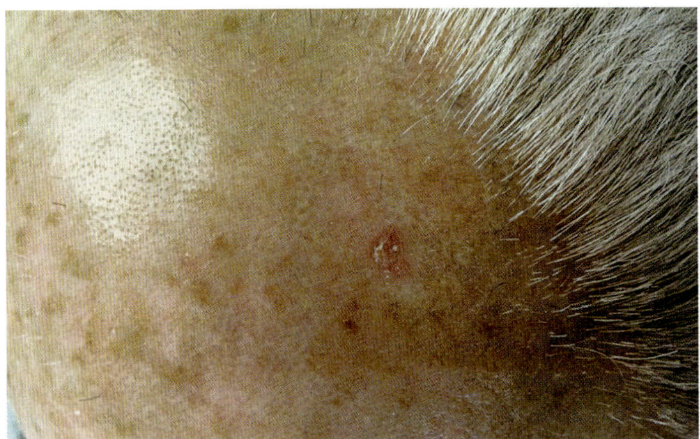

FIG. 3: Erythematous actinic keratosis with overlying scale on the scalp.

pigmented or reticulated appearance that can complicate prompt diagnosis. Lichenoid AKs demonstrate a dense inflammatory infiltrate and atrophic AKs have an atrophic epidermis.

Histologically, the atypia, when present, is usually limited to the lower epidermis and is accompanied by parakeratosis alternating with orthokeratosis over adnexal structures. This may progress into squamous cell carcinoma (SCC) gradually over time.

### Treatment

A variety of treatment options, including 5-fluorouracil (5-FU) alone, salicylic acid followed by 5-FU, imiquimod, diclofenac, tretinoin, and cryotherapy are available. We recommend cryotherapy to treat single AKs, and topical 5-FU for multiple lesions.

## LEUKOPLAKIA AND ERYTHROPLAKIA

Oral leukoplakia and oral erythroplakia are clinical diagnoses that raise suspicion of oral SCC. Oral leukoplakia is linked to both tobacco and alcohol usage and can affect any part of the oral cavity. Homogeneous leukoplakia is uniformly thin, flat, and white in appearance, whereas nonhomogeneous leukoplakia may have mixed erythema and either a speckled or nodular look. As leukoplakia may be a premalignant condition or representative of lichen planus, diagnosis should be made by biopsy or noninvasive staining techniques, such as methylene blue.

Histopathological examination of oral leukoplakia may demonstrate varying degrees of epithelial dysplasia. Depending on the cellular changes seen, treatment can range from observation and behavioral modifications to surgical excision and/or $CO_2$ laser ablation.

Erythroplakia is flat or depressed erythematous change of the oral mucosa, typically occurring in elderly men. Lesions are usually less than 1.5 cm in diameter, but unlike oral leukoplakia, nearly always show at least moderate-to-severe dysplasia on biopsy and occasionally *in situ* or invasive carcinoma. Prompt diagnosis with surgical excision, $CO_2$ laser ablation, or cryosurgery is recommended, with regularly scheduled follow-up.

## BASAL CELL CARCINOMA

Basal cell carcinoma (BCC) is the most common cancer in fair-skinned individuals, especially those with light hair or eyes and sun-damaged skin.

### Pathogenesis

Basal cell carcinomas are believed to originate from pluripotent stem cells in the basal layer of the epidermis or skin adnexae. Their development is primarily linked to mutations in the *PTCH1* gene, whose protein, PTCH1, normally functions to inhibit the smoothened (SMO) protein on the cell surface. "Hedgehog" signaling ligands normally inhibit PTCH1 and allow upregulation of hedgehog genes via SMO. When the *PTCH1* or *SMO* genes are mutated, however, there may be uncontrolled downstream hedgehog signaling that leads to the development of basal cell carcinoma.

The main risk factor for BCC development is exposure to ultraviolet radiation, followed by environmental exposures, such as arsenic, ionizing radiation, X-rays, and immunosuppressive treatments. Ultraviolet B (UVB) and chronic radiation exposure are more strongly associated with basal cell carcinomas than their ultraviolet A (UVA) or intense, intermittent radiation counterparts.

### Clinical Features

The prototypical lesion is a nodular BCC that appears as a raised, pearly nodule with telangiectasias and central ulceration. Less common variants include superficial BCC characterized by an erythematous thin plaque, and the often pedunculated or sessile fibroepithelial form on the trunk.

Pathological findings vary according to the tumor subtype, but generally include aggregates of basaloid keratinocytes often with peripheral clefting, peripheral palisading, and focal necrosis or apoptosis (Figs 4 to 6).

### Treatment

Better understanding of the role hedgehog signaling plays in BCC pathogenesis has led to the development of hedgehog pathway inhibitors as a novel systemic therapy for widespread or metastatic tumors. Initial studies of the drug vismodegib demonstrated clearance of pre-existing BCCs in patients with the basal cell nevus (Gorlin) syndrome. Studies regarding the use of hedgehog inhibitors in topical formulations are currently underway.

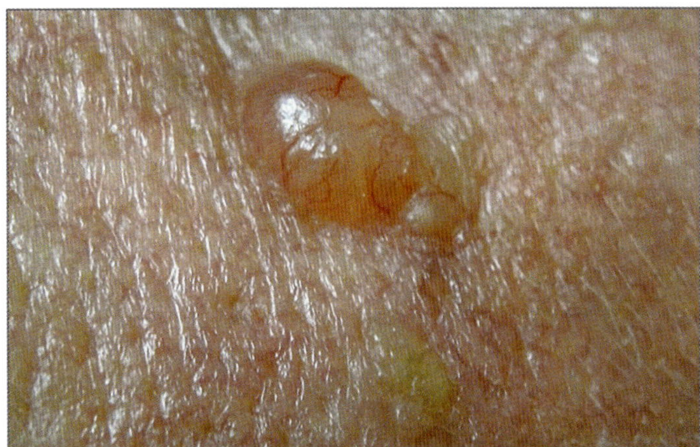

FIG. 4: Nodular basal cell carcinoma located on the face. Note translucent, pearly quality and prominent telangiectasia.

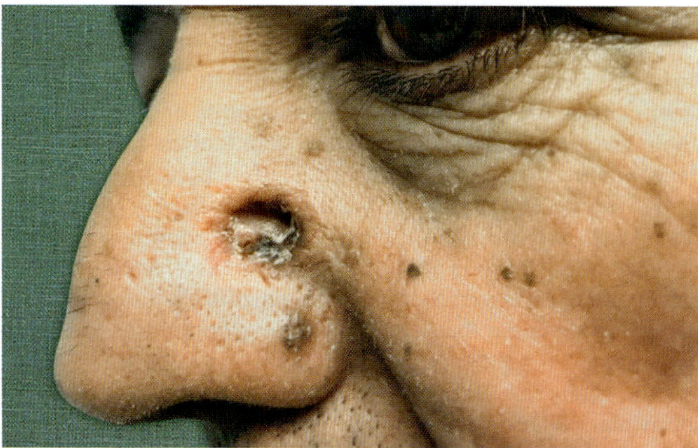

FIG. 5: Crater form basal cell carcinoma infiltrating left nasal side wall.

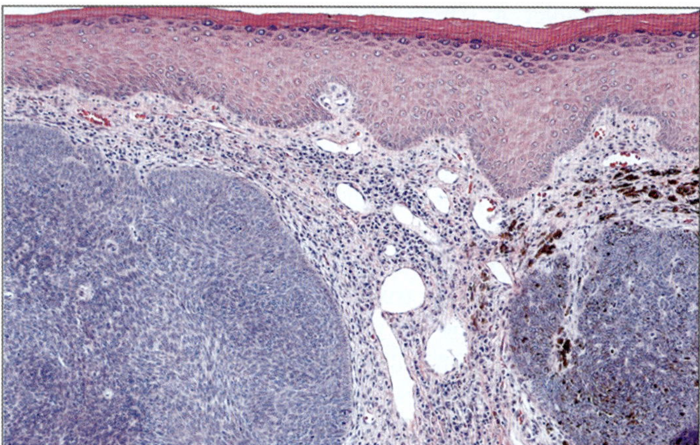

FIG. 6: Basal cell carcinoma, with nests of basaloid cells in the dermis. Note peripheral palisading and dilated blood vessels.

Traditional treatments for BCC include surgical excision, Mohs surgery, electrodessication and curettage, and topical chemotherapy. A recent study comparing topical chemotherapy agents and photodynamic therapy found that those patients treated with 5% imiquimod were most likely to have sustained BCC clearance at 3 and 12 months post-treatment, followed by those treated with 5% 5-FU.

## SQUAMOUS CELL CARCINOMA IN SITU (BOWEN'S DISEASE)

Squamous cell carcinoma *in situ* tends to first present as a slow-growing, irregular, erythematous plaque with overlying scale or crust. Risk factors for SCC include chronic sun exposure, carcinogen toxicity, human papillomavirus infection, and immunosuppression. Bowen's disease usually appears on sun-exposed areas of the body, such as the head and neck, and may arise from a pre-existing actinic keratosis or *de novo*.

### Clinical Features

It can range from several millimeters to several centimeters in size and may transform into invasive SCC over time.

Several variants of SCC *in situ* exist, including erythroplasia of Queyrat, bowenoid papulosis, pigmented SCC *in situ*, and verrucous SCC *in situ*. Erythroplasia of Queyrat refers to the clinical presentation of SCC *in situ* involving the penis, whereas bowenoid papulosis describes histological changes suggestive of SCC within a wart.

Regardless of the exact type, histologic examination of SCC *in situ* demonstrates full-thickness atypia of the epidermis, overlying confluent parakeratosis, keratinocyte necrosis, and acanthosis.

### Treatment

Treatment of SCC *in situ* varies from topical medications, such as 5-FU to Mohs micrographic surgery, depending on the location, histopathology, and severity. Photodynamic therapy has better cosmesis compared to cryotherapy and 5-FU, but is associated with a high recurrence rate. Electrodessication with curettage has been shown to have a 99% cure rate for Bowen's disease, and may be considered when other treatment modalities are unavailable.

## Invasive Squamous Cell Carcinoma

Invasive SCC represents the spread of full-thickness atypia limited to the epidermis into the dermis and subcutaneous tissue.

### Pathogenesis

Risk factors for invasive SCC include chronic exposure to UV radiation, chronic ulcerated scars, predisposing genetic conditions such as xeroderma pigmentosum, and immunosuppression. Approximately 60% of invasive SCCs arise from pre-existing actinic keratoses and expand by invading neighboring tissue. Although the overall rate of hematogenous metastasis is low, patients with invasive SCC involving the lip, ear, or ulcer and immunosuppressed patients are at much greater risk for disseminated disease.

### Clinical Features

The classic SCC is an erythematous papule or plaque on sun-exposed skin with secondary scaling or crusting. It may present, however, as an erosion, ulceration, or hyperkeratotic plaque with pain or tenderness at the tumor site, especially if perineural invasion has occurred.

On histological examination, invasive SCC demonstrates full-thickness atypia of the epidermis with downward keratinocyte spread into the dermis and below. The degree of atypia can vary from one section to the next and individual cells can exhibit a number of other suggestive features, such as nuclear pleomorphism, mitosis, and apoptosis. Keratin pearls may be seen in well or partially differentiated tumors. Overall staging should be based on a combination of histological findings, clinical tumor size, and presence of lymph node or distant metastases.

### Treatment

Surgical excision and Mohs micrographic surgery remain the first line of therapy for invasive SCC. Small or thin SCCs may be treated with topical chemotherapy agents or electrodessication with curettage as well. Histological findings suggestive of further spread, such as perineural invasion, warrant close follow-up evaluations or even sentinel lymph node biopsy (Fig. 7).

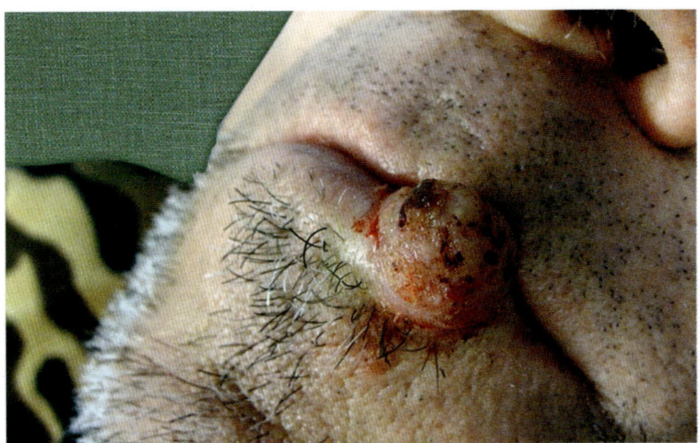

FIG. 7: Invasive squamous cell carcinoma involving the left lower lip.

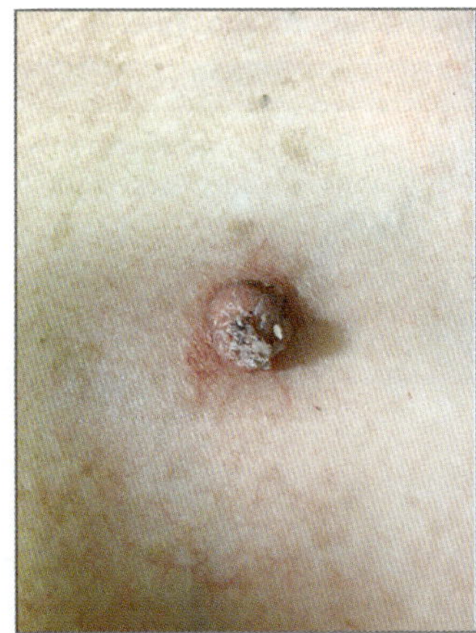

FIG. 8: Keratoacanthoma, a crateriform nodule with keratinous center.

## KERATOACANTHOMA

Keratoacanthoma (KA) is a rapidly growing cutaneous neoplasm that often presents as a solitary erythematous crateriform nodule filled with keratinous material on sun-exposed skin.

Risk factors for KA development include ultraviolet radiation, carcinogen toxicity, history of trauma, and tobacco use.

Keratoacanthomas usually grow rapidly over several weeks before regressing slowly over many weeks to months, frequently leaving behind an atrophic scar. Despite reports of KAs metastasizing to other organs, there remains considerable debate whether a KA is best classified as a pseudomalignancy or pseudo-benignity.

Histological evaluation of keratoacanthoma reveals a large tumor composed of well-differentiated keratinocytes filled with cornified material and surrounded by an inflammatory infiltrate. Cellular atypia, including nuclear pleomorphism and abnormal mitoses, may suggest a diagnosis of KA-like squamous cell carcinoma. Treatment options vary from surgical excision to radiotherapy and intralesional methotrexate (Figs 8 to 10).

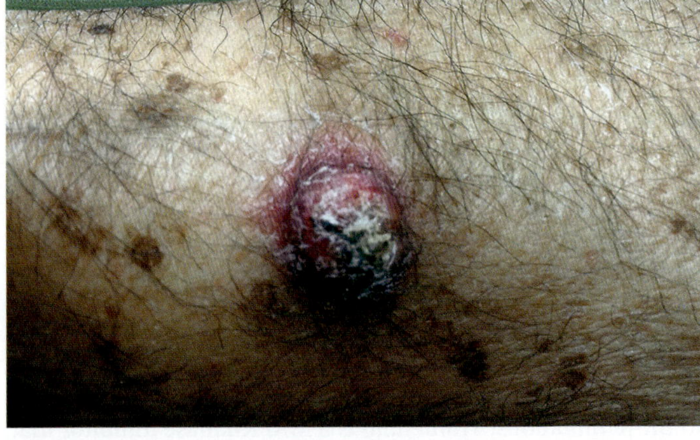

FIG. 9: Keratoacanthoma on the upper extremity.

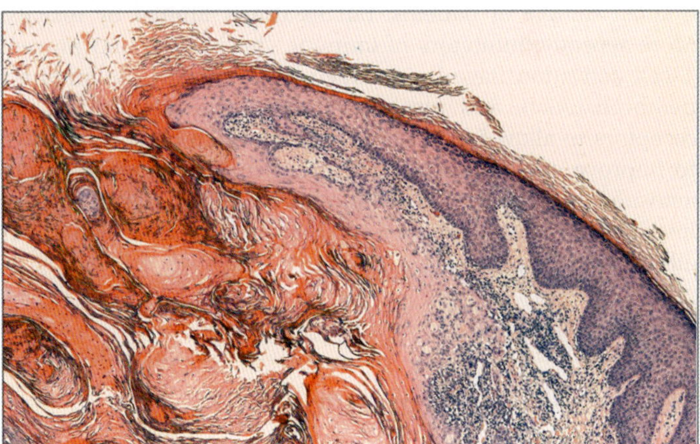

FIG. 10: Keratoacanthoma, with well-differentiated keratinocytes filled with cornified material and surrounded by inflammatory infiltrate.

## MALIGNANT MELANOMA

As one of the deadliest skin cancers, malignant melanoma warrants immediate identification and treatment. Risk factors for development include fair skin, freckling, significant sun exposure, use of tanning beds, history of blistering sunburns, immunocompromised state, predisposing genetic conditions, such as Wiskott–Aldrich syndrome and xeroderma pigmentosum, and personal or family history of melanoma. Clinical features include asymmetry, uneven borders, multiple colors, diameter greater than 6 mm, and changing color and shape over time. Of note, up to 10% of melanomas are not pigmented but instead amelanotic.

The pathogenesis of malignant melanoma involves multiple mutations and genetic abnormalities. Point mutations in the *BRAF* and *NRAS* genes are found in high frequency and are the most common mutations associated with melanoma. Pigment-related, tumor suppressor, and oncogenes may also demonstrate high rates of mutation. This rapid mutation rate is mostly due to exposure to ultraviolet A and B radiation, age, and chemotherapeutics.

Diagnosis of melanoma is established with a full-thickness biopsy, allowing for classification into several subtypes, as shown in table 1. Histological features of malignant melanoma include cytological atypia, melanocytes at varying stages of maturation, pagetoid spread, and high mitotic activity (Fig. 11). Poor prognostic factors on histological analysis include evidence of vertical growth, ulceration, infiltrative growth into surrounding nerves and vessels, and increased Breslow thickness.

Other essential tools in the work-up include sentinel lymph node biopsy, chest X-ray, and 18-fluorodeoxyglucose positron emission tomography/computed tomography. Ultrasound exam-

**TABLE 1: Malignant melanoma subtypes**

| Subtype | Clinical features | Histology |
|---|---|---|
| Lentigo maligna melanoma | May look like age spots; arises from premalignant flat lesions on sun-exposed surfaces | Melanocyte proliferation and extension into adnexa; melanophages and lymphocytes present in dermis |
| Superficial spreading melanoma | Relatively flat lesion demonstrating radial and vertical growth; located on legs or back | Epithelioid melanocytes in the epidermis with evidence of melanocyte proliferation; cytological atypia with thinning of epidermis |
| Acral lentiginous melanoma | Occurs more frequently in darkly-pigmented individuals on acral surfaces and mucous membranes | Spindle or epithelioid cells with atypical melanocytes; elongation of rete ridges with epidermal acanthosis |
| Mucosal melanoma | On mucous membranes; covered by squamous cells | Spindle and epithelioid cells in cell-like pattern with melanin pigment |
| Nodular melanoma | Early vertical growth with little radial growth; smooth texture with uniform black or blue coloration | Round tumor cells with hyperchromatic nuclei demonstrating vertical growth |
| Desmoplastic melanoma | Slow growing lesion on head or neck | Spindle cells with atypical melanocytes in mucinous matrix with evidence of infiltrative growth and presence of lymphocytes |
| Pediatric atypical Spitzoid tumor | – | Melanocytes in a spindle or epithelioid shape. Cells with intranuclear inclusions and prominent nucleoli |
| Uveal melanoma | Melanoma of the uvea or conjunctiva | Presence of epithelioid and spindle cells |

ination of lymph nodes is not recommended and should not serve as a substitute for sentinel node biopsy. Obtaining baseline and follow-up values of lactate dehydrogenase can help predict prognosis and determine the need for metastatic work-up and S100-B levels may predict prognosis in patients requiring lymph node dissection.

Treatment option vary, ranging from surgical excision for early stage lesions to targeted drug and immunotherapies. Vemurafenib and dabrafenib are competitive BRAF inhibitors and show much promise in patients with melanoma secondary to BRAF mutations. Trametinib is a MAPK-kinase inhibitor that, when combined with a BRAF inhibitor, allows for increased tumor regression. Interleukin-2 has resulted in remission in a small sample of patients, but its use is limited by toxicity. More recently, inhibitors of immune checkpoints that prevent T-cell activation have been targeted. Specifically, ipilimumab, pembrolizumab, and nivolumab antagonize inhibitory T-cell receptors to allow for T-cell activation, which has been shown to improve overall survival. Cell transfer of autologous T-cells activated in a laboratory is another potential therapy under investigation. Despite these and other treatments, melanoma is all too often a fatal cancer.

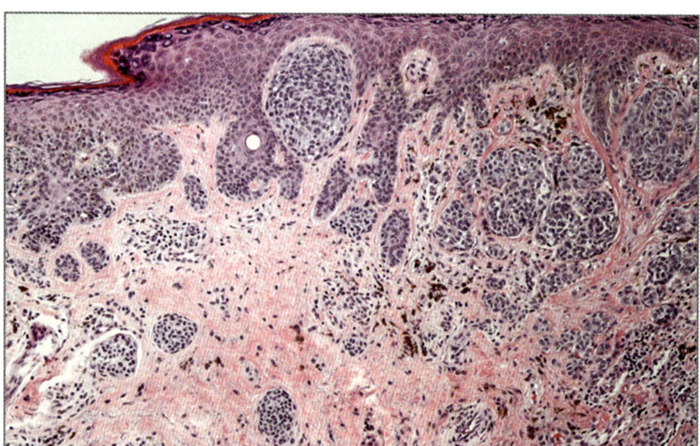

**FIG. 11:** Malignant melanoma, showing irregular nests of atypical melanocytes in the dermis.

## NEOPLASMS

### Sebaceous Gland Neoplasms

Neoplasms of adnexal structures, such as the sebaceous gland, are important to identify and treat early. Sebaceous adenoma is a benign proliferation of sebocytes and seboblasts, whereas sebaceoma refers to deep dermal sebaceous growths. Sebaceous adenomas and sebaceomas present as papules or nodules on the head, neck, and trunk, occasionally with a yellowish color. One or more sebaceous adenomas in a single patient can be indicative of Muir–Torre syndrome, an autosomal dominant condition characterized by sebaceous adenomas, keratoacanthomas, and visceral cancer, particularly colonic adenocarcinoma. Microscopically, sebaceous adenomas show an abundance of mature seboblasts and sebocytes without significant mitosis or necrosis (Fig. 12).

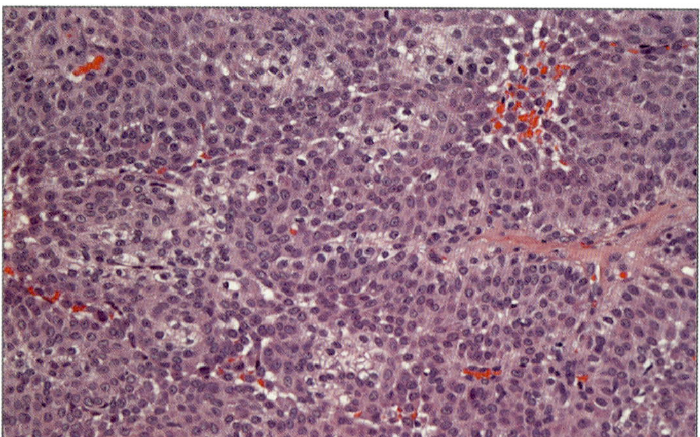

**FIG. 12:** Sebaceous adenoma, with proliferation of sebocytes and seboblasts.

Sebaceous nevi are epidermal nevi with both sebaceous and sweat gland components that primarily arise on the scalp. They are hairless flesh-colored to yellow plaques thought to derive form *HRAS* and *KRAS* gene mutations. Basal cell carcinoma may develop within sebaceous nevi, but this is much less common than benign superimposed follicular or sweat gland neoplasms such as trichoblastoma. Treatment of choice for both cosmetic and medical reasons is local excision, best done prior to the onset of puberty.

Sebaceous carcinoma is an adenocarcinoma that is typically divided into ocular and extraocular types. Clinically, it may appear similar to sebaceous adenoma, but with increased erythema and secondary changes like crusting and ulceration. Depending on the exact morphology, its histologic appearance may vary from nests and lobules to thin strands of atypical cells. Given the risk of metastatic spread, surgical excision remains the primary form of treatment.

## Follicular Neoplasms

Most follicular neoplasms are benign and treated with surgical excision. These benign tumors, however, often have malignant counterparts that are locally aggressive with metastatic potential. In addition, some follicular neoplasms are indicative of inherited syndromes, which must be considered when assessing these lesions.

Table 2 classifies major benign follicular neoplasms based on pathogenesis, clinical features, and histopathology. Treatment consists of excision or electrosurgery for cosmesis.

Trichilemmal carcinoma may result from malignant transformation of benign trichilemmoma. Risk factors for transformation include ultraviolet or ionizing radiation exposure, trauma to the area, immunosuppression, and genetic disorders, including xeroderma pigmentosum and Cowden disease. Clinically, this presents as a 0.5–7.5 cm, exophytic or polypoid mass, located on sun-exposed surfaces, specifically the scalp, forehead, and neck. The lesion may present with ulceration, telangiectasias, scaling, or rolled borders. Histologically, the tumor consists of lobules of atypical keratinocytes with clear cell change and palisading keratinocytes at the borders. Even though metastatic potential is low, although complete surgical excision with 2–3 cm margins or Mohs surgery is considered for treatment. Recurrence is rare, but local destruction by the tumor warrants early identification and treatment.

Trichoblastic carcinoma is another rare tumor, which may result from malignant transformation of a benign trichoblastoma. Pathogenesis is unknown, although immunosuppression may be a risk factor for development. Clinically, trichoblastic carcinoma presents as a rapidly growing nodule with pruritus and erythema, occurring most often on the face and scalp. Histologically, the tumor consists of follicular germinative cells with peripheral palisading, small keratin cysts, calcification, high mitotic activity, and follicular papillae. Complete surgical excision with uninvolved tissue margins or Mohs surgery is suggested for treatment. In addition, radiotherapy and chemotherapy can serve as adjuvant treatment for metastases.

Pilomatrix carcinoma may occur after malignant transformation of benign pilomatricoma. The pathogenesis is believed to result from mutations in the *CTNNB1* gene that encodes β-catenin,

**TABLE 2: Follicular neoplasms**

| Name | Pathogenesis/Associations | Clinical Features | Pathology |
|---|---|---|---|
| Basaloid follicular hamartoma | Mutation in *PTCH* gene; generalized basaloid follicular hamartoma syndrome; myasthenia gravis; systemic lupus erythematosus | 1–3 cm lesions; skin-colored to brown, located on face and scalp | Strands or branching cords of small basaloid cells intermixed with squamous cells |
| Pilar sheath acanthoma | – | Solitary papule up to 5 mm in diameter with central depression; located on upper lip, face, or head | Lobular proliferation of keratinocytes with clear cytoplasm surrounding cystic spaces |
| Trichofolliculoma (Fig. 13) | – | Solitary skin-colored or white lesion with central pore with multiple hairs that may exude sebum; located on nose | Loculated cystic cavities, filled with keratin and surrounded by multiple small follicles, often intermixed with Merkel cells and sebocytes |
| Trichoepithelioma | Mutation in tumor suppressor genes on short arm of chromosome 9 and *CYLD* gene; Brooke–Spiegler syndrome | Firm, round, shiny tumors of yellow, pink, brown, or blue color; presents after puberty on cheeks, eyelids, or around the nose | Uniform basaloid cells with peripheral palisading, surrounded by cellular stroma containing fibroblasts; contains small horn cysts, hair follicles, and calcifications |
| Trichoblastoma | Pre-existing sebaceous nevus or coexistent basal cell carcinoma | Solitary lesion 1–2 cm in diameter; skin-colored, brown, blue, or black papules or nodules commonly occurring on face or scalp | Cords and nests of basaloid germinative cells with peripheral palisading and abundant mitotic activity; follicular papillae, small keratin cysts, and melanocytes with melanin pigment |
| Trichilemmoma | Coexistent with trichoblastoma, sebaceous adenoma, and sebaceous nevus; presence of multiple lesions is associated with Cowden disease | Solitary lesion of 1–5 cm in diameter; skin-colored papule that grows slowly and forms small plaques resembling warts; located on face, ears, neck, forearms, and hands | Lobules of uniform clear cells with basophilic cells at the periphery; may have overlying hyperkeratosis |
| Pilomatricoma | Overactive Bcl-2 and mutations in CTNNB1, resulting in loss of regulation of β-catenin; myotonic dystrophy, Rubinstein–Taybi syndrome, and Turner syndrome | Skin-colored or purple solitary lesion arising on the head and neck; hard and bony texture with angulated shape ("tent sign") | Uniform basaloid cells lining cystic cavity with pale eosinophilic anucleated cells, intermixed with keratin and calcium deposits |

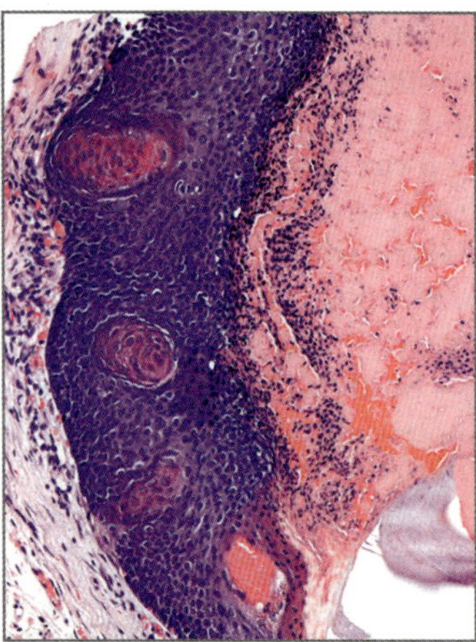

FIG. 13 Trichofolliculoma, demonstrating multiple small follicles surrounding cells filled with keratin.

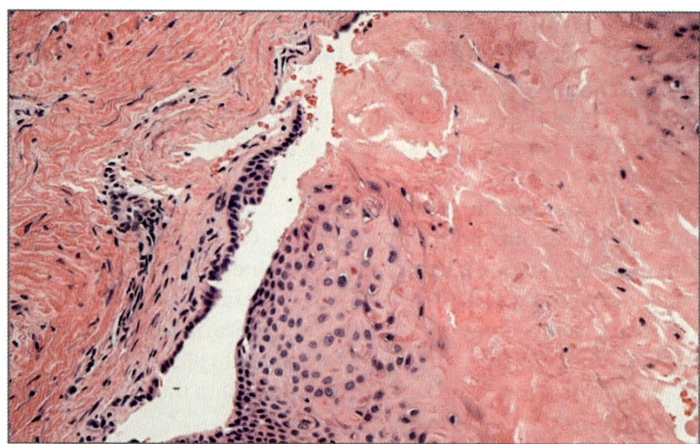

FIG. 14: Combined apocrine and trichilemmal cyst, with apocrine cells on the left and trichilemmal cells on the right.

and the lesion presents as a rapidly growing or ulcerative nodule from 0.5–20 cm, most often located on the head, neck, upper limbs, and buttocks. Pilomatrix carcinoma has a high rate of local recurrence and may metastasize to regional lymph nodes and distant organs, including the lungs and liver. Histological examination exhibits poor borders, cytonuclear atypia, high mitotic activity, tumor necrosis, calcification, ossification, and occasionally lymphovascular or perineural invasion. Treatment includes complete surgical excision with wide margins or Mohs surgery. Radiographic imaging is suggested to assess for metastasis and radiotherapy is recommended for cases of recurrence or metastasis.

Malignant proliferating trichilemmal cyst may occur after malignant transformation of a benign trichilemmal cyst likely due to the loss of *P53* tumor suppressor gene activity. This diagnosis should be considered when presented with rapid growth of a smooth, rounded, intradermal swelling with overlying alopecia. Involvement of regional lymph nodes and distant metastases may be present. Histologically, an infiltrative growth pattern coupled with cytonuclear atypia and high mitotic activity differentiate this neoplasm from its benign counterpart. The characteristic transition of classic epithelial cells to anucelated, keratinized cells should warn pathologists of the presence of malignant proliferating trichilemmal cyst. Treatment involves surgical excision with uninvolved tissue margins or Mohs surgery.

## Cysts

Although there are many types of cysts, the overwhelming majority consists of two types of hair follicle cysts: the trichilemmal, or pilar, cyst and the epidermal inclusion cyst.

The proliferating trichilemmal cyst, also known as a pilar tumor, usually arises from a trichilemmal cyst (Fig. 14). It ranges from 1 to 10 cm in size, and is believed secondary to trauma or inflammation. The cyst presents as a solitary, firm to soft, painless nodule, often with ulceration and purulent discharge, and is usually located on the scalp. Microscopic evaluation reveals a lobulated mass of proliferating squamous epithelium with central keratinization and peripheral palisading of basaloid cells. Focal necrosis and calcification is often found. Treatment is surgical excision with clear tissue margins or Mohs surgery.

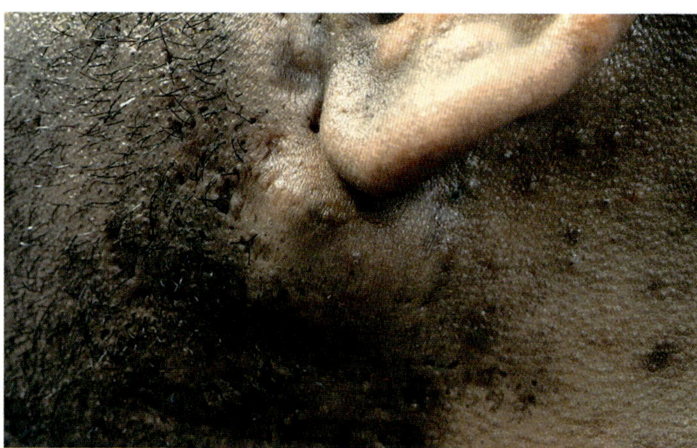

FIG. 15: Epidermal inclusion cyst located below the left ear, within a background of moderate-severe acne vulgaris.

Epidermoid cysts are cutaneous dome-shaped cysts usually found on the scalp and face. They have a black center filled with keratin, range in size from 0.5 to 5 cm, and often arise near a hair follicle and remain attached to the underlying skin (Fig. 15). These benign lesions can easily become infected and may even rupture, releasing a yellow sebaceous material with a foul odor. Histologically, the cyst walls are comprised of squamous epithelium and the sebaceous material consists of keratinocytes shed from the cyst lining. While these lesions are benign, there have been cases of SCC, BCC, and melanoma developing within the cysts, especially when they are allowed to grow without treatment. Of note, multiple epidermoid cysts located in uncharacteristic areas can indicate an underlying systemic disorder, such as Gardner syndrome and basal cell nevus syndrome. Treatment consists of complete surgical excision to prevent recurrence.

## Sweat Gland Neoplasms

Sweat gland neoplasms represent a range of benign and malignant tumors of "clear" sweat (eccrine) and "body" sweat (apocrine) tissue. Table 3 delineates benign sweat gland neoplasms along with associated malignant transformations. Treatment options include excision, electrosurgery, and Mohs surgery depending on cosmetic appearance, associated symptoms, and potential for spread.

**TABLE 3: Sweat gland neoplasms**

| Name | Clinical features | Pathology | Malignant transformation | Pathology (malignancy) |
|---|---|---|---|---|
| Poroma (Figs 16 and 17) | Solitary or multiple clusters of nodules with ulceration and bleeding often located on acral surfaces; red in color | Sheets of basaloid cells with centrally located nuclei and sharp distinction from keratinocytes; squamous differentiation and clear cell change; high vascularity | *Porocarcinoma*: Usually on lower extremities; potential for nodal and distant metastases (Fig. 18) | Clear cell change with cellular atypia, tumor necrosis, infiltrative growth, and high mitotic activity; squamous and spindle cell differentiation present |
| Hidradenoma | Solitary, skin-colored nodule or cyst producing watery discharge | Basaloid cells with small ductular lumens; clear cell change and squamous metaplasia; demarcated border | *Hidradenocarcinoma*: Multinodular solid neoplasm that may have local recurrence, distant metastases, and nodal spread | Ductal structures with tubular vacuoles and tumor necrosis, cellular atypia, and increased mitotic activity; most similar to nodular hidradenoma |
| Syringoma | Multiple firm papules of yellow to skin color, located near eyes or eyelids, sometimes associated with Down syndrome | Epithelial cells in nests, cords, or tubules; may have clear cell change; ducts shaped like commas or tadpoles | *Syringoid eccrine carcinoma*: Lymphovascular and perineural invasion with risk of recurrence and metastasis | Infiltrative growth, cytonuclear atypia, increased mitotic activity |
| Chondroid syringoma | Slow-growing, painless nodule, usually on the nose, cheek, or upper lip | Epithelial cells in cords, ducts, or tubules with a stromal component of Chondromyxoid material | *Malignant chondroid syringoma*: Hematologic and lymphatic metastases to nodes, lungs, and bone | Cellular atypia, high mitotic activity, infiltrative growth, tumor necrosis, and presence of satellite tumor nodules |
| Spiradenoma | Solitary, painful nodule in the trunk or upper extremities; may be associated with Brooke-Spiegler syndrome | Lobulated mass of two epithelial cell types in vascular stroma: Large cells with round nuclei and prominent nucleoli; small cells with hyperchromatic nuclei | *Spiradenocarcinoma*: High recurrence rate with lymphatic invasion and distant metastases | Loss of nodular growth pattern with infiltrative growth, rapid mitoses, and tumor necrosis |
| Cylindroma | Solitary or multiple (turban tumor) lesions affecting the scalp and face; may be associated with familial cylindromatosis and Brooke–Spiegler syndrome | Nodules of epithelial cells that are well-circumscribed and arranged in "jigsaw puzzle" pattern; large and small basaloid cells present | *Malignant cylindroma*: Rapid growth, ulceration, bleeding, and aggressive course; local recurrence and distant metastases | Infiltrative growth with cytonuclear pleomorphism, peripheral palisading, and loss of jigsaw puzzle appearance |
| Syringocystadenoma papilliferum | Solitary or multiple hamartomatous lesions on the face of scalp; may occur in a nevus sebaceous | Numerous papillary structures with a fibrovascular core and lined by two layers of epithelial cells | Syringocystadenocarcinoma papilliferum | Disorderly arrangement of papillary structures with loss of the two layers of epithelial cells in the benign form |
| Hidradenoma papilliferum | Solitary lesions with ulceration and bleeding, found in vulva and perianal region | Solid or cystic nodule formed with papillary structures lined by two cell layers; clear cell change | None | – |

Microcystic adnexal carcinoma is a rare neoplasm associated with ultraviolet radiation exposure, radiation therapy, and immunosuppression. Clinically, this tumor presents as a flesh-colored, smooth, solitary nodule most commonly located on the upper or lower lip. Histologically, the tumor consists of epithelial cells in sclerotic stroma with infiltrative growth and perineural and intraneural invasion. There is little cytological atypia and mitotic activity, but microcysts of keratin and tubular/ductal structures are often present. Metastasis is rare, but recurrence rates of up to 60% as well as extension into subcutaneous and adjacent tissue make complete excision difficult. Mohs surgery is therefore the treatment of choice to ensure adequate normal tissue margins.

## Fibrous Neoplasms

Dermatofibromas are benign firm, skin-colored or hyperpigmented papules believed to be often secondary to trauma that are characteristically positive for factor XIIIa and CD68, but negative for CD34. There is often benign hyperplasia (pseudoepitheliomatous hyperplasia) of the overlying epidermis. The highly malignant dermatofibrosarcoma

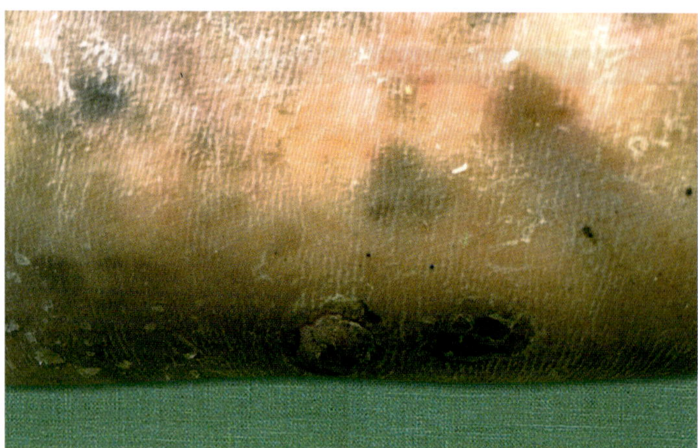

**FIG. 16:** Poroma (central inferior nodule) involving the acral surface of the lower extremity.

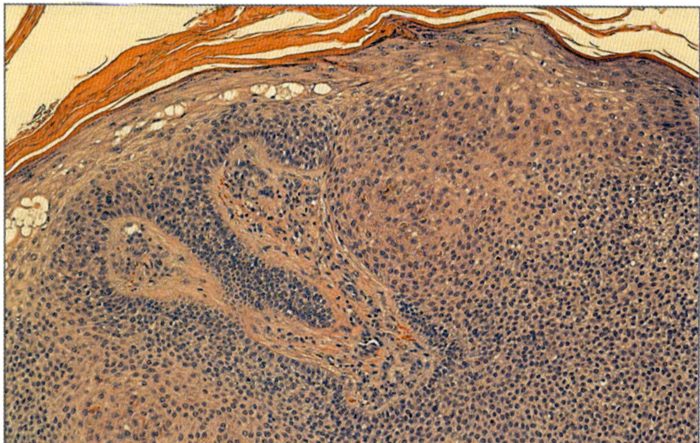

**FIG. 17:** Eccrine poroma, demonstrating sheets of basaloid cells with centrally located nuclei and high vascularity.

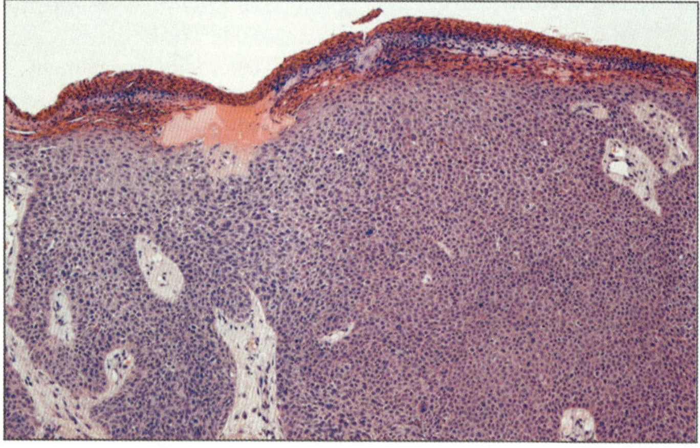

**FIG. 18:** Histology of porocarcinoma, with sheets of basaloid cells exhibiting cellular atypia, high mitotic activity, and infiltrative growth.

protuberans, however, is CD34 positive and has ringed fusions of chromosomes 17q22 and 22q13. They present as pink nodules and are treated via wide excision, sometimes with adjuvant radiotherapy if surgical margins are inadequate. In contrast, dermatofibromas do not require treatment unless symptomatic.

## Neural Neoplasms

Growths of peripheral nerves and their individual components frequently involve the skin and should always be on the clinician's differential diagnosis.

Neuromas are benign neoplasms with approximately equal parts of Schwann cells and axonal pieces. They may form secondary to injury, infection, or amputation, as in traumatic neuromas, or arise without any identifiable precipitating factors. Traumatic neuromas present as small, firm, tender papules that are characterized histologically by cross-linking nerve fascicle bundles within a fibrous background. The Schwann cells present stain positive for S100 and the accompanying perineural cells stain positive for epithelial membrane antigen.

Solitary circumscribed neuroma, otherwise known as palisaded encapsulated neuroma, is a tumor of the peripheral nerve sheath and often appears as an asymptomatic papule on the head and neck. Microscopic examination reveals Schwann cells and axons with varied nuclear palisading confined within a capsule.

Like solitary circumscribed neuromas, neurofibromas are peripheral nerve sheath tumors and are frequently encountered in practice. Though usually associated with neurofibromatosis type I (*NF1* gene mutation on 17q11.2), neurofibromas need not be multiple or grouped and may appear as solitary lesions. Most are soft, flesh-colored papulonodules that are often pedunculated and occasionally symptomatic (Fig. 19). They are formed by a mixture of Schwann cells, perineurial cells, fibroblasts, and blood vessels, and have wavy, spindle cell proliferations that may stain positive for S100 and CD34 on histological and immunohistochemical analysis. Multiple neurofibroma subtypes exist, including plexiform, diffuse, pigmented, dendritic cell, and lipomatous. Excision is the treatment of choice.

Schwannomas are nerve sheath tumors composed of proliferations of Schwann cells that present as individual, asymptomatic nodules. Multiple lesions may appear in individuals with predisposing factors, such as neurofibromatosis type II. All schwannomas form secondary to *NF2* (22q12.2) gene mutations resulting in loss of function of the merlin protein. Malignant transformation and local recurrence after excision are rare.

Although neurofibromas and schwannomas are usually benign, they may occasionally transform into malignant peripheral nerve sheath tumors. The evolution of neurofibromas to malignant peripheral nerve sheath tumors is not fully understood as they demonstrate a variety of genetic mutations, including alterations in NF1 and *P53*. They may differentiate to one of several nerve cells, including Schwann cells, perineural cells, and fibroblasts and must be surgically excised early to prevent metastasis.

Merkel cell carcinoma is a relatively rare tumor, most often found in white men. Risk factors for its development are believed to include ultraviolet exposure and immunosuppression. Pathogenesis involves mutations in the P53 tumor suppressor gene and infection by Merkel cell polyomavirus. Clinically, this tumor presents as a rapidly growing, flesh-colored nodule on a sun-exposed surface, especially the head and neck. The nodule is firm in consistency and non-tender to palpation, often has telangiectasias, and has a presentation similar to that of actinic keratosis and SCC. Diagnosis is made by biopsy and immunohistochemical staining for CK20 and NFP

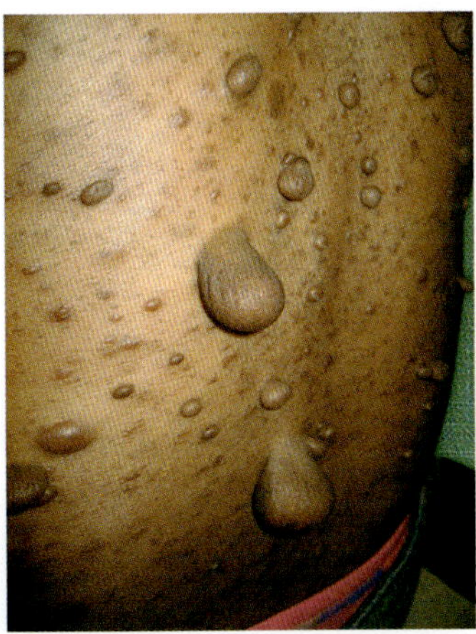

**FIG. 19:** Multiple neurofibromas of varying sizes and shapes involving the back in a patient with neurofibromatosis type I.

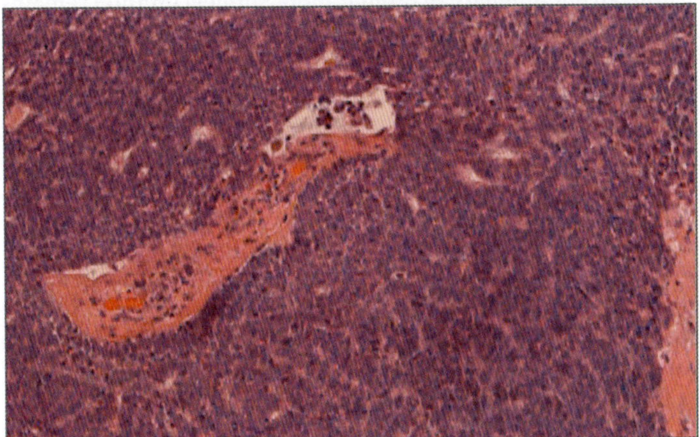

**FIG. 20:** Merkel cell carcinoma, with densely populated small blue cells demonstrating high mitotic activity.

neuroendocrine markers. Histological analysis shows densely populated small blue cells, resembling lymphocytes, with high mitotic activity, necrosis, and lymphovascular invasion (Fig. 20).

High recurrence rates, regional lymph node involvement, and metastatic potential characterize Merkel cell carcinoma as an aggressive tumor with an increased mortality rate. First-line treatment is wide local excision with 1–2 cm margins or Mohs procedure for improved border management. Evidence of metastasis is not necessarily an indication for radiotherapy because of the lack of proven survival benefit. A mucosal variant, most often affecting the larynx, has a much poorer prognosis.

## Adipose Neoplasms

Tumors of fat range from benign to malignant and may present in both genders and all age groups. Clinically, adipose neoplasms are usually soft, mobile masses and many can be treated with simple excision. Differences between them, however, are apparent on histologic examination and chromosomal analysis. Table 4 notes characteristics of adipose neoplasms.

# MUSCLE NEOPLASMS

Tumors of muscle are primarily limited to leiomyoma and its malignant counterpart, leiomyosarcoma. Leiomyomas are benign growths of the arrectores pilorum muscle, dartoic, vulvar, or mammary muscles, or blood vessel musculature. They clinically present as red-purple papules or nodules that vary in size from several millimeters to a few centimeters, and typically appear on the face, back, or extensor extremities. Most leiomyomas are extremely tender, a symptom often incited by cold or trauma.

The development of multiple leiomyomas is a characteristic of hereditary leiomyomatosis renal cell carcinoma (HLRCC) syndrome, an autosomal dominant disorder secondary to a loss of function mutation in the fumarate hydratase gene. Individuals with HLRCC have single or multiple cutaneous and uterine leiomyomas, as well as an increased risk of type II papillary renal cell carcinoma. Histological examination reveals smooth muscle proliferations without significant mitotic activity coalescing into nodules. Those with excessive mitotic activity may be labeled as an atypical smooth muscle tumor or leiomyosarcoma, depending on the extent of invasion. Treatment ranges from excision to cryotherapy and even botulinum injections.

Leiomyosarcomas are smooth muscle neoplasms with cellular atypia and high mitotic activity. Loss of the retinoblastoma protein and P53 mutations are common findings among the many complex genetic alterations seen in leiomyosarcomas. Those limited to the dermis are often identified as atypical smooth muscle tumors as they have limited metastatic potential. Subcutaneous leiomyosarcomas have metastatic potential varying from 0 to 39%, but can be up to 60% for deep intramuscular tumors. They present as firm, solitary, skin-colored or red nodules or plaques, especially on the extremities.

**TABLE 4: Adipose neoplasms**

| Name | Pathogenesis | Clinical features | Pathology | Treatment |
|---|---|---|---|---|
| Lipoma | Associated with translocations of 12q13-15 | Soft, mobile, subcutaneous masses | Uniform mature fat cells with eccentric nuclei | Excision and liposuction |
| Hibernoma | Unknown | Soft, mobile, subcutaneous masses | Brown fat cells encased by vascularized septa | Excision |
| Nevus lipomatosus superficialis | Unknown | Soft, clustered, yellowish papules and nodules | Mature adipocytes within the dermis | Excision |
| Lipoblastoma | Immature adipose accumulations, associated with 8q rearrangements | Soft, mobile masses | Immature to mature fat cells with lobulated and myxoid characteristics | Excision |
| Liposarcoma | De novo neoplasm with translocation of chromosomes 12 and 16 | Large, dome-shaped, subcutaneous masses | Well-differentiated, myxoid, round cell, pleomorphic, and dedifferentiated variants | Excision, oncology and/or surgical oncology evaluation |

Biopsies of leiomyosarcoma demonstrate irregularly interspersed bundles of spindle cells with focal pleomorphism and mitoses. Tumors with fewer mitoses are associated with longer recurrence-free periods. Leiomyosarcomas are usually positive for alpha smooth muscle actin and desmin, although neither is specific for the cancer. Wide excision with definite clear margins is the mainstay of treatment and patients should be closely monitored for recurrences or metastases.

## VASCULAR TUMORS

Vascular tumors may present early in infancy or well into adulthood with either benign or very malignant growth patterns. Childhood hemangiomas are benign growths often derived from an in utero transplant of placental tissue, that undergo a rapid proliferation phase within the first few months of life, followed by involution several years later, occasionally leaving behind an atrophic scar. Depending on their location within the dermis or subcutaneous tissue, they may be bright red or nearly flesh-colored. Noninvoluting variants, hemangiomas close to vital regions such as the eye or lips, and those to succumb to ulceration or superinfection require intervention to prevent secondary complications. Management options include intralesional and topical corticosteroids, topical β-blockers, surgical excision, and laser therapy.

Angiokeratomas are uncommon dermal malformations that can affect many regions of the body as solitary or multiple lesions. Clinically, they are small red to blue or purple papules that bleed with trauma, which may have dark lacunae or a white veil on dermoscopy. Dilated dermal vessels with overlying hyperkeratosis are seen on histological examination.

Cherry or senile angiomas are benign capillary neoplasms usually no more than several millimeters in size that largely affect the trunk and extremities. They are smooth, bright red papules that may be successfully managed with laser therapy or electrosurgery (Fig. 21).

Like angiokeratomas and cherry angiomas, pyogenic granulomas are vascular growths that present as red to blue papulonodules. In contrast, however, they are usually larger, grow faster, and may bleed more aggressively with trauma. They demonstrate an overexpression of vascular endothelial growth factor, basic fibroblast growth factor, and MAP kinases, and have even been recently linked to use of vemurafenib for malignant melanoma. Biopsy shows multiple clustered small blood vessels within an endothelial cell proliferation. Surgical excision remains the mainstay of treatment, although other options are available.

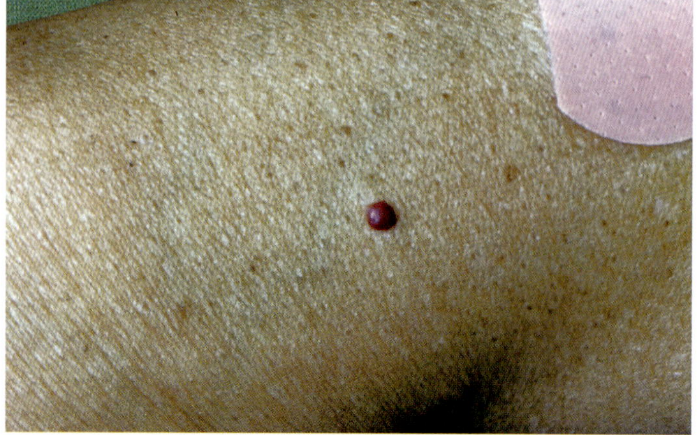

**FIG. 21:** Cherry angioma in an elderly patient over the upper extremity.

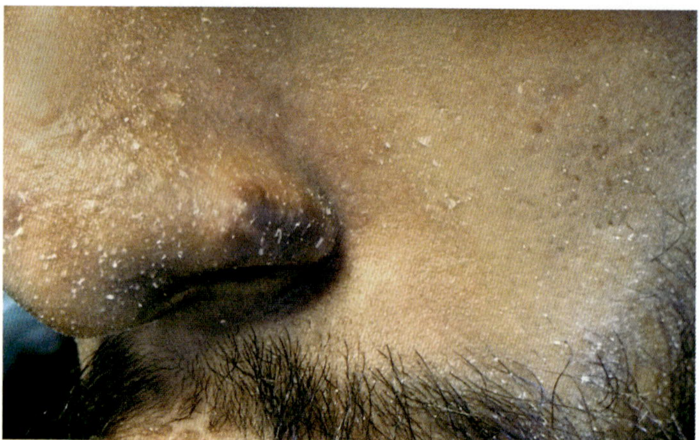

**FIG. 22:** Kaposi sarcoma over the left nasal ala in a newly-diagnosed AIDS patient.

Kaposi sarcoma (KS) is one of the major vascular malignancies that involve the skin. Though commonly associated with HIV/AIDS, the disease can be seen in iatrogenic or age-related immunodeficiency as well. Human herpes virus 8 (HHV-8) infection is necessary, but not sufficient to develop KS, linked in classic form to people of Italian, Greek and Jewish lineage. HHV-8 activates c-kit, which helps transform microvascular endothelial cells into the spindle cells characteristic of Kaposi sarcoma on histology. KS presents as blue-purple patches, nodules, or plaques with a predilection for the lower extremities (Fig. 22). Those secondary to HIV/AIDS immunodeficiency are usually responsive to antiretroviral therapy, but if not, then cryosurgery, intralesional chemotherapy, or even systemic chemotherapy may be attempted.

Cutaneous angiosarcoma is a rare and highly malignant neoplasm often arising on the head and neck of older male patients. Risk factors for angiosarcoma include radiation therapy and vascular and lymphatic insufficiency. Angiosarcomas vary in clinical appearance from red or blue/purple patches and plaques to papulonodules. Stewart–Treves syndrome has historically denoted angiosarcoma arising within a site of chronic lymphedema, such as the ipsilateral upper extremity following a radical mastectomy. Microscopically, angiosarcomas have epithelioid or spindle cell proliferations that stain positive for certain immunohistochemical markers including CD31, CD34, vascular endothelial growth factor, and factor VIII. 5-year survival rate ranges between 12% and 24%, and up to 94% of patients with cutaneous angiosarcoma have disease recurrences. Local invasion, lymph node spread, and metastasis are indicators of poor prognosis. Treatment options include surgical resection, radiotherapy, chemotherapy, and combinations of the above.

## SUGGESTED READINGS

1. Alsaad KO, Obaidat NA, Ghazarian D. Skin adnexal neoplasms--part 1: an approach to tumours of the pilosebaceous unit. J Clin Pathol. 2007;60(2):129-44.
2. Benmansour A, Laanaz S, Bougtab A. Stewart-Treves syndrome: a case report. Pan African Med J. 2014;19:2.
3. Chao MM, Schwartz JL, Wechsler DS, et al. High-risk surgically resected pediatric melanoma and adjuvant interferon therapy. Pediatr Blood Cancer. 2005;44(5):441-8.

4. Cruz MA, Cho E-F, Schwartz RA, Janniger CK. Congenital neurocutaneous melanosis. Cutis. 1997;60:178-81.
5. Dodds A, Chia A, Shumack S. Actinic keratosis: rationale and management. Dermatol Ther (Heidelb). 2014;4(1):11-31.
6. Firnhaber JM. Diagnosis and treatment of Basal cell and squamous cell carcinoma. Am Fam Physician. 2012;86(2):161-8.
7. Hamman MS, Brian Jiang SI. Management of trichilemmal carcinoma: an update and comprehensive review of the literature. Dermatol Surg. 2014;40(7):711-7.
8. Hamm H, Höger PH. Skin tumors in childhood. Dtsch Arztebl Int. 2011;108(20): 347-53.
9. Happle R. Nevus sebaceus is a mosaic RASopathy. J Invest Dermatol. 2013;133: 597-600.
11. Hegedus F, Matthew LM, Schwartz RA. Radiation dermatitis: An overview. Int J Dermatol. 2017;56(9):904-14..
10. Ibrahim A, Asuku ME. Nodular swelling on the lower lip; pyogenic granuloma. Eplasty. 2014;14:ic45.
12. Jadotte YT, Schwartz RA. Solar cheilosis: an ominous precursor: part I. Diagnostic insights. J Am Acad Dermatol. 2012;66(2):173-84; quiz 85-6.
13. Jadotte YT, Schwartz RA. Solar cheilosis: an ominous precursor part II. Therapeutic perspectives. J Am Acad Dermatol. 2012;66(2):187-98; quiz 99-200.
14. John A, Schwartz RA: Basal cell naevus syndrome: an update on genetics and treatment. Br J Dermatol 2016; 174: 68-76.
15. John A, Schwartz RA. Muir-Torre syndrome: An update and approach to diagnosis and management. J Am Acad Dermatol. 2016;74:558-66.
16. Kaminska-Winciorek G, Calik J, Wydmanski J, et al. Primary melanoma in rare locations: clinical and dermatoscopic features. Indian J Dermatol Venereol Leprol. 2014;80(4):369-71.
17. Kauffmann RM, Chen SL. Workup and staging of malignant melanoma. Surg Clin North Am. 2014;94(5):963-72, vii.
18. Kim JH, Kim MR, Lee S, et al. Dermoscopy: a useful tool for the diagnosis of angiokeratoma. Ann Dermatol. 2012;24(4).
19. Korkolis DP, Liapakis IE, Vassilopoulos PP. Dermatofibrosarcoma protuberans: clinicopathological aspects of an unusual cutaneous tumor. Antican Res. 2007;27: 1631-4.
20. Kwiek B, Schwartz RA. Keratoacanthoma: Update and review. J Am Acad Dermatol. 2016;74:1220-33.
21. Lobato-Berezo A, Chirruca-Grijelmo M, Martínez-Pérez M, et al. Dermatofibroma arising within a black tattoo. Case Rep Dermatol Med. 2014;2014:745304
22. Lo JA, Fisher DE. The melanoma revolution: from UV carcinogenesis to a new era in therapeutics. Science. 2014;346(6212):945-9.
23. Marek L, Grzanka A, Chmielowska E, et al. Merkel cell carcinoma: an illustrative case and review. Postepy Dermatol Alergol. 2014;31(5):325-8.
24. Micali G, Lacarrubba F, Nasca MR, et al. Topical pharmacotherapy for skin cancer: part I. Pharmacology. J Am Acad Dermatol. 2014;70(6):965.e1-12; quiz 77-8.
25. Micali G, Lacarrubba F, Nasca MR, et al. Topical pharmacotherapy for skin cancer: part II. Clinical applications. J Am Acad Dermatol. 2014;70(6):979.e1-12; quiz 9912.
26. Miettinen M. Smooth muscle tumors of soft tissue and non-uterine viscera: biology and prognosis. Mod Pathol. 2014;27(Suppl 1):S17-29.
27. Musumeci ML, Schlecht K, Perrotta R, et al. Management of cutaneous hemangiomas in pediatric patients. Cutis. 2008;81(4):315-22.
28. Obaidat NA, Alsaad KO, Ghazarian D. Skin adnexal neoplasms--part 2: an approach to tumours of cutaneous sweat glands. J Clin Pathol. 2007;60(2):145-59.
29. Papadopoulos AJ, Schwartz RA, Lefkowitz A, et al. Extragenital bowenoid papulosis associated with atypical human papillomavirus genotypes. J Cutan Med Surg. 2002;6(2):117-21.
30. Patel GA, Ragi G, Krysicki J, et al. Subungual melanoma: a deceptive disorder. Acta Dermatovenerol Croat. 2008;16(4):236-42.
31. Raju S, Vazirnia A, Totri C, et al. Treatment of Merkel cell carcinoma of the head and neck: a systematic review. Dermatol Surg. 2014;40(12):1273-83.
32. Regauer S, Beham-Schmid C, Okcu M, et al. Trichoblastic carcinoma ("malignant trichoblastoma") with lymphatic and hematogenous metastases. Mod Pathol. 2000;13(6):673-8.
33. Reinstadler DR, Sinha UK. Uncommon cutaneous neoplasms of the head and neck. Facial Plast Surg Clin North Am. 2012;20(4):483-91.
34. Rodriguez-Peralto JL, Riveiro-Falkenbach E, Carrillo R. Benign cutaneous neural tumors. Semin Diagn Pathol. 2013;30(1):45-57.
35. Sammut SJ, Tomson N, Corrie P. Pyogenic granuloma as a cutaneous adverse effect of vemurafenib. N Engl J Med. 2014;371(13):1265-7.
36. Satyaprakash AK, Sheehan DJ, Sangueza OP. Proliferating trichilemmal tumors: a review of the literature. Dermatol Surg. 2007;33(9):1102-8.
37. Schwartz RA, Blaszczyk M, Jablonska S. Generalized eruptive keratoacanthoma of Grzybowski: follow-up of the original description and 50-year retrospect. Dermatology. 2002;205(4):348-52.
38. Schwartz RA, Bridges TM, Butani AK, et al. Actinic keratosis: an occupational and environmental disorder. J Eur Acad Dermatol Venereol. 2008;22(5):606-15.
39. Schwartz RA, De Jager RL, Janniger CK, et al. Giant basal cell carcinoma with metastases and myelophthisic anemia. J Surg Oncol. 1986;33(4):223-6.
40. Schwartz RA, Janniger CK. Bowenoid papulosis. J Am Acad Dermatol. 1991;24(2 Pt 1):261-4.
41. Schwartz RA, Kist JM, Thomas I, et al.Ocular melanoma metastatic to skin: the value of HMB-45 staining. Dermatol Surg. 2004;30(6):942-4.
42. Schwartz RA, Lambert WC. The Merkel cell carcinoma: a 50-year retrospect. J Surg Oncol. 2005;89(1):5.
43. Schwartz RA, Micali G, Nasca MR, et al. Kaposi sarcoma: a continuing conundrum. J Am Acad Dermatol. 2008;59(2):179-206.
44. Schwartz RA, Tarlow MM, Lambert WC. Keratoacanthoma-like squamous cell carcinoma within the fibroepithelial polyp. Dermatol Surg. 2004;30(2 Pt 2):349-50.
45. Schwartz RA, Torre DP. The Muir-Torre syndrome: a 25-year retrospect. J Am Acad Dermatol. 1995;33(1):90-104.
46. Schwartz RA. Keratoacanthoma. J Am Acad Dermatol. 1994;30(1):1-19; quiz 20-2.
47. Schwartz RA. Keratoacanthoma: a clinico-pathologic enigma. Dermatol Surg. 2004;30(2 Pt 2):326-33; discussion 33.
48. Schwartz RA. Sign of Leser-Trelat. J Am Acad Dermatol. 1996;35(1):88-95.
49. Schwartz RA. Skin Cancer: recognition and management. Oxford: Blackwell Publishers; 2008.
50. Sharma A, Bialynicki-Birula R, Schwartz RA, et al. Lichen planus: an update and review. Cutis. 2012;90(1):17-23.
51. Sharma A, Schwartz RA. Stewart-Treves syndrome: pathogenesis and management. J Am Acad Dermatol. 2012;67(6):1342-8.
52. Tarlow MM, Nemlick AS, Rothenberg J, et al. Pseudoglandular-type melanoma: a rare melanoma variant. J Cutan Pathol. 2008;35(6):588-90.
53. Tenjarla S, Sheils LA, Kwiatkowski TM, et al. Cutaneous angiosarcoma of the foot: a case report and review of the literature. Case Rep Oncol Med. 2014;2014:657876.
54. Thomas I, Kihiczak NI, Rothenberg J, et al. Melanoma within the seborrheic keratosis. Dermatol Surg. 2004;30(4 Pt 1):559-61.
55. Thway K, Fisher C. Malignant peripheral nerve sheath tumor: pathology and genetics. Ann Diagn Pathol. 2014;18(2):109-16.
56. Uzarska M, Czajkowski R, Schwartz RA, et al. Chemoprevention of skin melanoma: facts and myths. Melanoma Res. 2013;23(6):426-33.
57. Winship IM, Dudding TE. Lessons from the skin--cutaneous features of familial cancer. Lancet Oncol. 2008;9(5):462-72.
58. Wong SY, Dlugosz AA. Basal cell carcinoma, Hedgehog signaling, and targeted therapeutics: the long and winding road. J Invest Dermatol. 2014;134(e1):E18-22.
59. Yagnik VD. Giant epidermoid cyst over the male breast. Clin Pract. 2011;1(1):e2.
60. Yardimci G, Kutlubay Z, Engin B, et al. Precancerous lesions of oral mucosa. World J Clin Cases. 2014;2(12):866-72.
61. Zargaran M, Baghaei F. A clinical, histopathological and immunohistochemical approach to the bewildering diagnosis of keratoacanthoma. J Dent (Shiraz). 2014;15(3):91-7.

# 74 CHAPTER Malignant Lymphoproliferative Disorders of Skin

*Nilendu Sarma, Anupam Das*

## INTRODUCTION

Lymphoproliferative disorders, which refer to monoclonal lymphocytosis of either T- or B-cell types, may be caused by diverse conditions. Acquired and genetic factors and even insect bite or drugs may induce this. These may be seen in benign (parapsoriasis and pityriasis lichenoides) or in malignant condition (leukemia and lymphoma). The differentiation is frequently difficult. There is another variant, called pseudolymphoma, caused by arthropod bites, nodular scabies, or drugs.

## CUTANEOUS PSEUDOLYMPHOMA

Cutaneous pseudolymphomas are basically benign proliferation of lymphocytes but mimick lymphomas clinically and histologically. These are also known as cutaneous lymphoid hyperplasia.

Common triggering factors are tattoo dye, trauma and acupuncture, insect and spider bites, vaccinations, gold, aluminum, liquid silicone, infections (varicella-zoster virus, *Borrelia burgdorferi, Leishmania panamensis*, molluscum contagiosum, scabies, *Helicobacter pylori*), acupuncture sites, folliculitis, and drugs. Anticonvulsants (mainly phenytoin and carbamazepine), zoledronic acid, and cyclosporine are known to induce pseudolymphoma.

Differentiation from malignant proliferation is important. Important histological features of pseudolymphoma are presence of prominent epidermal spongiosis, less dense yet well-circumscribed collection of lymphocytes that is mostly present in upper dermis along with other cells (mixed infiltration) like histiocytes, eosinophils, and plasma cells. Other important findings include tingible body macrophages, preserved and evenly spaced follicular dendritic cells (CD21+), and lack of Bcl-2 staining.

Clinical correlation is most crucial for diagnosis.

Removal of offending agents is very important. Topical imiquimod, subcutaneous injection of interferon-alpha (IFN-$\alpha$), fractional resurfacing, and subsequent Q-switched Nd:YAG (neodymium-doped yttrium aluminum garnet) 532-nm laser are used for treating this condition.

## CUTANEOUS LYMPHOMA

Cutaneous lymphoma (CL) constitutes 4% of all non-Hodgkin's lymphoma and mycosis fungoides (MF) is the major type. Skin is the second most common organ, second only to gastrointestinal tract of extranodal non-Hodgkins' lymphoma. CL can be of two types. Primary CL and secondary CL. Primary CL is defined as lymphoma that originates in the skin or at least restricted at the skin at the time of diagnosis and is generally remains confined to the skin for a longer period of time. Secondary CL, as the name suggests, originates in some other tissues and involves the skin secondarily.

### Classification

Cutaneous lymphoma is now understood to have significant difference from systemic lymphoma in its prognosis and response to treatment. Classification of CL has seen continuous updating reflecting our improvement in the knowledge of its intricate behavior. Earlier systems of classification were Rappaport classification, the Kiel classification, Working Formulation for the Non-Hodgkin Lymphomas, and the first global classification called Revised European–American Classification of Lymphoid Neoplasms (REAL classification).

Knowledge in the field of immunopathology of lymphoma especially on different CD markers, T-cell receptors (TCRs), molecular and genetic abnormality in the causation of individual subtypes has reached a never before level. Having said that, it is now also understood that clinical behavior of the lymphoma (e.g., site) has more valuable implication in diagnosis and evaluation of prognosis than it was though earlier.

As per the recent joint European Organization for Research and Treatment of Cancer (EORTC) and World Health Organization (WHO) classification, CLs with primary cutaneous manifestations have been divided into three major classes, these are called:

1. Cutaneous T-cell and natural killer (NK)-cell lymphomas
2. Cutaneous B-cell lymphomas (CBCLs)
3. Precursor hematologic neoplasm.

Cutaneous T-cell and NK-cell lymphomas have been subclassified into nine subtypes as follows:

1. Mycosis fungoides
2. Mycosis fungoides variants and subtypes (three subtypes)
3. Sézary syndrome
4. Adult T-cell leukemia or lymphoma
5. Primary cutaneous CD30+ lymphoproliferative disorders (two subtypes)
6. Subcutaneous panniculitis-like T-cell lymphoma (SPTL)

7. Extranodal NK or T-cell lymphoma, nasal type
8. Primary cutaneous peripheral T-cell lymphoma, unspecified (two subtypes)
9. Primary cutaneous CD4+ small or medium-sized pleomorphic T-cell lymphoma (provisional).

Three variants of MF have been proposed; these are folliculotropic MF, pagetoid reticulosis, and granulomatous slack skin. Primary cutaneous anaplastic large cell lymphoma and lymphomatoid papulosis have been placed under primary cutaneous CD30+ lymphoproliferative disorders and primary cutaneous aggressive epidermotropic CD8+ T-cell lymphoma (provisional) and cutaneous γ/δ T-cell lymphoma (provisional) have been mentioned as two variants of primary cutaneous peripheral T-cell lymphoma, unspecified.

Following five subclasses of CBCLs have been described:

1. Primary cutaneous marginal zone BCL
2. Primary cutaneous follicle center lymphoma (PCFCL)
3. Primary cutaneous diffuse large BCL, leg type (PCDLBCL-LT)
4. Primary cutaneous diffuse large BCL, other
5. Intravascular large BCL.

CD4+/CD56+ hematodermic neoplasm (blastic NK-cell lymphoma) is the sole type of neoplasia under of precursor hematologic neoplasm.

Cutaneous T-cell lymphoma (CTCL) group is dominated by MF (including its subtypes). The second most common is primary cutaneous CD30+ lymphoproliferative disorders. The remaining disorders (<10% of all T-cell lymphoma) were initially grouped under a group called CD30- large T-cell lymphoma.

Some of the important features of WHO/EORTC classification are:

- Separation of extranodal NK or T-cell lymphoma, nasal type, and CD4+/CD56+ hematodermic neoplasm (blastic NK-cell lymphoma) and keeping them as two separate entities
- Identification of prognostic markers and classification of disease are based on prognosis. Lymphoma with α/β phenotype was found to have better prognosis than γ/δ phenotype that was found to be highly aggressive
- Small-medium cells had better prognosis than larger cells
- CD4+ T-cell phenotype had better prognosis than CD8+ T-cell phenotype.

On this ground, the broader group, peripheral T-cell lymphoma (PTL), was subdivided into three provisional subtypes. Thus, γ/4+ T-cell lymphoma (some SPTL, some NK or T-cell lymphoma, and other) was made a separate group to highlight its aggressive behavior. Now SPTL means only α/β T-cell phenotype. The remaining entities that do not fit into any of these three provisional groups will now fall under the original term, PTL, unspecified.

## CUTANEOUS T-CELL LYMPHOMA

Cutaneous T-cell lymphoma refers to a group of lymphoproliferative disorders which is essentially characterized by cutaneous localization of neoplastic T-cells. MF and Seźary syndrome (SS) constitute about 50% of all CLs.

### Epidemiology

The disease is distributed worldwide with a predilection for the individuals working in industries. The disease is more common in men (M:F = 2:1). Presently, the age-adjusted incidence of CTCL is about six cases per 1 million in a year. The incidence and survival of CTCL has been increasing steadily for over 25 years. The overall incidence has stabilized since 1998, with an annual percent change (APC) of 5.7% from 1973 to 1998 and an APC of 0.1% from 1998 to 2009. The incidence of CTCL is no longer increasing. This may be attributed to real incidence stabilization, stabilization of physician detection, and/or artifact. The disease predominantly affects middle aged to elderly population with an average onset between 50 years and 60 years. However, all ages including children can be affected rarely.

### Classification

The latest classification is according to the new WHO or EORTC consensus classification for primary CLs (see earlier).

Mycosis fungoides and three of its variants like follicular MF, pagetoid reticulosis and granulomatous slack skin, CD30+ lymphoproliferative diseases (anaplastic large cell lymphoma and lymphomatoid papulosis), SPTL, and CD4+ small or medium pleomorphic T-cell lymphoma have been mentioned as indolent variant.

Other conditions like SS, cutaneous peripheral T-cell lymphoma, unspecified, cutaneous aggressive CD8+ T-cell lymphoma, and cutaneous γ/δ T-cell lymphoma have been grouped as aggressive variant.

### Mycosis Fungoides

#### Pathogenesis

Cutaneous T-cell lymphoma is a T-cell malignancy that originates in the skin-homing memory CD4+ CD45RO+ T lymphocyte. This is why CTCL starts as various T-cell-mediated dermatoses and clinically mimicks those conditions in the initial stages. Skin in these inflammatory dermatoses is infiltrated with the dendritic cells, reactive T-cells, macrophages, mast cells, and plasma cells. Differentiating the malignant T-cells from the normal benign T-cells is frequently a difficult task.

Very indolent growth of MF indicates that the malignant T-cells have less proliferating potential even lesser than normal skin-homing T-cell.

Proliferation may be an orchestrated event through stimulatory signals from microenvironment. Proneopalstic role of mast cells in CLs has been established.

It has been observed that the stimulating signal for proliferation may come from CD28. The overexpression IL10, Fas ligand, PD1, and CTLA4 may lead to disseminated disease beyond skin.

Early lesions of CTCL show infiltration of both malignant CD4+ and reactive CD8+ T-cells along with Th1 cytokine profile. Gradually decreasing density of CD8+ T-cells relative to the atypical CD4+ tumor cells in the CTCL lesions is typical and signifies role of specific immunogenic mechanism. With advancing stages, there is a loss of Th1 cytokines, [decreased interleukin (IL)-2, IFN-γ, and IL12], and an increase in Th2 cytokines, such as IL4, IL5, IL10, and IL13.

In accordance with these findings, studies have detected upregulation of genes associated with Th2 phenotype like *GATA3* and downregulation of genes associated with Th1 phenotype like *STAT4*. Genes related with proliferation of T-cell like *JUNB* and *JUND* are also increased. This supports the view that MF and CTCL is a genetically controlled disease.

Th17 subset of CD4+ T-cells might play role in recruiting T-cells and also neutrophils into the skin through its action on keratinocytes. IL17A is detected in the skin in about 50% of MF patients but not in the blood indicating absence of its role in SS.

Role of other cytokines like IL15 and IL16 is also suggested in various stages of CTCL development. The presence of FOXP3+ regulatory T-cells (Treg) correlates with improved survival, because these cells suppress the proliferation of malignant cell proliferation.

## Clinical Features

The presentation of MF, the prototype of CTCL, has been described in details. It is divided into three stages: patch, plaque, and tumor. All three lesion types can be seen concomitantly. 30% of patients may present with skin tumors or erythroderma at the onset. Erythroderma is often considered as fourth stage (*see* Seźary syndrome).

The first stage (patch) may go unnoticed and uneventful in the form of a nonspecific dermatitis. In fact various inflammatory dermatoses may transform to patch stage MF. Patches of various size and number, preferentially distributed over covered areas of the lower trunk, buttocks, and upper thigh (bathing trunk distribution), develop insidiously, persist for long period, progress to plaque or sometimes improve. Patches are may be asymptomatic or intensely pruritic. Patches appear as erythematous or brownish, scaly eczematous lesions and may also have hypo- or hyperchromasia, lichenification, atrophy, telangiectasia, and poikiloderma (Figs 1 and 2).

Plaque type MF is often asymmetrically distributed annular, polycyclic or horseshoe-shaped with well-demarcated margin and may ulcerate. Size and number may increase from existing lesions. Face and scalp may also be affected.

Tumor stage MF is characterized by presence of erythematous papules and nodules that progress to form larger lesions. Common sites are face and flexures-like axilla, inguinal folds, inframammary folds, and antecubital folds. Involved face may appear as "leonine facies". Oral and genital mucosae are also affected.

Mycosis fungoides may have unusual presentations such as hypo- or hyperpigmented patches, hyperkeratosis, follicular, syringotropic, bullous/vesicular/pustular, and rarely pigmented purpura-like eruption. Some cases show abrupt onset of tumors without preceding patches or plaques of MF. This has been termed d'emblee MF. Now this is known that most of these cases belong to the group of primary cutaneous CD30+ pleomorphic, medium or large cell T-cell lymphomas. The disease can spread to almost all the organs, including the central nervous system. Viscera are involved in 50–75% of such cases.

## Differential Diagnosis

*Patch stage*: Patch stage MF may be mimicked by different dermatitis like eczema, psoriasis, ichthyosiform dermatoses, small and large plaque parapsoriasis, the later one actually may transform to MF in 7.5–14% cases.

Plaque and nodular MF may be mimicked by leprosy, sarcoidosis, tinea, and lupus (subacute cutaneous lupus erythematosus, tumid lupus).

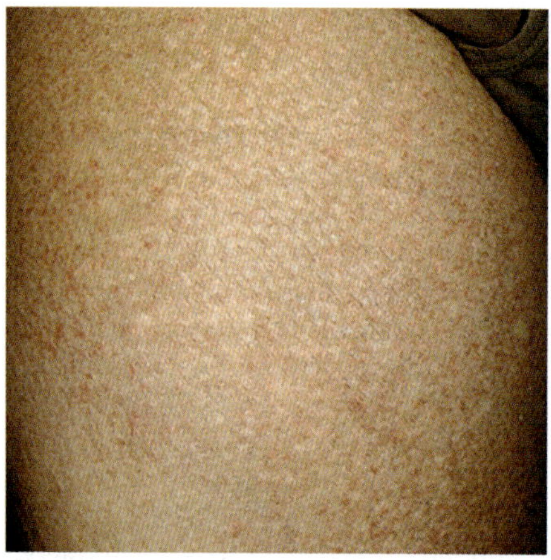

**FIG. 1:** Patch stage mycosis fungoides showing erythema, scaling, telangiectasia, and mild atrophy on the thigh of a young man.

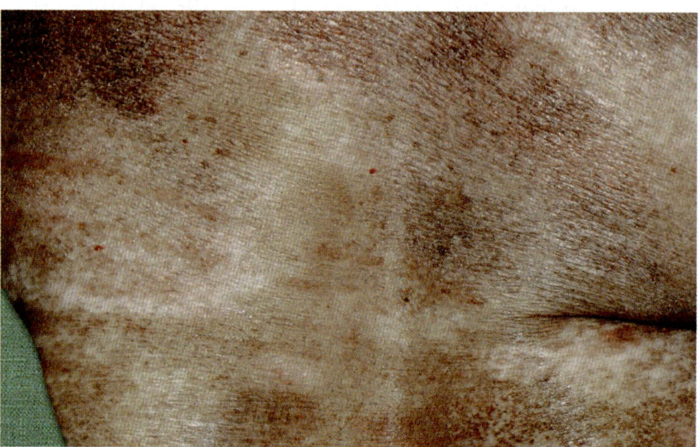

**FIG. 2:** Mycosis fungoides presenting as widespread scaly eczematous patches, poikiloderma developed over long-standing hypopigmentation in an old lady.

Malignant T-cells may disseminate, generally in tumor stage and involve regional lymph node or even other organs. However, bone marrow is much rarely involved.

## Variants of Mycosis Fungoides

- *Pagetoid reticulosis*: It is a histological subtype of CTCL with characteristic clinical presentation. This is another example where clinical presentation indicates the disease severity. It has been found that all cases with multifocal and widespread disease (Ketron–Goodman type) basically represented more aggressive disease and mostly showed CD8+, or γ/δ-positive T-cell lymphoma; they have been excluded from classical pagetoid reticulosis as per latest disease classification. Thus, pagetoid reticulosis, presently is defined as disease manifesting as single or localized disease (Woringer–Kolopp type) on the acral areas. It appears as scaly and psoriasiform plaque. It has a favorable prognosis with rare occurrence of death.

Typically, the T-cells show CD3+, CD4+, and CD8- but cases with CD3+, CD4-, CD8+, and also CD30+ T-cells are also found.

Histologically, the hallmark features are presence of pagetoid spread of atypical haloed lymphoid cells (single or nest) in the epidermis and dermis showing no malignant cells. The atypical cells have larger, hyperchromatic, and cerebriform nuclei.

- *Folliculotropic mycosis fungoides*: Neoplastic, atypical appearing T-cells surround the deep follicular and perifollicular areas (folliculotropism) frequently sparing the epidermis (absence of epidermotropism). There may be follicular mucinous alteration. Clinically, this presents as follicular papules, keratosis pilaris-like lesions, comedo-like papules, epidermal cysts, and plaques involving head and neck area. Area around the eye and eyebrow are affected and typically leads to alopecia. Pruritus is often severe. Sometimes, malignant T-cells show syringotropism (distributed around eccrine glands). Prognosis is worse than classical plaque stage MF mostly because difficulty in accessing the deeper neoplastic cells.
- *Granulomatous mycosis fungoides and granulomatous slack skin*: Major folds of the body develop pendulous and lax skin. Histopathology shows presence of granulomatous infiltration with neoplastic T-cells. Granuloma may appear as sarcoidal, tuberculoid granuloma or periadnexal and granuloma annulare-like. It is very rare and associated with a poorer prognosis in comparison to classic MF.

## Other Types of Cutaneous T-cell Lymphoma

### Subcutaneous Panniculitis-like T-cell Lymphoma

Solitary or multiple nodules and plaques over the legs, clinically appearing as panniculitis for many years may turn malignant and widespread lesions many develop. However, systemic dissemination is generally rare as is ulceration of the skin lesions. It may be associated with constitutional symptoms. Systemic symptoms such as fever, fatigue, and weight loss may be present. Patient may suddenly worsen frequently associated with hemophagocytic syndrome.

Histopathological investigations show subcutaneous infiltrates of small, medium-sized, or large pleomorphic T-cells without involvement of dermis and epidermis. Immunophenotype study shows α/β+, CD3+, CD4-, and CD8+ type of T-cells. This has an indolent behavior. Some cases (25%) that showed features like epidermal or dermal infiltration, γ/δ+, CD3+, CD4-, CD8-, and CD56+ T-cells having much worse prognosis have now been separated from this group in the recent classification and classified as cutaneous γ/δ-positive T-cell lymphoma (Fig. 3).

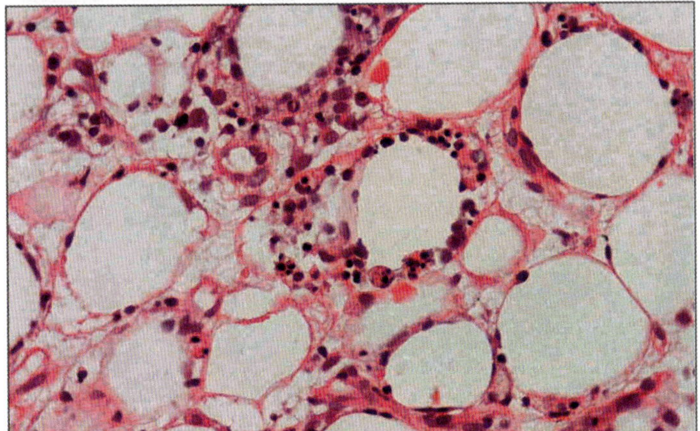

**FIG. 3:** Infiltration with atypical lymphocytes of the subcutaneous fat (rimming of the fat cells) (H&E, 400x).

*Courtesy*: Dr M Ramam, Professor, Department of Dermatology, All Indian Institute of Medical Science, Delhi.

### Cutaneous γ/δ-Positive T-cell Lymphoma

It is an extremely rare, highly malignant and rapidly fatal (average survival of 15 months after diagnosis) lymphoma and resistant to treatment, such as polychemotherapy and radiotherapy. It manifests with disseminated plaques, ulceronecrotic nodules or tumors, on the extremities and characteristically involves mucosal sites. Immunocompromised status is an important predisposing factor.

Medium to large neoplastic T-cells are present in epidermis, dermis, and subcutis.

Immunophenotypical characteristics include CD3+, CD2+, CD7+/–, and β-F1–.

### Primary Cutaneous Aggressive Epidermotropic CD8+ Cytotoxic T-cell Lymphoma

It appears as localized or disseminated papulonodules and tumors with central ulceration and necrosis. Other findings include superficial, hyperkeratotic patches, and plaques.

### Nasal-type Extranodal NK or T-cell Lymphoma

Tumors are most common in the nasal cavity but other sites may include the skin, gastrointestinal tract, testis, kidney, upper respiratory tract, and rarely the eye or orbit.

### Transformed Mycosis Fungoides

Large cell transformation (LCT) is characterized by a morphologic change of small- to medium-sized atypical T-cell lymphocytes to a large cell variant. The three patterns of LCT include a new solitary nodule within a long standing classic MF patch or plaque, the abrupt onset of multiple nodules that persist, and a new or enlarging tumor.

## Seźary Syndrome

Seźary syndrome is a form of CTCL characterized by erythroderma with leukemic involvement of peripheral blood [Seźary cells (SCs)]. Some cases of MF may progress to erythroderma and SS (SS preceded by MF). Although there has been lot of controversies regarding their differences with SS that has started and *de novo*, it is generally accepted that SS can develop in both the ways.

By definitions, SS will have leukemic involvement of atypical SCs in the blood in addition to erythroderma. SC is an atypical mononuclear cell with large, convoluted nucleus and scanty cytoplasm containing vacuoles. This is present in peripheral blood. This stains positively with periodic acid-Schiff stain (Fig. 4).

Atypical SCs were detected in blood even in normal individual and some other benign diseases.

In 2007, the tumor burden was refined by International Society for Cutaneous Lymphomas and the EORTC. Method of documentation of a dominant *TCR* gene rearrangement in the blood was done specifically with polymerase chain reaction or Southern blot method to avoid false interpretation that was a problem of earlier peripheral buffy coat smear method.

$B_0$ is defined as SC less than or equal to 5%, $B_1$ more than 5% but less than 1,000 cells/mm$^3$ or absence of a clonal rearrangement of the TCR or both and $B_2$ is defined as presence of dominant T-cell clone in addition to one or more of the following findings of:

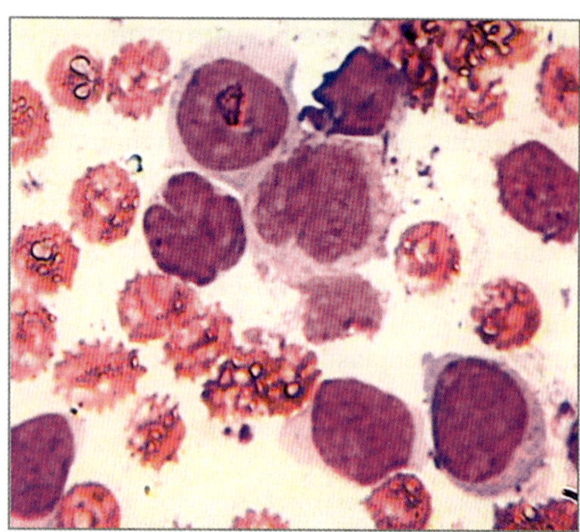

**FIG. 4:** Convoluted nucleus of Seźary cells (H&E, oil x1,000)
*Courtesy*: Dr Abhay Mani Martin, Senior Consultant and Head, Department of Dermatology, Baby Medical Hospital, Kozhikode, Kerala.

- An absolute SC count of 1,000 cells/mm$^3$ or higher
- Expanded CD3+ or CD4+ cells with a CD4/CD8 ratio of 10 or higher
- Expanded CD4+ T-cells with abnormal immunophenotype including loss of CD7 (≥40%) or CD26 (≥30%).

Presence of $B_2$ along with erythroderma was made mandatory for a diagnosis of SS. This included SS that developed from MF as well.

## Clinical Presentations

Seźary syndrome develops much faster except when SS is preceded by MF. Erythema may range from mild-to-severe exfoliative dermatitis. Pruritus is frequently severe. Other common associated findings are palmoplantar keratoderma, alopecia, ectropion, and lymphadenopathy. Complications of erythroderma like dyselectrolytemia and hypothermia are often noticed.

## Quantitative Assessment of Sézary Cells

For SS (including SS preceded by MF), assessment of blood involvement is necessary for diagnosis as well as staging and planning for treatment. Quantitative methods for SCs have been used to classify SS in $B_0$–$B_2$ stages. Additionally, more than 20% SC is also used by other as one important criteria for diagnosis of $B_2$ and this is known to have prognostic importance.

## Immunophenotype

CD4+ CD7- and CD4+ CD26- are considered typical phenotypic markers of MF or SS. As loss of CD7 may be found in some other conditions, absence of CD26 is now considered a more sensitive and specific marker.

# Diagnosis of Mycosis Fungoides and Sézary Syndrome

Diagnosis and staging of MF is based on clinical, histopathological, and laboratory investigations. Diagnosis at early stage may be extremely difficult.

Complete examination of skin associated with assessment of extent of involvement of lymph node, blood, and systemic organs is necessary for this purpose. Immunophenotyping, clonality assessment with TCR gene analysis, and more advanced tests may be required.

Mycosis fungoides can have varied clinical presentation. Thus, it is of paramount importance to differentiate it from many other conditions (Box 1).

The recommended protocols for assessment for diagnosis and initial staging of MF/SS are as follows:

- *Physical examination*: Involvement by patch, plaque, and erythroderma should be assessed in terms of body surface area (BSA). For tumors, number of lesions, aggregate volume, largest size lesion, and regions of the body involved have to be assessed
- *Lymph nodes (LNs)*: Identification of any LN of size more than or equal to 1.5 cm having a firm consistency, or irregular, clustered and fixed
- Histopathological findings in MF are abnormal T-cells in the epidermis (epidermotropism) or follicular epithelium without spongiosis and basal cell liquefaction (Fig. 5). Frequently, there is a band-like lymphocytic infiltration in the upper dermis. Atypical lymphocyte may also be seen in dermis (Fig. 6). Atypical lymphocyte is defined as cells with small to medium hyperchromatic nuclei with irregular or convoluted (cerebriform) nuclear contours. In early stages, atypical lymphocytes are seen in the basal layers (lentiginous pattern). This is described as "tagging". In advanced plaque

**BOX 1** Differential diagnosis of mycosis fungoides (all stages)

- Actinic reticuloid
- Air borne contact dermatitis
- Atopic dermatitis
- Early vitiligo
- Hodgkin's disease
- Leprosy
- Nonspecific eczema
- Pityriasis alba
- Pityriasis versicolor
- Postinflammatory hypopigmentation
- Post kala-azar dermal leishmaniasis
- Psoriasis
- Sarcoidosis
- Sarcoma
- Adult T-cell leukemia lymphoma
- Sézary syndrome

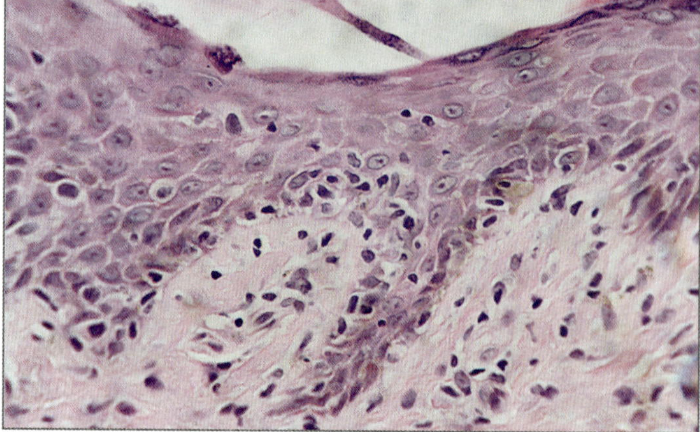

**FIG. 5:** Scattered atypical lymphocytes in epidermis and upper dermis without spongiosis or any signs of cytotoxicity (H&E, x400).

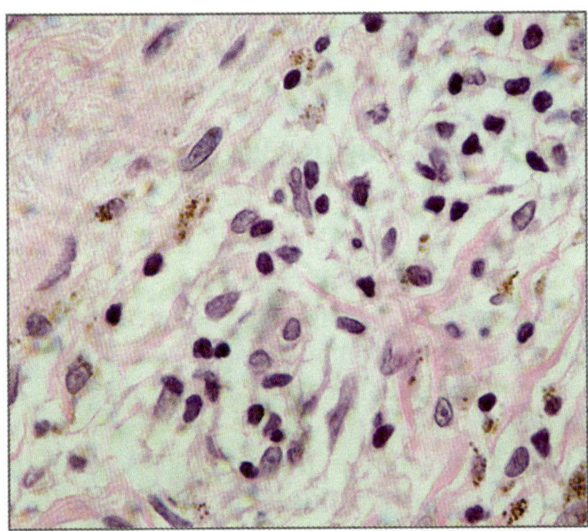

FIG. 6: Atypical lymphocytes in the dermis in early mycosis fungoides (H&E, x1,000 oil immersion view).

and nodular stages, they spread as single cell within the epidermis or are seen as cluster of many cells (Pautrier's microabscess). It should be remembered, however, that cerebriform morphology is not specific for neoplastic T-cells. Excessive inflammatory cells may mask the finding and hamper confident diagnosis especially in early stage as well as in erythroderma.

- *Immunophenotyping*: CD2, CD3, CD4, CD5, CD7, and CD8. B-cell markers like CD20. CD30 may also be included in suspected cases of lymphomatoid papulosis, anaplastic lymphoma, or large-cell transformation is considered
  - Clonality assessment through *TCR* gene rearrangement
- *Blood tests*: Total and differential white blood cell count, liver function tests, lactate dehydrogenase, and all routine biochemistry
  - Clonality assessment through of *TCR* gene rearrangement and relatedness to any clone in skin
  - *Sézary cell*: Assessment and absolute number count with flow cytometry (including CD4+/CD7- or CD4+/CD26-)
- *Radiologic tests*: Only chest X-ray or ultrasound of the peripheral nodal groups in T1 or T2 (N0M0). In most of the advanced cases—CT scans of chest, abdomen, and pelvis alone ±FDG-PET [fluorodeoxyglucose (FDG)-positron emission tomography] scan
- *Lymph node biopsy*: Excisional LN biopsy (≥1.5 cm in diameter and/or is firm, irregular, clustered, or fixed) and evaluation with light microscopy, flow cytometry, and TCR gene rearrangement.

## Staging and Classification

Staging is important for treatment planning and prognosis assessment. A detailed discussion of staging is beyond the scope of this book.

## Treatment of Mycosis Fungoides or Sézary Syndrome

Treatment of MF or SS is different from other forms of CTCL. Here a short outline of treatment for MF or SS is mentioned. Treatment is divided into two parts, skin-directed therapy (SDT) and systemic therapy (Table 1).

**TABLE 1. Treatment of mycosis fungoides or Sézary syndrome**

| Skin directed therapy | Systemic therapy |
|---|---|
| • Topical corticosteroids<br>• Topical nitrogen mustard<br>• Topical carmustine (BCNU)<br>• Psoralen ultraviolet A, ultraviolet B<br>• Total skin electron beam therapy<br>• Superficial X-irradiation | • *Chemotherapy*: Methotrexate, CHOP, chlorambucil, doxorubicin (liposome-encapsulated), purine analog (deoxycoformycin, 2-chlorodeoxyadenosine, fludarabine)<br>• *Biological response modifiers:*<br>  ○ Interferon-α<br>  ○ Retinoids<br>  ○ Rexinoids—bexarotene<br>  ○ Denileukin diftitox<br>• *Immunotherapy*: Alemtuzumab<br>• Extracorporeal photoimmunotherapy |

### Early Disease (A-IIA)

Early start of therapy does modify survival. So, expectant therapy is best at this stage. SDT is the initial treatment of choice in most cases. The options are highly potent topical corticosteroids like betamethasone dipropionate 0.05% or mometasone furoate 0.1%. Intralesional steroids are used for thicker lesions. Topical corticosteroids can induce apoptosis of malignant T-cells and Langerhans cells and can successfully treat patch stage MF. For more widespread disease, psoralen ultraviolet A (PUVA), UVB (narrow band), and total skin electron beam therapy is frequently used with success. Other options are topical chemotherapy (mechlorethamine and carmustine). Bone marrow suppression is a known side effect of topical carmustine. This is available as solution of 10 mg BCNU dissolved in 60 mL 95% alcohol or as 20–40% ointment.

Second-line therapies at this stage are retinoids like bexarotene and IFN-α, low-dose oral methotrexate (MTX), denileukin diftitox, and radiotherapy. These are highly effective and should always be used before systemic chemotherapy. Denileukin diftitox should be avoided in poorly controlled hypertension, heart failure, or in patients with renal or hepatic dysfunction. After the monotherapy regime fails, SDTs can be used in combination with systemic chemotherapy.

### Advanced Stage (IIB-IVB) MF

Sequential therapy with single drug at a time is not inferior to multidrug combination chemotherapy and thus is preferred. SDT or biologic response-modifying agents like IFN-α, bexarotene, vorinostat, and the fusion toxin denileukin diftitox are considered as first line even at this stage. Aggressive systemic chemotherapy and transplantation strategies are started early in the course in stage IVB.

### Skin Assessment and Scoring

For assessment of treatment response, modified Severity Weighted Assessment Tool (mSWAT) can be utilized. This is recommended for any therapeutic trials on MF or SS. It involves direct assessment of the BSA of each type of MF or SS lesion. Complete response, partial response, stable disease, progressive disease, and relapse have been defined for skin, lymph node, and blood.

## CUTANEOUS B-CELL LYMPHOMA

Primary cutaneous B-cell lymphoma is defined as BCL of the skin, in the absence of any evidence of internal or nodal involvement at the time of diagnosis. It constitutes about 20–25% of CLs. The latest classification system considers three types of CBCL: primary cutaneous marginal zone lymphoma (PCMZL), PCFCL, and PCDLBCL-LT.

### Primary Cutaneous Follicle Center Lymphoma

It constitutes more than 50% of primary CBCL. Clinically, it presents as a solitary or multiple papulonodules or plaques, most commonly distributed over the trunk and upper extremities. The median age at diagnosis is 60 years. Uncommon clinical presentations include military papulopustules over the face and forehead; rosacea-like lesions; rhinophyma-like presentation; annular erythematous plaques, etc.

Closest clinical differential diagnoses are cystic acne, inclusion cyst, arthropod bites, cutaneous lymphoid hyperplasia, basal cell carcinoma, Merkel cell carcinoma, folliculotropic MF, etc. The 5-year survival rate of PCFCL is 95%; however, there are 40% chances of cutaneous relapse.

Histopathologically, it is characterized by dermal and subcutaneous proliferation of centrocytes (small and cleaved cells) and centroblasts (large and intact cells). The pattern of growth can be follicular, diffuse and/or nodular. The follicle center cells generally express CD20+, CD79a+, Bcl-6+, and Bcl-2- immunophenotype. Bcl-2 positivity is a more common finding in the nodal variant. Expression of forkhead box P1 (FOX-P1) is associated with a poor prognosis.

### Primary Cutaneous Marginal Zone Lymphoma

Previously designated as immunocytomas and plasmacytomas, it is now considered a member of the spectrum of extranodal marginal zone BCL involving mucosae. So, it is also known as mucosa-associated lymphoid tissue or skin-associated lymphoid tissue lymphomas. It usually presents as solitary, multiple or grouped violaceous papulonodules and plaques distributed over the arms, trunk, and head neck region. It has a predilection for males, with the median age at presentation around 55 years. Elderly patients are more likely to have an underlying nodal disease and this mandates an extensive work-up of the patient. Overall, the prognosis of PCMZL is excellent with the 5-year survival rate being 99%. Atypical presentation includes association with fibrotic nodules in a teenager. Differential diagnoses include arthropod bites, urticaria, leukemia cutis, drug-induced pseudolymphoma, etc. Histopathology shows nodular to diffuse dermal infiltrate of marginal zone B cells (small to medium in size, irregular nuclei, inconspicuous nucleoli, and abundant pale cytoplasm), lymphoplasmacytoid cells, plasma cells, and centroblasts.

The immunophenotype of PCMZL is CD20+, CD43+, CD10-, CD5-, Bcl-2+, Bcl-6-, MUM1/IRF4+, and CD138+. A unique feature of PCMZL is overexpression of microRNAs 155 and 150, and this could be responsible for the extraordinarily good survival rates of the patients.

### Primary Cutaneous Diffuse Large B-cell Lymphoma, Leg Type

It presents as solitary to multiple red or blue papulonodules and plaques over the legs. Elderly females are commonly affected with the median age at diagnosis being 76 years. Atypical presentations include verrucous plaque-like, multiple nodules with widespread garland-like, and a blue to red multicolored rainbow pattern.

The 5-year survival rate is poor (50%). Poor prognostic factors include location on the leg and multiple skin lesions. Histopathology shows a diffuse dermal proliferation of centroblasts and immunoblasts. The cells have a round nucleus, the size of which is twice that of a lymphocyte. Nucleoli are prominent and mitotic figures are abundant. The immunophenotype is CD20+, CD79a+, CD10-, and Bcl-2-. PCDLBCL-LT strongly expresses Bcl-2, MUM1/IRF4, and FOX-P1. These three markers distinguish this entity from PCFCL. Moreover, there is monotypic surface or cytoplasmic immunoglobulin expression in PCDLBCL-LT whereas PCFCL is negative for immunoglobulin M. The t(14;18) translocation is not found in PCDLBCL-LT which is a common finding in PCFCL.

### Diagnostic Work-up

Biopsy is necessary for the diagnosis of CBCL and the prerequisite is the presence of reticular dermis and fatty tissue in the specimen. Besides, a complete history, skin examination, laboratory parameters like hemogram, hepatic profile, renal profile, metabolic profile, lactate dehydrogenase, antinuclear antibody, Lyme titer, rapid plasma reagin, serology for HBV, HCV, HIV; PET/CT and flow cytometry are required for a concrete diagnosis of CBCL.

### Treatment

The management of PCBCL depends on the type of the disease and the extent of involvement. Localized therapies are meant for indolent disease like PCFCL and PCMZL. Localized or solitary lesion of these tumors can be managed with excision, local radiotherapy and cryotherapy, topical corticosteroids, imiquimod, nitrogen mustard and bexarotene, intralesional injections of corticosteroids, IFN-$\alpha$, and rituximab. More extensive diseases of these types are treated with intravenous rituximab, chlorambucil and/or rituximab, and CVP (cyclophosphamide, vincristine, and prednisone).

However, aggressive types like primary cutaneous diffuse large BCL-leg or other/non-leg require to multiagent chemotherapy and immune-based modalities like R-CHOP (cyclophosphamide, doxorubicin, oncovin/vincristine, and prednisone with rituximab) ± local radiotherapy, and cryotherapy.

Some of the treatment options under trial are *IFN-$\gamma$* gene transfer with TG1042 (adenovirus-IFN-$\gamma$), lenalidomide, aurora kinase inhibitors, ofatumumab—human monoclonal antibody, lumiliximab (anti-CD23), and dacetuzumab—anti-CD40.

## SUGGESTED READINGS


1. Altamura D, Calonje E, Liau JL, et al. Diffuse cutaneous pseudolymphoma due to therapy with medicinal leeches. JAMA Dermatol. 2014;150(7):783-4.
2. Barzilai A, Feuerman H, Quaglino P, et al. Cutaneous B-cell neoplasms mimicking granulomatous rosacea or rhinophyma. Arch Dermatol. 2012;148:824-31.
3. Baumgartner-Nielsen J, Lorentzen H. Imiquimod 5%: a successful treatment for pseudolymphoma. Acta Derm Venereol. 2014;94(4):469
4. Belousova IE, Vanecek T, Skreg SV, et al. Unusual clinicopathological presentation of primary cutaneous diffuse large B-cell lymphoma, leg type, with multiple nodules and widespread garland-like lesions. Am J Dermatopathol. 2009;31:370-4.
5. Berger CL, Tigelaar R, Cohen J, et al. Cutaneous T-cell lymphoma: malignant proliferation of T-regulatory cells. Blood. 2005;105:1640-7.
6. Burg G, Dummer R, Nestle FO, et al. Cutaneous lymphoma consist of a spectrum of nosologically different entities including mycosis fungoides and small plaque parapsoriasis. Arch Dermatol. 1996;132:567-72.
7. Camilot D, Arnez ZM, Luzar B, et al. Cutaneous pseudolymphoma following tattoo application: report of two new cases of a potential lymphoma mimicker. Int J Surg Pathol. 2012;20(3):311-5
8. Cho-Vega JH, Tschen JA, Duvic M, et al. Early-stage mycosis fungoides variants: case-based review. Ann Diagn Pathol. 2010;14:369-85.
9. Chong BF, Wilson AJ, Gibson HM, et al. Immune function abnormalities in peripheral blood mononuclear cell cytokine expression differentiates stages of cutaneous T-cell lymphoma/mycosis fungoides. Clinical Cancer Research. 2008;14:646-53.
10. Ciree A, Michel L, Camilleri-Broet S, et al. Expression and activity of IL-17 in cutaneous T-cell lymphomas (mycosis fungoides and Sezary syndrome). Int J Cancer. 2004;112:113-20.
11. Demirkesen C, Tuzuner N, Esen T, et al. The expression of IgM is helpful in the differentiation of primary cutaneous diffuse large B cell lymphoma and follicle center lymphoma. Leuk Res. 2011;35:1269-72.
12. Dummer R, Eichmuller S, Gellrich S, et al. Phase II clinical trial of intratumoral application of TG1042 (adenovirus-interferon-gamma) in patients with advanced cutaneous T-cell lymphomas and multilesional cutaneous B-cell lymphomas. Mol Ther. 2010;18:1244-7.
13. Foley C, Leonard N, Wynne B. Cutaneous pseudolymphoma: a rare side effect of cyclosporine. J Am Acad Dermatol. 2015;72(3):e85-6.
14. Gallardo F, Garcia-Muret MP, Servitje O, et al. Cutaneous lymphomas showing prominent granulomatous component: clinicopathological features in a series of 16 cases. J Eur Acad Dermatol Venereol. 2009;23:639-47.
15. Gazdar AF, Carney DN, Russell EK, et al. In vitro growth of cutaneous T-cell lymphomas. Cancer Treatment Rep. 1979;63:587-90.
16. Ghatalia P, Porter J, Wroblewski D, et al. Primary cutaneous marginal zone lymphoma associated with juxta-articular fibrotic nodules in a teenager. J Cutan Pathol. 2013;40:477-84.
17. Girardi M, Heald PW, Wilson LD. The pathogenesis of mycosis fungoides. New Engl J Med. 2004;350:1978-88.
18. Gjerdrum LM, Woetmann A, Odum N, et al. FOXP31 regulatory T cells in cutaneous T-cell lymphomas: association with disease stage and survival. Leukemia. 2007;21:2512-8.
19. Gokdemir G, Ari S, Altunay I, et al. Primary cutaneous diffuse large B-cell lymphoma of the leg, with an atypical clinical picture of verrucous plaques associated with stasis dermatitis. Clin Exp Dermatol. 2010;35:e87-9.
20. Goteri G, Filosa A, Mannello B, et al. Density of neoplastic lymphoid infiltrate, CD81 T cells, and CD1a1 dendritic cells in mycosis fungoides. J Clin Pathol. 2003;56:453-8.
21. Haghighi B, Smoller BR, LeBoit PE, et al. Pagetoid reticulosis (Woringer-Kolopp disease): an immunophenotypic, molecular, and clinicopathologic study. Mod Pathol. 2000;13:502-10.
22. Herrmann JL, Hughey LC. Recognizing large-cell transformation of mycosis fungoides. J Am Acad Dermatol. 2012;67:665-72.
23. Huang CT, Yang WC, Liu YC, et al. Primary cutaneous diffuse large B-cell lymphoma, leg type, with unusual clinical presentation of bluish-reddish multicolored rainbow pattern. J Clin Oncol. 2011;29:e497-8.
24. Hwang ST, Janik JE, Jaffe ES, et al. Mycosis fungoides and Sezary syndrome. Lancet. 2008;371:945-57.
25. Jones G, Wilson LD, Fox-Goguen L. Total skin electron beam radiotherapy for patients who have mycosis fungoides. Hematol Oncol Clin North Am. 2003;17:1421-34.
26. Jones GW, Kacinski BM, Wilson LD, et al. Total skin electron radiation in the management of mycosis fungoides: consensus of the European Organization for Research and Treatment of Cancer (EORTC) Cutaneous Lymphoma Project Group. J Am Acad Dermatol. 2002;47:364-70.
27. Kempf W, Ostheeren-Michaelis S, Paulli M, et al. Granulomatous mycosis fungoides and granulomatous slack skin: a multicenter study of the Cutaneous Lymphoma Histopathology Task Force Group of the European Organization For Research and Treatment of Cancer (EORTC). Arch Dermatol. 2008;144:1609-17.
28. Kennedy-Crispin M, Myskowski PL. Cryotherapy for primary cutaneous B-cell lymphoma. J Am Acad Dermatol. 2012;67:e292-4.
29. Kim YH, Liu HL, Mraz-Gernhard S, et al. Long-term outcome of 525 patients with mycosis fungoides and Sezary syndrome: clinical prognostic factors and risk for disease progression. Arch Dermatol. 2003;139:857-66.
30. Kitagawa KH, Grassi M. Zoledronic acid-induced cutaneous B-cell pseudolymphoma. J Am Acad Dermatol. 2011;65(6):1238-40.
31. Kluk J, Charles-Holmes R, Carr RA. Primary cutaneous follicle centre cell lymphoma of the scalp presenting with scarring alopecia. Br J Dermatol. 2011;165:205-7.
32. Koch R, Jaffe ES, Mensing C, et al. Cutaneous gamma/delta T-cell lymphoma. J Dtsch Dermatol Ges. 2009;7(12):1065-7.
33. Koens L, Vermeer MH, Willemze R, et al. IgM expression on paraffin sections distinguishes primary cutaneous large B-cell lymphoma, leg type from primary cutaneous follicle center lymphoma. Am J Surg Pathol. 2010;34:1043-8.
34. Korgavkar K, Xiong M, Weinstock M. Changing incidence trends of cutaneous T-cell lymphoma. JAMA Dermatol. 2013;149(11):1295-9.
35. Li J, Pulitzer MP, Myskowski PL, et al. A case-control study of clinicopathologic features, prognosis, and therapeutic responses in patients with granulomatous mycosis fungoides. J Am Acad Dermatol. 2013;69:366-74.
36. Lozzi GP, Massone C, Citarella L, et al. Rimming of adipocytes by neoplastic lymphocytes: A histopathologic feature not restricted to subcutaneous T – Cell lymphoma. Am J Dermatopathol. 2006;28:9-12.
37. Lucinda TS, Hazel OH, Joyce LS, et al. Successful Treatment of Tattoo-Induced Pseudolymphoma with Sequential Ablative Fractional Resurfacing Followed by Q-Switched Nd: YAG 532 nm Laser. J Cutan Aesthet Surg. 2013;6(4):226-8.
38. Magro CM, Yang A, Fraga G. Blastic marginal zone lymphoma: a clinical and pathological study of 8 cases and review of the literature. Am J Dermatopathol. 2013;35:319-26.
39. Massone C, Fink-Puches R, Laimer M, et al. Miliary and agminated-type primary cutaneous follicle center lymphoma: report of 18 cases. J Am Acad Dermatol. 2011;65:749-55.
40. McCusker ME, Garifallou M, Bogen SA, et al. Sezary lineage cells can be induced to proliferate via CD28-mediated costimulation. J Immunol. 1997;158:4984-91.
41. Metgud RS, Doshi JJ, Gaurkhede S, et al. Extranodal NK/T-cell lymphoma, nasal type (angiocentric T-cell lymphoma): A review about the terminology. J Oral Maxillofac Pathol. 2011;15:96-100.
42. Monsalvez V, Montes-Moreno S, Artiga MJ, et al. MicroRNAs as prognostic markers in indolent primary cutaneous B-cell lymphoma. Mod Pathol. 2013;26:171-81.
43. Muniesa C, Estrach T, Pujol RM, et al. Folliculotropic mycosis fungoides: clinicopathological features and outcome in a series of 20 cases. J Am Acad Dermatol. 2010;62:418-26.
44. Olsen E, Vonderheid E, Pimpinelli N, et al.; for the ISCL/EORTC. Revisions to the staging and classification of mycosis fungoides and Sézary syndrome: a proposal of the International Society for Cutaneous Lymphomas (ISCL) and the cutaneous lymphoma task force of the European Organization of Research and Treatment of Cancer (EORTC). Blood. 2007;110:1713-22.
45. Park JH, Shin HT, Lee DY, et al. World Health Organization-European Organization for Research and Treatment of Cancer classification of cutaneous lymphoma in Korea: a retrospective study at a single tertiary institution. J Am Acad Dermatol. 2012;67:1200-9.
46. Pimpinelli N, Olsen EA, Santucci M, et al. Defining early mycosis fungoides. J Am Acad Dermatol. 2005;53:1053-63.
47. Rabenhorst A, Schlaak M, Heukamp LC, et al. Mast cells play a protumorigenic role in primary cutaneous lymphoma. Blood. 2012;120:2042-54.
48. Riyaz N, Sasidharanpillai S, Aravindan KP, et al. Phenytoin induced cutaneous B cell pseudolymphoma. Indian J Dermatol. 2015;60:522.
49. Roschewski M, Dunleavy K, Wilson WH. Diffuse large B cell lymphoma: molecular targeted therapy. Int J Hematol. 2012;96:552-61.
50. Samimi S, Benoit B, Evans K, et al. Increased programmed death-1 expression on CD4 + T cells in cutaneous T-cell lymphoma: implications for immune suppression. Arch Dermatol. 2010;146:1382-8.
51. Sequeira FF, Jayaseelan E, Stephen J. Paraphenylenediamine-induced cutaneous pseudolymphoma. Indian J Dermatol. 2014;59:424

52. Singletary HL, Selim MA, Olsen E. Subcutaneous interferon alfa for the treatment of cutaneous pseudolymphoma. Arch Dermatol. 2012;148(5):572-4.
53. Slater DN. The new World Health Organization – European Organization for Research and Treatment of Cancer classification for cutaneous lymphomas: a practical marriage of two giants. Brit J Dermatol. 2005;153:874-80.
54. Sokol L, Naghashpour M, Glass LF. Primary cutaneous B-cell lymphomas: recent advances in diagnosis and management. Cancer Control. 2012;19:236-44.
55. Soon CW, Pincus LB, Ai WZ, et al. Acneiform presentation of primary cutaneous follicle center lymphoma. J Am Acad Dermatol. 2011;65:887-9.
56. Suárez AL, Pulitzer M, Horwitz S, et al. Primary cutaneous B-cell lymphomas: part I. Clinical features, diagnosis, and classification. J Am Acad Dermatol. 2013;69(3):329.e1-13; quiz 341-2.
57. Swerdlow SH, Campo E, Harris NL, et al. WHO classification of tumours of haematopoietic and lymphoid tissues, 4th edition. Lyon: IARC Press; 2008.
58. Toro JR, Beaty M, Sorbara L, et al. Gamma delta T-cell lymphoma of the skin; a clinical, microscopic, and molecular study. Arch Dermatol. 2000;136:1024-32.
59. Toro JR, Liewehr DJ, Pabby N, et al. Gamma-delta T-cell phenotype is associated with significantly decreased survival in cutaneous T-cell lymphoma. Blood. 2003;101(9):3407-12.
60. van Doorn R, Scheffer E, Willemze R. Follicular mycosis fungoides, a distinct disease entity with or without associated follicular mucinosis: a clinicopathologic and follow-up study of 51 patients. Arch Dermatol. 2002;138:191-8.
61. Vermeer MH, van Doorn R, Dukers D, et al. CD81 T cells in cutaneous T-cell lymphoma: expression of cytotoxic proteins, Fas ligand, and killing inhibitory receptors and their relationship with clinical behavior. J Clin Oncol. 2001;19:4322-9.
62. Vonderheid EC, Bernengo MG, Burg G, et al. Update on erythrodermic cutaneous T-cell lymphoma: Report of the International Society for Cutaneous Lymphomas. J Am Acad Dermatol. 2002;46:95-106.
63. Wilcox RA. Cutaneous B-cell lymphomas: 2013 update on diagnosis, risk-stratification, and management. Am J Hematol. 2013;88(1):73-6.
64. Willemze R, Jaffe ES, Burg G, et al. WHO-EORTC classification for cutaneous lymphomas. Blood. 2005;105:3768-85.
65. Willemze R, Kerl H, Sterry W, et al. EORTC classification for primary cutaneous lymphomas: a proposal from the Cutaneous Lymphoma Study Group of the European Organization for Research and Treatment of Cancer. Blood. 1997;90:354-71.
66. Zinzani PL, Quaglino P, Pimpinelli N, et al. Prognostic factors in primary cutaneous B-cell lymphoma: the Italian Study Group for Cutaneous Lymphomas. J Clin Oncol. 2006;24:1376-82.

# 75 CHAPTER Graft-versus-host Disease

Tanumay Raychaudhury

## INTRODUCTION

Graft-versus-host disease (GVHD) is a constellation clinical manifestation evoked by reaction of transplanted cells from an immunocompetent donor individual with a histoincompatible immunosuppressed host. It is a multisystem disorder that commonly involves skin and is found as common complications of hematopoietic cell transplantation (HCT), however, blood transfusion, fetomaternal transfusion and solid organ transplantation may lead to GVHD. Cutaneous involvement often serves as the flagging sign to diagnose GVHD and may often be severe enough contributing to great morbidity and mortality. Because these disorders share clinical and histopathological features with a variety of other skin diseases, thorough consideration of the differential diagnosis is essential for the management of post-HCT patients with lesions suggestive of cutaneous GVHD.

## CLASSIFICATION

Classically, GVHD has been divided into acute and chronic forms based upon the time of onset of disease:

- *Acute GVHD*: Manifestations of GVHD occurring within 100 days after HCT
- *Chronic GVHD*: Manifestations of GVHD occurring more than 100 days after HCT.

However, this conventional division has been challenged by the recognition that signs of acute and chronic GVHD may occur outside of these designated periods.

## ACUTE CUTANEOUS GRAFT-VERSUS-HOST DISEASE

Acute GVHD is common after allogeneic HCT, and can lead to disorders of the skin, gastrointestinal tract, liver, and hematopoietic system. Cutaneous involvement is often the earliest manifestation of acute GVHD; skin lesions frequently appear within 2–4 weeks of HCT, but may occur anytime after hematopoietic cell engraftment.

### Clinical Manifestations

#### Skin Lesions

Acute cutaneous GVHD typically begins with erythematous, blanchable macules on the ears, palms, or soles. The lateral neck, cheek, and upper back are additional common sites of early involvement. Follicular lesions may be seen.

As acute cutaneous GVHD progresses, lesions become generalized and morbilliform (measles-like) in appearance. Smooth or hyperkeratotic papules and postinflammatory hyperpigmentation may occur. In severe cases, patients develop generalized erythroderma, bullae, or extensive skin sloughing.

Acute cutaneous GVHD may complain of pruritus or a burning sensation in the skin. In some patients, skin pain or pruritus precedes the onset of visible skin lesions.

- *Stage 1*: Less than 25% body surface area (BSA) involvement
- *Stage 2*: 25–50% BSA involvement
- *Stage 3*: Greater than 50% BSA involvement
- *Stage 4*: Erythroderma with bullae.

The combined stages of skin, liver, and gastrointestinal disease are used to determine the overall severity (grade) of acute GVHD.

#### Oral Lesions

Erythema, erosions, ulcers, lichenoid lesions, xerostomia, and pain involving the oral cavity have been attributed to acute GVHD. However, it is difficult to distinguish this disorder from mucositis secondary to chemotherapy administered in preparation for HCT. Some authors have suggested that lesions that persist for longer than 3 weeks after HCT or involve the hard palate (an uncommon site for chemotherapy-induced mucositis) may be more likely to represent acute GVHD.

### Diagnosis

In the absence of concomitant extracutaneous manifestations, making a definitive diagnosis of acute cutaneous GVHD may be challenging since clinical or histological features are nonspecific.

### Skin Biopsy

Key histopathological findings on skin biopsy in acute cutaneous GVHD include interface dermatitis (vacuolization of the basal layer of the epidermis and a lymphocytic infiltrate in the superficial dermis) and epidermal apoptotic keratinocytes. Apoptotic keratinocytes may also be present in the follicular epithelium.

The lymphocytic infiltrate can be sparse and perivascular or more extensive. Migration of lymphocytes into the epidermis (lymphocyte exocytosis) is common. The presence of satellite cell necrosis (two or more lymphocytes surrounding an apoptotic keratinocyte) also supports a diagnosis of acute GVHD. Fulminant lesions demonstrate subepidermal clefting and full-thickness necrosis of the epidermis.

Immunofluorescence testing may demonstrate nonspecific immunoglobulin M and complement deposits at the basement membrane zone, but generally is not indicated.

### Histological Grading

- *Grade 0*: Normal skin or changes not referable to GVHD
- *Grade 1*: Vacuolization of the basal layer at the dermal-epidermal junction
- *Grade 2*: Basal layer vacuolization, necrotic epidermal cells, lymphocytic infiltrate
- *Grade 3*: Grade 2 changes plus cleft formation at the dermal-epidermal junction
- *Grade 4*: Grade 2 changes plus separation of the epidermis from the dermis.

The presence of erythroderma and bullae is sufficient to diagnose grade 4 GVHD, and is associated with a poor prognosis.

The sensitivity and specificity of skin biopsy for acute GVHD has not been definitively established. Despite the lack of strong evidence to support performing a skin biopsy in patients with suspected GVHD, a biopsy may provide information that can be used in conjunction with other clinical findings to support a diagnosis of acute GVHD or to establish an alternative cause of the skin eruption.

The differential diagnosis of acute cutaneous GVHD is given in table 1.

## CHRONIC CUTANEOUS GRAFT-VERSUS-HOST DISEASE

Chronic GVHD is a major cause of morbidity and mortality in long-term survivors of allogeneic HCT. The skin is the most common site of involvement.

### Clinical Manifestations

#### Skin

Traditionally, chronic cutaneous GVHD has been classified as lichen planus-like or sclerotic (resembling scleroderma); however, many different clinical presentations of chronic GVHD are now recognized, reflecting a spectrum of epidermal and dermal (sclerotic) changes.

- *Lichen planus-like lesions*: Lichen planus-like chronic GVHD presents as erythematous to violaceous papules or plaques

**TABLE 1: Differential diagnosis of acute cutaneous graft-versus-host disease**

| Disease | Clinical feature | Histological feature |
|---|---|---|
| • Drug eruptions<br>• *Common*: Sulfonamides, beta-lactams-morbilliform rash voriconazole-phototoxic drug reaction | • Rash starts on trunk and spreads to extremities unlike GVHD with cephalocaudal/acral involvement<br>• Reappears rapidly on restarting offending drug-rechallenge not indicated | More likely to have tissue eosinophilia though GHVD may also show eosinophilic infiltrate |
| Erythema multiforme | Target or targetoid lesions | Necrotic keratinocytes, subepidermal clefts, and vacuolization of basal keratinocytes—again seen in cGVHD |
| Viral infections (e.g., HHV-6, HHV-7, cytomegalovirus, others) | Maculopapular or morbilliform variants in both | Sparse perivascular lymphocytic infiltrate |
| Eruption of lymphocyte recovery | Self-limited exanthema with transient fever; concomitant gastrointestinal and hepatic involvement do not occur | Superficial perivascular mononuclear cell infiltrate-may imitate grade 1 cGVHD |
| Chemotherapy-induced acral erythema | Symmetric edema, erythema, or blistering mostly acral | Interface dermatitis with variable keratinocyte necrosis, dilation of the superficial vascular plexus, and limited inflammatory infiltrate |
| Toxic–epidermal necrolysis | Starts as dusky erythematous macules that become confluent to progress to extensive blistering and denudation | Subepidermal bullae and full-thickness epidermal necrosis- mimics grade 4 disease |
| Engraftment syndrome | Rash, fever, signs of capillary leak syndrome, commonly seen after autologous HCT | Dominance of CD4+ cells and a decreased number of CD1a+ cells in the epidermis are specific features for the skin lesions of ES |
| Acute radiation dermatitis | Cutaneous erythema, desquamation, blistering, or cutaneous necrosis—limitation of involvement points in favor of radiation dermatitis | Vacuolization of the basal layer, apoptotic keratinocytes, satellite cell necrosis, and a superficial perivascular lymphocytic infiltrate—all seen in cGVHD |

GVHD, graft versus host disease; cGVHD, chronic graft-versus-host disease; HHV-6, human herpesvirus 6; HHV-7, human herpesvirus 7; HCT, hematopoietic cell transplantation; ES, engraftment syndrome.

with a predilection for the dorsal hands and feet, forearms, and trunk. Lichen planus-like chronic GVHD also can occur in a follicular distribution

- *Sclerotic manifestations*: Sclerosis is a common manifestation of chronic GVHD.

The depth at which cutaneous sclerosis occurs determines the clinical presentation:

- *Lichen sclerosus-like*: When sclerosis occurs in the superficial dermis, lesions resemble lichen sclerosus. Lichen sclerosus-like lesions are typically found on the upper back as white or gray thin plaques with accentuated dermatoglyphics
- *Morpheaform*: Morphea-like chronic GVHD results from sclerosis that primarily involves the dermis. This variant usually presents with firm, hyperpigmented, hypopigmented, or skin-colored plaques. Affected skin often has a shiny appearance and demonstrates hair loss secondary to elimination of adnexal structures.
  Unlike systemic sclerosis, BSA involvement in sclerotic GVHD often is discontinuous
- *Deep sclerosis/eosinophilic fasciitis-like*: Deep sclerosis may also occur. Subcutaneous fibrosis results in a cellulite-like rippled appearance to the skin due to thickening of the fibrous septae within fat, particularly on the medial arms and thighs. Fascial involvement tends to occur late in the chronic period, and may lead to the appearance of prominent linear demarcations, often referred to as the "groove sign," and contractures that limit range of motion
  Calcinosis universalis may be presented in rare cases of chronic GVHD
- *Poikiloderma*: It describes the combination of atrophy, hypopigmentation, and hyperpigmentation in the skin. Poikilodermatous skin changes in chronic GVHD appear as patches with mottled pigmentation and telangiectasias
- *Other cutaneous findings*: In addition to poikiloderma, other pigment disorders may occur in chronic GVHD, including the appearance of depigmented, hypopigmented, and hyperpigmented areas. Hyperpigmentation may occur in a widespread, leopard-skin like pattern.

Widespread eczematous lesions and malar eruptions resembling systemic lupus erythematosus have been reported as histopathologically confirmed chronic GVHD. Other cutaneous findings associated with chronic GVHD include hypohidrosis, ichthyosis, erythema, pruritus, and maculopapular eruptions.

### Oral Lesions

The National Institute of Health Consensus Development Project classified oral lichen planus-like changes, hyperkeratotic plaques, and restriction of mouth opening due to sclerosis as diagnostic features of oral chronic GVHD.

Lacy or reticulated white plaques that resemble Wickham's striae of lichen planus may occur on the tongue, buccal mucosa, lips, or palate. Hyperkeratotic plaques, mucosal erythema, erosions, and ulceration can also occur.

Patients may suffer from sicca symptoms resembling those that occur in Sjögren's syndrome secondary to impairment of salivary gland function. Mucoceles and oral verruciform xanthoma have been also reported.

### Hair Disorders

Scarring or nonscarring alopecia or scaly papules on the scalp may occur in chronic GVHD, but are not sufficient to establish the diagnosis in the absence of other findings consistent with GVHD. Thinning hair, patchy hair loss, coarse or dull hair, and premature graying have also been associated with this disorder.

### Nail Disorders

A variety of nail abnormalities ranging from mild nail dystrophy to total nail loss (anonychia) may occur. Nail abnormalities include longitudinal ridging, splitting or brittle nails, onycholysis (separation of the nail plate from the nail bed), and pterygium (abnormal adherence of the nail plate to the proximal nail fold or hyponychium).

### Ocular and Genital Mucosa

Inflammation of the conjunctiva, pseudomembranous or cicatricial conjunctivitis, and keratoconjunctivitis sicca (dry eye) syndrome may occur in patients with chronic GVHD. Vulvar or vaginal erosions, lichen planus-like lesions, or sclerosis leading to labial resorption or tissue agglutination also may occur in affected women.

## Diagnosis

The diagnosis of chronic cutaneous GVHD is described in table 2.

## Diagnostic Procedures

The histopathological changes in chronic GVHD vary according to the type of skin involvement.

A 4 mm punch biopsy is sufficient for the evaluation of lichen planus-like, lichen sclerosus-like, and most morpheaform lesions. Deep incisional biopsy is often necessary to evaluate for fascial involvement. Magnetic resonance imaging (MRI) also may have value for the diagnosis of subcutaneous disease and fasciitis.

### Scoring Systems Used

- National Institutes of Health composite 0–3 skin score
- Lee skin symptom score, a scale based on the patient's assessment
- National Institutes of Health chronic GVHD Oral Mucosal Score.

**TABLE 2: Diagnosis of chronic cutaneous Graft-versus-host disease**

| Organ | Diagnostic (sufficient to establish diagnosis of chronic cutaneous GVHD) features |
|---|---|
| Skin | Poikiloderma, lichen planus-like features, sclerotic features, morphea-like features, and lichen sclerosus-like features |
| Oral mucosa | Lichen type features, hyperkeratotic plaques, and restricted mouth opening from sclerosis |
| Genitalia | Lichen planus-like features, vaginal scarring or stenosis |

**TABLE 3: Differential diagnosis of chronic cutaneous Graft-versus-host disease**

| Disease | Differentiating clinical feature |
|---|---|
| Lichen planus | • Lesions of GVHD may be less angular and may have less well-defined margins than lichen planus<br>• Flexural wrists and shins are classic sites for true lichen planus unlike GVHD |
| Lichenoid drug eruptions | Systemic involvement absent |
| Pityriasis lichenoides chronica | Systemic involvement absent, oral and nail changes rare |
| Scleroderma | Distal to proximal progression of cutaneous sclerosis on the extremities not observed in chronic GVHD |
| Radiation-induced sclerosis | History of radiation, usually not bilateral |
| Nephrogenic fibrosing dermopathy | Associated with renal failure, gadolinium use |
| Poikiloderma | • Poikiloderma of Civatte—chronic sun exposure in fairer skin types, present before SCT<br>• Poikiloderma of collagen vascular disorders like dermatomyositis, SLE—other systemic features<br>• Parapsoriasis, CTCL- other features<br>• Bloom syndrome, Rothmund–Thomson syndrome—younger age of onset, photoexposed sites |

GVHD, graft-versus-host disease; SLE, systemic lupus erythematosus; CTCL, cutaneous T-cell lymphoma; SCT, stem cell transplant.

## Differential Diagnosis

The differential diagnosis of chronic cutaneous GVHD is described in table 3.

# MANAGEMENT

Systemic therapy is generally required for the management of patients with acute GVHD, under the purview of a hematologist. High potency topical corticosteroids may provide improvement in patients with limited skin disease and no internal involvement.

Phototherapy options for acute cutaneous GVHD include psoralen plus UVA (PUVA) and narrow band UVB phototherapy and have been associated with improvement in acute cutaneous GVHD that was refractory to systemic glucocorticoid therapy or that flared upon glucocorticoid tapering.

Topical corticosteroids and topical calcineurin inhibitors may have some benefit for patients with limited nonsclerotic chronic GVHD. Phototherapy and systemic therapies are the mainstays of treatment for patients with sclerotic lesions.

Extracorporeal photopheresis if available may be helpful in cases which become nonresponsive to corticosteroids. Halofuginone and thalidomide are two other emerging drugs in chronic GVHD. Halofuginone helps in reversing sclerodermoid features in chronic GVHD.

## Ancillary Measures in Chronic GVHD

Recommendations include:
- Photoprotection
- Regular use of emollients on intact skin
- Careful use of topical corticosteroids to reduce risk for cutaneous atrophy
- Use of topical or systemic antipruritic agents when needed
- Wound management.

Cutaneous squamous cell carcinoma (SCC) is a potential long-term complication of HCT.

Patients should be educated regarding early signs of skin sclerosis, such as skin tightness, edema, and reduced range of motion, and should be instructed to seek care if these symptoms occur.

## Oral Lesions

Topical high potency corticosteroids are often used for the treatment of oral GVHD. Encouraging good oral hygiene and utilizing of topical anesthetic agents, such as viscous lignocaine, to reduce pain and facilitate oral intake.

Leukoplakia and oral SCC should be looked for and biopsied.

Patients with xerostomia may benefit from salivary stimulants (sugarless gum or candy), oral lubricants or saliva substitutes, and topical fluoride to prevent tooth decay.

No therapy is necessary for small, superficial mucoceles. Deep lesions that cause discomfort can be surgically excised.

# SUGGESTED READINGS

1. Cheng H, Tian J, Zeng L, et al. Halofugine prevents cutaneous graft versus host disease by suppression of Th17 differentiation. Hematology. 2012;17(5):261-7.
2. Feldstein JV, Bolaños-Meade J, Anders VL, et al. Narrowband ultraviolet B phototherapy for the treatment of steroid-refractory and steroid-dependent acute graft-versus-host disease of the skin. J Am Acad Dermatol. 2011;65(4):733-8.
3. Ferrara JL, Levine JE, Reddy P, et al. Graft versus-host disease. Lancet. 2009;373(9674):1550-61.
4. Filipovich AH, Weisdorf D, Pavletic S, et al. National Institutes of Health consensus development project on criteria for clinical trials in chronic graft-versus-host disease: I. Diagnosis and staging working group report. Biol Blood Marrow Transplant. 2005;11(12):945-56.
5. Flowers ME, Inamoto Y, Carpenter PA, et al. Comparative analysis of risk factors for acute graft-versus-host disease and for chronic graft-versus-host disease according to National Institutes of Health consensus criteria. Blood. 2011;117(11):3214-9.
6. Hausermann P, Walter RB, Halter J, et al. Cutaneous graft-versus-host disease: a guide for the dermatologist. Dermatology. 2008;216:287-304.
7. Man J, Kalisiak M, Birchall IW, et al. Chronic cutaneous graft-versus-host disease manifesting as calcinosis cutis universalis on a background of widespread sclerodermatoid changes. J Cutan Med Surg. 2010;14(5):249-53.
8. Pines M, Snyder D, Yarkoni S, et al. Halofuginone to treat fibrosis in chronic graft-versus-host disease and scleroderma. Biol Blood Marrow Transplant. 2003;9(7):417-25.
9. Pines M, Snyder D, Yarkoni S, et al. Halofuginone to treat fibrosis in chronic graft-versus-host disease and scleroderma. Biol Blood Marrow Transplant. 2003;9(7):417-25.
10. Shulman HM, Kleiner D, Lee SJ, et al. Histopathologic diagnosis of chronic graft-versus-host disease: National Institutes of Health Consensus Development Project on Criteria for Clinical Trials in Chronic Graft-versus-Host Disease: II. Pathology Working Group Report. Biol Blood Marrow Transplant. 2006;12(1):31-47.

# 20 SECTION Emergencies in Dermatology

# 76 CHAPTER Adverse Drug Reactions

*Sandipan Dhar, Sahana M Srinivas*

## INTRODUCTION

Adverse drug reactions (ADRs) are undesirable clinical manifestations resulting from administration of a particular drug. It is defined "an appreciably harmful or unpleasant reaction, resulting from an intervention related to the use of a medicinal product, which predicts hazard from future administration and warrants prevention or specific treatment, or alteration of the dosage regimen, or withdrawal of the product". World Health Organization defines drug reactions as "a response to a medicine which is noxious and unintended, and which occurs at doses normally used in man for the prophylaxis, diagnosis or therapy of disease, or the modification of physiological function.

## EPIDEMIOLOGY

The epidemiological features of drug reactions are varied. Many cases of ADRs are under reported or failed to be recognized. The frequency and clinical pattern of cutaneous drug reactions are determined by the drug use, underlying specific conditions and the pharmacogenetic traits of a population. Studies of drug reactions in various cohorts revealed incidence rates ranging from 1 out of 1,000 to 2 out of 100 in hospitalized patients. In adults, ADRs have been reported to occur in 10–20% of all hospitalized patients and are thought to be the fourth leading cause of death.

The overall incidence of ADRs varies from 6–30%. A meta-analysis of prospective studies showed overall incidence in hospitalized children was 9.5% and in outpatient setting the incidence was between 1.5% and 2.5%. Many studies have shown there is no gender predisposition for the development of drug reactions. Asian studies have shown younger age group affected than older group with ADRs as compared to Europe and US. The incidence of different clinical pattern of drug reaction and the causative drug varies with different studies. Antibiotic-associated eruptions are among the most commonly reported reactions. Indian studies have shown maculopapular eruptions to the most common clinical pattern.

## ETIOPATHOGENESIS

The pathogenesis of most of the drug eruptions is not clearly understood. Drug eruptions occur due to immunological and nonimmunological mechanism.

### Risk Factors

Factors influencing the risk of cutaneous eruptions include constitutional factors like pharmacogenetic variation in drug-metabolizing enzymes, human leukocyte association (HLA), and acquired factors like number of drugs taken, age of patient, active viral infection [human herpesvirus (HHV-6)], renal insufficiency, concurrent use of other medication, and drug interaction. Reactivation of HHV-6 is associated with relapse in drug hypersensitivity reaction. Older age group is associated with higher mortality rate.

### Genetics

Human leukocyte association alleles play an important association in development of severe cutaneous adverse reactions (SCARs). Several genetic studies have been performed to discover the genetic predisposition to drug hypersensitivity and gain insight into phenotypic diversity. These include hypersensitivity to abacavir associated with HLA-B*57:01, carbamazepine-induced Steven-Johnson syndrome (SJS), and toxic epidermal necrolysis (TEN) with HLA-B*15:02. Different studies of HLA alleles associated with drug hypersensitivity are summarized in table 1. HLA-DR4 is significantly associated with hydralazine-related drug-induced lupus. With the genetic research findings

**TABLE 1: Human leukocyte association alleles associated with hypersensitivity reactions**

| Drug | Association with HLA | Hypersensitivity reactions |
|---|---|---|
| Abacavir | HLA-B*57:01 | Abacavir hypersensitivity |
| Allopurinol | HLA-B*58:01 | SJS/TEN/DRESS |
| Carbama-zepine | HLA-B*15:02, HLA-B 15:08, HLA-B*15:11, HLA-B*15:18, HLA-A*31:01 | SJS/TEN/DRESS |
| Nevirapine | HLA DR B1*01:01, HLA-B*14:02, HLA-B*35:05 | DRESS/MPE |
| Dapsone | HLA-B*13:01 | DRESS |
| Lamotrigine | HLA-B*15:02 | SJS/TEN |
| Phenytoin | HLA-B*15:02, CYP2C9*3 | SJS/TEN |

HLA, human leukocyte association; SJS, Steven–Johnson syndrome; TEN, toxic epidermal necrolysis; DRESS, drug reaction with eosinophilia and systemic symptoms; MPE, maculopapular eruption.

SCARs which are currently unpredictable could be predictable and preventable in the future.

Human leukocyte association genes contribute to the genetic susceptibility of the cross reactivity of ADRs among aromatic antiepileptic drugs. HLA-A*2402 and HLA-B*1502 are associated with cross allergic reactions in Hans Chinese population. HLA allele varies in different ethnic population. HLA-B*1502 is present in 4.8–12.8% in southeast Asians in contrast to 0–1% in white people.

### Immunological

Drug eruptions due to hypersensitivity reactions are due to immunologic mechanism. Drugs or their metabolites may act as haptens, inducing a specific cell-mediated or humoral response. The stimulated cytotoxic CD8+ T-cells clonally expand and along with perforin, granzyme B, granulysin, and cytokines mediate the keratinocyte apoptosis leading to epidermal necrolysis. Immunological reactions result from immunoglobulin E (IgE)-dependent, cytotoxic, immune complex-mediated or cellular mechanisms that are Gell-Coombs classification of immunological reactions (Table 2). Idiosyncratic drug eruptions are unpredictable and are due to immunological mechanisms. Nonspecific dysbalance of cytokines and inflammatory mediators contribute to drug eruptions.

### Nonimmunological

Adverse drug reactions due to nonimmunological reactions are not uncommon. They occur due to activation of overdose, pharmacologic side effects, cumulative toxicity, delayed toxicity, interactions between drugs, metabolic alterations, and exacerbation of the disease.

Recently extensive studies have been done on the pathogenesis of cutaneous drug reactions due to targeted therapies. These include inhibitors acting on the cell membrane and inhibitors of intracellular molecular signaling pathways. These cell membrane inhibitors include epidermal growth factor receptor inhibitors, angiogenesis, and multikinase inhibitors.

## CLASSIFICATION

Adverse drug reactions can be classified based on pathogenesis and clinical morphology. Pharmacologically they are classified into two basic types: type A and type B. Type A ADRs are due to pharmacological actions of drug which are dose dependent and predictable. Type B are hypersensitivity reactions which are less dependent on dose, unpredictable, and primarily based on host genetics (Table 2). Morphological classifications of ADRs are depicted in table 3.

## CLINICAL FEATURES

Cutaneous drug reactions vary from mild eruptions to widespread skin involvement with life-threatening complications. Once the morphology has been established, a specific diagnosis can be made. Severe ADRs can be associated with fever, lymphadenopathy, and joint pains. Pruritus is present in majority of the drug reactions. Persistence of reactions depends on half-life of drugs. The drugs causing different morphological reactions are summarized in table 3.

### Exanthematous Eruptions

These eruptions account for 95% of skin reactions. They occur as maculopapular, morbilliform or scarlatiniform eruptions. Initially occur on the trunk and spreads peripherally (Fig. 1). They start within 1 week of initiation of therapy and resolve within 7–14 days with desquamation. Drug hypersensitivity syndrome (DHS) occurs as maculopapular rash along with fever and organ involvement (hepatitis, nephritis, vasculitis, pneumonia, and meningitis). Mucosal involvement is rare (Figs 2 and 3). DHS also known as drug reaction with eosinophilia and systemic symptoms (DRESS) is most commonly seen with anticonvulsants. It occurs in 1:3,000 exposures and is seen on first exposure to the drug with initial symptoms starting 1–6 weeks later. Recurrences can occur even though the offending drug is removed. Mortality rate is around 8%.

### Urticarial Eruptions

Urticaria and angioedema induced by drug are usually IgE-mediated immediate hypersensitivity reactions. Drug-induced urticaria occurs in 10% cases and is often associated with acute rather than chronic urticaria. Urticaria presenting as wheals are usually migratory and transient and lasts less than 24 hours (Fig. 4). Angioedema is most commonly caused by ACE-inhibitors. Serum sickness-like reaction is characterized by fever, urticarial rash, and arthralgia and begins 1–3 weeks after initiation of drugs.

### Pustular Eruptions

Drug-induced acne occurs at atypical sites and is often monomorphous. Acute generalized exanthematous pustulosis (AGEP) develops in less than 24 hours and is most commonly associated with beta-lactam and macrolide antibiotics. It is

**TABLE 2: Pharmacological classification of drug reactions**

| | | |
|---|---|---|
| Type A reactions (predictable) | • Toxic effects • Secondary effects<br>• Side effects • Drug interactions | |
| Type B reactions (unpredictable) | Immune-mediated reactions (Gell and Coombs classification)<br>• *Type 1*: Immunoglobulin E dependent<br>• *Type II*: Cytotoxic mediated<br>• *Type III*: Immune complex mediated<br>• *Type 1V*: T-cell mediated<br>Nonimmunological-mediated reactions (sometimes predictable) | • Urticaria, angioedema, anaphylaxis<br>• Drug-induced thrombocytopenia<br>• Vasculitis, serum sickness-like reaction<br>• Exanthematous, Steven–Johnson syndrome, toxic epidermal necrolysis<br>• Photosensitivity reactions, pigmentary changes, warfarin necrosis, pruritus |

**TABLE 3: Morphological classification of adverse drug reactions and implicated drugs**

| Clinical morphology | Types | Few causative drugs |
|---|---|---|
| Exanthematous | • Simple eruptions | Penicillin, sulfonamides, amoxicillin, and antiepileptics |
| | • Hypersensitivity syndromes | Phenytoin, phenobarbitone, carbamazepine, dapsone, allopurinol, minocycline, and lamotrigine |
| Urticarial | • Urticaria/angioedema | Penicillins, NSAIDs, cephalosporins, sulfonamides, and ACE inhibitors |
| | • SSLR | Cefaclor, cefprozil, minocycline, infliximab, and rituximab |
| Pustular | • Acneiform eruptions | Corticosteroids, iodides, isoniazid, androgens, lithium, and phenytoin |
| | • AGEP | Beta-lactam antibiotics and macrolides |
| Bullous eruptions | • Bullous FDE | Phenolphthalein, NSAIDs, sulfonamides, tetracyclines, and lamotrigine |
| | • EM/SJS/TEN | Anticonvulsants, sulfonamides, antibiotics, NSAIDs, and dapsone |
| | • Pseudoporphyria | Tetracycline, furosemide, and naproxen |
| | • Pemphigus/BP/LAD | Penicillamine, captopril, penicillin, rifampin, vancomycin, diclofenac, and piroxicam |
| Miscellaneous | NEH, FDE, drug-induced lupus, photosensitivity reactions, lichenoid eruptions, cutaneous pseudolymphoma, drug-induced vasculitis, pigmentary changes, nonscarring alopecia, psoriasiform reactions, pruritus, peripheral neuropathy, hair and nail changes, eruptions from biological therapies, anticoagulant-induced skin necrosis, TNF antagonists | Procainamide, hydralazine, isoniazid, minocycline, phenytoin, penicillin, sulfonamides, chloramphenicol, dopamine, mannitol, sodium bicarbonate, warfarin, antineoplastic drugs, and antiretroviral drugs |

SSLR, serum sickness-like reaction; AGEP, acute generalized exanthematous pustulosis; FDE, fixed drug eruption; EM, erythema multiforme; BP, bullous pemphigoid; LAD, linear IgA disease; NEH, neutrophilic eccrine hidradenitis; TNF, tumor necrosis factor; NSAIDs, nonsteroidal anti-inflammatory drugs; ACE, angiotensin converting enzyme.

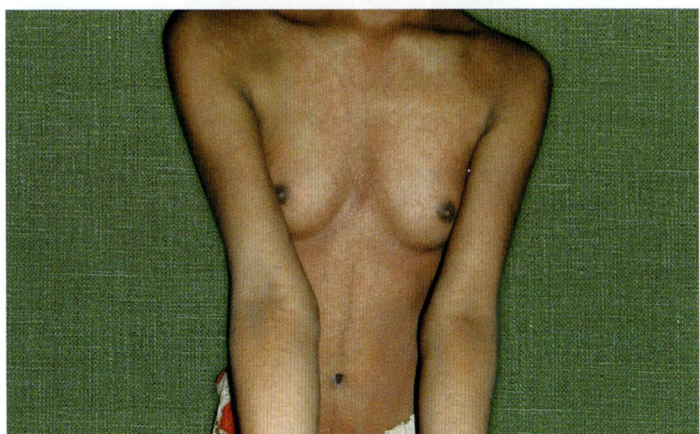

**FIG. 1:** Morbilliform eruption due to amoxicillin.

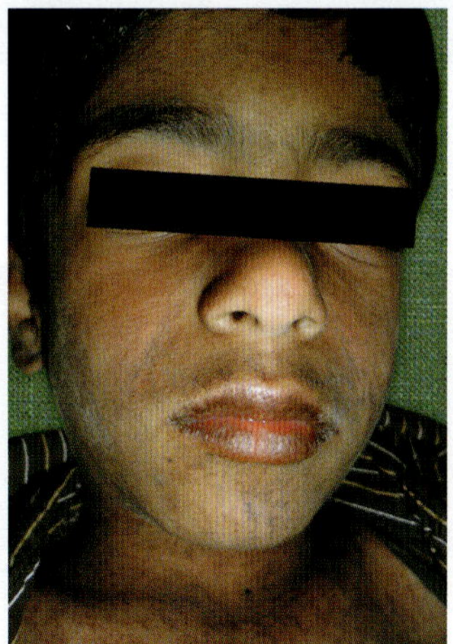

**FIG. 2:** An 11-year-old boy with drug hypersensitivity rash, mucous membrane is spared.

characterized by sterile nonfollicular pustules associated with fever and leukocytosis (Fig. 5).

## Bullous Eruptions

Erythema multiforme (EM) major, SJS, and TEN (SCARs) represent spectrum of same disease in varying severity. Many studies have shown there is not much distinction between SJS and EM major (Fig. 6). EM is a distinctive clinical reaction characterized by presence of target lesions. Target lesions are distributed more on acral regions and presents as central vesicle surrounded by edematous zone with a peripheral ring of erythema. Epidermal detachment less than 10% defines SJS and more than 30% defines TEN. Sometimes there may be an overlap between SJS and TEN (10–30%).

Stevens-Johnson syndrome-TEN presents as severe form of drug reaction characterized by skin and mucous membrane involvement and are described as epidermal necrolysis. Prodromal symptoms are severe and start few days to 3 weeks after the initiation of drug. Prodromal symptoms include fever, arthralgia, malaise, headache, vomiting, diarrhea, and myalgia. In TEN, there is skin tenderness. Atypical target lesions, blisters, and erosions are seen in SJS (Fig. 7). Clinically, SJS-TEN is characterized by symmetrical, erythematous or purpuric

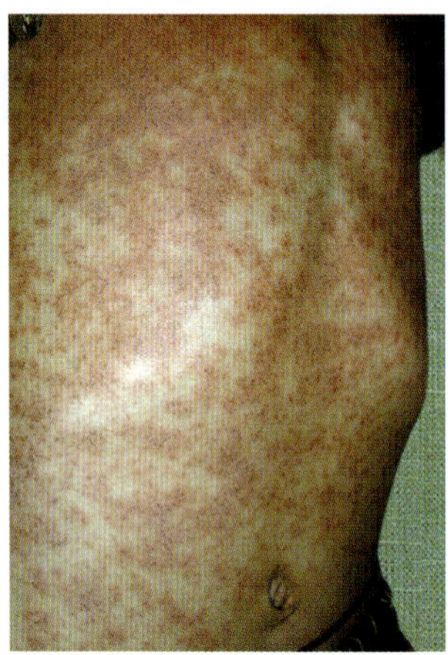

FIG. 3: Drug hypersensitivity eruption due to phenytoin.

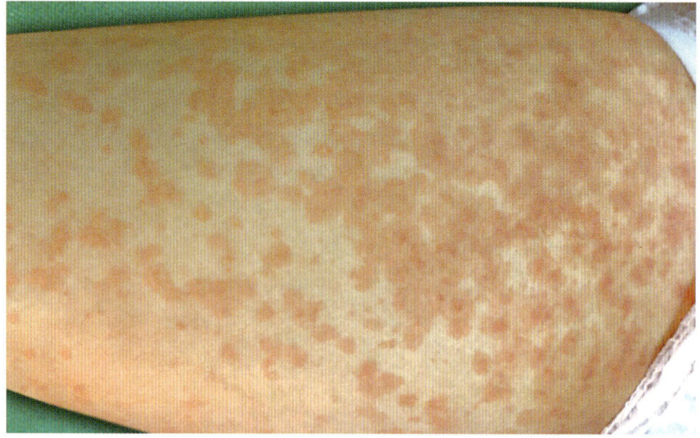

FIG. 6: Multiple target lesions in erythema multiforme.

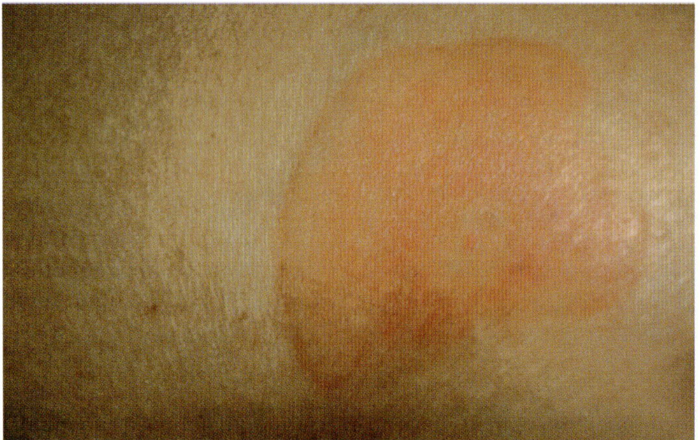

FIG. 4: Weals in drug-induced urticarial.

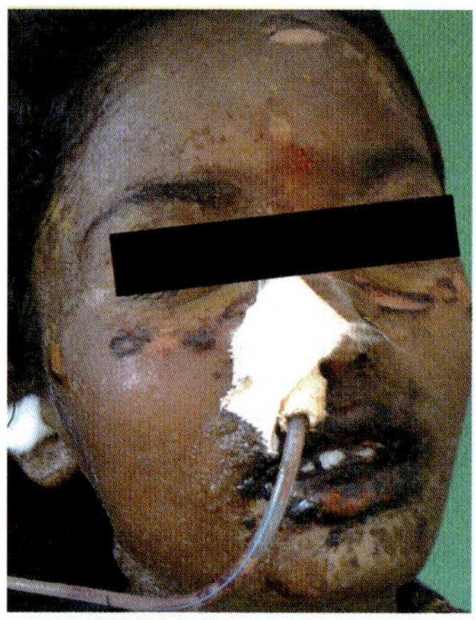

FIG. 7: An overlap case of Steven–Johnson syndrome or toxic epidermal necrolysis due to phenobarbitone. Severe mucosal involvement is present.

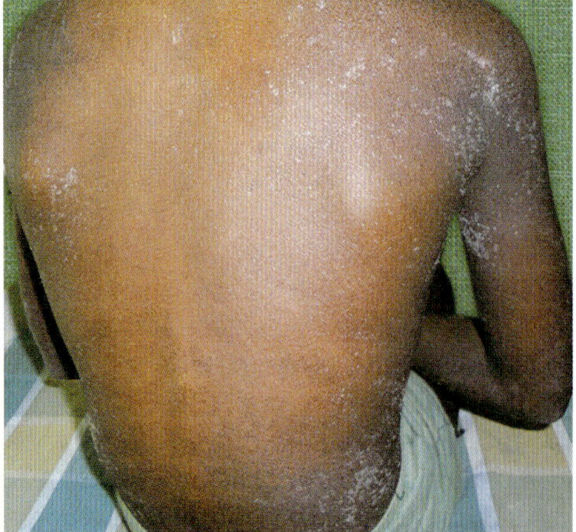

FIG. 5: Multiple sterile nonfollicular pustules in acute generalized exanthematous pustulosis.

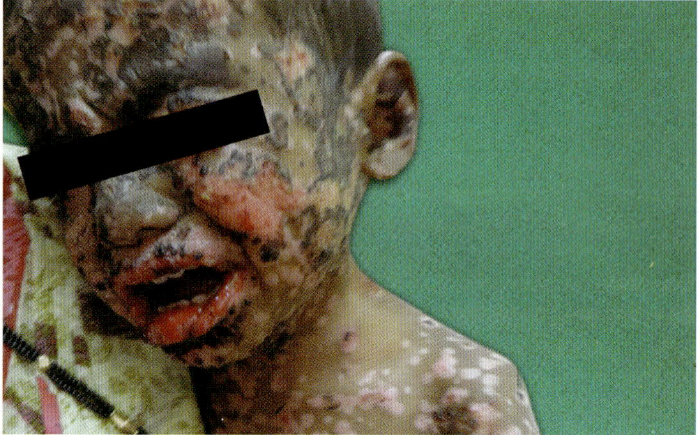

FIG. 8: Toxic epidermal necrolysis showing diffuse necrosis and crusting.

macules on trunk and extremities that gradually becomes generalized with epidermal necrosis leading to exfoliative dermatitis (Figs 8 and 9). Nikolsky's sign is positive. Scalp, palms, and soles are often not involved. Mucous membrane is involved in 90% cases and includes conjunctivitis, keratitis, photophobia, and erosions on the lips, stomatitis, and urethritis. Visceral involvement is seen in hepatitis, nephritis, colitis, and respiratory distress. Long-term complications include xerophthalmia, trichiasis, subconjunctival fibrous scarring, symblepharon, and anogenital strictures. Mortality rate is more in TEN due to gastrointestinal bleeding, colonic perforation, and sepsis.

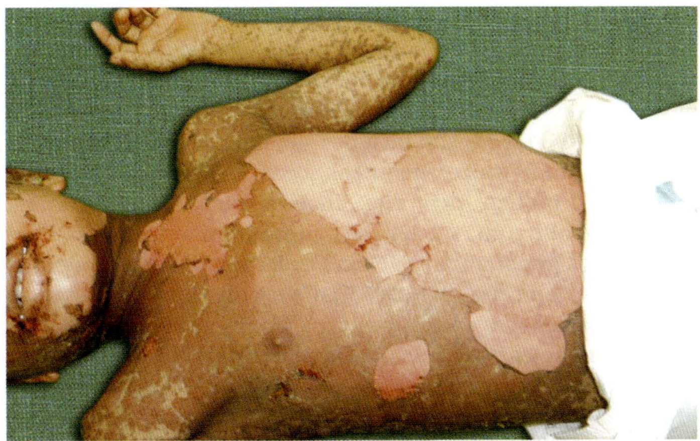

FIG. 9: Epidermal detachment in toxic epidermal necrolysis.

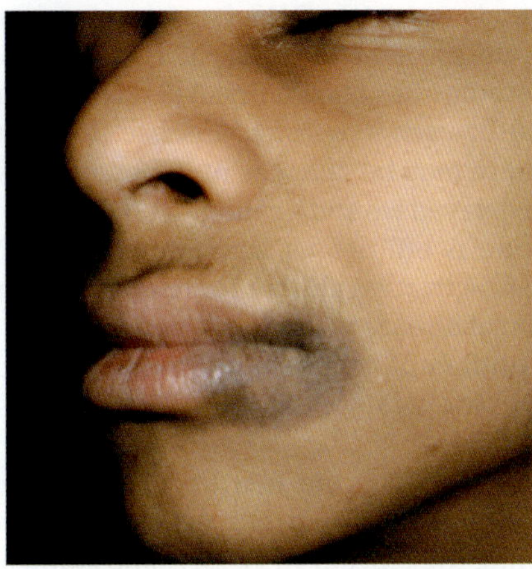

FIG. 10: A well-defined hyperpigmented macule in fixed drug eruption.

## Miscellaneous

There are various miscellaneous clinical patterns of drug reactions (Table 3), but only few of them have been emphasized. More than 100 drugs have been implicated in causing fixed drug eruption (FDE) (Fig. 10). FDE develops 30 minutes to 8–16 hours after initiation of drugs. FDE presents as well-defined solitary to multiple erythematous plaque or bullous lesions that resolves with persistent hyperpigmentation. Sites more commonly involved are oral mucosa, glans penis, and extremities. Recurrent FDE occurs on the same site of previous reaction. Lichenoid drug eruptions present as eczematous or purplish plaque and are seen more on trunk without involving mucous membrane and nails. Drug-induced vasculitis is difficult to diagnose and is often a diagnosis of exclusion. Clinically manifests as palpable purpura, urticaria, nodules, and ulcers. Drug-induced lupus may manifest many years after taking the drug. Clinically, symptoms are similar to systemic lupus but there is no cutaneous involvement. Antihistone antibodies are present in 95% cases of drug-induced lupus but they are not specific for this syndrome. There are several reports of drug-induced lupus attributed to minocycline. Anticoagulant-induced skin necrosis is a rare, sometimes life-threatening reaction induced by warfarin or heparin. Initially starts as painful purpuric lesion which later becomes necrotic. Chemotherapeutic agents induced reactions vary from benign to life-threatening complications. Anagen hair loss occurs due to cytotoxic chemotherapeutic agents and is often dose related. This hair loss is reversible and may take several weeks to months for the hairs to grow.

## DIAGNOSIS

A methodological approach is necessary for diagnosing ADRs. A detailed history regarding all the drugs taken chronologically by the patient, time interval between initiation of drug and skin eruption, previous history of drug reactions, and morphological pattern should be noted and the causative drug must be identified. Naranjo et al. put forward the diagnostic criteria of drug eruptions (Box 1). The most common differential diagnosis is viral exanthem especially for exanthematous reactions.

## PROGNOSIS

SCORTEN predicts the severity of illness in severe drug reactions like SJS and TEN. This scoring is applicable to adults and not to children. Poor prognostic markers include age more than 40 years, total body surface area more than 10%, serum urea more than 28 mg/dL, serum glucose level more than 252 mg/dL, serum bicarbonate level less than 20 mEq/L, heart rate more than 120 beats/min, and presence of visceral or hematological malignancies. Mortality is high with increasing score.

## INVESTIGATIONS

There is no gold standard investigation for diagnosing drug reactions. The diagnosis is done on clinical assessment. High eosinophil count, lymphocytosis, atypical lymphocytes, and abnormal liver functions tests are present in DHS. Rechallenge can be used to eliminate suspicion of a low probability drug reaction. Role of intradermal tests and patch testing is very limited. Skin biopsy can be done in severe reactions with systemic involvement for confirmation and to rule out other differential diagnosis (Fig. 11). Other *in vitro* tests like migration inhibition factor test, lymphocyte toxicity assay, lymphocyte transformation test, and basophil degranulation test have been used but their true sensitivity and specificity is not known. Radioallergosorbent test (RAST) is sensitive for immediate type of hypersensitivity reactions but is not much used. Recently fluorescence enzyme immunoassays (ImmunoCAP) have been used to detect drug-specific IgE antibodies in serum, but their sensitivity is only 40–75%.

## MANAGEMENT

There are many treatment protocols but there are no specific guidelines or randomized control trials for management of different types of drug reactions. Majority of ADRs is not serious. Withdrawal of offending drug, supportive therapy, and specific therapy forms the main important treatment strategies for management of drug reactions. All suspected drugs should be

**BOX 1 Diagnostic criteria for drug reactions**

Diagnostic criteria:
- Temporal relationship
- Recognized response to the suspected drug
- Confirmed by improvement after drug withdrawal
- Reaction on rechallenge

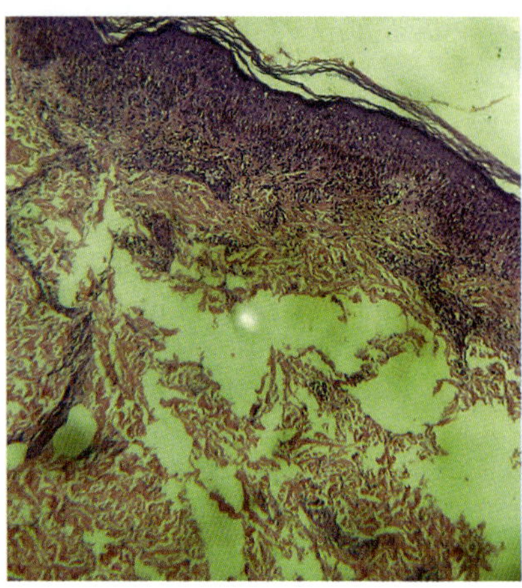

FIG. 11: Histopathology of severe drug reaction showing spongiotic epidermis with lymphocytic exocytosis. Basal layer vacuolation noted with occasional necrotic keratinocytes. Papillary dermis is edematous with moderated lymphohistiocytic infiltrate (H&E x10).

**TABLE 4: Management of drug reactions**

| | |
|---|---|
| Mild ADRs | • Withdrawal of offending drug<br>• Symptomatic treatment (emollients, calamine lotion)<br>• Oral antihistamines |
| Moderate ADRs | • Withdrawal of offending drug<br>• Emollients + topical corticosteroids (mid potency)<br>• Oral antihistamines |
| Severe ADRs | • Withdrawal of offending drug<br>• Supportive therapy<br>• Systemic corticosteroids (dose: 1–2 mg/kg body weight)<br>• Intravenous immunoglobulin (in TEN, dose: 2 g/kg given as 0.4 g/kg per day for 5 consecutive days, given within 72 hours<br>• Cyclosporine (dose: 3–6 mg/kg per day for 2–3 weeks)<br>• Second-line drugs: Cyclophosphamide, plasmapheresis, pentoxifylline, and infliximab |

ADRs, adverse drug reaction.

withdrawn immediately. However, it is important to weigh the risk-benefit ratio of the drug if it is necessary. The management protocols are outlined in table 4.

## Mild Adverse Drug Reactions

Mild ADRs subside with removal of offending drug. Bland emollients like white soft paraffin and antihistamines for pruritus are advised.

## Moderate Adverse Drug Reactions

Mild to moderate topical corticosteroids have been used to decrease the skin lesions in moderate ADRs like maculopapular rash and AGEP. Systemic corticosteroids are preferred in severe cases.

## Severe Adverse Drug Reactions

Studies have shown that withdrawal of drug on first appearance of skin lesions decreases the mortality from 26 to 5%. Supportive care in DHS and SCARs includes emollients, bland dressings like petrolatum gauze, maintenance of fluid and electrolyte imbalance, protein rich diet, maintenance of temperature, prevention of trauma to skin, and prevention of infection. Care of the eye is important in TEN and drug-induced erythroderma. Lubricants, topical antibiotics, and steroids should be used to prevent infections and adhesions. Immunosuppressants are specific therapies in treatment of severe drug reactions.

Systemic corticosteroids are indicated in severe DHS, drug-induced erythroderma not responding to conservative therapy, SJS, severe AGEP, and angioedema. Use of systemic corticosteroids in TEN is still controversial. Steroid has immunosuppressive, anti-inflammatory, and antiapoptic effects. It is given at the dose of 1-2 mg/kg body weight. In DHS, it can be given for 2-3 months with tapering doses. Short term for 2-3 weeks can be given in AGEP. Some studies has shown first 3-5 days of steroids in TEN may be useful in early control of disease. Precautions should be taken as there may be chances of infections, gastrointestinal bleeding, and delayed wound healing.

Cyclosporine is efficacious in treatment of TEN. It acts by inhibiting T-cell activation and tumor necrosis factor-α. It arrests the progression of disease in 24-36 hours. Dose used is 3-6 mg/kg body weight until complete resolution and then followed with tapering doses for 2-3 weeks. Renal parameters should be monitored regularly.

Intravenous (IV) Ig is the first treatment of choice in TEN based on clinical and laboratory evidence. There are many studies regarding the efficacy of IV Ig. Some studies have shown beneficial effects with few no benefits. It arrests the progression of disease and hastens re-epithelialization. It possesses anti-Fas activity and inhibits keratinocyte apoptosis by blocking the binding of Fas ligand to Fas receptors. It also has anti-infective properties and corrects protein and fluid loss. Various studies have shown that cumulative dose of 1.5-3.5 g/kg can be used. Small doses of 0.1-0.5 g/kg daily for 4 days are sufficient to treat TEN. It should be avoided in patients with thromboembolism, renal insufficiency, and cardiac abnormalities.

Few anecdotal case reports have shown cyclophosphamide in management of TEN. Initially, it is started at the dose of 300 mg and later tapered. Pentoxifylline, plasmapheresis, and infliximab have been tried in few studies but there is no proper evidence of its efficacy.

# COUNSELING

Education of the patient about the avoidance of offending drug and other cross-reacting drugs forms the corner stone of management in prevention of drug reactions. Counseling family members about the potential risk in DHS is necessary. Patients should carry small dairy regarding his drug allergies and should intimate the treating physician. All drug reactions and any newly observed side effects should be promptly reported to regulatory authorities.

## SUGGESTED READINGS


1. Byrne P, Williams B, Pritchard M. Minocycline-related lupus. Br J Rheumatol. 1994;33:674-6.
2. Cheng CY, Su SC, Chen CH, et al. HLA associations and clinical implications in T-cell mediated drug hypersensitivity reactions: an updated review. J Immunol Resp. 2014;2014:565320.
3. Choon SE, Lai NM. An epidemiological and clinical analysis of cutaneous adverse drug reactions seen in a tertiary hospital in Johor, Malaysia. Indian J Dermatol Venereol Leprol. 2012;78:734-9.
4. Chung WH, Chang WC, Lee YS, et al. Genetic variants associated with phenytoin-related severe cutaneous adverse reactions. JAMA. 2014;312:525-34.
5. Coombs PR, Gell PG. Classification of allergic reactions responsible for clinical hypersensitivity and disease. In: Gell RR (Ed). Clinical Aspects of Immunology. Oxford: Oxford University Press; 1968. pp. 575-96.
6. Dhar S, Banerjee R, Malakar R. Cutaneous drug reactions in children. Indian J Pediatr Dermatol. 2014;15:5-11.
7. Dhar S, Malakar S. Stevens-Johnson Syndrome: an update. Ind J Dermatol. 1997;42:204-10.
8. Dhar S, Sharma VK. Fixed drug eruptions to ciprofloxacin. Br J Dermatol. 1996;134:156-8.
9. Dhar S. Role of blood transfusion in the management of SJS and TEN. Ind J Dermatol Venereol Leprol. 1998;64:250-1.
10. Dhar S. Systemic corticosteroids in toxic epidermal necrolysis. Indian J Dermatol Venereol Leprol. 1996;62:270-1.
11. Drake LA, Dinehart SM, Farmer ER, et al. Guidelines of care for cutaneous adverse drug reactions. J Am Acad Dermatol. 1996;35:458-61.
12. Edwards IR, Aronson JK. Adverse drug reactions: definitions, diagnosis and management. Lancet. 2000;356:1255-9.
13. Impicciatore P, Choonara I, Clarkson A, et al. Incidence of adverse drug reactions in pediatric in/out patients: a systematic review and meta-analysis of prospective studies. Br J Clin Pharmacol. 2001;52:77-83.
14. International drug monitoring: the role of national centres. Report of a WHO meeting. World Health Organ Tech Rep Ser. 1972;498:1-25.
15. Lazarou J, Pomeranz B, Corey P. Incidence of adverse drug reactions in hospitalized: a meta-analysis of prospective studies. JAMA. 1998;279:1200-5.
16. Macdonald JB, Macdonald B, Golitz LE, et al. Cutaneous adverse effects of targeted therapies: Part II: Inhibitors of intracellular molecular signaling pathways. J Am Acad Dermatol. 2015;72:221-36.
17. Naldi L, Crotti S. Epidemiology of cutaneous drug-induced reactions. G Ital Dermatol Venereol. 2014;149:207-18.
18. Naranjo CA, Busto U, Sellers EM, et al. A method of estimating the probability of adverse drug reactions. Clin Pharmacol Ther. 1981;30:239-45.
19. Nayak S, Acharjya B. Adverse cutaneous drug reaction. Indian J Dermatol. 2008;53:2-8.
20. Neuman MG, Malkiewicz IM, Shear NH. A novel lymphocyte toxicity assay to assess drug hypersensitivity syndromes. Clin Biochem. 2000;33:517-24.
21. Patel RM, Marfatia YS. Clinical study of cutaneous drug eruptions in 200 patients. Indian J Dermatol Venereol Leprol. 2008;74:430.
22. Pereira FA, Mudgil AV, Rosmarin DM. Toxic epidermal necrolysis. J Am Acad Dermatol. 2007;56:181-200.
23. Pudukadan D, Thappa DM. Adverse cutaneous drug reactions: Clinical pattern and causative agents in a tertiary care centre in South India. Indian J Dermatol Venereol Leprol. 2004;70:20-4.
24. Roujeau JC, Stern R. Severe adverse cutaneous reactions to drugs. N Engl J Med. 1994;331:1272-85.
25. Rütter A, Luger TA. High-dose intravenous immunoglobulins: An approach to treat severe immune-mediated and autoimmune diseases of the skin. J Am Acad Dermatol. 2001;44:1010-24.
26. Sharma VK, Dhar S, Gill AN. Drug related involvement of specific sites in fixed eruptions: a statistical evaluation. J Dermatol (Tokyo). 1996;23:530-4.
27. Sharma VK, Dhar S. Clinical pattern of cutaneous drug eruption among children and adolescents in north India. Pediatr Dermatol. 1995;12:178-83.
28. Sidoroff A. Acute generalized exanthematous pustulosis. Hautarzt. 2014;65: 430-5.
29. Sukasen C, Puangpetch A, Medhasi S, et al. Pharmacogenomics of drug-induced hypersensitivity reactions: challenges, opportunities and clinical implementation. Asian Pac J Allergy Immunol. 2014;32:111-23.
30. Wang W, Hu FY, Wu XT, et al. Genetic susceptibility to the cross-reactivity of aromatic antiepileptic drugs-induced cutaneous adverse reactions. Epilepsy Res. 2014;108:1041-5.
31. Warin RP, Champion RH. Urticaria. Major problems in dermatology. 1974;1:10-4.
32. Worswick S, Cotliar J. Steven-Johnson syndrome and toxic epidermal necrolysis: a review of treatment options. Dermatol Ther. 2011;24:207-18.

# 77 CHAPTER Dermatologic Emergencies

*Amanjot Kaur Arora, Dipankar De*

## INTRODUCTION

Emergency, according to Oxford Dictionary is defined as "a serious, unexpected and often dangerous situation which needs immediate action". Emergencies in dermatology can be due to primary skin diseases and cutaneous manifestation of systemic diseases. The magnitude of dermatological emergencies was recently studied by George et al., who found that out of 476,224 admissions to 178 intensive care units in England, Wales, and Northern Ireland in between December 1995 and September 2006, 2,245 (0.47%) admissions due to dermatological disorders were identified.

## DERMATOLOGICAL EMERGENCIES

Conditions leading to an emergency situation in dermatology can be summarized as follows (Box 1). Most of these conditions give rise to acute skin failure which should be managed in an intensive care set up with a multispecialty approach, well equipped with gadgets to maintain appropriate environmental temperature and humidity and patient's vitals, fluid, and electrolyte balance.

### Acute Skin Failure

Irvine described skin failure as "inability of skin to maintain core body temperature, failure to prevent percutaneous loss of fluid, electrolytes, and protein with resulting imbalance, and failure of mechanical barrier to prevent penetration of foreign materials."

#### Consequences of Acute Skin Failure

As skin is a vital organ, its failure to perform its normal function is associated with a myriad of consequences which adversely affects patient survival. The consequences have been tabulated in box 2.

#### Fluid and Electrolyte Imbalance

Barrier dysfunction leads to increased transepidermal water losses (TEWL), which in conditions like toxic epidermal necrolysis (TEN) and other vesiculobullous conditions is accompanied by electrolyte loss.

Fluid loss occurs by transpiration and also by leaky capillaries. It is much increased and is roughly proportional to the basal metabolic rate. Acute erythrodermic patients seemed to have a higher TEWL than chronic erythrodermic patients. The usual total water loss through the skin is 400 mL/day (600–1,000 mL/day in temperate climates). In patients with acute skin failure, the daily percutaneous water loss far exceeds this, reaching a magnitude of 3–4 L in adult TEN patients with approximately 50% body surface area (BSA) involvement. In such a situation, inadequate fluid supplementation may lead to a state of dehydration, decreased urine output, and can

**BOX 1 Dermatological emergencies**

***Erythroderma*:**

- Primary (idiopathic)
- *Psoriasis*
  - *Psoriatic erythroderma*
  - Acute generalized pustular psoriasis of von Zumbusch
- *Dermatitis*: Atopic, seborrheic, and contact dermatitis
- Pityriasis rubra pilaris
- *Disorders of keratinization*: Lamellar ichthyosis, bullous and nonbullous ichthyosiform erythroderma
- *Vesiculobullous disorders*: Immunobullous and mechanobullous disorders
- Cutaneous T-cell lymphoma
- *Other solid organ malignancies*: Prostate, lung, thyroid, liver, breast, ovary, fallopian tube, rectum, esophagus, stomach, and melanoma
- Graft-versus-host disease (GVHD)
- *Infections*: Dermatophytosis, toxoplasmosis, histoplasmosis, leishmaniasis, and candidiasis
- *Infestations*: Norwegian scabies
- *Systemic disease*: Systemic lupus erythematosus, dermatomyositis, acute GVHD, postoperative transfusion induced, sarcoidosis, and thyrotoxicosis
- *Drug reactions*: Stevens–Johnson syndrome/toxic epidermal necrolysis, exfoliative dermatitis, drug rash eosinophilia and systemic symptoms
- *Miscellaneous*: Lichen planus, mastocytosis, Reiter's syndrome, and sarcoidosis
- Idiopathic

***Adverse drug reactions*:**

- Urticaria or angioedema
- Serum sickness
- Drug-induced anaphylaxis

*Continued*

*Continued*

**BOX 1 Dermatological emergencies**

***Collagen vascular disorder*:**
- Acute cutaneous lupus erythematosus

***Infections*:**
- Necrotizing fasciitis
- Congenital cutaneous candidiasis
- Meningococcemia
- Scarlet fever
- Disseminated gonococcal infection
- Rocky mountain spotted fever
- Dengue hemorrhagic fever
- Dengue shock syndrome

***Bacterial toxin-mediated illness*:**
- Staphylococcal scalded skin syndrome
- Toxic shock syndrome

***Severe form of type 2 lepra reaction*:**
- Acute neuritis with nerve abscess or impending nerve palsy

***Metabolic/nutritional (usually in children)*:**
- Disorders of biotin metabolism
- Essential fatty acid deficiency
- Kwashiorkor
- Acrodermatitis enteropathica
- Cystic fibrosis
- Leiner's disease
- Maple syrup urine disease

***Miscellaneous disorders*:**
- Kawasaki's disease
- Dermatomyositis
- Sarcoidosis
- Diffuse cutaneous mastocytosis

*With permissions from*: Inamadar AC, Palit A. Critical Care in Dermatology. 1st ed. Jaypee Brothers Medical Publishers (P) Ltd.

**BOX 2 Consequences of acute skin failure**

- Altered thermoregulation
- Metabolic abnormalities
- Loss of barrier function
- Altered immune function
- Loss of nutrient
- Fluid—electrolyte imbalance
- Pulmonary complications
- High output cardiac failure
- Development of multiorgan failure
- Infections

lead to a state of prerenal azotemia. Electrolyte imbalance in the form of low $Na^+$, high $K^+$, hypocalcemia (secondary to hypoalbuminemia) is seen in conditions of acute skin failure. Hypophosphatemia is seen in these patients as well which aggravates insulin resistance and leads to increased blood sugar levels.

### Altered Hemodynamics and Thermoregulation

There is increased TEWL, hypothermia, and tachycardia leading to compensatory hypermetabolism and a raised basal metabolic rate with resultant weight loss. Excessive scaling causes clogging of sweat glands and a consequent hypohidrotic state leading to risk of hyperthermia. Necrotic keratinocytes producing interleukin (IL)-1 can also lead to hyperthermia.

### Immune Dysfunction and Infections

There is a high degree of immune dysfunction, impaired chemotaxis, and decreased phagocytic activity of granulocytes and low serum gamma globulin levels are common. Sequestration of the lymphocytes in the skin may lead to CD4+ T-lymphocytopenia.

Defective barrier function and altered immune function lead to infection by harmful exogenous pathogens. Itching, fissuring, and excoriation increase the chances of staphylococcal sepsis in these patients. Patients with cutaneous T-cell lymphoma and HIV positivity have all the more increased chances of developing sepsis due to further lower immunity.

### Peripheral Edema

Peripheral edema occurs due to shifting of water in the extravascular compartment because of hypoalbuminemia and increase leakiness of blood vessels due to increased cutaneous synthesis of vascular permeability factor or vascular endothelial growth factor. Complications like acute respiratory distress syndrome and capillary leak syndrome may develop.

### Management

Acute skin failure may be fatal for a patient and demands intensive care. Intensive care in dermatology involves the management of the primary skin disorder as well as the associated systemic complications, such as vitals, fluid, and electrolyte imbalance in a multispecialty set-up. Patients with acute skin failure have a high mortality rate and a longer stay in intensive care unit than the average for the nondermatological adult intensive care patients.

## Erythroderma

First described by Hebra in 1868, erythroderma, or exfoliative dermatitis, is an inflammatory disorder in which erythema, scaling, and induration occur in a generalized distribution involving more than 90% of the BSA. This is associated with significant risk of morbidity and mortality.

### Epidemiology

The incidence of erythroderma was first estimated by Sehgal and Srivastva, in a prospective study from the Indian subcontinent, where the incidence was recorded as 35 per 100,000 dermatology outpatients. In another study from the Netherlands annual incidence has been estimated to be approximately 1 per 100,000 in the adult population. Erythroderma can occur at any age and in both sexes, but is more frequent in older adults (mean age 42–61 years) and in males with a male:female = 4:1. In a South African study on 138 patients of erythroderma, it was found that 75% were black, 22.5% Indian, and 2.5% white. Erythroderma is uncommon but seen in pediatric age group. In two Indian studies, the incidence of erythroderma among children was found out to be around 0.11%. The mean age of onset in children is around of 3.3 years, with a male to female ratio of 0.89:1.

## Etiology

Pre-existing dermatosis is the single most common cause of adult erythroderma, of which psoriasis is the commonest. Drug is an important etiology in both adults and children (Box 3). In neonates and infants infections or immunodeficiency may be the most common cause. However, cause of erythroderma remains unknown in 9–47% of the cases.

## Histopathology

Histopathology can help to identify the cause of erythroderma in up to 50% of cases, particularly if multiple skin biopsies are examined. Clinicopathologic correlation in erythroderma is difficult because the specific features of a dermatosis are masked by nonspecific features of erythroderma. However, multiple skin biopsy specimens submitted simultaneously enhanced diagnostic accuracy. For example, in erythroderma due to lymphoma, the infiltrate may gradually become polymorphic until it acquires specific diagnostic features. Best clinicopathological correlation, provided biopsies are taken from characteristic clinical lesions, is seen in psoriasis, pityriasis rubra pilaris (PRP), ichthyosiform erythroderma, or pemphigus foliaceus.

The histological appearances vary depending upon the severity and duration of the inflammatory process. In the acute stage, spongiosis and parakeratosis are prominent, and a nonspecific inflammatory infiltrate permeates, to a variable depth with a grossly edematous dermis. In the chronic stage, acanthosis and elongation of the rete ridges become more prominent.

**BOX 3 Important drugs causing erythroderma**

- Allopurinol
- Amiodarone
- Antimalarials
- Barbiturates
- Captopril
- Carbamazepine
- Chloroquine
- Chlorpromazine
- Cisplatin
- Clofazimine
- Dapsone
- Diltiazem
- Fluorouracil
- Indinavir
- Interferon
- Isoniazid
- Minocycline
- Phenobarbital
- Phenothiazines
- Phenylbutazone
- Phenytoin
- Retinoids
- Sulfasalazine
- Sulfonamides
- Sulfonylurea
- Terbinafine
- Tetracycline
- Thiazide
- Vancomycin
- Zidovudine

## Pathogenesis

There is intense dermal inflammation which gives rise to increased adhesion molecule expression (VCAM-1, ICAM-1, E-selectin, and P-selectin), leading to increased epidermal proliferation and increased production of inflammatory mediators like interleukins (IL-1,2,8) and tumor necrosis factor. This leads to significantly elevated epidermal turnover rate, and decrease in transit time of keratinocytes through the epidermis.

## Clinical Features

Erythroderma is characterized by the presence of erythema and scaling involving more than 90% of the skin surface. Majority of the manifestations are common in all cases. Duration of the disease and etiologies have some role in the presentation.

Rapidity of onset [faster with drug hypersensitivity, superficial pemphigus, staphylococcal scalded skin syndrome (SSSS), and PRP], severity and quality of scaling, pruritus, and many other clinical parameters may assist clinically in identifying the etiology (Table 1).

The associated scaling varies extensively in size and color depending upon the stage of erythroderma. In acute cases, the scales are large and crusted, whereas in chronic cases the scales are small and drier.

Loss of hair, eyelashes and discoloration, various nail changes (more common in psoriasis) like brittleness, dullness, paronychia, pitting, subungual hyperkeratosis, Beau's lines, shininess, onycholysis, onychauxis, splinter hemorrhages, and palmoplantar keratoderma are often associated.

**TABLE 1: Typical clinical findings in various secondary erythroderma**

| Cause | Major differentiating features |
|---|---|
| Psoriasis | • Typical psoriasiform plaque in early stage present on elbows, knees, sacrum or such lesions present at the margin of the erythroderma. Large lamellar scales usually silvery white, collarette of scales indicative of exfoliating pustules<br>• Nail changes<br>• Arthritis<br>• History of withdrawal of steroids, methotrexate or use of tar products or high dose of phototherapy |
| Pityriasis rubra pilaris | • Initial seborrheic dermatitis like eruption in scalp<br>• Cephalocaudal progression<br>• Salmon orange colored erythema<br>• Islands of sparing<br>• PRP sandal on palms and soles<br>• Follicular papules on dorsal surface of fingers, elbows, and wrists<br>• Characteristic histopathological findings—checkerboard appearance of alternating orthokeratosis and parakeratosis in both horizontal and vertical directions |

*Continued*

*Continued*

| Cause | Major differentiating features |
|---|---|
| ***Eczemas:*** | |
| Atopic dermatitis | • Personal or family history of atopy<br>• History of localized disease, most often moderate to severe<br>• Marked pruritus with lichenification and excoriation<br>• Criteria fulfillment<br>• Lesions in characteristic flexural distribution on antecubital and popliteal fossae<br>• Usually elderly patient<br>• Yellowish greasy scales involving seborrheic areas predominantly |
| Seborrheic dermatitis | • Sparing of palms and soles<br>• History of recurrent episodes of seborrheic dermatitis |
| Contact dermatitis | • History of pre-existing dermatosis and particular site<br>• History of contact with plant allergen or cement or photoexacerbation |
| Ichthyosis and related syndromes | • Present since or soon after birth<br>• History of collodion membrane at birth<br>• Family history of disease or consanguineous marriage of parents<br>• Brown adherent scales |
| ***Immunobullous disorders*:** | |
| Pemphigus foliaceus | • Flaccid blisters<br>• Erosions with collarette of scales<br>• Nikolsky's sign may be positive<br>• Positive Tzanck smear<br>• Subcorneal split in histopathology with positive direct immunofluorescence showing "fishnet pattern"<br>• Elderly patient |
| Bullous pemphigoid | • Tense blisters<br>• Urticarial plaques<br>• Histopathology—subepidermal bulla with eosinophilic infiltrate<br>• History of a known malignancy |
| Paraneoplastic pemphigus | • Severe mucosal involvement |
| Drug reaction | • Rapid progression of erythroderma<br>• Temporal relationship with a newly started drug or a frequently implicated drug<br>• Facial edema<br>• Systemic involvement like hepatitis, pneumonitis, and nephritis<br>• Organomegaly<br>• Lymphadenopathy |
| Cutaneous T-cell lymphoma or Sézary syndrome | • Leonine facies<br>• Marked pruritus<br>• Organomegaly<br>• Lymphadenopathy<br>• Presence of Sézary cells >5% or more of peripheral blood<br>• Lymphocytes |
| Dermatomyositis | • Heliotrope rash<br>• Poikiloderma<br>• Gottron's papules<br>• Proximal muscle weakness<br>• Raised muscle enzymes<br>• Electromyography |
| ***Infestations*:**<br>Norwegian scabies | • Poor hygiene<br>• Hospitalized or mentally challenged<br>• Physically severely incapacitated<br>• Burrows<br>• Demonstration of mites on KOH mount<br>• Keratoderma<br>• Markedly thickened nails |
| ***Infections*:** | |
| Staphylococcal scalded skin syndrome | • Skin tenderness<br>• Sloughing and erosions |
| Scarlet fever | • Positive Nikolsky's sign<br>• Perioral<br>• History of fever, pharyngitis, or skin staphylococcal infection<br>• Age <10 years<br>• Constitutional symptoms<br>• Caudal progression |
| Congenital cutaneous candidiasis | • Widespread macules, papules, and pustules which become confluent and generalize into an erythroderma<br>• Palms and soles involved<br>• KOH examination shows budding yeasts and pseudohyphae |

PRP, pityriasis rubra pilaris.

*With permissions from*: Inamadar AC, Palit A. Critical Care in Dermatology. 1st ed. Jaypee Brothers Medical Publishers (P) Ltd.

Palmoplantar keratoderma appears in approximately 30% of erythrodermic patients. It is often an early sign in pityriasis rubra pilaris. It is also a pointer towards Norwegian scabies when associated with scale and crusts on hands, and painful and fissured keratoderma is usally seen in Sezary syndrome

The "nose sign" in erythroderma that is, sparing of nose of erythema and scaling in patients with erythroderma, has been reported by Pavithran. It has been hypothesized that it is either due to greater exposure of the area to sunlight with its presumptive antimitotic activity or nervous habit of frequent rubbing of nose leading to removal of scales.

Generalized lymphadenopathy (also known as dermatopathic lymphadenopathy or lipomelanotic reticulosis of Pautrier) may be present. Lymphadenopathy with organomegaly points to a diagnosis of drug hypersensitivity or malignancy.

## Complications

Nutritional imbalance, especially of proteins, in erythroderma is multifactorial. Dermatopathic enteropathy, exfoliation, and exudation are major causes. Dermatopathic enteropathy also leads to impaired absorption of iron and vitamin B12 and an increased cellular turnover rate gives rise to relative folate deficiency. Thus anemia, both due to nutritional deficiencies and anemia of chronic disease, occurs in erythrodermic patients (Box 4).

## Prognosis

The prognosis of erythroderma is determined by its cause. Despite best efforts, mortality rates of up to 18–64% have been documented in initial studies. Sepsis, cardiac failure, pneumonia, dyselectrolytemia, and renal failure are the common causes of mortality in patients of erythroderma. Relapse is a common problem with erythroderma of eczematous, psoriatic or of unknown origin and may continue for months or years.

## Management

Identification and removal etiology is of prime importance. Proper history with focus on onset, duration, progression pattern, associated diseases, initial complaint, and detailed drug history often aid in identification of the etiology. Clinical examination should be meticulous to identify any suggestive finding that may indicate the associated or primary condition.

Routine and specific investigations should be done in all cases to identify the primary causes and extent of involvement of systemic organs. Commonly, complete hemogram, total and differential leukocyte counts, absolute eosinophil count, erythrocyte sedimentation rate, liver and kidney function tests, including serum electrolytes, urine macro- and microscopic examination, electrocardiogram (ECG), and chest radiograph should be done in all cases.

Swab from the breeched area of skin should be sent for culture. A foul smell is generally indicative of skin infection.

Investigations like skin scrapings/KOH, serum immunoglobulin E levels, serum and urine protein electrophoresis (multiple myeloma), CD4+ T-cell count or CD8+ T-cell count, human immunodeficiency virus 1 and 2 testing, antinuclear antibody, anti-double-stranded DNA, rheumatoid factor, fine needle aspiration cytology from lymph nodes, bone marrow examination (lymphoma or leukemia) and work-up for malignancy can be done as per suspicion in individual case. Serum lactate dehydrogenase may be higher especially in malignancy.

**BOX 4 Complications of erythroderma**

- Skin failure
- Nutritional imbalance
- Fluid electrolyte imbalance
- Temperature dysregulation
- Dermatopathic enteropathy
- Hypoproteinemia
- Renal failure

Skin biopsy with routine histopathology and direct immunofluorescence is very important.

## Basic Care

Management of acute skin failure requires a dermatological intensive care set up with a multispecialty approach. A clean, separate room, with barrier nursing facility is required. Air conditioning should be there to maintain temperature at 30–32°C which is required to keep the patient comfortable, minimize evaporative loss from the body, and reduce the patient's effort to maintain core body temperature. Room heater may be used. Burn unit can be used if available. Regular handwashing and aseptic handling of the patient is a must.

Parenteral access to body, central line insertion and catheterization, regular dressing and cleaning of oral and nasal cavities, eyes, and vagina is required especially in patients with TEN. Although, oral intake must be encouraged, a nasogastric tube should be considered in the presence of severe oral erosions or severely ill patients.

Frequent record of the pulse, respiratory rate, blood pressure, and urine volume and a body temperature and gastric emptying is important. An accurate daily intake-output chart should be maintained.

## Topical Therapy

Bland emollients, vapor permeable dressings (gauze), and physiologic lipids (component mixture of cholesterol, ceramide, and free fatty acids in an optimized ratio of 3:1:1) accelerate the barrier repair. Biological dressings like amniotic membranes, collagen-based dressings, and autograft and allograft epidermal sheets can also be used to provide barrier and at the same time accentuate the healing of raw areas.

## Specific Therapy

The status of steroids in management of erythroderma is still debatable.

## Management of Hemodynamic Changes, Fluid, Electrolyte, and Nutritional Support

Blood pressure, urine output, and pulse rate are important markers of fluid balance. A urine output of 50–100 mL/h and an osmolality lower than 1,020 are indicative of adequate tissue perfusion. A decrease in urine output is the first sign of hypovolemia and dehydration.

Adequate fluid intake must be maintained. Intravascular fluids and electrolytes levels need to be corrected. Fluid overload and eventual pulmonary edema should be avoided. For this, the previous day's urine output is an important measure. The initial fluids of choice are colloids (human albumin or fresh-frozen plasma) and normal saline (NS). Human albumin is a better choice than plasma, because there is no risk of infections and takes care of the patient's protein needs as well. Protein intake of at least 2–3 g/kg in adults and 3–4 g/kg body weight per day in children has to be ensured.

## Urticaria and Angioedema

Urticaria and angioedema have been discussed in another chapter. Management of severe acute urticaria and angioedema that has progressed to an emergency situation is covered here.

### Management of Acute Attacks of Urticaria and Angioedema

Management algorithm for an episode of acute urticaria and angioedema has been summarized in flowchart 1. Nonsedating antihistamines are the drug of choice and their dose can be increased to four times the usual, in case of no response to standard dose. The emergency treatment for histaminergic nonhereditary angioedema causing respiratory embarrassment from oropharyngeal-laryngeal angioedema is intramuscular epinephrine. Treatment should be repeated if there is no improvement after 10–15 minutes and injection hydrocortisone 100 mg intramuscular/intravenous (IM/IV) 8 hourly till acute stage is over can be given.

First episode of hereditary angioedema can be rarely fatal. Options for treatment of established swellings include replacement of C1-inhibitor with plasma-derived products (i.e., cinryze or berinert P), bradykinin receptor and kallikrein antagonists, and a recombinant C1 inhibitor. Long-term prophylaxis is done with 17-α-alkylated attenuated androgens, such as danazol, stanozolol, oxandrolone, and tibolone and (unattenuated) methyl testosterone, reduce the frequency and severity of attacks in most patients. International consensus now recommends reduced doses, i.e., a maximum of 200 mg danazol or 2 mg stanozolol daily.

A recombinant protein that acts as a reversible inhibitor of kallikrein, ecallantide, is currently indicated for acute attacks of hereditary angioedema in adult patients. The efficacy of the drug in the treatment of hereditary angioedema has been proven in two randomized, double-blind, placebo-controlled, multicenter trials, EDEMA3 and EDEMA4, where treatment with 30 mg of ecallantide resulted in statistically significant improvement in symptoms compared to placebo. In addition to its use in the treatment for hereditary angioedema, ecallantide has also been used in the management of nonhistaminergic angioedema, not due to hereditary angioedema, though the indication is off-label in this case.

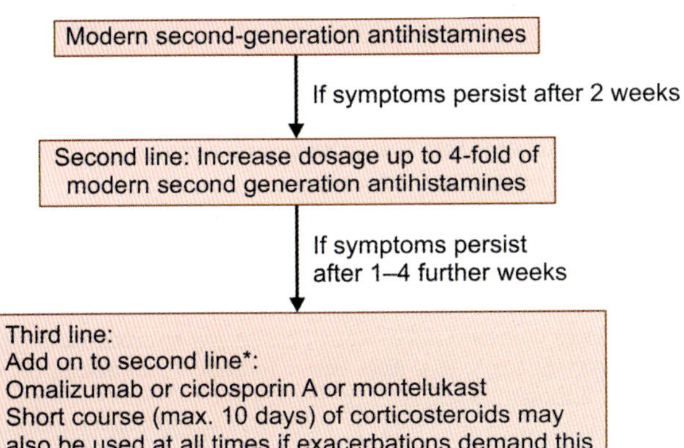


*The order of third line treatments does not reflect the order of preference.

**FLOWCHART 1:** Management protocol in urticaria and angioedema.

### Management of Anaphylaxis

Patients with airway and breathing problems should be made to sit up as this will make breathing easier. Lying flat with or without leg elevation is helpful for patients with a low blood pressure. If the patient feels faint, do not sit or stand them up—this can cause cardiac arrest. Any drug suspected of causing an anaphylactic reaction should be stopped (e.g., stop IV infusion of a gelatin solution or antibiotic). Remove the stinger after a bee sting. Early removal is more important than the method of removal.

Adrenaline in a dose of 0.5 mL of 1:1,000 (0.01 mg/kg) intramuscularly, should be given and repeated after 5 minutes, if no improvement is seen. Adrenaline should be given intravenously only if the administrator is sufficiently experienced. An IV fluid challenge of 500–1000 mL (NS/5% dextrose solution/colloidal volume expanders) should be given, particularly, in patients with persistent hypotension in spite of adrenaline dosage.

Despite limited evidence, antihistamines are considered important treatment for an anaphylactic reaction. They may help counter histamine-mediated vasodilation and bronchoconstriction. Injection chlorphenamine slowly intravenously or intramuscularly, in a dose 10–20 mg is preferred.

Given their slow onset of action, corticosteroids have not been evaluated and are unlikely to contribute substantially to the acute treatment of anaphylaxis, although they are routinely used to prevent delayed or biphasic allergic manifestations.

All patients with episode of anaphylaxis must be kept under supervision for a minimum period of 4–6 hours and must be counseled thoroughly for the avoidance of causative agent and the patient must be advised to carry a card with mention of anaphylaxis and its management.

# TOXIN-MEDIATED DISEASES

## Staphylococcal Scalded Skin Syndrome (Ritter Disease)

*Staphylococcus aureus* is an important pathogen of humans. Among multiple virulence factors, staphylococci secrete several exotoxins directly associated with particular disease symptoms. These include toxic shock syndrome toxin 1 (TSST-1), enterotoxins, and exfoliative toxins (ETs). The latter are produced by some strains of *S. aureus* belonging to phage group II, usually strain 71 and 55 and are the sole agents responsible for SSSS. Two antigenically distinct forms of enterotoxins have been identified: toxin A (ET A) and toxin B (ET B). SSSS is seen most commonly in neonates, who have decreased renal excretion of the toxin due to immature renal function and lack of immunity to toxins. Thus, outside the early pediatric population also, any person with decreased renal function, such as a patient on dialysis or a poorly controlled diabetic, is at risk for developing SSSS, though less frequently.

The initial event is usually a localized staphylococcal infection of skin, pharynx, conjunctiva, nares, etc. This is followed by development of widespread erythema and tenderness, which progresses rapidly to blister formation. Since, the bulla are very thin walled, it is rare to find intact bulla but numerous superficial painful erosions at the sites of previously intact blisters. In well-established disease, there is separation of the perioral crusts leaving behind radial fissures around the mouth, which is typical of SSSS. The condition usually heals within 7–14 days. Since, there is widespread denudation of skin, the patient who is usually a child can succumb to the consequences of acute skin failure like fluid, electrolyte imbalance, hypothermia, and sepsis.

### Diagnosis

Swabs from denuded areas do not grow *S. aureus*, since it is a toxin-mediated disorder. Tzanck preparation from a freshly denuded area reveals many acantholytic cells without inflammatory cells. Clinically, absence of mucosal involvement in SSSS separates it from TEN. In addition to Tzanck smear, a frozen section can help to differentiate between SSSS and TEN as the treatment options are diametrically opposite. Frozen section will show the split in the granular layer in SSSS whereas all the epidermal layers will show necrosis in TEN.

### Treatment

Supportive care is same as in cases of acute skin failure. Early institution of antibiotic helps in treating the primary infection and halts the progression of disease. However, prior to the first dose of antibiotic being given, it is important for blood cultures to be drawn so that the presence or absence of methicillin resistant *S. aureus* (MRSA) can be established. Based on local resistance patterns, it is appropriate to start treatment with IV vancomycin, or other drugs that can cover MRSA. Clindamycin is often chosen, especially in neonates, due to its ability to inhibit additional toxin production. If cultures show methicillin-sensitive *S. aureus*, then the patient could be switched over from the initial IV antibiotic to either a penicillinase-resistant penicillin, or a first or second generation cephalosporin, to complete the course of antibiotics orally at home. IV immunoglobulin has also been recommended to combat SSSS, but a recent study associates its use with prolonged hospitalization.

### Prognosis

The prognosis of this condition is better in children as compared to adults with a mortality rate of less than 10% in children, but between 40% and 63% in adults, despite therapy. The high mortality rate in adults is ascribed to presence of underlying immunocompromised state and other comorbidities in adults suffering from SSSS.

## Staphylococcal Toxic Shock Syndrome

It is an, mostly staphylococcal sometimes streptococcal, exotoxin-mediated multisystem illness characterized by fever, desquamation, and circulatory shock. Though historically TSS was frequently menstrual in origin due to usage of super-absorbent tampons, most cases of TSS occurring in recent times are of nonmenstrual origin. Nonmenstrual TSS is associated with upper airway infections, burns, postpartum infections, cutaneous infections, surgical procedures, and nasal packing. Staphylococcal TSS is mediated by TSST-1 and staphylococcal enterotoxins A, B, and C which act as superantigens, resulting in massive cytokine release from T-cells (*see* Chapter on Bacterial Skin Infection).

## Streptococcal Toxic Shock Syndrome

Streptococcal TSS is associated with a more fulminant course and greater mortality as compared to staphylococcal TSS. It is caused by infection with particular toxin-producing strains of *Streptococcus pyogenes*, including M protein types 1, 3, 12, and 28. Streptococcal pyrogenic exotoxin A, B, and C, streptococcal superantigen, and mitogenic factor are toxins usually associated with this type of TSS.

### Clinical Features

Patients typically present with excruciating pain, most commonly affecting a leg that may be succeeded by necrotizing fasciitis or myonecrosis. Soon after presentation, patients develop shock and multiorgan failure, such as renal failure, respiratory distress syndrome, and disseminated intravascular coagulation, thus leading to a higher risk of mortality.

Center for Disease Control and Prevention has defined criteria for diagnosis of staphylococcal as well as streptococcal TSS.

### Management

Positive blood cultures are uncommon (<15%), and mortality is less than 3%. Due to protracted complications, it is better to manage these patients in an ICU set up and give supportive care as in acute skin failure. The mainstay of treatment of staphylococcal TSS includes rapid identification and drainage/removal of focus of infection. Appropriate antibiotic cover is required. Clindamycin can also be used as it reduces the production of staphylococcal toxin.

## CONCLUSION

Dermatological emergencies, though rare, carry a high incidence of morbidity and mortality. Skin is the largest organ of the body. Undoubtedly, its failure is associated with a number of complications that require a multidisciplinary, intensive care approach. In the present scenario, when incidence of medical litigation is high, the present day dermatologists need to have adequate knowledge about monitoring these patients and work in liaison with other specialties to manage these patients appropriately.

## SUGGESTED READINGS

1. Agarwal S, Khullar R, Kalla G, et al. Nose sign of exfoliative dermatitis: A possible mechanism. Arch Dermatol. 1992;128:704.
2. Akhyani M, Ghodsi ZS, Toosi S, et al. Erythroderma: a clinical study of 97 cases. BMC Dermatol. 2005;5:5.
3. Berk DR, Bayliss SJ. MRSA, staphylococcal scalded skin syndrome, and other cutaneous bacterial emergencies. Pediatr Ann. 2010;10:627-33.
4. Berth-Jones J. Eczema, lichenification, prurigo and erythroderma. In: Burns T, Breathnach S, Cox N, et al (Eds). Rook's Textbook of Dermatology, 8th edition. Oxford: Blackwell-Science; 2010. pp. 23.1-23.51.
5. Bukowski M, Wladyka B, Dubin G. Exfoliative toxins of *Staphylococcus aureus*. Toxins (Basel). 2010;2:1148-65.
6. Centers for Disease Control and Prevention. Streptococcal Toxic Shock Syndrome (STSS) (Streptococcus pyogenes) 2010 Case Definition [Internet] [cited 2018

Aug 27]. Available from: http://wwwn.cdc.gov/nndss/conditions/streptococcal-toxic-shock-syndrome/case-definition/2010/

7. Centers for Disease Control and Prevention. Toxic Shock Syndrome (Other Than Streptococcal) (TSS) 2011 Case Definition [Internet] [cited 2018 Aug 27]. Available from: http://wwwn.cdc.gov/nndss/conditions/toxic-shock-syndrome-other-than-streptococcal/case-definition/2011/
8. Cicardi M, Bork K, Caballero T, et al. Evidence-based recommendations for the therapeutic management of angioedema owing to hereditary C1 inhibitor deficiency: Consensus report of an International Working Group. Allergy. 2012;67: 147-57.
9. Cicardi M, Bork K, Caballero T; for the HAWK (Hereditary Angioedema International Working Group). Evidence-based recommendations for the therapeutic management of angioedema owing to hereditary C1 inhibitor deficiency: consensus report of an International Working Group. Allergy. 2012;67:147-57.
10. Elias PM, Feingold KR. Does the tail wag the dog? Role of the barrier in the pathogenesis of inflammatory dermatoses and therapeutic implications. Arch Dermatol. 2001;137:1079-81.
11. Empinotti JC, Uyeda H, Ruaro RT, et al. Pyodermitis. An Bras Dermatol. 2012;87: 277-84.
12. George SM, Harrison DA, Welch CA, et al. Dermatological conditions in intensive care: a secondary analysis of the Intensive Care National Audit and Research Centre (ICNARC) Case Mix Programme database. Crit Care. 2008;12Suppl 1:S1.
13. Grant-Kels JM, Fedeles F, Rothe MJ. Exfoliative dermatitis. In: Goldsmith LA, Katz SI, Gilchrest BA, et al (Eds). Fitzpatrick's Dermatology in General Medicine, 8th edition. New York: McGraw-Hill; 2012. pp. 266-79.
14. Haemodynamics of extensive skin disease. Lancet. 1983;1(8334):1144.
15. Handler MZ, Schwartz RA. Staphylococcal scalded skin syndrome: diagnosis and management in children and adults. J Eur Acad Dermatol Venereol. 2014;28:1418-23.
16. Inamadar AC, Palit A. Acute skin failure: concept, causes, consequences and care. Indian J Dermatol Venereol Leprol. 2005;71:379-85.
17. Inamadar AC, Palit A. Critical Care in Dermatology, 1st edition. New Delhi: Jaypee Brothers Medical Publishers; 2013.
18. Itin PH. Dermatologic Consultations in the Hospital Ward: The skin, an Interdisciplinary Organ. Dermatology. 2009;219:193-4.
19. Junkins-Hopkins JM. Biologic dressings. J Am Acad Dermatol. 2011;64:e5-7.
20. Järvinen KM, Celestin J. Anaphylaxis avoidance and management: educating patients and their caregivers. J Asthma Allergy. 2014;7:95-104.
21. Kress DW. Pediatric dermatology emergencies. Curr Opin Pediatr. 2011;23:403-6.
22. Levine N. Exfoliative dermatitis–skin biopsy is required to determine the cause of this pruritic eruption. Geriatrcs. 2000;55:25.
23. Li J, Zheng HY. Erythroderma: a clinical and prognostic study. Dermatology. 2012;225(2):154-62.
24. Longhurst H, Cicardi M. Hereditary angio-oedema. Lancet. 2012;379(9814):474-81.
25. McCormick JK, Yarwood JM, Schlievert PM. Toxic shock syndrome and bacterial superantigens: an update. Annu Rev Microbiol. 2001;55:77-104.
26. Mohd Noor N, Hussein SH. Transepidermal water loss in erythrodermic patients of various aetiologies. Skin Res Technol. 2013;19(3):320-3.
27. Pavithran K. Nose sign of exfoliative dermatitis. Indian J Dermatol Venereol Leprol. 1988;54:42.
28. Pruszkowski A, Bodemer C, Fraitag S, et al. Neonatal and infantile erythroderma: A retrospective study of 51 patients. Arch Dermatol. 2000;136:875-80.
29. Rothe MJ, Bialy TL, Grant-Kels JM. Erythroderma. Dermatol Clin. 2000;18:405-15.
30. Sarkar R, Basu S, Sharma RC. Neonatal and infantile erythroderma. Arch Dermatol. 2001;137:822-3.
31. Sarkar R, Sharma RC, Koranne RV, et al. Erythroderma in children: A clinico-etiological study. J Dermatol. 1999;26:507-11.
32. Sehgal VN, Srivastava G, Sardana K. Erythroderma/exfoliative dermatitis: A synopsis. Int J Dermatol. 2004;43:39-47.
33. Sentis HJ, Wallemze R, Scheffer E. Histopathologic studies in Sezary's syndrome and erythroderma mycosis fungoides: a comparison with benign forms of erythroderma. J Am Acad Dermatol. 1986;15:1217-26.
34. Sigurdsson V, de Vries IJ, Toonstra J, et al. Expression of VCAM-1, ICAM-1, E-selectin, and P-selectin on endothelium in situ in patients with erythroderma, mycosis fungoides and atopic dermatitis. J Cutan Pathol. 2000;27:436-40.
35. Sigurdsson V, Toonstra J, Bihari IC, et al. Interleukin-4 and interferon-gamma expression of the dermal infiltrate inpatients with erythroderma and mycosis fungoides–an immunohistochemical study. J Cutan Pathol. 2002;27: 429-35.
36. Tarbox JA, Gutta RC, Radojicic C, et al. Utility of routine laboratory testing in management of chronic urticaria/angioedema. Ann Allergy Asthma Immunol. 2011;107:239-43.
37. Walsh NMG, Prokopetz R, Tron VA, et al. Histopathology in erythroderma: review of a series of cases by multiple observers. J Cutan Pathol. 1994;21:419-23.
38. Zuberbier T, Aberer W, Asero R, et al. Methods report on the development of the 2013 revision and update of the EAACI/GA2 LEN/EDF/WAO Guideline for the definition, classification, diagnosis, and management of urticaria. Allergy. 2014;69(7):e1-29.
39. Duffey H, Firszt R. Management of acute attacks of hereditary angioedema: Role of ecallantide. J Blood Med. 2015;6:115-23.

21 SECTION

# Dermatologic Therapy

78 CHAPTER

# Principles of Topical Therapy

*Vishalakshi Viswanath, Poonam Pund*

## INTRODUCTION

Skin is the largest organ of the body and the largest interface between internal milieu and external environment and an important barrier for exogenous substances. Efficacy of topical formulation depends on method of delivering particular drug. The skin offers a number of penetration routes through the "stratum corneum" (SC) barrier; the intercellular, intracellular, follicular and eccrine pathways, and these penetration routes form the basis of topical therapy in dermatology. The advantages of topical therapy are outlined in box 1.

## SKIN AS A BARRIER

To be effective; an active drug or principle must cross the SC barrier to achieve therapeutic efficacy. SC is a composite material made of proteins and lipids that is crucial for life. The SC consists of dead cells called as corneocytes. SC is structurally organized as brick and mortar model. The corneocytes (the bricks: about 85% of the mass of horny mass) and intercellular lipids (15%) are arranged in approximately 15–20 layers. It consists of about 70% proteins, 15% lipids, and only 15% water. The lipids in the extracellular space are made up of three chief constituents: ceramides, cholesterol, and free fatty acids that are present in the molar ratio: 1:1:1. This ratio is also critical to maintain the barrier integrity. The bricks and mortar structure provide efficient protection against the penetration of foreign substances.

## PERCUTANEOUS ABSORPTION OF DRUGS

It involves three steps:

1. Penetration, the entry of a substance into a particular skin layer
2. Permeation, the penetration through one layer into another, and finally
3. Resorption, the uptake into the vascular system.

**BOX 1 Advantages of topical therapy**

- Elimination of gastrointestinal adverse effects
- Elimination of hepatic first pass metabolism
- Reduced toxicity since doses less than that for oral administration are required
- Slow and continuous release possible resulting in improved efficacy
- Decrease in costs due to dosing frequency
- Improved patient compliance

### Factors Influencing Percutaneous Drug Absorption

These are related to the individual, drug vehicle, and environmental influences (Table 1). Absorption is greatly regulated by age, gender, and site that influence through SC thickness, pH, number of sebaceous glands, and hydration state. The hydrophobic lipids in the extracellular spaces in SC are not uniformly distributed but they are sequestered into lamellar membranes that surround corneocytes. One important function of the lamellar membranes is to act as reservoirs of lipid soluble drugs (e.g., topical steroids) that can accumulate and be released slowly in the viable epidermis.

Percutaneous drug delivery is a passive process governed by Fick's law, that is, the rate of absorption or flux (J) of any substance across a barrier is proportional to its concentration difference across that barrier.

**TABLE 1: Host factors affecting percutaneous absorption**

| Factors | Salient features |
|---|---|
| Age | The skin barrier function is significantly less in infants. This can result in increased permeability |
| Gender | Not significant however skin barrier was weakest in the few days just before the onset of menses in one Caucasian study |
| Regional difference | A rule of thumb is that the absorption of drug is in the following order nail < palm/sole < trunk/extremities < face/scalp < scrotum |
| Skin hydration | Occlusion of an intact skin can lead to increase in hydration of the skin and this will increase the penetration of a topically applied substance |
| Skin pH | Maintenance of acid mantle is essential for homeostasis of the SC and its barrier function |
| Skin disease state | Human studies have shown increased penetration of active drugs in psoriatic and atopic dermatitis skin |
| Massaging | It increases the absorption, as it increases the blood supply to the part |

SC, stratum corneum.

**TABLE 2: Drug factors that can affect absorption**

| Factors | Salient features |
|---|---|
| Potency | Concentration of soluble drug in the vehicle is the key for percutaneous absorption. However higher concentrations does not always mean greater absorption. Higher the concentration of the drug in the topical formulation better is the absorption and therapeutic effect |
| Molecular weight | Topical medications with a molecular weight less than 1,000 are effective |
| Vehicle | The vehicle is the link between drug potency and therapeutic effectiveness. Choice of vehicle is important as the choice of active drug. Ointments have better penetration than creams, lotions, gels, or pastes. A vehicle which irritates the skin would alter the skin barrier and may increase drug absorption |
| Frequency of application | It does not significantly affect the absorption. Except in case of emollients where efficacy increases by frequent applications |
| Partition coefficient (PC) | It describes the ability of drug to move from the vehicle into the stratum corneum. PC can be improved by various methods such as hydration, or with penetration enhancers |

**TABLE 3: Steps in percutaneous absorption of topical agent**

| Factors | Salient features |
|---|---|
| Diffusion | Movement of molecules along the concentration gradient between the vehicle in which the medication is embedded and the stratum corneum |
| Adsorption | Adhesion of topically applied substances to skin |
| Absorption | Uptake and storage of topically applied substances inside the skin |
| Resorption | Uptake of topically applied substances with transfer to blood vessels or lymphatics. In the case of most dermatologic agents, resorption is not desirable |
| Metabolism | Process by which an absorbed agent is enzymatically degraded and removed from the circulation |

$$J = K_p C_v$$

where $K_p$ is the permeability coefficient and $C_v$ is the concentration of the drug in the vehicle. Various parameters govern the permeability coefficient such as the partition coefficient ($K_m$), diffusion coefficient (D), and length of diffusion pathway (L).

$$K_p = DK_m/L$$

The parameters related to the drug that can affect absorption are listed in table 2.

Steps in percutaneous absorption of topical agent or what happens to a topical drug when it enters body is described in table 3.

## GENERAL PRINCIPLES OF TOPICAL THERAPY

### Vehicles

Vehicle is defined as all the constituents of the formulation apart from the active pharmaceutical agent. It is the composition of vehicle that can significantly influence rate and extent of absorption. According to Fick's law $J = K_p C_v$ rate of absorption, i.e., J can be modified by vehicle where $K_p$ is the permeability coefficient and $C_v$ is the concentration of the drug in the vehicle. The various types of vehicles are summarized in box 2.

### Penetration Enhancers

An ideal penetration enhancer should be nontoxic, nonirritating, and non-allergenic and should not have pharmacological activity within the body. They should be unidirectional, rapid in action and the activity and duration of effect should be both predictable and reproducible.

Penetration enhancers can be chemical, physical, and biochemical in nature.

- *Chemical enhancers* interact with the lipid matrix of SC to alter the barrier structure and increase transdermal drug delivery. They are typically of low cost and do not require battery power devices as in physical enhancers but major disadvantage is irritation to skin when present in high concentration. Water is the most common chemical enhancer. Other substances include dimethyl sulfoxide, pyrrolidones, fatty acids, essential oil, terpenes and terpenoids, oxazolidinones, urea, surface active agents such as sodium lauryl sulfate and benzalkonium chloride and chelating agents such as ethylenediaminetetraacetic acid and citric acid salicylates
- *Physical enhancement* is done by a variety of devices to increase drug delivery. Stripping of SC layers by using a micropore tape or cyanoacrylate glue reduces the layers that the drug has to penetrate. Other techniques include fractional photothermolysis and microneedling (creation of microchannels). Electroporation uses very short (microsecond to milliseconds) and high voltage electrical pulses to induce structural rearrangements of SC lipids leading to pore formation. Iontophoresis uses electrophoresis principle to drive the similarly charged drug with the help of low current electrode across the SC. Ultrasound and radiofrequency uses the principle of heating the deeper tissues for better penetration
- *Biochemical enhancers* are new modalities of drug delivery where they directly increase permeability of SC lipid matrix in addition to altering lipid metabolism. Peptides disrupt and penetrate the SC and prevent the repair response of the skin and thereby prevent barrier recovery. These two mechanisms help in drug delivery.

Natural substances and agents such as basil oil, clove oil, and capsaicin have been used as enhancers in various drug delivery systems.

### Dispensing Methods and Instructions

The quantity of medication to be applied is a very important aspect governing efficacy and side effects. A single gram of cream covers roughly surface area of about 100 $cm^2$ and forms a 100 µm thick layer. An equal amount of ointment covers 5–10% greater area. The amount of topical medication required for single or multiple application is as mentioned in table 4.

**BOX 2 Types of vehicles**

**Liquids**

- *Solution*: Monophasic vehicle, the liquid vehicle, may be water based or nonwater based (e.g., alcohol and oil). Alcoholic solutions evaporate rapidly, e.g., tinctures and paints
- *Lotions*: Monophasic vehicle, thicker than solution. There are two phase systems, consisting of a finely divided insoluble drug dissolved in a liquid, it needs to be rubbed when applied, e.g., calamine lotion
- *Wet dressings*: Used in oozing or crusted lesions seen in different types of eczema, e.g., potassium permanganate compresses, normal saline compresses. They act as anti-infectives and astringents
- *Baths*: Used in inflammatory disorders, e.g., starch bath in erythroderma, tar bath in psoriasis

**Semisolids**

- *Creams*: There are two phase systems involving one or more immiscible liquids dispersed in another with the help of an emulsifying agent

| Phase systems | Continuous phase | Dispersed phase |
|---|---|---|
| Water in oil (cold creams) | Oil | Water |
| Oil in water creams (vanishing creams) | Water | Oil |

Water in oil creams also called as cold creams which provide a soothing effect to the skin and are more moisturizing in effect. Oil in water creams however are easier to wash off. Creams may contain preservatives and are therefore prone to produce allergic reactions

- *Ointments*: Semisolid, greasy preparations of hydrocarbons (petrolatum, mineral oil, paraffins, and synthetic hydrocarbons), e.g., betamethasone ointment. They provide more occlusion and hence better penetration of the medication. They do not contain preservatives and are therefore less allergenic. Four types of ointment bases:
  - Hydrophobic anhydrous hydrocarbon base, e.g., petrolatum
  - Hydrophilic anhydrous absorption base, e.g., anhydrous lanolin
  - *Emulsion base*: Water in oil, e.g., lanolin or oil in water, e.g., stearyl alcohol
  - Water soluble base. This can absorb water soluble drugs, e.g., polyethylene glycol
- *Pastes*: They are prepared by incorporating powders into ointments or creams, e.g., anthralin incorporated in Lassar's paste for psoriasis, zinc oxide paste used as sunscreen. They are occlusive and hence provide hydration.
- *Gels*: Transparent preparations containing polymers (cellulose ethers or carbomer) in water or a water-alcohol mixture. They liquefy on contact with the skin, dry and leave a thin film of active medication, e.g., clindamycin gel for acne. They are especially useful on hairy areas

**Solids**

- *Powders*: They help in minimizing friction, improving hygiene, and providing a cooling effect, e.g., clotrimazole powder. They should not be used in oozing conditions in the flexures as they may cause maceration

**TABLE 4: Amount of topical medication**

| Area treated | Single application (g) | Total amount required for three applications per day for 2 weeks (g) |
|---|---|---|
| Hands, head, face, anogenital region | 2 | 90 |
| One arm, anterior or posterior trunk | 3 | 120 |
| One leg | 4 | 180 |
| Entire body | 25 | 1,125 |

**TABLE 5: Fingertip units (FTU) and hand areas required for application in various sites**

| Site (for an adult) | Quantity in FTU | No. of hand areas |
|---|---|---|
| Face and neck | 2.5 | 5 |
| Front and back of trunk | 14 | 28 |
| One arm | 4 | 8 |
| One hand | 1 | 2 |
| One leg | 8 | 16 |
| One foot | 2 | 4 |

FTU, fingertip unit.

## Fingertip Unit

If a cream or ointment is squeezed out of a tube which has a nozzle of 5 mm, over the distal section of an index finger from distal skin crease to tip of finger, the amount is roughly equal to 0.5 g (0.49 g in males and 0.43 g in females). One fingertip unit (FTU) covers the surface area of the flat of two hands, i.e., two hand areas. Table 5 enumerates the FTUs and number of hand areas required for covering different body sites.

## Factors Determining Choice of Topical Preparation

Efficacy of topical preparation depends on factors such as type of vehicle, type of lesion, site of lesion, and body surface area (BSA). For oozing lesions dressings are preferred. For body folds like the axilla and groin, preparations like the creams and lotions are preferred. An occlusive vehicle like an ointment enhances penetration of the active ingredient and improves efficacy. Generally, ointments and water in oil creams are less irritating, while gels may be irritating. Depending on the drug used, the acceptable BSA on which the drug can be applied safely without causing side effects varies. Potent steroids are not used more than 50 g weekly for 2 weeks such as clobetasol propionate cream 0.05% to avoid hypothalamic pituitary adrenal (HPA) suppression.

## Instructions for Topical Therapy

To achieve maximum efficacy with minimum side effects, the patient should be given proper instructions regarding the topical application (Box 3).

**BOX 3 Instructions provided to patients regarding topical therapy**

- Frequency of application
- Timing of application
- Quantity for every application
- Common side effects seen with the medication
- Total duration of use
- Not to self-treat

## Side Effects of Topical Therapy

Allergic (gentamicin, neomycin, and bacitracin) and irritant reactions are most common. Topical steroids can cause atrophy, acne, acneiform eruptions, hirsutism, hyperpigmentation, vascular fragility, and purpura.

Retinoid dermatitis manifests as erythema, scaling, pruritus, burning, stinging, and dryness.

Systemic side effects can occur rarely especially when large amount of medication is used or when used over inflammatory lesions or on abraded skin.

# NEWER DRUG DELIVERY SYSTEMS

Various drug delivery and drug targeting systems are currently under development. Targeting is the ability to direct the drug. These newer drug delivery systems find a role in delivery of the active drug in various antiacne preparations, antifungals, and antipsoriatic drugs. Most importantly these have been used in various cosmetics and cosmeceutical preparations. These cause sustained release of the dug, thereby reducing the side effects and improve the efficacy and tolerability of the topical formulation (Box 4).

**BOX 4 Newer drug delivery systems**

- *Vesicular system*: Liposomes, silicone vesicles and matrices, and multi-walled delivery systems
- *Emulsions*: Microemulsions, liquid crystals, multiple emulsions, nanoemulsions, and pickering emulsions
- *Particulate systems*: Microparticulates, porous polymeric systems, nanoparticulates, and cyclodextrin complexes
- *Nanodelivery systems*: Nanospheres and nanocapsules
- Peptides and growth factors

Liposomes are spherical vesicles with diameter between 25 and 5,000 nm whose membrane consists of amphiphilic lipids (i.e., lipids that are hydrophilic on one side and lipophilic on the other side) that enclose an aqueous core, similar to the bilayer membranes of living cells (Fig. 1). Because liposomes offer an amphiphilic environment, they may encapsulate hydrophilic substances in their aqueous core and lipophilic substances in their lipid bilayer. This unique dual release capability enables the delivery of two types of substances once they are applied on the skin; each differs in its effects on skin permeability, which may enhance the desired therapeutic benefit. The commonly used liposomal systems are natural lecithins (egg or soybean lecithin) or synthetic lecithin (dipalmitoyl lecithin). The most common lecithin is mixture of phosphatidylcholine, phosphatidylethanolamine, phosphatidylinositol, phosphatidylserine, and phosphatidic acid. Conventional liposomes remain confined to SC building a reservoir in it. Specially designed vesicles are required for drug transfer.

Multiple other forms of liposomal vesicular systems include niosomes, sphingosomes, marinosomes, transfersomes, ethosomes, asymmetric oxygen carrier system, ultrasomes, phytosomes, and photosome.

Silicones and the other classes of delivery systems are commonly used in cosmetic, personal care, and cosmeceutical products.

# IMPORTANT TOPICAL THERAPIES

## Corticosteroids

These are one of the most widely used medications in dermatology. Corticosteroids are naturally occurring or synthetic compounds with a cyclopentanoperhydrophenanthrene ring. Mechanisms of action of steroids include anti-inflammatory action, antiproliferative action on keratinocytes, and immunosuppressive action. The drug active, vehicle affects the potency of the compound. The potency of various corticosteroids is assessed by the vasoconstrictor assay. Fluorinated compounds and lipid esters like butyrate are more potent. Classes of topical corticosteroids (TCSs) based on the potency are outlined in table 6.

Corticosteroids can be applied topically, under occlusion or be given intralesionally. TCS are the mainstay in eczemas, such as atopic dermatitis, allergic contact, and irritant contact dermatitis, lichen simplex chronicus, and prurigo nodularis. Other TCS responsive disorders include lichen planus, psoriasis, vitiligo, alopecia areata, and localized bullous disorders.

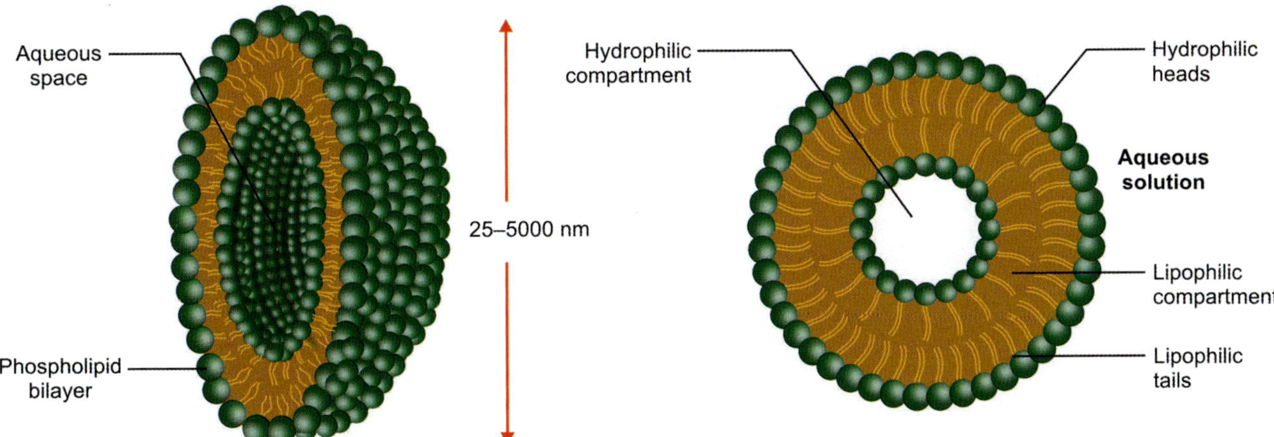


FIG. 1: Liposome structure with phospholipid bilayer.

**TABLE 6: Classes of corticosteroids**

| Class | Corticosteroids |
|---|---|
| 1 (super potent) | Clobetasol propionate 0.05%, halobetasol propionate 0.05% |
| 2 (very potent) | Betamethasone dipropionate 0.05%, mometasone furoate 0.1% ointment |
| 3 (potent) | Fluticasone propionate 0.05% ointment |
| 4 (mid strength) | Fluocinolone acetonide 0.025% ointment, mometasone furoate 0.1% cream |
| 5 (mid strength) | Hydrocortisone butyrate 0.1% cream |
| 6 (mild) | Desonide 0.05% cream |
| 7 (least potent) | Hydrocortisone acetate 0.1–1% cream |

**BOX 5 Common side effects of corticosteroids when used for topical therapy**

- Skin atrophy, telangiectasia, striae, and hypopigmentation
- Steroid acne, rosacea, and perioral dermatitis
- Hypertrichosis
- Folliculitis, poor wound healing
- Tachyphylaxis, rebound phenomenon
- Cataract and glaucoma
- Hypothalamic–pituitary–adrenal axis suppression

Intralesional steroids are indicated in keloids, hypertrophic scars, lichenified eczemas, hypertrophic lichen planus, and alopecia areata.

Side effects of topical steroids are given in box 5. HPA axis suppression can occur if potent steroids are used for long duration.

Potent TCS should preferably be avoided in children, on the face, in body folds, for prolonged periods and over a large area. Duration and side effects should be monitored and the patient should be educated about the same.

## Antifungals

The older preparations include Whitfield's ointment (3% salicylic acid and 6% benzoic acid) and Castellani's paint (resorcinol, acetone, magenta, phenol, boric acid, and methylated spirit). Various classes of topical antifungals available are described in table 7 and the newer antifungals with improved delivery systems are described in table 8. AN2690 is a novel oxaborole broad-spectrum antifungal designed with properties required to allow for easier penetration through the nail plate, has been shown to have superior *in vitro* penetration compared to ciclopirox olamine.

## Antibacterials

Topical antibacterials are mainly used in acne, superficial bacterial infections like impetigo and after minor surgical procedures to prevent infection. Various antibacterials and their spectrum of action have been enumerated in table 9.

## Antiparasitic Agents

*Permethrin*: It is the topical drug of choice for scabies and pediculosis. It acts on the nerve cell membranes of the parasite causing paralysis and death of the mite. Available as a 5% cream for scabies, it is safe for children above 2 months of age and also in pregnancy as a single application for 10–12 hours. In pediculosis capitis, 1% permethrin used as a hair rinse is kept for 10 minutes. It is also useful in rosacea by acting on the demodex mites. Repeat application after 1 week improves treatment efficacy. Other antiparasitic agents include gamma benzene hexachloride 1%, crotamiton 10%, malathion 0.5% solution, benzyl benzoate 25% preparation, and sulfur 6%.

**TABLE 7: Classification of topical antifungals**

| Antifungal class | Examples | Effective against | Mechanism of action | Comments |
|---|---|---|---|---|
| Azoles | Miconazole, clotrimazole, oxiconazole, sertaconazole, bifonazole, ketoconazole, econazole, and sulconazole | Dermatophytes, candida, pityrosporum, and erythrasma | • Act by blocking ergosterol incorporation in the fungal cell membrane.<br>• Antibacterial<br>• Activity<br>• Anti- inflammatory activity (few azoles) | Clotrimazole is available in powder form for tinea pedis and as oral troches for oral candidiasis. Ketoconazole is available as 2% shampoo for tinea capitis |
| Allylamines and benzylamines | Terbinafine 1%, butenafine, and naftifine | Dermatophyte infection and pityriasis versicolor | Inhibiting the enzyme squalene epoxidase | • Shorter duration of therapy requirement as compared to azoles<br>• Narrower spectrum compared to azoles |
| Morpholines | • Amorolfine 5%<br>• As nail lacquer | – | – | – |
| Polyenes | – | Oral and vaginal candidiasis | – | • Fungistatic and fungicidal<br>• Not effective against dermatophytes |
| Ciclopirox olamine | Nail lacquer, cream, and shampoo | Antibacterial activity | – | Broad-spectrum antifungal |
| Tolnaftate 1% | Cream | Dermatophytes and *Malassezia* species | – | – |

**TABLE 8: Newer drug delivery for antifungals**

| Newer drug delivery system | Example |
|---|---|
| Liposomes and niosomes | • Fluconazole loaded with liposomes<br>• Ciclopirox olamine liposome<br>• Ketoconazole on niosomes |
| Ethosomes, transfersomes ketoconazole | Econazole, fluconazole, and griseofulvin |
| Water soluble biopolymer technology (more effective than conventional lacquer) | Ciclopirox hydrolacquer |
| Iontophoresis | Terbinafine nail solution |
| AN2690 novel oxaborole | Used for onychomycosis |

## Antivirals

Various topical agents are used for the treatment of viral infections of skin though many of these agents may not be actually viricidal.

- *Acyclovir*: 5% cream can be used for treatment of herpes labialis and herpes genitalis. It requires phosphorylation by the viral enzyme thymidine kinase for its action. Penciclovir 1% cream, idoxuridine, cidofovir, and foscarnet are other topical antivirals.

## Antiacne Agents

Various topical antiacne agents and novel drug delivery systems are summarized in tables 10 and 11.

## Topical Therapies for Psoriasis

Besides topical steroids and keratolytic agents, other therapies which are used in psoriasis include coal tar, anthralin, and calcipotriol. Calcipotriol inhibits epidermal proliferation, induces differentiation, and has anti-inflammatory effects; it is used in other condition such as morphea.

## Topical Calcineurin Inhibitors

Tacrolimus and pimecrolimus are the chief drugs. Indications include atopic dermatitis (especially in children and facial lesions), eczemas, oral lichen planus, vitiligo, psoriasis, and alopecia areata. Adverse effects include irritation and local infections.

## Topical Cytotoxic Agents and Immunomodulators

These include fluorouracil, bleomycin, imiquimod, and topical interferon-α. These are chiefly indicated in viral warts and various premalignant and malignant tumors. Other therapies useful in warts include podophyllin, trichloroacetic acid, cantharidin, and salicylic acid. Candida antigen is also used as intralesional therapy.

## Depigmenting Agents

Hydroquinone is a commonly used skin lightening agent. Other skin lightening agents are azelaic acid, glycolic acid, arbutin, kojic acid, resorcinol, and monobenzone. They act by inhibiting tyrosinase enzyme. Kligman's regime is used in melasma and contains 5% hydroquinone, 0.1% tretinoin, and 0.1% dexamethasone in a hydrophilic ointment. Various newer preparations with modifications have been formulated. They are used for various melasma, freckles, and postinflammatory hyperpigmentation.

## Cosmetics and Cosmeceuticals

Cosmetics are substances applied to the human body for cleansing, beautifying, promoting attractiveness, or altering appearance. The main cosmetics used in daily life are fragrances, deodorants, moisturizers, cleansers, depilatories, bleaching agents, shampoos, conditioners, hair dyes, and nail polish. Cosmeceuticals are products which belong to a category between

**TABLE 9: Topical antibacterial drugs**

| Class of antibiotics | Spectrum of action | Comments |
|---|---|---|
| Mupirocin 2% cream/ointment | *Staphylococcus aureus*, *Streptococcus pyogenes*, *Staphylococcus epidermidis*, and methicillin resistant *Staphylococcus aureus* | • For prophylaxis against recurrent staphylococcal infections<br>• Low rate of sensitization |
| Sodium fusidate (Fusidic acid) 2% | Antistaphylococcal activity | • Sensitization rare<br>• So combined with steroids for treating infected eczema |
| Aminoglycosides neomycin, gentamicin, framycetin | Gentamicin is effective against Pseudomonas aeruginosa | Contact allergy is common with neomycin |
| Pleuromutilin, retapamulin (1%) | *Staphylococcus aureus* and *Streptococcus pyogenes* | Less resistance |
| Sulfonamides, silver sulfadiazine 1% | Broad-spectrum for Gram-positive and negative organisms | Useful for ulcers |
| Metronidazole (0.75–1%) | Anaerobic infections | • Additional immunomodulatory properties<br>• Used in rosacea, decubitus ulcers |
| Quinolones 1% nadifloxacin | Broad-spectrum of action | • Antifungal and antibacterial properties<br>• Resistance uncommon<br>• Used in acne |
| Lincosamides like clindamycin and macrolides like erythromycin | *P. acnes* | Used in acne |

drugs and cosmetics. Various botanicals, antioxidants, vitamins, peptides, and sunscreens fall in this category.

## Miscellaneous Agents

These are used in various dermatological diseases and are summarized in table 12.

## CONCLUSION

Topical therapy forms the mainstay of treatment in various dermatological diseases. Newer drug delivery systems in topical therapy ensure enhanced penetration, good therapeutic efficacy, lesser side effects, and better patient compliance.

**TABLE 10: Antiacne agents**

| Agent | Class | Mechanism of action | Effective on type of acne |
|---|---|---|---|
| Benzoyl peroxide (2.5–10%) | Anti-inflammatory antibiotic | Bactericidal effect against *Propionibacterium acnes* with reduction of free fatty acid. It has effect on inflammatory and noninflammatory lesions | Inflammatory and noninflammatory lesions |
| Tretinoin (0.025%, 0.05%, and 0.01%) | Topical retinoids | It enhances epithelial turnover, loosens keratin debris, is comedolytic and prevents formation of new lesions | All grades of acne, comedolytic, anti-inflammatory, and antiproliferative activity |
| Adapalene 0.1% | Topical retinoids | Synthetic derivative of naphthoic acid with retinoid-like activity | ALL grades of acne, comedolytic, anti-inflammatory, and antiproliferative activity |
| Erythromycin and clindamycin | Antibiotics | Effective against *P. acnes* | Inflammatory acne |
| Nadifloxacin 1% | Antibiotics | Broad-spectrum antifungal | Inflammatory acne |
| Azelaic acid 10% and 20% | Dicarboxylic acid | • Bacteriostatic against *P. acnes* and inhibits tyrosinase enzyme<br>• Comedolytic | Inflammatory acne |
| Nicotinamide 4% | Anti-inflammatory | Anti-inflammatory properties | Inflammatory acne |

**TABLE 11: Newer drug delivery systems in acne**

| Topical acne treatments | Potential novel systems for agent delivery |
|---|---|
| Clindamycin phosphate | Aerosol foams, polymers, and nanoemulsions |
| Retinoids (e.g., adapalene and tretinoin) | Microsponges, liposomes, nanoemulsions, and aerosol foams |
| Benzoyl peroxide | Polymers and fullerenes |

**TABLE 12: Miscellaneous agents used in dermatology**

| Type | Mechanism of action | Indications | Side effects |
|---|---|---|---|
| **Astringents** | | | |
| • Aluminum acetate 5% (diluted 1:40)<br>• Potassium permanganate 1:10,000<br>• Silver nitrate 0.5–1%, etc. | • Used to reduce local pain and destroy granulation tissue<br>• They act by causing precipitation of protein | Weeping conditions like acute eczema and exudative ulcers | Irritation, contact dermatitis |
| **Chemical Cauterizing agents** | | | |
| • Trichloroacetic acid (10–20%)<br>• Phenol 88%<br>• Silver nitrate 1%<br>• Ferric chloride, etc. | Local tissue destruction and sloughing with denaturation of proteins used to cauterize various growths and tissues | Removal of moles, warts, papillomas, molluscum contagiosum | Irritation, contact dermatitis |
| Soothing agents | • Inert substance, provides physical protection and has mild astringent and antiseptic action<br>• Reduce itching, burning, and discomfort in the skin | Sunburn, urticaria, contact dermatitis, and insect bite | – |
| **Emollients** | | | |
| • Petrolatum<br>• Extract of aloe vera plant<br>• Mustard and olive oil<br>• Cetyl and stearyl alcohol and glycerin<br>• Propylene glycol | These agents are used to soothe the dry skin. Retain moisture by decreasing evaporation and drawing moisture to the skin | Dry scaly dermatoses like psoriasis, ichthyosis, keratoderma, atopic dermatitis (to be applied after hydration/bath for optimal effect) | Petrolatum is messy to use, folliculitis (chemical or bacterial) |
| **Keratolytics** | | | |

*Continued*

*Continued*

| Type | Mechanism of action | Indications | Side effects |
|---|---|---|---|
| • Salicylic acid 3–40%<br>• Resorcinol 2–10%<br>• Urea 10–40%<br>• Hydroxy acids (like glycolic acid and lactic acid) | Promote desquamation of scales or for thickened stratum corneum. Contraindicated in acute or subacute inflammation | Ichthyosis, palmoplantar keratoderma, acne, and palmoplantar warts | Irritation and salicylism (if salicylic acid is used >6% over large area for prolonged period especially in infants) |
| **Cleansing agents** | | | |
| • Normal saline<br>• Povidone iodine (for clean uninfected wounds)<br>• Cetrimide<br>• Hydrogen peroxide (for cleaning infected and dirty wounds) | Antimicrobial action, effervescent quality of $H_2O_2$ helps to debride | For cleaning wounds prior to dressing | Iodinated compounds may cause irritation |
| **Antipruritic agents** | | | |
| • Menthol 0.1–2% in cream or ointment base<br>• Camphor 1–3%<br>• Capsaicin<br>• Phenol 0.5–2%<br>• Crotamiton 10% in lotion or ointment form and antihistamines | Menthol and camphor act by local cooling and soothing effect. Capsaicin acts through counter-irritation | For relief of local pruritus and pain | Contact dermatitis |
| **Antiperspirants** | | | |
| • Aluminum chloride hexahydrate<br>• Formaldehyde soaks<br>• Botulinum toxin | Acts by blocking the sweat glands | Hyperhidrosis of palms, soles, and axilla | |

## SUGGESTED READINGS


1. Aggarwal N, Goindi S. Preparation and evaluation of antifungal efficacy of griseofulvin loaded deformable membrane vesicles in optimized guinea pig model of Microsporum canis-Dermatophytosis. Int J Pharm. 2012;437(1-2):277-87.
2. Bansal S, Kashyap CP, Aggarwal G, et al. A comparative review on vesicular drug delivery system and stability issues. IJRPC. 2012;2(3):704-13.
3. Baran R, Tosti A, Hartmane I, et al. An innovative water-soluble biopolymer improves efficacy of ciclopirox nail lacquer in the management of onychomycosis. J Eur Acad Dermatol Venereol. 2009;23:773-81.
4. Bhalaria MK, Naik S, Misra AN. Ethosomes: A novel delivery system for antifungal drugs in the treatment of topical fungal diseases. Indian J Exp Biol. 2009;47(5):368-75.
5. Chiang A. Percutaneous absorption in diseased skin: an overview. J Appl Toxicol. 2012;32(8):537-63.
6. Denet AR, Vanbever R, Preat V. Skin electroporation for transdermal and topical delivery. Adv Drug Deliv Rev. 2004;56:659-74.
7. Fireman S. A look at emerging delivery systems for topical drug products. Dermatologic Therapy. 2011;24:477-88.
8. Giusti F. Skin barrier, hydration, and pH of the skin of infants under 2 years of age. Pediatr Dermatol. 2001;18(2):93-6.
9. Hougeir FG. A review of delivery systems in cosmetics. Dermatologic Therapy. 2012;25:234-7.
10. Hui X, Baker SJ, Wester RC, et al. In vitro penetration of a novel oxaborole antifungal (AN2690) into the human nail plate. J Pharm Sci. 2007;96:2622-31.
11. Inayat BK, Setty CM. Chemical penetration enhancers for transdermal drug delivery systems. Trop J Pharma Res. 2009;8(2):173-9.
12. Kielhorn J, Melching-Kollmu S, Mangelsdorf I. Dermal Absorption. WHO/IPCS Environmental Health Criteria, Draft February 2005 [Internet] [Cited May 2018]. Available from: http://www.who.int/ipcs/methods/dermal_absorption/en/
13. Kleesz P. Full-body skin mapping for six biophysical parameters: baseline values at 16 anatomical sites in 125 human subjects. Skin Pharmacol Physiol. 2012;25(1):25-33.
14. Muizzuddin N. Effect of systemic hormonal cyclicity on skin. J Cosmet Sci. 2005;56(5):311-21.
15. Nino M, Calabrò G, Santoianni P. Topical delivery of active principles: the field of dermatological research. Dermatol Online J. 2010;16(1):4.
16. Patravale VB, Mandawgade SD. Novel cosmetic delivery systems: an application update. Int J Cosmet Sci. 2008;30(1):19-33.
17. Prausnitz, Mark R, Elias PM, et al. Skin barrier and transdermal drug delivery. Dermatology, 3rd edition. Philadelphia, PA: Elsevier Saunders; 2012. pp. 2065-74.
18. Proksch E. The skin: an indispensable barrier. Exp Dermatol. 2008;17(12):1063-72.
19. Rajan R, Deepa T. Vasudevan. Effect of permeation enhancers on the penetration mechanism of transferosomal gel of ketoconazole. J Adv Pharm Technol Res. 2012;3(2):112-6.
20. Saini S, Chauhan SB, Agrawal SS. Recent development in penetration enhancers and techniques in transdermal drug delivery system. J Adv Pharm Edu Res. 2014;4(1):31-40.
21. Verma P, Pathak K. Nanosized ethanolic vesicles loaded with econazole nitrate for the treatment of deep fungal infections through topical gel formulation. Nanomedicine. 2012;8(4):489-96.
22. Wolverton SE. Basic principles of pharmacology. In: Wolverton SE (Ed). Comprehensive Dermatologic Drug Therapy, 2nd edition. Philadelphia, PA: Saunders Elsevier; 2007. pp. 3-14.

# 79 CHAPTER Systemic Dermatological Therapy

*Sujay Khandpur, Vishal Gupta, Riti Bhatia*

## INTRODUCTION

Topical medications form the mainstay of dermatological therapy. Systemic agents are however, indicated when the disease fails to respond adequately to topical agents, is extensive, invasive or deep-seated or associated with systemic manifestations. This chapter outlines the mechanism of action, indications, adverse effects, and monitoring recommendations for some of the commonly used systemic agents in dermatological practice.

## ANTIMALARIALS

The antimalarial drugs commonly used in dermatological practice are hydroxychloroquine (HCQ), chloroquine (CQ), and quinacrine. HCQ and CQ structurally belong to the class of 4-aminoquinolines and are derivatives of quinine, an alkaloid derived from the bark of South American cinchona tree. Quinacrine is a synthetic acridine compound having an extra-benzene ring, and is not available in India. Antimalarials are almost completely absorbed from the gastrointestinal (GI) mucosa, widely distribute, and have strong affinity for skin and melanin-containing retinal cells, where concentrations are between 100 times and 200 times that of plasma concentration. The half-lives of CQ and HCQ are 40 and 50 days, respectively. They have a slower onset of action it takes 4–6 weeks for these drugs to reach a steady-state plasma concentration. Excretion is through both the liver and kidneys. Antimalarials accumulate in the lysosomes and lead to inhibition of function of the lysosomal acidic proteases and even, alteration of the lysosomal morphology. The various mechanisms by which antimalarials exert their effects are summarized in table 1.

**TABLE 1: Antimalarials mechanism of action**

| | |
|---|---|
| Immunomodulatory effects | • *Lysomotropic effect*: Interference in effective antigen processing and presentation to T-cells<br>• Inhibition of cytokine release<br>• Inhibition of endosomal toll-like receptors (TLRs) like TLR9<br>• Inhibition of phospholipase A2 leading to decrease in prostaglandin and leukotriene levels<br>• Decreased cell functioning such as chemotaxis, phagocytosis, and superoxide production by neutrophils |
| Photoprotective effects | • Absorption of ultraviolet (UV) light<br>• Prevention of UV light-induced keratinocyte apoptosis through exertion of anti-inflammatory response<br>• Upregulation of c-Jun transcription leading to photoprotection |
| Others | • Excretion of porphyrins from the hepatocytes into circulation ultimately leading to urinary excretion<br>• Anticoagulant effect<br>• Lipid-lowering effect<br>• Hypoglycemic effect |

### Indications

Lupus erythematosus (LE) is the only Food and Drug Administration (FDA)-approved indication of antimalarials in dermatology. The list of indications is summarized in table 2.

**TABLE 2: Indications of antimalarials in dermatology**

| | |
|---|---|
| Photosensitive dermatoses | Lupus erythematosus, cutaneous manifestations of dermatomyositis, porphyria cutanea tarda, solar urticaria, and polymorphous light eruption |
| Granulomatous dermatoses | Sarcoidosis, granuloma annulare, and erythema nodosum (chronic) |
| Others | Lichen planus (lichen planopilaris, oral lichen planus), Jessner's lymphocytic infiltrate, chronic ulcerative stomatitis, accelerated rheumatoid nodulosis, subcutaneous panniculitis-like T-cell lymphoma, cutaneous small vessel vasculitis, erythema nodosum leprosum, cutaneous leishmaniasis (intralesional injection) |

### Adverse Effects

Gastrointestinal intolerance (most common) and various ocular toxicities (most well-known) are the side effects with antimalarials like CQ and HCQ. Quinacrine is considered to be safe in this regard. CQ is considered to be more oculotoxic than HCQ. The major adverse effects are listed in table 3.

**TABLE 3: Adverse effects of antimalarials**

| | |
|---|---|
| Ocular | • Reversible<br>  ○ *Neuromuscular in-coordination*: Accommodation defects, diplopia<br>  ○ *Corneal deposits*: Asymptomatic or can cause visual blurring/halos around lights<br>• Irreversible<br>  ○ Retinopathy (Bull's eye appearance on fundoscopy) |
| Gastrointestinal | Anorexia, nausea, vomiting, diarrhea, and transaminitis |
| Hematologic | Hemolytic anemia, agranulocytosis or pancytopenia (more common with quinacrine as compared to chloroquine and hydroxychloroquine) |
| Cutaneous | Blue-gray to black pigmentation (resembles ecchymoses and usually affects face, hard palate, forearms, and shins), progressive bleaching of hair roots, transverse melanonychia on nails, psoriasis flare-ups (debatable), lichenoid eruption due to quinacrine is known to precede aplastic anemia, others: pruritus, urticaria, eczema, alopecia, morbilliform rash, exfoliative dermatitis, and erythema annulare centrifugum |
| Others | Psychosis, irritability, depression, insomnia, nightmares, lowering of seizure threshold in predisposed individuals, peripheral neuropathy, proximal myopathy (due to accumulation in vacuoles of striated muscles), conduction disorders, and hypertrophic cardiomyopathy (controversial) |

## Dosing and Monitoring Guidelines

For LE (and most of the other indications), the maximum daily dose of HCQ and CQ is 3 mg/kg and 6.5 mg/kg (up to 400 mg/day), respectively. The onset of effect takes about 4–8 weeks. In cases not responding to HCQ, it can be substituted by CQ. In case of unsatisfactory response to both of these after 12 weeks, quinacrine (100 mg daily) may be added. It is not advisable to use HCQ and CQ in combination because of the increased risk of retinal toxicity.

The pregnancy prescribing status is category C. The benefits of continuing HCQ in pregnancy (to prevent a flare-up of systemic lupus erythematosus in pregnancy) outweigh the risks posed to the fetus. Although not supported by subsequent studies, it has been shown that cigarette smoking is associated with decreased efficacy of antimalarials. The monitoring guidelines for antimalarials are summarized in table 4.

The American Academy of Ophthalmology recommends categorizing patients on CQ and HCQ into low-risk and high-risk groups (Table 5). The recommended tests include visual acquity, fundoscopy, and automated threshold visual field testing. In addition, one of the following objective tests should be performed: fundus autofluorescence, spectral domain-optical coherence tomography, and multifocal electroretinogram.

**TABLE 4: Antimalarials monitoring guidelines**

| | |
|---|---|
| Complete blood counts | Every month for the first 3 months, followed by every 4–6 months |
| Serum biochemistry (liver and renal function tests) | Every month for initial 3 months followed by every 4–6 months |
| Glucose-6-phosphate dehydrogenase (G6PD) | Not advised to routinely perform G6PD screening |

**TABLE 5: Low- and high-risk category of patients for use of chloroquine (CQ) and hydroxychloroquine (HCQ)**

| Low-risk group patients | High-risk group patients |
|---|---|
| • HCQ ≤6.5 mg/kg/day (cumulative dose 1,000 g)<br>• CQ ≤3 mg/kg/day (cumulative dose 460 g)<br>• *Duration*: 5 years or less | • Higher daily dose<br>• Duration more than 5 years<br>• Age ≥60 years<br>• Comorbidities like diabetes, renal or liver disease<br>• Pre-existing retinopathy |
| Baseline eye examination<br>Repeated after 5 years | Baseline eye examination<br>Repeated annually |

# DAPSONE

Structurally, dapsone is 4,4'-diamino-diphenyl sulfone (4,4'-DDS). It is well-absorbed from the gut, having an oral bioavailability of more than 86%. Peak concentrations in plasma are reached within 2–8 hours after administration. Twenty-four hours after oral ingestion of 100 mg, plasma concentrations range from 0.4 to 1.2 µg/mL, and a dose of 100 mg/day produces steady-state plasma concentrations of free dapsone of 2–6 µmol/L. It is metabolized both by the liver and activated polymorphonuclear leukocytes or mononuclear cells. In the liver, dapsone is metabolized by two distinct routes, N-acetylation (by N-acetyltransferase) and N-hydroxylation (by cytochrome P-450 enzymes), resulting in formation of monoacetyldapsone and dapsone hydroxylamine, respectively. The mean half-life of elimination is about 20-hour, allowing for its once-a-day dosing. Dapsone and its metabolites are conjugated with glucuronide to form water-soluble metabolites which are primarily excreted through the kidneys.

It is a bacteriostatic drug similar to other sulfonamides, this inhibits folic acid pathway in susceptible organisms by inhibiting the synthesis of dihydrofolic acid through competition with para-amino benzoate for the active site of dihydropteroate synthetase. Some alternate unknown mechanisms play role for its anti-inflammatory activity (Box 1).

## Indications

The FDA-approved indications of dapsone are leprosy and dermatitis herpetiformis. The list of indications is given in table 6.

## Adverse Effects

Methemoglobinemia and hemolytic anemia are dose dependent caused by the N-hydroxylated metabolite of dapsone (dapsone hydroxylamine), a strong oxidant. The hemoglobin level in

**BOX 1 Mechanisms of action of dapsone in noninfectious inflammatory dermatoses**

- Inhibition of neutrophil myeloperoxidase leading to suppression of "neutrophil respiratory burst"
- Scavenging of reactive oxygen intermediates generated by neutrophils
- Stabilization of neutrophil lysosome enzymes
- Inhibition of neutrophil chemotaxis:
  - Suppression of integrin (CD11b/CD18)-mediated neutrophil adherence function
  - Inhibition of chemoattractant-induced signal transduction
- Inhibition of generation of 5-lipoxygenase products (e.g., leukotriene B4, 12-hydroxyeicosatetrenoate)
- Inhibition of leukotriene B4 receptor binding of polymorphonuclear neutrophils
- Inhibition of interleukin-8 production or releasing of peripheral blood stimulated with lipopolysaccharide

**TABLE 6: Dapsone indications**

| | |
|---|---|
| Dapsone as monotherapy | Dermatitis herpetiformis, bullous systemic lupus erythematosus, erythema elevatum diutinum, prurigo pigmentosa, linear immunoglobulin A dermatosis |
| Dapsone as adjuvant | Subcorneal pustular dermatosis, bullous pemphigoid, pemphigus vulgaris, Sweet's syndrome, pyoderma gangrenosum, relapsing polychondritis, leukocytoclastic vasculitis or urticarial vasculitis, loxoscelism, Ofuji's disease, subacute lupus erythematosus, and lupus panniculitis |
| Others | Urticaria, eosinophilic cellulitis, Behcet's syndrome, granuloma faciale, granuloma annulare, granulomatous rosacea, erosive oral lichen planus, benign lymphocytic infiltrates of the skin, mycetoma, nodulocystic acne, pustular psoriasis or acrodermatitis continua |

**BOX 2 Idiosyncratic adverse effects of dapsone**

- *Hematologic*:
  - *Agranulocytosis or leukopenia*: Usually within the first 12 weeks
- *Hepatic*:
  - Cholestatic, mixed or hepatocellular pattern of liver injury, can also be a part of dapsone hypersensitivity syndrome
- *Gastrointestinal*:
  - Anorexia, nausea, and vomiting
- *Nervous system*:
  - Primarily a distal motor peripheral neuropathy with some degree of sensory involvement. Recovery occurs on discontinuation of therapy. Permanent retinal damage with optic atrophy, acute psychosis
- *Cutaneous*:
  - *Dapsone hypersensitivity syndrome*: Usual latency is 2–6 weeks; manifests as fever, generalized cutaneous eruption, peripheral eosinophilia and hepatitis, Stevens–Johnson syndrome or toxic epidermal necrolysis (SJS-TEN), erythroderma, maculopapular rash, erythema multiforme, and urticaria

**TABLE 7: Dapsone monitoring guidelines**

| | |
|---|---|
| Complete blood counts | Weekly for first month, two-weekly in the next 2 months, followed by every 3 months |
| Serum biochemistry (liver and renal function tests) | Every 3–4 months |
| Glucose-6-phosphate dehydrogenase levels | Baseline |
| Methemoglobin levels | Only in patients who become symptomatic |

patients treated with dapsone generally decreases by 1–2 g/dL, reticulocyte count increases by 2–12%, and erythrocyte life span is shortened. Clinically insignificant methemoglobinemia (to the extent of 15%) may develop even in normal patients treated with standard doses (100 mg/day) for long term but adaptive increase in the activity of NADH-dependent reductase in the erythrocytes occurs on continued treatment leading to improvement of methemoglobinemia.

Dyspnea, nausea, and tachycardia usually occur at levels of 30% or above, while lethargy, stupor, and deteriorating consciousness occur as methemoglobin levels approach 55%. Levels of 70% are usually fatal. The idiosyncratic side effects of dapsone are summarized in box 2.

### Dosing and Monitoring Guidelines

The usual adult dosage is 50–100 mg/day that may be increased (up to 150–300 mg/day) if response is insufficient. Minimum effective dose should be continued. Some recommend taking dapsone in the evening. This is because the maximum level of methemoglobin in peripheral blood is usually reached 4–6 hours after ingestion of dapsone. Prophylactic administration of ascorbic acid, folate, iron, vitamin E, and cytochrome P450 inhibitors has been tried. Dapsone is a pregnancy category C drug. It is generally considered that the benefits outweigh the risk in case of leprosy and many other infectious and noninfectious diseases. However, since dapsone is excreted in breast milk and there are reports of hemolytic anemia in infants of mothers taking dapsone, it is recommended that breastfeeding be discontinued while on dapsone therapy. The recommended monitoring guidelines for dapsone are summarized in table 7.

## COLCHICINE

Colchicine is the active principle of the plant, *Colchicum autumnale*, and other plants of Colchiaceae family. It oxidizes to dark color on exposure to ultraviolet light and is transformed into different photo-isomers. Hence, colchicine must be shielded from sunlight. Peak plasma levels are reached between 30 minutes and 120 minutes after ingestion. It is metabolized in the liver, and the majority is eliminated through bile in the feces. Overall, 10–20% of the dose is eliminated unchanged in the urine. Mechanisms by which colchicine acts are shown in table 8.

### Indications in Dermatology

Currently, there are no FDA-approved indications of colchicine in dermatology practice. It is often used in primarily neutrophilic dermatoses (Table 9).

**TABLE 8: Colchicine mechanism of action**

| | |
|---|---|
| Anti-inflammatory | • Reduces mobility, adhesiveness, and chemotaxis of polymorphonuclear cells<br>• Interferes with intercellular adhesion molecules and selectins<br>• Inhibits T-lymphocyte activation and its adhesion to endothelial cells |
| Antimitotic | Mitotic arrest at metaphase phase, interfering with cell motility |

## Adverse Effects

Most patients are able to tolerate 0.5 mg twice a day, while increasing to three-times a day often lead to GI side effects. The adverse effects of colchicine are summarized in table 10.

## Dosing and Monitoring Guidelines

The usual dose of colchicine is 0.5 mg 2–3 times daily (start with a lower dose to avoid GI irritation), which is slowly tapered as the disease activity improves. It is avoided during pregnancy (pregnancy category C; risk of teratogenicity). Complete blood counts and serum biochemistry should be monitored monthly for the initial few months, followed by every 3 months.

# THALIDOMIDE

Thalidomide was first introduced in 1956 in Germany as an over-the-counter sedative and antiemetic in pregnancy. Following reports of phocomelia in infants born to women who ingested thalidomide during pregnancy, it was withdrawn in 1961. Thalidomide has made a remarkable comeback since then, and in 1998 was US-FDA approved for erythema nodosum leprosum.

Chemically, it is an α-N-phthalimido-glutarimide. The phthalimide ring is considered responsible for the teratogenic effects whereas the glutarimide ring (structurally similar to other sedatives) causes sedation. It is lipid soluble, crosses the placental barrier easily, is distributed extensively in the body, including semen, making it necessary for male patients taking the medication to wear condoms even if they have undergone vasectomy, and is partially excreted in the bile, whereas less than 1% is excreted in the urine. Peak values after oral dose are reached within 2–6 hours. High-fat meal can delay absorption by approximately 2 hours. The half-life of thalidomide is approximately 10 hours. It has been shown to have sedative, anti-inflammatory, immunomodulatory, and antiangiogenic activity (Table 11).

## Indications

The various dermatological indications have been summarized in table 12.

## Contraindication

Based on limited but alarmingly compelling data, toxic epidermal necrolysis should not be treated with thalidomide.

## Adverse Effects

Teratogenicity is the most severe adverse effect. It is classified as pregnancy category X. Possibly this may be related to its antiangiogenic properties, cell injury, negative action on chondrogenesis, growth factors, integrins, or mesonephric signals for limb growth. Safety and prescribing information on thalidomide is presented in box 3.

The major adverse effects of thalidomide are summarized in table 13.

The monitoring guidelines for patients on thalidomide are given in box 4.

# RETINOIDS

Retinoids are natural and synthetic compounds which have biological activity similar to vitamin A. Vitamin A molecule consists of a benzene ring, a polyene chain, and a carboxylic end group. Modification of the polyene side chain and the polar end group leads to formation of first generation retinoids or nonaromatic retinoids {tretinoin [all-trans retinoic acid (RA)], isotretinoin (13-cis-RA), and alitretinoin (9-cis-RA)}. Substitution of the cyclic group of vitamin A by various ring systems leads to production of second generation or monoaromatic retinoids (etretinate and acitretin). The third generation or polyaromatic retinoids (bexarotene, tazarotene, and adapalene) are formed through cyclisation of the polyene side chain of the vitamin A molecule.

**TABLE 9: Colchicine indications**

| Indications | | Remarks |
|---|---|---|
| Neutrophilic dermatoses | Recurrent aphthous stomatitis, Behcet's disease, Sweet's syndrome, pyoderma gangrenosum, and relapsing polychondritis | In Behcet's disease, beneficial effects are seen on orogenital aphthae as well as ocular and articular symptoms, and erythema nodosum |
| Immunobullous diseases | Dermatitis herpetiformis, linear immunoglobulin A disease or chronic bullous disease of childhood, subcorneal pustular dermatosis, and epidermolysis bullosa acquisita | Colchicine is usually an alternative to dapsone in these disorders |
| Vasculitis | Leukocytoclastic vasculitis, urticarial vasculitis | |
| Psoriasis | Plaque psoriasis, pustular psoriasis or palmoplantar pustulosis, psoriatic arthritis, and topical colchicine (1%) for recalcitrant plaque psoriasis | Overall, colchicine has a limited role in psoriasis and seems to work for thin psoriatic lesions or as maintenance therapy after remission is obtained through another modality |
| Urticaria | Chronic spontaneous urticaria, delayed pressure urticaria | |
| Others | Severe cystic acne, erythema nodosum, erythema nodosum leprosum, calcinosis cutis, scleroderma, pachydermoperiostosis, condyloma acuminate, fibromatosis, primary anetoderma, scleredema, and actinic keratosis | |

**TABLE 10: Colchicine adverse effects**

| | |
|---|---|
| Gastrointestinal | • Diarrhea, nausea, vomiting, and abdominal pain<br>• *Long-term therapy*: Steatorrhea, reduced absorption of vitamin B12, fat, sodium, potassium, nitrogen, xylose, and other actively transported sugars |
| Hematological | Agranulocytosis, thrombocytopenia, and aplastic anemia occurs after prolonged treatment |
| Others | *Neuromuscular*: Proximal myopathy, axonal neuropathy, azoospermia, cutaneous: urticaria, alopecia, toxic epidermal necrolysis, and precipitation of porphyria cutanea tarda |

**TABLE 11: Thalidomide: Mechanism of action**

| | |
|---|---|
| Anti-inflammatory | • Inhibition of chemotaxis of neutrophils and lymphocytes<br>• Inhibition of macrophage phagocytosis<br>• Stabilization of lysosomal membranes<br>• Decrease in the generation of superoxide and hydroxyl radicals |
| Immunomodulatory | • Inhibition of tumor necrosis factor (TNF)-α by enhancing the degradation of TNF-α mRNA<br>• Conversion of lymphocyte response from Th1–Th2 |
| Antiangiogenic | Inhibition of vascular endothelial growth factor |
| Sedative | Activation of sleep center in the forebrain |

**TABLE 12: Summary of indications of thalidomide in dermatology**

| | |
|---|---|
| Very effective | Erythema nodosum leprosum (the only FDA-approved indication in dermatology), recurrent aphthous stomatitis, Behcet's disease, lupus erythematosus, and prurigo nodularis |
| Moderately effective | Actinic prurigo, Langerhans cell histiocytosis, cutaneous sarcoidosis, erythema multiforme, graft-versus-host disease, Jessner's infiltrate, and uremic pruritus |
| Possibly effective | Kaposi's sarcoma, lichen planus, melanoma, and pyoderma gangrenosum |
| Contraindicated | Toxic epidermal necrolysis (paradoxical increase in tumor necrosis factor-α activity) |

Food intake enhances the bioavailability of retinoids. Retinoids are stored in the liver. Etretinate is also stored in adipose tissue due to its lipophilicity (50 times more than its metabolite acitretin), from where it is slowly released and persists for several years in fatty tissues of the body. Isotretinoin and bexarotene are undetectable in serum 1 month after stopping therapy due to the higher water solubility.

Retinoids are oxidized into biologically inactive water soluble metabolites in the liver by inducible enzyme cytochrome P-450 3A4 isoform. Acitretin is re-esterified into etretinate when ethanol is coadministered. This finding led to the recommendation of prolonged period of contraception after acitretin therapy, which is 2 years in Europe and 3 years in the United States (Table 14).

Cytosolic retinoic acid binding protein-1 (CRABP-I) modulates levels of RA in various tissues, CRABP-II predominates in the epidermis. High levels of CRABP may indicate a greater sensitivity to retinoids and it is found in the lesional skin in psoriasis, ichthyosis, Darier's disease, pityriasis rubra pilaris, and keratosis pilaris. Retinoid receptors are members of the steroid-thyroid hormone superfamily and are classified into two families, the RA receptors and the retinoid X receptors, each having three isoforms (α, β, and γ) encoded by separate genes. Mechanism in various dermatological disorders is described in table 15.

**BOX 3 System for Thalidomide Education and Prescribing Safety**

Main goal is to prevent fetal exposure to thalidomide

The three-step approach is to:

- Control access to the drug
- Educate and register prescribers, pharmacists, and patients
- Monitor compliance

Thalidomide can be prescribed for only 28 days at a time with no refills and prescriptions are valid for 1 week only

**Female patients:**

- Blood or urine pregnancy test before starting treatment
- Pregnancy tests must be repeated every month while taking thalidomide and 4 weeks after the last dose
- More frequent pregnancy tests may be needed if the patient has an irregular menstrual period or vaginal bleeding
- Sexual abstinence or
- Use two highly effective birth control methods simultaneously for at least 1 month before receiving thalidomide. These methods must be continued until 1 month after the last dose

**Male patients:**

- Sexual abstinence or
- Use a condom during intercourse while, and for 1 month after, taking thalidomide

**TABLE 13: Thalidomide adverse effects**

| | |
|---|---|
| Teratogenicity | Deformities of the upper and lower extremities (amelia, phocomelia, bone hypoplasia, and absence of bones), abnormalities of the external ear (anotia, micro pinna, and small or absent auditory canals), abnormalities of the eye (enophthalmos and microphthalmos), neural tube abnormalities, and defects of the internal organs |
| Peripheral neuropathy | Symmetric painful paresthesias of extremities with sensory loss in the lower extremities with or without muscle cramps or weakness. Considered to be reversible following drug discontinuation, but in some cases, it can be slow to resolve or even irreversible. Though no definite correlation between neuropathy and cumulative dose; probably the risk increases after cumulative dose of 20 g |
| Others | Neutropenia, drowsiness, headache, mood changes, nausea, constipation, dizziness, ankle edema, weight gain, myxedema, diabetes, deep vein thrombosis, sinus bradycardia, decreased libido, erythematous and papulovesicular transient eruptions, allergic vasculitis, and toxic epidermal necrolysis |

**TABLE 14: Systemic retinoids: Pharmacology**

| Retinoid | Absorption | | Elimination | | | Standard dosage |
|---|---|---|---|---|---|---|
| | Peak levels (h) | Bioavailability (%) | Half-life | Metabolism | Excretion | |
| **First generation/nonaromatic retinoids** | | | | | | |
| Tretinoin (all-trans retinoic acid) | 1–2 | – | 40–60 min | Hepatic | Bile, urine | 0.5–1 mg/kg/day |
| Isotretinoin (13-cis-retinoic acid) | 3 | 25 | 10–20 h | Hepatic | Bile, urine | 0.5–2 mg/kg/day |
| Alitretinoin (9-cis-retinoic acid) | – | No data available | 2–10 h | Hepatic | Urine, feces | 10–30 mg/day |
| **Second generation or monoaromatic retinoids** | | | | | | |
| Etretinate | 4 | 44 | 80–160 days | Hepatic | Bile, urine | 0.25–1 mg/kg/day |
| Acitretin | 4 | 60 | 50 h | Hepatic | Bile, urine | 0.5–1 mg/kg/day |
| **Third generation/polyaromatic retinoids (arotinoids)** | | | | | | |
| Bexarotene | 2 | No data available | 7–9 h | Hepatic | Hepatobiliary | 300 mg/m$^2$/day |

**TABLE 15: Mechanism of action of retinoids in dermatological diseases**

| Disorder | Effect and mechanism |
|---|---|
| Disorders of keratinization | • Induce differentiation and inhibit proliferation<br>• Decrease in keratins 1, 2, 10 and collagenase<br>• Increase in keratins 4, 6, 13, 16, 17, 19, type 1 transglutaminase, loricrin, involucrin and filaggrin<br>• Reduction of tonofilaments, corneocyte adhesiveness, impaired permeability barrier, and increased transepidermal water loss |
| Disorders of sebaceous glands | • Sebum suppression (isotretinoin >> tretinoin> acitretin >> other retinoids) by:<br>○ Reduced expression of promatrix metalloproteinase (MMP)-9 and MMP-13<br>○ Cell cycle arrest and apoptosis of sebocytes by a retinoic acid receptor-independent mechanism<br>○ 90% decrease in sebaceous gland size by decreasing proliferation of basal sebocytes and 70–90% decrease in sebum production<br>• *Altered sebum composition*: Marked decrease in wax esters, slight decrease in squalene, and a relative increase in levels of cholesterol, free sterols and total ceramides in skin surface lipids. Decrease in triglyceride fraction<br>• Decreased androgen synthesis by competitive inhibition of 3α-hydroxysteroid activity of retinol dehydrogenase which results in about 80% decrease of local dihydrotestosterone production and also decreases androgen receptor binding capacity |
| Malignancies (chemoprevention) | • Induction of apoptosis by:<br>○ Regulation of expression of apoptosis linked gene products: Bcl-2, tissue transglutaminase<br>○ Activation of tumor suppressor genes, viz. *p21, p38, p53*<br>○ Stimulating caspase proteolytic activity<br>○ Elevating reactive oxygen species<br>○ Rendering tumor cells more susceptible to effector cell lysis by affecting ICAM-1 expression on tumor cells |
| Inflammatory disorders | • Suppression of cyclooxygenase-2 expression and prostaglandin E2 synthesis leading to reduced cell proliferation<br>• Increased levels of ceramide inducing apoptosis<br>• Inhibition of leukotriene B4, nitric oxide, and tumor necrosis factor alpha |

## Indications in Dermatology

Psoriasis, acne, and cutaneous T-cell lymphoma (CTCL) are the FDA-approved indications of systemic retinoids in dermatology. The list of indications is given in table 16.

Various regimens of systemic retinoids recommended in psoriasis are shown in table 17.

Isotretinoin is the only retinoid approved for systemic use by the FDA, for severe, recalcitrant, nodular acne. However, this is also used in less severe forms of acne include in following situations:

- Acne that improves less than 50% after 6 months of oral antibiotic therapy
- Acne associated with significant scarring or psychological distress
- Antibiotic-resistant strains of *Propionibacterium acnes*
- Dosage regimens are described in table 18.

## Adverse Effects

Teratogenicity is the major adverse effect of retinoids. Other adverse effects seen are mucocutaneous, musculoskeletal, hepatic, and lipid abnormalities (Table 19).

**TABLE 16: Indications of systemic retinoids in dermatology**

| FDA-approved indications | Off label indications |
|---|---|
| • *Psoriasis (acitretin)*:<br>○ Pustular psoriasis (localized and von Zumbusch psoriasis)<br>○ Erythrodermic psoriasis<br>○ Severe and recalcitrant psoriasis<br>• *Acne (isotretinoin)*:<br>○ Nodulocystic acne<br>○ Recalcitrant acne<br>• *Cutaneous T-cell lymphoma (bexarotene)* | • *Rosacea and acne-related disorders*: Hidradenitis suppurativa, Ofuji's disease, AIDS-associated eosinophilic folliculitis, pyoderma faciale (rosacea fulminans), acne with solid facial edema, dissecting cellulitis of the scalp<br>• *Disorders of keratinization and related disorders*: Ichthyosis, Darier's disease, keratoderma, and Papillon–Lefèvre syndrome<br>• *Inflammatory disorders*: Chronic hand eczema, pityriasis rubra pilaris, lupus erythematosus, and lichen planus<br>• *Chemoprophylaxis of neoplastic processes*: Xeroderma pigmentosum, nevoid basal cell carcinoma syndrome, skin cancer in solid organ transplant patients<br>• *Miscellaneous*: Atrophoderma vermiculatum, ulerythema ophryogenes, confluent and reticulated papillomatosis of Gougerot and Carteaud, Bazex paraneoplastic acrokeratosis, follicular mucinosis, and sarcoidosis |

**TABLE 17: Regimens of retinoids used in psoriasis**

| | |
|---|---|
| Plaque psoriasis | 0.3–1.0 mg/kg/day for 4–12 weeks |
| Combination with psoralen and ultraviolet A (PUVA) or UVB | 0.3–0.5 mg/kg for 6 weeks |
| Erythrodermic psoriasis | Started at 0.3 mg/kg/day and increased to 0.5–0.6 mg/kg/day for 3 month<br>Maintenance therapy required for up to 6 months |
| Pustular psoriasis | Started at 1 mg/kg/day, tapered to 0.5–0.6 mg/kg/day over 3–6 month<br>Maintenance therapy required for up to 6–12 months |

**BOX 4 Thalidomide monitoring guidelines**

*Complete blood counts*:
- Monthly for first 3 months followed by every 3 months
- Discontinue treatment if absolute neutrophil count falls below 750/mm

*Nerve conduction studies*:
- Sensory nerve action potential amplitudes in at least three peripheral nerves, usually the median, radial, or sural
- A fall from baseline values of more than 40% on repeat testing should lead to discontinuation of the treatment, and a decrease of 30–40% should lead to a review of its use
- Follow-up testing is recommended after every 10 g cumulative dose or every 6 months

*Pregnancy tests*:
- Monthly in women having regular menstrual cycles
- Two weekly in women having irregular menstrual cycles

**TABLE 18: Regimens of isotretinoin for acne vulgaris**

| Conventional regimen | Low-dose regimen | Intermittent regimen |
|---|---|---|
| 0.5–1.0 mg/kg/day until a cumulative dose of 120–150 mg/kg is reached | 0.25–0.4 mg/kg/day | 0.5–1 mg/kg/day, given for 1 week every month |

**TABLE 19: Retinoids adverse effects**

| | |
|---|---|
| Teratogenicity | • Spontaneous abortions in one-third cases<br>• Cranial and facial anomalies, defects in cardiovascular system, central nervous system, and thymic abnormalities |
| Mucocutaneous adverse effects | Dryness and cheilitis (dose related), acne fulminans, and pyogenic granulomas |
| Deranged lipid profile | • Reversible; elevated triglycerides seen most commonly<br>• Most commonly caused by bexarotene followed by isotretinoin and acitretin |
| Hepatic effects | Severe hepatic derangement rare. Transaminitis is dose related, seen in few patients |
| Others | Psychosis, depression and rarely, suicidal ideation. Black box warning issued by the FDA for use of isotretinoin in patients with depression. Hyperostosis and premature epiphyseal closure in children, myalgias, dryness of eyes and blepharoconjunctivitis, transient headaches, pseudotumor cerebri seen with concomitant tetracycline administration, hypothyroidism with bexarotene and alitretinoin |

## Monitoring Guidelines

Periodic monitoring of liver function, lipid profile, pregnancy, and other parameters is done as mentioned in table 20.

## Investigational Retinoids

Systemic retinoids which selectively target individual retinoid receptors are being investigated in order to circumvent the adverse effects (Box 5).

# ANTIHISTAMINES

The H1 and H2 antihistamines are inverse agonists as they work by downregulating the constitutive activated state of corresponding receptor.

## H1 Antihistamines

First-generation antihistamines contain aromatic rings and alkyl substituents which render them lipophilic, thus explaining

**TABLE 20: Retinoids monitoring guidelines**

| Systemic retinoids—laboratory monitoring guidelines | |
|---|---|
| **Baseline** | **Follow-up** |
| • Serum or urine pregnancy test (in women of childbearing years). Two pregnancy tests done before initiating isotretinoin therapy in females<br>• The federal registry iPLEDGE risk evaluation and mitigation strategy (REMS) by FDA requires:<br>  ○ All patients on isotretinoin be enrolled and the wholesalers, prescribing physicians, and pharmacies be a part of this program<br>  ○ Females should practice contraception 1 month prior to starting the medication; contraception should be continued till 1 month after the therapy has been stopped<br>  ○ Pregnancy test should be done monthly and at the end of therapy<br>  ○ For acitretin, a longer period of contraception of 1 year is recommended<br>• Complete blood count<br>• Liver function (AST, ALT, ALP, bilirubin)<br>• Fasting lipid profile (triglycerides, total cholesterol, LDL, and HDL cholesterol)<br>• Renal function (blood urea nitrogen, creatinine) | • Monthly for 3 months, then every 3 months<br>• Complete blood count<br>• Liver function (AST, ALT)<br>• Fasting lipid profile<br>• Renal function<br>• Serum or urine pregnancy test monthly (in women of childbearing years)<br>• X-ray wrists, ankles, thoracic spine in case of long-term retinoid therapy was initially recommended. However, recent British Association of Dermatologists guidelines do not recommend routine radiological investigations due to risk of unnecessary radiation exposure. This may be decided on case to case basis, as indicated by symptoms |

Bexarotene, alitretinoin: Additional thyroid function testing (baseline, every 1–2 months after initiating therapy)

FDA, food and drug administration; AST, aspartate transaminase; ALT, alanine transaminase; ALP, alkaline phosphatase; LDL, low-density lipoproteins; HDL, high-density lipoproteins.

**BOX 5 Investigational retinoids**

- *Temarotene (Ro 15-0778)*: This retinoid has some immunosuppressive activity like cyclosporine. But no sebosuppressive or antikeratinizing property
- *Arotinoid ethyl ester*: It is analogous to etretinate. It is highly effective in treating etretinate-resistant disorders of keratinization. Side effect profile is similar to etretinate
- *Fenretinide*: It is a highly selective activator of retinoid receptors. It is available as oral preparation, dose of 200 mg/day. This drug can be used for actinic keratoses, chemoprevention of basal cell carcinoma, and oral leukoplakia. Drug allergy and nyctalopia (night blindness) are the side effects reported.

their ability to cross the blood brain–barrier. Second generation antihistamines are less sedative due to their high H1 selectivity and low lipophilicity. These drugs are free from anticholinergic and antiserotonergic side effects. Based on the structural characteristics, the H1 receptor antagonists have been historically classified into six chemical families (Table 21).

Most antihistamines show good absorption when administered via the oral route, effective plasma concentrations are reached within 3 hours after dosing (Table 22).

## Dosing of Antihistamines

Dosage and frequency of administration of H1 antihistamines are given in table 23.

## Indications

The H1 antihistamines are the largest class of drugs useful in allergic diseases like urticaria. Indications of first- and second-generation H1 antihistamines are listed in table 24.

## Adverse Effects

First-generation H1 antihistamines potentially cause an array of adverse effects involving many body systems. Adverse effects of H1 antihistamines are shown in table 25.

**TABLE 21: Antihistamines: structural classes**

| Chemical class | First (old) generation | Second (new) generation |
|---|---|---|
| Alkylamines | Chlorpheniramine | Acrivastine |
| Piperazines | Hydroxyzine | Cetirizine, levocetirizine |
| Piperidines | Cyproheptadine | Astemizole, desloratadine, ebastine, fexofenadine, loratadine, mizolastine, and terfenadine |
| Ethanolamines | Diphenhydramine | – |
| Ethylenediamines | Tripelennamine | – |
| Phenothiazines | Promethazine | – |
| Others | | Azelastine and olopatadine |

## H2 Antihistamines in Dermatology

Likewise the former, they are also inverse agonists of H2 receptor. More recently there is evidence of presence of H2 receptors on mast cells mediating vascular permeability and release of inflammatory mediators. They are rapidly absorbed from GI tract peak level at 1–2 hours then usually metabolized by liver extensively and excreted through kidney. A recent Cochrane review in 2012 concluded that evidence for use of H2 antihistamines was weak and unreliable. Combination of H1 and H2 antihistamines has been found to be helpful in reducing pruritus and whealing in urticaria pigmentosa and mastocytosis. H4 antihistamines might play an important role in the downregulation of inflammation in patients with atopic dermatitis, asthma, and other chronic inflammatory diseases.

# ANTIANDROGENS IN DERMATOLOGY

These include drugs which block the androgen receptor and those that inhibit the effect of androgens without an effect on androgen receptor. These are called androgen inhibitors. Other

**TABLE 22: Pharmacology of antihistamines**

| Drug | Onset of action (hrs) | Duration of action (hrs) | Dose adjustment |
|---|---|---|---|
| Chlorpheniramine | 3 | 24 | Elimination is prolonged in renal dysfunction, hence monitoring may be done for excessive sedation |
| Diphenhydramine | 2 | 12 | none |
| Hydroxyzine | 2 | 24 | Liver and kidney failure |
| Bilastine | 2 | ≥24 | Not needed. Avoid concomitant administration of bilastine with P glycoprotein inhibitors in renal dysfunction |
| Cetirizine | 0.7–1 | ≥24 | Liver and kidney failure |
| Desloratadine | 2–2.6 | 24 | Liver and kidney failure |
| Loratadine | 2 | 24 | Kidney and liver failure |
| Fexofenadine | 1–3 | >24 | Kidney failure |
| Levocetirizine | 0.7–1 | 24 | Adjust according to creatinine clearance |
| Rupatadine | 2 | 24 | Liver and kidney failure |
| Mizolastine | 1 | 24 | Contraindicated in liver failure, data not available for kidney failure |
| Ebastine | 2 | 8 | No dose adjustment needed in renal dysfunction and up to moderate liver derangement. Dose up to 10 mg can be given in severe liver failure |

**TABLE 23: Dosing of H1 antihistamines**

| Drug | Dose (mg/kg/day) | Adult dose | Pediatric dose |
|---|---|---|---|
| Chlorpheniramine | 0.35 | 4 mg tid, qid, 8–12 mg bid | 6–11 year: 2 mg qid 4–6 h |
| Hydroxyzine | 2 | >6 year: 25–50 mg qid 6–8 h/qhs | <6 year: 25–50 mg qid |
| Pheniramine | 0.5 | • Oral 25 mg qid 8–12 h, 50 mg qid 12 h<br>• Injectable 22.75 mg–45.5 mg intramuscularly 12 hourly | – |
| Cyproheptadine | 0.25–0.5 | 4 mg 3–4 times/day, highest 32 mg | 2–6 year: 12 mg/day, 7–14 year: 16 mg/day |
| Cetirizine | | >6 year: 5–10 mg qid | 2–6 year: 5 mg qid; 6 month to 2 year: 2.5 mg qid |
| Desloratadine | | >12 year: 5 mg qid | 6–12 year: 2.5 mg qid, 1–6 year: 1.25 mg qid, 6–12 month: 1 mg qid |
| Loratadine | | >6 year: 10 mg qid | 2–6 year: 5 mg qid |
| Fexofenadine | | >12 year: 60 mg qid, bid 120–180 mg qid | 2–12 year: 30 mg qid, bid, 6 month to 2 year: 15 mg bid |
| Levocetirizine | 0.125 | 5 mg qid | 6 month to 5 year: 1.25 mg qid, 5–11 year: 2.5 mg qid |
| Ebastine | | > 6 year: 10–20 mg qid | 6–12 year: 5 mg qid, 2–5 year: 2.5 mg qid |

**TABLE 24: Indications of H1 antihistamines in dermatology**

| Nonsedating antihistamines | Indications (evidence level) | Sedating antihistamines | Indications (evidence) | Intravenous antihistamines | Indications (evidence) |
|---|---|---|---|---|---|
| • Cetirizine<br>• Desloratadine<br>• Fexofenadine<br>• Levocetirizine<br>• Loratadine<br>• Mizolastine<br>• Rupatadine | • Chronic urticaria (A)<br>• Angioedema (A)<br>• Dermographism (A)<br>• Solar urticaria (D)<br>• Other urticarias (E)<br>• Mastocytosis (A) | • Alimemazine<br>• Chlorpheniramine<br>• Hydroxyzine<br>• Cyproheptadine<br>• Promethazine | • Pruritus (C) | • Chlorpheniramine<br>• Pheniramine | • Acute anaphylaxis (A)<br>• Angioedema (A) |

drugs may be both antiandrogens and androgen inhibitors, like progesterone. Table 26 shows the classification of these agents.

## Mechanism of Action

Testosterone has minimal biological activity until it is converted to dihydrotestosterone (DHT) by the enzyme 5α-reductase. Type 1 5α-reductase is located in nongenital skin mostly sebaceous lobules, hair follicles, liver, spleen, and kidney. Type 2 5α-reductase is located primarily in hair follicles over scalp (frontal scalp to vertex), sebaceous ducts, genital skin of both men and women, and genital tract of men. Type 2 5α-reductase has larger effect on hair follicles as it produces DHT at a faster rate. Antiandrogens reverse the effect of androgens at the peripheral level, at cutaneous sites.

**TABLE 25: Adverse effects of H1 antihistamines**

| | |
|---|---|
| Central nervous system effects | Altered circadian rhythm, daytime somnolence, sedation, drowsiness, fatigue and impaired concentration and memory with first-generation H1-antihistamines |
| Cardiac effects | Dose-related sinus tachycardia, reflex tachycardia, prolonged atrial refractive period, and supraventricular arrhythmias can occur with first-generation H1-antihistamines |
| Anticholinergic effects | Mydriasis, blurred vision, dry eyes, dry mouth, urinary retention and hesitancy, constipation, erectile dysfunction, and memory deficits (with first-generation antihistamines) |
| Antiadrenergic effects | Peripheral vasodilation, orthostatic hypotension, and dizziness (seen with promethazine) |
| Substance abuse | Euphoria, hallucinations, and "getting high" reported with cyclizine, diphenhydramine, dimenhydrinate with first-generation H1-antihistamines |
| Antiserotonergic effects | Include appetite stimulation and weight gain (especially with cyproheptadine) |
| Drug reactions | Urticaria, anaphylactic reaction, and maculopapular drug rash (rare) |

**TABLE 26: Antiandrogens: Classification**

| Antiandrogens (block androgen receptor) | Androgen inhibitors (act by pathways other than androgen receptor blockade) |
|---|---|
| • Spironolactone<br>• Progesterone<br>• Cyproterone acetate<br>• Cimetidine | • *5α-reductase inhibitors*:<br>○ Finasteride<br>○ Dutasteride<br>○ Ketoconazole<br>○ Progesterone<br>• *Gonadotropin-releasing hormone agonists*:<br>○ Leuprolide<br>○ Nafarelin |

## ANDROGEN INHIBITORS

### Finasteride

It is a specific type 2 5α-reductase inhibitor. Its indication is primarily due to its inhibitory effect on DHT levels in the scalp hair follicles (Table 27).

**TABLE 27: Indications of finasteride in dermatology**

| FDA-approved indications | Non-FDA-approved indications |
|---|---|
| Male pattern androgenetic alopecia | • Female pattern androgenetic alopecia<br>• Hirsutism<br>• Hidradenitis suppurativa<br>• Acne vulgaris |

FDA, Food and Drug Administration.

#### Adverse Effects

Finasteride is a category X drug, causing genitourinary abnormalities in the male offspring. Sexual dysfunction and altered immune surveillance are infrequent adverse effects (Table 28).

#### Monitoring Guidelines

No specific laboratory tests are required in patients receiving finasteride for male pattern androgenetic alopecia (AGA). Oral contraception is required in premenopausal women receiving finasteride.

### Dutasteride

Dutasteride is a dual inhibitor of 5α-reductase. The affinity for type 1 5α-reductase is due to a trifluorophenyl group on the 21-carbon position of the main structure of finasteride. It should therefore be avoided in females of reproductive age group due to its longer half-life (approximately 5 weeks). Dutasteride is about three times as potent as finasteride at inhibiting type 2 5α-reductase and more than 100 times as potent at inhibiting type 1 5α-reductase. Dutasteride is used off label for similar indications in dermatology as finasteride. Side effects seen with dutasteride are same as that with finasteride, such as, sexual dysfunction. The association with breast malignancy is not proven.

### Ketoconazole

Ketoconazole is an azole antifungal agent which has a secondary androgen inhibitory effect due to inhibition of CYP enzymes. Ketoconazole has been used off label in hirsutism in doses of 400–800 mg/day effectively with few side effects. Hepatic toxicity is seen in 5–10% of patients receiving ketoconazole. Nausea, vomiting, headache, and thrombocytopenia are other side effects reported.

### Spironolactone

Spironolactone is an aldosterone antagonist containing the basic steroid nucleus of four rings. Spironolactone acts by blocking androgen synthesis as well as androgen receptor and decreases the response of luteinizing hormone (LH) to gonadotropin-releasing hormone (GnRH). Bioavailability of spironolactone is 90%. Canrenone is the active metabolite of spironolactone formed in the liver. Half-life of the drug is around 12.5 hours. Spironolactone has been used off-label to treat acne, hirsutism, and AGA. The most significant side effects of spironolactone are teratogenicity, feminization of male fetus, and hyperkalemia, seen more often in patients with renal failure. Other adverse effects reported are GI disturbance and gynecomastia. Spironolactone should not be given to women with risk factors for breast malignancy. Periodic monitoring of potassium, blood pressure, and weight is advised.

### Cimetidine

Cimetidine blocks the androgen receptor. There are anecdotal reports of its use in acne, hirsutism, and AGA in doses of 800–1600 mg/day. Other uses include eosinophilic dermatoses,

**TABLE 28: Adverse effects of finasteride**

| | |
|---|---|
| Teratogenicity | Finasteride is contraindicated in women of child bearing potential as it has been shown to cause genitourinary abnormalities in the male offspring. Blood donation by a patient receiving finasteride is contraindicated for 6 months for the same reason |
| Sexual dysfunction | Loss of libido, erectile dysfunction, gynecomastia, and ejaculatory dysfunction are infrequently found. Sexual dysfunction has been found to be significantly higher (43.6% vs. 15.6%) in patients who were informed of side effects of finasteride (nocebo effect) |
| Altered immune function | Altered Th1/Th2 balance leading to decreased immune surveillance, in elderly males |
| Decreased prostate specific antigen | Around 50% reduction of prostate-specific antigen occurs in males >50 years of age and 20–30% reduction is seen in males aged 18–49 years |

urticaria, warts, and inhibition of dapsone toxicity. Adverse effects include dizziness, mild somnolence, reversible transaminitis, loss of libido, erectile dysfunction, and gynecomastia.

## Hormonal Agents

Oral contraceptive pills (OCPs) decrease the level of androgens and therefore sebum production. This effect is produced by suppression of LH production by the pituitary gland, which in turn decreases androgen synthesis by the ovaries. Oral contraceptives also reduce the androgen production by the adrenal glands and peripheral androgen production. The estrogen component of hormonal contraceptives increases levels of sex hormone-binding globulin, thereby decreasing levels of free testosterone. OCPs also inhibit 5α-reductase in hair follicles and skin.

Low dose OCPs have been shown to be effective in mild-to-moderate acne.

Drospirenone is a novel progestin that has antiandrogenic properties that has shown significant improvement in acne compared to placebo.

The most serious potential adverse effects of OCPs are venous and arterial complications. Contraindications to the use of OCPs include venous thromboembolic disease, heart disease or genetic clotting disorder, hypertension, smoking in women older than 35 years, severe obesity, liver disease, diabetes mellitus, migraine headaches, current pregnancy or breastfeeding, prolonged immobilization, hypersensitivity to any component of the OCPs, and history of malignancy, such as breast, endometrial, or liver.

## Cyproterone Acetate

It inhibits GnRH and blocks androgen receptor. Its uses include AGA, severe acne, and hirsutism. It has been found to be more useful in cases with underlying hyperandrogenism. Treatment dose is 100 mg/day on days 5–15 of the menstrual cycle supplemented by 50 µg ethinyl estradiol on days 5–25. The side effects include menstrual disturbances, loss of libido, weight gain, breast tenderness, depression, and GI upsets.

# PHOSPHODIESTERASE INHIBITORS

Phosphodiesterase (PDE) inhibitors increase the intracellular levels of cyclic adenosine monophosphate (cAMP), which results in various downstream effects in different cell types. Increased cAMP in macrophages results in inhibition of proinflammatory mediators [tumor necrosis factor (TNF)-α, interleukin (IL)-6, IL-12]. PDE isoenzyme-5 (PDE-5) selectively breaks down the cyclic guanosine monophosphate (cGMP), a smooth muscle tone regulator. Nitric oxide (NO) signals the conversion of GMP into cGMP which accumulates inside the cell. Inhibition of the PDE-5 enzyme increases the available intracellular cGMP which leads to vasodilatation. There are 11 families of PDEs that have different tissue specificity. Dermatologically useful PDE inhibitors can be classified according to the selectivity of inhibition of PDE enzyme (Table 29).

## Sildenafil Citrate

Sildenafil is an inhibitor of PDE type 5. PDE-5 receptors are located in the vasculature, smooth muscle cells of the heart, vagina, urethra, bladder, and prostate. Inhibition of PDE-5 causes an increase in cGMP and leads to vasodilatation. Recently, PDE-5 inhibitors have been shown to have antiproliferative action. Sildenafil has been found to be useful in patients who have obtained inadequate benefit from a calcium channel blocker (CCB) or who are unable to tolerate CCBs (Table 30).

Most common adverse effects are headache, nasal congestion, and dyspepsia. Sildenafil is contraindicated in patients on nitric oxide donors. It must be used with caution in patients with history of or risk factors of unstable angina, myocardial infarction, or arrhythmias.

**TABLE 29: Phosphodiesterase (PDE) inhibitors used in dermatological disorders**

| Selective PDE inhibitors | Nonselective PDE inhibitors |
|---|---|
| • Sildenafil<br>• Tadalafil<br>• Vardenafil | • Pentoxifylline |

**TABLE 30: Indications and contraindications of sildenafil**

| Indications | Contraindications |
|---|---|
| • Raynaud's phenomenon<br>• Nonhealing skin ulcers | • *Absolute*:<br>○ Patient receiving concomitant nitrates or nitric oxide donors<br>• *Relative*:<br>○ Patients with history or risk of:<br>– Myocardial infarction<br>– Unstable angina<br>– Hypotension<br>– Hypertension<br>– Arrhythmias<br>– Vascular disorders |

## Tadalafil

The longer half-life made tadalafil an attractive option as a daily dose treatment for systemic sclerosis-related peripheral vasculopathy. Trials comparing tadalafil with placebo in patients of systemic sclerosis with digital ulcers show contradictory results in terms of efficacy. However, the tolerability has been shown to be uniformly good in all trials.

## Vardenafil

Vardenafil is similar to sildenafil in terms of pharmacokinetic properties, with rapid onset of action, maximal benefit at 1 hour, and a half-life of about 4 hours. Vardenafil has been shown to increase peripheral blood flow, measured by Doppler laser flowmetry, in a dose of 10 mg twice daily given for 2 weeks.

## Apremilast

Apremilast is a novel oral PDE-4 inhibitor. It is postulated to act by inhibiting production of TNF, IL-12, IL-2, interferon-$\gamma$, IL-5, IL-8, leukotriene B4 (LTB4), and the adhesion molecule CD18/CD11b (Mac-1). It also augments production of IL-10, an anti-inflammatory cytokine. In dosage of 20–30 mg twice daily apremilast seems to be efficacious, safe, and tolerable for patients with moderate to severe plaque psoriasis and atopic dermatitis.

## Pentoxifylline

Pentoxifylline is a methylated xanthine derivative. It is a nonselective inhibitor of more than one subtype of PDE. It acts by increasing intracellular cAMP, activating protein kinase A, and has downstream effects blocking the nuclear factor-$\kappa\beta$ pathway in addition to inhibition of TNF-$\alpha$ production. Pentoxifylline is also a rheological agent. Pentoxifylline is FDA approved for intermittent claudication. It is used off label in venous leg ulcers and vasculopathies. The side effects are dose related and the most common are those of the GI tract and central nervous system (dizziness, headache, anxiety, and confusion). Rarely, it can lead to edema, hypotension, nasal congestion, urticaria, brittle nails, thrombocytopenia, and fatal hemorrhage.

## CONCLUSION

The scope of systemic therapy in dermatology has increased considerably in the recent past, especially in light of the emerging off-label uses of many systemic agents. Dermatologists need to continuously update themselves not only on the new systemic agents being introduced, but also on the new uses of the old drugs. The readers of this chapter are likely to benefit by developing a better understanding of the common systemic drugs used in dermatology.

## SUGGESTED READINGS


1. Bird ST, Brophy JM, Hartzema AG, et al. Male breast cancer and 5$\alpha$-reductase inhibitors finasteride and dutasteride. J Urol. 2013;190(5):1811-4.
2. Caglayan E, Huntgeburth M, Karasch T, et al. Phosphodiesterase type 5 inhibition is a novel therapeutic option in Raynaud disease. Arch Intern Med. 2006;166(2):231-3.
3. Callen JP, Camisa C. Antimalarial agents. In: Wolverton SE (Ed). Comprehensive Dermatologic Drug Therapy, 2nd edition. Philadelphia, PA: Saunders Elsevier; 2007. pp. 259-73.
4. Coleman MD, Coleman NA. Drug-induced methaemoglobinaemia. Treatment issues. Drug Saf. 1996;14(6):394-405.
5. Dinh QQ, Sinclair R. Female pattern hair loss: Current treatment concepts. Clin Interv Aging. 2007;2(2):189-99.
6. Fedorowicz Z, van Zuuren EJ, Hu N. Histamine H2-receptor antagonists for urticaria. Cochrane Database Syst Rev. 2012;3:CD008596.
7. Frangos JE, Alavian CN, Kimball AB. Acne and oral contraceptives: update on women's health screening guidelines. J. Am. Acad. Dermatol. 2008;58(5):781-76.
8. Fung-Leung WP, Thurmond RL, Ling P, et al. Histamine H4 receptor antagonists: the new antihistamines? Curr Opin Investig Drugs Lond Engl. 2004;5(11):1174-83.
9. Hassan I, Dorjay K, Anwar P. Pentoxifylline and its applications in dermatology. Indian Dermatol Online J. 2014;5(4):510-6.
10. Kaidbey KH, Petrozzi JW, Kligman AM. Topical colchicine therapy for recalcitrant psoriasis. Arch Dermatol. 1975;111(1):33-6.
11. Koltun W, Lucky AW, Thiboutot D, et al. Efficacy and safety of 3 mg drospirenone/20 mcg ethinylestradiol oral contraceptive administered in 24/4 regimen in the treatment of acne vulgaris: a randomized, double-blind, placebo-controlled trial. Contraception. 2008;77(4):249-56.
12. Konda C, Rao AG. Colchicine in dermatology. Indian J Dermatol Venereol Leprol. 2010;76(2):201-5.
13. Leonard JN, Fry L. Treatment and management of dermatitis herpetiformis. Clin Dermatol. 1991;9(3):403-8.
14. Marmor MF, Kellner U, Lai TYY, et al; American Academy of Ophthalmology. Revised recommendations on screening for chloroquine and hydroxychloroquine retinopathy. Ophthalmology. 2011;118(2):415-22.
15. Orfanos CE, Zouboulis CC, Almond-Roesler B, et al. Current use and future potential role of retinoids in dermatology. Drugs. 1997;53(3):358-88.
16. Ormerod AD, Campalani E, Goodfield MJD. British Association of Dermatologists guidelines on the efficacy and use of acitretin in dermatology. Br J Dermatol. 2010;162:952-63.
17. Patton TJ, Zirwas MJ, Wolverton SE. Systemic Retinoids. In: Wolverton SE (Ed). Comprehensive Dermatologic Drug Therapy, 2nd edition. Philadelphia, PA: Saunders Elsevier; 2007. pp. 275-300.
18. Radomsky CL, Levine N. Thalidomide. Dermatol Clin. 2001;19(1):87-103.
19. Rodriguez-Caruncho C, Bielsa Marsol I. Antimalarials in dermatology: mechanism of action, indications, and side effects. Actas Dermo-Sifiliográficas. 2014;105(3):243-52.
20. Sagorin C, Ertel NH, Wallace SL. Photoisomerization of colchicine. Loss of significant antimitotic activity in human lymphocytes. Arthritis Rheum. 1972;15(2):213-7.
21. Sawaya ME. Antiandrogens and androgen inhibitors. In: Wolverton SE (Ed). Comprehensive Dermatologic Drug Therapy, 2nd edition. Philadelphia, PA: Saunders Elsevier; 2007. pp. 417-35.
22. Schafer PH, Parton A, Gandhi AK, et al. Apremilast, a cAMP phosphodiesterase-4 inhibitor, demonstrates anti-inflammatory activity in vitro and in a model of psoriasis. Br J Pharmacol. 2010;159(4):842-55.
23. Schiopu E, Hsu VM, Impens AJ, et al. Randomized placebo-controlled crossover trial of tadalafil in Raynaud's phenomenon secondary to systemic sclerosis. J Rheumatol. 2009;36(10):2264-8.
24. Schmitt-Hoffmann AH, Dittrich S, Saulnier E, et al. Mechanistic studies on the ethyl-esterification of acitretin by human liver preparations in vitro. Life Sci. 1995;57(26):407-12.
25. Siegenthaler G, Saurat JH, Salomon D, et al. Skin cellular retinoid-binding proteins and retinoid-responsive dermatoses. Dermatologica. 1986;173(4):163-73.
26. Stirling D, Sherman M, Strauss S. Thalidomide. A surprising recovery. J Am Pharm Assoc (Wash). 1997;NS37(3):306-13.
27. Strauss JS, Krowchuk DP, Leyden JJ, et al. Guidelines of care for acne vulgaris management. J Am Acad Dermatol. 2007;56(4):651-63.
27. Takimoto E, Champion HC, Li M, et al. Chronic inhibition of cyclic GMP phosphodiesterase 5A prevents and reverses cardiac hypertrophy. Nat Med 2005;11(2):214-22.
28. Uetrecht J, Zahid N, Shear NH, et al. Metabolism of dapsone to a hydroxylamine by human neutrophils and mononuclear cells. J Pharmacol Exp Ther. 1988;245(1):274-9.
29. Wahie S, Daly AK, Cordell HJ, et al. Clinical and pharmacogenetic influences on response to hydroxychloroquine in discoid lupus erythematosus: a retrospective cohort study. J Invest Dermatol. 2011;131(10):1981-6.
30. Wilson J. Androgens. In: Hardman JG, Limbird LE, Molinoff PB, et al (Eds). Goodman & Gilman's: The Pharmacological Basis of Therapeutics, 9th edition. New York: McGraw-Hill; 1996. pp. 1441-57.
31. Wolf R, Matz H, Orion E, et al. Dapsone. Dermatol Online J. 2002;8(1):2.
32. Wolkenstein P, Latarjet J, Roujeau JC, et al. Randomised comparison of thalidomide versus placebo in toxic epidermal necrolysis. Lancet. 1998;352(9140):1586-9.
33. Wozel VE. Innovative use of dapsone. Dermatol Clin. 2010;28(3):599-610.
34. Wu JJ, Huang DB, Pang KR, et al. Thalidomide: dermatological indications, mechanisms of action and side-effects. Br J Dermatol. 2005;153(2):254-73.
35. Zouboulis CC. Retinoids--which dermatological indications will benefit in the near future? Skin Pharmacol Appl Skin Physiol. 2001;14(5):303-15.

# 80 CHAPTER

# Lasers and Lights in Dermatology

*Imran Majid*

## INTRODUCTION

Lasers and light sources have revolutionized the way dermatology as a subject is being looked at in the present era. Use of lasers and light sources in dermatology has been increasing exponentially over the past two decades. Ranging from infective disorders to those with a presumed autoimmune pathogenesis lasers and light sources are being used in the treatment of a large number of dermatological disorders. This is in addition to the revolutionary role of lasers in aesthetic dermatology where lasers have been utilized most commonly and most efficiently till now. This chapter will outline the utility of different lasers and light sources in the field of dermatology.

## PRINCIPLES OF LASER THERAPY

Lasers are light sources which deliver light energy at a single specific wavelength that is typical of each laser device. When laser light is delivered to the tissue some amount of it gets reflected while the major portion gets either absorbed or scattered in the tissue after penetrating the surface vertically. Therapeutically, it is the absorbed part of the laser light that is important for the treating clinician. Which particular portion of the tissue irradiated with the laser absorbs, depends upon the characteristics of the laser light and presence of specific chromophores in the tissue. For example, in the skin there are three main chromophores in the form of melanin, hemoglobin, and water each of which absorbs light over a particular range of wavelengths known as its absorption spectrum (Fig. 1). When a particular chromophore absorbs laser energy of a specific wavelength the tissue containing the chromophore gets heated up and is usually destroyed. This is the principle of "selective photothermolysis" which forms the basis of all laser-based treatments in medicine including dermatology.

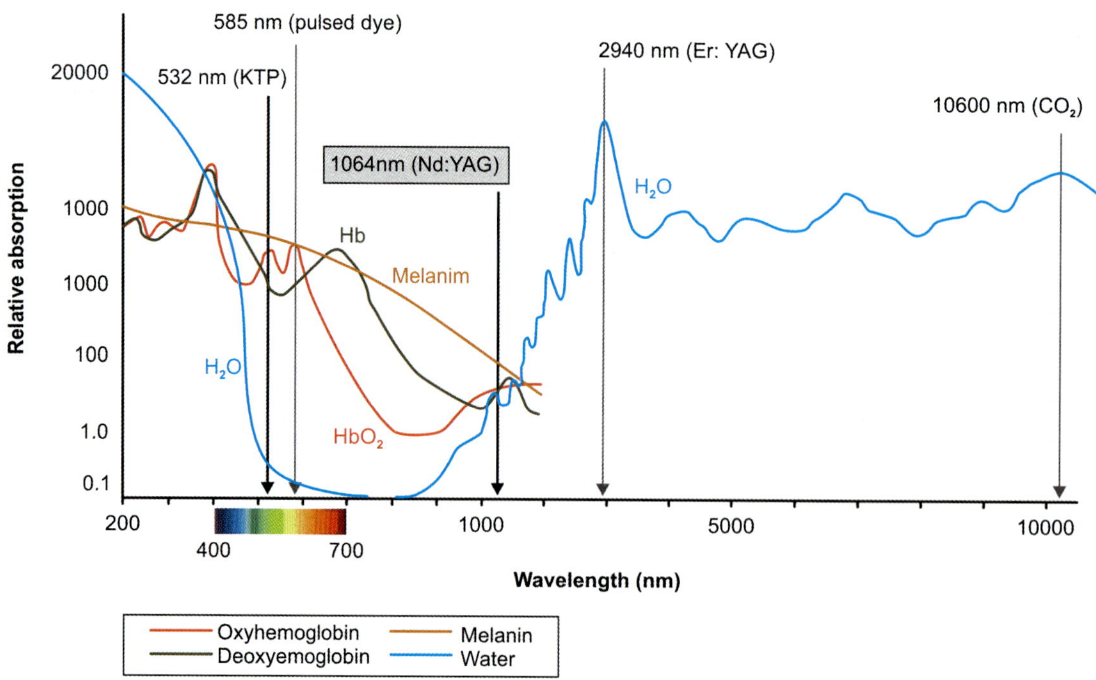


**FIG. 1:** Laser tissue interaction showing the absorption spectrum of different chromophores.

**BOX 1 Laser parameters of therapeutic importance**

- *Fluence*: Means the laser energy delivered per unit of surface area; measured in J/cm$^2$
- *Pulse duration*: Means the time over which one pulse of laser energy is delivered to tissue; measured in milliseconds to nanoseconds
- *Frequency*: Means the number of lesser pulses delivered per second
- *Spot size*: The area of the tissue which can be irradiated during a single laser pulse; measured in micrometers to centimeters

## LASER PARAMETERS AND THEIR IMPORTANCE

While using lasers for any skin condition there are certain parameters that are selected by the operator for proper utilization of laser energy to achieve a therapeutic benefit (Box 1). These parameters include:

- *Fluence*: It is defined as the amount of energy delivered per unit area. The unit for measuring fluence is J/cm$^2$. Each laser device is capable of a certain range of energy that it can deliver per unit area of the tissue
- *Pulse duration (pulse width)*: It is the time duration over which a pulse of laser energy is delivered to the tissue. It varies from picoseconds (pigment lasers) to milliseconds (hair removal lasers) depending upon the chromophore to be targeted
- *Frequency*: It means the number of pulses of laser energy delivered per second. It can vary from one to about a hundred pulses per second
- *Spot size*: This is the size of the spot over which the laser delivers light energy. It is measured in mm$^2$ or cm$^2$.

## SPECIFIC INDICATIONS FOR LASERS IN DERMATOLOGY

### Hair Reduction

Permanent hair reduction is the most common indication for laser treatment as far as Indian dermatology is concerned. Permanent hair reduction basically refers to a stable long-term reduction in hair regrowth after one or multiple laser treatment sessions. Epilation with lasers leads to a long-term reduction in hair counts for a time beyond the duration of hair cycle at a particular body site. Laser systems that are used in hair reduction employ a laser wavelength in the range of 600–1100 nm which is the spectrum that can reach the depth of the hair follicle and that gets absorbed most preferentially by melanin in the hair bulb area. In patients with darker skin, melanin in the epidermis competes in this absorption and this makes laser assisted hair removal more difficult to perform in such patients. Fair skin with dark black hair is thus considered "ideal" for laser assisted hair removal.

The efficacy of this hair reduction depends upon many factors, the most important of which is probably the diameter and pigmentation of the hair being treated. As melanin is the specific chromophore involved in hair reduction, the efficacy does increase with increase in the melanin content of the hair being treated with lasers. Another factor that is important while treating females with hirsutism is the treatment of any underlying cause. If the etiology of hirsutism is treated alongside the laser treatment the outcome is almost always rewarding (Figs 2 and 3).

There are four main laser- and light-based systems that have been employed in hair removal. These are the 800-nm diode laser, the 685-nm Alexandrite laser, the 1,064-nm Nd:YAG (neodymium-doped yttrium aluminum garnet) laser, and the intense pulse light (IPL) system (Box 2). All of these devices have demonstrated varying degrees of permanent hair reduction in clinical studies.

The efficacy of laser-based hair reduction increases with repeated treatments and on an average, a person needs an average of 5–10 sessions of laser treatment to achieve a significant level of hair reduction on the face. Number of sessions required on extrafacial sites is usually less than that required on the face. Interval between consecutive laser sessions depends upon the hair cycle duration at that particular site where the effect is desired. As an example, laser sessions on face are spaced at 4–6 week intervals as the duration of anagen phase on face is in the same range.

### Adverse Effects

Adverse effects associated with laser hair removal are usually temporary and include crusting that can remain for few days after the procedure, postinflammatory hyperpigmentation that is more common in people with darker skin, and also hypopigmentation. However, the most important adverse effect associated with laser-based hair removal is "paradoxical hypertrichosis" which is seen especially in females with facial hirsutism. Many of these females have been seen to be suffering from an underlying hormonal disorder like polycystic ovarian syndrome.

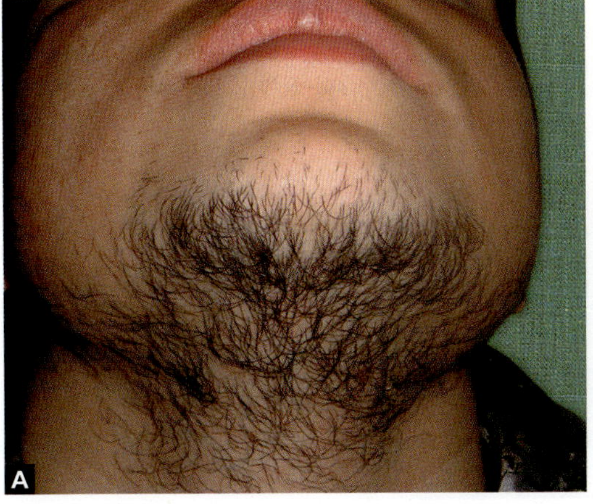


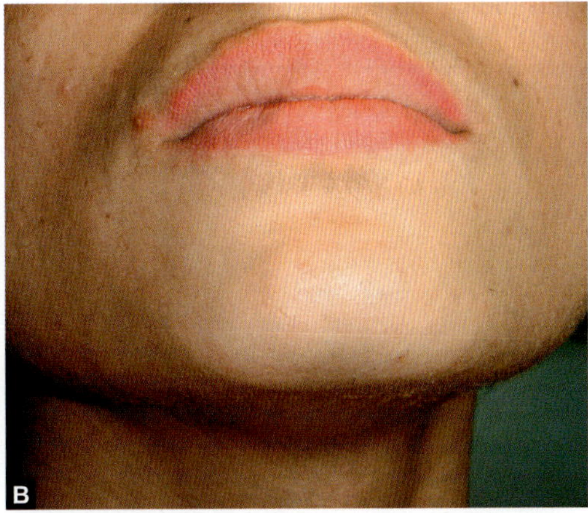


**FIG. 2:** Laser hair reduction: response 6-months after 8 sessions of diode laser treatment.

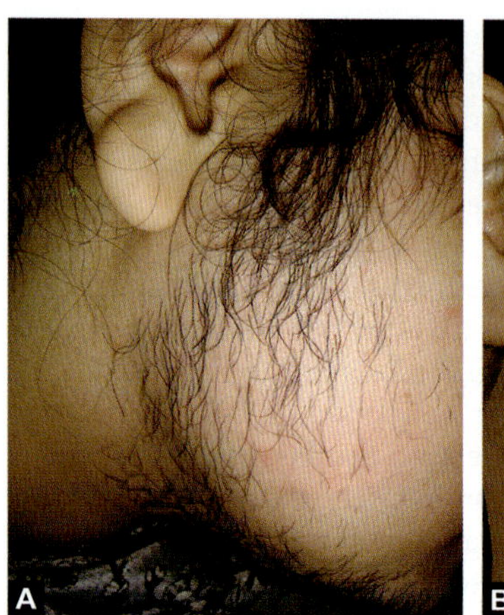
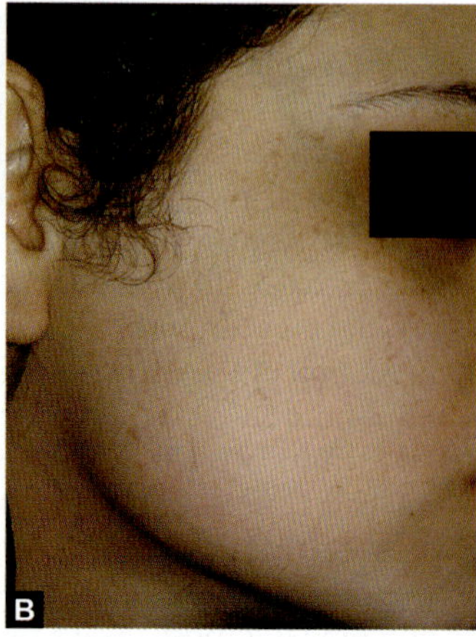

FIG. 3: Excellent response after 8 sessions of diode laser hair reduction.

**BOX 2 Laser hair reduction**

- Efficacy increases with more sessions of laser treatment
- For the face one needs an average of 5–10 sessions
- Four main devices are effective in laser assisted hair removal. These are:
  - Diode laser—claimed to be among the most effective devices
  - Alexandrite laser—reported to be as effective as diode laser
  - Nd:YAG laser—safer in darker skin but a bit less efficacious
  - Intense pulse light—a multipurpose device which can be used for hair reduction as well

Nd:YAG, neodymium-doped yttrium aluminum garnet.

### Home-based Laser Hair Removal Devices

A new development in the arena of laser-based hair removal is the advent of home-based laser devices. These devices are smaller hand-held devices that employ similar techniques as the above-mentioned lasers and light sources. The efficacy of these home-based devices in causing a long-term hair reduction has however not been proven with certainty till date.

## TREATMENT OF PIGMENTED LESIONS

After laser-based hair removal, the next most common indication for lasers in Indian context is the treatment of pigmented lesions like ephelides, melanocytic nevi, nevus of Ota, pigmented tattoos, and other pigmentary disorders. Two main lasers that have been extensively used in this indication are Q-switched Nd:YAG laser and Q-switched ruby laser. In addition, Q-switched Alexandrite laser and IPL systems have also been used in the treatment of pigmented lesions.

Melanin obviously forms the target chromophore in laser-based treatment for pigmented lesions. Melanin-containing melanosomes in the skin are approximately 0.5 microns in diameter and have a thermal relaxation time of about 50–500 nanoseconds. This is the primary reason for using Q-switched lasers which provide pulse widths in nanosecond segment. Recently, picosecond pulse-width lasers have become available which are claimed to be even more effective than nanosecond lasers for treatment of pigmented lesions. An interesting feature about melanin is its wide absorption spectrum ranging from 300 nm to 1,100 nm. It needs to be remembered however that longer the wavelength used, deeper is the penetration of laser and less is the energy delivered. Thus, for dermal lesions longer wavelengths are employed while for more superficial epidermal lesions shorter wavelengths are preferred.

### Epidermal Pigmented Lesions

These include ephelides, lentigines, café-au-lait macules (CALM), and other epidermal pigmentary lesions. These lesions respond really well to Q-switched lasers like 694 nm Q-switched ruby, 532 nm Q-switched Nd:YAG, and also Q-switched Alexandrite lasers (Fig. 4). Another way by which these lesions can be treated is by ablating the lesional portion of epidermis by means of an ablative $CO_2$ or Er:YAG erbium-doped yttrium aluminum garnet (Er:YAG) laser. The only adverse effect that can occur is postinflammatory pigmentation which is sometimes even darker than the primary lesion. This needs to be explained to the patient before the treatment is started (Box 3). Another important practical consideration is the recurrence of lesions which sometimes occurs with CALM and some nevoid conditions like nevus spilus.

#### Nevus of Ota

Lasers have been particularly impressive in the management of this dermal melanosis. As the pigment in nevus of Ota is primarily dermal, longer wavelengths are needed to reach the target melanin. Q-switched Nd:YAG laser at 1064 nm, Q-switched ruby at 694 nm, and Q-switched Alexandrite at 755 nm have all been used with success in the treatment of this condition. Multiple sessions are required to achieve therapeutic benefit and clearing of the lesion is directly related to the number of treatment sessions (Fig. 5).

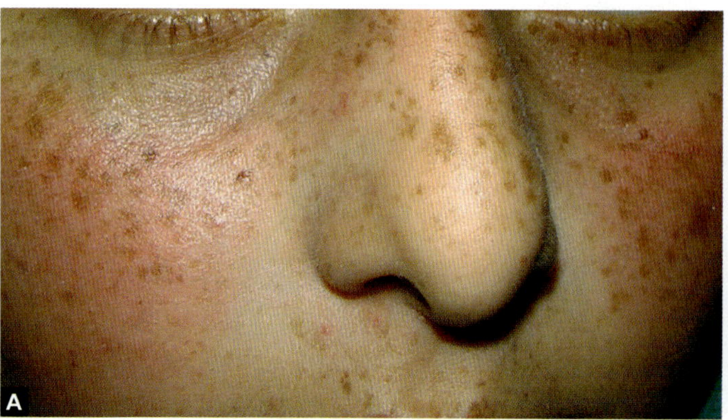
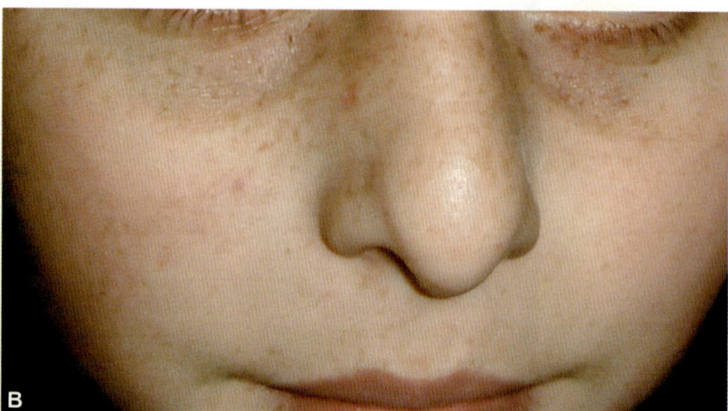

FIG. 4: Ephelides show an excellent response to Q-switched ND:YAG laser treatment.

## Melasma

Use of lasers in melasma is still controversial and there are no well-documented clinical studies that favor the use of lasers or light sources in this condition. The most important concern here is the propensity of melasma to recur following any treatment and also the chances of superimposed postinflammatory hyperpigmentation that can aggravate the pigmentation already present.

## Tattoos

Tattoos made of blue or black ink are satisfactorily treated by any of the Q-switched lasers. The number of sessions required depends upon whether the tattoo is professional or amateur as the amount of ink present varies a lot between these two types of tattoos (Fig. 6).

**BOX 3 Treatment of pigmented lesions**

- Q-switched lasers with pulse duration in nanoseconds or even picoseconds are the most commonly used
- Some lesions have a propensity to recur after laser treatment, e.g., café-au-lait macules and nevus spilus
- Dermal melanocytic lesions like nevus of Ota respond really well to treatment
- For melanocytic nevi, vaporizing lasers like $CO_2$ or Er:YAG laser are claimed to be safer than Q-switched lasers

## Facial Rejuvenation

One of the most fascinating areas where lasers have made their mark most prominently is the field of facial rejuvenation. In fact, this field has contributed the most to the popularity of lasers as therapeutic devices. Lasers that are employed in facial rejuvenation are divided into ablative and nonablative types. While the former are claimed to be more effective, the latter group is thought to be safer with less downtime. Among the ablative lasers, $CO_2$ laser at 10,600 nm and Er:YAG laser at 2,940 nm are the most commonly used. Both of these lasers give excellent results when used in the treatment of aging skin. The only drawback with these lasers is the possibility of prolonged erythema lasting for weeks to months, oozing and crusting, and postinflammatory pigmentation especially in darker skin. Recent advancement in this field in the form of fractional laser technology has solved many of these issues. Fractional photothermolysis is a relatively new concept in laser rejuvenation wherein the laser system, instead of causing a photo-injury to the whole skin, produces longitudinal arrays of microscopic thermal injury to specific depths in the dermis. These longitudinal thermal wounds are known as microscopic treatment zones and they are separated from each

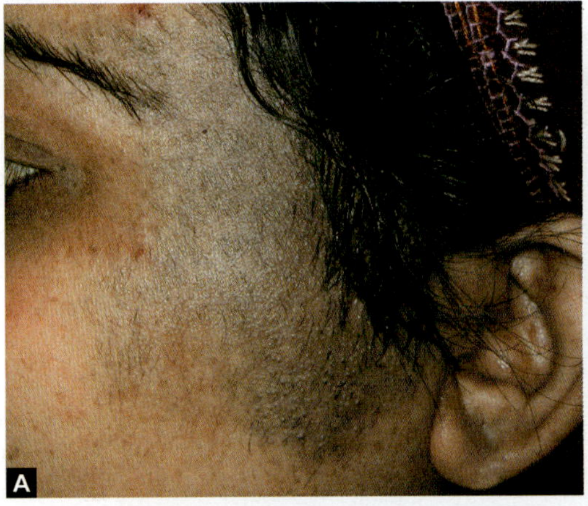


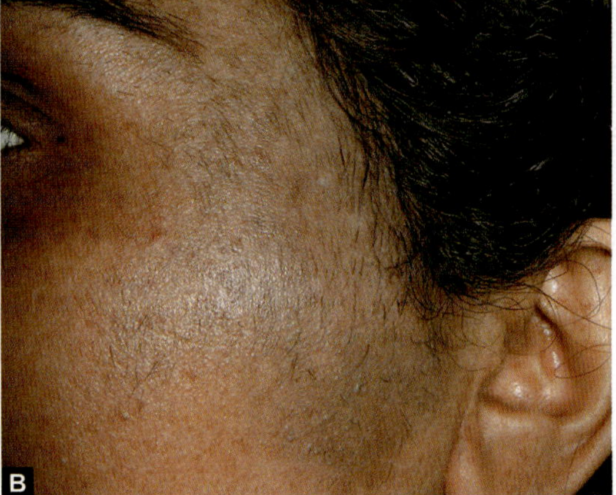


**FIG. 5:** Nevus of Ota shows excellent response to Q switched Nd:YAG laser.

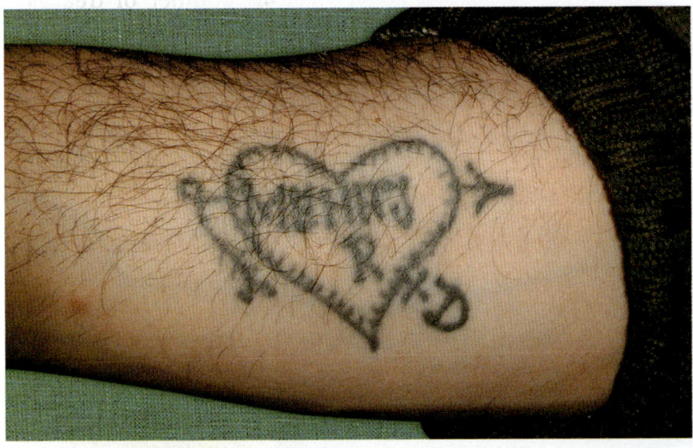

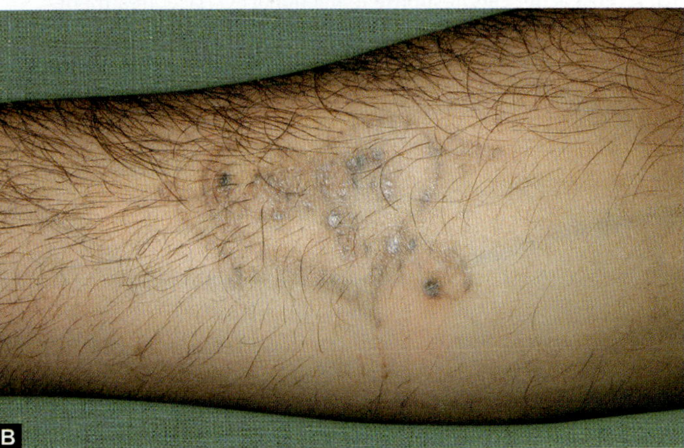


**FIG. 6:** Blue-black ink tattoo: successful treatment with Q switched Nd:YAG laser.

other by normal, noninjured skin. Thus, fractional lasers treat only a "fraction" of the whole skin keeping the integrity of epidermis intact. As the microscopic wound created by a fractional laser is surrounded by normal, healthy tissue, the healing is rapid and the adverse effects are reduced to a considerable degree.

Nonablative lasers used for skin rejuvenation include 1,450-nm diode laser, 1,320-nm Nd:YAG laser, 1,540-nm erbium glass laser, IPL, and pulsed dye laser (PDL) (Box 4). The biggest advantage with the nonablative lasers and light sources is that there is almost no or minimal downtime after the use of these devices. However, the efficacy is supposed to be less than that of ablative devices.

## Acne Scars

For the treatment of acne scars both ablative as well as nonablative skin rejuvenating laser devices have been used with varying degrees of success. In fact, fractional ablative laser resurfacing with $CO_2$ laser or Er:YAG laser is currently rated as one of the most effective treatment options in this indication. In addition, nonablative lasers like erbium glass laser and even IPL also give modest response in atrophic acne scars. Among the different morphological types of acne scars the rolling and superficial boxcar scars respond better than ice-pick scars or deep boxcar scars (Fig. 7).

**BOX 4 Lasers for skin rejuvenation and scars**

- Fractional photothermolysis is currently the most popular technology in this indication
- Fractional ablative lasers like $CO_2$ and Er:YAG are claimed to be more effective than nonablative lasers
- Downtime associated with ablative laser resurfacing is much more than with nonablative laser treatment
- Acne scars, traumatic scars, and burn scars can also be treated successfully with fractional laser photothermolysis

## Thermal and Traumatic Scars

Ablative laser resurfacing has emerged as an effective treatment in postburn and post-traumatic scar management. Both hypertrophic as well as atrophic traumatic and burn scars are treated with varying degree of success with laser resurfacing. Fractional laser resurfacing is in fact claimed to be the most effective nonsurgical modality for treatment of traumatic and burn scars at present (Fig. 8).

# Vascular Lesions

Vascular lesions amenable to laser treatment include the following described further.

## Vascular Malformations

The most common and most important vascular malformation treated with lasers is the port-wine stain (PWS) which are

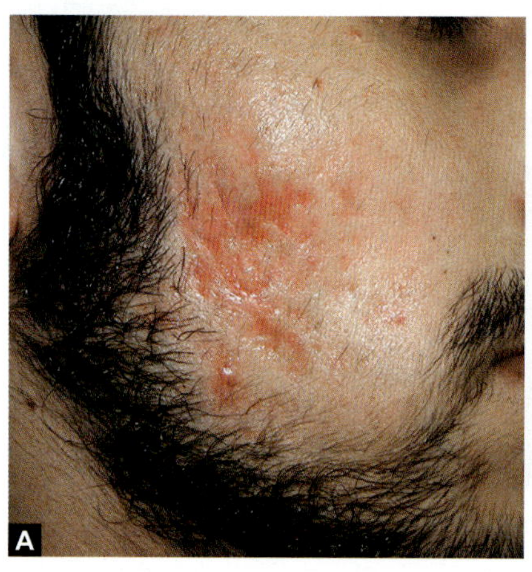


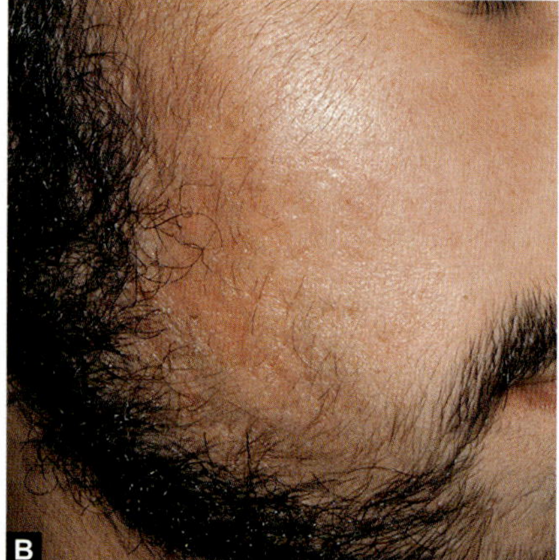


**FIG. 7:** Post acne scars: response to fractional $CO_2$ laser treatment.

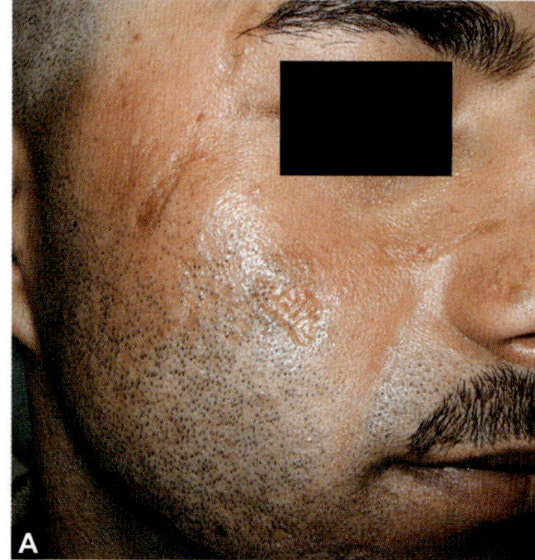


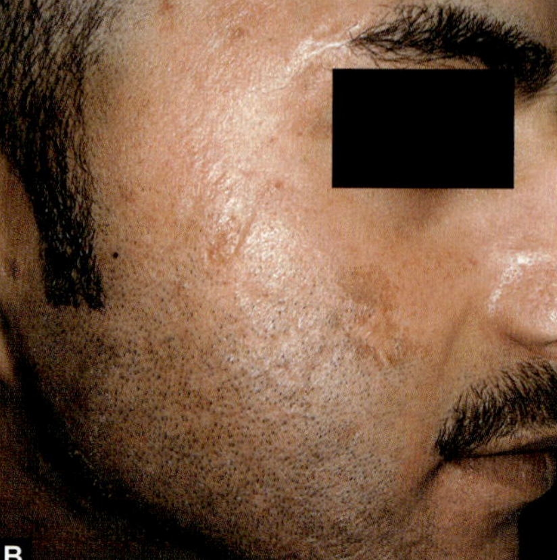


**FIG. 8:** Post-traumatic scars can also show good response to fractional $CO_2$ laser.

basically capillary malformations usually seen on the face and scalp. A PDL at 585 nm or 595 nm is the specific laser device used to treat PWS. Other lasers that have anecdotally been used are the Nd:YAG laser and IPL device. However, PDL is the only laser device that achieves the most significant therapeutic benefit in PWS. What needs to be remembered is that nodular or hypertrophic PWS do not show the same response as flat and superficial PWS. Similarly, children younger than 1 year of age and head-and neck PWS respond better than older age patients and distal extremity lesions.

### Infantile Hemangioma

The role of lasers in infantile hemangiomas is limited to those lesions which are flat and superficial. It is important to note that a vascular laser like PDL has a maximum depth of penetration of 1.2 mm and thus it cannot practically treat and hemangiomas are more than 1.2 mm in thickness. Other lasers like Nd:YAG and IPL have also been used in infantile hemangiomas with inconsistent results. PDL is often used in combination with topical timolol to improve therapeutic results in infantile hemangiomas.

### Telangiectasia and Dilated Veins

Facial telangiectasias are successfully treated with vascular lasers like PDL, potassium tritanyl phosphate (KTP) laser, and IPL. While smaller telangiectasias need nonpurpuric doses, the larger vessels do need higher energies causing purpuric end points. Facial telangiectasias in the setting of rosacea also do respond with fair amount of success to IPL and PDL devices. For dilated veins, Nd:YAG and diode lasers are also effective in addition to PDL (Box 5).

## OTHER LIGHT SOURCES IN DERMATOLOGY

Apart from lasers the other light sources that are used in dermatological practice are ultraviolet A light (UVA) usually used in combination with psoralens and ultraviolet A (PUVA), narrowband UVB (NBUVB), ultraviolet A1 (UVA1), and excimer laser or light. These light sources are effectively employed in the treatment of many immune-mediated skin disorders like vitiligo (Fig. 9), psoriasis, eczemas, cutaneous T-cell lymphomas, alopecia areata, etc.

**BOX 5 Lasers for vascular lesions**

- Pulsed dye lasers are the most effective in this category of skin lesions
- Flatter and thinner lesions respond better than thicker or deep-seated lesions
- Multiple sessions at regular intervals are needed to achieve the therapeutic effect

### PUVA

In PUVA therapy, oral psoralens are administered and the body is exposed to UVA light from high energy UVA sources 2 hours after the ingestion of the oral psoralen. Light sources utilized in this form of treatment emit the whole UVA spectrum with wavelength ranging from 320 to 400 nm. PUVA is a useful treatment option in many skin diseases like psoriasis, vitiligo, eczemas, cutaneous T-cell lymphomas, etc. Important adverse effects of PUVA include acute phototoxicity, lentiginosis, ageing of the skin, and even cutaneous malignancies after long-term use.

### NBUVB

This is another form of phototherapy that scores over PUVA in many respects as it is considered to be much safer than the latter. Here, NBUVB light is utilized with an emission spectrum mainly at or around 311 nm. While the efficacy of NBUVB is the same as that of PUVA, the safety is certainly better as no oral drugs are needed and no sun protection to eyes is needed after NBUVB exposure. This form of phototherapy is recommended even in pregnant females and also in children and no reports of any skin malignancies after the use of NBUVB are there in the world literature. Indications of NBUVB are almost the same as for PUVA. NBUVB is also combined with many topical or oral agents to increase its therapeutic efficacy in skin diseases like psoriasis and vitiligo.

### Targeted Phototherapy

This is another recent and exciting field of phototherapy wherein high-intensity UVA, UVB, or excimer light or laser is used particularly on the skin lesions while the rest of skin remains protected. Indications for targeted phototherapy include vitiligo (<5% body surface area involvement), psoriasis, alopecia areata, discoid eczema, etc. The most important advantage of targeted phototherapy is that unaffected skin is not irradiated and thus

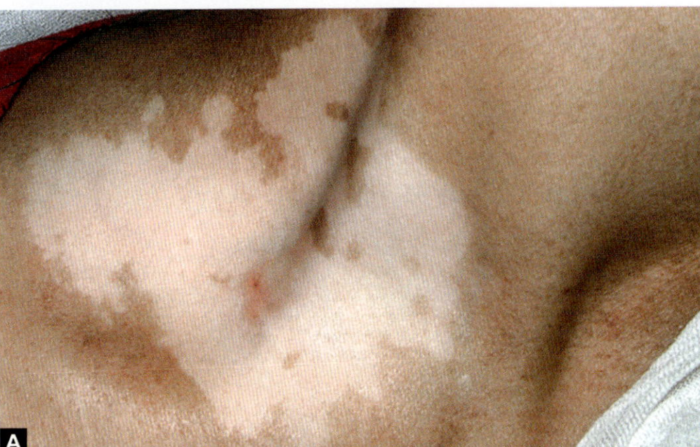


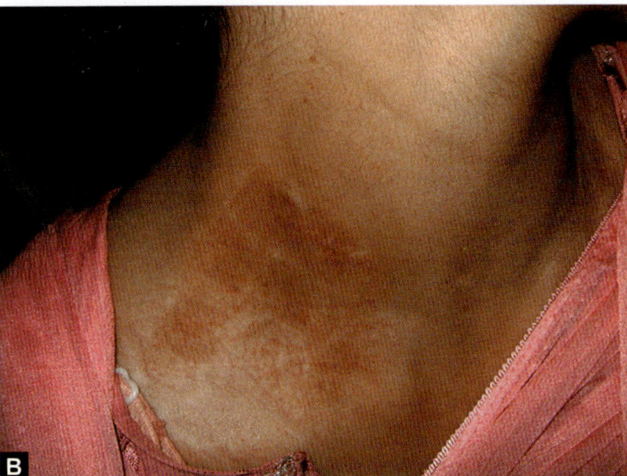


**FIG. 9:** Vitiligo can be safely managed with Targeted UVB device. **A,** Before; **B,** After.

**BOX 6 Phototherapy in dermatology**

- Indicated in treatment of psoriasis, vitiligo, eczemas, and cutaneous T-cell lymphomas mainly
- Divided into three main types:
  - PUVA: Utilizes UVA light (320–400 nm) in addition to oral psoralens
  - NBUVB: Safer than PUVA and recommended even in pregnancy and childhood. Here, 311 nm wavelength is utilized
  - Targeted phototherapy: Includes excimer laser or light at 308 nm, targeted UVA, and targeted UVB devices. Safest and the most rapidly acting of all phototherapy devices

PUVA, psoralen and ultraviolet A; UVA, ultraviolet A; NBUVB, narrowband ultraviolet B; UVB, ultraviolet B.

much higher energies can be delivered to the involved skin. It usually shows therapeutic effects much faster than traditional phototherapy regimens and is also safer than the latter. The most popular targeted phototherapy source is excimer laser or excimer light which provides light energy around 308 nm wavelength. The other two forms of targeted phototherapy are targeted UVA and targeted UVB light (Box 6).

## SUGGESTED READINGS


1. Anderson RR, Parish JA. Selective Photothermolysis: Precise microsurgery by selective absorption of pulsed radiation. Science. 1983;220:524-7.
2. Aurangabadkar S. Q-switched Nd:YAG laser for nevus of Ota: An Indian study of 50 patients. J Cutan Aesthet Surg. 2008;1:80-4.
3. Battle E, Suthamjariya K, Alora B. Very long-pulsed diode laser for hair removal on all skin types. Lasers Surg Med. 2000;12:85.
4. Dawe RS. Comparing narrowband ultraviolet B treatment regimens for psoriasis. Br J Dermatol. 2009;161:1215-6.
5. Fontana CR, Bonini D, Bagnato VS. A 12-month follow up of hypopigmentation after laser hair removal. J Cosmet Laser Ther. 2013;15:80-4.
6. Gan SD, Graber EM. Laser hair removal: a review. Dermatol Surg. 2013;39:823-38.
7. Graber EM, Tanzi EL, Alster TS. Side effects and complications of fractional laser photothermolysis: experience with 961 treatments. Dermatol Surg. 2008;34(3):301-5.
8. Hamzavi I, Lui H. Using light in dermatology: An update on lasers, ultraviolet phototherapy, and photodynamic therapy. Dermatol Clin. 2005;23:199-207.
9. Karsai S, Czarnecka A, Jünger M, et al. Ablative fractional lasers (CO2 and Er:YAG): a randomized controlled double-blind split-face trial of the treatment of peri-orbital rhytides. Lasers Surg Med. 2010;42:160-7.
10. Kilmer SL, Anderson RR. Clinical uses of Q-switched ruby and Q-switched Nd:YAG lasers for treatment of tattoos. J Dermatol Surg Oncol. 1993;19:330-8.
11. Laubach H-J, Tannous Z, Anderson RR, et al. Skin responses to fractional photothermolysis. Lasers Surg Med. 2006;38:142-49.
12. Lowe NJ, Lask G, Griffin ME. Laser skin resurfacing: pre- and post-treatment guidelines. Dermatol Surg. 1995;21:1017-19.
13. Majid I, Imran S. Fractional CO2 laser resurfacing as monotherapy in the treatment of atrophic facial acne scars. J Cutan Aesthet Surg. 2014;7:87-92.
14. Mysore V. Targeted phototherapy. Indian J Dermatol Venereol Leprol. 2009;75:119-25.
15. Railan D, Kilmer S. Laser treatment of benign pigmented cutaneous lesions. In: Goldman MP (Ed). Cutaneous and Cosmetic Laser Surgery. California: Elsevier Mosby; 2006. pp. 93-106.
16. Ross EV, Anderson RR. Laser-tissue interactions. In: Goldman MP (Ed). Cutaneous and Cosmetic Laser Surgery. California: Elsevier Mosby; 2006. p. 1-26.
17. Vachiramon V, Brown T, McMichael AJ. Patient satisfaction following laser hair removal in ethnic skin. J Drugs Dermatol. 2012;11:191-5.

# INDEX

Page numbers followed by *b* refer to box, *f* refer to figure, *fc* refer to flowchart, and *t* refer to table.

## A

## B

## C

## D

## E

## F

## G

## J



## K

## L

## M

## O



## P

## Q

## R



## S

## T

## U



## V

## W



## X



## Y



## Z